LEXICON of Psychiatry, Neurology, and the Neurosciences

LEXICON of Psychiatry, Neurology, and the Neurosciences

FRANK J. AYD, JR., M.D.

Editor, International Drug Therapy Newsletter
Emeritus Director, Professional Education and Research
Taylor Manor Hospital
Ellicott City, Maryland

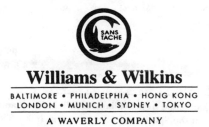

Williams & Wilkins

BALTIMORE • PHILADELPHIA • HONG KONG
LONDON • MUNICH • SYDNEY • TOKYO

A WAVERLY COMPANY

Editor: David C. Retford
Project Manager: Barbara J. Felton
Copy Editor: John M. Daniel
Designer: Wilma E. Rosenberger

Copyright © 1995
Williams & Wilkins
428 East Preston Street
Baltimore, Maryland 21202, USA

Accurate indications, adverse reactions, and dosage schedules for drugs are provided
in this book, but it is possible that they may change. The reader is urged to review the
package information data of the manufacturers of the medications mentioned.

Printed in the United States of America

Library of Congress Cataloging-in-Publication Data

Ayd, Frank J.
    Lexicon of psychiatry, neurology, and the neurosciences / Frank J.
  Ayd, Jr.
      p. cm.
    Includes bibliographical references and index.
    ISBN 0-683-00298-8
    1. Psychiatry—Dictionaries.   2. Neurology—Dictionaries.
  3. Neurosciences—Dictionaries.
    [DNLM: 1. Psychiatry—dictionaries.   2. Neurology—dictionaries.
  3. Neurosciences—dictionaries. WM 13 1995]
    RC334.A96 1995
    616.8803—dc20
DNLM/DLC
for Library of Congress

94-38956
CIP

95 96 97 98
2 3 4 5 6 7 8 9 10

To Rita Corasaniti Ayd
My loving, sharing, and supporting wife for fifty years,
mother of our twelve children, grandmother, and great grandmother.

Foreword by David J. Kupfer, M.D.

Frank Ayd's *Lexicon of Psychiatry, Neurology, and the Neurosciences* is clearly a book that will remain on my desk as a primary resource—until it is replaced by the second edition. Both clinicians and researchers have experienced a huge intellectual explosion in biological psychiatry, as well as in clinical and basic neuroscience. Since these advances have dramatically increased over the past decade, all of us now need extensive roadmaps and information trees to comprehend the importance of these developments for our clinical practice. While there are no quick ways to achieve such an understanding, this lexicon does offer several shortcuts. For example, the encyclopedic nature of this lexicon provides a comprehensive yet selective primary glossary. This glossary covers clinical assessment and nosology as well as issues of treatment. It provides an important set of guidelines in understanding basic biological and neuroscientific concepts. It even aids us in appreciating the complexity and importance of biostatistical design and analytic issues. It literally has the potential of becoming the *Webster's* of biological psychiatry. I therefore recommend this volume highly for students, practitioners, and clinical and basic scientists.

David J. Kupfer, M.D.
Professor and Chairman
Department of Psychiatry
University of Pittsburgh School of Medicine
Pittsburgh, Pennsylvania

Foreword by David Skupny A.D.

Foreword by Charles B. Nemeroff, M.D.

To pen a glossary of any field is a monumental task, and one that must, by definition (no pun intended), be a labor of love. To prepare a glossary of a relatively narrowly, well-defined area is difficult but certainly achievable—for example, a glossary of psychoanalysis (Moore BE, Fine BD [eds]. *Psychoanalytic Terms and Concepts*. New Haven and London: American Psychoanalytic Association and Yale University Press, 1990). However, to put together a glossary of a very large field such as psychiatry and then to include neurology and neuroscience is unfathomable for most of us, but obviously and thankfully not to Frank Ayd. At a time when most people are enjoying the perquisites of retirement, Ayd has accepted, and accomplished, this daunting task. What follows in this tome is a thoughtful alphabetical listing of definitions of terms that we utilize daily, but frequently without fully grasping their exact meaning. Not only are the definitions comprehensive and understandable, but they are referenced with the vast majority of the relevant publications of the last 7–8 years. Moreover, the references are made to what are generally acknowledged to be the very best journals and books in their fields. All of this precision is, of course, a testimony to the healthy obsessive qualities of Ayd and to his never-ending search for knowledge in this and other fields of inquiry. Moreover, many of the leading investigators in the field agreed to peer-review various letters in the glossary—largely a testimony to Frank Ayd's stature in the field—and he, as always, listened to the critics. The result, I believe, is most remarkable.

As noted above, the breadth of material contained is astounding. Where else can one find definitions in the same source, for example, of "satyriasis," "savoxepine," "Scatchard plot," "Scheffé procedure," "secondary mania," "segregation analysis," and "selegiline"? The fields of neuroscience, psychiatry, and neurology have witnessed remarkable advances in the last two decades, particularly in the areas of psychopharmacology, brain imaging, epidemiology, nosology, molecular neurobiology, genetics, and neurochemical pathology. No single investigator or practitioner could possibly remain well informed in each of these areas—hence the need for this volume. As Samuel Johnson set the framework in place for subsequent generations of dictionaries, so too does Ayd provide the foundation for subsequent volumes.

As an aside, in preparing this foreword, I have wondered when a Boswell will step forward to document the remarkable career of Frank Ayd, which would undoubtedly parallel the growth and development of modern psychiatry.

It is, of course, my hope—and I am now speaking for myriad colleagues—that this volume, once used and reused by a generation of clinicians and investigators, will see a subsequent edition, one revised by none other than the irrepressible Dr. Ayd.

Charles B. Nemeroff, M.D., Ph.D.
Professor and Chairman
Department of Psychiatry and Behavioral Sciences
Emory University School of Medicine
Atlanta, Georgia

Preface

In the four decades since the advent of chlorpromazine inaugurated modern psychopharmacotherapy and the subsequent introduction of a host of psychoactive drugs, there has been an unprecedented revolution in psychiatry. Concurrent with these developments, there have been significant refinements and improvements in nosology and in defining reliable diagnostic criteria for all major psychiatric illnesses. This is attested to by the successive editions of the American Psychiatric Association's *Diagnostic and Statistical Manual of Mental Disorders* and the World Health Organization's *International Classification of Diseases*.

Psychiatrists have been collaborating with biostaticians to design better-controlled trials. In addition, they have, alone or in association with psychologists, devised hundreds of rating scales, diagnostic scheduled interviews, questionnaires, and other methods of gathering clinical data to enhance diagnostic accuracy, to gather baseline data, and to measure, as objectively as possible, treatment outcomes.

In the past quarter century, psychiatrists have become medical intranauts, exploring the inner spaces of man. They are studying drug pharmacokinetics, pharmacodynamics, and plasma concentrations to correlate with mechanisms of action, treatment response, adverse effects, and optimal dosage. They are using increasingly sophisticated neuroimaging techniques—EEG, QEEG, CT, PET, SPECT, MRI, MRS, and others—to determine what goes on and where and why in the brains of psychotic, nonpsychotic, demented, cognitively impaired patients. They are using pharmacological probes and other means of gathering data to add to our understanding of the neurochemistry, neurophysiology, neuroendocrinology, neuropathology, and genetics of the psychiatric ills with which people can be afflicted. They are using a variety of analytical methods to quantitate the amount of drug or other substances in the body. Along with these trends, molecular psychiatry and the neurosciences have spawned and grown dramatically. These unprecedented innovations and developments have generated a new psychiatric language and vocabulary that have expanded exponentially and rapidly, and with which anyone reading contemporary psychiatric journals or attending psychiatric lectures or seminars must be familiar.

This book is intended to make communications of psychiatric knowledge and research comprehensible and meaningful for all physicians and, in particular, psychiatrists, psychiatric residents, psychologists, PharmDs, social workers, mental health workers, and science writers. Its goal is to enhance understanding of psychiatry, biological psychiatry, and the neurosciences so clinicians, researchers, and other scientists can communicate better with each other for the good of all.

This volume contains definitions of words that did not exist a few decades ago. It provides descriptions of psychiatric, neurological, and genetic disorders, as well as concise information on psychoactive drugs; their classification, pharmacology, pharmacokinetics, and pharmacodynamics; adverse reactions; and beneficial and adverse drug-drug interactions. The majority of entries in this lexicon contain references to articles and books for more information. More than 350 peer-reviewed journals are cited, as are over 150 books. Most citations were published since 1987.

This lexicon is the product of many minds. Numerous colleagues in Europe, Israel, North America, and Australia graciously peer-reviewed sections on which they are recognized experts. They have helped me immeasurably. I am pleased to acknowledge their valuable contributions, my indebtedness to them, and my sincere gratitude. I am very blessed to have so many friends and colleagues who without hesitation agreed to peer-review segments of this volume. I also thank David Kupfer and Charles Nemeroff, each of whom has written a foreword to this first edition. I acknowledge my gratitude to Fred Goodwin, Ross Baldessarini, and James Jefferson for their endorsements of this lexicon.

Finally, I thank Ann Lovelace, Mary Ann Ayd, and Joan Kennedy, without whose expert secretarial assistance, patience, and assiduous efforts on my behalf this lexicon would not be. They deserve the appreciation of all who find this lexicon a valuable source of information.

To keep the lexicon as up-to-date as possible, material for a second edition is being gathered. I am proud that Philip Janicak has accepted my invitation to join me as Associate Editor for future editions. A limited number of highly qualified experts will be our consultants and will critique new material as it is written.

I have striven to make the lexicon as user-friendly as possible. Since its conception, it has been structured so that any user would have the information needed at his or her fingertips. As I mentioned, the lexicon is the product of many minds. It would not be the work it is without the gracious feedback from scores of colleagues. Because we are human, however, errors and oversights are inevitable. As I asked for critiques from numerous reviewers, I ask for help from all lexicon users. Any pertinent information that may have been overlooked, any errors, any comments and suggestions, and any queries or compliments would be greatly appreciated. You may write me at: Ayd Medical Communications, 1130 East Cold Spring Lane, Baltimore, Maryland 21239-3931 (FAX 410-532-5419).

Frank J. Ayd, Jr., M.D.

How to Use the Lexicon

Prehistoric humans discovered they could accomplish more in a day's work with the use of tools, so they fashioned tools to be extensions of their limbs. These tools became invaluable resources to make efficient use of time. With the recent phenomenal growth in the medical field, burgeoning new subdisciplines creating voluminous studies, new medications, and new and modified treatments, scientists, researchers, and clinicians are confronted daily with a new medical/scientific language. Hence, a new tool is needed. Standard medical dictionaries are a necessity for general reference, but more is needed to aid the psychiatrist, neurologist, and neuroscientist to remain current with evolving terminology. This lexicon is fashioned to be used as a foraging tool for fast, effective reference.

→ You will find psychiatric drug interactions cross-referenced. For example: to find the interaction between lithium and a benzodiazepine, you need only turn to either reference; the definition will be under each citation. However, nonpsychiatric drug interactions such as ibuprofen and alprazolam will be listed only under the psychiatric drug, alprazolam.

→ As many timely journal and book references as possible are cited within the definition, providing additional sources for users wanting more information.

→ Proprietary names are listed in parentheses directly after the generic citation.

→ Cross-references are added at the end of the definition in bold after the word "See."

→ Synonyms are placed at the end of the definition in quotation marks.

→ Chemicals starting with numbers are listed alphabetically starting with the first letter. 2,5-dimethylamphetamine appears in the letter "D" after dimethracin.

→ Acronyms and abbreviations are used within the definition for brevity.

How to Use the Lexicon

Contents

A

A   Street name for amphetamines.

A₄   See **beta-amyloid**.

A-71623   (Boc-Trp-Lys[e-N-2-methylphenylami-nocarbonyl]-Asp-[NMe]Phe-NH₂)   Novel cholecystokinin (CCK) tetrapeptide that exhibits high affinity and selectivity (more than 1,000 times that of regular CCK) for CCK-A type receptors. It has potent anorectic actions.

ABAC   See **nomogram**.

ABA design   Experimental trial design in which condition A is presented first, B second, and A third. Frequently, a placebo is used in the control treatment first, active treatment second, and placebo or control treatment third. Unlike counterbalanced design, such as ABBA, in which patients can be randomly assigned to conditions ABBA and BAAB, the ABA design does not allow random assignment to two or more balanced orderings of treatment. To some degree it does allow a placebo or otherwise controlled condition. It is very easy for evaluators to guess when the patient is on medication.

ABBA design   Counterbalanced order of presentation of independent variables. The independent variable condition A is followed by the second independent variable condition B, followed by conditions B and A.

ABB crossover design   New designs and statistical methods make it possible to estimate true treatment effects, even if there are carryover effects. For example, if one is comparing treatments A and B, and if patients can receive three treatments, only two treatment sequences are needed, ABB and BAA. If only two treatment periods are possible, the four treatment sequences AB, BA, AA, and BB are used. These designs allow the carryover effect of each treatment to be estimated using a within-patient analysis.

abecarnil   (ZK 112-119) Novel ligand for central benzodiazepine (BZD) receptors, possessing anxiolytic and anticonvulsant properties, but with considerably reduced muscle relaxant effects in comparison to BZDs. It is the first beta-carboline in clinical development with partial agonist properties at BZD receptors; preliminary testing suggests it will be a clinically useful anxiolytic. Early clinical trials indicate that 6–9 mg/day is safe and efficacious and that after abrupt withdrawal there is minimal evidence of withdrawal symptoms. See **beta-carboline**.

aberrant gene   See **gene, aberrant**.

"A-bomb"   Street name for heroin, marijuana, or heroin and marijuana.

abreaction   See **catharsis**.

abscissa   Distance along the horizontal coordinate, or x axis, of a point P from the vertical, or y axis, of a graph.

absence, epileptic   Clouding or loss of consciousness lasting 2–15 seconds accompanied by generalized epileptic discharge. It is the principal sign of petit mal epilepsy. During the seizure, facial expression is blank and there may be rhythmical eye movements. After the ictal period (the actual seizure), post ictal events are minimal, and return to normal is prompt. It is called "simple absence" when there are no other signs (e.g., the patient does not fall or have a convulsion); if other signs occur the absence is called complex. The classic electroencephalogram (EEG) pattern is 3 Hz spike and wave, which is bilateral, synchronous, and symmetrical. When other EEG patterns occur, the condition is called "atypical absence," although it is the EEG pattern, not the clinical picture, that is atypical.

absence seizure   See **seizure, absence**.

absence status   State characterized by a spectrum from subtle consciousness alterations to obvious torpor or stupor, accompanied by periorbital movements with rapid eye blinking in phases and myoclonic jerks. Patients are disoriented, may perseverate, and appear apathetic. Absence status usually occurs in patients with a known history of generalized seizures; most episodes are seen under age of 20, but sudden onset in later life has been reported, in some cases with no seizure history. It can be induced by co-administration of clonazepam with valproate or carbamazepine. Also called "petit mal status."

absolute risk   Observed or calculated risk of an event in a population under study.

absolute value   Positive value of a positive or negative number.

absorption   Process by which a drug proceeds from the site of administration to the site of measurement (generally plasma or whole blood) within the body. The symbol F, the fraction of administered drug absorbed, represents the extent of absorption or the fraction of the dose that reaches general circulation after drug administration (also called bioavailability). Following intravenous administration, F is always 1.0 (100%). F can vary between 0 and 1.0 (Javaid JI, Janicak PG, Holland D. Blood level monitoring of antipsychotics and antidepressants. *Psychiatr Med*

1991;9:168–187). Absorption is concerned with how a drug or substance gets from the point of entry (usually gastrointestinal [GI] tract, muscle, or subcutaneous tissue) into the blood circulatory compartment. There are many routes of drug administration and absorption. These include mucosal surfaces (ophthalmic, nasal, oral, gastrointestinal, rectal, and vaginal) and, for a few drugs, the dermis. Oral medication must be absorbed from the gastrointestinal tract or from the oral mucosa. The percentage of the drug absorbed from the GI tract depends on its acid/base and lipophilic properties, as well as the physiology of the GI tract. The degree to which a drug is ionized affects its solubility. Subcutaneously or intramuscularly injected medications must be absorbed from these tissues into the main circulation. Dissociation constant (pKa), lipid solubility, and pH at the site of absorption all affect the absorption of a given drug. The rate and/or extent of absorption of a number of drugs can be markedly influenced by factors such as antacids and other drugs, gastric motility, pH at the absorption site, and dosing relative to mealtime. The rate of absorption of a drug determines the rapidity of onset of its effects.

absorption/intramuscular injection   Rate of absorption after intramuscular (IM) injection may vary widely depending on vascularity of the injection site, degree of ionization and lipid solubility of the drug, volume of the injection, and osmosity of the injected solution. These factors account for the variability of absorption of IM injection of benzodiazepines. For example, absorption of IM diazepam is slow and less complete, resulting in peak plasma concentrations that are lower than those following oral dosing. In contrast, IM lorazepam is rapidly absorbed, with an approximate time to peak concentration of 1.5 hours and more than 90% complete absorption within 2 hours of administration.

abstinence   Discontinuation and complete avoidance of further use of a drug of dependency by a drug-dependent person. It is distinct from sobriety in the terminology of Alcoholics Anonymous.

abstinence syndrome   See **withdrawal syndrome**.

abstraction ability   Capacity to make valid generalizations. Considered important in evaluating the presence of psychiatric illness, it is frequently assessed by proverbs testing. Evaluation must take into account patients' ethnic, socioeconomic, and educational backgrounds.

abstract thinking   Cognitive processes involving ability to classify, form generalizations, and

proceed beyond concrete or egocentric thinking in problem-solving tasks. Difficulty in abstract thinking is a common symptom of schizophrenia. See **schizophrenia/negative symptoms**.

abulia   Profound apathy due to severe bilateral prefrontal lobe disease. It may be severe enough to produce a state of akinetic mutism.

abuse   Use of a legal or illicit substance or medication for nonmedical or pleasurable purposes unconnected to approved medical indications. Abuse is present whenever drug use results in adverse effects to self or others, even though the user may be unwilling or unable to acknowledge that such adverse effects are occurring. Drug or substance abuse is also a legal term used in certain federal, state, and local statutes. It is also used as a psychiatric diagnosis. The meaning of drug or substance abuse depends on the context. Abuse should be distinguished from addiction and dependency, and is not defined by a "majority opinion." See **medical abuser; street abuser**.

abuse liability   Capacity of a compound to produce physiological or psychological dependence and alter behavior in a manner detrimental to the individual or his or her environment. It is defined, at least in part, in terms of a drugs capacity to function as a positive reinforcer in animals and humans. The higher a compound's capacity to function as a positive reinforcer, the greater is its abuse liability. In animals, drug discrimination and drug self-administration procedures have been shown to predict the abuse liability of drugs. Most drugs that are abused by humans are self-administered by animals.

Acamprosate   See **calcium acetyl homotaurinate**.

"Acapulco gold"   Street name for a potent variety of cannabis (marijuana) plant that reputedly has a higher content of alpha-9-tetrahydrocannabinol.

"accelerator"   Street name for amphetamine.

accelerometer   Miniature piezoelectric or strain-gauge device responsive to acceleration in a single plane that can be used to measure muscle movement. Accelerometers weigh only a few grams, do not significantly obstruct movement, or impose a significant exertional load. Accelerometric studies of tardive dyskinesia are being done with increasing frequency.

acceptable drinking   See **drinking, acceptable**.

acceptable risk   See **risk, acceptable**.

acceptor   Tissue constituent that binds a ligand without necessarily producing an effect.

accident, cerebrovascular   See **stroke** (preferred term).

accumulation Phenomenon in which repeated administration of a drug, especially one with a long elimination half-life, results in protracted build-up in plasma/tissue concentration.

accumulation index Relative extent of drug accumulation, a function of half-life and dosing interval.

accuracy Ability to obtain a standard value and reproduce it repeatedly; degree to which a measurement represents the true value of the attribute being measured; validation of an assay by comparison of the actual amount of drug in the control sample with the amount recovered.

"ace" Street name for marijuana.

acebutolol (Sectral) Cardioselective beta-blocker with a half-life of 3–4 hours. Daily dosage range is 400–800 mg. It has some local anesthetic activity. Pregnancy risk category B. See **beta-adrenergic blocking agent**.

acemetacin (Emflex) Glycolic acid ester of indomethacin that is a weaker inhibitor of prostaglandin synthesis than other nonsteroidal anti-inflammatory drugs. Side effect profile is similar to that of indomethacin, its main metabolite.

acemetacin + lithium See **lithium + acemetacin**.

Acepril See **captopril**.

acetaldehyde Highly toxic product of the first phase of alcohol metabolism that is thought to play an important role in alcohol-induced liver damage and may also contribute to the pathogenesis of alcohol dependence. Alcohol dehydrogenase, which accounts for over 90% of alcohol metabolism in the liver and determines the rate of acetaldehyde formation, is implicated in genetic susceptibility to alcoholic liver disease (Sherman DIN, Ward RJ, Warren Perry M, et al. Association of restriction fragment length polymorphism in alcohol dehydrogenase 2 gene with alcohol-induced liver damage. *Br Med J* 1993;307:1388–1390).

acetaminophen (Datril; Tempra; Tylenol) Clinically proven analgesic and antipyretic that produces some of its analgesic effects by elevation of the pain threshold and antipyresis through action at the hypothalamic heat-regulating center. It is a weak inhibitor of prostaglandin. Probably equal to aspirin in analgesic and antipyretic effectiveness, it is unlikely to produce many of the side effects associated with aspirin and aspirin-containing products, particularly gastric and duodenal irritation. It is often combined with other analgesics. It is the principal constituent of many over-the-counter products for headaches, minor pains and aches, and colds.

acetaminophen + alcohol Alcohol enhances diversion of acetaminophen to the quinonim-

ide. In large enough doses, severe pathology can result from formation of toxic intermediates of acetaminophen and reduction of hepatic glutathione (Hathcock JN, Metabolic mechanisms of drug-nutrient interactions. *Fed Proc* 1985;44[1]:124–129).

acetaminophen + carbamazepine See **carbamazepine + acetaminophen**.

acetaminophen + fluoxetine See **fluoxetine + acetaminophen**.

acetaminophen + lithium See **lithium + acetaminophen**.

acetaminophen + nicotine transdermal system See **nicotine transdermal system + acetaminophen**.

acetaminophen + oxycodone See **oxycodone + acetaminophen**.

acetaminophen + zidovudine See **zidovudine + acetaminophen**.

acetazolamide (Diamox) Inhibitor of carbonic anhydrase, an enzyme involved in the transport of CO_2 across membranes. It is a diuretic used for the adjunctive treatment of edema associated with congestive heart failure and drug-induced edema. It also is used as adjunctive therapy for chronic open-angle and acute angle-closure glaucoma. It sometimes possesses anticonvulsant activity. Pregnancy risk category C.

acetazolamide + lithium See **lithium + acetazolamide**.

acetophenazine (Formerly Tindal) Piperazine phenothiazine neuroleptic used as an antipsychotic. It is similar in action to other piperazine phenothiazine neuroleptics (perphenazine, trifluoperazine, fluphenazine). It is weakly anticholinergic, mildly sedative, and unlikely to cause hypotension. It causes a high incidence of acute early onset extrapyramidal reactions and photosensitivity reactions. Pregnancy risk category C.

acetophenazine + antacid Aluminum- and magnesium-containing antacids may decrease absorption of acetophenazine, decreasing therapeutic response to it.

acetophenazine + beta-blocker Beta-blockers may inhibit acetophenazine metabolism, raising plasma level of acetophenazine and increasing risk of toxicity.

acetophenazine + phenytoin Acetophenazine may inhibit metabolism of phenytoin, increasing risk of phenytoin toxicity.

acetorphan Parenterally active enkephalinase inhibitor that significantly reduces objective signs and subjective symptoms of opiate withdrawal. It does not produce drug dependence. Efficacy is comparable to that of clonidine for treating subjective symptoms of opiate withdrawal and perhaps even greater in relieving objective signs of withdrawal (e.g., anor exia, mydriasis), which shows that enkephalinase inhibition may be a novel and safe therapeutic approach to the opioid withdrawal syndrome (Hartmann F, Poirier M-F, Bourdel M-C, et al. Comparison of acetorphan with clonidine for opiate withdrawal symptoms. *Am J Psychiatry* 1991;148:627–629).

acetylation Phase II or "synthetic" hepatic metabolic pathway in which conjugation of an active drug or its metabolites occurs, making them biologically inactive and water soluble or "polar." The hepatic enzyme N-acetyltransferase is responsible for acetylation. About half the U.S. population has reduced N-acetyltransferase activity ("slow acetylators"). Rapid acetylators require higher doses of some drugs to attain the desired therapeutic response. Slow acetylators tend to be more susceptible to adverse reactions when treated with certain drugs (e.g., isoniazid, phenelzine).

acetylator phenotype Genetic expression in a given person of the ability to acetylate (introduce an acetyl group to) different organic compounds. Individuals can be divided into normal, rapid or extensive, and slow or poor acetylators.

acetylator, rapid Person whose hepatic N-acetyltransferase function is hyperactive, resulting in rapid metabolism of certain drugs. Rapid acetylators are more likely to require larger doses of some drugs (e.g., phenelzine) to obtain a therapeutic response and maintain the same average plasma concentration as slow acetylators. They are more likely to respond unpredictably to usual doses of a drug and to develop hepatotoxicity due to acetylhydrazine accumulation. Also called extensive metabolizer. See **acetylator, slow**.

acetylator, slow Person whose hepatic N-acetyltransferase function is hypoactive, resulting in slow metabolism and elevated plasma concentration of certain drugs, and increased susceptibility to adverse drug effects. Also called poor metabolizer. See **acetylator, rapid**.

acetylcholine (ACh) Neurotransmitter synthesized from choline and acetyl coenzyme A in the presence of choline acetyltransferase. ACh is important for memory and other functions and peripherally for neuromuscular functioning. There are two types of ACh receptors, nicotinic and muscarinic. ACh concentration is reduced in the brains of Alzheimer patients. ACh mechanisms may be involved in affective disorders.

acetylcholine antagonist Atropine and related drugs.

acetylcholine precursor Choline or lecithin (a phosphatidylcholine), according to activation by either muscarine or nicotine.

acetylcholine receptor Nicotinic or muscarinic receptors.

acetylcholine receptor agonist Substance (e.g., arecoline, oxotremorine, pilocarpine) that acts like acetylcholine when attached to muscarinic acetylcholine receptors, either by direct action on the receptor or by increasing ACh release.

acetylcholinesterase (AChE) Principal enzyme that metabolizes acetylcholine. AChE converts acetylcholine into an acetyl group and choline. It provides the only means of inactivating acetylcholine. Many "nerve gases" are acetylcholinesterases.

acetyl-l-carnitine (ALCAR) Acetylic derivative of L-carnitine, a natural substance in the human body with some cholinergic properties. ALCAR has been assumed to fulfill a regulating role in neuronal transmission. It is being studied for the treatment of pathological or age-dependent conditions characterized by cognitive impairment. When given to patients with degenerative or vascular pathology, it induces some improvement in performance. Placebo-controlled studies indicate that treatment with ALCAR significantly reduces severity of depressive symptoms in senile depression.

achalasia Neurogenic esophageal disorder of unknown etiology causing impairment of esophageal peristalsis and of lower esophageal sphincter relaxation; sometimes called "cardiospasm." It may occur at any age, but usually begins between 20 and 40. Onset is insidious, and progression is gradual over months or years. The major symptom is dysphagia for both solids and liquids. Some patients complain of chest pain, regurgitation, or nocturnal cough. Nocturnal regurgitation of undigested food occurs in about one-third of patients and may cause aspiration. Weight loss is usually mild to moderate. Achalasia must be differentiated from dysphagia induced by neuroleptics and other dopamine-blocking drugs.

achievement age Educational age. It is established by standard achievement tests consisting of a series of educational, rather than intelligence, tests.

"acid" Street name for lysergic acid diethylamide (LSD).

"acid dropper" Street name for a person who uses lysergic acid diethylamide (LSD).

"acid freak" Street name for a habitual user of lysergic acid diethylamide (LSD).

"acid head" Street name for a habitual user of lysergic acid diethylamide (LSD).

acquired immunodeficiency syndrome (AIDS) Illness caused by infection of T-lymphocytes with human immunodeficiency virus (HIV).

HIV can directly infect the central nervous system and cause a spectrum of syndromes ranging from subtle behavioral changes to fulminating encephalitis. Physical disorders are frequently associated with psychiatric disorders including depression, mania, manic-depressive illness, schizophrenia, paranoid psychoses, personality problems, adjustment reactions, dementia, and a variety of organic mental disorders. Affective disorders, especially depressive illness, are the most frequently encountered psychiatric illnesses; they can be treated effectively with medication and supportive psychotherapy. Because AIDS patients are more susceptible to neuroleptic-induced extrapyramidal reactions than patients without AIDS, neuroleptics should be used cautiously and in lower doses in AIDS patients.

acrocentric   Chromosome with a nearly terminal centromere so that one arm is very short.

acrophase   Peak of a sine function fitted to the raw data of a rhythm; time of peak daily activity in circadian rhythms.

Actibine   See **yohimbine**.

actigraph   Biomedical instrument that measures body movement.

acting-out   Acting without reflection or apparent regard for negative consequences (DSM-IV). See **defense mechanism**.

action dystonia   See **dystonia, action**.

action potential   Wave of electrical impulses that travels down an axon to start release of a neurotransmitter.

active placebo   Placebo that may mimic the side effects, but does not have the specific and assumed therapeutic pharmacologic actions of, the drug under investigation. Presence or absence of side effects may allow patients to identify whether they are receiving drug or placebo (for example, dry mouth may be associated with amitriptyline), necessitating the use of an active placebo in a well-designed and well-controlled study.

active sleep   See **sleep, active**.

aculalia   Nonsensical or jargon speech seen with Wernickes type of aphasia.

Acuphase   See **zuclopenthixol**.

acute   Rapid onset and abrupt cessation of expressed symptoms.

acute brain syndrome   See **delirium**.

acute confusional state   (ACS) Disorder characterized by clouding of consciousness, impairment of short-term memory, disorientation, and visual hallucinations or misinterpretations. Often there is fluctuation in symptom severity, which is frequently worse in the evening. If confusion is of recent origin and accompanied by some diminution of consciousness, possible causes include (a) drug toxicity—many prescription and some over-the-counter drugs (e.g., antihistamines, drugs for nighttime sedation), alcohol, tranquilizers of all kinds, and polypharmacy can cause confusion; (b) infections—respiratory and urinary infections may be an occult cause of confusion in the elderly; (c) cerebral anoxia resulting from heart failure or silent myocardial infarction, which may present as confusion; (d) metabolic states such as dehydration and hypoglycemia; and (e) environmental change or bereavement, especially in individuals with some prior mental impairment. In an already demented patient, deviations from the expected pattern of deterioration or abrupt change in condition should prompt a search for an ACS-producing medical condition. Drugs with anticholinergic actions (neuroleptics, antidepressants, antiparkinson agents, and some sedative/hypnotics), alcohol, and benzodiazepines are particularly toxic in the elderly and can be responsible for development of an ACS (Aujoulat O, Habib M, Braguer D, et al. Acute confusional state: retrospective study among 207 cases in a neurological unit. *J Pharm Clin* 1992;11:140–145). See **delirium**.

acute dystonia   See **dystonia, acute**.

acute persistent akathisia   See **akathisia, acute persistent**.

acute phase plasma protein   Alpha-1-antichymotrypsin (AAC), alpha-1-antitrypsin (AAT); haptoglobin (HAPT), alpha-1-acid glycoprotein (AGP), ceruloplasmin (CPM), prealbumin, transferrin, immunoglobulin G (IgG), immunoglobulin A (IgA), and immunoglobulin M (IgM). Depressed patients have elevated levels of a number of acute phase plasma proteins compared with control subjects. Depressed men have significantly elevated levels of HAPT, AAC, and IgG. Elevations in HAPT and AAC are highly correlated with each other and with depression severity. They are negatively correlated with thyroid stimulating hormone response to thyrotropin. These findings provide further evidence for an inflammatory response during depression (Joyce PR, Hawes CR, Mulder RT, et al. Elevated levels of acute phase plasma proteins in major depression. *Biol Psychiatry* 1992;32:1035–1041).

acute psychotic agitation/drug-induced   Impaired state, usually seen in an emergency room, often caused by cocaine, phencyclidine (PCP), amphetamine, or alcohol. It is manifested by severe agitation and delusions, dilated pupils, slurred speech, nystagmus, ataxia, elevated blood pressure, tachycardia, and some pyrexia. These signs and symptoms should prompt a search for needle tracks, nasal septum erosion, and other evidence of illicit drug use.

acute psychotic agitation/drug therapy Rapid symptomatic control can be achieved with an antipsychotic or benzodiazepine (BZD) alone or in combination orally or intramuscularly. Combined neuroleptic/BZD therapy can be more effective than either drug alone; advantages include efficacy with lower doses of each drug and lower risk of adverse effects due to either drug (Easton MS, Janicak PG. The use of benzodiazepines in psychotic disorders: a review of the literature. *Psychiatric Ann* 1990; 20:535–544; Horst WD, Preskorn SH. The role of benzodiazepines in the treatment of psychotic disorders. *Psychiatric Ann* 1993;23:317–324).

acute stress reaction Transient disorder of significant severity that develops in an individual without any other apparent mental disorder in response to exceptional physical and/or mental stress and that usually subsides within hours or days. The stressor may be an overwhelming traumatic experience involving serious threat to the security or physical integrity of the subject or loved person(s) (e.g., natural catastrophe, accident, battle, criminal assault, rape), or an unusually sudden and threatening change in the social position and/or network of the individual (e.g., multiple bereavement, domestic fire). The risk of developing an acute stress reaction is increased if physical exhaustion or organic factors (e.g., advanced age) are also present. Individual vulnerability and coping capacity play a role in occurrence and severity, as evidenced by the fact that not all persons exposed to exceptional stress develop the disorder. Symptoms show great variation, but typically include an initial state of "daze" with some constriction of the field of consciousness and narrowing of attention, inability to comprehend stimuli, and disorientation. The state may be followed either by further withdrawal from the surrounding situation (to the extent of a psychogenic stupor) or by agitation and overactivity (flight reaction or fugue). Autonomic signs of panic anxiety (tachycardia, sweating, flushing) are commonly present. Symptoms usually appear within minutes of the impact of the stressful stimulus or event and disappear within 2 or 3 days (often within hours). Partial or complete amnesia for the episode may be present. Acute stress reaction is not the same as post-traumatic stress disorder (International Classification of Diseases-10, World Health Organization, 1990). See **post-traumatic stress disorder**.

Adalat See **nifedipine**.

"Adam" Street name for 3,4-methylenedioxymethamphetamine (MDMA).

"Adam and Eve" Street expression for simultaneous consumption of 3,4-methylenedioxymethamphetamine (MDMA) and 3,4-methylenedioxyethamphetamine (MDEA).

Adapin See **doxepin**.

adaptive randomization Computer-assisted method of keeping prognostic variables in balance by adapting the probabilities of allocation of treatment to the characteristics and the prognostic features of the current patient, based on those patients who have already completed the study.

addict Term used in so many ways that it is meaningless except in context. *JAMA* defined it as a person physically dependent on one or more psychoactive substances, whose long-term use has produced tolerance, who has lost control over intake, and who would manifest withdrawal phenomena if discontinuance occurs. *Addict* is often used interchangeably with drug or alcohol dependence. However, in DSM-IV, physical dependence and tolerance are not criteria for addiction.

addiction Disease process characterized by continued use of a specific psychoactive substance despite physical, psychological, or social harm (American Society of Addiction Medicine,1990); complex behavioral disorder, the result of reward or liking and not physical dependence, characterized by loss of control over substance use, continuing use despite problems caused by it, and denial of drug use and the problems it causes (DuPont RL. Thinking about stopping treatment for panic disorder. *J Clin Psychiatry* 1990;51[suppl A]: 38–45). Addiction usually connotes a more serious problem than abuse, but there is no sharp line that defines when impaired volitional capacity equals addiction. DSM-IV suggests nine criteria for inferring decreased volitional control. At one time addiction implied that if a drug were suddenly withdrawn there would be a full-blown withdrawal syndrome. It also implied that original drug effects wore off more rapidly as a result of tolerance if used continuously. Addictive drugs have been associated with euphoric effects and therefore linked to pleasure-seeking. In addition to drug-related consequences to health and functioning, addicts experience irresistible craving and compulsion to use the drug. Addiction is characterized by (a) inability to control amount and frequency of use; (b) irresistible cravings and urges; (c) continued use despite adverse effects; (d) denial of indisputable negative consequences; and (e) tendency to abuse other mood-altering drugs or alcohol, either concomitantly or in the absence of the abused substance (a common but not defining characteristic). The relationship of addiction to changes in numbers, structure, or avidity of receptors for the drug in question is unclear. The words *dependence* and *addiction* are frequently used interchangeably. The concept of "physiological dependence" as applied to cocaine addiction is controversial, although some typical physiologic changes are associated with abrupt withdrawal following heavy use. See **dependence**.

addiction psychiatry   Subspeciality formally recognized in 1992, with the American Board of Medical Specialists approval of a certification process, including fellowships and an examination through the American Board of Psychiatry and Neurology. There is growing support for other medical specialties to develop American Board of Medical Specialists credentials in addiction medicine. Guidelines for postgraduate training have been developed; in 1991, there were 48 postresidency addiction fellowship programs, with 161 graduates and 122 fellows in training.

additive drug interaction   See **drug interaction, additive**.

additive genetic variance   See **genetic variance, additive**.

add-on study   Clinical drug trial in which new medication or placebo is added to current medications.

adenine   White crystalline base, 6-aminopurine found in various animal and vegetable tissues.

adenosine   Major neuromodulator that acts at two different receptor subfamilies: the A_1 receptor, which inhibits adenylate cyclase through G_i; and the A_2 receptor, which stimulates adenylate cyclase through G_s (Barraco RA, El-Ridi MR, Ergene E, Phillis JW. Adenosine receptor subtypes in brainstem mediate distinct cardiovascular response patterns. *Brain Res Bull* 1991;26:59–84; Stein MB, Black B, Brown TM, Uhde TW. Lack of efficacy of the adenosine reuptake inhibitor dipyridamole in the treatment of anxiety disorders. *Biol Psychiatry* 1993;33:647–650).

adenosine-3,5-cyclic monophosphate   (cAMP) See **cyclic adenosine monophosphate**.

adenosine triphosphatase   (ATPase) "Sodium pump" enzyme responsible for maintaining electrical gradient across cell membranes in erythrocytes and other cells.

adenylate cyclase   See **adenylylcyclase** (preferred term).

adenylylcyclase   (AC) Enzyme that generates cAMP. It is linked to many different receptors and can be a second messenger. When receptors are activated, there may be an increase or decrease in the second messenger cAMP. Ac-

tivation and inhibition of AC in lymphocytes and platelets resembles signal transduction processes in brain tissue. These cells, therefore, can be used as a model to study some aspects of psychiatric disorders, especially major depressive disorder (MDD) and post-traumatic stress disorder (PTSD). It has been reported, but not confirmed, that in both MDD and PTSD, receptor-mediated activation of AC is lower than in matched normal control groups. Also called "adenylate cyclase."

adiadokokinesis   Inability to perform rapid alternating movements, indicating a disorder of the cerebellum or its tracts. Such symptoms are called "neurological soft signs."

Adifax   See **dexfenfluramine**.

adinazolam   (Deracyn CT) Triazolobenzodiazepine and dimethylamino derivative of alprazolam (ALP) that binds to GABA receptors. It has anxiolytic and reputedly antidepressant effects and is reported to be as effective as ALP in the treatment of agoraphobia with panic attacks. Adinazolam is rapidly absorbed after oral administration with a mean T_{max} of 0.8 hours. Because it has a short half-life (approximately 2–4 hours) and a very short duration of therapeutic action (approximately 3 hours), it is usually given in a slow-release form. The major adinazolam metabolite, N-desmethyladinazolam (NDMAD), is more than 25 times as potent as adinazolam as a benzodiazepine agonist, suggesting that the metabolite, and not the parent drug, may mediate antianxiety actions. Elimination half-life of NDMAD also is short (about 3.7 hours). Adinazolam and NDMAD are not affected by consumption with food. At present (1994), nothing is known about the possible relationship between adinazolam/NDMAD plasma levels and clinical response. Like tricyclic antidepressants, adinazolam has effects on both norepinephrine and serotonin neurotransmitter systems. Effective antidepressant dosages range from 30 to 120 mg/day. Like other effective antidepressants, it has been reported to induce hypomania and mania (Hicks F, Robins E, Murphy G. Comparison of adinazolam, amitriptyline and placebo in the treatment of melancholic depression. *Psychiatry Res* 1987;23:221–227). Adinazolam may have problems associated with other benzodiazepines: potential for undue sedation, dependence, abuse, and withdrawal symptoms. Adinazolam should always be tapered slowly; a grand mal seizure has been reported during rapid tapering. See **n-desmethyladinazolam**.

adinazolam SR   (Deracyn SR) Sustained release formulation of adinazolam designed to lengthen duration of action.

adinazolam + cimetidine Cimetidine significantly decreases oral clearance of adinazolam and its metabolite n-desmethyladinazolam, and prolongs its half-life because of inhibition of oxidative metabolism (N-demethylation). The interaction may enhance adinazolam's central nervous system depressant effects.

adinazolam + ranitidine Ranitidine does not alter adinazolam pharmacokinetics or pharmacodynamics (Suttle AB, Songer SS, Dukes GE, et al. Ranitidine does not alter adinazolam pharmacokinetics or pharmacodynamics. *J Clin Psychopharmacol* 1992;12:282–287).

Adipex-P See **phentermine**.

Adipost See **phendimetrazine**.

adjunctive thyroid hormone therapy Augmentation of antidepressant response with thyroid hormone, first reported in 1969 (Prange AJ Jr, Wilson IC, Rabon AM, Lipton MA. Enhancement of imipramine antidepressant activity by thyroid hormone. *Am J Psychiatry* 1969;126:39–51). Since then, some clinicians have reported that addition of thyroid hormone, in particular triiodothyronine (T_3), can benefit as many as 50% of antidepressant nonresponders, particularly women. Treatment usually is initiated with liothyronine, 10–25 g/day, with increments up to 50 or 75 g if necessary. Adjunctive thyroid hormone may begin to enhance antidepressant response in as little as a few days. If no response occurs with 50 g/day, higher doses are unlikely to be beneficial. Adjunctive therapy has been especially recommended for patients with subnormal thyroid function or evidence of subclinical dysfunction (e.g., blunted thyroid-stimulating hormone [TSH] response to thyrotropin-releasing hormone [TRH] testing); however, abnormal thyroid function is not necessary for treatment response. Thyroxine (T_4) can be a beneficial adjuvant, but T_3 appears to have a faster onset of action.

adjusted rate Rate adjusted so that it is independent of the distribution of a possible confounding variable. For example, age-adjusted rates are independent of the age distribution in the population to which they apply.

adjustment disorder Brief maladaptive reactions to life's stresses or crises. Symptoms and behavior are beyond the expected normal range of reactions to such stresses. Symptoms may include depressed or anxious mood. conduct disturbances, employment or academic difficulties, withdrawal, or physical complaints. Adjustment disorders usually remit when the stressor no longer exists. Patients meeting criteria for a specific syndrome (e.g. major depression) are categorized as having the disorder appropriate to that syndrome.

adjuvant Addition to a drug that affects the drug's action in a predictable way, usually therapeutically.

Admon See **nimodipine**.

adolescence Period between puberty and maturity during which sexual and reproductive capabilities reach full maturity. It begins with the appearance of secondary sexual characteristics at about age 12 and terminates at about age 20.

adoption study Study in which adopted-apart biological relatives are compared to estimate the influence of heredity. They are based on three principal designs: (a) the adoptees family method, used to determine the risk for a particular condition to the biologic and adoptive parents of index cases versus control subjects; (b) the adoptees study method, concerned with the adopted-away children of affected parents; and (c) the crossfostering method, which compares adoptees who have an affected biologic parent with adoptees whose biologic parents are normal but who are reared by an adoptive parent affected with the condition under study.

adrenaline See **epinephrine**.

adrenergic Relating to nerve fibers, tracts, or pathways in which synaptic transmission is mediated by epinephrine or norepinephrine. See **adrenergic nerve**.

adrenergic agent See **sympathomimetic**.

adrenergic-cholinergic imbalance hypothesis of affective disorders Postulation that there is overactivity of central cholinergic relative to noradrenergic neurotransmission in depression, and the converse in mania. It is based on depressiogenic and antimanic effects of central cholinomimetics such as physostigmine, opposing and antagonistic effects of physostigmine and psychostimulants, and antidepressant effects of cholinolytics (Janowsky DS, El-Yousef MK, Davis JM, Sekerkl MJ. A cholinergic-adrenergic hypothesis of mania and depression. *Lancet* 1972;2:632–633).

adrenergic nerve Nerve that releases the neurotransmitter epinephrine, or norepinephrine.

adrenergic receptor Receptor that recognizes and initiates the actions of catecholamines such as epinephrine and norepinephrine (noradrenaline). Based on pharmacological criteria, several distinct types of adrenergic receptors have been classified (alpha-1, alpha-2, beta-1, beta-2). Also called "adrenoceptor"; "noradrenergic receptor."

adrenergic system Bodily system in which epinephrine is the neurotransmitter.

adrenoceptor See **adrenergic receptor**.

adrenocortical hormone See **adrenocorticotropic hormone**.

adrenocorticotropic hormone   (ACTH) One of the anterior pituitary hormones; a single chain polypeptide containing 39 amino acids. ACTH also is a neuromodulator in the central nervous system. Its release is stimulated primarily by corticotropin-releasing hormone (CRH). ACTH stimulates the adrenal cortex to secrete cortisol and several weak androgens. The CRH-ACTH-cortisol axis is central to the response to stress. There is evidence that some ACTH analogs may improve attention, motivation, or mood. ACTH may be related to at least some neuropeptides.

adrenoleukodystrophy   (ALD) X-linked recessive disorder that mainly affects nervous system white matter, the adrenal cortex, and the Leydig cells in the testes. It is associated with abnormal accumulation of saturated very long chain fatty acids because of impaired capacity to degrade these substances, a reaction that normally takes place in the peroxisome. The disorder has been mapped to Xq28. Clinical manifestations vary markedly from a rapidly progressive childhood cerebral form, to an adult form called adrenomyeloneuropathy that progresses slowly over decades, to a form that manifests as Addison's disease without neurological involvement. The various phenotypes occur frequently within the same family and even sibships; segregation analysis suggests the existence of a modifier gene. ALD presents commonly as a psychiatric disorder. Therapeutic interventions include a promising dietary approach and bone marrow transplantation.

adrenomyeloneuropathy   (AMN) Adult form of adrenoleukodystrophy that progresses slowly over decades to a form that manifests as Addison's disease without neurological involvement.

Adroyd   See **oxymetholone**.

adult attention deficit hyperactivity disorder (AADHD) Criteria are (a) meet DSM-IV criteria for attention deficit hyperactivity disorder (ADHD) by age 7; (b) have at least five DSM-IV symptoms of the disorder at the time of assessment; and (c) have a history of chronic symptoms of ADHD from childhood to adulthood.

Adult Children Anonymous   Self-help group to assist co-dependents and adult children of dysfunctional families.

Adult Children of Alcoholics   (ACOAs) Self-help group consisting of adults who in their view continue to reflect adverse effects of being offspring of alcoholics. Many consider themselves alcoholics who often marry alcoholics and also often have alcoholic relatives. They are at higher risk for divorce, their sons often are problem drinkers, and they are at risk for depression. Their behavior often is a manifestation of psychopathology generated by a disruptive, traumatic, and very unhappy childhood in which they were deprived of a stable family life.

adulteration   Common practice of illicit drug producers that consists of mixing the drug with another substance to expand the volume. Adulterants commonly found in illicitly purchased cocaine include talc, flour, cornstarch, and various sugars. Adulterants can be responsible for unpleasant and serious adverse reactions if inhaled or injected.

advance sleep phase syndrome   See **circadian phase sleep disorder**.

adverse drug experience   (ADE) Any adverse event associated with use of a drug in humans, whether or not considered drug-related. Included are: (a) adverse events during the use of a drug product in professional practice; (b) adverse events occurring from drug overdose, whether accidental or intentional; (3) adverse events occurring from drug withdrawal; and (4) any significant failure of expected pharmacological action. A serious ADE is life-threatening or results in or prolongs hospitalization, death, congenital anomaly, cancer, overdose, or permanent disability. An unexpected ADE is one not found in current labeling (Collins GE. Adverse drug experience communications and reporting industry perspective: regulations and practice. *Drug Infect J* 1991;25:131–137).

adverse drug interaction   One drug reducing the efficacy of another, or one drug increasing the toxicity of another.

adverse drug reaction   (ADR) Any noxious and unintended response to a drug that occurs at doses used in humans for prophylaxis, diagnosis, or therapy, excluding failure to accomplish the intended purpose (Karch FE, Lasagna L. Adverse drug reactions. *JAMA* 1975; 234:1236–1241). The term implies a causal relationship with the drug, yet many ADRs are based on allergy or hypersensitivity; their occurrence seems entirely unpredictable. Many have a much higher concordance among monozygous than dizygous twins, suggesting a genetic basis. ADRs that occur in therapeutic situations may or may not be dose-related. Drug inefficacy is not an ADR, nor are toxic responses to accidental or deliberate overdose. ADRs are usually classified as mild (no treatment necessary); moderate (requires change in drug therapy and may require additional or special treatment); severe (potentially life-threatening and requiring specific treatment of the ADR); and lethal (directly or indirectly contributes to the patient's death). In an elderly population, patients with frailty arising from multiple pathologies are more likely to have ADRs than the more robust elderly, even when their therapeutic regimens are simplified. ADRs can be divided into types A and B. The former are the normal but augmented pharmacological effects of a drug, and the latter are abnormal, bizarre effects. See **adverse drug experience; adverse drug reaction, type A; adverse drug reaction, type B**.

adverse drug reaction, idiosyncratic   Unpredictable drug side effect, including hypersensitivity reactions, that often develops suddenly and without warning. Such reactions may be genetically determined; they are neither related to a drug's known pharmacological effects nor are obviously allergic in nature. They occur in less than 0.1% of patients, and are not detected by toxicology testing in animals or in early clinical testing, and thus are virtually impossible to prevent. The most common clinical manifestations of idiosyncratic reactions include fever and disorders of the lungs, bone marrow, peripheral blood cells, heart, and serous membranes. They may be serious medical problems, depending on how extensively the drug is used and the severity of the reaction. Often there is a history either of prior exposure to the drug or a lag period of more than a week between starting the drug and the development of toxicity. When a patient who has had an idiosyncratic reaction is re-exposed to the offending drug, there may be immediate recurrence of the idiosyncratic symptoms.

adverse drug reaction, predictable   Exaggeration of a drug's normal pharmacologic effects.

adverse drug reaction, serious   Adverse drug reaction that may result in death, prolonged or new hospitalization, or permanent or severe disability (U.S. Food and Drug Administration).

Adverse Drug Reactions Reporting System   Postmarketing source of early warnings of toxic drug reactions available to the Food and Drug Administration (FDA). The system receives information from around the world, covers all drugs, is relatively inexpensive, and is a viable method to detect adverse drug reactions. See **MEDWatch**.

adverse drug reaction, type A   Result of an exaggerated but normal pharmacological action of a therapeutic dose of a drug (e.g., dry mouth produced by the anticholinergic action of a tricyclic antidepressant [TCA] or drowsiness induced by a benzodiazepine). Most type A reactions are common, predictable, and usually dose-dependent. Their morbidity is high but their mortality is generally low. Usual treatment is dosage reduction. Many are not due to the pharmacological action that mediates therapeutic effects, but to some other property. For example, most TCAs have anticholinergic effects causing atropine-like effects. Type A reactions occur at the extremes of dose-response curves for pharmacological and toxicological effects. They tend to occur in individuals who (a) may receive more drug than is customarily required; (b) may receive a conventional drug dose, but metabolize or excrete it slowly, resulting in high plasma levels; or (c) may be unusually sensitive to the drug. Time to onset of a type A reaction depends on the drug's pharmacokinetics and the tissue threshold necessary for the reaction. For an oral drug, onset will probably be between half an hour and the time to reach steady state (five times the drug's half-life). For intravenous drugs, onset may be instantaneous. Also called "type I."

adverse drug reaction, type B   Aberrant, unexpected, unpredictable, and potentially serious reaction inexplicable in terms of the drug's normal pharmacology. Such reactions may be due to hypersensitivity or immunologic reactions and usually require cessation of the drug. They are the most difficult drug reactions to predict or even detect and are generally associated with high mortality, although incidence and morbidity are usually low. They are a major focus of pharmacoepidemiologic studies of adverse drug reactions. Type B reactions require a minimum of 5 days on treatment before the cells become hypersensitive to the drug, but there is no maximum time for these reactions to have occurred; although most will have occurred by 12 weeks, some may be delayed as long as a year (e.g., tardive dyskinesia with neuroleptics). Reactions may appear after the drug has been stopped (e.g., agranulocytosis). Also called "type II."

adverse effect   See **adverse drug experience; adverse drug reaction**.

adverse event   (AE) Injury caused by medical management (rather than the *disease*) that prolongs hospitalization, produces a disability at the time of discharge, or both. AEs do not necessarily indicate low-quality care, nor does their absence necessarily indicate high-quality care. For example, a drug reaction occurring in a patient who has been appropriately prescribed a drug for the first time is an AE, but one that is unavoidable given today's technology. By contrast, if the reaction occurs in a patient who is given a drug despite known sensitivity to it, the AE may be due to negligence. Sometimes there are no good alternatives and the sensitivity may be judged to be a lower risk than the use of the drug. Negligence is more frequent in patients who have had more severe AEs. Drug complications are the most common type of AE. AEs result from the interaction of the patient, the patient's disease, and a complicated, highly technical system of medical care.

adverse event, serious   See **adverse drug reaction, serious.**

adverse reaction   See **adverse drug experience; adverse drug reaction.**

Advil   See **ibuprofen.**

aerophagia   Swallowing of air to such an extent as to cause abdominal distention, persistent belching, flatulence, and/or symptoms of hyperventilation.

affect   Feeling tone, pleasurable or unpleasurable, that accompanies and/or determines the general attitude toward an idea. It includes inner feelings and their external manifestations. *Affect* and *emotion* are often used interchangeably. Sustained affect is a mood. See **mood.**

affect, blunted   Diminished emotional responsiveness manifested by reduction in facial expression (barren or "wooden" expression), modulation of feelings, and reduction in communicative gestures. It is seen more frequently in schizophrenia than in classic affective disorder. In schizophrenia, it is considered a negative symptom. See **schizophrenia/negative symptoms.**

affect, flattened   Global inability to experience, or at least to express, emotions. It is seen primarily in schizophrenia or dementia and should be distinguished from anhedonia. Also called "emotional blunting."

affect, inappropriate   Emotional response incompatible with the demands of a particular situation, expressed thought, or mood.

affective disorder   One of a group of clinical conditions, the common and essential feature of which is mood disturbance, either depression or elation, accompanied by related cognitive, psychomotor, psychophysiological, and interpersonal difficulties. Some psychiatrists define the term "affective disorder" as including both mood and anxiety disorders. Also called "mood disorder."

affective disorder/circadian shift   Partial sleep deprivation may induce an antidepressant response in unipolar depression. In bipolar patients, sleep deprivation (whether due to physical illness, emotional stress, or events disrupting sleep schedules such as transmeridian flights) may induce mania. Bipolar patients are particularly vulnerable to circadian shifts, especially when they involve sleep deprivation, and must recognize such disruptive challenges as significant and important events that can precipitate manic symptoms and severely exacerbate their illness.

affective disorder, seasonal   See **seasonal affective disorder.**

affective disorder/treatment resistant, thyroid function   See **adjunctive thyroid hormone therapy.**

affective lability   Rapid changes in affect, usually short-lived and fluctuating.

affective psychosis   Affective disorder with psychotic symptoms. The illness is severe and recurrent, but it does not generally lead to deterioration between episodes. It can be treated, and relapses can be minimized by the use of prophylactic (maintenance) drug therapy and cognitive or interpersonal therapy. Life-time risk is approximately 1% for the adult population.

affective spectrum disorder   Term proposed by Hudson and Pope to denote disorders of affect and its clinical spectrum. Disorders identified as members of this family are responsive to treatment with tricyclic antidepressants and chemically similar agents (e.g., maprotiline, viloxazine), monoamine oxidase inhibitors, serotonin uptake inhibitors, and atypical agents (e.g., bupropion, mianserin, and trazodone), suggesting they have a common pathophysiology. These disorders include major depression, bulimia, panic disorder, attention deficit hyperactivity disorder, cataplexy, migraine, and irritable bowel syndrome. Several other disorders (e.g., posttraumatic stress disorder, atypical facial pain) nearly meet the criteria of the model as well. There may be other disorders in the family that cannot be identified by antidepressant response (e.g., bipolar disorder, schizoaffective disorder), but that nevertheless share an etiologic feature with affective spectrum disorder. Identified forms of affective spectrum disorder, including major depression, afflict a large proportion of the population (Hudson JI, Pope HG Jr. Affective spectrum disorder: does antidepressant response identify a family of disorders with a common pathophysiology? *Am J Psychiatry* 1990;147:552–564; Hudson JI, Pope HG Jr. Affective spectrum disorder? *Am J Psychiatry* 1991;148:548–549).

affective style   (AS) Measure of emotional-verbal behavior of relatives in direct interaction with the patient. Family communication may help to predict the course of schizophrenia.

affect reaction   Danish diagnostic term applied to histrionic or panicky behavior or an impulsive suicidal attempt in response to an identifiable event, usually rejection.

affinity   Tightness with which a neurotransmitter or antagonist binds to a receptor. It may be quantified by the affinity constant (K_m or B_{max}). Drug affinity for a particular receptor is a major predictor of the drug's milligram potency and also may predict its likelihood to cause certain adverse effects.

affinity chromatography Procedure used to purify antibodies directed against a specific protein (antigen). Usually, crude serum from an inoculated animal contains many different antibodies. One can bind the antigen used in the immunization to a column support and pass the crude serum over the column. The antibodies directed against the specific protein will bind to the column, and the unbound antibodies will be washed through. The specific antibodies are removed from the column under conditions that reverse binding. These antibodies are considered affinity-purified by the fact that they had affinity for the protein on the column. The technique can also be used to purify enzymes by attaching the enzyme substrate to the column.

"African black" Street name for a potent variety of marijuana.

aftercare Continuing rehabilitation treatment and support provided for a patient following release from an institution. Aftercare should be planned and arranged before discharge and maintained as long as necessary.

agarose gel Gel made of extract of seaweed (agar), used to separate molecules by size via migration through an electric field.

age-associated memory impairment (AAMI) Disorder (existence of which is debated) alleged to occur in patients over age 60 in the absence of clinical evidence for dementia. It is characterized by gradual onset, slow decline, and selective memory loss (diminished ability to remember names, think of the correct word, recall location of objects, and concentrate). Although it may represent the earliest symptoms of dementia, most patients do not develop dementia when followed-up for as long as 10 years. In most cases, symptoms are benign. AAMI is a nonprogressive, "normal" variant of aging that should be distinguished from the earliest stages of Alzheimer's dementia (Crook T, Bartus RT, Jervis SH, et al. Age-associated memory impairment: proposed diagnostic criteria and measures of clinical change. Report of a National Institute of Mental Health work group. *Dev Neuropsychol* 1986;2:261–276). Also called "benign amnesia"; "benign senescent forgetfulness." See **neurocognitive disorder, mild**.

ageism Stereotyping of children or the elderly because of age, in such a way as to create negative expectations of them in order to discriminate against them and avert dealing with their social and physiological problems.

age-specific mortality rate Mortality rate in a specific age group.

aggregate data Information concerning a population as a whole, but in which little if any specification is possible as to which individuals in the group carry the phenomena of interest. Aggregate data may be used for prediction once a direct link between the variables of interest has been established.

aggression Behavior with physical and/or verbal concomitants in which actual physical harm to others, self, or property would result if the behavior is carried to its completion.

aggression, interictal Irritability that often occurs in temporal lobe epilepsy. It manifests intermittently during hours or days of dysphoric moods, with little provocation, in the form of angry or furious outbursts. Patients tend to be predominantly good-natured, highly ethical, and often very religious; they typically will not injure someone else and will be deeply remorseful for their ill-tempered behavior. The behavior should be contrasted with the more persistent aggressivity characterized by shallow mood and affect that occurs in frontal lobe disease, which may become unbearable to the next-of-kin. By contrast, patients with interictal aggression show deepened emotionality.

aggression, nonsituational Unprovoked, directed, or nondirected aggression attributed to no known cause; general irritability.

aggression, passive Mechanism in which the person indirectly and unassertively expresses aggression toward others.

aggression, physical Aggressive physical contact with another person or object (e.g., biting, throwing an object, slapping). Threatening behavior, such as raising a hand as if to hit, is not considered an act of physical aggression.

aggression, situational Aggression that may be provoked by physical abuse or verbal taunts of others, or by heightened physiological arousal sparked by participation in competitive sports, vigorous exercise, or provocative films.

aggressive behavior Behavior ranging from normal assertive and coping behavior to acts of violence. It may be expressed overtly (cursing) or covertly (gossiping), directly (physical assault), or indirectly (verbal hostility). Aggression also includes diverse motivational, emotional, and behavioral aspects. When aggressive behavior is excessive or inappropriate, suppression may be necessary. Lithium, beta blockers, clonazepam, buspirone, fluoxetine, eltoprazine, carbamazepine, and valproic acid have been used successfully in the treatment of aggressive behavior in some patients. Androgen antagonists or antiandrogens (cyproterone acetate and depomedroxyprogesterone) can be useful in reducing violent tendencies of highly aggressive males.

agitation Inability to sit still, pacing, fidgeting, movements of legs or fingers, wringing hands, and/or pulling at clothes, not limited to isolated periods, when discussing something upsetting. Subjective feelings of tension or restlessness are often incorrectly called agitation (Spitzer RL, Antacid J. *Schedule for Affective Disorders and Schizophrenia.* New York: New York State Psychiatric Institute, 1978). Agitation also must be differentiated from akathisia. See **akathisia**.

agnosia Loss of ability to identify, comprehend the meaning of, or recognize the importance of various types of sensory stimulation. It is not attributable to sensory loss, language impairment, or cognitive dysfunction.

agnosia, auditory Inability to recognize sounds that is not attributable to a hearing defect.

agnosia, visual Inability to recognize objects visually. See **prosopagnosia**.

agonist Substance (drug, transmitter, toxin) that binds to and stimulates a receptor, initiating a series of events leading to a biologic response. Agonists act on a receptor to produce effects similar to the natural ligand, whereas antagonists block the action of neurotransmitter ligands. All known neurotransmitters are receptor agonists, although some are also functional antagonists. Drugs may be direct or indirect agonists: the former are effective at the postsynaptic receptor; the latter work by enhancing effects of the natural neurotransmitter at its receptor.

agonist/antagonist Opioid analgesic with mixed actions, usually antagonist at the mu receptor and agonist at the kappa receptor.

agonist, direct Agonist effective at the postsynaptic receptor.

agonist, indirect Agonist that works by enhancing the effects and/or quantity of the natural neurotransmitter at its receptor. Enhancement can occur by increasing the presynaptic release of the neurotransmitter.

agonist, inverse Substance that produces effects at a receptor that are opposite to those produced by the usual agonist. For example, inverse agonists at benzodiazepine receptors have anxiogenic, proconvulsant, and promnestic properties and are interesting probes for the study of molecular receptor mechanisms.

agonist, partial Agent that acts as an agonist at low concentrations of the endogenous ligand, but which at higher concentrations displaces it from its recognition sites, diminishes its effects, and becomes an antagonist. Its intrinsic efficacy is between that of a pure agonist and the zero intrinsic efficacy of a pure antagonist. Partial agonists mimic natural neurotransmitter ligands in that they stimulate a receptor, yet do it only partially (like a rheostat that partially turns on the lights, whereas the natural ligand turns them on all the way). This fixed quality is engineered into the molecule and cannot be increased by raising the concentration of the partial agonist. Partial agonists are net agonists in the absence of the natural ligand that are less effective than the natural ligand; in the presence of the natural ligand they are net antagonists. RO 16-6028 is an example of a benzodiazepine partial agonist; buspirone is an example of a serotonin$_{1A}$ partial agonist.

agonist, partial inverse Substance whose profile mirrors that of the partial agonist (i.e., that induces functionally opposite effects). RO 15-4513 is an example of a partial inverse benzodiazepine agonist.

agoraphobia Term introduced by Westphal (1871) meaning "fear of the marketplace," now used to describe a phobia characterized by the need to avoid being in a "trapped" situation, usually a public place. It occurs most often in women and usually begins between the ages of 18 and 35, with a central symptom of anxiety that appears only in clearly defined situations. Agoraphobics fear losing control in a public place where they may become embarrassed; some with extreme agoraphobia do not leave their homes for any reason. Treatments include psychotherapy, cognitive therapy, pharmacotherapy, and behavior therapy. Agoraphobics often claim they are "very sensitive" to medicines and frequently give a history of having "side effects to almost every drug I have taken." Hence, they are often reluctant to take any medicine that may cause adverse effects and prefer to get along without it. They elect to suffer an untreated or inadequately treated illness because of an unwarranted fear of "addiction" or loss of control they associate with treatment with any psychoactive drug. Because agoraphobic patients are often disturbed by the side effects of medicines, treatment should be initiated with low doses followed by gradual dosage increments to achieve patient compliance and the benefits of a drug.

agranulocytosis White blood cell count of less than 2000 cells/mm^3, a polymorphonuclear leukocyte count of less than 500 cells/mm^3, and relative lymphopenia; erythrocyte and platelet values are normal. The blood dyscrasia is often iatrogenic; the two basic categories of drug-induced agranulocytosis are immunologic and toxic. In the immune-mediated type (allergic reaction), the drug triggers development of an antibody against antigens on granulocytes or on their immediate bone marrow precursors. The toxic type of agranulocytosis is mediated by biochemical rather than immune events in which the drug kills precursor cells directly, resulting in depletion of bone marrow cells. Toxic depression of the granulocyte cell line in marrow is related to cumulative drug dose. The two mechanisms have been presented as distinct entities, but it is possible that many drugs damage both compartments. Drugs also may trigger development of a "lupus-like" syndrome. Agranulocytosis has been caused most often by piperidine and aliphatic phenothiazine neuroleptics, by the atypical neuroleptic clozapine, and by the anticonvulsants carbamazepine, valproate, phenytoin, and ethosuximide. It also has been caused infrequently by mianserin, some tricyclic antidepressants (e.g., amitriptyline, desipramine, imipramine), benzodiazepines, chlorpromazine, cimetidine, hydrochlorothiazide, meprobamate, propranolol, and ranitidine. Onset of drug-induced agranulocytosis is generally gradual, occurring most often between 6 weeks and 6 months, although some cases have developed after a year or more of treatment with the causative agent. When agranulocytosis is induced by drug allergy, onset of symptoms is abrupt, although the time of onset varies between a few days to several weeks from the start of drug therapy and occasionally occurs later. Patients treated with drugs known to induce agranulocytosis should have regular hematological monitoring, weekly at first and then every 2 to 3 months until the end of the second treatment year. They should be counseled to report promptly any physical signs and symptoms. If agranulocytosis is suspected, a full blood count should be done immediately. The causative drug should be stopped immediately at the onset of agranulocytosis, since it is often fatal if not detected and treated early with aggressive antibiotic therapy to prevent infection. Retreatment with the same causative agent carries a high risk of recurrence of agranulocytosis. If necessary, treatment with another neuroleptic or tricyclic antidepressant should be initiated cautiously, with weekly hematological monitoring for the first 6 months. Agranulocytosis and neutropenia occur more frequently than aplastic anemia. In acute neutropenia, fever, sore throat, and painful mucosal ulcers are the common first symptoms. The incidence is highest in elderly females. Withdrawal of the drug may be followed by complete recovery in 2 or 3 weeks; however, the patient has been sensitized to the drugs and any further administration will result in prompt recurrence. Agranulocytosis must not be confused with the more common transient benign leukopenia. See **aplastic anemia; blood dyscrasia; thrombocytopenia.**

agraphia Impairment of the ability to communicate ideas in writing. It may involve individual letters, syllables, words, or phrases. It is usually due to a cerebral disorder.

AIDS delirium Medication side effects are a common cause of delirium in AIDS patients, particularly with anticholinergic drugs such as tricyclic antidepressants (amitriptyline), low-potency antipsychotics (chlorpromazine), antiemetics (scopolamine), antiparkinson agents (benztropine), and antihistamines (diphenhydramine). Other drugs that have caused delirium in central nervous system (CNS)-compromised AIDS patients are meperidine and short-acting benzodiazepines (midazolam and triazolam). Discontinuation of the responsible drug and discussing the cause of the symptoms to reassure the patient are often all that AIDS delirium patients require. In cases of extreme agitation secondary to delirium, a small dose of lorazepam, starting with 0.5 mg intravenously (slow push) or intramuscularly, may be beneficial (Gilman WS, Busch KA. Neuropsychiatric aspects of AIDS and psychopharmacologic management. *Psychiatr Med* 1991;9:313–329). Low doses of haloperidol also may be effective with minimal side effects (Weisman H, Platt M, Schindledecker R. Standardized diagnosis and clinical use of haloperidol for delirium symptoms in 58 AIDS patients. Poster presented at 3rd European Conference on Clinical Aspects and Treatment of HIV Infection, Paris, 1992).

AIDS dementia complex (ADC) Neuropsychologic dysfunction similar to subcortical dementia that occurs in AIDS. First symptoms are memory and concentration impairment and reduced psychomotor speed. Later, behavioral disturbances appear, with symptoms such as social withdrawal, apathy, depression, hallucinations, and neuromotor deficits such as ataxia, tremor, and affected handwriting. In the terminal state, AIDS patients can become completely apathetic and mute, and in some cases may be incontinent of urine and feces.

AIDS/mania Approximately 8% of AIDS patients are susceptible to having both manic and hypomanic episodes that may occur either early or late in the course of human immunodeficiency virus (HIV) infection. Hypomanic episodes occur after treatment with antidepressants and require substitution of lithium to induce remission. Patients with no family or personal history of mood disorder are more likely to develop mania late in the course of HIV infection and to have a higher prevalence of comorbid dementia (Lyketsos

C, Hanson AL, Fishman M, et al. Manic syndrome early and late in the course of HIV. *Am J Psychiatry* 1993;150:326–327).

AIDS psychosis/neuroleptic treatment Neuroleptic treatment of psychotic symptoms in patients with human immunodeficiency virus (HIV) infection or AIDS is effective, particularly for positive psychotic symptoms such as psychomotor agitation, hallucinations, and delusions (Vogel-Scibilia SE, Mulsant BH, Keshavan MS. HIV infection presenting as psychosis: a critique. *Acta Psychiatr Scand* 1988;78: 652–656). In a study of AIDS-related organic mental syndromes, bromperidol produced significant remission of positive psychotic symptoms with minimal side effects; "negative" symptoms were less sensitive or insensitive to bromperidol treatment. Because AIDS patients are quite susceptible to extrapyramidal side effects of antipsychotic drugs (e.g., dystonia, rigidity, and akathisia), they are best treated with low doses (Perretta P, Nisita C, Zaccagnini E, et al. Diagnosis and clinical use of bromperidol in HIV-related psychoses in a sample of seropositive patients with brain damage. *Int Clin Psychopharmacol* 1992;7:95–99).

AIDS-related complex (ARC) Presence of a human immunodeficiency virus (HIV)-positive state, fatigue, and diminished resistance to infections, without the symptoms of complete AIDS. Psychostimulants (e.g., methylphenidate 2.5–5 mg twice a day, not exceeding 90 mg/day; dextroamphetamine not exceeding 60 mg/day) have been shown to be effective in the treatment of cognitive impairment due to ARC, even in the absence of significant affective symptoms. The dosages may cause some involuntary dyskinetic movements. Pemoline has also been used, but efficacy has not been well documented (Fernandez F, Adams F, Levy JK, et al. Cognitive impairment due to AIDS-related complex and its response to psychostimulants. *Psychosomatics* 1988;29:38–46; Holmes V, Fernandez F, Levy JK. Psychostimulant response in AIDS-related complex patients. *J Clin Psychiatry* 1989;50:5–8).

akathisia Term derived from the Greek verb *akathemi* ("never to sit down"), first used by Haskovec (1902) to describe patients with restlessness and inability to sit still. Akathisia has been reported to occur naturally in child psychiatric patients and in nonpsychotic children treated for Tourette's disorder. A universally accepted definition of akathisia still does not exist, but most researchers emphasize two components: (a) a subjective or psychological feeling of inner restlessness distinct from anxiety or dysphoria that results in an inability to

remain still and a compulsion to move; and (b) objective, observable restless movements. It may present with a wide range of subjective complaints and behavioral disturbances. Patients frequently call akathisia "the jitters" because they feel compelled to walk or pace the floor. When sitting, they constantly shift their legs or tap their feet. When standing, they may continuously rock forward, backward, and side-to-side, or constantly shift their weight from one foot to the other. Shortly after the introduction of neuroleptics, akathisia was recognized as one of their most common and distressing early-onset side effects. Drug-induced akathisia has also been reported with lithium, methysergide, tricyclic antidepressants, and trazodone. In some patients, fluoxetine has induced an akathisia-like reaction manifested by agitation, restless motor movement, dysphoria, pacing, and an internal sense of desperation. However, these descriptions differ significantly from those given by patients with naturally occurring or neuroleptic-associated akathisia. Akathisia is often considered an extrapyramidal reaction, but pathophysiology is unknown; some evidence suggests dopamine neurons in the ventral tegmental area may be involved. Estimates of akathisia prevalence in neuroleptic-treated patients range between 20% and 75%. It is usually related not only to acute administration of a neuroleptic, but also to a recent dosage increase. It is often associated with severe parkinsonism, but not tardive dyskinesia. Neuroleptic-induced akathisia (NIA) has been associated with behavioral deterioration, worsening of psychosis, and treatment noncompliance. Akathisia may be difficult to distinguish from psychotic agitation or anxiety, especially if a patient describes a subjective experience of akathisia in terms of being controlled by an outside force. If the akathisia is mistaken for psychosis, the physician may increase the neuroleptic dose and actually worsen the condition, causing the patient to suffer more and ultimately become noncompliant. Beta-blockers, particularly propranolol, are effective in the treatment of NIA. A central site of action appears likely, because several studies have shown that hydrophilic beta-blockers (e.g., nadolol, atenolol, and sotalol) are less effective than propranolol, which is highly lipophilic. Recent research (1992) suggests that $beta_1$-adrenoceptor blockade is sufficient to improve NIA. Comparisons of two highly lipophilic beta-blockers—propranolol, which is a nonselective $beta_1$ and $beta_2$ blocker, and betaxolol, which is highly $beta_1$ selective—revealed no difference in antiakathisia effects. Treatment-resistent akathisiahas been treated successfully in some patients with the selective irreversible monoamine oxidase-B inhibitor selegiline (5 mg twice a day). Ritanserin, a 5-HT$_2$ antagonist, also has been effective, indicating involvement of the serotonergic system in the pathophysiology of the syndrome (Fleischhacker WW. Propranolol for fluoxetine-induced akathisia. *Biol Psychiatry* 1991;30:531–532). Anticholinergic drugs are not consistently effective.

akathisia, acute persistent Form of chronic neuroleptic-induced akathisia that persists in some patients. See **akathisia; akathisia, tardive**.

akathisia/agitation Agitation can be a manifestation of major depression, mania, generalized anxiety disorder, and other psychiatric disorders. It can be manifested by significant restlessness or motor movements similar to those of akathisia. Although it may be very difficult to distinguish neuroleptic-treated agitation from neuroleptic-induced akathisia, a pattern of worsening agitation with increasing neuroleptic dosage warrants suspicion of akathisia.

akathisia, chronic Neuroleptic-induced extrapyramidal reaction characterized by motor restlessness and an inability to sit still. It can be subdivided into (a) acute persistent akathisia, (b) withdrawal akathisia, and (c) tardive akathisia.

akathisia, tardive Drug-induced akathisia that develops after months or years of treatment with an antipsychotic or non-neuroleptic dopamine-blocking agent such as metoclopramide. It is characterized by a relatively mild sense of restlessness and lack of response to conventional anticholinergic treatment. Observable features in standing patients include rocking from foot to foot, walking on the spot, walking/pacing, inability to remain seated, changing stance. Observable features in seated patients include trampling/shuffling legs, fidgeting arms/hands, shifting position, repeated knee crossing, swinging leg, crossing/uncrossing legs, trunk shifting, and pumping legs up and down. Tardive akathisia may be associated with parkinsonism and tardive dyskinesia. Tardive akathisia and tardive dyskinesia have similar pharmacologic characteristics in that both may be evoked or may worsen following withdrawal or reduction of neuroleptic treatment; restarting or increasing the neuroleptic dose will alleviate the symptoms.

akathisia, withdrawal Symptoms that occur when chronic antipsychotic drug treatment is withdrawn for more than 2 weeks.

Akatinol See **memantine**.

akinesia Movement disorder manifested by diminution or loss of initiation of voluntary muscle movement. Complete loss is called "bradykinesia." Akinesia is a well known but often unrecognized neuroleptic side effect that produces the mask-like facial expression, absent arm swing, slow initiation of motor activity, and soft monotonous speech that are so common among neuroleptic-treated patients. It can be the only manifestation of an extrapyramidal reaction in patients receiving antipsychotic drugs. It is thought to be attributable to dopamine receptor blockade by neuroleptics. Neuroleptic-induced akinesia is often indistinguishable from deficit (negative) symptoms of schizophrenia. The patient's reduced spontaneity may be mistaken for depression. Quite often the patient seems drowsy and acts "washed-out." Muscle rigidity, cogwheeling, and tremor may be present. Akinesia may be devastating to the patients subjective and psychosocial progress. Akinesia characteristically is responsible for a reduction in leg-crossing, a symptom that can help to distinguish it from nonakinetic patients. Most persons (80%) (except those with parkinsonism) cross their legs when seated in a comfortable chair; only 10% of patients with mild akinesia cross their legs (Van Putten T. Adverse psychological [or behavioral] responses to antipsychotic drug treatment of schizophrenia. *In* A Rifkin [ed], *Schizophrenia and Affective Disorders: Biology and Drug Treatment*. Boston: John Wright, 1983, pp 323–341). Akinesia can be alleviated by antiparkinson medication or by dosage reduction or discontinuation of the neuroleptic. It also can be treated with methylphenidate and pemoline. Akinesia should be distinguished from bradykinesia, a distinct clinical syndrome marked by impaired initiation and maintenance of motor activity that appears to be associated with blue mood (at least in vulnerable persons), anhedonia, bradyphrenia (slowed cognition), and perhaps stereotyping of thought. There is evidence suggesting that a functional reduction in dopaminergic neurotransmission may play an important role in the pathophysiology of the akinesia syndrome in three conditions in which it appears commonly: Parkinson's disease, retarded depression, and the negative symptom state of schizophrenia (Bermanzohn PC, Siris SG. Akinesia: a syndrome common to parkinsonism, retarded depression, and negative symptoms of schizophrenia. *Compr Psychiatry* 1992;33:221–232). See **bradykinesia**.

akinesia, early morning See **akinesia, end of dose**.

akinesia, end of dose   Akinesia due to a "wearing off" of the effect of levodopa in Parkinson's disease patients. It occurs as the disease progresses and/or after two or more years of levodopa (L-dopa) treatment, during which levodopa's duration of action shortens and symptoms appear before the next dose is due. When wearing off of the prior evening's dose occurs each morning, it is called "early morning akinesia." Common symptoms are slowness, stiffness, freezing, and falls. Wearing off is a sign of proceeding degeneration and an indication of changes in pharmacokinetics of L-dopa and of the responsiveness of dopaminergic receptor sites to it. Also called "wearing off."

akinetic-abulic syndrome   Group of symptoms frequently occurring in the course of neuroleptic therapy, such as pseudoparkinsonism, bradykinesia, rigidity, decreased mental drive, and disinterest.

akinetic depression   See **depression, postpsychotic**.

akinetic mutism   See **mutism, akinetic**.

Akineton   See **biperiden**.

Alamix   See **cisapride**.

alanine aminotransferase   (ALT) Hepatic enzyme formally known as serum glutamic pyruvic transaminase (SGPT). Normal range is 5–40 IU/ml. Marked elevations (500–2000 IU/ml) occur with hepatitis, but correlation with clinical severity is poor. Increased serum ALT also is associated with cirrhosis, liver metastases, obstructive jaundice, infectious mononucleosis, hepatic congestion, pancreatitis, renal disease, and ethanol ingestion.

AL-ANON   Self-help group composed of spouses, children, relatives, and significant others of alcoholics, who are usually Alcoholics Anonymous (AA) members. AL-ANON was developed as a movement parallel to but separate from AA in the late 1940s.

alaproclate   Relatively specific serotonin uptake inhibitor being tested as an antidepressant in Europe. Testing to date has not provided evidence of efficacy in the treatment of dementia of the Alzheimer's type.

ALATEEN   Support group for teenaged children of alcoholics.

albumin   Major protein of plasma and its principal drug-binding protein. For most drugs as much as 80–95% is protein-bound. Many pathological conditions can affect albumin concentrations, which can affect drug dosing whenever total drug concentrations are a guide to dosage adjustment.

alcohol   Short-acting sedative that by pharmacological classification shares certain properties with sedative/hypnotic drugs, including a similar withdrawal syndrome. Alcohol is readily absorbed from the gastrointestinal tract. More than 90% is metabolized by the liver through oxidative mechanisms involving mainly alcohol dehydrogenase (ADH). ADH produces acetaldehyde, which in turn is oxidized to acetate. Acetaldehyde is toxic to the liver and other organs. Alcohol induces the microsomal ethanol oxidizing system (MEOS), which is responsible in part for alcohol metabolism, and induces the microsomal P450 involved in drug metabolism. Chronic alcohol ingestion results in increasing tolerance to alcohol and drugs, resulting in a complex interaction among drugs, other chemicals, and alcohol. Acute alcohol ingestion generally interferes with a drug's metabolism, increasing plasma concentration. Ingestion of alcohol over several weeks stimulates hepatic enzymes, accelerating metabolism of many other drugs.

alcohol abuse   Use of alcohol in a quantity and with a frequency that causes the individual significant physiological, psychological, or sociological distress or impairment.

alcohol abuse and dependence   Manifestations of alcohol use disorders (DSM-IV) that may be episodic or continuous. Anxiety and depression commonly arise as a result of chronic alcohol use. Anxiety may take the form of generalized anxiety, panic attacks, and phobias, such as agoraphobia. Depression may be minor or severe; the latter may produce disturbed mood, vegetative symptoms, and suicidal thoughts and actions that are similar to the symptoms of major depression.

alcohol + acetaminophen   Alcohol enhances the diversion of acetaminophen to the quinonimide. In large enough doses, severe pathology can result from the formation of toxic intermediates of acetaminophen and reduction of hepatic glutathione (Hathcock JN, Metabolic mechanisms of drug-nutrient interactions. *Fed Proc* 1985;44[1]:124–129).

alcohol addiction   Physiological and psychological dependence on alcohol.

alcohol + amitriptyline   See **amitriptyline + alcohol**.

alcohol amnestic disorder   Syndrome thought to be due to nutritional deficiency that occurs with varying intensity in chronic alcoholics. It is manifested by marked deterioration in short-term memory, varying degrees of retrograde amnesia, nystagmus, ataxia, and confusion associated with cognitive deficits and often confabulation (not required for the diagnosis). Onset is frequently preceded by an acute episode of Wernicke's syndrome. In its acute phase, alcohol amnestic disorder is characterized by mental confusion and disorientation to time, place, and/or person; in its chronic stages, the confusional state subsides and patients again become alert, but typically apathetic and lacking in spontaneity or self-direction; memory function is severely disturbed. See **Wernicke's syndrome**. Also called "Korsakoff's psychosis"; "Korsakoff's syndrome."

alcohol + benzodiazepine See **benzodiazepine + alcohol**.

alcohol blood level See **blood alcohol concentration**.

alcohol/breast milk Alcohol is excreted in breast milk. When maternal alcohol blood levels are high or when alcohol is consumed in large quantities during breast feeding, intoxication can occur in the neonate, and the flow of breast milk can be inhibited. Short-term alcohol consumption by lactating women significantly and uniformly increases the odor of breast milk, causing infants to consume significantly less breast milk than when the mother is not drinking alcohol (Mennella JA. Transfer of alcohol to human milk: effects on flavor and the infant's behavior. *N Engl J Med* 1991;325:981–985).

alcohol + bromocriptine See **bromocriptine + alcohol**.

alcohol + bupropion See **bupropion + alcohol**.

alcohol + buspirone See **buspirone + alcohol**.

alcohol + chlordiazepoxide See **chlordiazepoxide + alcohol**.

alcohol + citalopram See **citalopram + alcohol**.

alcohol + clobazam See **clobazam + alcohol**.

alcohol + clomipramine See **clomipramine + alcohol**.

alcohol + clorazepate See **clorazepate + alcohol**.

alcohol + clovoxamine See **clovoxamine + alcohol**.

alcohol + cocaine See **cocaine + alcohol**.

alcohol/cognitive deficits Chronic alcohol abuse causes deficits in cognitive functioning that may vary from mild to profound. In some cases they are so mild they can be detected only by psychological tests. Even when mild, they can be disabling, but not usually enough to meet diagnostic criteria for dementia associated with alcoholism. Profound cognitive deficits, especially when accompanied by nutritional deficiency, may signal Korsakoff's syndrome. Usually, however, cognitive deficits that accompany chronic alcohol abuse are not severe enough in and of themselves to justify a separate diagnosis and are simply seen as correlates or consequences of a long period of (generally) abusive drinking (Anon. Alcohol and cognition. *Alcohol Alert* 1989, No. 4, pp 1–3). See **alcohol dementia**.

alcohol dehydrogenase (ADH) Liver enzyme that metabolizes a number of drugs such as chloral hydrate. It plays a major role in alcohol detoxification and participates in metabolism of neurotransmitters and fatty acids and clearance of biogenic toxic metabolites. ADH shows considerable polymorphism; it has over 20 different isoenzymes with greatly differing kinetic properties in vitro. The enzyme is encoded by three gene loci, ADH_1, ADH_2, and ADH_3, which lie adjacent to each other on chromosome 4. Polymorphism is present only at ADH_2 and ADH_3 (Hittle JB, Crabb DW. The molecular biology of alcohol dehydrogenase: implications for the control of alcohol metabolism. *J Lab Clin Med* 1988;112:7–15).

alcohol dehydrogenase isozyme (ADH_2) Hepatic isoenzyme with a high capacity to convert alcohol into acetaldehyde. Alcohol oxidation occurs chiefly in the liver, initiated principally by ADH_2. Like many hepatic enzymes, it is polymorphic, which may account in part for variations in rate of alcohol metabolism among different individuals and may contribute to the sensitivity of many Asians to small amounts of alcohol.

alcohol dementia Organic syndrome that follows prolonged and heavy alcohol use. It is diagnosed by persistence of dementia for at least 3 weeks after drinking ceases and exclusion of all other causes of dementia. Characteristic features include deterioration in previous intellectual abilities; short- and long-term memory deficits; and impairment in abstract thinking, judgment, and impulse control of sufficient magnitude to interfere significantly with work, usual social activities, or relationships with others. Severity can vary from mild impairment in functioning to impairment requiring custodial care. Alcohol dementia must be differentiated from mild cognitive deficits related to alcohol dependence that are revealed only by neuropsychological evaluation.

alcohol dependence Chronic loss of control over consumption of alcoholic beverages despite obvious psychological or physical harm. Increasing amounts are required over time, and abrupt discontinuance may precipitate a withdrawal syndrome. Morning relief drinking may occur to counteract withdrawal symptoms. Following abstinence, relapse is frequent. See **alcohol dependence syndrome**.

alcohol dependence syndrome Cluster of symptoms secondary to alcohol misuse: tolerance, craving, morning withdrawal, drinking to relieve or avoid withdrawal, drink-seeking behavior, loss of control over alcohol intake, drinking increasingly unaffected by ordinary social conventions and as a key feature, the feeling of compulsion to drink.

alcohol + desipramine   See **desipramine + alcohol**.

alcohol + diazepam   See **diazepam + alcohol**.

alcohol + diphenhydramine   See **diphenhydramine + alcohol**.

alcohol + disulfiram   After ingestion of a small amount (about 50 mg) of disulfiram, within 10 minutes of drinking, alcohol flushing and a sensation of facial warmth occurs; by 20–30 minutes vasodilation of peripheral blood vessels is manifested by a red appearance; between 30 and 90 minutes the patient may have a throbbing headache, chest tightness, difficulty breathing, weakness, vertigo, nausea and vomiting, pallor, hypotension, and tachycardia. Other interactions include blurred vision, sweating, thirst, and confusion. More severe reactions include hypotension, cardiovascular collapse, and, sometimes, convulsions.

alcohol/elderly   Alcohol misuse and abuse in those 65+ years of age has increased in recent years, even though the elderly appear to drink less because (a) they have less money to spend on alcohol; (b) despite metabolizing alcohol as efficiently as younger persons, they experience higher levels of peak alcohol concentrations with similar doses of alcohol (older persons can experience the effects of alcohol while imbibing less); and (c) they are more sensitive to alcohol. There is an increased risk for drug interactions in the elderly, especially adverse drug reactions, that may be aggravated by alcohol. Older alcoholics have a high incidence of illnesses and problems not caused by alcohol (e.g., chronic obstructive pulmonary disease, peptic ulcer disease, psoriasis, tobacco dependence, organic brain syndrome, affective disorder, abuse of or dependence on legal prescription drugs). The potential for drug interactions increases with greater reliance on prescription drugs, multiple prescriptions, difficulty in correct self-administration, and age-related changes in physiology. Alcohol abuse in the elderly can mimic and/or contribute to major depression. Some apparent dementia is actually a form of drug-induced cognitive impairment, reversible in the absence of the drugs. Reduced alcohol consumption could improve treatment outcomes.

alcohol + femoxetine   See **femoxetine + alcohol**.

alcohol + fluoxetine   See **fluoxetine + alcohol**.

alcohol + fluvoxamine   See **fluvoxamine + alcohol**.

alcohol-free beer + monoamine oxidase inhibitor (MAOI)   See **monoamine oxidase inhibitor + alcohol-free beer**.

alcohol hallucinosis   Persistent auditory and/or visual hallucinations after recovery from delirium tremens. They are more common in men. Hallucinations are more prominent at night and may be threatening and frightening, commanding the patient to do things against his or her will (suicide, bizarre behavior). Some hallucinations, however, may be pleasant. Alcohol hallucinosis may respond to antipsychotic drug therapy. Some clinicians use electroconvulsive therapy to rapidly terminate hallucinations persisting for several weeks.

alcohol hot flush syndrome   Type of alcohol sensitivity prevalent among Asians. It is believed to be due to a structural mutation in the gene that codes for an enzyme involved in alcohol metabolism (aldehyde dehydrogenase). The enzyme is thus unable to metabolize acetaldehyde, a toxic product of alcohol metabolism.

alcohol + hypnotic   See **hypnotic + alcohol**.

alcohol idiosyncratic intoxication   See **intoxication, pathological**.

alcohol + imipramine   See **imipramine + alcohol**.

alcohol intoxication   Common, alcohol-induced organic mental disorder characterized by varying stages of behavior alteration, depending on the amount of alcohol used and individual variation in tolerance. Maladaptive behavior effects most commonly seen are impaired judgment, shortened attention span, inappropriate emotional responses, mood lability, disinhibition of aggressive impulses, and social or occupational dysfunction. At lower levels of alcohol ingestion, stimulant properties may predominate. A blood alcohol level of 30 mg% will produce a euphoric effect in most individuals who do not have an established tolerance. At 50 mg%, central nervous system depressant effects become more prominent, with associated motor coordination problems and some cognitive deficits. In the United States, the legal limit of intoxication ranges from 80 mg% to 100 mg% (i.e., levels of 100 mg% or more are deemed to indicate impaired function even in the absence of testing of that function). If the person is excited or assaultive, diazepam (5 mg orally every 30–60 minutes) can be helpful, although paradoxical worsening of irritability and hostility may occur. If the person refuses oral medication or is very agitated, lorazepam (1–2 mg/hour) can be given intramuscularly until the patient is calm. Those with coexisting psychoses are best treated with individualized doses of high-potency neuroleptics given as oral concentrate or intramuscularly.

alcohol + lithium   See **lithium + alcohol**.

alcohol/liver disease   About 15% of heavy drinkers eventually develop liver disease. The proportion of patients with liver disease who have alcohol problems is more variable, depending on the characteristics of the population studied. Psychiatric morbidity is higher among patients who have alcoholic liver disease than among other liver disease patients; two-thirds of inpatients with alcoholic liver disease had diagnosable psychiatric disorders, compared with one-third of a control group with nonalcoholic liver disease. Depression and anxiety disorders were more common in patients with alcoholic liver disease than in the normal control group. In 20%, psychiatric illness appeared to be secondary to the patient's drinking habits or to ill health; in the majority, the psychiatric disorder predated the alcohol problem. Alcoholics recognize that their liver damage is self-induced, and onset of liver disease can motivate them to control their drinking (Collis I, Lloyd G. Psychiatric aspects of liver disease. *Br J Psychiatry* 1992;161: 12–22).

alcohol + lorazepam   See **lorazepam + alcohol.**

alcohol + maprotiline   See **maprotiline + alcohol.**

alcohol + marijuana   Combined use in variable amounts, frequencies, and settings is well established. Acute administration of tetrahydrocannabinol (THC), the primary psychoactive component of marijuana, in combination with alcohol results in additive or superadditive effects on psychomotor performance, enhanced impairment of mental performance, and marked effects such as a greater increase in pulse rate and conjunctival congestion compared to ingestion of either drug alone. Marijuana smoking reduces the peak plasma alcohol level attained after drinking a standard alcohol beverage; the attenuation parallels a delay in the time-to-peak levels but does not significantly delay the appearance of alcohol-induced intoxication. However, there is a substantial decrease in the duration of *subjective* effects consistent with a reduction of the maximum and a delay in the peak plasma alcohol levels (Lukas SE, Benedikt R, Mendelson JH, et al. Marihuana attenuates the rise in plasma ethanol levels in human subjects. *Neuropsychopharmacology* 1992;7:77–81).

alcohol + metoclopramide   See **metoclopramide + alcohol.**

alcohol + moclobemide   See **moclobemide + alcohol.**

alcohol + nefazodone   See **nefazodone + alcohol.**

alcohol/neurological disorders   Chronic alcohol consumption may be responsible for development of the following neurological/neuropsychiatric disorders: (a) Wernicke-Korsakoff syndrome; (b) cerebral cortical atrophy (alcohol-associated dementia); (c) cerebellar degeneration; (d) polyneuropathy; (e) alcohol myopathy; and (f) the Pellagra syndrome (dementia, dermatitis, diarrhea, and death).

alcohol + nifedipine   In healthy volunteers, the area under the plasma concentration-time profile of nifedipine increased 54% in the presence of alcohol. The maximum pulse rate was achieved more rapidly in the presence of alcohol, but neither increase in pulse rate nor change in blood pressure index reached significance between treatments. Patients should be warned of the potential consequences of alcohol consumption during nifedipine treatment (Qureshi S, Langaniere S, Mcgilveray IJ, et al. Nifedipine-alcohol interaction. *JAMA* 1990;264:1660–1661).

alcohol + nortriptyline   See **nortriptyline + alcohol.**

alcohol + orphenadrine   See **orphenadrine + alcohol.**

alcohol + other drugs   Alcohol may interact harmfully with more than 100 medications, including some sold over the counter. Alcohol effects are especially augmented by medications that depress central nervous system (CNS) function (e.g., sedatives, sleeping pills, anticonvulsants, antidepressants, antianxiety drugs, and certain analgesics). There is a consequent increased danger of driving an automobile after even moderate drinking if such medications are taken. In advanced heart failure, alcohol may not only worsen the disease, but interfere with the function of medications to treat it (Anon. Moderate drinking. *Alcohol Alert* 1992, No. 16, pp 1–4). Many drugs (e.g., benzodiazepines, antidepressants, opioid analgesics, antihistamines, hypoglycemics) may impair driving, especially in the elderly whose vision, attention, information processing ability, and motor coordination may be adversely affected by drug CNS effects (Ray WA, Thopa PB, Shorr RI. Medications and the older driver. *Clin Geriatr Med* 1993;9:413–438).

alcohol + oxazepam   See **oxazepam + alcohol.**

alcohol + paroxetine   See **paroxetine + alcohol.**

alcohol + phenothiazine   See **phenothiazine + alcohol.**

alcohol + phenytoin   See **phenytoin + alcohol.**

alcohol + prazepam   See **prazepam + alcohol.**

alcohol + propranolol   See **propranolol + alcohol.**

alcohol + psychotropic drug   See **psychotropic drug + alcohol.**

alcohol-related birth defects   (ARBDs) Abnormalities that occur in the children of women who drink seven drinks per week of any alcohol beverage (beer, wine, wine coolers, liquor) during pregnancy. Over 2000 scientific reports (1993) confirm that alcohol is a teratogenic drug capable of producing lifelong disabilities after intrauterine exposure. Defects include facial, cardiac, renal-genital, skeletal, and other congenital abnormalities such as hernias. Approximately 5% of all congenital abnormalities may be attributable to prenatal alcohol exposure (Sokol RJ. Alcohol and abnormal outcomes of pregnancy. *Can Med Assoc J* 1981;125:143–148). See **fetal alcohol effects; fetal alcohol syndrome**.

alcohol + remoxipride   See **remoxipride + alcohol**.

alcohol + sertraline   See **sertraline + alcohol**.

alcohol/sleep   Alcohol affects sleep onset, duration, and architecture, reducing the amount of rapid eye movement (REM) sleep and increasing slow wave sleep. Like other short-acting sedative/hypnotics, it is metabolized fairly quickly. As the night progresses, blood alcohol concentrations fall, resulting in some rebound and heightened arousal, an increase in REM sleep, and recurrent awakenings associated with tachycardia, sweating, headaches, and intense dreams or nightmares. Alcohol also affects sleep indirectly. It can compromise the activity of the dilator muscles of the upper airway, thereby causing or worsening snoring and sleep apnea that results in increased arousals during the night. Alcohol-caused gastritis, esophageal reflux, and polyuria also contribute to arousals. Chronic alcohol drinkers often experience various types of sleep disturbance, ranging from acute sedative effects to fragmented, nonrestful sleep. Withdrawal after heavy alcohol consumption may cause "terminal sleep" associated with late delirium tremens, during which sleep may be continuous for 24–36 hours. Possibly the most troublesome alcohol-related sleep disturbance is disrupted sleep during the first year or two of alcohol abstinence. Sleep is fragmented during abstinence, and the amounts of REM and slow-wave sleep are reduced. There is some evidence that benzodiazepines worsen these symptoms.

alcohol/sleep apnea   Alcohol is a respiratory suppressant. When consumed in moderate amounts, it may greatly enhance respiratory impairment in patients with sleep apnea syndrome.

alcohol/suicide   Suicide attempts and suicide are strongly associated with excessive drinking and alcohol-related problems. Between 15% and 26% of those who kill themselves are alcoholic, and as many as 55% of suicide attempters have consumed alcohol at the time of the attempt (Merrill J, Milner G, Owens J, Vale A. Alcohol and attempted suicide. *Br J Addict* 1992;87:83–89). Alcohol misuse alone

can induce depression, suicidal behavior, and suicide through its depressant and disinhibitory effects. Schizophrenic and affective disorder patients also have high rates of alcohol abuse, depression, and suicidal behavior. Schizophrenics have a lifetime prevalence of alcohol dependence/abuse of 47%. Patients with co-morbid alcohol misuse and schizophrenia are at high risk of suicide, especially if they become depressed (Regier DA, Farmer MD, Rae DS, et al. Comorbidity of mental disorders with alcohol and other drug abuse. *JAMA* 1990;264:2511–2518). Alcohol abuse is common among cocaine users; prevalence of conjoint use of cocaine and alcohol among persons who commit suicide is high. In the San Diego Suicide Study, 84% of substance users also drank alcohol regularly (Fowler RC, Rich CL, Young D. San Diego Suicide Study, II: substance abuse in young cases. *Arch Gen Psychiatry* 1986;43;962–965). In 1985, a survey in New York City revealed that in one in every five cases studied, the person who committed suicide had used cocaine within days of his or her death. In addition, alcohol was detected in one-half of all the cocaine users at autopsy (Marzuk PM, Tardiff K, Leon AC, et al. Prevalence of cocaine use among residents of New York City who committed suicide during a 1-year period. *Am J Psychiatry* 1992;149:371–375). See **alcoholism/suicide**.

alcohol/tolerance   State following alcohol consumption that may be metabolic and functional. Metabolic tolerance follows prior exposure to alcohol and results in changes in the distribution, metabolism, or excretion of alcohol, producing lower blood and brain alcohol levels after alcohol ingestion. Functional tolerance is an increase in cellular resistance to the effects of alcohol in the central nervous system. Tolerance also can be acute or chronic. Alcohol tolerance can be influenced by conditioning and learning.

alcohol, unit of   Each unit of alcohol contains 10 ml or 8.0 g of absolute alcohol. A unit of alcohol is: one single whiskey; one glass of sherry or fortified wine; one glass of table wine; one half pint of beer; one quarter pint of strong lager. A bottle of brandy, whiskey, gin, or other "hard liquor" contains 30 units of alcohol.

alcohol + verapamil   See **verapamil + alcohol**.

alcohol + warfarin   See **warfarin + alcohol**.

alcohol withdrawal   Acute alcohol withdrawal can be divided into two phases. Phase I typically begins 24–36 hours after the last drink and is manifested by increasing anxiety, irritability, and feeling "shaky" inside. The phase generally requires no treatment beyond reassurance. Phase II can occur 2–14 days after the last drink as blood alcohol drops. During this period there is increased risk for generalized tonic-clonic seizures ("rum fits"), for which anticonvulsant therapy may be necessary. See **delirium tremens.**

alcohol withdrawal/gamma-hydroxybutyric acid (GHB) GHB inhibits voluntary alcohol consumption in rats having a strong preference for it and suppresses the alcohol withdrawal syndrome in rats physically dependent on it. In a double-blind study of oral, nonhypnotic doses of GHB in the treatment of withdrawal symptoms in alcoholics, GHB effect was rapid and devoid of negative side effects (Gallimberti L, Canton G, Gentile N, et al. Gamma-hydroxybutyric acid for treatment of alcohol withdrawal syndrome. *Lancet* 1989;2:787–789).

alcohol withdrawal/neonate Alcohol misuse during pregnancy is responsible for a neonatal withdrawal syndrome within 48 hours of birth. It is manifested by sleep disturbances, tremor, hyper-reflexia, and feeding difficulties.

alcohol withdrawal seizures Generalized toxic-clonic (grand mal) seizures that occur in chronic alcoholics following heavy drinking. Hypomagnesemia and blood alkalosis are found at this stage. In general, every stage of alcohol tolerance and withdrawal from simple irritability and autonomic instability through delirium tremens to seizures represents a progressive, more serious decrease in seizure threshold.

alcohol withdrawal syndrome State characterized by reduced GABAergic functioning, noradrenergic hyperactivity, and activation of the hypothalamic-pituitary-adrenal axis that develops after cessation of or reduction in prolonged, heavy alcohol ingestion. It is followed within several hours by coarse tremor of the hands, tongue, and eyelids, accompanied by such symptoms as nausea, vomiting, weakness, diaphoresis, fast heart rate, anxiety, and irritability. The spectrum of symptoms includes seizures (rum fits), hallucinations, autonomic hyperactivity (e.g., fever, sweating, tachycardia, elevated blood pressure and respiratory rate), and insomnia (delirium tremens). Mild cases can be managed with simple support and vitamins. Benzodiazepines (chlordiazepoxide, diazepam, alprazolam, lorazepam, oxazepam) attenuate withdrawal syndrome severity and are now the standard approach to medically supervised withdrawal. Phenobarbital is used if benzodiazepines are contraindicated. Routine use of phenytoin to prevent seizures is unnecessary. If hallucinosis develops, low doses of high-potency neuroleptics (intramuscular [IM] or oral concentrate) may be indicated. Treatment also involves aggressive use of vitamin B_{12}, folic acid (1 mg), thiamine (100 mg IM), and magnesium sulfate to prevent onset of irreversible nutritionally based neurological damage such as Wernicke-Korsakoff syndrome. Intravenous electrolytes and dextrose and water may be needed, but overhydration is more likely in these patients than dehydration. Central venous pressures should be monitored if large amounts of intravenous fluids and electrolytes are needed.

alcohol + zopiclone See **zopiclone + alcohol.**

alcoholic One who meets criteria for alcohol dependence or has experienced physical, psychological, social, or occupational impairment as a consequence of habitual, excessive consumption of alcohol.

alcoholic, recovering Alcoholic who is successfully abstaining from drinking. The term emphasizes the concept that alcoholism has no cure and that recovery must be continuously worked at.

Alcoholics Anonymous (AA) Self-help group formed in 1935 by two recovering alcoholics (one a physician) for the purpose of rehabilitating alcoholics. AA has expanded into an international movement. Members try to live by the 12 principles of AA to achieve and maintain sobriety through self-help and mutual support. AA has been a major contributor to effective assessment and treatment of primary alcoholism, but AA counselors, as a rule, have trouble with alcoholism secondary to primary psychiatric illness. Sometimes these counselors resist needed treatment of primary disorders with proper medications, often misleading the person into believing that all medications are addictive and equivalent to alcohol.

alcoholism **1.** Primary chronic disease with genetic, psychosocial, and environmental factors influencing its development and manifestations. Often progressive and fatal, it is characterized by impaired control over drinking, preoccupation with alcohol, use of alcohol despite adverse consequences, and distortions in thinking, most notably denial. Symptoms may be continuous or periodic (Morse RM, Flavin DK, for the Joint Committee of the National Council on Alcoholism and Drug Dependence and the American Society of Addiction Medicine to Study the Definition and Criteria for the Diagnosis of Alcoholism: Definition of alcoholism. *JAMA* 1992; 268: 1012–1014). **2.** Incurable disease that manifests itself as an inability to drink normally; an alcoholic is one whose life has become intolerable because of alcohol (Alcoholics Anonymous). There is no one best definition of alcoholism, and the different criteria overlap a great deal.

alcoholism, acute Obsolete term meaning only severe intoxication by alcohol.

alcoholism/biological markers Measurable indicators of chronic alcohol intake. Although most are indicative of alcohol's toxic effects and tend to normalize on abstinence, they offer a useful index of remission and relapse. They include elevations of hepatic enzymes (e.g., alanine aminotransferase and aspartate aminotransferase), increased mean corpuscular volume, and presence of isotransferins. Studies of alcoholics also suggest that alterations in noradrenergic function such as low cerebrospinal fluid 3-methoxy-4-hydroxyphenylglycol (MHPG) or blunted growth hormone response to clonidine may be a vulnerability marker. Some peripheral markers have also been reported (e.g., increased Km of platelet 5-HT uptake, low platelet monoamine oxidase activity, reduced platelet G-protein sensitivity, and increased production of butanedioles after alcohol intake). Some studies of high-risk groups (sons of alcoholics) indicate important differences on a range of variables. High-risk males have been reported to have reduced endocrine and physiological responses to alcohol; they may have altered P300 evoked potentials and a hyper-responsive heart rate response to stressors that is normalized by alcohol. Such data may someday delineate the basic biological processes that predispose to alcoholism, and may lead to screening for vulnerability, which could in turn lead to directed intervention.

alcoholism/blood markers Screening tests that indicate at least moderate alcohol misuse. Many alcoholics have (a) mild uric acid elevation; (b) elevated free fatty acids; (c) a mean corpuscular volume of 95–100 g; and (d) gamma-glutamyl transferase (GGT) levels of 30–50+. Alcohol also decreases production of all types of blood cells, resulting in a macrocytic anemia, decreased white cell production, decreased thymus-derived lymphocytes, and decreased production of platelets and clotting factors. Existence of these markers should raise suspicion of alcoholism, especially in patients complaining of insomnia, dysphoria, nervousness, or work and interpersonal problems.

alcoholism, chronic Obsolete term synonymous with alcoholism.

alcoholism, dually diagnosed Alcoholism plus another major psychiatric disorder that alone would warrant treatment. There are three "pure" types: alcoholism plus drug abuse; alcoholism plus antisocial personality; and alcoholism plus depression or schizophrenia.

alcoholism, familial Pattern of alcoholism occurring in more than one generation within a family, due to genetic or environmental factors.

alcoholism/physical and laboratory findings Hypertension without other apparent cause plus signs and symptoms of alcohol liver disease is a frequent physical manifestation of alcohol misuse. Laboratory tests (red blood cell, mean corpuscular volume, and the liver transaminases, including gamma-glutamyl transferase [GGT], serum glutamic oxaloacetic transferase [SGOT], and serum glutamic pyruvic transaminase [SGPT]) may help to establish the diagnosis of alcohol abuse. Other abnormalities found in alcoholics include elevated uric acid, depressed platelet count, anemia, and elevated triglycerides. None alone would make the diagnosis of alcoholism, but combined with other data they can help to detect alcohol abuse.

alcoholism, primary Development of alcohol dependence before the onset of any other type of psychiatric illness.

alcoholism, secondary Misuse of alcohol as a consequence of anxiety or some other type of psychiatric disorder; or onset of alcoholism after emergence of signs and symptoms of another psychiatric disorder (causality is not necessarily implied).

alcoholism/suicide Alcoholism accounts for about one-fourth of suicides studied from a diagnostic perspective. Risk factors that predict suicide in alcoholism include continued drinking, major depressive episode, suicidal communication, poor social support, serious medical illness, unemployment, and living alone. As the number of risk factors increases, so does the likelihood of suicidal outcome. Any four factors identify about 70% of alcoholics who commit suicide; all seven identify up to 83%. These percentages hold for alcoholic women and blacks. Major depression does not account for accumulation of other risk factors. Depression is found in nearly 75% of alcoholics who commit suicide. Whether as a complication of alcoholism or occurring alone, depression is the single most responsible factor in suicide. Treatment of the accompanying depression reduces risk of suicide (Murphy GE, Wetzel RD, Robins E, McEvoy L. Multiple risk factors predict suicide in alcoholism. *Arch Gen Psychiatry* 1992;49:459–463). See **alcohol/suicide**.

alcoholism, type I One of two genetically distinct forms of alcoholism. Type I, the more common, affects 75% of male alcoholics and almost all women alcoholics. It is characterized by late onset (after age 25) and rapid development of tolerance to and dependence on the anxiolytic effects of alcohol. It is relatively mild and influenced by environmental factors (e.g., low socioeconomic status and alcohol use by relatives and peers). Although fighting and arrests are usually not associated with the natural history of type I alcoholism, guilt and fear about dependence on alcohol are typically present. Type I alcoholics free of other mental disorders may not benefit from any pharmacotherapy. Those who exhibit symptoms or have a history of other mental disorders should be divided into primary and secondary alcoholics, depending on the relative times of onset of alcoholism and other mental disorders. See **alcoholism, type II; alcoholism, primary; alcoholism, secondary.**

alcoholism, type II   One of two genetically distinct forms of alcoholism that afflicts almost only men. Approximately 25% of alcoholic men have the disorder. Although some type II alcoholics have no genetic history, it is usually inherited by sons from their fathers, but not by daughters, and the gene effect is less influenced by environmental factors. Excessive consumption of alcohol starts at an early age, and antisocial personality disorder and criminality co-exist with alcoholism in the families. Women with a genetic background often have other symptoms of somatization. Type II alcoholics are a more severely affected group, with a lower frequency of abstinence and social drinking and a greater tendency to drinking bouts compared with type I alcoholics. Persistent seeking of alcohol for its euphoriant effects leads to early onset of inability to abstain entirely from alcohol, as well as fighting and arrests when drunk. Type II alcoholics are twice as likely to be depressed, four times as likely to have attempted suicide, and also twice as likely to have been incarcerated for crimes involving physical violence. Untreated, the disorder may be fatal. If psychotropic drugs are indicated in type II alcoholics to treat symptoms such as poor impulse control and dysthymia, carbamazepine and lithium probably are preferable. Type II alcoholics are unlikely to benefit from benzodiazepines. See **alcoholism, type I.**

Aldactazide   See **spironolactone.**

Aldactone   See **spironolactone.**

aldehyde dehydrogenase   (ALDH) Liver enzyme that catalyzes oxidation of acetaldehyde (the major metabolic product of alcohol) to acetate. It plays a major role in alcohol detoxification and participates in the metabolism of neurotransmitters and fatty acids, and in clearance of biogenic toxic metabolites.

Aldomet   See **methyldopa.**

Aldoril   See **hydrochlorothiazide.**

aldosterone   Steroid isolated from the adrenal cortex that causes sodium retention and potassium loss. Secretion is regulated by the renin-angiotensin mechanism and to a lesser extent by adrenocorticotropic hormone.

alexia   Loss of ability to understand the meaning of written or printed words or sentences. It results from organic brain damage and does not involve impairment in vision or intelligence. Also called "word blindness"; "visual aphasia."

alexia, acquired   Loss of previous ability to read. See **alexia.**

alexia, congenital   Inability to learn to read not consistent with the individuals mental age and other intellectual achievement. See **alexia.**

alexithymia   Disturbance in affective and cognitive functions in patients with diagnoses including somatic illness, substance abuse, and post-traumatic stress disorder (from the Greek for "no words for feelings"). Salient features include difficulty recognizing and verbalizing feelings, paucity of fantasy life, descriptions of physical symptoms instead of emotions, and speech and thought that are concrete and closely tied to external events. Alexithymic people have few dreams. Alexithymia has long been associated with substance abuse. It may play a role in the etiology and treatment of alcoholism.

Alfenta   See **alfentanil.**

alfentanil   (Alfenta) Opioid analgesic derivative of fentanyl used primarily as an anesthetic. It is considerably less potent than fentanyl, acts more rapidly, and has a markedly shorter duration of action. It permits use of reduced doses of barbiturates such as thiopental for anesthesia induction for electroconvulsive therapy. Pregnancy risk category C.

algorithm   Graphic representation of a sequence of steps to follow for solving a problem, wherein each step depends on the result of the previous one. See **clinical algorithm; decision tree.**

algorithm, clinical   See **clinical algorithm.**

alignment chart   See **nomogram.**

aligodeoxynucleotide   Small synthetic piece of DNA with a nucleotide sequence that is the reverse of a complementary part of messenger RNA (mRNA). It binds (hybridizes) to the mRNA, under suitable conditions, according to the rules of the genetic code. The hybridization prevents translation of the mRNA, and the encoded protein cannot be synthesized (Helene C, Toulme JJ. Specific regulation of the gene expression by antisense, sense and antigene nucleic acids. *Biochem Biophys Acta* 1990;1049:99–125).

Alimix   See **cisapride.**

aliphatic phenothiazine   See **phenothiazine, aliphatic.**

alkaloid   Complex nitrogen-containing organic base of plant origin (e.g. morphine).

alkalosis   Disorder characterized by hydrogen ion loss or base excess in body fluids (metabolic alkalosis) or by carbon dioxide loss due to hyperventilation (respiratory alkalosis).

alkyl group   Radical derived from an open chain hydrocarbon. It is often referred to as an aliphatic group (e.g., a methyl or ethyl group).

"Allah"   Street term for opium.

allele   (allelomorph) Alternative form of a gene, found in the corresponding loci on homologous chromosomes, that determines alternative characteristics in inheritance. Only two alleles—one derived from each parent— that have segregated at meiosis can be present in any individual.

allele, multiple   More than two alleles existing for a given locus in the population. Each allele carries contrasting Mendelian characteristics and goes to different mature germ cells. Though only two alleles at a locus can be present in any one normal individual, there may be more than two different alleles at that locus in the population as a whole.

allele, silent   Amorph; allele with no detectable product.

allelic   Having the characteristics of an allele. Eye color is an allelomorphic characteristic.

allelomorph   See **allele.**

Allergan   See **atropine.**

allograft   Tissue graft from a donor of one genotype to a host of another genotype, host and donor being members of the same species.

allosteric negative modulator   Specific inductor able to bring out negative modifications at an allosteric site.

allosteric positive modulator   Specific inductor able to bring out positive modifications at an allosteric site.

allostery   Influencing enzyme activity by a change in conformation of the enzyme induced by the noncompetitive binding of a nonsubstrate at a site other than the active site of the enzyme.

allotype   Genetically determined difference in antigens (e.g., the Gm and Inv variants), that are detected by their antigenic properties.

alogia   Marked poverty of speech or speech content.

alopecia   Hair loss. Many psychotropic drugs may induce alopecia after prolonged administration; mode of action is unknown. Alopecia (usually a partial diffuse hair loss) has been infrequently attributed to antidepressants (amitriptyline, amoxapine, bupropion, desipramine, fluoxetine, imipramine, maprotiline, nortriptyline, protriptyline, and trimipramine); anxiolytics (buspirone); antipsychotics (haloperidol, loxapine, and perphenazine); anticonvulsants (carbamazepine, clonazepam, phenytoin, and valproic acid); lithium; and methylphenidate. Alopecia also may be due to hypothyroidism.

alpha$_1$-acid glycoprotein   (AGP) Major protein like albumin that binds cationic drugs such as chlorpromazine, thioridazine, fluphenazine, loxapine, thiothixene, carbamazepine, triazolam, imipramine, and other tricyclic antidepressants. AGP is a putative endogenous inhibitor of the site labeled by tritiated imipramine. Plasma concentration can be measured by radioimmunodiffusion assay. Significant elevations occur in some patients with major depression, after surgery and trauma, and in inflammation, celiac disease, Crohn's disease, malignancy, myocardial infarction, renal failure, rheumatoid arthritis, and stress. Levels are decreased in the nephrotic syndrome, in the fetus, and with oral contraceptive use. See **albumin.**

alpha-adrenergic antagonist   See **clonidine.**

alpha adrenergic blockade   Effects of some antidepressants and neuroleptics that lead to orthostatic hypotension and consequently to syncope, falls, and hip fractures, especially in the elderly.

alpha$_1$ adrenergic receptor   Type of catecholamine receptor present throughout the body. On smooth muscle of arterioles, they bring about vasoconstriction if stimulated. Their inhibition by neuroleptics and antidepressants may produce postural hypotension, dizziness, and reflex tachycardia.

alpha$_2$ adrenergic autoreceptor   Presynaptic or somatodendric receptor that regulates release of norepinephrine from the locus ceruleus through a negative feedback mechanism.

alpha$_2$ adrenergic receptor   Presynaptic receptor that further reduces norepinephrine output when stimulated, thus acting as a negative feedback to the release of norepinephrine. The receptors are now classified into at least four pharmacologically distinct subtypes: alpha$_2$-A, alpha$_2$-B, alpha$_2$-C and alpha$_2$-D. Three human alpha$_2$-gene products have been cloned: alpha$_2$-C$_{10}$, alpha$_2$-C$_2$ (alpha$_2$-B), and alpha$_2$-C$_4$ (a possible alpha$_2$-B variant).

alpha-delta sleep   See **sleep, alpha** (preferred term).

alpha electroencephalogram   Electroencephalogram (EEG) that is predominantly 8–13 Hz (alpha activity) in all recorded leads. It is usually characterized by moderate to high amplitude and rhythmical nature. Alpha waves are elicited from a resting subject with closed eyes. See **alpha rhythm**.

alpha electroencephalogram activity Continuous 10 Hz-cycle/second activity that appears over the occipital region when subjects rest with closed eyes. It is diminished when the eyes are opened or subjects are alerted by a cognitive task. Alpha activity is generally decreased in schizophrenics and may also be decreased in their offspring.

alpha error See **error, alpha**.

alpha half-life See **half-life, alpha**.

alpha-haptoglobin Type of alpha$_2$ globulin with a specific affinity for hemoglobin. It is often elevated in diabetics.

alpha-helical CRF Synthesized peptide antagonistic to corticotropin-releasing factor (CRF) that is 10 times less potent than CRF in binding to central nervous system CRF receptors. It is useful for examining the functional significance of endogenous CRF systems in behavior.

alpha-hydroxytriazolam (AHT) Major metabolite of triazolam that contributes little to the overall drug effect in humans because it reaches peak plasma concentrations of less than 20% of triazolam and its activity is 6 times less than the parent drug.

alpha intrusion Brief superimposition of electroencephalographic alpha activity on sleep activities during a stage of sleep.

alpha-methyldopa Competitive inhibitor of dopa decarboxylase, the enzyme essential for converting dopa to dopamine. It is metabolized to a false neurotransmitter, alpha-methylnorepinephrine, that theoretically may compete with dopamine at postsynaptic striatal dopamine receptors. There are a few reports of de novo, reversible parkinsonism in patients treated with alpha-methyldopa, usually in individuals in their 60s after treatment with 1–2 g/day for 3–8 weeks. Following drug withdrawal, parkinsonian symptoms resolve within a few days to weeks. Attempts to treat tardive dyskinesia with alpha-methyldopa have not been very successful (Huang CC, Wang RIH, Hasegawa A, et al. Reserpine and alpha-methyldopa in the treatment of tardive dyskinesia. *Psychopharmacol Bull* 1981;73:359–362).

alpha-methylfentanyl Homolog of fentanyl developed in 1980 to be sold to heroin addicts as a very potent form of heroin. It is a designer drug with a very narrow margin between the euphoric dose and the dose that causes respiratory depression; fatalities among abusers are not uncommon. See **3-methylfentanyl**.

alpha-methylparatyrosine (AMPT) Potent, specific inhibitor of tyrosine hydroxylase, the rate-limiting enzyme in the synthesis of dopamine and noradrenaline. It has some

antimanic efficacy. It has also been reported to induce depression, cause panic attacks, and evoke acute dystonic reactions in healthy male volunteers (McCann UD, Penetar DM, Belenky G. Acute dystonic reaction in normal humans caused by catecholamine depletion. *Clin Neuropharmacol* 1987;13:565–568). Attempts to treat tardive dyskinesia with alpha-methylparatyrosine have produced equivocal results (Nassrallah HA, Dunner FJ, McCalley-Whitters, et al. Pharmacologic probes of neurotransmitter systems in tardive dyskinesia: implications for clinical management. *J Clin Psychiatry* 1986;47:56–59).

alpha-methylserotonin (AM5-HT) Substance formed in vivo from administered alpha-methyltryptophan. It displaces most of the cerebral serotonin (5-HT) and mimics the behavior of endogenously synthesized cerebral 5-HT.

alpha-noradrenergic receptor Presynaptic (alpha$_2$) or postsynaptic (alpha$_1$) receptor for noradrenaline.

alpha-propyldopacetamide Catechol that inhibits tryptophan hydroxylation and other tetrahydropterin-requiring enzymes such as tyrosine hydroxylase.

alpha rhythm Electroencephalographic (EEG) rhythm with a frequency of 8–13 Hz in human adults. It is most prominent over the parieto-occipital cortex when the eyes are closed. The rhythm is blocked by eye opening or other arousing stimuli. It indicates the awake state in humans; is present in most, but not all, normal individuals; and is most consistent and predominant during relaxed wakefulness, particularly with reduction of visual input. It often slows by 0.5–1.5 Hz and becomes more diffuse during drowsiness. Frequency varies with age; it is slower in children relative to young and middle-aged adults. EEG slowing does not appear to be part of normal healthy aging (Thorpy MJ. *Handbook of Sleep Disorders*. New York: Marcel Dekker, 1990).

alpha sleep See **sleep, alpha**.

alpha-tocopherol Potent antioxidant that is a biologically active component of vitamin E. It has been tested in placebo-controlled double-blind studies in doses of 400 IU 3 times a day for the treatment of tardive dyskinesia, but has no consistent systematic benefit at doses tested. A combination of selegiline and alpha-tocopherol is being evaluated in early untreated Parkinson's disease in a large, multicenter trial (DATATOP) by The Parkinson Study Group in the United States. See **vitamin E**.

alpha value Level of alpha selected in a hypothesis test; tolerable probability value of declaring a hypothesis is not true when it actually is true. The value should be set before doing statistical tests.

alpha wave training Type of biofeedback in which subjects use information from their electroencephalogram as a means of achieving a relaxed state. A tone sounds in the absence of alpha waves and disappears when the subject produces them.

alpidem (Amaxyl; Ananxyl) Imidazopyridine anxiolytic that binds to omega$_1$ and omega$_3$ benzodiazepine receptors. It is not a benzodiazepine (BZD), but has anxioselective activity and anticonvulsant activity. It was synthesized in an attempt to find an alternative to the BZDs with fewer sedative and addictive properties. In humans, doses of 25–100 mg are well absorbed orally and well tolerated clinically. Plasma concentrations peak on average at 2.5 hours, and half-life is estimated to be 21 hours, although there is marked interindividual variation. Side effects include lightheadedness, drowsiness, and daytime tiredness, but gastrointestinal upset is most difficult for patients to tolerate. Alpidem has been shown to be an effective and safe treatment for generalized anxiety disorder. Alpidems anxiolytic properties are reversed by the BZD antagonist, flumazenil. Abrupt withdrawal of alpidem therapy to date has not caused serious withdrawal reactions, suggesting that it may have a low potential for inducing dependence. Alpidem is undergoing clinical trials in Europe.

alpidem + clomipramine In one study, co-administration had a slightly superior effect on depression and anxiety compared to clomipramine + bromazepam and was well tolerated (Cottraux J, Riant N. Alpidem versus bromazepam in depressed outpatients treated with clomipramine. A controlled comparison. *Clin Neuropharmacol* 1992;15[suppl 1/B]: 521B).

alprazolam (Xanax) (ALP) First triazolobenzodiazepine introduced into clinical practice as an anxiolytic. It is classified as a short- to intermediate-acting benzodiazepine (BZD) because its elimination half-life, including metabolites, is 6–20 hours. It is metabolized mainly by hydroxylation, yielding two metabolites (alpha- hydroxyalprazolam and 4-hydroxyalprazolam). Alpha-hydroxyalprazolam is pharmacologically active (though less so than the parent drug), as indicated by high affinity for binding to BZD receptors; 4-hydroxyalprazolam is not pharmacologically active. Since the metabolites are rapidly conjugated and excreted, unconjugated concentrations are considerably lower than those of the parent compound. ALP kinetics are af-

fected by age, even though it has a short half-life. A study of the pharmacokinetics of ALP and its active metabolite showed they are normal in hemodialysis patients but not in continuous ambulatory peritoneal dialysis patients. End-stage renal disease is associated with changes in absorption, distribution, and/or elimination of ALP (Schmith VD, Piraino B, Smith RB, et al. Alprazolam in end-stage renal disease. Part 1. Pharmacokinetics. *J Clin Pharmacol* 1991;31:571–579). Groups of patients receiving dialysis showed enhanced sensitivity to some psychomotor and memory effects of ALP (Schmith VD, Piraino B, Smith RB, et al. Alprazolam in end-stage renal disease. Part 2. Pharmacodynamics. *Clin Pharmacol Ther* 1992;51:533–540). ALP is widely used for generalized anxiety disorder and panic disorder. It has also been tested as an antidepressant, but with no clear evidence of this action. Its principal disadvantage for the treatment of depression and panic disorder is its propensity for abuse, physiologic dependence, and the attendant withdrawal syndrome many patients experience when trying to discontinue active treatment. This is more of a problem in the treatment of depression and panic disorder than of anxiety, as the doses used tend to be higher and the duration of treatment longer. Results of limited clinical trials indicate that ALP addition to the neuroleptic therapy of treatment-resistant chronic schizophrenics diminishes core psychotic symptoms and, to a lesser extent, "negative" symptoms and anxiety/depression. Patient-administered as-needed (PRN) doses of ALP should be avoided, because its relatively short half-life can contribute to the problem of interdose breakthrough anxiety. ALP discontinuation is associated with greater distress than is discontinuation of diazepam treatment. Several studies have documented that ALP discontinuation may be associated with more intense rebound anxiety and/or withdrawal symptoms and that psychological dependence, reinforced by these phenomena, may occur more often as a consequence. These greater effects may reflect ALP's considerably tighter binding to BZD receptors. There have been a number of reports of ALP-induced dyscontrol or emergence of hostility during ALP therapy (Arana GW, Pearlman C, Shader RI. Alprazolam-induced dyscontrol in borderline personality disorder. *Am J Psychiatry* 1985;142:369). Pregnancy risk category D.

alprazolam/breast milk Infant withdrawal symptoms have been reported after abrupt weaning or rapid cessation of long-term alprazolam use during nursing (Anderson PO,

Mcguire GG. Neonatal alprazolam withdrawal—possible effects of breast-feeding. *Drug Intell Clin Pharm* 1990;23:614).

alprazolam + carbamazepine Carbamazepine (CBZ) may enhance alprazolam (ALP) metabolism, significantly lowering (> 50%) plasma ALP concentration and increasing the risk of causing ALP withdrawal symptoms. CBZ may not only contribute to ALP withdrawal syndrome, but its continued administration may not prevent its worsening (Arana GW, Epstein S, Molloy M, et al. Carbamazepine-induced reduction of plasma alprazolam concentrations: a clinical case report. *J Clin Psychiatry* 1988;49:448–449).

alprazolam + cimetidine Co-administration inhibits alprazolam hydroxylation, but clinical significance of the interaction has not been fully established (Abernathy DR, Greenblatt DJ, Divoll M, et al. Interaction of cimetidine with the triazolobenzodiazepines alprazolam and triazolam. *Psychopharmacology* 1983;80: 275–278).

alprazolam + clomipramine Study of co-administration kinetics in 45 healthy male volunteers indicates no significant changes (Carson SW, Wright CE, Millikin SP, et al. Pharmacokinetic evaluation of the combined administration of alprazolam [ALP] and clomipramine [CMI]. *Clin Pharmacol Ther* 1992;51:154).

alprazolam + desipramine Alprazolam can raise desipramine (DMI) plasma level and increase risk of DMI toxicity.

alprazolam + dextropropoxyphene A study showed that dextropropoxyphene significantly prolonged alprazolam half-life from 12 to 18 hours and reduced total clearance from 0.08 to 0.05 L/hour/kg (Abernathy DR, Greenblatt DJ, Morse DS, Shader RI. Interaction of propoxyphene with diazepam, alprazolam, and lorazepam. *Br J Clin Pharmacol* 1985;19:51–57).

alprazolam + disulfiram No serious interactions have been reported (Diquet B, Gujadhur L, Lamiable D, et al. Lack of interaction between disulfiram and alprazolam in alcoholic patients. *Eur J Clin Pharmacol* 1990;38: 157–160).

alprazolam + electroconvulsive therapy (ECT) Therapeutic response to unilateral electroconvulsive therapy (ECT) is much diminished in patients receiving concurrent alprazolam. In addition, there can be difficulties in evoking seizures. Alprazolam offers little benefit and may predispose patients to adverse effects during ECT. There also should be concern about provoking further impairment of cognitive and memory function (Jarvis MR, Goewert AJ, Zorumski CF. Novel antidepressants and maintenance electroconvulsive

therapy. A review. *Am Clin Psychiatry* 1992;4: 275–284).

alprazolam + fluoxetine Co-administration may increase psychomotor impairment, but usually it is insufficient to warrant modifying the dose of either agent if the combination is clinically effective. Clinical studies show decreased alprazolam (ALP) clearance. In vitro studies suggest that the oxidative metabolite norfluoxetine is responsible for inhibition of ALP metabolism, thus explaining the lag in recovery of ALP clearance after fluoxetine levels have fallen to almost zero with norfluoxetine levels remaining high. In one double-blind parallel study, co-administration increased ALP plasma levels about 30%. No significant changes were observed in mood status (Anon. *A pharmacokinetic/pharmacodynamic evaluation of the combined administration of alprazolam and fluoxetine*. Kalamazoo, MI: The Upjohn Company, 1990).

alprazolam + haloperidol In a double-blind study, alprazolam (ALP) plus haloperidol (HAL) was effective in the management of 28 agitated acutely psychotic schizophrenic patients, particularly in the first 48 hours. Subjects were randomly assigned to receive oral HAL 5 mg and ALP 1 mg or HAL 5 mg plus placebo. Patients treated with the combination generally require significantly less HAL to achieve similar results than when treated with HAL alone. The combination also may result in fewer dystonic reactions (Barbee JG, Mancuso DM, Freed CR, et al. Alprazolam as a neuroleptic adjunct in the emergency treatment of schizophrenia. *Am J Psychiatry* 1992; 149:506–510).

alprazolam + imipramine Co-administration decreases imipramine (IMI) clearance, with continued therapeutic improvement and reduction in IMI side effects after alprazolam is added (Wells BG, Evans RL, Ereshefsky L, et al. Clinical outcome and adverse effect profile associated with concurrent administration of alprazolam and imipramine. *J Clin Psychiatry* 1988;49:394–399).

alprazolam + lithium Therapeutic doses of alprazolam for patients on maintenance lithium therapy (900–1500 mg/day) may produce a statistically significant reduction in renal lithium clearance without any change in lithium plasma level or any adverse effects (Evans RL, Nelson MV, Melethil S, et al. Evaluation of the interaction of lithium and alprazolam. *J Clin Psychopharmacol* 1990;10: 355–359).

alprazolam + methadone Since its introduction in 1983, alprazolam (ALP) has become more popular than diazepam (Valium) among methadone maintenance patients who use a benzodiazepine to "boost" methadone effects. They take 20–40 mg after ingesting methadone to produce a "high" without sedation (Weddington WW, Carney AC. ALP abuse during methadone maintenance therapy. *JAMA* 1987;257:3363). Many patients typically take a large dose in the morning prior to receiving their methadone, then engage in sporadic use throughout the day. ALP's greater addiction liability, shorter half-life, and more intense withdrawal symptoms make addiction to it more likely and its management in methadone patients more complicated (McDuff DR, Schwartz RP, Tommasello A, et al. Outpatient benzodiazepine detoxification procedure for methadone patients. *J Subst Abuse Treat* 1993;10:297–302).

alprazolam + neuroleptic Neuroleptic augmentation with alprazolam has been reported to be effective and safe (Donyon R, Angrist B, Peselow E, et al. Neuroleptic augmentation with alprazolam: clinical effects and pharmacokinetic correlates. *Am J Psychiatry* 1989;146:231–234).

alprazolam + oral contraceptive Oral contraceptives can decrease alprazolam's clearance, but clinical significance of the interaction is unknown.

alprazolam + phenelzine Alprazolam enhances the therapeutic effect of phenelzine with no significant adverse effects and no effect on phenelzine's platelet monoamine oxidase activity (Fawcett J. Targeting treatment in patients with mixed symptoms of anxiety and depression. *J Clin Psychiatry* 1990;51[11, suppl]:40–43).

Alprazolam SR See **alprazolam, sustained release form**.

alprazolam, sustained release form (Alprazolam SR) (ALP-SR) Alprazolam (ALP) formulation with a prolonged T_{max} plateau that permits once-a-day dosing. In patients with panic disorder with or without agoraphobia, a mean maximal daily dose of 4.7 mg was effective across almost all measures of anxiety, panic, and phobic avoidance. The formulation has been compared with ALP and placebo in panic disorder and agoraphobia, and has been found to be effective. ALP-SR is generally well tolerated; sedation is the most commonly reported side effect. Absorption is minimally affected by food (Schweizer W, Patterson W, Rickels K, Rosenthal M. Double-blind, placebo-controlled study of a once-a-day, sustained-release preparation of alprazolam for the treatment of panic disorder. *Am J Psychiatry* 1993;150:1210–1215).

alprazolam + tranylcypromine Co-administration has been reported effective in treatment-resistent panic disorder, without serious adverse drug interactions.

alprostadil (prostaglandin E_1) Drug that is self-administered for the treatment of impotence.

altanserin Primary serotonin (5-HT)$_2$ antagonist that distinguishes between 5-HT$_2$ and 5-HT$_{1C}$ receptors. It is being evaluated for anxiety and depression.

alternative hypothesis See **hypothesis, alternative**.

altruism In group therapy, therapeutic factor in which patients feel better about themselves or learn something positive about themselves through the help they extend to fellow group members (Bloch S, Crouch E: *Therapeutic Factors in Group Psychotherapy*. Oxford: Oxford University Press, 1985).

Alurate See **aprobarbital**.

Alzheimer's disease (AD) Progressive neurodegenerative disease that affects approximately 10% of those over age 65 and 20% of those over 80. Currently, clinical diagnosis is one of exclusion; the only widely accepted risk factors are age and family history of the disorder. AD is characterized by gradually worsening cognitive deficits (notably in memory, abstraction, and reasoning) frequently accompanied by personality and behavioral changes (e.g., depression, agitation, paranoid symptoms, insomnia, sundowning, wandering, and aggression). Language disorder is a core symptom, the earliest sign of which is impaired category fluency. Expressive speech becomes circumlocutory, with extensive use of incomplete and prepositional phrases and indefinite words; as severity increases, there is progressive reduction in verbal complexity. In the early stages of AD there usually are no motor, gait, or coordination disturbances. Neurological signs such as primitive reflexes, extrapyramidal symptoms, and myoclonus occur late in the illness and are considered a consequence of advanced cerebral damage. A snout reflex and extrapyramidal signs are the most common neurological features in elderly AD patients presenting to psychiatrists, confirming the need for neurological examination in elderly demented patients. Recent data suggest that a quantitative electroencephalograph (EEG) measure (absolute alpha power) is related to rate of cognitive decline (Kuskowski MA, Mortimer JA, Morley GK, et al. Rate of cognitive decline in Alzheimer's disease is associated with EEG alpha power. *Biol Psychiatry* 1993;33:659–662). AD patients have multiple neurotransmitter deficits; marked reduction in acetylcholinesterase enzymes (AChE) and acetylcholine (ACh) in the brain have been consistently reported. Up to 50% of patients demonstrate nonsuppression of cortisol following dexamethasone administration. Numerous other abnormalities have been reported, but none with sufficient consistency or specificity to qualify as a clinical diagnostic marker. Psychopharmacologic and psychotherapeutic treatments may be useful when symptoms become disturbing to caregivers. Psychopharmacologic treatment can ease the burden on the caregiver and postpone institutionalization. Neuroleptics are often used for some of the more disturbing behavioral symptoms. When starting neuroleptic treatment, clinicians should use dosages that might be homeopathic in younger patients. Incremental dosage adjustments should ideally be made very gradually (at biweekly intervals or even less frequently with outpatients) and continued in accordance with the patient's and caregiver's needs. AD is now seen as a degenerative process with distinctive biochemical changes underlying the neuropathologic features of senile plaques and neurofibrillary tangles (Selkoe DJ. The molecular pathology of Alzheimer's disease. *Neuron* 1991;6:487). It also has been hypothesized that impairment of the microtubule (MT) system, regardless of cause, leads to impaired cellular functioning; the effects accumulate with time and eventually reach threshold levels for symptomatic behavioral manifestations, neurochemical changes, and neuropathological lesions. MTs are ubiquitous cellular components present in the highest concentration in the brain, the organ most prominently affected in AD. The MT system is vital to numerous cellular functions, including axonal transport of neurotransmitters, cell division, and goal-directed motion. MTs are present in nondividing cells (such as neurons) as well as actively dividing cells (such as skin fibroblasts). Impairment in each of these functions has been reported for AD patients. AD may have a genetic etiology. Chromosome 21 produces an amyloid precursor protein that may be snipped in two, which is thought to result in the beta-amyloid (or A_4 peptide) deposits commonly found in the brains of AD patients. Three gene defects resulting in three different amino acid substitutions in the amyloid precursor protein have been identified in familial AD, a rare, inherited form of the disorder. Chromosome 19 damage has also been identified. Another possible etiology may be a slow virus, but attempts to demonstrate it have generally been frustrating.

Alzheimer's Disease and Related Disorders Association (ADRDA) Association that in conjunction with the National Institute of Neurological and Communicative Disorders Stroke (NINCDS) has established criteria for probable Alzheimer's disease (McKhann G, Drachman D, Folstein M, et al: Clinical diagnosis of Alzheimer's disease: report of the NINCDS-ADRDA work group. *Neurology* 1984;34:939–944).

Alzheimer's disease/aggression Physical aggression may occur during the course of Alzheimer's disease. There may be (a) "situational" episodes, as when a caregiver attempts to help during grooming or stop the patient from "going home," or (b) "spontaneous" episodes unrelated to caregiver activity. Delusions, hallucinations, and misidentification are often associated with aggressive episodes.

Alzheimer's disease, familial Form of Alzheimer's disease (AD) that occurs before age 65, is associated with mutation of an amyloid precursor protein gene, and seems to be transmitted as an autosomal dominant trait. A family history and age of onset are the most useful clinical features that can be related to etiology. In late-onset disease, chromosome 19 is implicated at the apolipoprotein E locus (APOE), which has three alleles: APOE-2, -3, and -4. A study of 42 families with a history of AD showed that the proportion of those affected varied from 18.8% for APOE-2/3 to 91.3% for APOE-4/4; the 4/4 genotype was associated with earlier age at onset and more rapid progression (Corder E, Saunders M, Strittmer W, et al. Gene dose of apolipoprotein E type 4 allele and the risk of Alzheimer disease in late onset families. *Science* 1993;261:921–923). Genetic studies with early-onset familial disease initially showed linkage to chromosome 21 (St George Hyslop PH, Tanzi RE, Polinsky RJ, et al. The genetic defect causing familial Alzheimer's disease maps on chromosome 21. *Science* 1987; 235:885–890). This was followed by identification of the gene coding for the amyloid precursor protein on chromosome 21. Inheritance of one of these rare mutations completely predicts occurrence of the disease. Subsequently, a second gene for early-onset AD linked to markers on chromosome 14 was identified (Schellenberg G, Bud T, Wijsman E, et al. Genetic linkage evidence for a familial Alzheimer's disease locus on chromosome 14. *Science* 1992, 258:668–671). Several genes localized to chromosome 14 influence the metabolism or processing of amyloid precursor protein, and further genetic analysis may define which genes are important.

Alzheimer's disease, type I Alzheimer's disease characterized by late onset and absence of loss of cells from subcortical nuclei. A biochemical deficit in presynaptic nerve cells of the cholinergic systems occurs and is reflected by a deficiency of choline acetyl transferase. Deficits in other neurotransmitter systems, including cholecystokinin and vasoactive-intestinal peptide, have been identified.

Alzheimer's disease, type II   Alzheimer's disease characterized by early onset and loss of cells from subcortical nuclei. A biochemical deficit in presynaptic nerve cells of the cholinergic systems occurs and is reflected by a deficiency of choline acetyl transferase. Other biochemical abnormalities (deficits) in noradrenergic, serotonergic, and dopaminergic systems and in cholecystokinin and vasoactive-intestinal peptide also may occur.

Alzipam   See **lorazepam**.

amantadine   (Paritrel; PK Mez; Symadine; Symmetrel) Indirect dopamine agonist with antiviral and antiparkinson properties. It is rapidly absorbed after oral ingestion. Half-life, typically about 12 hours, is largely determined by kidney function. It has been used in the prophylaxis and treatment of influenza A. It is used to treat mild Parkinson syndrome, by itself or in addition to other antiparkinson drugs. Because amantadine is thought to exert a protective effect on striatal dopamine receptors, it has also been used to treat tardive dyskinesia, but without effects on psychiatric symptoms. Amantadine has infrequently exacerbated schizophrenia in patients being treated with antipsychotic drugs. It also can produce mental and behavioral side effects in normal subjects not taking other medications (e.g., those taking amantadine for antiviral prophylaxis and patients with Parkinson's disease). These side effects include jitteriness, agitation, insomnia, disorientation, anorexia, depression, visual hallucinations, paranoid delusions, and thought disorders, all of which resolve within 36–72 hours of amantadine discontinuation (Nestelbaum Z, Siris SG, Rifkin A, et al. Exacerbation of schizophrenia associated with amantadine. *Am J Psychiatry* 1986;143:1170–1171). Oral doses of about 200 mg/day may cause minor side effects such as insomnia, nervousness, dizziness, and headache. Higher doses have been associated with mood changes, delirium, hallucinations, drowsiness, and convulsions. Amantadine also may cause hyponatremia, the mechanism of action of which is probably inappropriate secretion of antidiuretic hormone (Lammers GJ, Roos RAC. Hyponatremia due to amantadine hydrochloride and L-dopa/carbidopa. *Lancet* 1993;342:439). These behavioral effects must be carefully considered when amantadine is given as protection against pseudoparkinsonism produced by neuroleptics in the treatment of patients already vulnerable to

psychosis. Amantadine has been shown in controlled, double-blind studies to attenuate craving and dysphoria during cocaine withdrawal (Tennant FS Jr, Sagherian AA. Double-blind comparison of amantadine and bromocriptine for ambulatory withdrawal from cocaine dependence. *Arch Intern Med* 1987; 147:109–112). It is probably as effective as bromocriptine in the treatment of cocaine withdrawal and is perhaps less toxic, but its effectiveness in maintaining short-term abstinence may decrease with time (Thompson DF. Amantadine in the treatment of cocaine withdrawal. *Ann Pharmacother* 1992;26:933–935). Pregnancy risk category C.

amantadine + benztropine   Co-administration may enhance anticholinergic effects, causing peripheral adverse reactions (dry mouth, blurred vision, severe constipation, and delayed micturition) and central anticholinergic effects (disorientation, restlessness, agitation, confusion, hallucinations, and delirium).

amantadine/breast milk   Amantadine is excreted in breast milk, but effects in neonates and infants are not known.

amantadine + bupropion   Bupropion (BUP) inhibits dopamine reuptake; amantadine facilitates release of presynaptic dopamine. Co-administration may cause dopaminergic overdrive, resulting in delirium. Caution during concurrent use of BUP and dopamine agonists, even at the lowest doses, is advisable (Liberzon I, Dequardo JR, Silk KR. Bupropion and delirium. *Am J Psychiatry* 1990;147:1659–1690).

amantadine + central nervous system stimulant   Co-administration may result in additive stimulation and should be used with caution.

amantadine + fluoxetine   Fluoxetine may elevate amantadine plasma levels, which may produce delirium (Baker RW. Fluoxetine and schizophrenia in a patient with obsessional thinking. *J Neuropsychiatry Clin Neurosci* 1992; 4:232–233).

amantadine/neuroleptic malignant syndrome   Oral amantadine (200–300 mg/day in divided dosages) has been used in the treatment of neuroleptic malignant syndrome (NMS), with results ranging from positive benefits to no benefit. There has been no correlation between dosage and effectiveness. Development of NMS has been reported following amantadine withdrawal.

amantadine/parkinsonism   Amantadine may reduce tremor, rigidity, and bradykinesia. It seldom causes toxicity, but benefits may wane in as many as 50% of patients after short-term treatment (2–3 months). When this happens, amantadine should be discontinued, since further treatment is unlikely to be beneficial.

Long-term therapy (1 or more years) may cause swelling of the legs and livedo reticularis that are not manifestations of systemic illness. These side effects usually do not worsen with continued treatment and disappear after amantadine is discontinued. Most Parkinson's disease patients need amantadine plus a levodopa drug.

amantadine + phenelzine A patient taking amantadine, haloperidol, and flurazepam developed hypertension after taking four doses of phenelzine (Jack RA, Daniel DG. Possible interaction between phenelzine and amantadine. *Arch Gen Psychiatry* 1984;41:726).

Amaxyl See **alpidem**.

Ambien See **zolpidem**.

amentia Mental retardation present from birth. It includes the more severe forms of mental retardation, but not borderline intellectual capacity.

American Board of Psychiatry and Neurology, Inc. (ABPN) Official agency to examine and certify physicians as diplomates (specialists) in psychiatry, child psychiatry, neurology, and neurology with special competence in child neurology, administrative psychiatry, geriatric psychiatry, forensic psychiatry, and addiction psychiatry.

American College of Neuropsychopharmacology (ACNP) Interdisciplinary professional organization founded in 1961, composed of leading North American psychiatrists, neuroscientists, psychologists, pharmacologists, and research-related health care professionals engaged in promotion of health and research on causes and treatment of diseases affecting emotions and behavior, including addictive disorders. Members are elected primarily on the basis of original research contributions to the field of neuropsychopharmacology, which includes evaluation of the effects of natural and synthetic compounds on the brain, mind, and human behavior.

American Psychiatric Association (APA) Founded in 1844 as the Association of Medical Superintendents of American Institutions for the Insane, its name was changed in 1891 to American Medico-Psychological Association, and in 1921 to the American Psychiatric Association. Membership totals more than 37,000 psychiatrists and psychiatrists-in-training.

Amfebutamone See **bupropion**.

Amfetamone See **bupropion**.

amfonelic acid (AFA) Nonamphetamine stimulant that can facilitate impulse-induced release of dopamine in the striatum with haloperidol or clozapine administration in the presence or absence of ritanserin (Brougham LR, Conway PG, Ellis DB. Effect of ritanserin on the interaction of amfonelic

acid and neuroleptic-induced striatal dopamine metabolism. *Neuropharmacology* 1991;30: 1137–1140).

Amidate See **etomidate**.

amiflamine Alphamethylamine derivative that is a reversible inhibitor of monoamine oxidase-A selective for serotonin (5-HT) neurons. It acts as a prodrug. Although an effective monoamine oxidase inhibitor itself, its metabolism to form FLA (+) gives rise to a compound of greater potency that also appears to be actively transported into serotonergic nerve terminals.

amiloride (Midamor) Potassium-sparing diuretic.

amiloride + lithium See **lithium + amiloride**.

amine hypothesis of depression Postulation that depressive symptoms are due to a decrease in functional concentrations of noradrenaline and/or serotonin (5-HT) receptor sites in the brain. It is based on the observation that monoamine oxidase inhibitors impair catabolism of the biogenic amine neurotransmitters and that imipramine reduces their reuptake into nerve terminals, thereby prolonging their action at the postsynaptic receptor site. It was widely assumed that depletion of biogenic amines is associated with symptoms of depression and that a rise in amine concentrations is associated with elevation of mood, drive, and motivation. The hypothesis became the basis of a theory that is somewhat reductionistic.

amine neurotransmitter See **neurotransmitter, amine**.

amineptine (Survector 100) Antidepressant that differs from classic tricyclics (TCAs) because of an amino-acidic chain of seven carbon atoms attached to the central nucleus. It increases release and reduces reuptake of dopamine. It is virtually devoid of anticholinergic, serotonergic, and adrenergic effects at therapeutic doses. An effect on serotonin can be observed at high doses. It has a rapid onset of effect without the characteristic time-lag of TCAs. It has reversible hepatic toxicity. Several cases of amineptine abuse/addiction have been reported. Presently available only in France and Italy, amineptine is being studied in other sections of the world (Mendis N, Hanwella DR, Weerasinghe C, et al. A double-blind comparative study: amineptine [Survector 100] versus imipramine. *Clin Neuropharmacol* 1992;12[suppl 2]:58–65).

2-amino-5-phosphonovalerate (AP5) N-methyl-D-aspartate (NMDA) receptor antagonist that blocks long-term potentiation in vivo at doses shown to impair performance in a special learning task.

amino acid   One of 20 different molecules that are the building blocks of protein, including glycine, leucine, cysteine, phenylalanine, tryptophan, and asparagine. They are strung together in a precise linear order, specified by information contained in the DNA genetic code, to create the many proteins found in living organisms.

amino acid neurotransmitter   See **neurotransmitter, amino acid**.

aminoglutethimide   (Cytadren) Steroid suppressive agent that interferes with biosynthesis and metabolism of many steroids, including cortisol and dehydroepiandrosterone (DHAS). It has been found effective in some patients with treatment-resistant major depression. Pregnancy risk category D.

Aminophyllin   See **aminophylline**.

aminophylline   (Aminophyllin) Mixture of theophylline and base, with the action of theophylline alone, used in the treatment of asthma and reversible bronchospasm associated with chronic bronchitis and emphysema.

aminophylline + lithium   See **lithium + aminophylline**.

amiodarone   (Cordarone) Di-ionated benzofurane derivative used in the treatment of cardiac arrhythmias. It may cause a bilateral 6- to 10-Hz postural and action tremor of the arms similar to essential tremor. It was described as a coarse, parkinsonian resting tremor in the left leg in a single patient treated for 4 days with 1.2–1.6 g daily. It resolved within 5 days of drug withdrawal and returned again on re-exposure (Werner EG, Olanow CW. Parkinsonism and amiodarone therapy. *Ann Neurol* 1989;25:630–632). Uncommon movement disorders reported with amiodarone include myoclonus, hemiballism, dyskinesias of the extremities, and orofacial dyskinesias (Lang AE. Miscellaneous drug-induced movement disorders. *In* Lang AE, Weiner WJ [eds], *Drug-Induced Movement Disorders*. Mt Kisco, NY: Futura, 1992). Pregnancy risk category C.

amiodarone + midazolam   See **midazolam + amiodarone**.

amisulpiride   (Deniban; Enordin; Socian; Sofian; Solian) Orthomethoxy benzamide compound with a higher affinity for dopaminergic receptors, especially D_2, than sulpiride. It also binds to D_3 receptors. It is a low-potency, atypical, sedative neuroleptic with low propensity to cause extrapyramidal symptoms. It has an unusual dose-dependent behavioral profile: high doses have marked antipsychotic properties, and low doses produce direct stimulant effects. In double-blind studies, it is as effective an antidepressant as amitriptyline.

It has also been shown effective for maintenance antidepressant treatment up to 1 year.

Amitril   See **amitriptyline**.

amitriptyline   (Amitril; Elatrol; Elavil; Emitrip; Endep; Enovil; Laroxyl; Lentizol; Levate; Mevaril; Novotriptyn; Saroten; Tryptal; Tryptizol) (AMI) Tricyclic antidepressant (TCA) that is the most anticholinergic of all antidepressants. It is about 5% as potent as atropine and has a very high affinity for muscarinic receptors compared with other TCAs. At therapeutic doses it may produce as much cholinergic blockade as classic anticholinergic drugs. In clinically effective doses, AMI may significantly increase heart rate when prescribed alone and/or in combination with tranylcypromine. Because of its anticholinergic effects, it should be prescribed cautiously for the elderly. Its sedating effects have been beneficial for depressed human immunodeficiency virus (HIV)-infected patients who also suffer from agitation and severe insomnia. In patients unable to take oral medication, intramuscular administration is effective (Bloomingdale LM, Bressler B. Rapid intramuscular administration of tricyclic antidepressants. *Am J Psychiatry* 1979;136:8). Pregnancy risk category D.

amitriptyline + alcohol   Amitriptyline (AMI) plasma concentrations are increased in the presence of alcohol; there is a probable decrease in first-pass metabolism and also an increase in nortriptyline concentrations. Alcohol has no effect on steady-state concentrations of AMI and nortriptyline in individuals ingesting low levels of alcohol intermittently. In recently abstinent alcoholics, there may be increased concentrations of hydroxylated amitriptyline (OHAMI) and decreased concentrations of nortriptyline and 10-hydroxylated nortriptyline (Ciraulo DA, Shader RI, Greenblatt, DJ, Creelman W [eds], *Drug Interactions in Psychiatry*. Baltimore: Williams & Wilkins, 1989).

amitriptyline/breast milk   Infants of nursing mothers treated with amitriptyline (AMI) had nondetectable blood levels of AMI/nortriptyline and no adverse effects (Brixen-Rasmussen L, Halgrener J, Jorgensen A. Amitriptyline and nortriptyline excretion in human breast milk. *Psychopharmacology* 1982;76:94–95).

amitriptyline + buprenorphine   In normal subjects, sublingual buprenorphine 0.4 mg and oral amitriptyline 50 mg mildly impaired performance on a number of psychomotor tests. The combination can be used with reasonable safety (Saarialho-Kere U, Mattila MJ, Paloheimo M, Seppala T. Psychomotor, respiratory and neuroendocrinological effects of buprenorphine and amitriptyline in healthy volunteers. *Eur J Clin Pharmacol* 1987;33:139–146).

amitriptyline + carbamazepine Co-administration reduces serum amitriptyline (AMI) and nortriptyline plasma levels about 40%, undermining AMI's therapeutic efficacy unless dosage is increased and serum levels are monitored (Leinonen E, Lillsunde P, Laukkanen V, Ylitalo P. Effects of carbamazepine on serum antidepressant concentration in psychiatric patients. *J Clin Psychopharmacol* 1991;11:313–318).

amitriptyline + chlordiazepoxide (Limbitrol) Combination of a benzodiazepine (chlordiazepoxide) and a tricyclic antidepressant (amitriptyline) marketed for the relief of moderate to severe depression associated with moderate to severe anxiety. Both components exert their action on the central nervous system. Adverse reactions are those associated with use of either component alone. Most frequently reported are drowsiness, dry mouth, constipation, blurred vision, dizziness, and bloating.

amitriptyline + chlordiazepoxide/pregnancy Safe use during pregnancy and lactation has not been established because of the chlordiazepoxide component. According to the manufacturer: "An increased risk of congenital malformations associated with the use of minor tranquilizers (chlordiazepoxide, diazepam, and meprobamate) during the first trimester of pregnancy has been suggested in several studies. Because the use of these drugs is rarely a matter of urgency, their use during this period should almost always be avoided. The possibility that a woman of childbearing potential may be pregnant at the time of institution of therapy should be considered. Patients should be advised that if they become pregnant during therapy or intend to become pregnant they should communicate with their physicians about the desirability of discontinuing the drug." (*Physician's Desk Reference* 1993, pp 20–23).

amitriptyline + citalopram Addition of citalopram to previously initiated amitriptyline therapy has no influence on plasma amitriptyline and nortriptyline (Baumann P. Clinical pharmacokinetics of citalopram and other selective serotonergic reuptake inhibitors [SSRI]. *Int Clin Psychopharmacol* 1992;6[suppl 5]:13–20; Baettig D, Bondolfi G, Montaldi S, et al. Tricyclic antidepressant plasma levels after augmentation with citalopram. *Eur J Clin Pharmacol* 1993;44:403–405).

amitriptyline + fluoxetine Fluoxetine inhibits hepatic metabolism of amitriptyline (AMI), producing elevated AMI plasma levels and side effects consistent with AMI toxicity.

amitriptyline + fluvoxamine Co-administration markedly enhances amitriptyline (AMI) plasma level due to inhibition of demethylation by fluvoxamine (FLV). AMI produces a higher plasma level of FLV than occurs with FLV monotherapy. Increased plasma levels of each drug may potentiate antidepressant effects in some patients, but also may cause adverse reactions; serum level monitoring is indicated (Bertschy G, Vandel S, Vandel B, et al. Fluvoxamine-tricyclic antidepressant interaction: an accidental finding. *Eur J Clin Pharmacol* 1991; 40:119–121). Inhibitory effects of FLV on AMI metabolism disappear within 1–2 weeks of FLV discontinuation (Haertter S, Wetzel H, Hammes E, Hiemke C. Inhibition of antidepressant demethylation and hydroxylation of fluvoxamine in depressed patients. *Psychopharmacology* 1993;110:302–308).

amitriptyline + guanfacine Co-administration can result in clinically significant increased blood pressure in hypertensive patients. Blood pressure may return to former levels within 2 weeks of amitriptyline discontinuation.

amitriptyline + isocarboxazid Co-administration has precipitated mania (Ramon de la Fuente J, Berlanga C, León-Andrade C. Mania induced by tricyclic-MAOI combination therapy in bipolar treatment-resistant disorder: case reports. *J Clin Psychiatry* 1986;47:40–41).

amitriptyline + methadone Amitriptyline potentiates opioid-associated respiratory depression and sedation (Hasten PD, Horn JR. *Drug Interactions*, 6th ed. Philadelphia: Lea & Febiger, 1990).

amitriptyline + moclobemide Possible interactions were investigated in 21 female inpatients. After 2 weeks treatment with moclobemide (300 mg/day), amitriptyline (up to 150 mg/day) was given to seven patients after a treatment-free interval of 0–3 days. In four patients, AMI was added to current moclobemide treatment after 2 weeks, and in 10 patients combined moclobemide and AMI therapy was given from the beginning. In all three groups tolerance was excellent and there were no signs of incompatibility (Amrei R, Guntert TW, Dingemanse J, et al. Interactions of moclobemide with concomitantly administered medication: evidence from pharmacological and clinical studies. *Psychopharmacology* 1992;106:S24–S31). No clinically relevant interactions have been reported (Priest R. Therapy-resistant depression. *Int Clin Psychopharmacol* 1993;7:201–202).

amitriptyline + monoamine oxidase inhibitor (MAOI)   Amitriptyline may help protect against tyramine-induced hypertensive reactions associated with MAOI therapy (Pare CMB, Kline N, Hallstrom C, et al. Will amitriptyline prevent the "cheese" reaction of monoamine-oxidase inhibitors? *Lancet* 1982;2: 183–186; Kline NS, Pare M, Hallstrom C, Cooper TB. Amitriptyline protects patients on MAOI from tyramine reactions. *J Clin Psychopharmacol* 1982;2:434–435).

amitriptyline + morphine   Co-administration increases morphine bioavailability and degree of analgesia. Although a useful interaction, it also may increase morphine toxicity (Ventafridda V, Ripamonti C, DeConno F, et al. Antidepressants increase bioavailability of morphine in cancer patients. *Lancet* 1987;1: 1204). Amitriptyline also potentiates opioid-associated respiratory depression and sedation (Hasten PD, Horn JR. *Drug Interactions*, 6th ed. Philadelphia: Lea & Febiger, 1990).

amitriptyline-N-oxide   Pro-drug of amitriptyline (AMI) used therapeutically in Europe. Mode of action is believed to be conversion into AMI. It produces adequate concentrations of AMI in the brain at low plasma concentration and has a lower incidence of adverse side effects compared to AMI.

amitriptyline + paroxetine   Co-administration may necessitate use of lower doses than usually prescribed for either drug, since each inhibits the other's metabolism, raising the plasma level of each.

amitriptyline + perphenazine   (Etrafon; Etrafon-A; Etrafon-D; Etrafon-F; Etrafon-M; Etrafon-2-10; Longopax; Longopox Mite; Mite; Mutabase-2-10; Mutabon-A; Mutabon Ansiolittico; Mutabon Antidepressivo; Mutabon-D; Mutabon-F; Mutabon-M; Mutabon Mite; Triavil) Combination product composed of the piperazine phenothiazine neuroleptic perphenazine and the tricyclic antidepressant amitriptyline (AMI). Each inhibits the others metabolism. AMI may block the extrapyramidal effects of perphenazine; combined therapeutic effects are greater than those of either component alone. It is prescribed for moderate to severe anxiety/depression, agitation and depression, and psychotic depression.

amitriptyline + sulpiride   Co-administration may be useful in the treatment of severe depression (Bonceir C, Masquin A, Omieux MC. Indications psychiatriques du sulpiride. A propos de 60 observations. *J Med Lyonnais* 1971;52:519–533).

amitriptyline + tranylcypromine   Co-administration may cause a hypertensive crisis, significant increase in heart rate, and significant lengthening of the PR interval.

amitriptyline + valproate   Amitriptyline (100 mg/day) increased valproate half-life, but the change was not clinically significant (Pisani F, Primerano G, D'Agostino AA, et al. Valproic acid amitriptyline interactions in man. *Ther Drug Monit* 1986;8:382–383).

amnesia   Loss of memory; inability to recall past experiences. Amnesia may be anterograde, retrograde, or mixed. See **amnestic syndrome**.

amnesia, anterograde   Inability to recall events occurring after administration of a drug or because of other significant pathology. It is a potential effect of all benzodiazepines and a well documented side effect of electroconvulsive therapy (ECT) more likely to occur with bilateral than unilateral ECT. It also may occur at the onset of delirium and with anesthetic agents (e.g., midazolam). See **amnesia, anterograde/benzodiazepine**.

amnesia, anterograde/benzodiazepine   Potential effect of all benzodiazepines (BZDs) and a recognized effect of high-potency BZDs, especially the triazolobenzodiazepine triazolam (TZL). It depends on dose and route of administration. With hypnotics, dose is the major determinant of the degree to which a drug is associated with memory problems. Anterograde amnesia may be beneficial when BZDs (e.g., midazolam) are used as premedication for surgery, endoscopy, or cardioversion, but could have undesirable consequences in other situations. Patients taking a BZD hypnotic such as TZL, for example, have forgotten actions performed under the drug's influence. Clinical reports on TZL-caused amnesia suggest it may be a primary effect (i.e., not simply secondary to sedation). Prevalence of anterograde amnesia caused by BZD hypnotics is probably grossly under-reported, because patients are usually unaware of memory impairment and report only more pronounced instances of amnesia. Projections from the Food & Drug Administration's Adverse Effects Reporting System suggest that amnesia is more than 100 times more prevalent after TZL use than with other BZD hypnotics.

amnesia, psychogenic   Dissociative disorder characterized by inability to recall important aspects of a traumatic event; probably mediated by dissociative processes. Essential feature is sudden inability to recall important personal information. There is often a history of organic amnesia due to a head injury, for example. It usually is time-limited but, in rare cases, may last a lifetime. The patient may display perplexity and disorientation and may wander aimlessly. In many if not all cases, semantic (conceptual) memory and memory of skills remain intact (Lipowski ZJ: *Delirium: Acute Confusional States.* New York: Oxford University Press, 1990). Also called "dissociative amnesia". See **dissociative disorder**.

amnesia, retrograde   Loss of memory for events that occurred prior to the amnesia-causing incident.

amnesia, transient global   (TGA) Syndrome, first clearly recognized in 1964, that typically occurs in middle-aged or elderly persons who suddenly develop a memory disorder, often regarded as confusion, that lasts from 15 minutes to up to 48 hours. During this time, registration and recall of current events are impaired, and although seemingly healthy, the person is often distressed and unaware of what is wrong. Afterwards, the person cannot remember any events during the confused period. Electroencephalogram usually is normal. Personality, problem-solving, language, and visuospatial function remain intact. There is no loss of personal identity, and complex functions such as driving may be performed without difficulty. Recovery is complete, and recurrences are unusual. It is widely held that the cause of TGA lies within the temporal lobe, although its etiology is an enigma. The most widely accepted view is that TGA is due to thromboembolic cerebrovascular disease with ischemia in the territory of the posterior cerebral arteries, which supply the medial temporal lobes. TGA should not be mistaken for delirium.

amnestic "hangover"   Amnesia produced by many benzodiazepine hypnotics and sedatives.

amnestic syndrome   Impaired short- and long-term memory occurring in a state of clear awareness. It may be due to head trauma, hypoxia, thiamine deficiency, or encephalitis.

Amoban   See **zopiclone**.

amobarbital   (Amytal; Dexamyl) 5-ethyl-5-isoamyl-barbituric acid, a barbiturate sedative-hypnotic and anticonvulsant. Schedule II; pregnancy risk category D.

amobarbital + paroxetine   Paroxetine does not potentiate the sedative effects of amobarbital. No clinically significant interactions have been reported (Boyer WF, Feighner JP. An overview of paroxetine. *J Clin Psychiatry* 1192; 53[suppl]:3–6).

amobarbital + secobarbital   (Tuinal) Combination sedative/hypnotic product marketed in three strengths: 25 mg secobarbital and 25 mg amobarbital; 50 mg secobarbital and 50 mg amobarbital; and 100 mg secobarbital and 100 mg amobarbital. It is used for preanesthetic sedation and more often to treat insomnia. Often abused, it is known by the street name "rainbows." Dependence can be produced by

taking 500–600 mg/day for 30 days. Schedule II; pregnancy risk category B.

amobarbital sodium   Sodium derivative of amobarbital, a central nervous system depressant producing sedation or hypnosis, depending on the dose given. Schedule II; pregnancy risk category D.

amodiaquine   Quinine-based antimalarial drug known to be capable of producing dystonia and other dyskinesias (Akindele O, Odejide AO. Amodiaquine-induced involuntary movements. *Br Med J* 1976;6029:214–215).

Amopax   See **amoxapine**.

amorph   Silent allele; gene that has no detectable product; an apparently inactive gene.

amotivational syndrome   Term coined in 1968 to describe a group of subtle yet reliable behavioral sequelae to chronic marijuana use. Symptoms include deterioration in personal appearance; apathy; passivity; lethargy; loss of effectiveness; and inability or unwillingness to concentrate, follow routines, and engage in meaningful goal-directed behavior. Its existence as a direct effect of marijuana use is considered doubtful by many, although patients who voluntarily seek treatment for marijuana abuse typically complain of amotivational effects.

Amoxan   See **amoxapine**.

amoxapine   (Amopax; Amoxan; Asendin; Asendis; Defanyl; Demelox; Demolox; Moxadil; Omnipress) N-desmethyl analog of loxapine, a dibenzoxazepine antipsychotic, marketed as an antidepressant. Biochemical and clinical profiles are similar to those of tricyclic antidepressants (TCAs). Like conventional TCAs, it blocks neuronal reuptake of noradrenaline and, to a lesser extent, of serotonin. Like neuroleptics, it elevates prolactin and has some dopamine receptor blocking properties. Many patients who initially seem to have dramatic and rapid positive response to amoxapine lose their response between the 3rd and 12th week of treatment, an outcome labeled by some as "therapeutic fade." It has been associated with almost all types of early-onset extrapyramidal reactions induced by neuroleptics and dopamine receptor blocker antiemetics, including acute dystonia, akinesia, akathisia, and parkinsonism, as well as tardive dyskinesia (TD) in some patients. Apart from amoxapine, there are no convincing reports of TD caused by antidepressant therapies. Amoxapines extrapyramidal effects are most likely related to antidopaminergic effects exerted by its metabolite 7-hydroxyamoxapine, which has been shown to have greater affinity for postsynaptic receptors than the neuroleptic loxapine, a characteristic shared by neither amoxapine nor its 8-hydroxymetabolite. Therapeutic doses of amoxapine have been associated with hyperthermia, rigidity, and rhabdomyolysis. Some cases of amoxapine toxicity resemble neuroleptic malignant syndrome. Dopamine radioreceptor bioassay indicates that patients on amoxapine have plasma levels similar to those of patients on neuroleptics. Pregnancy risk category C.

amoxapine/breast milk Amoxapine (250 mg/day) produces low concentrations in human milk, but effects on infants have not been studied (Gelenberg AJ. Amoxapine, a new antidepressant, appears in human milk. *J Nerv Ment Dis* 1979;167:635–636).

amoxapine + central nervous system (CNS) depressant Combined use increases CNS depression beyond that caused by either drug alone.

amoxapine + cimetidine Cimetidine increases amoxapine serum level.

amoxapine + electroconvulsive therapy (ECT) Amoxapine's predilection to cause seizures raises concern that serious adverse effects could occur if it is taken during ECT (Jarvis MR, Goewert AJ, Zorunski CF. Novel antidepressants and maintenance electroconvulsive therapy. A review. *Am Clin Psychiatry* 1992;4:275–284).

amoxapine + epinephrine Co-administration may cause a pressor response and arrhythmia.

amoxapine + methadone Amoxapine prolongs and potentiates methadone's analgesic effects, and potentiates methadone-induced respiratory depression (Hasten PD, Horn JR. *Drug Interactions*, 6th ed. Philadelphia: Lea & Febiger, 1990).

amoxapine + monoamine oxidase inhibitor Co-administration may cause hyperpyrexia, excitability, convulsions, coma, and death.

amoxapine + morphine Amoxapine prolongs and potentiates morphine's analgesic effects, and potentiates morphine-induced respiratory depression (Hasten PD, Horn JR. *Drug Interactions*, 6th ed. Philadelphia: Lea & Febiger, 1990).

amoxapine + pergolide Co-administration has been used to treat patients refractory to amoxapine alone. Response is usually rapid (within a week), but without incremental improvement over the next month. Some patients tolerate the combination well; others develop nausea and vomiting that may or may not respond to lowering pergolide dosage.

amoxapine/seizures Amoxapine has been reported to cause seizures at therapeutic doses (Jefferson JW. Convulsions associated with amoxapine. *JAMA* 1984;251:603). Seizures have been reported in 36.4% of amoxapine overdoses, compared to 4.3% for heterocyclic antidepressant poisonings. Seizures due to

amoxapine overdose are often persistent and difficult to control (Litovitz TL, Troutman WG. Amoxapine overdose: seizures and fatalities. *JAMA* 1983;250:1063–1071).

"amp" Street term for amphetamine.

amperozide Atypical neuroleptic that belongs to a category of new antipsychotics with antidopaminergic and other receptor activity. It has a high affinity for serotonin $(5\text{-HT})_2$ receptors, moderate affinity for alpha$_1$ receptors, and minimal affinity for dopamine D_1 and D_2 receptors. In a pilot trial, 6 of 10 schizophrenics showed improvement in positive and negative symptoms; only one developed an extrapyramidal reaction (mild tremor). Prolactin level was not increased during treatment. Electrocardiographic changes included T-wave morphology and prolongation of QT time. A major double-blind trial has been completed in the United States (Gerlach J. New antipsychotics: classification, efficacy, and adverse effects. *Schizophr Bull* 1991;17:289–309; Christeneson E, Bjork A. Amperozide: a new pharmacological approach in the treatment of schizophrenia. *Pharmacol Toxicol* 1990:66[suppl 1]:5–7; Lindenmayer JP. Recent advances in pharmacotherapy of schizophrenia. *Psychiatr Ann* 1993;23:201–208).

amphetamine (Benzedrine; Biphetamine; Dexamyl) (AMPH) Potent catecholaminergic agonist that causes release of biogenic amines and blocks their reuptake. It is a stimulant that causes release of catecholamine by a Ca^{2+} independent effect on the vesicle membrane that may involve effects on pH gradients (Sulzer D, Rayport S. Amphetamine and other psychostimulants reduce pH gradients in midbrain dopaminergic neurons and chromaffin granules: a mechanism of action. *Neuron* 1990; 5:797–808). The D optical isomer is biologically several times more active than the L form. AMPH is an indirect dopamine agonist for D_1, D_2, and some NA receptors. Reinforcing effects are similar to those of cocaine. It may improve symptoms in some schizophrenics; it also may cause or exacerbate psychotic symptoms, especially paranoid schizophrenia, in a manner consistent with the dopamine hypothesis of schizophrenia (i.e., through dopaminergic overactivity in the limbic system and striatum). Adverse side effects include insomnia, fever, headaches, confusion, irritability, hostility, and visual hallucinations. AMPH and its derivatives suppress rapid eye movement (REM) sleep and in higher doses increase vigilance and disturb sleep continuity. Oral administration of 10–15 mg d-amphetamine just before bedtime decreases REM period time and prolongs REM latency.

Oral administration of 10 mg d-amphetamine 20 minutes before bedtime increases waking and decreases total sleep time. Acute AMPH use causes tachycardia, elevated blood pressure, pupillary dilation, agitation, elation, and hypervigilance. Chronic use often produces tolerance that causes these symptoms to subside, although agitation and hypervigilance may remain. Dyskinetic and dystonic reactions to chronic AMPH use also have been reported (Ellinwood EH. Amphetamine psychosis: individuals, settings and sequences. *In Current Concepts on Amphetamine Abuse.* Washington, DC: US Government Printing Office; 1972. National Institute of Mental Health Publication HSM 72-9085:143–157). After about 10 years, AMPH abusers and addicts tend to markedly diminish use, possibly because of central nervous system signs and symptoms such as paranoia, auditory or visual hallucinations, and choreoathetosis. Suggested modes of action of AMPH are (a) partial agonist, mimicking action of norepinephrine at the receptor; (b) inhibition of catecholamine uptake; (c) inhibition of monoamine oxidase; and (d) displacement of norepinephrine, releasing it onto receptors. All temporarily increase norepinephrine at the receptor or have a direct stimulatory action at the receptor and are consistent with the catecholamine hypothesis of depression. Schedule II; pregnancy risk category D.

amphetamine challenge test   Test dose of 10–30 mg dextroamphetamine given to a patient with major depression; if symptomatic relief occurs a noradrenergic antidepressant (desipramine, maprotiline) may be effective (Fawcett J, Kravitz H, Sabelli H. Stimulant challenge test. *In* Hall RCW, Beresford TP [eds], *Handbook of Diagnostic Procedures*, vol 1. New York: Spectrum, 1984, pp 223–251). Amphetamine challenge is also used in separating subtypes of schizophrenia.

amphetamine + clonidine   Combined use may be effective in children with attention deficit disorder refractory to either drug alone (Mandoki MW. Clonidine d-amphetamine combination in the treatment of children with attention deficit hyperactivity disorder. *Neuropsychopharmacology* 1993;9:183S).

amphetamine + fluoxetine   Fluoxetine (FLX), 60 mg/day, plus amphetamine, 45 mg 3 times a day (well in excess of conventional doses), potentiated FLX's antidepressant effects in a patient refractory to FLX alone and combined imipramine/amphetamine. Relapse occurred on four occasions when d-amphetamine was not used (Linet LS. Treatment of refractory depression with a combination of fluoxetine

and d-amphetamine. *Am J Psychiatry* 1989;146: 803–804).

amphetamine + lithium   Lithium may antagonize amphetamine central stimulant effects (Van Kammen DP, Murphy D. Attenuation of the euphoriant and activating effects of d- and l-amphetamine by lithium carbonate treatment. *Psychopharmacologia* 1975;44:215).

amphetamine + monoamine oxidase inhibitor (MAOI)   The psychostimulant dextroamphetamine combined with an MAOI can be safe and effective in depressed patients. However, concurrent use of amphetamine with an MAOI, including furazolidone, procarbazine, and selegiline, may prolong and intensify amphetamine's cardiac stimulant and vasopressor effects and produce symptoms such as headaches, cardiac arrhythmias, vomiting, and sudden and severe hypertensive and hyperpyretic crises. Recreational drug users, especially those who abuse amphetamines, risk hypertensive crises if they abuse these drugs while being treated with an MAOI or within several weeks of discontinuation of MAOI therapy (Devabhaktuni RV, Jampala VC. Using street drugs while on MAOI therapy. *J Clin Psychopharmacol* 1987;7:60–61). See **monoamine oxidase inhibitor + dextroamphetamine**.

amphetamine + morphine   Co-administration is synergistic in producing analgesia and euphoria, but not additive side effects or toxicity. It produces fewer unwanted adverse effects than morphine alone (Jasinski DR, Preston K. Evaluation of mixtures of morphine and d-amphetamine for subjective and physiological effects. *Drug Alcohol Depend* 1986;17:1–13).

amphetamine/pregnancy   Amphetamine use throughout pregnancy has been reported to cause a high perinatal mortality rate, high incidence of obstetric and pregnancy-related complications, increase in congenital malformations, and high rate of neonatal neurologic abnormalities (e.g. disordered sleep patterns, tremors, poor feeding, hyperactive reflexes, abnormal crying, and hyperirritability) (Oro AS, Dixon SD. Perinatal cocaine and methamphetamine exposure. Maternal and neonatal correlates. *J Pediatr* 1987;111:571–578).

amphetamine psychosis   Possibly the most common stimulant-induced psychosis, with onset following long-term use of increasing oral or intravenous doses. It is characterized by gradual evolution of paranoia with delusions of persecution, ideas of reference, feelings of omnipotence associated with hyper-reactivity to environmental stimuli, and loss of insight. It may culminate in a confused, panicky, fugue-like state that can result in violent behavior. There also may be compulsive stereotyped behavior (e.g., disassembling and reassembling gadgets) that may be difficult to stop; if forced to, the person may become irritable and anxious. Recovery from even prolonged amphetamine psychosis is slow, but usually complete. More florid symptoms fade within a few days or weeks, but some confusion, memory loss, and delusions often persist for months. Acute florid symptoms may respond rapidly to oral or intramuscular antipsychotic drug therapy (e.g., haloperidol). Agitation, anxiety, and early symptoms of psychosis can be treated with short-term benzodiazepine therapy.

amphetamine/street names A, accelerator, amp, bean, benny, black beauty (dextroamphetamine), blue angel, bombit (methamphetamine), brownie (dextroamphetamine), candy, cartwheel, Christmas tree (dextroamphetamine), crank (methamphetamine), crossroads, crosstop (with caffeine and ephedrine), crystal (intravenous methamphetamine), dexy (dextroamphetamine), double cross, glass (methamphetamine), greenie (with amobarbital), heart, ice (methamphetamine), jelly bean, meth (methamphetamine), peach, red devil, rose, snow pellet, speed, upper, wakeup, white, white cross.

amphetamine + tranylcypromine Co-administration is generally considered contraindicated because of the risk of a hypertensive crisis or hyperthermia. Some investigators have suggested that combined use could be safe and effective for treatment-resistant depression (Sovner R. Amphetamine and tranylcypromine in treatment-resistant depression. *Biol Psychiatry* 1990;28:1011–1013). A transient response to dextroamphetamine in treatment-resistant depression may predict response to the combination of dextroamphetamine and tranylcypromine. Although some patients have been safely treated with this combination, in view of the potentially fatal adverse reactions that have occurred, it should be reserved for patients with truly drug-resistant depressive disorders.

amphetamine + tricyclic antidepressant Co-administration may produce therapeutic effects, but because of release of norepinephrine may also potentiate cardiovascular effects including arrhythmias, tachycardia, severe hypertension, or hyperpyrexia.

Amplit See **lofepramine**.

amplitude Magnitude of measured activity. Types of measurements include (a) range of oscillations; (b) peak-to-peak (i.e., peak to preceding trough or trough to preceding peak); (c) peak to pre-activity baseline; (d) difference between the range's maximum or minimum value and the mean; and (e) area under the curve.

"Amy" Street name for amyl nitrite.

amygdala One of the components of the basal ganglia located deep within each cerebral hemisphere.

amygdaloidectomy Psychosurgical procedure that ablates the amygdaloid nucleus. It is particularly used in hallucinating patients.

amyl nitrate (Vaposole) Volatile nitrite that is a systemic vasodilator. It is inhaled, relaxing smooth muscles in blood vessels and promptly dilating large coronary vessels. It is indicated for rapid relief of angina pectoris due to coronary artery disease. Amyl nitrate is abused for sexual stimulation, frequently causing headaches. It may interact with alcohol, phenothiazine neuroleptics, beta blockers, or antihypertensives, causing excessive hypotension. Pregnancy risk category C.

amyloid Variety of polypeptide molecules defined by their standing properties and tendency to arrange in a twisted beta-pleated fibrillar structure. It is a proteinaceous material, deposits of which occur in the brains of Alzheimer's disease and older Down syndrome patients, and to a much lesser degree, in association with normal aging. It consists primarily of a highly aggregated 42-amino-acid polypeptide called beta-amyloid, or A4. Its precursor, cloned in 1989, is a larger protein known as the amyloid precursor protein (APP), which has been implicated in Alzheimer's disease. APP fragments have been shown to have both a neurotoxic and a neurotrophic effect.

amyloid beta-protein Amorphous deposits with or without neuritic plaques and neurofibrillary tangles have been demonstrated in the brains of Alzheimer's disease patients, in several non-neuronal tissues (skin and intestines) of Alzheimer's and Down syndrome patients, and in some healthy elderly people (Joachim CL, Mori H, Slekoe DJ. Amyloid beta-protein deposition in tissues other than brain in Alzheimer's disease. *Nature* 1989;341:226–230). Current research is seeking ways to block the enzyme that cleaves amyloid precursor protein (APP, the parent molecule of amyloid beta-protein) into its fragments, the putative receptor that may take up APP into the brain, and ways to thwart damaging effects of amyloid beta-protein on nerve cells.

amyloid precursor protein (APP) Parent molecule of amyloid beta-protein.

amyotrophic lateral sclerosis (ALS) Devastating, adult-onset paralytic disorder caused by degeneration of large motor neurons of the brain and spinal cord. It causes generalized and progressive wasting and weakness of skeletal muscles and usually results in death from respiratory complications within 5 years. No cause, cure, or preventive means have been found. Approximately 5–10% of cases are inherited as an autosomal dominant trait with age-dependent penetrance. Research on nerve growth factors has progressed to the point (1992) that therapeutic trials in ALS are being planned. Autoimmunity has been proposed as a possible cause. A recent study demonstrating lymphocytic infiltrates in about two-thirds of cases lends some credence to an autoimmune relationship (Engelhardt JI, Tafti J, Appel SH. Lymphocytic infiltrates in the spinal cord in amyotrophic lateral sclerosis. *Arch Neurol* 1993;50:30–36). Defects in glutamate metabolism also have been demonstrated (Rothestein JD, Martin LJ, Kuncl RW. Decreased glutamate transport by the brain and spinal cord in amyotrophic lateral sclerosis. *N Engl J Med* 1992;326:1464–1468). Also called "Charcot's disease"; "Lou Gehrig's disease"; "motor neuron disease."

Amytal See **amobarbital**.

Amytal interview Procedure to facilitate patient communication of thoughts and previously repressed memories, affects, and conflicts. The patient is interviewed after being given intravenous doses of amobarbital, which induce a completely relaxed and serene state.

Intravenously administered amobarbital may be superior to saline in relieving catatonic mutism (McCall WV, Shelp FE, McDonald WM. Controlled investigations of amobarbital interview for catatonic mutism. *Am J Psychiatry* 1992;149:202–206). See **narcotherapy**.

anabasine Alkaloid, derived from *Anabasis aphylla*, a plant growing in the Caucasus and Central Asia, that competitively inhibits nicotine. Chewing gum containing 3-mg doses is used to help smoking cessation in Russia. In clinical trials, more than 70% of 1,214 smokers stopped smoking.

anabolic Relating to a constructive metabolic process by which simple substances are converted by living cells into living tissue.

anabolic/androgenic steroid (AAS) Natural or synthetic derivative of testosterone. Most steroids were developed in the 1950s in an attempt to separate the hormone's masculinizing effects (androgenic) and skeletal muscle-building (anabolic) effects. Not to be confused with adrenal corticosteroids, AASs are prescription drugs with legitimate medical uses. They are, however, most frequently used by persons in good health for body-building, skeletal muscle enlargement, and/or increased strength. Such use has been con-

demned by many medical and athletic associations because of known adverse effects and unknown long-term damage to health. AASs are widely used among adolescents; one study estimated that 7% of 12th-grade male students had used them (Buckley WE, Yesalis CE, III, Friedl KE, et al. Estimated prevalence of anabolic steroid use among male high school seniors. *JAMA* 1988;260:3441–3445). Athletes using AASs for muscle strength enhancement are predisposed to mood changes, hepatotoxicity and adverse changes in lipid profiles, cardiac mechanical dysfunction, and death.

Steroids, even in limited quantities, may induce or precipitate changes in behavior that continue past the period of use. Psychiatric sequelae can be manifested in a number of ways. Most users have relatively mild subjective symptoms, but a small subgroup may experience severe psychiatric disturbances, including depressed mood and suicidal ideation. Schedule III.

anabolic steroid/abuse liability Over time, anabolic steroid users may use larger doses, increase the number of different steroids used per cycle, lengthen their cycles of use, shorten the time between cycles, and feel that steroids increase sexual drive, prowess, or pleasure. Despite disturbing side effects, three of four study subjects had no plans to stop steroid use and would not stop even if their peers did. Over a third would not stop even if concerned that steroids were harmful to their health (Kuscerow RP. *Adolescents and steroids: a user perspective*. Washington, DC: Office of Inspector General. Office of Evaluations and Inspections. Department of Health & Human Services, 1990).

anabolic steroid abuse/violence Steroid abuse has been associated with psychosis and organic manic syndromes, irritability, dysphoria, paranoia, violent outbursts, child abuse, spouse battery, and other forms of domestic violence (Schulte HM, Hall MJ, Boyer M. Domestic violence associated with anabolic steroid abuse. *Am J Psychiatry* 1993;150:348).

anabolic steroid/dependence Anabolic androgenic steroid (AAS) use can lead to a full spectrum of dependency symptoms. Manifestations include withdrawal symptoms (84%), withdrawal-related fatigue (43%), depressed mood (41%), restlessness (29%), anorexia (24%), and insomnia (20%). Dependent men use larger doses, have more cycles of use, are more dissatisfied with their body size, and have more aggressive symptoms than nondependent users. Drug dosage and dissatisfaction with body size are highly predictive of dependency. Increased use of alcohol and stimulants such as cocaine and amphetamines is associated with steroid dependence (Brower KJ, Blow FC, Young JP, Hill EM. Symptoms and correlates of anabolic-androgenic steroid dependence. *Br J Addict* 1991;86:759–768).

Anabolic Steroids Act of 1990 Legislation enacted by the U.S. Congress as part of the Omnibus Crime Control Act of 1990. It added 27 anabolic steroid substances to Schedule III of the Controlled Substance Act and established criminal penalties under the Federal Food, Drug and Cosmetic Act for distribution of human growth hormone without a physician's prescription (Interagency Task Force on Anabolic Steroids Report. Washington DC: U.S. Department of Health & Human Services, Public Health Services, 1991).

anabolic steroid/injectable nandrolone decanoate, nandrolone phenpropionate, testosterone cypionate, testosterone enanthate, testosterone propionate.

anabolic steroid/oral ethylestrenol, fluoxymesterone, methandrostenolone, methyltestosterone, norethandrolone, oxandrolone, oxymetholone, stanozolol.

anabolic steroid/street names d-ball, d-bol, deca, depo, maxi, prime, primo, roid.

Anabolin IM See **nandrolone phenpropionate**.

Anabolin LA 100 See **nandrolone decanoate**.

Anadrol-50 See **oxymetholone**.

Anafranil See **clomipramine**.

analeptic Stimulant such as caffeine or amphetamine, particularly agents that reverse depressed central nervous system function.

analysis Separation of the whole into its parts to ascertain their nature, proportion, function, inter-relationship, etc.

analysis of covariance (ANCOVA) Statistical method to determine if two or more related dependent variables exposed to two or more experimental conditions differ significantly from what would be expected by chance, while controlling the intercorrelation of the various variables. ANCOVA is always inappropriate when treatment groups differ significantly at baseline.

analysis of residuals In regression, an analysis of the differences between Y and Y to evaluate assumptions.

analysis of secular trends Study of the relationship and adjustment of human groups to the environment. These studies evaluate correlations or trends based on information derived from groups. They are most useful in raising hypotheses, but lack data on individuals and cannot identify a factor as a true cause, since other factors may account for the association. Inappropriate conclusions about associations identified from ecological data are often referred to as the ecological fallacy (Grisso JA. Making comparisons. *Lancet* 1993;342:157–160). Trends can be examined over time or across geographic boundaries. Analyses of secular trends rapidly provide evidence for or against a hypothesis. Also called "ecologic study."

analysis of variance (ANOVA) Statistical test to compare means from two or more groups. It is used with continuous data measured over multiple time-points across study subjects. The independent variable, controlled by the experimenter, is studied in relation to an outcome or dependent variable, the phenomenon of interest. Differences are commonly assigned to three aspects: individual differences among subjects or patients studied; group differences, however classified (e.g., by sex); and differences according to the various treatments. ANOVA can assess both the main effects of a variable and its interaction with other variables studied simultaneously. Also known as the ANOVA-F test, because the calculated statistic is called the F ratio. Variants of basic ANOVA include one-way ANOVA, multifactor ANOVA, analysis of covariance (ANCOVA), multivariate ANOVA (MANOVA), and ANOVA with repeated measures.

analysis of variance-covariance (AVACOV) Statistical method (modification of MANOVA) to perform analyses of variance on models consisting of four factors each with 10 levels. It can analyze repeated measures on one factor only.

analytic study Research design classified in two major ways: by how subjects are selected into the study and by how data are collected for the study. Analytic studies include case control and cohort studies and randomized clinical trials.

analytical toxicology Detection and identification of minute amounts of drugs or alcohol in body fluids. It has expanded tremendously in the last few decades. Qualified drug testing laboratories, providing objective qualitative and quantitative urinalysis results, are easily accessible to physicians. Laboratory accreditation must be checked by the physician, however, because low-quality laboratories still exist.

Anaprox See **naproxen**.

anarthria Complete inability to speak due to neural or muscular bulbar dysfunction.

Anavar See **oxandrolone**.

Anaxyl See **alpidem**.

anchor sleep In somnology, a minimum of at least 4 hours sleep at the same time everyday during a shift rotation.

Andro 100 See **testosterone aqueous**.

Andro Cyp See **testosterone cypionate**.

Andro LA 200 See **testosterone enanthate**.

Androcur   See **cyproterone.**

androgen   Sex hormone present in both sexes, but in greater quantity in males, that influences structural and behavioral characteristics associated with maleness. Androgen administration, as in use of anabolic steroids for muscle building, may inhibit gonadotropin secretion. It can also cause atrophy of interstitial tissue and the tubules of the normal testes, leading to a decline in spermatogenesis and suppression of endogenous testosterone.

androgenic   Causing or contributing to maleness. See **androgen.**

Android   See **methyltestosterone.**

Android F   See **fluoxymesterone.**

Androl - 50   See **oxymetholone.**

Androlone   See **nandrolone phenpropionate.**

Androlone D 100   See **nandrolone decanoate.**

Andronaq 50   See **testosterone aqueous.**

Andronaq-LA   See **testosterone cypionate.**

Andronate   See **testosterone cypionate.**

Andropository 100   See **testosterone enanthate.**

anecdotal observation   Quality of results from isolated observations not yet verified by statistical analysis of a larger body of data. The observation may be a coincidence; causation or statistical association cannot be implied.

Anectine   See **succinylcholine.**

anemia, aplastic   See **aplastic anemia.**

anesthetic + lithium   See **lithium + general anesthesia.**

aneuploidy   Abnormal number of chromosomes that are not an exact multiple of the haploid number. Examples are D trisomy, E trisomy, Down syndrome, and XXX, XXY, and XXYY syndromes.

Anexate   See **flumazenil.**

"angel dust"   Street name for phencyclidine (PCP).

"angel hair"   Street name for phencyclidine (PCP).

"angel mist"   Street name for phencyclidine (PCP).

anger   Strong feeling elicited by real or supposed injury that is often accompanied by desire to take vengeance.

anger attack   Sudden spell of anger inappropriate to the situation, having physical features resembling panic attacks, but lacking the affects of fear and anxiety. Anger attacks are experienced as uncharacteristic and occur frequently among depressed patients. Criteria include occurrences of the following over the previous 6 months: (a) irritability; (b) overreaction with anger to minor annoyances; (c) episodes in which the person inappropriately becomes angry and enraged with other people; (d) at least four of the following experienced during at least one of the anger attacks: (1) accelerated heart rate, heart pounding, or palpitations; (2) hot flashes or face reddening; (3) tightness of the chest, chest pain, or pressure; (4) numbness or tingling sensations of arms and legs; (5) lightheadedness, dizziness, or feelings of unsteadiness; (6) shortness of breath or difficulty breathing; (7) sweating; (8) shaking or trembling; (9) intense fear, panicky feelings, or anxiety; (10) feeling out of control or about to explode; (11) feeling like physically attacking or yelling at people; (12) physically or verbally attacking people; (13) throwing around or destroying objects; and (e) one or more anger attacks over the previous month. Fluoxetine (20 mg/day) may be an effective treatment (Fava M, Rosenbaum JF, McCarthy M, Pava J, Steingard R, Bless E. Anger attacks in depressed outpatients and their response to fluoxetine. *Psychopharmacol Bull* 1991;27:275–279).

angiotensin-converting enzyme inhibitor   (ACE inhibitor) **See captopril; enalapril; isinopril.**

anhedonia   Inability to derive pleasure from situations and stimuli that usually induce pleasure (Klein DF. Endogenomorphic depression. *Arch Gen Psychiatry* 1974;31:447–454). It profoundly affects quality of life in a wide range of human experiences and psychiatric disorders. It directly affects human motivation, reinforces lack of drive, tends to aggravate mood lowering, erodes hopefulness, and in certain psychiatric disorders affects choices toward life or death. Anhedonia is a pathognomonic feature of major depressive disorder and some severe personality disorders and postpsychotic states. It also can be induced by many psychopharmacological agents, especially neuroleptics. Anhedonia that often follows recovery from the florid phase of acute schizophrenia may respond to antidepressant drugs.

anhidrosis   Reduction in, or absence of, perspiration. It may be caused by antiparkinson drugs, atropine, and atropine-like compounds.

"animal"   Street name for lysergic acid diethylamide (LSD).

aniracetam   Nosotropic drug tested in Alzheimer's disease (Sourander LB, Portin R, Molsa P, et al. Senile dementia of the Alzheimer type treated with aniracetam: a new nootropic agent. *Psychopharmacology* 1987;91:90–95).

annual incidence   Number of new cases of a disorder occurring in the population per year.

anomia   Difficulty finding words. It is the most frequent language complaint of patients with temporal lobe epilepsy, who describe frustration in being unable to articulate a word for which they are looking, often settling for a poor semantic substitute. Frequent pauses and stereotypic utterances ("umm," "you know") tend to fill gaps in spontaneous speech. Often exacerbated by stress or performance anxiety, anomia can be tested by the Boston Naming Test and the Controlled Word Association Task.

anorectic   Drug that reduces appetite and is used for weight reduction. The majority are central nervous system stimulants. In descending order of approximate potency they are dexamphetamine, phentermine, chlorphentermine, mazindol, diethylpropion, and fenfluramine.

Anorex   See **phenmetrazine.**

anorexia nervosa   (AN) Heterogeneous, multifactorial eating disorder that occurs most commonly in prepubertal, adolescent, and young women. Distortion of body image is considered central to the diagnosis by most experts, hence the German name *magersuchuerheit*, the persistent pursuit of thinness. AN also is characterized by morbid fear of fat, refusal to maintain normal body weight, and obsession with dieting to the point of inducing profound weight loss, leading to body weight at least 15% below expected. Most weight loss is accomplished in secret. Patients often limit food intake to vegetables and fruit and avoid meats, milk products, and most calorie-rich foods. Although attributed to carbohydrate phobia, food avoidance isnow believed to be due to fat aversion (Drewnowski A. Taste responsiveness in eating disorders. *In* Schneider LH, Cooper SJ, Halmi KA [eds], The psychobiology of human eating disorders. *Ann N Y Acad Sci* 1989;575:399–409). AN patients suffer from hypotension, hypothermia, and abnormal electrocardiograms, all of which occur with starvation. Cardiovascular complications are the most common and most likely to result in fatalities, particularly in patients who vomit, purge, or abuse diuretics, because of induced electrolyte abnormalities (Sharp CW, Freeman CPL. The medical complications of anorexia nervosa. *Br J Psychiatry* 1993;162:452–462). Osteoporosis is an early and perhaps irreversible consequence of severe weight loss. Amenorrhea is common in menstruating women. Like patients with depression, AN patients have high cerebrospinal fluid concentrations of corticotropin-releasing hormone (CRH). Excessive endogenous secretion of CRH may play an important role in pathogenesis. AN has been divided into two distinct entities—bulimic type and restrictive type—depending on the presence of classic bulimic symptoms of cycles of bingeing and purging (Kennedy S, Garfinkle P. Advances in diagnosis and treatment of anorexia nervosa

and bulimia nervosa. *Can J Psychiatry* 1992;37: 309–315). There are apparently enough differences between the types in both diagnosis and management to warrant separate classifications, although long-term outcomes do not appear to be markedly different. See **bulimia nervosa; eating disorder/pregnancy.**

anorexiant   Substance that reduces appetite or induces aversion to food. See **anorectic.**

anorgasmia   Failure to achieve orgasm. Etiology is usually psychological or interpersonal, but it may be iatrogenic, due to antipsychotics, benzodiazepines, and antidepressants (heterocyclics, monoamine oxidase inhibitors [MAOIs], and serotonin uptake inhibitors). The only antidepressant that apparently does not cause anorgasmia is bupropion. Antipsychotics appear to interfere with orgasm through alpha-adrenergic blockade. Cyproheptadine may counteract anorgasmia due to tricyclic antidepressants, MAOIs, and fluoxetine.

anosmia   Loss of the sense of smell. Significantly impaired smell perception may occur in Parkinson's disease (Hawkes CH, Shephard BC. Selective anosmia in Parkinson's disease? *Lancet* 1993;341:435–436). Olfactory nerve damage also may impair the sense of taste; patients with anosmia complain of an inability to taste food unless it is highly seasoned.

anosognosia   Denial of hemiplegia by patients with a nondominant parietal syndrome, who insist nothing is wrong with the affected musculature and offer multiple excuses for impaired or absent limb function. Anosognosia is due to organic brain dysfunction and not to a psychological defense mechanism.

Anquil   See **benperidol.**

Ansaid   See **flurbiprofen.**

Antabuse   See **disulfiram.**

antacid + acetophenazine   See **acetophenazine + antacid.**

antacid + neuroleptic   See **neuroleptic + antacid.**

antacid + prazepam   See **prazepam + antacid.**

antagonism   Interference of one chemical or drug with the action of another.

antagonism, chemical   Reaction between two drugs that neutralizes their effects.

antagonism, functional   Production by two drugs of opposite effects on the same physiological function.

antagonism, receptor   Interaction with a receptor to inhibit or block the action of an agonist at the same site.

antagonist   Compound that binds to a receptor, but does not activate it; opposite of agonist. Antagonists reduce or block the action of neurotransmitters or other substances acting as agonists, thereby preventing the agonist from eliciting a physiological response. Antagonists are often desirable as antidotes. Also called "receptor blocker."

antecedent In behavior modification, event that precedes behavior causing concern. Most important types are setting events and discriminative stimuli. A setting event is a relatively stable feature of the environment that affects a substantial number of subsequent events. Discriminative stimuli are more transient events such as instructions or cues. Antecedents set the occasion for most behaviors but do not produce them automatically, with the exception of reflex involuntary responses known as respondents. Voluntary responses are known as operants. Behavior may be modified by changing the antecedents.

anterior pituitary See **pituitary, anterior**.

anterocollis See **dystonia, cervical**.

anterograde amnesia See **amnesia, anterograde**.

antiaggressive agent Drug that can be used to treat some patients with aggressive and self-injurious behavior. A number of new antiaggressive agents (e.g., eltropazine) are serotonin (5-HT)1_A and 5-HT1_B antagonists. Also called "serenic."

antiandrogen Agent (e.g., estrogens, progesterone, benperidol, cyproterone acetate) that blocks the action of testosterone and affects central sexual behavior mechanisms. Cyproterone acetate is used in the treatment of hypersexuality, pedophilia, and other sexual delinquencies in men. In daily doses of 100–200 mg, sexual desire virtually disappears within 2 weeks. Libido returns to its former state within 2 weeks of withdrawing the drug. See **cyproterone**.

antiandrogenous Relating to the lessening of androgen (the male sex hormone) production.

antianxiety drug See **anxiolytic**.

antiarrhythmic + maprotiline See **maprotiline + antiarrhythmic**.

antiarrhythmic + pimozide See **pimozide + antiarrhythmic**.

antibipolar therapy Treatment characterized by its ability to prevent or treat both mania and depression, such as lithium, carbamazepine, valproate, and electroconvulsive therapy. They differ from antidepressant drugs, which are effective *only* in the acute treatment and prevention of depression and can precipitate hypomanic or manic "switches" or "rapid cycling" between mania and depression.

antibody Complex protein molecule in the blood created by the immune response to the presence of an antigen. Each antibody fits a specific antigen and leads to its destruction.

anticholinergic drug Agent that antagonizes the action of acetylcholine at muscarinic receptor sites, commonly used for treatment of parkinsonism and neuroleptic-induced extrapyramidal side effects. Anticholinergics are sometimes administered from the onset of antipsychotic therapy with the aim of preventing extrapyramidal reactions. They also may have mildly antidepressant effects. Acute discontinuation can cause withdrawal symptoms—nausea, restlessness, diaphoresis, diarrhea, abdominal pain, dizziness, and insomnia, as well as marked dysphoria. Overdose can produce delirium and is a frequent cause of confusional episodes in younger patients. Anticholinergics may have stimulant and euphoriant properties and may be misused and/or abused. Also called "antimuscarinic."

anticholinergic/antiparkinson drug Classified into three groups: (a) antihistamines, including orphenadrine, promethazine, and diphenhydramine; (b) piperidines, which are the most potent and include benzhexol or trihexyphenidyl, procyclidine, and biperiden; and (c) tropines, the prototype of which is benztropine. Amantadine is not usually classified with anticholinergic drugs, even though one of its several possible modes of action is as an anticholinergic agent.

anticholinergic/antiparkinson drug abuse Since the late 1970s, abuse has increased steadily, especially of trihexyphenidyl. Abusers include schizophrenics, antisocial personality and borderline personality disorder patients, alcoholics, and multiple substance abusers. Many had the drug prescribed for treatment of neuroleptic-induced extrapyramidal reactions. Their histories include poor social relationships; prolonged periods of unemployment; and abuse of several drugs including alcohol, marijuana, hallucinogens, opiates, amphetamines, cocaine, benzodiazepines, neuroleptics, cough mixtures, and solvents. Those who abuse other drugs by injecting them usually take anticholinergics orally. Frequency of abuse ranges from daily ingestion to every 2 or 3 weeks, depending on availability. Dosages vary (e.g., 15–60 mg trihexyphenidyl per "trip"). Most patients cite a "buzz," "kick," or "high" as the reason for abuse. Schizophrenics report abusing the anticholinergics to counteract affective blunting. Effects of the abuse include a toxic-confusional state with visual hallucinations, distorted time sense, dehydration, tachycardia, pronounced thirst, and blurred vision. Some abusers report difficulties in recent memory, new learning, attention, and concentration that may persist for weeks after the acute intoxication clears (Ayd FJ Jr. Abuse of anticholinergic drugs: an under-recognized problem. *Int Drug Ther Newsl* 1985;20:1–2; Dilsaver SC. Antimuscarinic agents as substances of abuse: a review. *J Clin Psychopharmacol* 1988;8:14–22).

anticholinergic + antipsychotic   Anticholinergics are frequently prescribed, sometimes prophylactically, to counteract antipsychotic-induced extrapyramidal effects. Several double-blind studies, however, have shown that in some antipsychotic-treated patients, adjunctive anticholinergics may worsen symptoms, particularly thought disorganization, uncooperativeness, bizarre and unusual thoughts, suspiciousness and paranoid ideation, delusions, disorientation, and sleeplessness. Co-administration may (a) decrease absorption of the antipsychotic, interfering with its therapeutic effects; and (b) produce additive anticholinergic effects that may lead to anticholinergic toxicity.

anticholinergic + benzodiazepine   Co-administration may induce more severe cognitive impairment than either drug alone. Because many antidepressants, antipsychotics, and antiparkinson agents possess anticholinergic properties, interactions of this type may be common, particularly among the elderly.

anticholinergic + clomipramine   Co-administration increases risk of adverse anticholinergic effects. To avoid toxicity, careful dosage adjustment of clomipramine and/or the anticholinergic may be necessary.

anticholinergic + clozapine   Co-administration can cause moderate to severe anticholinergic toxicity.

anticholinergic delirium   See **delirium, anticholinergic**.

anticholinergic + diphenhydramine   Co-administration may cause severe anticholinergic symptoms or intoxication.

anticholinergic effect   Result of drug blockade of cholinergic nerves. Blurred vision, dry mouth, sweating, constipation, delayed micturition, and exacerbation of "narrow angle" glaucoma are common anticholinergic symptoms caused by some neuroleptics, tricyclic antidepressants, and antiparkinson agents. Sexual dysfunctions also may occur. More severe anticholinergic toxicity is manifested by seizures, hyperthermia, delirium, central nervous system depression, and coma.

anticholinergic + hydromorphone   Co-administration may produce additive peripheral and central anticholinergic toxic effects. See **anticholinergic toxicity**.

anticholinergic + hydroxyzine   Co-administration may produce severe anticholinergic symptoms or intoxication.

anticholinergic intoxication   Drugs with anticholinergic effects, both central and peripheral, produce dose-related blockage of acetylcholine receptors in the brain. Even in therapeutic doses, these drugs have subtle, unwanted anticholinergic effects. Increasing doses, or co-administration of usual therapeutic doses of several different anticholinergic medications, can be toxic and cause brain dysfunction. Impaired acquisition of new learning is the earliest detectable toxic central nervous system effect. Dosage increases and/or cumulative effects of several different anticholinergic medications cause more obvious impairments in attention and cognitive function. Continued administration of the same doses results in the progressive evolution of signs and symptoms of peripheral and central anticholinergic toxicity, including (a) diminished salivation and dry mouth; (b) diminished sweating; (c) hot, dry skin; (d) dilated pupils and impaired accommodation; (e) photophobia and changes in visual acuity; (f) difficulty in initiating urination and bladder distention; (g) tachycardia; (h) constipation and decreased bowel sounds; (i) confusion and impaired memory and learning; and (j) delirium, stupor, and coma. In most cases, anticholinergic toxicity is best treated by discontinuing the causative agents and waiting for the toxic effects to wane gradually over hours or days. Severe anticholinergic intoxication can be treated with a test dose of 1 mg physostigmine subcutaneously to confirm the diagnosis. If the test dose increases salivary flow, sweating, and intestinal hyperactivity, the diagnosis of anticholinergic toxicity is confirmed. Since physostigmine is metabolized more quickly than most anticholinergic drugs, treatment should consist of repeated doses (1–2 mg) given intravenously every 15–30 minutes, until clinical improvement or signs of cholinergic toxicity appear (e.g., bradycardia, hypersalivation, emesis, or defecation). Physostigmine should not be used without awareness of its contraindications and proper use.

anticholinergic + meperidine   Co-administration increases antimuscarinic effects, including the risk of paralytic ileus, and other manifestations of anticholinergic toxicity.

anticholinergic + neuroleptic   See **anticholinergic + antipsychotic**.

anticholinergic + orphenadrine   Co-administration may increase anticholinergic effects and risk of anticholinergic toxicity.

anticholinergic/tardive dyskinesia   Anticholinergic drug efficacy in the treatment of tardive dyskinesia (TD) is limited, and the drugs may in fact worsen TD. Withdrawal of anticholinergic drugs has been reported to improve TD in some patients. These drugs should be prescribed only for cases of tardive dystonia, in which relatively high doses are efficacious (*Tardive Dyskinesia. A Task Force Report of the American Psychiatric Association.* Washington, DC: American Psychiatric Association, 1992, pp 103–120).

anticholinergic toxicity　Syndrome associated with antihistamines, antiparkinson drugs, atropine, scopolamine, amantadine, antipsychotics, antidepressants, antispasmodics, mydriatic agents, skeletal-muscle relaxants, and many plants (notably jimson weed and *Amanita muscaria*). It is manifested by delirium with mumbling speech, tachycardia, dry flushed skin, dilated pupils, myoclonus, elevated temperature, urinary retention, and decreased bowel sounds. Seizures and dysrhythmias may occur in severe cases.

anticholinergic withdrawal　Syndrome that may occur following rapid discontinuation of anticholinergic drugs. Manifestations include bradykinesia, motor retardation, slowed thinking and speech production, lassitude, sleep disruption, nightmares, emotional withdrawal, irritability, dysphoria, nausea, vomiting, and diarrhea. The cause is believed to be central and peripheral cholinergic hyperfunction secondary to regulatory changes in muscarinic receptors due to sudden removal of sustained anticholinergic blockade.

anticipation　In genetics, increase in severity and progressively earlier age of onset of a genetic disease in successive generations. It is attributed to a type of genetic mutation wherein genes are unstable and expand or grow larger in subsequent generations, resulting in increasingly severe forms of the disease. The phenomenon occurs in dystrophia myotonica, the most common form of muscular dystrophy, and the fragile-X syndrome. A century ago, Vincent van Gogh wrote about what geneticists now label anticipation: "The root of the evil lies in the constitution itself, in the fatal weakening of families from generation to generation . . . the root of the evil certainly lies there, and there is no cure for it" (van gogh-Bonger [ed], *The Complete Letters of Vincent van Gogh* (vol 3, letter 521, August 1888). Boston: Little Brown, p 8).

anticoagulant + fluvoxamine　See **fluvoxamine + anticoagulant.**

anticonvulsant　Drug that prevents or controls seizures. Some also have antimanic and possibly antidepressant effects (e.g., carbamazepine, sodium valproate, clonazepam) and may be useful in controlling rage reactions and aggressive and combative behavior in the elderly and brain damaged (e.g., carbam-

azepine). Anticonvulsants are rarely stopped suddenly because of increased seizure risk.

anticonvulsant + electroconvulsive therapy (ECT)　An anticonvulsant should probably be discontinued, if possible, before starting ECT, because it can markedly increase the amount of current necessary to produce a seizure (Roberts MA, Attah JR. Carbamazepine + ECT. *Br J Psychiatry* 1988;153:418).

anticonvulsant + neuroleptic　Anticonvulsants that induce hepatic drug metabolizing enzymes may reduce neuroleptic blood levels and neuroleptic therapeutic efficacy.

anticonvulsant/pregnancy　Anticonvulsants, particularly phenytoin, valproic acid, and carbamazepine, as well as their combination, present a teratogenic risk to the fetus. The teratogenicity of phenytoin and probably of other anticonvulsants is mediated not by the parent compound but by toxic intermediary metabolites (e.g., epoxides) produced as a result of the biotransformation of the parent. See **fetal hydantoin syndrome.**

antidementia drug　See **nootropic drug.**

antidepressant　Drug that has been shown, in comparison with a placebo, to improve symptoms characteristic of the illness depression in at least a subgroup of patients with a depressive disorder of at least moderate severity. A drug effective only against nonspecific symptoms (e.g., insomnia) is not an antidepressant. There is no agreement on whether a drug that is superior to a placebo but inferior to a standard antidepressant, such as a tricyclic, should be called an antidepressant. Antidepressant drugs are now divided into the monoamine oxidase inhibitors (MAOIs) and the non-MAOIs, or cyclic antidepressants. The latter are subdivided into first-, second-, and third-generation antidepressants. The first generation includes original tricyclic antidepressants. The second generation comprises unrelated compounds, including trazodone, maprotiline, lofepramine, viloxazine, and mianserin. Many of the third-generation drugs are relatively selective inhibitors of serotonin uptake such as fluoxetine, fluvoxamine, sertraline, citalopram, and paroxetine; other third-generation antidepressants have more novel actions. Antidepressants are used in a wide variety of conditions besides depression, including obsessive-compulsive and other anxiety disorders, headache, chronic pain syndrome, enuresis, attention deficit disorders, bulimia, obesity, and cocaine withdrawal. They are also used to treat secondary depression in patients with psychotic illnesses, in mentally retarded patients with behavior disorders, and in mixed organic-affective disorders in the elderly.

antidepressant/anticholinergic potency All tricyclic antidepressants have significant anticholinergic effects. In descending order of potency, the tricyclic antidepressant amitriptyline is first, followed by protriptyline, doxepin, imipramine, nortriptyline, desipramine, maprotiline, and amoxapine. Trazodone and phenelzine are the least anticholinergic (Richelson E. Pharmacology of antidepressants in use in the United States. *J Clin Psychiatry* 1982;43:4–11).

antidepressant + beta-blocker Antidepressants have been shown to be safe and effective when used in combination with beta-blockers. Because beta-blockers significantly increase blood levels of certain psychotropic drugs, antidepressant serum levels should be monitored when used in combination with beta-blockers (Yudofsky SC. Beta-blockers and depression. The clinicians dilemma. *JAMA* 1992; 267:1826–1827).

antidepressant/breast milk Heterocyclic antidepressants have not been thoroughly studied during lactation. Maternal doses of amitriptyline (up to 150 mg/day), desipramine (300 mg/day), imipramine (200 mg/day), or nortriptyline (125 mg/day) have not caused observable effects in the few nursing infants studied. The tertiary amines produce late peaks of the corresponding secondary amine metabolite in breast milk. No agreement exists on the advisability of therapy with heterocyclics during lactation. Some recommend not using heterocyclics because of potential, but undemonstrated, long-term effects on the infants neurological development, although the American Academy of Pediatrics Committee on Drugs considers them acceptable during breast feeding. Infant exposure to tricyclic antidepressants can be minimized by using a secondary amine (i.e., nortriptyline or desipramine) and by giving the drug as a single dose at bedtime and skipping late-night feedings if possible. The infant should be monitored (Anderson PO. Drug use during breastfeeding. *Clin Pharm* 1991;10:594–624).

antidepressant, cyclic (CyAD) Antidepressant drug characterized by a cyclic chemical structure. CyADs include unicyclic compounds (bupropion), bicyclics (fluoxetine), tricyclics (amitriptyline, amoxapine, desipramine, dothiepin, doxepin, imipramine, maprotiline, nortriptyline, protriptyline), and tetracyclics (mianserin). See **antidepressant, heterocyclic**.

antidepressant, cyclic + moclobemide Co-administration seems to be safe if the drugs are gradually initiated together. A direct change can be made from moclobemide to a tricyclic antidepressant or second-generation antidepressant (e.g. maprotiline, mianserin) without an intervening wash-out period (Amrein R, Guntent TW, Dingemanse J, et al. Interactions of moclobemide with concomitantly administered medication: evidence from pharmacological and clinical studies. *Psychopharmacology* 1992;106[suppl]:S24–S31). See **moclobemide + tricyclic antidepressant**.

antidepressant, cyclic + procainamide Co-administration may produce hazardously prolonged cardiac conduction disturbances.

antidepressant, heterocyclic (HCA) Term coined by Baldessarini (1968) and recently adopted for all non–monoamine oxidase inhibitor (non-MAOI) antidepressants, ranging from the tricyclics to many newly introduced (second-generation) antidepressants that have either fewer or more rings. Most HCAs are about 80% protein bound, and only the unbound drug can enter the brain. Another definition is any non-MAOI antidepressant that has a noncarbon atom in any ring. This would make clomipramine an HCA, but not imipramine.

antidepressant/long-term side effects Long-term therapy with conventional tricyclics, monoamine oxidase inhibitors (MAOIs), and lithium is tolerated by the majority of patients. However, their side effects prompt some doctors to prescribe low maintenance doses, thereby risking undertreatment and/or relapse. Patients also may reduce dosages or simply stop taking the drug. Heterocyclic effects patients dislike include weight gain, chronic xerostomia contributing to dental caries, constipation or obstipation, and sexual dysfunction. Long-term MAOI therapy can cause distressing weight gain, edema, insomnia, and sexual dysfunction. Long-term lithium therapy can be complicated by weight gain, acne, diarrhea, polyuria, tremor, hypothyroidism, and, rarely, possible renal interstitial fibrosis. Little is known about long-term side effects of newer antidepressants such as maprotiline, trazodone, bupropion, serotonin uptake inhibitors, and selective reversible MAOIs (RIMAs).

antidepressant/Parkinson's disease Tricyclic antidepressants alleviate depression and some parkinson symptoms in depressed parkinson patients. However, their anticholinergic effects coupled with those of an antiparkinson drug often produce a peripheral and central anticholinergic syndrome, especially in the elderly, who are particularly prone to develop a toxic confusional state. Nevertheless, with judicious low-dose tricyclic therapy (50–75 mg daily; occasionally up to 150 mg daily), depression in Parkinson's disease patients can be effectively and safely treated. Newer antidepressants with fewer anticholinergic and cardiovascular effects also are effective and suitable for treating depressed Parkinson's disease patients, the majority of whom are elderly.

antidepressant preclinical screening tests   In addition to existing preclinical animal toxicology studies, efforts are being made to develop reliable tests in animals that may indicate whether a compound has antidepressant effects in humans. Current tests include (a) the Porsolt test; (b) antagonism of hyperactivity in olfactory-bulbectomized rats; and (c) antagonism of reserpine-induced hypothermia. Tricyclic antidepressants and serotonin uptake inhibitors antagonize behavioral despair in the Porsolt test. They also antagonize hyperactivity in olfactory-bulbectomized rats. The reserpine test detects antidepressant activity of drugs that mainly affect norepinephrine. Not surprisingly, serotonin uptake inhibitors do not antagonize reserpine-induced hypothermia.

antidepressant rating scales   Hamilton Depression Scale (HAM-D); Clinical Global Impressions (CGI); Depression Status Inventory (DSI); and Self Rating Depression Scale (SDS).

antidepressant/seizures   Seizures secondary to antidepressants given at therapeutic doses have been reported; most involve patients with a history of chronic epilepsy, acquired brain disorder, or recent electroconvulsive therapy. Seizures have characteristically occurred shortly after the drug was started or its dose was increased. At therapeutic doses, seizures do not seem to occur with monoamine oxidase inhibitors (MAOIs). By contrast, non-MAOI antidepressants lower seizure threshold. Risk, however, depends on (a) predisposing factors (personal or family history of seizures, organic brain disease, substance abuse or withdrawal); (b) amount and rate of dosage titration; and (c) the relative epileptogenic potential of the antidepressant. Seizures can occur at any time, but generally occur early in treatment. They are most common with sudden dosage changes or abrupt withdrawal of the antidepressant. Actual frequency is unknown for most antidepressants, but has been reported to be 1/1,000 patients (0.1%). In 1979, the British Committee on Safety of Medicines reported that the tricyclic antidepressants with epileptic potential, in increasing order, are desipramine, nortriptyline, trimipramine, imipramine, clomipramine, and amitriptyline (Edwards JG. Antidepressants and convulsions. *Lancet* 1979;2:1368–1369). Antidepressants can be used with relative safety in epileptic patients as long as initial dosages are low and titrated slowly. Available

evidence suggests that maprotiline, amoxapine, clomipramine, and bupropion should be avoided, and that trazodone and fluoxetine may be somewhat safer than tricyclic antidepressants (Skowron DM, Stemmel GL. Antidepressants and the risk of seizures. *Pharmacotherapy* 1992;12:18–22; Jick SS, Jick H, Knauss TA, Dean AD. Antidepressants and convulsions. *J Clin Psychopharmacol* 1992;12:241–245).

antidepressant/sexual dysfunction   Sexual side effects reported with antidepressants include decreased libido, impotency, anorgasmia, and delayed and retrograde ejaculation. Trazodone may cause priapism and serotonin uptake inhibitors seem more likely than other antidepressants to cause anorgasmia.

antidepressant therapy   There are five classes of antidepressant treatment: electroconvulsive therapy, monoamine oxidase inhibitors (MAOIs), non-MAOI antidepressants (heterocyclics and serotonin uptake inhibitors), dynamic psychotherapy, and cognitive therapy.

antidepressant (tricyclic) + electroconvulsive therapy   See **tricyclic antidepressant + electroconvulsive therapy.**

antidepressant (tricyclic)/withdrawal   See **tricyclic antidepressant/withdrawal.**

antidepressin   Putative hypothalamic peptide that relieves both neuroendocrine and behavior abnormalities of depression. It is hypothesized that repeated electroconvulsive therapy–induced seizures enhance production and release of antidepressin.

antidepressogenic   Drug that counteracts or blocks the capacity of a medicine to induce depression.

antidiabetic + moclobemide   See **moclobemide + antidiabetic.**

antidipsogenic   Capacity of a drug to attenuate water intake. Animal studies have shown that the opiate antagonist naloxone may exert a primary antidipsogenic effect.

antidipsotropic   Drug that produces either an adverse physical reaction when alcohol is consumed or antagonizes (reduces) the "high." Disulfiram, metronidazole, and citrated calcium carbamide fall into the first category, whereas naltrexone, which is also a serotonin uptake inhibitor, is in the second. Antidipsotropics are considered auxiliary treatments for alcoholism to be used in conjunction with psychosocial treatments. Much of their effectiveness is due to the patient's desire to avoid the violent physical reaction. Disulfiram acts more as an aid against impulsive drinking and calcium carbamide more as a preparation for countering risky circumstances.

antidiuretic hormone   (ADH) Vasopressin, an octapeptide hormone secreted by the supraoptic and paraventricular nuclei of the hypothalamus. ADH regulates water balance by stimulating resorption in the distal renal tubule.

antidyskinetic effect   Capacity of a drug to suppress and alleviate dyskinetic movements. Haloperidol has significantly greater antidyskinetic effects than thioridazine and clozapine.

antiestrogen   Group of drugs represented by tamoxifen, hydroxytamoxifen, and nafoxidine. They have mixed agonist and antagonist actions that differ from one tissue to another. They also differ in dose-response curves and pharmacokinetics. They may cross the blood-brain barrier and act on estrogen receptors in the central nervous system. By themselves, antiestrogens may not cause significant mood or behavior changes, but they could have a modulatory effect on some dopaminergic, serotonergic, and noradrenergic mechanisms.

antigen   Substance that can elicit antibody formation by immune-component cells and react specifically with the antibody so produced.

antiglutamatergic drug   Noncompetitive N-methyl-D-aspartate (NMDA) receptor antagonist (amantadine and memantine). They are used for the treatment of Parkinson's disease.

antihistamine   Drug that antagonizes the action of histamine, sometimes used as a sedative/hypnotic for the psychiatrically ill. Antihistamines often have anticholinergic effects and should be prescribed cautiously for the elderly and patients with prostatic hypertrophy, bladder neck obstruction, and narrow-angle glaucoma.

antihistamine/breast milk   Small amounts may be excreted in breast milk and cause central nervous system depression in nursing infants. Antihistamines also may inhibit lactation.

antihistamine + central nervous system depressant   Co-administration may cause drowsiness and impaired attention, resulting in accidents and/or falls.

antihormones   Estrogen and progesterone antagonists that may be important for the study of these hormones involvement in modulating mood and behavior.

antihypertensive   Drug that decreases blood pressure.

antihypertensive + bromocriptine   See **bromocriptine + antihypertensive**.

antihypertensive + clozapine   See **clozapine + antihypertensive**.

antihypertensive + levodopa   See **levodopa + antihypertensive**.

antihypertensive + maprotiline   See **maprotiline + antihypertensive**.

antihypertensive + moclobemide   See **moclobemide + antihypertensive**.

antihypoxydotic   Substance that protects against impairment of cerebral biological oxidation due to hypoxic, nutritive, histotoxic, ischemic, or metabolic causes. Some antihypoxydotics have been shown to selectively improve the noopsyche (intellectual and memory functions) and thus are called nootropics. See **nootropic drug**.

Antilirium   See **physostigmine**.

antimanic   Drug used to treat or prevent symptoms of mania. Lithium is the best known and most commonly prescribed antimanic drug. Others include anticonvulsants such as carbamazepine, valproic acid, clonazepam, and certain neuroleptics.

antimuscarinic   See **anticholinergic drug**.

antinociceptive   Substance capable of reducing or abolishing a painful stimulus (e.g., an analgesic).

antiobsessional drug   Antidepressant, often classified as serotonergic, that reduces obsessional symptoms in obsessive-compulsive patients.

antioxidant   Agent that inhibits oxidation, thereby preventing rancidity of oils or fats or deterioration of other materials through oxidative processes.

antioxidant/tardive dyskinesia   See **vitamin E**.

antipanic drug   Drug that blocks or reduces the frequency of panic attacks. Antipanic drugs include benzodiazepines, tricyclic and heterocyclic antidepressants, monoamine oxidase inhibitors, and some serotonin uptake inhibitors.

antiparkinson drug   One of a number of drugs used to treat symptoms of Parkinson's disease and extrapyramidal disorders other than tardive dyskinesia. They include anticholinergic agents (benztropine, benzhexol, biperiden, procyclidine, trihexyphenidyl), antihistamines (diphenhydramine, orphenadrine), and dopamine releasing agents (amantadine). They are equally effective, but patients differ widely in sensitivity to their side effects, and in some cases the gap between therapeutic and toxic doses may be narrow. Daily doses are as follows: benztropine 1–6 mg; benzhexol 5–15 mg; biperiden 2–6 mg; procyclidine 6–20 mg; trihexyphenidyl 5–15 mg; diphenhydramine 25–100 mg; orphenadrine 50–300 mg; amantadine 100–300 mg. Levodopa, the agent of choice for Parkinson's disease, does not antagonize the extrapyramidal effects of antipsychotic drugs. Anticholinergic agents such as benztropine and trihexyphenidyl effectively counteract drug-induced parkinsonism but are now secondary drugs in the treatment of Parkinson's disease. Neuropsychiatric side effects include: hallucinations, delusions, hypomania, and confusion. Hallucinations occur in approximately 30% of patients receiving levodopa, levodopa and carbidopa (Sinemet), or a dopamine receptor agonist. Delusions occur in 15–20% of patients receiving dopaminergic agents. Confusional episodes accompanied by disorientation, reduced attention, and memory impairment are induced more often by anticholinergic agents than by dopaminergic drugs. Depression has been attributed to levodopa, but frequency in treated patients is approximately the same as in patients with untreated Parkinson's disease.

antiparkinson drug therapy, maintenance Prophylactic and/or long-term use of antiparkinson drugs to preclude neuroleptic-induced extrapyramidal symptoms is controversial. Supporters stress its value in alleviating subtle extrapyramidal reactions such as bradykinesia, and some suggest that antiparkinson drugs exert their own therapeutic benefits in neuroleptic-treated patients. Others cite the fact that the majority of chronic neuroleptic-treated patients can withstand antiparkinson drug withdrawal, although some patients have increased extrapyramidal symptoms after discontinuation of antiparkinson drug therapy. In 1990, the World Health Organization reviewed prophylactic use of antiparkinson drugs. It concluded that although such drugs may be justified early in neuroleptic treatment (after which they should be discontinued), they should be used only when parkinsonism has actually developed and when other measures (e.g., neuroleptic dosage reduction or substitution of another neuroleptic less prone to induce parkinsonism) have proven ineffective. Long-term antiparkinson drug therapy should be discontinued gradually, not abruptly. There should be careful monitoring of extrapyramidal as well as behavioral effects in the postwithdrawal period.

antiparkinson drug therapy, prophylactic Administration of an antiparkinson drug during treatment with a neuroleptic drug for the purpose of preventing neuroleptic-associated extrapyramidal side effects. It can be divided into initial prophylaxis (administration of the antiparkinson drug at the onset of neuroleptic therapy) and maintenance prophylaxis (continuation of initial antiparkinson prophylactic therapy to prevent emergence or recurrence of extrapyramidal side effects). Prophylactic antiparkinson drug therapy is controversial. Some experts oppose it except for patients with a history of an extrapyramidal reaction during neuroleptic therapy. Otherwise, they believe, an antiparkinson drug should be prescribed only when a neuroleptic-induced extrapyramidal reaction occurs. Proponents of prophylactic therapy contend that both initial

and maintenance antiparkinson regimens are beneficial for some, if not most, neuroleptic-treated patients (Lavin MR, Rifkin A. Prophylactic antiparkinson drug use: I. Initial prophylaxis and prevention of extrapyramidal side effects. *J Clin Pharmacol* 1991;31:763–768; Lavin MR, Rifkin A. Prophylactic antiparkinson drug use: II. Withdrawal after long-term maintenance therapy. *J Clin Pharmacol* 1991; 31:769–777).

antipsychotic Term introduced about 1966 for drugs that are effective in treating psychoses. In low doses they can be useful antianxiety agents, but usually should be avoided for this indication because of the risk of tardive dyskinesia. They also are helpful with some features of depressed states and have applications in general medicine and surgery. Antipsychotics are divided into eight major chemical groups: butyrophenones, dibenzoxazepines, dihydroindolones, diphenylbutylpiperidines, phenothiazines, rauwolfia alkaloids, substituted benzamides, and thioxanthenes. Mesoridazine, loxapine, thiothixene, chlorpromazine, and thioridazine demonstrate potent affinities for the H_1 histaminic receptor and are more sedating than molindone and haloperidol, which have much lower affinities for the H_1 receptor. Patients with chronic aggression, especially the elderly and those with an organic brain disorder, should be treated cautiously with antipsychotics. They may dampen hedonic capacity, thereby causing or exacerbating negative symptoms, and may indirectly mimic negative symptoms of psychosis in the form of extrapyramidal side effects (especially akinesia).

antipsychotic + anticholinergic Anticholinergics are frequently prescribed, sometimes in a prophylactic manner, to counteract antipsychotic-induced extrapyramidal effects. Several double-blind studies, however, have shown that in some antipsychotic-treated patients, adjunctive anticholinergics may worsen symptoms, particularly thought disorganization, uncooperativeness, bizarre and unusual thoughts, suspiciousness and paranoid ideation, delusions, disorientation, and sleeplessness. Coadministration may (a) decrease absorption of the antipsychotic, interfering with its therapeutic effects; and (b) produce additive anticholinergic effects that may lead to anticholinergic toxicity. See **antiparkinson drug therapy, maintenance; antiparkinson drug therapy, prophylactic.**

antipsychotic/antidepressant + lithium Lithium augmentation has been found effective in bipolar, but not unipolar, depression unresponsive to antipsychotic/antidepressant therapy (Nelson; JC, Mazone CM. Lithium augmentation in psychotic depression refractory to combined drug treatment. *Am J Psychiatry* 1986;143:363–366).

antipsychotic/nonresponse   Most clinicians and researchers define poor or nonresponse to medication in schizophrenia as persistent, unchanged positive and negative psychotic symptoms that affect behavior (e.g., bizarre actions, poor self-care) despite treatment with full doses (over 500 mg chlorpromazine equivalents) of typical antipsychotics for at least 6 weeks.

antipsychotic/pregnancy   See **neuroleptic/ pregnancy**.

antipsychotic + tricyclic antidepressant   See **neuroleptic + tricyclic antidepressant**.

antisaccade task   Measurement of frontal lobe dysfunction in which subjects are required to suppress reflexive eye movements toward a cue they have been instructed not to look at, and to look in the opposite direction. Schizophrenic patients have more difficulty suppressing reflexive glances at the cue than do nonschizophrenic control subjects. Seventy-three percent of patients with impaired antisaccade performance have atrophy of the frontal cortex on computed tomography scans (Rosse RB, Schwartz BL, Kim SY, et al. Correlation between antisaccade and Wisconsin Card Sorting Test performance in schizophrenia. *Am J Psychiatry* 1993;150:333–335).

antisense   See **sense/antisense**.

antisense oligonucleotide   Short piece of DNA with a nucleotide sequence that is the reverse of complementary to part of a messenger RNA (mRNA). It binds (hybridizes) to the mRNA, under suitable conditions, according to the rules of the genetic code. Hybridization prevents translation of the mRNA, and the encoded protein cannot be synthesized (Helene C, Toulme J-J. Specific regulation of gene expression by antisense, sense, and antigene nucleic acids. *Biochem Biophys Acta* 1990; 1049:99–125). See **aligodeoxynucleotide**.

antisocial personality disorder   (APD) Very common psychiatric diagnosis among intravenous drug abusers that has been associated with poor treatment outcome in these patients. APD is also associated with significantly higher odds ratio of human immunodeficiency virus (HIV) infection independent of ethnicity, gender, and treatment status. Hence, APD is a risk factor for HIV infection among intravenous drug abusers (Brooner RK, Greenfield L, Schmidt CW, Bigelow GE. Antisocial personality disorder and HIV infection among intravenous drug abusers. *Am J Psychiatry* 1993;150:53–58).

Antivert   See **meclizine**.

Anxanil   See **hydroxyzine**.

anxiety   (From the Latin *anxietas* for "troubled in mind".) Subjective feeling of apprehension, dread, or foreboding ranging from excessive concern about the present or future to feelings of panic, accompanied by a variety of autonomic signs and symptoms in the absence of an obvious external stimulus. In pathological anxiety, these feelings occur without real external danger. Anxiety is the subjective, emotional description of what might objectively be called a stress reaction. Somatic manifestations are associated with arousal of the sympathetic nervous system and include palpitations, dry mouth, pupil dilation, panting, shortness of breath, sweating with skin pallor, anorexia and abdominal discomfort, choking or tight feeling in the throat, trembling, and dizziness. Symptoms may be persistent or occur in panic attacks. State anxiety, where the bounds of normality have been superseded, is extremely common. Anxiety is a common symptom but an uncommon illness, especially in the elderly. It should be differentiated from agitation, depression, hyperadrenergic states, toxicity from medication, secondary consequences of other illness, and neurologic or organic impairment. Late-onset, de novo anxiety may be the initial manifestation of an occult disease. A thorough medical and psychiatric evaluation is warranted before instituting treatment for anxiety. It is extremely difficult to measure effects of drugs on anxiety, especially in long-term studies. Levels of anxiety fluctuate greatly, rising or falling because of many factors other than drugs. Nor is it easy to define anxiety severity when so much depends on the patients own assessment and the doctors style of interpretation. Anxiety comes in many guises; different people see it and feel it in many different ways.

anxiety, breakthrough   Anxiety symptoms occurring between doses in patients treated with short elimination half-life benzodiazepines (BZDs) that produce large interdose fluctuations in blood concentrations and plasma concentrations falling below the minimum effective level. It has been reported with oxazepam, lorazepam, alprazolam, and triazolam. It can be the cause of "clockwatching" as patients anticipate the next dose of the anxiolytic. They describe a sudden and intense increase in anxiety, accompanied by a craving for the drug. These symptoms are interpreted as a worsening of the patients condition and may lead to requests for increased doses and occasionally to uncontrolled self-medication. Shortening interdose intervals is helpful in some patients; in others switching to a BZD with a long elimination half-life (e.g., diazepam, chlordiazepoxide, clorazepate) may be required. Symptoms may be interpreted as evidence of lack of efficacy or too low a dose of the drug rather than a need for more frequent dosing or a switch to another BZD with a longer half- life. A missed dose of a shorter-acting BZD is more likely to cause withdrawal or rebound symptoms than a missed dose of one with a longer half-life. Also called "interdose anxiety."

anxiety/depression States, symptoms, or syndromes that frequently co-exist clinically. Differentiating which is primary and which is secondary can be difficult without doing an in-depth mental status examination and taking a comprehensive history, especially of the onset, evolution, and clinical course of the patient's symptoms. If anxiety is primary, prominent symptoms would include loss of self-confidence in performing daily tasks; autonomic hyper-reactivity; difficulty falling asleep; and a sense that something must be done. If depression is prominent, feelings of guilt, worthlessness, anhedonia, loss of interest and motivation, psychomotor retardation, decreased libido, early-morning awakening, pessimism, and feelings of hopelessness are important differentiating symptoms.

Anxiety Disorders Association of America (ADAA) National, nonprofit organization founded in 1980 to promote awareness among professionals and the public of anxiety disorders. It is dedicated to early identification, prevention, and treatment of anxiety disorders and improvement of the lives of those who suffer from them (Ross J. Social phobia: the Anxiety Disorders Association of America helps raise the veil of ignorance. *J Clin Psychiatry* 1991;52:43–47).

anxiety, endogenous Anxiety that is postulated to have a biological cause and to follow a predictable developmental path from anxiety attacks to onset of agoraphobia and depressive illness (Sheehan DV, Sheehan KH. The classification of anxiety and hysterical states. Part 1. Historical review and empirical delineation. *J Clin Psychopharmacol* 1982;2:235–243).

anxiety, exogenous Anxiety that arises as a result of events in the environment and is psychological rather than biological in origin (Sheehan DV, Sheehan KH. The classification of anxiety and hysterical states. Part 1. Historical review and empirical delineation. *J Clin Psychopharmacol* 1982;2:235–243).

anxiety, free-floating Anxiety not attached to ideational content or an object of fear. It is characteristic of generalized anxiety disorder.

anxiety, interdose See **anxiety, breakthrough**.

anxiety, performance Form of social phobic anxiety characterized by fear of public speaking or "stage fright." Symptoms include dry mouth, palpitations, tremor, memory impairment, and at times overt panic attacks. Propranolol is effective given 10–30 minutes before performance is scheduled to begin. Beta-blockers do not impair cognition or recall, and therefore may be preferable to benzodiazepines for some patients. More severe forms of social phobic anxiety may be more effectively treated by the monoamine oxidase inhibitor (MAOI) phenelzine, or by the MAOI type A inhibitor moclobemide. See **social phobia**.

anxiety/pharmacotherapy The general guiding principle of pharmacotherapy for anxiety disorders is the lowest effective dose for the shortest possible time. This rule, however, should not interfere with judicious use of medications as long as the benefits justify it. Chronic psychiatric disorders may require long-term treatment, often with psychopharmacologic agents. Relapse is typical and should not be considered a treatment failure. Most antianxiety drugs are safe and have no or few long-term side effects, yet periodic drug discontinuation should be attempted to ascertain if drug therapy is still needed at the same or lower dosage.

anxiety, psychic Anxiety manifested predominantly by tension, apprehension, fear, irritability, and excessive worry, excluding panic attacks, that may or may not be accompanied by behavioral agitation. In the patient's perception, psychic symptoms overshadow any associated physical symptoms and signs of anxiety (Spitzer RL, Endicott J. *Schedule for Affective Disorders and Schizophrenia*. New York: New York State Psychiatric Institute, 1978). See **anxiety, somatic**.

anxiety, rebound Marked, temporary increase in anxiety above baseline levels following abrupt discontinuation of benzodiazepine (BZD) or other anxiolytic therapy. It is usually more serious with short-acting BZDs, particularly alprazolam, triazolam, midazolam, and temazepam. In some instances the anxiety may be a combination of relapse and withdrawal. Like rebound insomnia, rebound anxiety may be responsible for continued use and escalating doses of the anxiolytic. Unrecognized or untreated rebound anxiety may be the cause of drug dependence and "iatrogenic" treatment resistance. In some patients, rebound anxiety may be so severe that drug therapy needs to be resumed. Rebound anxiety may occur after abrupt cessation of daytime anxiolytic treatment, but it can also occur with rebound insomnia after discontinuation of regular nightly doses. Similarly, rebound anxiety following discontinuation of a daytime BZD anxiolytic may also be accompanied by rebound insomnia at night (Fontaine R, Chouinard G, Annable L. Rebound anxiety in anxious patients after abrupt withdrawal of benzodiazepine treatment. *Am J Psychiatry* 1984;141:848–853; Scharf MB, Jacoby JA. Lorazepam—efficacy, side effects, and rebound phenomena. *Clin Pharmacol Ther* 1982; 31:175–177). See **insomnia, rebound**.

anxiety, recurrent brief Diagnostic category with the same diagnostic requirements as generalized anxiety disorder but with a shorter time span. Anxious mood must be present for less than 2 weeks with a recurrence rate of at least once a month in the preceding year (Angst J, Wicki W. The Zurich Study XIII: recurrent brief anxiety. *Eur Arch Psychiatry Clin Neurosci* 1992;241:296–300).

anxiety, somatic Anxiety manifested predominantly by somatic signs and symptoms such as palpitations, shakiness, tremulousness, dizziness, headaches, chest pains, sighing, hyperventilation, sweating, rapid pulse, dyspepsia, nausea, urinary frequency and urgency, and diarrhea. Somatic symptoms are often considered the cause of the patient's anxiety, apprehension, nervousness, and worry. They are a prime motive for patients consulting a family physician or an internist rather than seeking psychiatric help. Somatic anxiety must be differentiated from the somatic symptoms of depression (Spitzer RL, Endicott J. *Schedule for Affective Disorders and Schizophrenia*. New York: New York State Psychiatric Institute, 1978). See **anxiety/depression**.

anxiety syndromes/depression Anxiety syndromes characterized by phobias, panic attacks, obsessions, or compulsions co-exist with major depression at rates far exceeding those explicable by chance. Depression may be complicated by obsessions, compulsions, phobias, or panic attacks, or the reverse may be true (i.e., anxiety disorders may give rise to depression). Alternatively, anxiety and depressive syndromes may be expressions of a common diathesis. Studies to determine whether anxiety symptoms in a depressed patient indicate coexistence of a separate disease process, and whether they have prognostic significance, indicate that when restricted to episodes of major depression, anxiety syndromes appear to be prognostically significant epiphenomena rather than indicators of an additional disorder. Depressed patients with anxiety symptoms experience more depressive morbidity during the ensuing 5 years (Coryell W, Endicott J, Winokur G. Anxiety syndromes as epiphenomena of primary major depression: outcome and familial psychopathology. *Am J Psychiatry* 1992;149:100–107).

anxiogen Compound that provokes anxiety (e.g., yohimbine, lactate, carbon dioxide, caffeine, beta-carbolines). Phenylethylamine may be an endogenous anxiogen.

anxiogenic Precipitating or perpetuating an anxiety disorder.

Anxiolit See **oxazepam**.

anxiolytic Substance that blocks or alleviates pathological anxiety and/or emotional tension, restoring the clinically anxious individual to tolerable levels of anxiety. Included are benzodiazepines, azapirones, meprobamate, barbiturates, and certain antihistamines such as diphenhydramine and hydroxyzine. Also called "antianxiety drug"; "minor tranquillizer."

anxiolytic, nonbenzodiazepine Substance that blocks or alleviates pathological anxiety, but that is not a benzodiazepine. There are two groups. Group 1 includes agents that bind to the GABA-BZ-Cl⁻ ionophore complex (beta-carbolines, cyclopyrrolones, triazolopyridazines). Group 2 compounds are agents that do not bind to the GABA-BZ-Cl⁻ ionophore complex (buspirone, gepirone, ritanserin).

anxiolytic + hydromorphone Co-administration increases central nervous system depression. Doses of one or both drugs should be reduced if used concomitantly or in close succession.

anxiolytic rating instruments Hamilton Anxiety Scale (HAM-A); Clinical Global Impressions (CGI); Anxiety Status Inventory (ASI); Self Rating Anxiety Scale (SAS); and Self Report Symptom Inventory (SCL-90).

Anxon See **ketazolam**.

"aotal" GABA-agonist that reduces voluntary alcohol consumption in rats and aids the maintenance of abstinence in chronic alcoholism. Its mechanism of action and efficacy are undergoing further investigation.

Aparkane See **trihexyphenidyl**.

apathy Want of feeling or absence of affect that often is a symptom of severe states of depression, certain forms of schizophrenia, and certain types of brain injury.

A₄ peptide See **beta-amyloid peptide**.

aphasia Deficit of language that may be due to motor or sensory dysfunction; loss of ability to speak or loss of ability to comprehend the meaning of written or printed words.

aphonia Loss of voice caused by laryngeal abnormalities. Also called "dysphonia."

aphrodisiac Substance that positively affects sexual functioning, enhances the responsiveness of the brain's sex centers and/or of the genitals, or facilitates the neurovascular-endocrine system's response to sex. Although many substances have been called aphrodisiacs, only a few truly are. Yohimbine and papaverine are aphrodisiacs for men.

Aphrodyne   See **yohimbine**.

Apilepsin   See **valproate**.

Aplacal   See **melperone**.

aplastic anemia   The most serious type of blood dyscrasia, resulting from suppression of all bone marrow function (hypoplasia). The defective production of red cells, white cells, and platelets results in low plasma counts for all cells (pancytopenia). Aplastic anemia is associated with a high incidence of mortality and protracted morbidity in patients who do recover. A small number of cases are congenital, but most are acquired. Anemia (reduced red cells) causes symptoms of weakness, fatigue, and shortness of breath on exertion. Thrombocytopenia (reduced platelets) can produce hemorrhage into the skin, menorrhagia, and bleeding from the gums and alimentary tract; death can occur from cerebral hemorrhage. Neutropenia or agranulocytosis (reduced white cells) can produce sore throat, ulceration of the mouth and pharynx, fever with sweating and chills, and infections of the skin and mucous membranes, often with secondary infections of candida. Pneumonia and septicemia are frequent causes of death. Acquired aplastic anemia is usually related to exposure to drugs or other chemicals. When it is not possible to identify a cause for the anemia, it is termed "idiopathic." Drug-induced aplastic anemia can be either acute or, more commonly, chronic. Acute cases present with severe bleeding and sometimes infection; in chronic cases signs of anemia occur over weeks or months following exposure to the toxin. Clinical features vary with severity. Drugs can induce aplastic anemia in one of two ways: (a) a direct, dose-related effect on cell division in the bone marrow; (b) an unpredictable "sensitivity" reaction that may be genetically determined. The classic example of drugs causing the first type of reaction is cytotoxic agents, which inhibit cell division in all patients in a dose-related manner. Their effect is immediate but reversible on drug withdrawal. The second type of reaction can be more serious because onset may be delayed, sometimes not becoming apparent until several months after the drug has been stopped. This reaction is not always reversible. The causative drug should never be readministered, as it sensitizes the patient and a second reaction could prove fatal. Some psychotropic drugs (e.g., clozapine and carbamazepine) can produce agranulocytosis and aplastic anemia, but usually not in the same patient. Also called "panmyelopathy." See **agranulocytosis, blood dyscrasia, thrombocytopenia**.

apnea   Cessation of airflow as measured by thermistor channels. See **sleep apnea**.

apnea-hypopnea index   Number of apneic episodes (obstructive, central, and mixed) plus hypopneas per hour of sleep as determined by all-night polysomnography.

apnea index   Number of apneic episodes (obstructive, central, and mixed) per hour of sleep as determined during all-night polysomnography.

Apo-Carbamazepine   See **carbamazepine**.

Apo-Diazepam   See **diazepam**.

Apo-Flurazepam   See **flurazepam**.

Apo-Haloperidol   See **haloperidol**.

Apo-Imipramine   See **imipramine**.

Apo-Lorazepam   See **lorazepam**.

Apo-Meprobamate   See **meprobamate**.

Apo-Oxazepam   See **oxazepam**.

Apo-Perphenazine   See **perphenazine**.

apomorphine   (APO) Dopaminergic agonist with a potent effect on D_1 and D_2 striatal receptors. Its effect is presumed to be biphasic: in large doses, it stimulates postsynaptic excitatory dopamine receptors, whereas small doses act preferentially on autoreceptors with resultant reduction in dopamine transmission. APO is administered subcutaneously and transported rapidly into the blood and central nervous system. It is rapidly metabolized in the liver. It induces a prompt and large elevation of serum growth hormone in humans when given in doses of 0.25–1.5 mg subcutaneously. Blunted response of growth hormone to APO challenge occurs in patients with endogenous depression and chronic schizophrenia. In some clinical trials, APO has decreased self-rating of craving for cocaine. APO is useful in Parkinson's patients with declining motor responses and intractable on/off fluctuations. Since it frequently causes vomiting, it is often preceded by the antiemetic domperidone, 20 mg orally twice a day. Low-dose APO has been used to investigate the dopamine supersensitivity hypothesis of tardive dyskinesia (Jeste DV, Cutler NR, Kaufman CA, Karoum F. Low-dose apomorphine and bromocriptine in neuroleptic-induced movement disorders. *Biol Psychiatry* 1983;18:1085–1091). Low-dose APO challenge (0.01 mg/kg subcutaneously) in seven patients with tardive akathisia in a placebo, double-blind, random design study revealed that APO caused a significantly greater reduction in the objective (movement) but not the subjective (distress) component of akathisia (Sachdev P, Loneragan C. Low-dose apomorphine challenge in tardive akathisia. *Neurology* 1993;43:544–547).

apomorphine (APO) challenge test   Measure of central nervous system dopamine activity used to determine pathophysiological changes in illnesses such as schizophrenia by measuring growth hormone response to apomorphine. The test is performed in subjects at bedrest. After an overnight fast an indwelling catheter is inserted in a forearm vein at 7:00 am. Blood samples of 10 ml are collected at −20, 0, +20, +40, +60, and +120 minutes after injection at 8:00 am of APO (0.5 mg diluted in saline to obtain 0.5 ml subcutaneously). A large number of studies have demonstrated that subcutaneous APO administration induces a reliable release of growth hormone in humans (Pitchot W, Ansseau M, Gonzalez Moreno A, Hansenne M, von Frenckell R. Dopaminergic function in panic disorder: comparison with major and minor depression. *Biol Psychiatry* 1992;32:1004–1011).

apoplexy   See **stroke** (preferred term).

Apo-Thioridazine   See **thioridazine**.

Apo-Trifluoperazine   See **trifluoperazine**.

A-Poxide   See **chlordiazepoxide**.

apparent volume of distribution   Proportional constant relating plasma concentration of a drug to total amount of drug in the body (Benet LZ, Sheiner LB. Pharmacokinetics: the dynamics of drug absorption, distribution and elimination. *In* Gilman AG, Goodman LS, Rall TW, Murad F [eds], *Goodman and Gilman's The Pharmacologic Basis of Therapeutics,* 7th ed. New York: Macmillan, 1985).

APP gene   See **gene, APP**.

applied relaxation   Type of psychological treatment used to reduce arousal and thereby enable patients to control panic attacks. Whether it is more effective than other psychological treatments for panic disorder has not been determined definitively, but it has been shown to be more effective than "progressive relaxation" used between attacks. It has been used to reduce the state of high arousal provoked by phobic stimuli with reasonably good results.

apraxia   Lack of ability to perform a pattern of movements, although the individual understands what is required and has no apparent physical reason for the inability. It is caused by damage to, or abnormality of, certain parts of the brain.

aprobarbital   (Alurate) Barbiturate sedative-hypnotic comparable to other drugs in its class. Schedule III; pregnancy risk category D.

Apropax   See **paroxetine**.

aprosodia   Speech lacking features of emotion, emphasis, and rhythm. It is a common symptom of Parkinson's disease.

APUD cell   Amine precursor, uptake and decarboxylation cell from which the platelet is derived.

arachidonic acid   See **eicosanoid**.

arachidonic acid metabolite   See **eicosanoid**.

Aramine   See **metaraminol**.

Arden ratio   See **EOG ratio**.

area under the curve   (AUC) Total amount of drug absorbed into the systemic circulation and available for distribution to the target organ and site of action. An important measure of bioavailability, AUC is directly proportional to the total amount of unchanged drug in the body. Accurate determination of AUC requires repeated blood samples obtained at frequent intervals over a period sufficiently long to assure virtually complete elimination of the drug and active metabolites.

arecoline   Acetylcholine receptor agonist that acts at both muscarinic and nicotinic receptor sites.

arginine vasopressin   (AVP) Neuropeptide that is contained and participates in all three avenues (i.e., via the anterior pituitary, posterior pituitary, and autonomic nervous system) through which the hypothalamus may initiate adaptive responses to stress. It stimulates adrenocorticotropic hormone (ACTH) release synergistically with corticotropin-releasing hormone and is thus involved in modulating activation of the hypothalamic-pituitary-adrenocortical axis during stressful stimuli. Animal studies indicate that AVP may play a role in the maintenance of alcohol tolerance. See **vasopressin**.

arginine vasotocin   (AVT) Nonapeptide found in the pineal gland that may play a role in sleep regulation.

arise time   Clock time when an individual gets out of bed after final awakening from the major sleep episode.

arithmetic mean   See **mean**.

"aroma of men"   Street name for volatile nitrites such as amyl nitrite sold in "head shops," pornography stores, and novelty shops, as well as through mail order houses.

Aropax   See **paroxetine**.

arousal   Abrupt change from a "deeper stage" of non–rapid-eye-movement (REM) sleep to a "lighter stage," or from REM sleep toward wakefulness, with the possibility of awakening as the final outcome. Arousal may be accompanied by increased tonic electromyogram activity and heart rate as well as by body movements.

arousal disorder   Parasomnia disorder characterized by an abnormal arousal mechanism in which forced arousal from sleep occurs. The classic arousal disorders are sleepwalking, sleep terror, and confusional arousals.

Artane See **trihexyphenidyl**.

Artane Sequels See **trihexyphenidyl**.

artificial association Spurious or false association that is one of several types of errors that can be made in performing a study. It can occur by chance or bias.

aryl Chemical group derived from, or related to, an aromatic hydrocarbon (e.g., a benzine-like molecule).

arylpiperazine See **azaperone**.

ascending dose design Study in which drug dosage is escalated until improvement or side effects intervene, obviating any need for further dose escalation. It tends to produce a curvilinear relationship between drug plasma level and efficacy.

ascending reticular activating system (ARAS) Diffuse network of nuclei and tracts located in the core of the brainstem that extends from the medulla to the thalamus. It mediates such responses as eye opening to painful stimuli, which is one clinical manifestation of intact arousal mechanisms. Other testable aspects of ARAS functioning are corneal reflexes, pupillary reactions, ocular motility, awareness, and arousal.

Asendin See **amoxapine**.

Asendis See **amoxapine**.

aspartate One of the most abundant amino acids in the brain. It acts as an excitatory neurotransmitter, but its precise role in brain function has not been ascertained.

aspartate aminotransferase (AST) Preferred name for glutamic oxaloacetic transferase (SGOT), an intracellular enzyme involved in amino acid catabolism and gluconeogenesis. Normal range is 5–40 IU/ml. AST is present in high concentrations in the heart, liver, kidney, and muscle tissue. Damage to any of these tissues results in elevated serum AST.

Asperger's syndrome (AS) Syndrome characterized by impaired social interaction, abnormal speech, impaired nonverbal communication, circumscribed interests, repetitive activities, and motor clumsiness. AS can coexist with Gilles de la Tourette's syndrome. Structural brain abnormalities are demonstrable on magnetic resonance imaging (MRI) scans (Berthier ML, Bayes A, Tolosa ES. Magnetic resonance imaging in patients with concurrent Tourette's disorder and Asperger's syndrome. *J Am Acad Child Adolesc Psychiatry* 1993;32:633–639).

asphyxiophylia Recurrent sexual behavior in which arousal and attainment of orgasm depend on and are heightened by asphyxiation up to, but not including, loss of consciousness. The male hangs himself, nude or seminude, with feet trussed and mouth and throat stuffed; he masturbates in this position. A narrow margin of time in which to release the noose and gag at the moment of orgasm heightens the excitement, danger, and extremely high risk of accidental death. Often found at the scene of an autoerotic death are women's underwear, pornographic material, alcohol, and inhalants such as nitrous oxide and isobutyl nitrite. See **autoerotic asphyxia**.

aspirin + lithium See **lithium + aspirin**.

aspirin + oxycodone See **oxycodone + aspirin**.

aspirin + valproate See **valproate + aspirin**.

aspirin + valproic acid See **valproic acid + aspirin**.

assay See **drug assay**.

assertiveness Affirmative and confident behavior that allows one to meet one's needs.

assessment Systematic, thorough evaluation of the strengths, weaknesses, and problems of a patient. It is carried out by a professional person or a team of staff members from different disciplines (multidisciplinary team assessment). It may be used to establish the nature or cause of disabilities, the most appropriate approach to treatment or educational placement, the patient's future potential, and/or the needs of the patient and his or her family. A number of questionnaires and interview schedules developed in recent years can be used with parents, teachers, or other key informants to aid assessments of all types. In assessing cognitive function, these may be used instead of or along with specific neuropsychological tests measuring mental age, or intelligence quotient.

Assival See **diazepam**.

association In genetics, a direct effect of a particular gene or genetic marker on a phenotype for individuals in a population. In statistics, a relation between two or more variables without any implication of causation or its absence from one variable to another.

assortative mating See **mating, assortative**.

assortment Random distribution to gametes of different combinations of chromosomes. At anaphase of the first meiotic division, one member of each pair passes to each pole, and the gametes thus contain one chromosome of each type. The chromosome may be of either paternal or maternal origin.

astasia-abasia Hysterical gait disorder characterized by bizarre staggering with abortive falls or collapse into the arms of medical staff personnel. Neurological examination confirms the absence of paralysis, ataxia, or sensory loss.

astereognosis Impairment of the ability to perceive the shape and texture of an object and identify it by tactile contact alone, although the peripheral sensory apparatus is intact. It frequently follows lesions of the parietal lobe.

asterixis   Inability to maintain a fixed posture against gravity accompanied by varying degrees of confusion. It can be due to short-lasting pauses of muscular activity causing postural lapses and may be regarded as a form of "negative myoclonus." Postural lapses are corrected immediately by sudden flapping of hand and arm, similar to the movement of a bird's wings. The symptom becomes most obvious when the patient stands still with outstretched arms and dorsiflexed wrists. The extremities are usually asynchronously affected, and the face and tongue are sometimes involved as well. The electroencephalogram is usually diffusely slowed. The involuntary movements are often a manifestation of metabolic encephalopathy, most frequently seen as part of hepatic encephalopathies and usually secondary to severe alcoholism. Without evidence of metabolic disturbance, asterixis suggests idiosyncratic vulnerability of the striatal system. Asterixis can be a neurologic side effect of high-potency neuroleptics. It may be induced by carbamazepine (CBZ), especially in patients receiving other psychotropic drugs in addition to CBZ (Rittmannsberger H, Leblhuber F. Asterixis induced by carbamazepine therapy. *Biol Psychiatry* 1992;32:364–368). It also has been reported during treatment with lithium, clozapine, and carbamazepine, and in severe hepatic or renal dysfunction, Wilson's disease, and thalamic or parietal lesions. Also called "flapping tremor."

asymmetry   Anatomic difference between the same structures on either side of the neuroaxis.

asymptotic   Pertaining to a limiting value when the independent variable approaches zero or infinity.

ataractic drug   Sedative/anxiolytic compound that relieves tension and anxiety without clouding of consciousness and without the pharmacological effects of barbiturates and neuroleptics. This term, suggested in 1955 by Fabing, is now seldom used.

Atarax   See **hydroxyzine**.

ataxia   Inability to coordinate muscles for the execution of voluntary movement. It may be due to a disorder in the brain or spinal cord.

atenolol   (Tenormin) Cardioselective, hydrophilic beta-adrenergic blocker that has been shown to suppress nocturnal melatonin secretion when administered in the afternoon. It effectively relieves neuroleptic-induced akathisia, but less effective than propranolol, which is highly lipophilic (Reiter S, Adler L, Angrist B, et al. Atenolol and propranolol in neuroleptic-induced akathisia. *J Clin Psycho-pharmacol* 1987;7:279–280). Pregnancy risk category C.

atenolol/breast milk   Atenolol is secreted in breast milk. Clinically significant bradycardia has been reported in breast-fed infants whose mothers are taking atenolol. Premature infants or those with renal impairment may be more likely to develop adverse effects. For more data, consult the manufacturer.

atenolol + clozapine   Atenolol has been used successfully to counteract clozapine-induced tachycardia with no adverse interactions.

atenolol + fluoxetine   Co-administration apparently produces no adverse interactions (Walley T, Pirmohamed M, Proudlove C, Maxwell D. Interaction of metoprolol and fluoxetine. *Lancet* 1993;341:967–968).

atenolol + fluvoxamine   Fluvoxamine apparently has no significant effect on serum levels, volume of distribution, elimination half-life, or total body clearance of atenolol (Benfield P, Ward A. Fluvoxamine: a review of its pharmacokinetic properties and therapeutic efficacy in depressive illness. *Drugs* 1986;32:313–334).

atenolol + sertraline   Sertraline has no effect on the beta-adrenergic blocking ability of atenolol. Aside from occasional mild headache, co-administration has evoked no serious adverse effects.

athetosis   Recurrent, slow, and continual change in position between two extremes, such as pronation and supination. The abnormal movements are called "athetoid movements". They usually involve the fingers and toes, although the face may also be affected. Athetoid movements of the fingers have been called "piano-playing" movements. Athetosis may coexist with chorea. It is caused by lesions of the putamen. Hypoxia and/or severe jaundice at the time of birth are possible causes. If the athetosis is caused by jaundice, it is often associated with deafness. It also may occur in people who have other forms of cerebral palsy and/or who are mentally handicapped. In the first year or two of life, athetotic babies are often floppy at first. The affected person has more control over movements if the nearest joint of the limb is held still (e.g., hand control is easier if the wrist is held in place). Movements are made worse by excitement or effort.

Ativan   See **lorazepam**.

Atozine   See **hydroxyzine**.

atracurium   Nondepolarizing curariform neuromuscular-blocking agent used to control muscle rigidity.

Atretol   See **carbamazepine**.

atropine (Allergan) Alkaloid extracted from atropa belladonna with anticholinergic, antispasmodic, antiperspirant, and mydriatic effects. It is frequently administered intramuscularly 30 minutes or intravenously 2 minutes prior to electroconvulsive therapy to decrease secretions and prevent vagal-induced bradycardia or asystole. It is a cholinergic antagonist that decreases brain acetylcholine content, presumably by blocking presynaptic muscarinic receptors and thereby increasing acetylcholine release due to loss of presynaptic inhibitory feedback.

atropine coma Used many years ago in the treatment of opiate addiction; now discredited.

"atropine equivalent" Concentration of atropine, in nanograms per milliliter, that would displace an equivalent amount of radioactively labeled compound in a radioreceptor assay.

attempted suicide See **suicide, attempted.**

attention Ability to focus in a sustained manner on one activity (DSM-IV). Disturbance in attention may be manifested by difficulty in finishing tasks that have been started, easy distractibility, or difficulty in concentrating on work.

attention-deficit disorder (ADD) Disorder consisting of two domains of dysfunction: one of attention and the other of impulsivity/hyperactivity. Clinical data indicate that the subtypes differ in gender ratio, presence of associated problems, possible outcome, and treatment needs. Some children with ADD have minor neurological abnormalities, minor physical anomalies, allergies, and physical and neurological illnesses such as seizure disorders. There may be significant psychiatric comorbidity, including poor peer relationships, social skills deficits, academic performance problems, communication disorders, other disruptive behavior disorders, substance abuse, mood disorders, anxiety disorders, tics and Tourette's syndrome, pervasive developmental disorders, and mental retardation. See **attention-deficit hyperactivity disorder.**

attention-deficit hyperactivity disorder (ADHD) Heterogeneous group of behavioral disorders of unknown etiology usually first evident in childhood. ADHD is generally characterized by behaviors that impair emotional, academic, and social development, including varying degrees of inattention, impulsiveness, and hyperactivity. Terms such as "hyperkinesis," "hyperkinetic syndrome," "minimal brain dysfunction (MBD)," "attention-deficit disorder (ADD)," and "attention-deficit disorder with hyperactivity (ADDH)" have been used to describe the condition. They are not synonymous and may describe patients with different disorders. Children with ADHD have difficulty organizing and completing tasks and chores involving multiple steps because they easily become distracted. They shift from one task to the next and are often careless and clumsy. They also have difficulty concentrating on what is said to them and consequently appear to intentionally forget or ignore established rules. They demonstrate their impulsiveness by interrupting conversations and speaking out of turn. Many are unable to consider the consequences of their actions; as a result, they may inadvertently embarrass others and occasionally injure themselves. Excessive talking and noisiness are commonplace, especially at school. These children have difficulty remaining seated, even in situations where they are expected to do so. They frequently squirm in their seats and are extremely fidgety. ADHD may occur in as many as 3–5% of children. It is from 3 to 6 times more common in boys than in girls. It appears to be more prevalent in first-degree biologic relatives and in siblings of girls with ADHD than in individuals with unaffected family members. Neuropharmacological investigations, genetic studies, and the association of ADHD with other neuropsychiatric syndromes indicate that it may be the result of central nervous system dysfunction. Psychostimulants (particularly dextroamphetamine, methylphenidate, and pemoline) are the mainstay of contemporary management of ADHD. Methylphenidate and dexamphetamine improve behavior in most hyperkinetic children. Dosage of both drugs is 0.3 mg/kg/day (total <20 mg/day) divided into two doses, one administered in the morning and one at mid-day. A low initial dose should be increased gradually to suit the needs of the individual child. Unwanted effects including anorexia, stomach pains and nausea, and suppression of growth have been reported in long-term use. To provide the greatest possible benefit, pharmacotherapy must generally be supplemented by behavioral, educational, psychosocial, and family interventions. ADHD may occur along with conduct, depressive, anxiety, and other disorders that may have differing risk factors, clinical courses, and pharmacological responses. Formerly called "hyperkinesia"; "hyperkinetic syndrome"; "minimal brain dysfunction."

attention-deficit hyperactivity disorder (ADHD)/adult outcome A longitudinal study to investigate adult sequelae of ADHD indicates that it predicts antisocial and drug abuse disorders. In addition, regardless of psychiatric status, ADHD appears to place children at relative risk for educational and vocational disadvantage. Childhood hyperactivity predisposes to adult maladjustment and continues to affect important functional domains in a substantial minority of subjects (Mannuzza S, Klein RG, Bessler A, et al. Adult outcome of hyperactive boys. Educational achievement, occupational rank, and psychiatric status. *Arch Gen Psychiatry* 1993;50:565–576).

attention, poor   Failure in focused alertness manifested by poor concentration, distractibility from internal and external stimuli, and difficulty in harnessing, sustaining, or shifting focus to new stimuli.

attributable risk   (AR) See **risk, attributable**.

atypical antipsychotic   See **neuroleptic, atypical**.

atrial natriuretic peptide   (ANP) Peptide hormone secreted by the atria that is involved in regulation of natriuresis and vascular smooth muscle relaxation. The peptide and its receptors are located in select brain areas, including central cardiovascular regulatory sites. Functionally, ANP may be involved in the central regulation of blood pressure fluid volume.

atypical bipolar II disorder   Condition characterized by recurrent hypersomniac-retarded major depressive episodes and occasional mild and brief periods of elation that fall short of the symptomatic threshold for mania. Because the hypomanic periods (which typically precede or follow the depressive episodes) are often pleasant, adaptive, and ego-syntonic, they are rarely reported, and the bipolar nature of the illness is often missed. When given tricyclic antidepressants, patients fail to respond, rapidly cycle out of a depression, or develop brief hypomanic excursions. Even then, the bipolar nature of the illness is often missed because the hypomanic shift may be labeled "flight into health" or "transference cures". Long-term exposure to heterocyclic antidepressants may adversely affect the course of the illness in the direction of rapid cycling and increased severity. Furthermore, repeated episodes of uncontrolled depression lead to much interpersonal havoc. Many patients meet criteria for borderline personality and are subjected to psychodynamic psychotherapies of one form or another. Gradual disappearance of borderline features has been observed in many bipolar patients on maintenance lithium carbonate. As many as 50% of patients with borderline conditions seem to represent the adverse characterologic sequelae of high-frequency affective disorders such as bipolar II (Akiskal HS. Subaffective disorders: dysthymic, cyclothymic, and bipolar II disorders in the "borderline realm." *Psychiatr Clin North Am* 1981;4:25–46).

atypical depression   See **depression, atypical**.

atypical neuroleptic   See **neuroleptic, atypical**.

atypical psychosis   See **psychosis, atypical**.

audit, psychiatric   See **psychiatric audit**.

auditory evoked potential   Electrophysiologic measure of central nervous system function. Evoked potential components are usually categorized into "exogenous" component, mainly controlled by the physical and temporal aspects of stimulation, and "endogenous" components, dependent on the allocation of attention to and cognitive processing of the stimuli P300 amplitude has been found to be decreased in a variety of psychiatric disorders, most notably schizophrenia. It is depressed by benzodiazepine sedation and can be used to monitor recovery of individuals sedated with benzodiazepines. See **brainstem auditory-evoked response; event-related potential**.

auditory hallucination   See **hallucination, auditory**.

aura   Sensory, motor, or psychic phenomena accompanied by electroencephalographic abnormalities that may precede a focal or partial seizure, but not a primary generalized seizure. An aura signals a stage prior to interictal synchronous, subconvulsive firing of epileptogenic tissue into a continuous discharge stage that recruits additional neuronal circuits. Unless the patient has multifocal disease, the aura, if present at all, is identical or at least highly similar in different attacks. Auras may suggest psychogenic epilepsy if they are highly complex, contain a great number of somatic or visceral sensations, and vary on different occasions.

"aurora"   Street name for phencyclidine (PCP).

"aurora borealis"   Street name for phencyclidine (PCP).

Aurorix   See **moclobemide**.

autism   Behaviorally defined syndrome of unknown etiology associated with poor social interaction, disordered language, and atypical responses to people, objects, and events. It is manifested by severe disturbances in cognition, language, and behavior that appear before 30 months of age. It is also associated with a hyperarousal state (e.g., hyperactivity, repetitive/stereotypic behavior, self-stimulation, hypervigilance). Autistic children often exhibit ritualized body movements, repeated touching and sniffing of objects, ritualistic ordering, checking and collecting, and insistence on precisely following routines. Follow-up studies indicate that the behaviors may change over time and that acquisition of communicative language prior to age 5 and level of intellectual functioning are the best prognostic indicators (Gonzalez NM, Alpert M, Shay J, Campbell M. "DSM-IV Field Trial: change of

diagnosis in autistic children on follow-up."
Presented at the 1992 annual meeting of the
American College of Neuropsychopharmacology). Psychophysiological studies of autism
have established deficiencies in information
processing, and increasing evidence suggests
some underlying brain pathology. Magnetic
resonance imaging (MRI) research indicates
hypoplasia of cerebellar lobules VI and VII,
the pons, and enlargement of the fourth
ventricle. Abnormalities found in the limbic
system including the hippocampus, amygdala,
mamillary body, anterior cingulate gyrus, and
septal nuclei (areas known to be related to
learning, memory, and behavior) may be related to clinical features of autism. Investigators also have found elevated norepinephrine
levels, decreased plasma activity of dopamine
beta-hydroxylase, and abnormalities in the
endogenous opioid system. Although fenfluramine, buspirone, levodopa, naltrexone,
lithium, and haloperidol have been tried in
autism, none has significantly reduced autistic
behaviors, and some cause treatment-limiting
adverse effects. Clonidine may reduce several
hyperarousal behaviors and improve social
relationships in some autistic subjects (Fank-
hauser MP, Karumanchi VC, German ML, et
al. A double-blind, placebo-controlled study of
the efficacy of transdermal clonidine in autism. *J Clin Psychiatry* 1992;53:77–82). Clomipramine is superior to desipramine in treating
obsessive-compulsive symptoms (Gorder CT,
Rapaport JL, Hamburger SD, et al. Differential response of seven subjects with autistic
disorder to clomipramine and desipramine.
Am J Psychiatry 1992;149:363–366).

autism, infantile   Severe developmental disorder first described by Kanner (1943) characterized by disturbances in motility, perception,
social interactions, speech, and language. Etiology is unknown, but infantile autism is
strongly suspected to have a neurological basis
(Kanner L. Autistic disturbances of affective
contact. *Nervous Child* 1943;2:217–250).

autistic fantasy   Mechanism in which the person substitutes excessive daydreaming for the
pursuit of human relationships, more direct
and effective action, or problem solving
(DSM-IV).

autistic thinking   Distorted, self-centered, fantastic thinking with no regard for reality.

autoerotic asphyxia   Self-induction of cerebral
anoxia, usually by means of ligatures or suffo-
cating devices, while the individual masturbates to orgasm. Found almost exclusively in
men, the activity may result in death if the
person's self-rescue plan fails or unconsciousness precludes its use. Mechanisms of asphyxiation include hanging, strangulation, suffoca-

tion, hanging and suffocation, strangulation
and suffocation, gas or volatile solvent, suffocation and gas or solvent, and chest compression. Plastic bags may be placed over the head
either for suffocation or as containers for
volatile substances or other intoxicating gases
(Hucker SJ. Sexual asphyxia. *In* Bowden P,
Bluglass R [eds], *Principles and Practice of Forensic Psychiatry*. London: Churchill Livingstone,
1990; Blanchard R, Hucker SJ. Transvestism,
bondage and concurrent paraphilic activities
in 117 fatal cases of autoerotic asphyxia. *Br J
Psychiatry* 1991;159:371–377). See **asphyxiophylia**.

autoimmunity   Immunity to self, exhibited in
conditions in which individuals form antibodies against one or more of their own antigens
from one or more of their own organ systems.

autoinduction   Stimulation of its own metabolism by a drug that stimulates the hepatic
microsomal enzyme oxidase system, causing a
decrease in the drug's plasma level after initial
achievement of steady state. Decrease in a
drug's plasma level after a few weeks of
therapy may be due to autoinduction and not
noncompliance. Carbamazepine is a well
known autoinducer (Macphee GJA, Brodie
MJ. Carbamazepine substitution in severe partial epilepsy: implication of autoinduction of
metabolism. *Postgrad Med J* 1985;61:779–783).

automated testing systems   Tests used in the
assessment of drug effects on cognitive functioning that have been transferred to a variety
of microprocessor-based computers. Best
known is the Perceptual Maze test, developed
from the Porteus Maze, which is designed
specifically to utilize computer programs in
both item design and performance analysis.
Others include digit span memory test; coding test from the Wechsler Digit Symbol Substitution Test; tracking test; memory test for
nonsense syllables and words; tapping test;
reaction time test; reading speed and vigilance
tasks; vocabulary test; and analog mood and
attitude scales, checklists, and questionnaires.

automatic behavior   Stereotyped, repetitive actions that apparently occur without awareness.
They may be a symptom of narcolepsy. See
automatism.

automatic epilepsy   See **seizure, complex partial** (preferred term).

automatic thoughts   Thoughts that occur without any apparent antecedent reflection or
reasoning. They are associated with depression and are characteristic of depressive cognition. Examples include (a) I'm no good; (b)
No one understands me; (c) I wish I were a
better person; (d) I'm so weak; (e) I'm so
disappointed in myself; and (f) I can't get

started (Beck AT. *Depression: Courses and Treatment*. Philadelphia: University of Pennsylvania Press, 1967).

automatism   Repetitive and stereotyped psychic, sensory, or motor phenomena resulting from brain dysfunction that occur in a confusional setting over which the individual has no control and for which there may be no memory. An automatism may be a result of an epileptic attack. Oral automatisms (e.g., lip smacking, chewing, swallowing) are ictal events, but most automatisms are postictal phenomena. Sleepwalking is an example of an automatism that is not ictal. See **automatic behavior**.

autonomic nervous system   See **nervous system, autonomic**.

autonomic side effects   Symptoms resulting from blockade or stimulation of the autonomic nervous system. See **anticholinergic effect**.

autoradiography   Technique that uses x-ray film to visualize radioactively labeled molecules or fragments of molecules to analyze length and number of DNA fragments after they are separated by gel electrophoresis for such qualities as receptor damage.

autoreceptor   Presynaptic receptor that controls synthesis and release of neurotransmitters within the neuron. It is located in the cell body, dendrites, and presynaptic position on the nerve terminal. It tends to be inhibitory.

autosomal dominant inheritance   See **inheritance, dominant**.

autosomal recessive inheritance   See **inheritance, recessive**.

autosome   Set of paired chromosomes (other than the sex chromosome) that are part of the chromosomal make-up of a karyotype. Humans normally have 22 pairs of autosomes and 2 sex chromosomes.

Avenol   See **ethchlorvynol**.

Aventyl   See **nortriptyline**.

average deviation   See **mean deviation**.

aversive conditioning   Method of behavior therapy that pairs a stimulus with a distasteful or repugnant reinforcement so that the patient learns to associate negative feelings with an undesirable behavior such as drug use or paraphilia.

aversive therapy   Controversial method of treating severe self-injurious behavior (SSIB) in developmentally disabled children with severe learning difficulties. Used in exceptional cases for patients whose SSIB is life-threatening and nonresponsive to nonaversive therapies, it incorporates unpleasant tastes and smells and especially electric shock. It may act speedily and have lasting effects, but should be used only by skilled staff members. The advent of microtechnology now allows smaller electric shocks to be administered remotely via a device worn by the patient (a sensor applied to the head to detect head banging is linked by radio to an electric shock stimulator on an arm or leg). Disadvantages of aversive methods include risk of causing harm or suffering if wrongly used; misapplication when other methods could perhaps have been introduced; and temptation for an over-stretched or inexperienced staff to turn to them as short-cuts. Nevertheless, with careful control, aversive therapy may bring substantial benefits with few side effects. Whenever aversive therapies are to be tried, both patients and staff must have safeguards, and the program should be reviewed by an independent ethical committee that could examine and agree on the need for treatment in individual cases. Such an approach could allay many fears about misuse, yet ensure availability for the very few people who might benefit from it.

avoidant personality   Personality characterized by a long-standing, pervasive, habitual and active withdrawal from social relationships; descriptive designation coined by Millon.

Avoxin   See **fluvoxamine**.

awakening   In polysomnography, return to the awake state from any non–rapid-eye-movement (non-REM) or REM sleep stages. It is characterized by alpha and beta electroencephalographic activity, rise in tonic electromyogram, voluntary rapid eye movements, and eye blinks. In addition, the polysomnogram must be paralleled by resumption of a reasonably alert state of awareness of the environment (Thorpy MJ. *Handbook of Sleep Disorders*. New York: Marcel Dekker, 1990).

axial dystonia   See **dystonia, axial**.

axial hyperkinesia   See **hyperkinesia, axial**.

axon   Part of the neuron consisting of a single fiber down which the action potential is transmitted to the nerve terminal.

Axoren   See **buspirone**.

azamianserin   (ORG-3770) Experimental antidepressant currently in phase III clinical trials in the United States.

azapirone   (AZP) Any of a structural class of anxiolytic compounds, the proposed mechanism of action of which is partial agonism of serotonin-1A ($5\text{-}HT_{1A}$) receptors and agonism of presynaptic $5\text{-}HT_{1A}$ receptors. Some also have a modest degree of activity at presynaptic dopamine receptors. Because of these actions, AZPs may be broad-spectrum psychotropics. Research and clinical data to date (1993) indicate that AZPs may effectively treat anxiety, depression, mixed anxiety-depression, behavioral dyscontrol in the developmentally disabled, and obsessive compulsive disorders.

Buspirone is the only marketed AZP. Others (gepirone, ipsapirone, tandospirone) are in various phases of clinical evaluation. Also called "arylpiperazine"; "azaspirodecanedi-one." See **buspirone; gepirone; ipsapirone; tandospirone.**

azaspirodecanedione   See **azaperone.**

Azurene   See **bromperidol**

B

Bacarate See **phendimetrazine**.

baclofen (Lioresal) Muscle relaxant and anti-spastic useful for alleviation of signs and symptoms of spasticity resulting from multiple sclerosis, particularly flexion or spasms and concomitant pain, clonus, and muscular rigidity. It contains gamma aminobutyric acid (GABA) and phenylethylamine moieties, producing dopaminergic agonism and antagonism and benzodiazepine-like agonism. It may act as a substance P antagonist. It has been used to reduce choreiform movements in Huntington's chorea and rigidity in Parkinson's disease. It has not been effective in the treatment of tardive dyskinesia or tardive dystonia. Its use should be carefully monitored and the dose increased gradually to reduce side effects. It is generally well tolerated; the most common side effect is sedation, which occasionally can be severe. Other side effects include nausea, vomiting, sedation, confusion, muscle weakness, and fatigue. Baclofen almost always causes confusion in patients with centrally determined spasticity. It should be used with great caution in epileptics, as it can make epilepsy worse. Agitation, confusion, psychosis, and mania have been reported upon abrupt discontinuation, and mania may occur during treatment (Stewart JT. A case of mania associated with high-dose baclofen therapy. *J Clin Psychopharmacol* 1992;12:215–216).

baclofen/breast milk Baclofen appears in milk in small amounts; it may be used by nursing mothers with caution (Eriksson G, Swahn C-G. Concentrations of baclofen in serum and breast milk from a lactating woman. *Scand J Clin Lab Invest* 1981;41:185–187).

baclofen + lithium Co-administration may aggravate hyperkinetic symptoms in patients with Huntington's chorea (Anden N-E, Dalen P, Johansson B. Baclofen and lithium in Huntington's chorea. *Lancet* 1973;2:93).

bacteriophage Virus that multiplies inside bacteria, often used by molecular geneticists to transfer foreign genetic information.

bactrim + warfarin See **warfarin + bactrim**.

"bad trip" Slang term for an acute adverse reaction to an hallucinogen or other pharmacological agents taken for pleasure. Although many drugs produce bad trips, the most common are lysergic acid diethylamide (LSD), mescaline, psilocybin, and marijuana. A bad trip may consist of an anxiety/panic reaction, dysphoric reaction, distorted perceptions, a paranoid hallucinatory state, or delirium. Bad trips are due to a combination of factors, including the user's pre-drug psychological state, the environment in which the drug is used, the purity and dose of the drug, the user's genetic vulnerability to the drug, and, possibly, the nature of the user's drug-induced distorted perceptions.

balanced placebo design Research technique that allows for the effect of subjects' beliefs about the treatment received by giving the experimental drug to subjects who believe it is a placebo and placebo to those who believe it is the experimental drug.

ballism Severe form of chorea involving proximal limb muscles. It is presumably due to lesions in the nucleus subthalamicus and is usually unilateral (hemiballism). The term "hemiballism/hemichorea" is often used to emphasize that any difference is a matter of degree.

ballismus Sudden, wild, jerky, darting movements of the arms and legs, with considerable rotary quality. It may occur spontaneously and also can follow abrupt discontinuation of neuroleptic therapy, particularly in children. If restricted to one side of the body, the disorder is called "hemiballismus."

band, chromosomal Development (1968) that allowed each chromosome to be identified individually for the first time. The International System for Human Cytogenetic Nomenclature (ISCN, 1981) identifies each chromosome band and sub-band in 400-, 550-, and 850-band preparations (Read A. *Medical Genetics. An Illustrated Outline.* London: Gower Medical Publishing, 1989).

banding technique Laboratory procedure that allows identification of an extra or missing chromosome and accurate localization of breakpoints in chromosome rearrangements. Each chromosome has a characteristic marking known as "banding." Technical developments have led to most laboratories recognizing between 400 and 800 bands on a chromosome, and in some cases up to 2,000 bands.

Banflex See **orphenadrine**.

"barb" Street name for barbiturates.

Barbased See **butabarbital**.

Barbita See **phenobarbital**.

Barbital See **phenobarbital**.

barbiturate Class of sedative hypnotic drugs introduced in the early part of the 20th century as replacements for paraldehyde and bromides. Named in honor of St. Barbara, on whose feast day in 1862 barbituric acid was first synthesized by Adolph von Bayer. Barbital was introduced into medical practice in 1903, and phenobarbital in 1912. Thereafter, over 2,500 derivatives of barbituric acid were synthesized, with more than 50 being used in medical practice. Barbiturates were widely prescribed as anxiolytics and sedatives/hypnotics until the 1970s, when the dangers of dependence and lethality in overdosage led to their replacement by the benzodiazepines.

barbiturate + carbamazepine Barbiturates can markedly lower carbamazepine (CBZ) serum concentrations and impede CBZ's therapeutic efficacy.

barbiturate + clomipramine Co-administration increases clomipramine (CMI) metabolism, resulting in lower levels of CMI and its active metabolite desmethylchlorimipramine and possibly interfering with CMI's therapeutic effects (Peters MD, Davis SK, Austin LS. Clomipramine: an antiobsessional tricyclic antidepressant. *Clin Pharm* 1990;9:165–178).

barbiturate intoxication Manifestations include headache, confusion, excitement, delirium, loss of corneal reflex, respiratory failure, and coma. Unabsorbed drug should be removed by lavage or catharsis, respiratory and cardiovascular systems should be stabilized, and drug elimination should be expedited by whatever techniques are feasible for each drug. Any dehydration should be corrected. Dialysis (rarely) may be needed with long-acting barbiturates for which alkalinization hastens excretion.

barbiturate + paroxetine Although paroxetine does not potentiate sedative or psychomotor effects of barbiturates, co-administration may increase adverse central nervous system effects (Cooper SM, Jackson D, Loudon JM, et al. The psychomotor effects of paroxetine alone and in combination with haloperidol, amylobarbitone, oxazepam or alcohol. *Acta Psychiatr Scand* 1989;80[suppl]:53–55).

barbiturate/street names barb, blue (amobarbital), blue angel (amobarbital), blue bird (amobarbital), blue devil (amobarbital), blue doll (amobarbital), candy Christmas tree (amobarbital + secobarbital), doll, double trouble (amobarbital + secobarbital), downer, goofball, goofer, lilly (amobarbital), nebbie (pentobarbital), nembie (pentobarbital), peanut, phennie (phenobarbital), pink (secobarbital), pink lady (secobarbital), purple heart (phenobarbital), rainbow (amobarbital + secobarbital), red (secobarbital), red and blue (amobarbital + secobarbital), red bird (secobarbital), red devil (secobarbital), red doll (secobarbital), seccy (secobarbital), sleeper, sleeping pill, t-bird (amobarbital + secobarbital), tooie (amobarbital + secobarbital), toolie (amobarbital + secobarbital), tootie (amobarbital + secobarbital), yellow (pentobarbital), yellow bullet (pentobarbital), yellow doll (pentobarbital), yellow football (pentobarbital), yellow jacket (pentobarbital).

barbiturate + tricyclic antidepressant (TCA) Barbiturates effectively lower TCA plasma levels (Alexanderson B, Price-Evans DA, Sjoqvist F. Steady-state plasma levels of nortriptyline in twins: influence of genetic factors and drug therapy. *Br Med J* 1969;4:764–768).

barbiturate + valproate Sodium valproate inhibits metabolism of phenobarbital by the liver, resulting in its accumulation in the body. Co-administration should be well monitored and suitable phenobarbital dosage reductions should be made when necessary to avoid excessive sedation and lethargy (de Gatta MRF, Gonzales ACA, et al. Effect of sodium valproate on phenobarbital serum levels in children and adults. *Ther Drug Monit* 1986;8:416–420).

"barb" Street name for barbiturates.

bar chart Graph used with nominal characteristics to display the numbers or percentages of observations for the variable of interest.

"barf tea" Street name for mescaline.

Barnetil See **sultopride.**

Barnotil See **sultopride.**

Barr body Chromosomal material seen at the edge of the nucleus of each cell of a normal human female, named after the discoverer of sexual dimorphism in somatic cells, Dr. Murray Barr. It can only be seen when stained with a special chemical and looked at under a microscope; Barr bodies are best studied by the buccal smear or oral mucosa techniques. The number of Barr bodies is always one less than the number of X chromosomes possessed. Barr bodies may be used in the diagnosis of abnormalities of the sex chromosomes in conditions associated with mental handicap (e.g., XXXX syndrome), although more sophisticated techniques for examining chromosomes have been developed. See **sex chromatin.**

basal ganglia Complex area of the brain that includes the corpus striatum (caudate nucleus, putamen, and globus pallidus), substantia nigra, claustrum, and subthalamic nucleus of Luys, which are concerned primarily with movement initiation and control. The basal ganglia contains the richest array in the central nervous system of neurotransmitters and their receptors. Basal ganglia disorders produce motor abnormalities characterized by rigidity, tremor, bradykinesia, and dyskinesia. They also may result in alterations of emotional expression or behavior, typically in association with movement disorders such as

Parkinson's disease, Wilson's disease, Huntington's disease, and Sydenham's chorea.

"base" Street name for cocaine freebase.

base See **nucleotide.**

"baseballer" Street name for a substance abuser who injects cocaine and heroin ("speedball").

base pair Two corresponding bases (adenosine-thyroinine or guanine-cytosine) inside an intact DNA molecule, held together by weak hydrogen bonds.

baseline Time prior to an intervention during which an initial measure is taken. Baseline observations should be continued until it is thought that the behavior is reliably represented and the treatment or intervention is started. Baseline measurements provide useful information and allow evaluation of the effects of the intervention.

bashful bladder syndrome See **paruresis.**

basuco See **coca paste.**

battered child syndrome Physical injuries and psychological trauma to children secondary to intentional acts of omission or repeated volitional excessive beatings by a parent or caretaker.

battered elder syndrome See **elder abuse.**

batterer Man who habitually beats women. Studies of batterers' clinical characteristics and personality traits show evidence of significant psychopathology including alcohol abuse, paranoid traits, and mild depression. They also appear to have borderline-antisocial personality traits, certain types of hostility, and histories of abuse as children (Else L., Wonderlich SA, Beatty WW, et al. Personality characteristics of men who physically abuse women. *Hosp Commun Psychiatry* 1992;44:54–58). There are also reports of men battered by women.

battery, quantitative electrophysiological See **electrophysiological test.**

"batu" Philippine slang term for dextroamphetamine ("ice").

Baye's theorem Formula for calculating the probability of an event's conditioning another event or events.

"bazooka" Street term for a cigarette made by adding 1/4 to 1/2 gram of coca paste to tobacco or marijuana. Coca paste, a grey-white or dull brown powder with a lightly sweet smell, is an intermediate product in the processing of cocaine hydrochloride. Also called "pasta."

B cell Lymphocyte subset that, although immunologically important, does not play a role in cell-mediated immunity.

"bean" Street name for amphetamine sulfate.

beat phenomenon Alternating coordination and interference between two uncoupled oscillators.

beclamide Drug used for treatment of behavior disorders and epilepsy in unstable, aggressive patients. Not widely used, it tends to be combined with other anticonvulsants. Side effects (e.g., weight loss, dizziness, and skin irritation) are mild and transient.

beclomethasone (Beconase) Potent corticosteroid used for the treatment of seasonal and perennial rhinitis and asthma. It has induced mania on rare occasions.

beclouded state See **delirium.**

Beconase See **beclomethasone.**

bedtime Clock time when one attempts to fall asleep (as distinguished from the clock time when one gets into bed).

befloxatone Selective, reversible pure competitive monoamine oxidase (MAO)-A inhibitor in phase II trials in Europe as an antidepressant. In clinical trials doses of 2.5 mg twice a day, 10 mg twice a day, and 40 mg twice a day were well tolerated. See **reversible inhibitor of monoamine oxidase type A.**

before-after trial Study in which individuals of one period and under one treatment are compared with individuals at a subsequent time, treated in a different fashion. If the disorder is not fatal and "before" treatment is not curative, the same subjects may be studied in the before and after periods, which strengthens the design through increased group comparability for the two periods (Anon. Glossary of methodologic terms. *JAMA* 1992;268:43–44). See **crossover design.**

behavior despair test See **Porsolt test.**

behavior modification Therapeutic approach based on the observation that an organism learns to repeat rewarding behaviors such as food-seeking and to avoid behaviors that produce a noxious response such as pain. In humans, social rewards are so important that an individual may tolerate unpleasant consequences to obtain even minor or negative social interaction. See **behavior therapy.**

behavior therapy Systematic application of learning theory principles to treat behavior disorders ranging from motor reflexes to complicated behavioral sequences. Treatment focus is on observable and measurable physiological or environmental events and on the patient's resultant behaviors rather than on mental states and constructs. Behaviors are analyzed, and an appropriate behavioral treatment technique is chosen. Indications include phobias, obsessions, compulsions, psychosomatic phenomena, and behavioral deficits. Techniques include (a) systematic desensitization; (b) flooding; (c) response prevention; (d) assertiveness training; (e) operant methods using positive and negative reinforcement; (f) aversion; (g) biofeedback; (h) social skills training; and (i) sex therapy. Behavior therapy is important for patients wishing to discontinue medication, because relapse rates with medication discontinuation are quite high. Behavior therapy alone can be effective when patients comply with exposure and ritual reduction instructions. The combination of a serotonin uptake inhibitor (e.g., clomipramine, fluoxetine, fluvoxamine, paroxetine, sertraline) with behavior therapy may be optimal treatment for many obsessive-compulsive disorder patients. It is effective and economical, and provides lasting reduction.

behavior therapy, dialectical (DBT) Combination of strategies from behavioral, cognitive, and supportive psychotherapies administered according to a treatment manual. It includes concomitant, weekly individual and group therapy for 1 year. Individual DBT uses directive, problem-oriented techniques (including behavioral skill training, contingency management, cognitive modification, and exposure to emotional cues) and supportive techniques (e.g., reflection, empathy, acceptance). Behavioral goals are prioritized according to importance. Problem focus of each individual is jointly determined by this hierarchy and the patient's behavior in each targeted area since the last session (Linehan MM. *Dialectical Behavior Therapy for Treatment of Parasuicidal Women: Treatment Manual.* Seattle: University of Washington, 1984; Linehan MM, Armstrong HE, Suarez A, et al. Cognitive-behavioral treatment of chronically parasuicidal borderline patients. *Arch Gen Psychiatry* 1991;48: 1060–1064).

behavioral disinhibition See **behavioral dyscontrol.**

behavioral dyscontrol Increase in hostility and aggressiveness ranging from feelings to overt behavior including rage reaction, paroxysmal excitement, irritability, and suicide attempts that can be provoked by alcohol and psychotropic drugs (e.g., the benzodiazepines, such as alprazolam) (Gardner DL, Cowdry RW. Alprazolam-induced dyscontrol in borderline personality disorder. *Am J Psychiatry* 1985;142: 98–100). Also called "behavioral disinhibition." See **disinhibition; paradoxical reaction.**

behavioral genetics See **genetics, behavioral.**

behavioral medicine Psychological interventions, prevention and treatment; application of behavioral theory and therapy to the treatment of medical disorders. Less than 20 years old, the term overlaps with "health psychology." Distinctions between the two are by no means clear, although health psychology is the more comprehensive, referring to all psychological aspects of illness and health care.

behavioral neurotoxicity Adverse effects of drugs on the central nervous system that induce abnormal behavior, including worsening of target symptoms, hyperactivity or hypoactivity, aggressivity, irritability, mood changes, and psychomotor retardation. See **behavioral toxicity.**

behavioral sensitization See **tolerance, reverse.**

behavioral teratogenicity See **teratogenicity, behavioral.**

behavioral tolerance See **tolerance, behavioral.**

behavioral toxicity Impairment of abilities necessary to perform psychomotor and cognitive tasks of everyday life induced by a variety of pharmacological agents, especially psychopharmaceuticals. Reactions may range from mild anxiety to severe psychotic symptoms. Symptoms that may occur singly or conjointly include (a) drowsiness; (b) insomnia; (c) vivid dreams; (d) nightmares; (e) depression; (f) excitement; (g) anxiety; (h) irritability; (i) hyperacusis; (j) listlessness; and (k) restlessness. Such symptoms may be precursors of a more florid psychiatric disorder (e.g., delirium). Behavioral toxicity manifested by akathisia and its subjective changes in affect may be erroneously attributed to illness-caused agitation and treated by increasing the dosage of the responsible drug, which worsens the drug-induced reaction. Behavioral toxicity generally occurs shortly after initiation of treatment with the causative drug. It is often, but not always, dose-dependent and usually remits after discontinuation of the etiologic agent. In some cases it can be severe, long-lasting, incapacitating, and possibly life-threatening. All types of psychoactive drugs have produced behavioral toxicity. Significant drug-induced behavioral toxicity can increase the risk of a drug-related accident and also be counter-therapeutic (Hindmarch I, Kerr J. Behavioral toxicity of antidepressants and particular reference to moclobemide. *Psychopharmacology* 1992;106:S49–S55). In child psychiatry, behavioral toxicity refers to some neuroleptic adverse effects, such as hypoactivity, apathy, social withdrawal, cognitive dulling, and sedation. See **acute confusional state; akathisia; psychotic exacerbation.**

Beldin See **diphenhydramine.**

bell-shaped distribution Shape of the normal (Gaussian) distribution.

Bell's mania Infrequent but severe form of mania manifested by sudden onset; severe insomnia; anorexia; disorientation; paranoia; bizarre hallucinations and delusions; confusion and bewilderment; delirium; and extremely disturbed and psychotic behavior (basis for the term *raving maniac*). Symptoms suggest that the mania may be due to an organic mental disorder. Electroconvulsive therapy is considered the treatment of choice. A combination of lithium and neuroleptics is more likely to be beneficial than lithium monotherapy. Also called "delirious mania."

benactyzine + meprobamate See **Deprol.**

Benadryl See **diphenhydramine.**

benapryzine Anticholinergic drug used in the treatment of Parkinson's disease.

beneficial effects of drugs Drug therapeutic efficacy against a given illness, condition, or target symptoms.

Benemid See **probenecid.**

benefit Therapeutic efficacy of drug or any therapy.

benefit-risk ratio Balance of a drug's therapeutic efficacy (benefit) with its liability to cause side effects (risk). The ratio should be determined both for the potential patient population as a whole and for each individual patient. An effective drug with serious side effects is more acceptable for a patient with a potentially fatal disease than a similarly toxic but effective drug in a patient with a self-limiting disease. Clinical trials characterize common side effects, but not those occurring more rarely.

"benny" Street name for amphetamines in general or specifically for the amphetamine benzedrine.

Benozil See **flurazepam.**

benperidol (Anquil; Concillium; Frenactil) Butyrophenone derivative antipsychotic that may be effective in reducing sexual interest. It has been used to treat deviant and antisocial sexual behavior, but efficacy has not been established by controlled trials. Benperidol should be introduced gradually to avoid drowsiness or insomnia. Most common side effects are muscle rigidity, spasms, and tremor (extrapyramidal signs) responsive to antiparkinson drugs. It can (rarely) cause hypotension, akathisia, and allergic reactions. Tardive dyskinesia also may occur.

benserazide Peripheral decarboxylase inhibitor that increases brain catecholamine levels when given simultaneously with levodopa. It potentiates and increases the duration of the effect of levodopa in parkinson patients, allowing significant (up to 75%) reduction of the effective dose of levodopa. Co-administration largely eliminates peripheral side effects of levodopa, but abnormal involuntary movements tend to develop earlier and in more severe form. See **co-beneldopa.**

bentazepam + clomipramine In a multicenter open study in patients with major depression, clomipramine (CMI) + bentazepam was better than CMI alone in reducing anxiety, with equal or better tolerability (Calcedo Ordonez A, Arosamene X, Otero Perez FJ, et al. Clomipramine/bentazepam in the treatment of major depressive disorders. *Hum Psychopharmacol* 1992;7:115–122).

Benylin See **dextromethorphan.**

Benzaline See **nitrazepam.**

benzamide Any of a new class of neuroleptics divided into four main categories of derivatives: aminoethyls (e.g., metoclopramide), 2-pyrolidyls (e.g., sulpiride) 3-pyrrolidyl, and 4-piperidyl. Benzamides are considered atypical neuroleptics because they are selective dopamine D_2 antagonists with a lower propensity to cause extrapyramidal effects than neuroleptics that have mixed D_1 and D_2 receptor antagonistic properties. The prototype is sulpiride; metoclopramide is an antiemetic.

Benzedrine See **amphetamine.**

Benzhexol See **trihexyphenidyl.**

benzodiazepine (BZD) Member of a group of drugs with sedative, anxiolytic, muscle-relaxant, and anticonvulsant effects. Fifteen are marketed in the United States (1993). BZDs vary widely in milligram potency and have qualitative differences in speed of onset of action and duration of clinical activity after single doses. Their pharmacokinetics also differ, particularly in respect to metabolic pathway, receptor affinity, lipid solubility, and elimination half-life. They can be divided into three general categories. *Ultrashort* (less than 5 hours) half-life BZDs (e.g., triazolam and midazolam) do not accumulate and are almost always used as hypnotics. *Short and intermediate* (5–24 hours) half-life BZDs (e.g., oxazepam, lorazepam, and alprazolam) have limited accumulation of parent drug and insignificant accumulation of active metabolites. *Long* (greater than 24 hours) half-life BZDs (e.g., chlordiazepoxide, diazepam, clorazepate, prazepam, clonazepam, and quazepam) frequently have active metabolites; both parent drugs and metabolites may accumulate during chronic therapy. BZDs are safe and effective treatments for a variety of anxiety states, but not for endogenous depression (Schatzberg AF, Cole JO. Benzodiazepines in depressive disorders. *Arch Gen Psychiatry* 1978;24:509–514; Klerman GL, Deltito J. The use of benzodiazepines in the treatment of depression. *Int Drug Ther Newsl* 1986;21:37–38). BZDs are ineffective in treating chronic aggressive behaviors and may aggravate aggression or precipitate rage attacks. They may be a cause of anxiety as a symptom of withdrawal. Four BZDs are available in parenteral formulations: chlordiazepoxide, diazepam, lorazepam, and midazolam. Intramuscular administration is not advisable except for lorazepam and midazolam. BZDs are not thought to stimulate hepatic microsomal oxidizing systems, but their metabolism may be altered by drugs that do affect hepatic function.

benzodiazepine/adjunctive therapy Acutely agitated psychotic patients may respond to the addition of a benzodiazepine (BZD) to antipsychotic drug therapy. The BZD is sedating and lessens acute agitation more rapidly than does the antipsychotic alone, allowing reduction in the neuroleptic dosage and lessening the risk and severity of early-onset extrapyramidal reactions, particularly dystonia and akathisia. Approximately one-third to one-half of chronic treatment–resistant patients respond to adjunctive BZD therapy. Lorazepam, clonazepam, diazepam, chlordiazepoxide, and alprazolam are used most often, in the same dosage ranges used for the treatment of anxiety. Doses at the upper end of the therapeutic range may be more effective than lower doses. Until more is known about the safety of long-term BZD adjunctive therapy, some experts advocate short-term use because of the risk of tolerance, dependency, and withdrawal reactions (Wolkowitz OM, Pickar D. Benzodiazepines in the treatment of schizophrenia: a review and reappraisal. *Am J Psychiatry* 1991;148:714–726). See **benzodiazepine + neuroleptic.**

benzodiazepine + alcohol Alcohol has no significant effects on benzodiazepine (BZD) pharmacokinetics, but has a clear influence on BZD pharmacodynamics. Central nervous system depressant effects of alcohol and BZDs are additive. Even in anxious subjects, the combination never improves driving performance and in most cases impairs driving ability to a greater extent than either substance taken alone. BZDs interact with low blood alcohol levels to produce greater impairment than would be expected from such a low blood level. Under no circumstances should a patient taking a benzodiazepine drink alcohol and then drive an automobile (Salzman C. Behavioral side effects of benzodiazepines. *In* Kane JM, Lieberman JA [eds], *Adverse Effects of Psychotropic Drugs.* New York: Guilford Press, 1992, pp 139–152). Reports of "traveler's amnesia" indicate that the amnestic effect of BZDs also is enhanced by alcohol.

benzodiazepine antagonist Chemical substance exerting an antagonistic action on benzodiazepine receptors. See **flumazenil.**

benzodiazepine + anticholinergic Co-administration may induce more severe cognitive impairment than either drug alone. Because many antidepressants, antipsychotics, and antiparkinson agents possess anticholinergic properties, adverse cognitive interactions may be common, particularly among the elderly.

benzodiazepine + beta-blocker Co-administration may be more effective than either class of drug alone in generalized anxiety disorder (GAD), especially in patients with treatment-resistant GAD.

benzodiazepine binding sites These are present in different densities throughout the central nervous system. Density is highest in the cerebral cortex, especially frontal cortex, structures of the limbic system, the cerebellar cortex, and a few specific regions of the brain stem. Benzodiazepine binding sites are part of a "supramolecular receptor complex" in the neuronal membrane that includes a binding site for the inhibitory amino acid neurotransmitter gamma-aminobutyric acid (GABA), a chloride channel, and binding sites for other modulators. When GABA binds to its binding site in this complex, it causes an "opening" of the chloride channel, allowing negatively charged chloride ions to enter the neuron, hyperpolarizing the neuronal membrane and making it more difficult for excitatory synaptic input to sufficiently depolarize the cell for the generation of an action potential. The efficiency of this inhibitory influence is potentiated by the binding of a benzodiazepine to its binding site, causing the chloride channels to open more frequently in response to GABA (Teboul E, Chouinard G. A guide to benzodiazepine selection. Part I: pharmacological aspects. *Can J Psychiatry* 1990;35:700–710).

benzodiazepine biotransformation See **benzodiazepine grouping.**

benzodiazepine/breast milk Benzodiazepines (BZDs) with long-acting metabolites can accumulate in breast-fed infants, especially neonates, because of their immature excretory mechanisms. Adverse effects include lethargy, jaundice, and weight loss. Long-acting BZDs should be avoided if possible during breastfeeding, particularly in the neonatal period. When BZD therapy is essential, the short-acting agents oxazepam and lorazepam appear to be preferable. Midazolam and its active metabolite attain low levels in milk only transiently after a 15-mg oral dose; intravenous administration has not been studied. Breast milk should be withheld for 6–8 hours after a single dose of diazepam for short procedures, such as dental work or endoscopy. Diazepam and several other BZD-like substances occur naturally in breast milk in very small, not necessarily meaningful amounts; their source and physiologic effects are not clear (Anderson PO. Drug use during breastfeeding. *Clin Pharm* 1991;10:594–624).

benzodiazepine + carbamazepine Carbamazepine (CBZ) can decrease plasma levels of benzodiazepines, reducing their efficacy. CBZ induces metabolism of clobazam and clonazepam (Brodie MJ. Established anticonvulsants and treatment of refractory epilepsy. *Lancet* 1990;336:350–354). See **carbamazepine + alprazolam.**

benzodiazepine + cimetidine   Because cimetidine inhibits hepatic microsomal enzymes, it may reduce hepatic clearance and increase plasma concentrations of benzodiazepines (BZDs) metabolized by oxidation (e.g., alprazolam, chlordiazepoxide, clorazepate, diazepam, estazolam, flurazepam, halazepam, prazepam, quazepam, temazepam, and triazolam). Dosage adjustment may be necessary to avert BZD toxicity during co-administration.

benzodiazepine + clomipramine   No pharmacokinetic interactions have been detected.

benzodiazepine + clozapine   Co-administration can produce severe sedation, hypersalivation, hypotension, toxic delirium, collapse, loss of consciousness and respiratory arrest. Symptoms usually occur within 1–2 days of starting high doses of clozapine (CLOZ) in patients taking long-acting benzodiazepines (BZDs) (Grohmann R, Ruther E, Sassim N, Schmidt LG. Adverse effects of clozapine. *Psychopharmacology* 1989;99[suppl]:S101–S104; Cobb CD, Anderson CB, Seidel DR. Possible interaction between clozapine and lorazepam. *Am J Psychiatry* 1991;148:1606–1607; Friedman LJ, Tabb SE, Sanchez CJ. Clozapine—a novel antipsychotic agent. *N Engl J Med* 1991;325:518). Although such reactions are rare, BZDs should be used cautiously when initiating CLOZ treatment. Whether BZDs increase frequency of respiratory arrest or sudden death due to other causes in CLOZ-treated patients, and whether risk is greater than with other drugs, are unclear. BZDs are sometimes needed to treat anxiety when initiating CLOZ in neuroleptic-free patients. Naber et al. report no additional adverse effects of the combination of BZDs and CLOZ (Naber D, Holzbach R, Perro C, et al. Clinical management of clozapine patients in relation to efficacy and side effects. *Br J Psychiatry* 1992;160[suppl 17]:54–59). Some therapists co-prescribe BZDs to treat agitation, anxiety, seizure disorder, or refractory psychotic symptoms in CLOZ-treated patients. In eight treatment-refractory patients, CLOZ (mean daily dose 860.50 mg) plus lorazepam (3.88 mg/day) or clonazepam (1.5 mg/day) for a mean duration of 15.44 months produced significant improvement without serious respiratory depression or arrest. Results suggest that CLOZ-BZD therapy, when carefully monitored, may be safe and clinically effective for some patients (Grace JJ, Priest B, Yadav M. Long-term clozapine and benzodiazepines: eight case reviews. Presented at the 146th annual meeting of the American Psychiatric Association, San Francisco, May 1993). Clinicians need to compare the risk-benefit ratio of combining a BZD and CLOZ with disadvantages of continued use of typical neuroleptic drugs. When the combination is first given, it may be desirable to have the patient hospitalized or observed in an outpatient setting for 2–4 hours (Meltzer HY. New drugs for the treatment of schizophrenia. *Psychiatr Clin North Am* 1993;16:365–385). See **clozapine + diazepam.**

benzodiazepine dependence   Despite the high incidence of benzodiazepine dependence, it is impossible to predict who is likely to become dependent, apart from those with a history of dependence on other drugs.

benzodiazepine dependence/secondary   State that arises in the context of multiple drug abuse and/or alcoholism. It often is a consequence of substance abusers using benzodiazepines (BZDs) (a) to counteract some unpleasant adverse effects associated with substance abuse; (b) to augment effects of other abused substances when they are in short supply; and (c) as a temporary substitute for an abused substance when its supply is exhausted. Secondary BZD dependence is much more frequent than primary BZD dependence.

benzodiazepine disinhibition   Agitation, belligerency, and assaultiveness that occasionally may be provoked by any benzodiazepine. Some reports suggest that the reaction is more likely to occur in patients with pre-existing brain damage (Salzman C. Anxiety in the elderly: treatment strategies. *J Clin Psychiatry* 1990;51[suppl]:18–21). Also called "paradoxical excitation." See **behavioral dyscontrol.**

benzodiazepine + disulfiram   Co-administration increases sedation and decreases benzodiazepine (BZD) clearance; BZD dosage adjustment may be necessary to avert toxicity. Disulfiram may also increase the half-lives of oxidatively metabolized BZDs. See **benzodiazepine grouping.**

benzodiazepine dose equivalents   Diazepam 5 mg is equivalent to: alprazolam 0.25 mg, chlordiazepoxide 25 mg, clonazepam 4 mg, clorazepate 3.75 mg, flurazepam 15 mg, halazepam 40 mg, lorazepam 1 mg, oxazepam 30 mg, prazepam 10 mg, temazepam 15 mg, and triazolam 0.5 mg.

benzodiazepine/elderly   Benzodiazepines (BZDs) are frequently prescribed for elderly patients, especially women, living in the community and for elderly patients in hospitals and nursing homes. There is abundant evidence that the elderly can benefit from the anxiolytic, sedative, and hypnotic activity of

BZDs. However, they are often prolonged BZD users not only for insomnia and anxiety, but for a range of nonspecific medical and psychiatric symptoms. Studies have documented durations of use of 1–5, 5–10, and more than 10 years. BZDs are relatively free of serious adverse effects in low doses for short periods, but the elderly are particularly prone to adverse reactions to both anxiolytic and hypnotic BZDs. Shorter-acting BZDs are better tolerated. Longer-acting BZDs are more likely to cause problems, however, because the elderly are prone to drug accumulation with unwanted sedative or central inhibitory effects that can cause cognitive changes. BZD clearance is delayed because of high lipid solubility and age-related increases in the proportion of adipose tissue. Delayed liver metabolism also plays a role in BZD accumulation, resulting in motor incoordination and delirium. Unwanted BZD effects, predominantly manifestations of central nervous system depression, are significantly increased in hospitalized elderly patients. These include excessive sedation, cognitive impairment, falls, and vulnerability to withdrawal symptoms. Hypnotics/sedatives as a group, and BZDs in particular, have been frequently implicated in drug-associated hospital admissions in elderly patients. The exact incidence of BZD dependency and withdrawal in the elderly is unknown, but since the risk of dependence and withdrawal is associated with prolonged use, the elderly may be at particular risk of dependence and withdrawal after the abrupt discontinuation of a BZD. Furthermore, since the clinical effects of BZDs are partly determined by their pharmacokinetics and pharmacodynamics, their alteration in the elderly are important and should not be overlooked by prescribers. Elderly patients are more sensitive to the side effects of BZDs because they excrete BZDs slowly, resulting in accumulation. They become more sedated and dependent at lower doses, and are more likely to appear demented because of medication-induced confusion, memory and other cognitive impairments, agitation, and disinhibition (Kruse WHH. Problems and pitfalls in the use of benzodiazepines in the elderly. *Drug Safety* 1990;5:328–334).

benzodiazepine + electroconvulsive therapy (ECT) It is often asserted that patients being treated with benzodiazepines (BZDs) should not be given ECT because the BZD's anticonvulsant properties might modify seizures and decrease the antidepressant efficacy of ECT. A BZD may shorten an ECT-induced seizure, but there are no substantive data indicating that BZD therapy diminishes ECT efficacy. On the other hand, BZD therapy may impede the full therapeutic effect of unilateral ECT and should be discontinued before unilateral ECT is administered (Pettinati HM, Stephens SM, Willis KM, Robin SE. Evidence for less improvement in depression in patients taking benzodiazepines during unilateral ECT. *Am J Psychiatry* 1990;147:1029–1036; Cohen SI, Lawton C. Do benzodiazepines interfere with the action of electroconvulsive therapy? *Br J Psychiatry* 1992;160:545–546).

benzodiazepine + erythromycin Erythromycin inhibits hepatic microsomal enzymes and may reduce hepatic clearance and increase plasma concentrations of benzodiazepines metabolized by oxidation (e.g., alprazolam, chlordiazepoxide, clorazepate, diazepam, estazolam, flurazepam, halazepam, prazepam, quazepam, temazepam, and triazolam).

benzodiazepine + fluoxetine Fluoxetine (FLX) inhibits hepatic microsomal enzymes and may reduce hepatic clearance and increase plasma concentrations of benzodiazepines metabolized by oxidation (e.g., alprazolam, chlordiazepoxide, clorazepate, diazepam, estazolam, flurazepam, halazepam, prazepam, quazepam, temazepam, and triazolam). FLX does not affect glucuronidated BZDs (e.g., lorazepam, oxazepam, and clonazepam).

benzodiazepine + fluvoxamine In open and controlled studies, fluvoxamine has been combined with benzodiazepines and lithium with no report of interactions (Stimmel GL, Skowron DM, Chameides WA. Focus on fluvoxamine: a serotonin reuptake inhibitor for major depression and obsessive-compulsive disorder. *Hosp Formul* 1991;26:635–643).

benzodiazepine/glucuronidation Benzodiazepines metabolized by glucuronidation include clonazepam, lorazepam, and oxazepam.

benzodiazepine grouping Benzodiazepines (BZDs) can be grouped according to their elimination half-lives, chemical structure, or method of biotransformation. Based on elimination half-life, BZDs can be divided into three groups: (a) Ultrashort-acting ($t_{1/2}$ <5 hours; triazolam and midazolam); (b) short- or short-to-intermediate-acting ($t_{1/2}$ 6–12 hours; oxazepam, lorazepam and alprazolam); (c) Long-acting ($t_{1/2}$ >12 hours; chlordiazepoxide, diazepam, clorazepate, prazepam, clonazepam, and quazepam). Patients receiving a short half-life BZD react more quickly to dosage changes than patients receiving long half-life agents. BZD grouping according to chemical structure includes (a) 1,4 BZDs that contain nitrogen atoms at positions 1 and 4 in the diazepine ring (bromazepam, chlordiazepoxide, clonazepam, clorazepate, diazepam, flunitrazepam, flurazepam, lorazepam, lormetazepam, midazolam, nitrazepam, oxazepam, prazepam, quazepam, and temazepam; (b) 1,5 BZDs that contain nitrogen atoms at positions 1 and 5 in the diazepine ring (clobazam); (c) triazolo-BZDs that often consist of the 1,4 BZD nucleus with an additional ring fused at positions 1 and 2 (alprazolam, loprazolam, midazolam, and triazolam). BZD grouping according to biotransformation includes (a) BZDs biotransformed by oxidative reaction in the liver, primarily N-demethylation or hydroxylation (adinazolam, alprazolam, bromazepam, chlordiazepoxide, clobazam, clonazepam, diazepam, estazolam, flunitrazepam, medazepam, and nitrazepam). These processes often yield pharmacologically active metabolites that must undergo further metabolic steps prior to excretion; (b) conjugated BZDs that do not have active metabolites (lorazepam, lormetazepam, oxazepam, and temazepam). Only the parent compounds account for clinical activity; (c) BZDs that undergo a high first-pass effect prior to reaching the systemic circulation and have a metabolic rate closely associated with hepatic blood flow (brotizolam, clotiazepam, midazolam, and triazolam). These agents may have short-lived active metabolites.

benzodiazepine holiday Drug-free interval during which need for continued benzodiazepine BZD therapy is assessed. For long-acting BZDs, drug-free periods should last a week or more to allow BZD metabolites to clear from the body. For intermediate- and short-acting BZDs, the drug holiday should be between 2 and 7 days. During the holiday, symptoms suppressed by the BZD as well as some early withdrawal symptoms may occur. Patients need to be encouraged to tolerate these symptoms, knowing that reinstitution of BZD therapy usually provides prompt relief. To ensure compliance, patients must be told of the purpose and benefits of a BZD holiday and be reassured that BZD therapy will be restarted when necessary.

benzodiazepine hypnotic See **hypnotic, benzodiazepine.**

benzodiazepine + isoniazid Isoniazid inhibits hepatic microsomal enzymes and may reduce hepatic clearance and increase plasma concentrations of benzodiazepines metabolized by oxidation (e.g., alprazolam, chlordiazepoxide, clorazepate, diazepam, estazolam, flurazepam, halazepam, prazepam, quazepam, temazepam, and triazolam).

benzodiazepine + levodopa Co-administration may decrease levodopa's therapeutic effects.

benzodiazepine + lithium Co-administration may be associated with sexual dysfunction in about 50% of patients. In men, it may be associated with difficulty in achieving an erection, decreased quality of orgasm in some patients, and improved quality of orgasm in others. In women, it may be associated with absence or change in quantity of menstrual blood. Because inhibition of sexual response with benzodiazepines (BZDs) alone has been reported, it is not known if sexual dysfunction occurring with lithium plus a BZD is due to the combination or to the BZD alone. It is also possible that lithium potentiates the effects of BZDs on sexual function (Ghadirian A-M, Annable L, Belanger M-C. Lithium, benzodiazepines, and sexual function in bipolar patients. *Am J Psychiatry* 1992;149:801–805).

benzodiazepine/mania High milligram potency benzodiazepines (BZDs) (e.g., clonazepam and lorazepam) in doses of 10–15 mg/day have been used alone or in combination with other antimanic drugs to treat acute mania. These drugs, especially clonazepam, have anticonvulsant and sedative properties that may be responsible for their antimanic efficacy. Clonazepam is more effective than placebo for acute mania (Edwards R, Stephenson V, Flewett T. Clonazepam in acute mania: a double-blind trial. *Aust N Z J Psychiatry* 1991; 25:238–242). Clonazepam is more effective than lithium in the first phase of treatment but less effective than lorazepam (Chouinard G, Young SN, Annable L. Antimanic effect of clonazepam. *Biol Psychiatry* 1982;18:451–466; Bradwejn J, Shiqui C, Koszycki D, et al. Double-blind comparison of the effects of clonazepam and lorazepam in acute mania. *J Clin Psychopharmacol* 1990;10:403–408). When combined with neuroleptics for treating acute mania, BZDs reduce the need for higher neuroleptic dosages. See **clonazepam; lorazepam.**

benzodiazepine + moclobemide In a meta-analysis, 467 patients received one or several benzodiazepines with moclobemide. Tolerance was rated as very good or good in over 83%, and there was no evidence of any relevant pharmacokinetic or pharmacological interactions (Amrein R, Guntert TW, Dingemanse J, et al. Interactions of moclobemide with concomitantly administered medication: evidence from pharmacological and clinical studies. *Psychopharmacology* 1992;106:S24–S31).

benzodiazepine + neuroleptic Co-administration is currently used as an adjunct in the treatment of partially unresponsive or nonresponsive schizophrenia and in acutely agitated, psychotic patients; as a substitute for neuroleptics alone in the acute treatment of mania; and as acute treatment for catatonia. There is no evidence that one benzodiazepine (BZD) is more effective than another, but many experienced clinicians recommend higher-potency BZDs (e.g., lorazepam, clonazepam, alprazolam). Although there is evidence that BZDs are efficacious in the treatment of acute mania, there is no evidence that they are equal or superior alternatives to neuroleptics alone or that co-administration of a BZD and a neuroleptic is more effective than a neuroleptic alone. There is some evidence that co-administration may allow use of a lower neuroleptic dose (Arana GW, Ornsteen ML, Kanter F, et al. The use of benzodiazepines for psychotic disorders: a literature review and preliminary clinical findings. *Psychopharmacol Bull* 1986;22:77–87; Salzman C, Green AI, Rodriquez-Villa F, et al. Benzodiazepines combined with neuroleptics for management of severe disruptive behavior. *Psychosomatics* 1986;27:17–21; Garza-Trevino ES, Hollister LE, Overall JE, et al. Efficacy of combinations of intramuscular antipsychotics and sedative-hypnotics for control of psychotic agitation. *Am J Psychiatry* 1989;146:1598–1601). Parenterally administered (intramuscular or intravenous) BZD has been found to be effective in the treatment of catatonia. The majority of patients have been treated with intramuscularly administered lorazepam or intravenously administered diazepam. If results are not seen quickly with lorazepam, aggressive treatment with a high-potency neuroleptic should be started (Easton MS, Janicak PG. Benzodiazepines for the management of psychosis. *Psychiatr Med* 1991;9:25–36). Of 16 double-blind studies assessing adjunctive BZD treatment in schizophrenia, 7 reported positive results and 4 reported mixed or transiently positive results. Overall response rate of patients is 30–50% (Wolkowitz OM, Pickar D. Benzodiazepines in the treatment of schizophrenia: a review and reappraisal. *Am J Psychiatry* 1991;148:714–726; Arana GW, Ornsteen ML, Kanter F, et al. The use of benzodiazepines for psychotic disorders: a literature review and preliminary clinical findings. *Psychopharmacol Bull* 1986;22:77–87). Therapeutic response to adjunctive BZDs usually occurs within hours or within 2–3 weeks. If it does not, BZDs should be withdrawn. In some cases, BZDs lose efficacy after several weeks as tolerance develops. New data suggest that severely refractory patients show little response other than sedation to BZD augmentation. In some patients, high doses are needed to achieve a therapeutic response. Close monitoring during dosage titration is necessary to avert behavioral disinhibition, a side effect that occurs in approximately 10% of patients and that responds to dosage lowering (Wolkowitz OM. Rational polypharmacy

in schizophrenia. *Ann Clin Psychiatry* 1993;5:79–90). See **benzodiazepine/adjunctive therapy.**

benzodiazepine + neuroleptic + valproate Combination frequently used when manic patients have psychotic symptoms such as hallucinations, threats to others, and insomnia not responsive to benzodiazepines (BZDs). Concomitant use of valproate, a neuroleptic, and a BZD (clonazepam, lorazepam) as clinically indicated is safe and effective and reduces drop-outs. Furthermore, a BZD can enhance sedation and reduce the amount of neuroleptic needed. As the manic episode comes under control, dosage of the neuroleptic and the BZD is reduced gradually until it has been discontinued totally. See **benzodiazepine/adjunctive therapy; benzodiazepine + neuroleptic.**

benzodiazepine + nicotine Data are conflicting. Smokers treated with benzodiazepines (BZDs) are reported to experience less drowsiness from their medication. Smokers showed a significantly shorter half-life and lower C_{max} (peak plasma concentration) of the active metabolites of clorazepate and desmethyldiazepam. Oxazepam clearance also has been found to be higher in smokers than in nonsmokers. However, no significant differences in clearance, volume of distribution, and half-life of diazepam, midazolam, lorazepam, and triazolam have been demonstrated between smokers and nonsmokers (Kim YJ. Tobacco smoking and psychotropic drug therapy. *Pharmacy News* 1992;21:1–11).

benzodiazepine + omeprazole Omeprazole inhibits hepatic microsomal enzymes and may reduce hepatic clearance and increase plasma concentrations of benzodiazepines metabolized by oxidation (e.g., alprazolam, chlordiazepoxide, clorazepate, diazepam, estazolam, flurazepam, halazepam, prazepam, quazepam, temazepam, and triazolam).

benzodiazepine + opioid analgesic Co-administration results in various and often contradictory pharmacological effects that depend principally on the pharmacodynamic action studied (i.e., sedation-hypnosis, respiratory depression, analgesia, hemodynamics), the interacting agents, and the route of administration. Different benzodiazepines can alter opioid-associated respiratory mechanics differently (Maurer PM, Bartkowski RR. Drug interactions of clinical significance with opioid analgesics. *Drug Safety* 1993;8:30–48).

benzodiazepine + oral contraceptive Oral contraceptives may decrease benzodiazepine clearance, leading to a slower peak in plasma levels (Abernethy DR, Greenblatt DR, Divoll M, Arendt R, Ochs HR, Shader RI. Impairment of diazepam metabolism by low-dose estrogen-containing oral-contraceptive steroids. *N Engl J Med* 1982;306:791–792).

benzodiazepine overdose Taken alone in overdose, benzodiazepines (BZDs) seldom produce serious effects, causing only mild to moderate signs of toxicity in most cases. Patients usually present with somnolence, diplopia, dysarthria, ataxia, and intellectual impairment. Prolonged deep coma (grade 3–4) or deep cyclic coma are rare. Stage 2 coma (unresponsive to painful stimuli) should provoke a search for other toxic substances, since severity of BZD poisoning is influenced by co-ingestion of other central nervous system (CNS) depressants. Other factors that could influence severity of CNS depression are dose ingested, type of BZD, and age and health of the patient before the overdose (Gaudreault P, Guay J, Thivierge RL, Verdy I. Benzodiazepine poisoning. Clinical and pharmacological considerations and treatment. *Drug Safety* 1991;6:247–265). In patients with obstructive pulmonary disease, BZDs in moderate doses can cause carbon dioxide narcosis because they depress ventilatory response to carbon dioxide. Depression of consciousness occurs after overdose; consciousness can return even though blood concentrations are still very high, presumably because of rapid development of tolerance. During recovery from BZD overdose, rebound insomnia and other BZD withdrawal effects occur.

benzodiazepine overdose/pregnancy Benzodiazepine (BZD) overdose during pregnancy rarely induces serious morbidity in the mother or fetus. However, large doses of BZDs administered to mothers near delivery can induce serious prolonged respiratory depression in neonates, especially if they are pre-term (Gaudreault P, Guay J, Thivierge RL, Verdy I. Benzodiazepine poisoning. Clinical and pharmacological considerations and treatment. *Drug Safety* 1991;6:247–265).

benzodiazepine + paroxetine Paroxetine does not potentiate the sedative or psychomotor effects of benzodiazepines, but co-administration may increase central nervous system adverse effects (Cooper SM, Jackson D, Loudon JM, et al. The psychomotor effects of paroxetine alone and in combination with haloperidol, amylobarbitone, oxazepam, or alcohol. *Acta Psychiatr Scand* 1989;80[suppl]:53–55).

benzodiazepine + phenobarbital Higher benzodiazepine doses may be required for anxiolysis (Stoudemire A, Moran MG. Psychopharmacologic treatment of anxiety in the medically ill elderly patient: special considerations. *J Clin Psychiatry* 1993;54[suppl 5]:27–33).

benzodiazepine + phenytoin Patients taking phenytoin require higher benzodiazepine (BZD) doses for anxiolysis than other patients (Stoudemire A, Moran MG. Psychopharmacologic treatment of anxiety in the medically ill elderly patient: special considerations. *J Clin Psychiatry* 1993;54[suppl 5]:27–33). Data on BZD effects on phenytoin metabolism are scanty and conflicting; in general they have no important effects (Pisani F, Perucca E, Di Perri R. Clinically relevant anti-epileptic drug interactions. *J Int Med Res* 1990;18:1–15).

benzodiazepine postwithdrawal syndrome Persistence of benzodiazepine (BZD) withdrawal symptoms for months or years after ordinary withdrawal (which usually subsides within a few days to a few weeks of drug discontinuation) has been reported. In the British literature, the phenomenon has been called the benzodiazepine postwithdrawal syndrome (BPWS). It may continue even if BZD therapy is reinstituted, although retreatment does not necessarily lead to continued dependence. There is considerable overlap between the symptoms of BPWS and the immediate withdrawal syndrome; BPWS symptoms are much more like those of clinical anxiety. Feelings of tension and threat, and bodily feelings such as unsteadiness, shaking, palpitations, and gastrointestinal symptoms are prominent with BPWS; symptoms that develop as secondary complications of anxiety, such as panic attacks and agoraphobia, also may occur. Whether symptoms that occur after BZD discontinuation represent re-emergence of anxiety or long-term complications of dependence is not known. If discontinuation of long-term therapeutic use of a BZD is being attempted or has been completed, clinical contact with the patient should continue for some time. Cognitive therapy is considered by some British researchers to be the treatment of choice for relieving anxiety that occurs after a BZD has been stopped (Tyler P. The benzodiazepine post-withdrawal syndrome. *Stress Med* 1991;7: 1–2). See **opioid abstinence syndrome, protracted.**

benzodiazepine/pregnancy Benzodiazepines (BZDs) cross the placenta and concentrate in fetal tissue because metabolism by the fetal liver is minimal. BZDs may cause fetal damage, especially during the first trimester. There is increased (but low) risk of cleft lip or palate, inguinal hernia, pyloric stenosis, and cardiocirculatory defects in the fetus. BZD use during the first trimester should therefore almost always be avoided. If given late in pregnancy, BZDs can cause neonatal depression. Fetuses exposed to BZDs during late pregnancy tend to accumulate BZDs and may have the "floppy infant syndrome" or neonatal withdrawal syndrome 2–3 weeks after birth. Intrauterine BZD dependency in the fetus and BZD withdrawal in the neonate may occur if a pregnant woman takes therapeutic doses of a BZD, especially during the last 4 weeks of pregnancy. See **benzodiazepine overdose/pregnancy; benzodiazepine withdrawal syndrome/neonatal; floppy infant syndrome.**

benzodiazepine + ranitidine Available evidence indicates ranitidine is less likely than cimetidine to interfere with disposition of any of the benzodiazepines (Abernathy DR, Greenblatt DJ, Eshelman FN, Shader RI. Ranitidine does not impair oxidative or conjugative metabolism: noninteraction with antipyrine, diazepam and lorazepam. *Clin Pharmacol Ther* 1984;35:188–192).

benzodiazepine receptor In 1977, benzodiazepine (BZD) receptors were identified, making it possible to map their location within the central nervous system (CNS). There is a high density of BZD receptors within the amygdala, which suggests that it is an important site for anxiolytic drug actions. Along with a subpopulation of gamma-aminobutyric acid (GABA)$_A$ receptors, BZD receptors form the GABA-benzodiazepine-chloride ion channel complex, which is an oligomeric protein consisting of at least four subunits that form a central chloride ion channel. GABA increases permeability of chloride ions through that chloride ion channel. When a BZD binds to its receptor, GABAergic neurotransmission is facilitated, and the rate of chloride ion transport across the neuronal membrane is increased. Heightened permeability of the cell to chloride ions decreases neuronal excitability by hyperpolarizing the neuronal membrane. Hyperpolarization of the neuronal membrane is believed to result in decreased activity of brain regions involved in emotional expression, such as the hippocampus and the amygdala, thus resulting in reduced arousal and anxiety (Paul SM. Anxiety and depression: a common neurobiological state? *J Clin Psychiatry* 1988; 49[S10]:13–16) There are two BZD receptor subtypes in the brain, BZ_1 (type 1 or omega$_1$) and BZ_2 (type 2 or omega$_2$). Type 1 receptors may be postsynaptic, and type 2 receptors may be presynaptic. Type 1 BZD receptors may mediate anxiolytic effects and have a high affinity for both BZDs and triazolopyridazines. Type 2 receptors mediate other BZD actions and have a high affinity for BZDs and a low affinity for triazolopyridazines. A peripheral BZD receptor (omega$_3$) is very abundant in peripheral tissues. Central binding sites are responsible for CNS effects; peripheral sites are normally associated with tumor growth or

as a marker for neuronal damage (Johnson EW, de Lanerolle NC, Kim JH, et al. "Central" and "peripheral" benzodiazepine receptors: opposite changes in human epileptogenic tissue. *Neurology* 1992;42:811–815).

benzodiazepine receptor ligand There are three types: (a) agonists, which include benzodiazepines (BZDs) that exert anxiolytic, hypnotic, and anticonvulsant effects and act as classic receptor agonists; (b) antagonists (e.g., flumazenil), which block BZD actions; and (c) inverse agonists (e.g, beta-carbolines and FG 7142), which are anxiogenic and proconvulsant.

benzodiazepine receptor, peripheral type (PBR) Type of drug receptor, first observed by Braestrup and Squires (1977), present in apparently all tissues, including the central nervous system. PBRs have been localized to kidney, lungs, ovaries, testes, adrenal glands, and blood cells. They are also found on neurons and glial cells and may regulate cell and cholesterol function (Diamond BI, Brown D, Wang J, et al. Altered plasma benzodiazepine receptors in patients with social phobia. *Neuropsychopharmacology* 1993;9:122S). They play a key role in the regulation of steroidogenesis by mediating the rate-limiting step in this biosynthetic pathway, which is transport of cholesterol to inner mitochondrial membranes. Once considered insignificant, PBRs are now viewed with renewed interest because certain benzodiazepines (BZDs), such as diazepam, may exert secondary effects on steroid production under appropriate physiologic conditions. The role of PBRs in steroid biosynthesis might help account for differences in pharmacological profiles and tolerance of various BZDs and may lead to alternative considerations in the therapeutic use of these drugs (Krueger KE. Peripheral-type benzodiazepine receptors: a second site of action for benzodiazepines. *Neuropsychopharmacology* 1991;4:237–244). Also called "mitochondrial receptor".

benzodiazepine/seizure Although apparently rare, seizures have been reported following abrupt withdrawal of both therapeutic and high doses of benzodiazepines (BZDs). There also have been a few case reports of seizures occurring at or near the end of a tapered withdrawal, and isolated reports of seizures occurring during BZD therapy. Most literature reports are anecdotal, often with relatively scant information. Other cases, information on which is not generally available, have been reported to individual pharmaceutical companies and/or the Food and Drug Aministration's Spontaneous Adverse Event Reporting System. True incidence is unknown, and it may be difficult for physicians to assess the risk involved.

benzodiazepine/seizure, risk factors Available data suggest that a seizure may be more likely to occur if, in addition to abrupt benzodiazepine (BZD) discontinuation, one or more of the following factors is present: (a) extended duration of ingestion (4 months to years); (b) high dosage; (c) concomitant or immediately subsequent ingestion of other drugs associated with seizure induction; (d) history of seizures; (e) history of alcohol abuse; (f) history of head trauma; and (h) abnormal electroencephalographic or brain scan results. Available data also suggest an elevated risk of seizures with individual BZDs (e.g., high milligram potency BZDs, lorazepam, alprazolam, and triazolam). Risk is enhanced in drug abusers, as BZDs have increasingly entered the repertoire of those who misuse a variety of substances for their euphoriant and sedative effects. Risk may be particularly high in abusers who inject BZDs in large doses and use deliberate seizure induction as a lever to induce physicians to prescribe a desired BZD.

benzodiazepine/sleep Benzodiazepines suppress some electroencephalographic features of stage 4 sleep and, in some cases, rapid eye movement (REM) sleep.

benzodiazepine/transient insomnia In the management of transient insomnia, the lowest dose of a hypnotic should always be used initially and as infrequently as possible. Hypnotics should not be prescribed for more than 2 weeks, and they need not be given every night. Patients can be allowed to use their own discretion, and ingestion can be limited to the nights of the week preceding a working day. If they are taken on alternate nights, the patient can recall the good sleep of the previous night or look forward to a good sleep during the coming night. If low doses are used frequently and for the shortest time, many problems associated with using hypnotics may be avoided. Rebound insomnia, in which sleep is more disturbed on withdrawal of a hypnotic than before treatment, and rebound anxiety, as reported with triazolam, are probably due to ingestion of unnecessarily high doses, whereas dependency arises with regular use over several months. Hypnotics must be given judiciously; patients must realize before treatment begins that their use is a temporary expedient and only for a limited period (Nicholson AN. Benzodiazepines and transient insomnia. *Prescribers J* 1983;23:100–105).

benzodiazepine + valproate See **diazepam + valproate.**

benzodiazepine + valproate + neuroleptic See **benzodiazepine + neuroleptic + valproate.**

benzodiazepine + warfarin Benzodiazepines have been used extensively and safely with warfarin (Stockley IH. *Drug Interactions: A Source Book of Drug Interactions, Their Mechanisms, Clinical Importance and Management,* 2nd ed. Oxford: Blackwell Scientific, 1991).

benzodiazepine withdrawal, interdose In many regular benzodiazepine (BZD) users, especially those using short-acting BZDs, symptoms of withdrawal can occur without dosage reduction (Cohen SI. Risks of dependence on benzodiazepine drugs. *Br Med J* 1989;208:456–457). Thus, some patients simultaneously complain of BZD adverse effects and BZD withdrawal phenomena. These merging symptoms might reflect uneven development of tolerance to the various actions of BZDs, with some types of BZD or gamma-aminobutyric acid (GABA) receptors undergoing adaptive changes more quickly than others (Ashton H. *Brain Function and Psychotropic Drugs.* New York: Oxford University Press, 1992). Research evidence suggests that a rebound hyperserotonergic state may contribute to withdrawal phenomenon, and that serotonin antagonists may be clinically useful in withdrawal from BZDs. De novo absence status has been reported in a 65-year-old woman following BZD withdrawal (Thomas P, Lebrun C, Chatel M. De novo absence status epilepticus as a benzodiazepine withdrawal syndrome. *Epilepsia* 1993;34:355–358).

benzodiazepine withdrawal syndrome, low-dose Syndrome that may occur with withdrawal from therapeutic doses of benzodiazepines (BZDs). It does not fit the pattern of other sedative-hypnotics, including alcohol, that have a "protracted withdrawal syndrome." Although it can be severe and disabling for many months, patients who remain completely abstinent from BZDs generally recover to their pre-BZD exposure level of symptoms. Signs and symptoms include anxiety, agitation, tachycardia, palpitations, anorexia, blurred vision, muscle cramps, insomnia, nightmares, confusion, muscle spasms, psychoses, increased sensitivity to sounds and light, and paresthesias. Patients at increased risk have a family or personal history of alcoholism, use alcohol daily, or concomitantly use other sedatives. For treatment, the phenobarbital conversion technique is inadequate to prevent occurrence of withdrawal symptoms. Propranolol, 20 mg every 6 hours, can be used alone or in combination with phenobarbital to reduce low-dose BZD withdrawal symptom intensity (Wesson DR, Smith DE, Seymour RB. Sedative-hypnotics and tricyclics. *In* Lowinson JH, Ruiz P, Millman RB [eds], Langrod JG [assoc ed],

Substance Abuse, A Comprehensive Textbook, 2nd ed. Baltimore: Williams & Wilkins, 1992).

benzodiazepine withdrawal syndrome/neonatal
Continuous use of benzodiazepines (BZDs) during pregnancy can lead to a neonatal BZD abstinence syndrome. Withdrawal signs in neonates have been attributed to intrauterine exposure to diazepam, alprazolam, and triazolam. Symptoms include tremulousness, hypertonicity, irritability, hyperactivity, restlessness, disturbed sleep, excessive crying, tremors, and/or hyper-reflexia. Although sucking may be vigorous, there may be episodes of vomiting. Indications for pharmacological treatment are seizures, poor feeding or failure to thrive, and severe hyperactivity or irritability. Initial doses of diazepam (0.1 mg/kg) should be administered intravenously. Larger or more frequent doses may be necessary to control symptoms. Once the child's condition has been stable for 1 week, daily doses can be reduced gradually over a 3- to 4-week period. If the child experiences serious abstinence symptoms, the dose should be held at the current level for a time before continuing the reduction (Gaudreault P, Guay J, Thivierge RL, Verdy I. Benzodiazepine poisoning. Clinical and pharmacological considerations and treatment. *Drug Safety* 1991;6:247–265).

benzodiazepine withdrawal, tapered Since the 1970s, there has been a steady rise in the number of persons who have become dependent on a BZD. Many have become long-term users, and some have become high-dose users. Because of the hazards of abrupt discontinuation (marked psychological and physical distress, seizures, and death), tapered withdrawal is preferred. Strategies include (a) gradual reduction of dose and frequency of the BZD currently used; (b) substitution of one BZD for another (e.g., a long-acting BZD [clonazepam, diazepam] for a short-acting one [alprazolam]), followed by taper of the longer-acting BZD; (c) converting the BZD to phenobarbital equivalents, followed by tapered withdrawal from phenobarbital; (d) use of adjunctive medication (i.e., carbamazepine) to effect a more rapid taper from the currently used BZD. See **carbamazepine/benzodiazepine withdrawal.**

benzomorphan One of a group of opioid analgesics and antagonists. Pentazocine, a kappa-agonist with weak mu-antagonist properties, is a well known benzomorphan. Some that interact with phencyclidine (PCP) and/or sigma binding sites have psychotomimetic effects, suggesting that such sites may be important in schizophrenia etiology. They may also act at opioid K receptors to produce dysphoria.

benzoyl-methylergonine See **cocaine.**

benzoylecgonine (BZE) Major, inactive metabolite of cocaine formed by hydrolysis by plasma pseudocholinesterases and liver esterases. It is not hepatotoxic. Plasma half-life is about 6 hours. It is excreted in urine at levels totalling approximately 45% of the dose. The enzyme multiplied immunoassay test can detect BZE at a sensitivity threshold of 50 ng/ml. It has been detected in the urine by chromatographic or enzyme immunological assays for 48–72 hours, and radioimmunoassays have detected it for 96–144 hours (Hamilton HE, Wallace JE, Shinek EL, et al. Cocaine and benzoylecgonine excretion in humans. *J Forens Sci* 1977;22:697–706).

benzphetamine (Didrex) Sympathomimetic amine with pharmacological activity similar to amphetamines (AMPHs) marketed as an anorectic agent. Like all AMPHs, it is subject to abuse. Schedule III; pregnancy risk category X.

benztropine (Cogentin) Anticholinergic, antihistaminic drug used in the treatment of Parkinson's disease and drug-induced early-onset extrapyramidal reactions (akathisia, akinesia, dystonia, and parkinsonism). Efficacy is attributed to its ability to reduce the functional activity of the excitatory cholinergic system in the basal ganglia. It is marketed in 2-mg-strength tablets or capsules and prescribed in doses of 1–8 mg/day. It also is available in parenteral form. Half-life is 24 ± 4 hours; thus it may be given once or twice daily. Benztropine is moderately selective for M_1 muscarinic receptors, with approximately 2 times higher affinity for M_1 than for M_2 receptors. It is beneficial in controlling hypersalivation and drooling and early tremor and rigidity. It is not as potent as levodopa in treating akinesia or bradykinesia and their associated slowness, stooping, and falls. Intravenous benztropine (0.5–2 mg) can dramatically and quickly relieve acute drug-induced dystonic reactions. Benztropine may cause dry mouth with associated adverse effects. This and other anticholinergic side effects (dilated pupils, urinary retention, and constipation) limit benztropine's usefulness in treating moderate and advanced states of parkinsonism. Given the variability in its pharmacokinetics, some individuals may be at greater risk for anticholinergic side effects, and small increases in dosage may result in clinically significant worsening of side effects. Elderly patients are particularly sensitive to its anticholinergic effects, resulting in impaired memory, impaired intellectual function, and a toxic confusional state or delirium. Some young people have perceived the subjective effects of benztropine as desirable, and a few have abused it. However, benztropine has rarely been abused by patients and by illicit drug users. Pregnancy risk category C.

benztropine + amantadine   Co-administration may enhance anticholinergic effects, causing peripheral adverse reactions (dry mouth, blurred vision, severe constipation, and delayed micturition) and central anticholinergic effects (disorientation, restlessness, agitation, confusion, hallucinations, and delirium).

benztropine + chlorpromazine   Benztropine is sometimes co-prescribed with chlorpromazine to treat or prevent acute early onset extrapyramidal reactions. The regimen may reverse some of chlorpromazine's therapeutic effects or may be responsible for additive anticholinergic toxicity (Singh MM, Smith JM. Reversal of some therapeutic effects of an antipsychotic agent by an antiparkinsonian drug. *J Nerv Ment Dis* 1973;50:157).

benztropine + clozapine   Benztropine has been used to successfully counteract clozapine-induced hypersalivation with no serious adverse interactions.

benztropine equivalent dose   (BZTE)   Benztropine 2 mg = 2 mg trihexyphenidyl = 2 mg biperiden = 25 mg diphenhydramine = 100 mg amantadine.

benztropine + fluoxetine   Fluoxetine may elevate benztropine plasma levels, possibly causing delirium (Baker RW. Fluoxetine and schizophrenia in a patient with obsessional thinking. *J Neuropsychiatr Clin Neurosci* 1992;2: 232–233).

benztropine + fluphenazine   A study reported that co-administration in a woman with tardive dyskinesia resulted in dysphagia. Attempts to decrease neuroleptic dosage worsened the dysphagia and produced acute dyspnea. When the fluphenazine dose was increased, symptoms quickly resolved (Weiden P, Harrigan M. A clinical guide for diagnosing and managing patients with drug-induced dysphagia. *Hosp Comm Psychiatry* 1986;37:396–398).

benztropine + haloperidol   Benztropine is sometimes co-prescribed with haloperidol to treat or prevent acute early-onset extrapyramidal reactions. The regimen may reverse some of haloperidol's therapeutic effects (Froemming JS, Lam YW, Jann MW. Pharmacokinetics of haloperidol. *Clin Pharmacokinet* 1989;17:396–423).

benztropine/hyperthermia   Benztropine can inhibit sweat gland activity, causing the skin to become hot and dry. Sweating may be depressed enough to raise body temperature, but notably so *only* after large doses or at high environmental temperatures. Under such conditions benztropine-induced hyperthermia may raise the body temperature to 43° C (109.4° F) or higher. Risk of serious and even fatal hyperthermia is enhanced in patients being treated with benztropine plus high doses of antipsychotics, especially those with potent antimuscarinic properties (e.g., aliphatic and piperidine phenothiazine neuroleptics). See **heatstroke.**

benztropine + molindone   A patient receiving both drugs began to find it difficult to swallow solids and liquids 1 month after the regimen was begun. Esophageal manometry revealed increased upper esophageal sphincter pressure and a poorly contractile esophagus that returned to normal 5 days after the medications were stopped (Moss HB, Green H. Neuroleptic-associated dysphagia confirmed by esophageal manometry. *Am J Psychiatry* 1982; 139:515–516).

benztropine + neuroleptic   Prophylactic benztropine effectively reduces occurrence of neuroleptic-induced dystonia in young patients receiving high-potency neuroleptic therapy for acute psychosis. However, not all patients require anticholinergics, and these drugs can produce cognitive deficits. Co-administration of benztropine with piperidine or aliphatic phenothiazines, which are anticholinergic, can lead to additive anticholinergic effects, including fecal compaction. The effect of benztropine on neuroleptic plasma levels is unresolved; some studies report lowering of plasma levels; one, an increase; most, no effect.

benztropine + thiothixene   There is a case report of esophageal atony with massive esophageal dilatation that disappeared after the drugs were discontinued and recurred when they were readministered. Esophageal dilatation was attributed to the anticholinergic effects of both drugs (Woodring JH, Martin CA, Keefer B. Esophageal atony and dilatation as a side effect of thiothixene and benztropine. *Hosp Comm Psychiatry* 1993;44:686–688).

Bercetina   See **flunarizine.**

bereavement, spousal   Loss of a spouse through death is common in late life and frequently leads to major depression in 10–30% of the widowed (Zisook S, Shuchter SR. Depression through the first year after the death of a spouse. *Am J Psychiatry* 1991;148:1346–1352). A study of electroencephalographic (EEG) sleep in bereaved subjects with major depression, bereaved subjects without depression, and normal healthy control subjects (neither bereaved nor depressed) showed that bereaved subjects with major depression had significantly lower sleep efficiency, more early morning awakening, shorter rapid eye movement (REM) latency, greater REM sleep percentage, and lower rates of delta wave generation in the first non-REM (NREM) period, compared with bereaved subjects without depression. Sleep of bereaved subjects with single-episode major depression resembled that of elderly patients with recurrent unipolar major depression. Sleep in bereavement without depression was similar to that of healthy control subjects. These data indicate that subjects who experience a first-episode depressive syndrome in the context of spousal bereavement have sleep-EEG characteristics that (a) distinguish them from bereaved persons without depressive syndromes and (b) are similar to sleep-EEG characteristics of recurrent depression (Reynolds CF, Hoch CC, Buysse DF, et al. Electroencephalographic sleep in spousal bereavement and bereavement-related depression of late life. *Biol Psychiatry* 1992;31:69–82). Some clinicians hold that early treatment of the sleep disturbance of acutely bereaved elders may lessen the risk of major depression. Others report that antidepressant drug therapy may alleviate symptoms of major depression (including sleep disturbance) in spousal bereavement with major depression (Pasternak RE, Reynolds CF, Schlernitzauer M, et al. Acute open-trial nortriptyline therapy of bereavement-related depression in late life. *J Clin Psychiatry* 1991; 52:307–310).

Bespar   See **buspirone.**

bestiality   Sexual deviation in which an individual derives gratification from sexual contact with animals.

beta activity   Beta electroencephalographic wave or sequence of waves with a frequency greater than 13 Hz.

beta$_1$-adrenergic receptor   Receptor for noradrenaline found in heart muscle, stimulation of which increases heart rate. Also present in the brain.

beta$_2$-adrenergic receptor   Receptor for noradrenaline found in vascular and uterine smooth muscle, stimulation of which relaxes the uterus and causes vasodilation in many tissues. Also present in the brain.

beta-adrenergic receptor kinase   (BARK) Cyclic AMP–independent kinase involved in regulation of adrenergic receptors.

beta-adrenergic blocking agent   (BABA) One of a group of drugs (e.g., propranolol, atenolol, metoprolol, nadolol, and acebutolol) that may play a valuable role in the treatment of certain anxiety disorders (e.g., social phobias). They were previously used in schizophrenia but without great success. They may produce depressive symptoms and psychotic symptoms, including visual hallucinations. See **beta-blocker.**

beta-amyloid   (A$_4$) Toxic substance found in the brain plaques of Alzheimer's disease patients. It is part of the larger amyloid precursor protein that resembles a membrane protein, with the beta amyloid partially embedded within the membrane. A defect in the regulating action of certain enzymes (lysosomal proteases) involved in the breakdown of protein may lead to release of beta-amyloid.

beta-amyloid peptide   A 43-amino-acid amyloidotic peptide that arises from abnormal processing of a normal cellular protein in the brain called the amyloid peptide precursor (APP). Although APP is not increased in brain or blood of Alzheimer patients, the A$_4$ peptide itself is overproduced in the brains of Alzheimer patients (Pardridge WM. Microvessels from Alzheimer's disease brain: biochemistry of amyloid peptides. *Ann Intern Med* 1988;109: 41–54). Also called A$_4$ peptide.

beta-amyloid protein   (beta-AP) Excessive accumulation of beta-amyloid in the brain is pathognomic of Alzheimer's disease. Beta-amyloid protein is neurotoxic to primary hippocampal neurons from rats and primary cortical neurons from humans. Preliminary data suggest that neurofibrillary changes and beta deposition may be causally related to Alzheimer's disease and potentially treated by substance P.

beta-blocker   One of a group of beta-adrenergic receptor agonists that are among the most commonly prescribed and useful of all medications. They have cardiovascular applications in the treatment of hypertension, arrhythmias, and angina pectoris; they are used prophylactically in those who have suffered a prior myocardial infarction. They are increasingly being used for performance anxiety, neuroleptic-induced akathisia, migraine headaches, glaucoma, hyperthyroidism, hand tremors, and treatment of rage and violent behavior associated with brain lesions or injury. After 1967, reports in the medical literature associated use of beta-blockers with clinical depression, although a later study found no causal connection between them and depression (Bright RA, Everitt DE. Beta-blockers and depression: evidence against an association. *JAMA* 1992;267:1183–1187). It is possible that depression occasionally occurs, but it has not been established with currently available investigative methods. When depression occurs in patients taking or being considered for beta-blockers, effective alternatives not prominently associated with depression should be considered (e.g., captopril instead of propranolol for a depressed patient being treated for hypertension). Antidepressants are effective and safe when used in conjunction with beta-blockers. However, since beta-blockers may significantly increase blood levels of certain psychotropic drugs, antidepressant serum levels should be monitored during co-administration (Yudofsky SC. Beta-blockers and depression. The clinician's dilemma. *JAMA* 1992;267: 1826–1827).

beta-blocker + acetophenazine Beta-blockers may inhibit acetophenazine's metabolism, raising its plasma level and increasing risk of toxicity.

beta-blocker/akathisia Following reports of benefits of propranolol therapy for neuroleptic-induced akathisia, atenolol, metoprolol, and nadolol were tested for this indication and found ineffective (Reiter S, Adler L, Angrist B, et al. Atenolol and propranolol in neuroleptic-induced akathisia. *J Clin Psychopharmacol* 1987;7:279–280; Zubenko GS, Lipinski JF, Cohen BM, Carreira PJ. Comparison of metoprolol and propranolol in the treatment of akathisia. *Psychiatry Res* 1984;11:143–148; Ratey JJ, Sorgi P, Polakoff S. Nadolol as a treatment for akathisia. *Am J Psychiatry* 1985; 142:640–642). Betaxolol, however, may be useful. See **propranolol/akathisia.**

beta-blocker + antidepressant Co-administration is effective and safe. However, since beta-blockers may significantly increase blood levels of certain psychotropic drugs, antidepressant serum levels should be monitored (Yudofsky SC. Beta-blockers and depression. The clinician's dilemma. *JAMA* 1992;267: 1826–1827).

beta-blocker + benzodiazepine Combined therapy may be more effective than either class of drug alone in generalized anxiety disorders, especially in patients with treatment-resistant generalized anxiety disorder.

beta-blocker + fluoxetine Fluoxetine may inhibit oxidative metabolism of metoprolol and other lipophilic beta-blockers that undergo extensive hepatic metabolism, resulting in higher plasma concentrations of the beta-blocker and adverse cardiovascular effects (Walley T, Pirmohamed M, Proudlove C, Maxwell D. Interaction of metoprolol and fluoxetine. *Lancet* 1993;341:967–968). Patients who require beta-blockade while on fluoxetine should be prescribed water-soluble drugs (e.g., atenolol, sotalol).

beta-blocker/psychiatric uses Although marketed for cardiovascular indications, some beta-blockers (atenolol, metoprolol, nadolol, propranolol) are useful for the treatment of a variety of psychiatric disorders, including akathisia, tremor (e.g., lithium-induced), performance anxiety, behavioral complications of brain damage, generalized anxiety disorders, as an adjunct to benzodiazepines in alcohol withdrawal, aggression/agoraphobia, mania, adjunctive treatment of schizophrenia, cocaine intoxication, adjunctive treatment of narcotic/benzodiazepine withdrawal, and tardive dyskinesia. Adverse reactions may include sedation, lethargy, dizziness, depression, nightmares, confusion, ataxia, hypotension, bradycardia, bronchospasm, nausea, and sexual dysfunction.

beta-carboline One of a group of active benzodiazepine (BZD) receptor inverse agonists that are reversible inhibitors of monoamine oxidase type A. They are condensation products of aromatic amino acids and aldehydes that bind with various degrees of affinity to the BZD recognition site and have been useful in exploring its function. They cause behavioral and neuroendocrine changes characteristic of anxiety and stress by reducing gamma-aminobutyric acid (GABA) neurotransmission.

beta-electroencephalogram Electroencephalogram (EEG) with predominantly 13-Hz and higher frequencies (beta activity) in all recorded leads. Beta-EEGs are usually low-voltage and very fast. They are associated with alert wakefulness. See **beta rhythm.**

beta-endorphin (BE, BEND) Polypeptide for the brain's endogenous opioid system that is found in the brain and anterior pituitary. It is the most potent of the natural opioids. It is a 31-amino-acid hormone released by the pituitary into the systemic circulation in response to various psychological and physiological stimuli. In some, but not all, depressed patients, high basal plasma levels and greater-than-normal secretion in response to cholinergic stimulation have been observed. Some studies have shown nonsuppression of plasma BE after dexamethasone administration in depressed patients in whom dexamethasone did not suppress cortisol, even in patients whose baseline BE levels were not higher than normal. In a test of the hypothesis that high degrees of specific clinical symptoms of depression are associated with higher-than-normal plasma levels of BE-like immunoactivity, high levels were associated with more severe anxiety, phobia, and obsessions/compulsions in depressed patients (Darko DF, Risch SC, Gillin JC, Golshan S. Association of beta-endorphin with specific clinical symptoms of depression. *Am J Psychiatry* 1992;149:1162–1167). BE levels appear to be lowered by short-acting opioid agonists (heroin, morphine) and raised by antagonists (naloxone) in humans, although with chronic administration of long-acting opioids such as methadone, these acute effects on BE decrease and levels return to normal (Kosten TR, Morgan C, Kreek M-J. Beta endorphin levels during heroin, methadone, buprenorphine, and naloxone challenges: preliminary findings. *Biol Psychiatry* 1992;32:523–528).

beta error See **error, beta.**

beta half-life See **half-life, beta.**

beta-lipotropin (B-LPH) Precursor to beta-endorphin and adrenocorticotropic hormone (ACTH).

beta-N-methylamino-L-alanine (BMAA) Low-potency, stereospecific excitatory amino acid and excitotoxant. See **excitotoxin.**

beta-N-oxalylamino-L-alanine (BOAA) Environmental excitotoxant implicated in neurolathyrism. It exerts excitotoxic activity exclusively through quisqualate receptors.

beta-phenylethylamine See **phenylethylamine.**

beta-phenyl-GABA (Phenibut) Tranquilizer with nootropic effects. It and baclofen are derivatives of gamma-aminobutyric acid (GABA) and beta-phenylethylamine (PEA).

beta rhythm In electroencephalography, a certain range of beta activity (13–35 Hz). Amplitude is variable, but usually under 35 uV. Beta rhythm is usually associated with alert wakefulness or vigilance and is accompanied by a high tonic electromyogram. It may be drug-induced. See **beta electroencephalogram.**

betaxolol (Kerlone) Lipophilic, beta$_1$-selective adrenergic blocker marketed for treatment of hypertension. It also can be used for the treatment of neuroleptic-induced akathisia (Adler LA, Angrist B, Rotrosen J. Efficacy of betaxolol in neuroleptic-induced akathisia. *Psychiatry Res* 1991;39:193–198).

bethanechol (Urecholine) Cholinergic/muscarinic receptor agonist that produces stimulatory effects on the parasympathetic nervous system (e.g., stimulation of smooth muscles of the gastrointestinal tract and particularly the urinary bladder). It is used to counteract anticholinergic effects of psychoactive drugs; 25 or 50 mg three or four times a day can often reduce intensity of peripheral anticholinergic drug effects, making continued treatment with the anticholinergic drug feasible (Siris SG. Pharmacological treatment of depression in schizophrenia. *In* LE DeLisi [ed], *Depression in Schizophrenia.* Washington, DC: American Psychiatric Press, 1990, pp 143–162). It also has been used to treat cognitive impairments associated with Alzheimer's disease, although there is little substantive evidence that it is effective.

bhang **1.** Least-potent grade of cannabis (marijuana) derived from uncultivated flowers and tops with a low resin content comprising 1–2% tetrahydrocannabinol. **2.** Term used in India for a tea drink made from cannabis.

bhang psychosis See **cannabis psychosis.**

bias Variation between the value used in the analysis and the true value. It could occur at any stage of a study. Bias may result in incorrect study conclusions. See **error, systematic.**

bias, experimenter Experimenter expectations inadvertently communicated to study subjects that may influence experimental findings and/or an approach to data analysis that produces inaccurate outcomes.

bias, publication Bias created by the fact that research with statistically significant results is more likely to be submitted and published than work with null or nonsignificant results. It has been noted in educational, psychological, and medical research circles. The most serious potential consequence may be an overestimate of treatment effects or risk-factor associations in published work, leading to inappropriate decisions about patient management or health policy. It may compromise the validity of conventional reviews as well as the quantitative overview techniques of meta-analysis and decision analysis, which often rely solely on published data. Conclusions based only on a review of published data should be interpreted cautiously, especially for observational studies. Distortions of the publication process can distort the scientific basis of medicine, typically in favor of new and controversial therapies (Rennie D, Flanagin A. Publication bias. The triumph of hope over experience. *JAMA* 1992;267:411–412).

bias, sampling Error caused by the sampling procedure that will produce biased estimations if no appropriate correction is applied. The error is due to selection of a nonrepresentative sample of subjects or observations. A classic example is a 1936 *Literary Digest* poll that predicted Landon's election over Roosevelt because telephone directories were used as a basis for selecting respondents. Also called "selection bias."

bias, selection See **sampling bias.**

bias, volunteer Phenomenon that may occur when study populations include volunteers. Individuals who volunteer for some procedures are not generally representative of the total population. Self-selected patients who seek out treatment based on newspaper publicity, for example, are likely to do significantly better than randomly selected patients who are simply offered the treatment.

bigarexia nervosa Pathological belief of users/abusers of anabolic-androgenic steroids that they appear small and weak when in fact they are large and muscular. Some "bigarexics" deliberately wear baggy sweatclothes even in summer to disguise their imagined smallness and may decline social invitations for fear they would be seen by others as too small. Many have a history of anorexia nervosa.

"big chief"   Street name for mescaline.

"big flake"   Street name for cocaine.

"big H"   Street name for heroin.

Bikalm   See **zolpidem.**

bilateral electroconvulsive therapy   See **electroconvulsive therapy, bilateral.**

bilineality   In genetics, existence in both parental lines of the same illness that affects the proband.

bimodal distribution   Distribution with two points at which the frequency is considerably greater than on either side of the points. The points need not be of the same frequency.

binding   Formation of a bond between one compound and another, usually a noncovalent attachment of a drug (ligand) to tissue constituents (plasma proteins or tissue binding sites).

binding constant   Measure of a drug's affinity for various uptake receptor sites, derived from how much drug is required to displace a given amount of a neurotransmitter (e.g., serotonin, or a serotonin-specific ligand). The lower the binding constant, the greater the affinity. The more affinity a drug has for the site, the lower the concentration required for displacement and the lower the binding constant.

binding site   Particular domain on the surface of the receptor molecule that has a characteristic spatial arrangement of functional groups that can recognize and bind specific ligands. Often a binding site and a receptor are effectively the same. However, in the gamma-aminobutyric acid (GABA)–benzodiazepine (BZD)–chloride ion channel complex, GABA binds to the GABA receptor and a BZD binds to an adjacent site, facilitating the GABA-induced inhibitory effect. Also called "recognition site."

binge   Discrepancies between lay and technical uses of this term require clarification. In the DSM-III-R, binge is "rapid consumption of a large amount of food in a discrete period of time." In the DSM-IV, it is an "episode of binge eating characterized by both: i.) eating, in a discrete period of time (e.g., in any 2-hour period), an amount of food that is definitely larger than most people would eat during a similar period of time; and, ii.) a sense of lack of control over eating during the episode (e.g., a feeling that one cannot stop eating or control what or how much one is eating)" (Wilson GT, Walsh BT. Eating disorders in the DSM-IV. *J Abnorm Psychol* 1991;100:362–365). A survey of young women with eating disorders, however, revealed they regard binging as a particular form of overeating in which a large amount of food is eaten with a sense of

loss of control and subsequent fullness and dysphoria (Beglin SJ, Fairburn CG. What is meant by the term "binge?" *Am J Psychiatry* 1992;149:123–124).

binge drinking   Consumption of large amounts of alcohol (five or more drinks in a row) on a single occasion. It involves drinking to get drunk and perception of the appropriateness of heavy drinking in social situations. Binge drinkers consume greater quantities, with greater regularity, and experience more intoxication and alcohol-associated problem behaviors than do non-binge drinkers. They are three times as likely as non-binge drinkers to indulge in unplanned sexual activity as a result of drinking; binge-drinking men are four times as likely to be involved in arguments or fights. Persons who drink more often than weekly are almost exclusively binge drinkers. In a 1990 survey, 41% of American college students were binge drinkers. In the latest survey, close to half of the binge drinkers (46.5% of men, 48.3% of women) were drunk twice or more in the prior month, compared with 5% or fewer of non-binge drinkers (Wechsler H, Isaac N. "Binge" drinkers at Massachusetts colleges. Prevalence, drinking style, time trends, and associated problems. *JAMA* 1992;267:2929–2931). Women are more likely to be binge drinkers than men. The majority of binge drinkers often have a family history of psychiatric disorder and/or alcohol misuse (Dunne FJ, Galatopoulos C, Schipperhiju JM, Gender differences in psychiatric morbidity among alcohol misusers. *Compr Psychiatry* 1993;34:95–101).

binomial distribution   Probability distribution that describes the number of successes observed in independent trials, each with the same probability of occurrence.

Binswanger's disease   Subcortical vascular disorder and form of dementia in which the cortex is spared and there are multiple small infarctions in the subcortical gray and white matter with demyelination in the latter. It was considered a result of arterial thickening associated with hypertension, but its origin has not been determined. It shares with other forms of hypertensive vascular disease the predominant involvement of the small penetrating arteries. Onset is typically in the 5th or 6th decade of life, with personality and intellectual deterioration, episodes of stroke and/or seizure, and a typical appearance on computed tomography (CT) scans. There may be delusional depression, which can be treated with a tricyclic antidepressant (e.g., amitriptyline, clomipramine) or a monoamine oxidase inhibitor (e.g., tranylcypromine) combined with an antipsychotic drug. Also called "subcortical atherosclerotic encephalopathy."

bioassay Quantitative assessment of the potency of a substance's effect on biological material (e.g., tissues, cells, experimental animals or humans).

bioavailability 1. Availability of a drug to the body after absorption from the gastrointestinal tract and first-pass metabolism through the liver. It is a function of completeness and rate of absorption of a given dose, plasma protein binding, and degree of first-pass metabolism. Bioavailability is presumably 100% when a drug is administered intravenously. Following oral or intramuscular administration it also may be 100%, although usually it is less; it will be high and close to 100% if an orally administered drug is completely absorbed and minimally metabolized on its first pass through the liver. Bioavailability can be influenced by (a) the drug's physiochemical properties; (b) the drug's formulation; (c) diseases that affect gastrointestinal function; (d) consumption with or immediately after food; and (e) gonadal hormones that change absorption rates (bioavailability of a drug administered to women may be altered, necessitating dosage adjustment in order to achieve a comparable plasma concentration in men). 2. Availability of drug at a given receptor site, which can be influenced by many factors.

biochemical genetics Study of physicochemical reactions associated with DNA replication and protein synthesis.

biofeedback System of detecting signals of previously imperceptible bodily functions (e.g, heart rate, skin temperature, or pressure in the colon) and bringing them under voluntary control. The signals can be transformed into a light or tone.

biogenic amine Member of a group of endogenous compounds that play an important role in brain function as central neurotransmitter substances, including catecholamines (epinephrine, norepinephrine, and dopamine), acetylcholine, histamine, and the indoleamine serotonin.

biogenic amine hypothesis of depression Postulations that depression is associated with an absolute or relative deficiency of catecholamines (norepinephrine) or indolamines (serotonin) at functionally important receptor sites in the brain. Elation, conversely, may be associated with an excess of such amines. The concept was derived originally from a serendipitous discovery that monoamine oxidase inhibitors and certain tricyclic drugs have mood-elevating properties and exert dramatic effects on brain monoamine functions. Disorders in norepinephrine and serotonin activity

have been implicated in the etiology of depression and mania.

biological rhythms Cyclical variations in physiological and biochemical function, level of activity, and emotional state repeated at regular intervals ranging from minutes to months. They include (a) circadian rhythms with a cycle of about 24 hours; (b) ultradian rhythms with a cycle shorter than 1 day; and (c) infradian rhythms with a cycle that may be weeks or months (*Biological Rhythms: Implications for the Worker.* Washington, DC: Office of Technology Assessment, U.S. Congress, 1991).

biological clock Neuromechanism that regulates internal temporal order and timing of hormonal, physiologic, and behavioral rhythms.

biological marker Test that may aid in differential diagnosis, usually a measure of biochemical abnormalities that reflect a disturbance in one biochemical system (e.g., a single enzyme; a single enzyme, and amount of the given substrate).

biological plausibility Whether an association makes sense in light of other types of information available in the literature (e.g., data from other human studies, studies of other related questions, animal studies, or in vitro studies) and the implications of scientific or pathophysiologic theory. For example, it is biologically plausible that cigarettes cause lung cancer. Also called "coherence with existing information."

biological psychiatry See **psychiatry, biological.**

biometrical genetics See **genetics, biometrical.**

bionics Use of information gained from the study of biological systems in the design and development of man-made engineering systems.

biopharmaceutics See **pharmacokinetics** (preferred term).

biopsychosocial Interface between and among the biological, behavioral, emotional, and social forces that influence health and well-being. Term coined by Engel, often used in a sloppy, fuzzy, and unhelpful way.

biopterin Cofactor in hydroxylation of phenylalanine, tyrosine, and tryptophan leading to production of the neurotransmitters dopamine, norepinephrine, and serotonin. Reduced quantities of biopterin have been reported in the cerebrospinal fluid of patients with Alzheimer's disease and Down syndrome.

Biorphen See **orphenadrine.**

biostatistics Application of statistics to biological and medical problems. Also called "medical statistics."

biotransformation See **drug biotransformation.**

biperiden (Akineton; Dekinet) Cholinergic mus muscarinic receptor antagonist used in the treatment of parkinsonism and early-onset drug-induced extrapyramidal reactions (akinesia, acute dystonia, akathisia, and parkinsonism). It may preferentially block the M_1 muscarinic receptor subtype. Compared with placebo, it significantly prolongs rapid eye movement (REM) latency and suppresses REM sleep time and REM percentage in a dose-dependent manner. On the hypothesis that centrally active anticholinergic substances may have an antidepressant effect, biperiden (12 mg/day) was tested in a small group of depressed patients for 4 weeks and found no more efficacious than placebo in alleviating depressive symptoms. However, hypomanic changes have been reported infrequently in patients treated with biperiden (Salin-Pascual RJ, Granados-Fuentes D, Galicia-Polo L, Nieves E. Rapid eye movement (REM) sleep increases by auditory stimulation reverted with biperiden administration in normal volunteers. *Neuropsychopharmacology* 1991;5:183–186). Pregnancy risk category C.

biperiden/breast milk Biperiden may be excreted in breast milk, may be toxic to an infant, and may reduce milk production. Treatment of nursing mothers with biperiden is inadvisable.

biperiden + remoxipride Neither drug influences the other's pharmacokinetics or pharmacodynamics (Yisak W, von Bahr C, Farde L, et al. Drug interaction studies with remoxipride. *Acta Psychiatr Scand* 1990;82[suppl 358]:58–62).

biperiden + zotepine Biperiden does not affect zotepine serum level.

biphasic half-life Drug half-life marked by two distinctly different rates of clearance from the blood.

biphasic response Symptom improvement following an initial period of symptom exacerbation. It is often observed during treatment with serotonin agonists in depressed patients.

Biphetamine See **amphetamine.**

bipolar See **bipolar disorder.**

bipolar disorder Affective illness characterized by mood swings between mania and depression. It may be subdivided into manic-, depressed, or mixed types on the basis of currently presenting symptoms. It is a fluctuating, chronic illness in which the same patient may manifest entirely different symptoms at various times. Clinical subtypes have been identified (e.g., rapid cycles, early vs. late onset in life, dysphoric components) that may have distinct biologic underpinnings and therefore may respond differently to pharmacological agents and have a different illness course. A mild form of bipolar disorder is sometimes labeled cyclothymic disorder. Formerly called manic depressive psychosis, circular or mixed type.

bipolar I disorder (BI) Manic depressive disorder with a history of both mania (as opposed to merely hypomania) and depression. BI is present when one or more manic episodes occur with a history of depressive episodes. Risk increases when family members have the disorder (about 60–65% of relatives have a positive history). It starts at an early age (late adolescence or early adulthood, mean age 30) and is equally divided between males and females.

bipolar II disorder (BII) Putative atypical subtype of depressive illness currently being defined and studied. It is characterized by manic depressive disorder preceded or followed by mild hypomania or hyperthymic temperament. BII is 2 times more frequent in females than in males. It starts at any age, but in 50% of patients onset is between 20 and 50 years of age, mean 40. Patients with bipolar II disorder apparently continue to have it over time, rather than developing bipolar I disorder. Clinical data indicate that bipolar II patients have a relatively good prognosis.

bipolar III disorder. (BIII) Disorder in which patients do not meet bipolar I or bipolar II criteria, but have first-degree relatives with bipolar illness. They may inadequately respond to tricyclic antidepressants (TCAs) alone, and may rapidly cycle on TCAs from depression into hypomania (sometimes termed "pharmacological mania"). Characteristics include onset before or at age 25, abrupt onset, psychotic depression, postpartum onset, hypersomnic retarded depressions, pharmacological hypomania, bipolar family history, loaded pedigree, and consecutive generation affective history. Also called "unipolar II depression"; "pseudo-unipolar depression."

bisexuality 1. Capability of achieving orgasm with a partner of either sex; 2. Freudian concept that components of both sexes could be found in the same person.

bitemporal electroconvulsive therapy See **electroconvulsive therapy, bilateral.**

bivariate plot Two-dimensional plot or scatterplot of the values of two characteristics measured on the same set of subjects.

"black" Street name for opium.

"black beauty" Street name for amphetamine.

"black Moroccan" Street name for hashish.

black-out Discrete episode of anterograde amnesia with no impairment of long-term memory resulting from ingestion of alcohol or other drugs (e.g, alprazolam, triazolam).

blepharoclonus Excessive, uncontrolled eye blinking that often precedes blepharospasms.

blepharospasm Focal dystonia manifested by intermittent or persistent involuntary closure of the eyes due to spasmodic bilateral contractions of the orbicularis oculi muscles. Initially it may present with nonspecific discomfort or excessive, uncontrollable blinking (blepharoclonus). Eyelid closure may be forceful, interfering with sight. Blepharospasm is sometimes seen in Parkinsons disease and torsion dystonia. Clonazepam, lorazepam, baclofen, and trihexyphenidyl provide symptomatic benefit in up to one-third of patients, but degree of improvement is often unsatisfactory and achieved at the expense of adverse reactions. Open and controlled studies indicate that botulinum toxin injections are beneficial (Grandas F, Elston J, Quinn N, Marsden CD. Blepharospasm: a review of 264 patients. *J Neurol Neurosurg Psychiatry* 1988;51:767–772). Blepharospasm combined with mouth movements is Meige's syndrome. See **Meige's syndrome.**

blind, blinded In research, condition in which the subject is unaware of the treatment being received (single-blind study), or both subject and investigator are unaware of it (double-blind study). Investigators also can be blind to each other's assessments to avoid influencing their observations. Placebo blinding is recommended in trials involving an untreated group when knowledge of the treatment assignment by either the patient or physician might affect perceived outcome or evaluation of possible toxicity. Blinding is especially desirable when subjective endpoints (e.g, pain, functional status, or quality of life) are studied, because such evaluations are open to substantial bias. The term *masked* is preferred in studies in which vision loss of patients is an outcome of interest (Anon. Glossary of methodologic terms. *JAMA* 1992;268:43–44). See **double-blind trial.**

blinded medications Two or more medications that appear identical in every way.

blink rate Number of eye blinks per minute counted by direct observation over a 3-minute period while the subject is sitting quietly. There is a putative correlation between blink rate and brain dopamine activity. Blink rate is increased in patients tolerant of alcohol and/or sedatives.

block design Study designed to eliminate the effect of nuisance factors when comparing effects of exposure factors on the dependent variable of interest by putting some homogeneous subjects into blocks and applying exposure factors within each block.

blocking Interruption of a train of speech before a thought or idea has been completed. After a period of silence that may last from a few seconds to minutes, the person indicates that he or she cannot recall what he or she has been saying or meant to say. Blocking should be judged present only if the person spontaneously describes losing the train of thought or, upon questioning, gives that as the reason for pausing.

blood alcohol concentration (BAC) Ratio of alcohol in the blood expressed as grams per deciliter. The U.S. National Highway Traffic Safety Administration defines BAC higher than 0.01 g/dl but lower than 0.10 g/dl as a low level of alcohol, and BAC higher than 0.10 g/dl (the legal level of intoxication in most states) as indicating intoxication. BAC produced by drinking a specific amount of alcohol is determined by factors such as body weight and rate of alcohol absorption from the gastrointestinal tract. Alcohol consumed on an empty stomach produces a higher BAC than the same amount drunk during or after a meal. After one or two drinks, nontolerant individuals experience minor changes in coordination, behavior, or mood. However, individuals vary greatly in sensitivity, depending on heredity and prior experience. As BAC increases above 100 mg% (approximately five drinks in 1 hour for a 160-lb man), most social drinkers manifest significant signs of intoxication: impaired speech, ataxia, mood lability, impaired judgment, and memory and attention deficits. When plasma levels exceed 100 mg%, symptoms intensify. Marked dysarthria and ataxia are accompanied by extensive impairment of judgment, psychomotor skills, attention, memory, and mood control. When plasma levels exceed 300 mg of alcohol per 100 ml of blood, the anesthetic action of alcohol predominates; the possibility of coma, respiratory failure, and death increases dramatically at BACs between 400 and 700 mg%.

blood-brain barrier (BBB) Extremely thin barrier that prevents many molecules and substances from freely diffusing or being transported into brain tissues or cerebrospinal fluid from the blood stream. It segregates brain interarterial fluid from the circulatory blood.

blood doping Intravenous infusion of blood to increase oxygen available for aerobic metabolic activity. Blood doping is thought to enhance performance by improving thermoregulation, buffering the inhibitory effect on muscle cells, and augmenting cardiac output secondary to increased blood volume and preload. Blood doping is done to enhance athletic endurance. Red blood cells (RBCs) from two units of the athlete's blood are frozen 8–12 weeks prior to the athletic event, the time needed for hemoglobin to return to pretransfusion levels and allow the body to surmount the detraining effect of blood donation. Blood is then infused 1 week before competition. Many adverse effects are associated with blood doping. If RBC concentration is increased too much, the corresponding elevation in blood viscosity can lead to decreased cardiac output, blood flow velocity, and peripheral blood-oxygen concentration, resulting in reduced aerobic capacity. Risk of blood clots, deep venous thrombosis, and pulmonary embolism is increased. Although a maximum safe hematocrit level has not been identified, most sources recommend keeping it below 0.5 to avoid these adverse effects (Smith DA, Perry PJ. The efficacy of ergogenic agents in athletic competition. Part II: other performance-enhancing agents. *Ann Pharmacother* 1992;26:653–659).

blood dyscrasia Blood cell abnormality ranging from reduction in the number of white blood cells (leukopenia or agranulocytosis), to increased fragility of red blood cells (hemolytic anemia), to more severe bone marrow aplasia resulting in aplastic anemia. Blood dyscrasias have been reported with use of carbamazepine, chlorpromazine, clozapine, and other drugs. They are among the most common serious adverse effects of drug therapy, with high morbidity and mortality. A diagnosis of drug-induced blood dyscrasia should be confirmed as quickly and accurately as possible. The diagnosis is made clinically and by blood tests. A drug cause is suggested by (a) previously reported associations between the drug and dyscrasia; (b) pattern of clinical association (e.g., dose, history of administration); (c) other manifestations of drug sensitivity; and (d) absence of other causes. In most cases, withdrawal of the drug responsible for the reaction improves the blood picture and returns it to normal, provided death does not occur from associated complications. Aplastic anemia, however, can be irreversible. See **agranulocytosis; aplastic anemia; thrombocytopenia.**

blood level Amount of drug that reaches the systemic circulation. Measurement of the concentration can indicate if the drug is within the therapeutic range, within an ineffective range, or within a toxic range. Maximum clinical responses to certain psychoactive drugs (lithium, antidepressants, carbamazepine) have been partially correlated with specific ranges of blood levels.

"blotter" Street name for lysergic acid diethylamide (LSD).

"blow" Street name for cocaine; street name in the United Kingdom for cannabis products.

"blowing smoke" Street name for marijuana.

"blue" Street name for amobarbital, glutethimide, or oxymorphone.

"blue angel" Street name for amobarbital or amphetamine.

"bluebird" Street name for amobarbital.

"blue bloater" Patient with chronic obstructive pulmonary disease who experiences more sleep-related hypoxemia than others. See **"pink puffer."**

"blue devil" Street name for amobarbital.

"blue doll" Street name for amobarbital.

"blue dot" Street name for lysergic acid diethylamide (LSD).

"blue heaven" Street name for lysergic acid diethylamide (LSD).

"blue velvet" Street name for paregoric plus antihistamine or elixir terpin hydrate.

blunted affect See **affect, flattened; schizophrenia/negative symptoms.**

blunting, emotional See **affect, flattened.**

B-mitten complex Electroencephalographic pattern consisting of a sharp wave followed by a higher voltage slow wave, so that the complexes resemble the thumb and hand of a mitten. B-mitten complexes are rare in normal control subjects and are primarily associated with psychiatric dysfunction. They occur bilaterally and synchronously over frontal and frontal-central areas during sleep stages 3 and 4. They are best seen in monopolar recordings. The B-mitten pattern is age-related, occurring mostly between 15 and 20 years of age.

"body bag" Street name for high-purity heroin.

body compartment In pharmacokinetics, the body is conceived as a collection of separate "compartments," each holding some fraction of an absorbed drug dose in a dynamic equilibrium with other compartments. The number of compartments and the rate at which a drug enters and leaves a compartment is largely a function of the drug's physicochemical properties, notably lipophilicity and pKa (dissociation constant). See **one-compartment model; two-compartment model.**

body dysmorphic disorder Type of obsessive-compulsive disorder (OCD) characterized by preoccupation with an imagined defect in physical appearance (e.g., a large nose, "elfish" ears, or small genitals), even in the absence of any outward appearance problems. It is not a delusion and patients can acknowledge that their feelings may be exaggerated. It is a chronic, often secret disorder that can cause significant distress and impairment. It may be seen in patients seeking plastic surgery. It has high co-morbidity with other psychiatric disorders (e.g., schizophrenia, mood disorders, anorexia nervosa, severe personality problems) and may respond to psychiatric treatment, especially with serotonin uptake inhibitors such as clomipramine and fluoxetine (Phillips KA, McElroy SL, Keck PE, et al. Body dysmorphic disorder: 30 cases of imagined ugliness. *Am J Psychiatry* 1993;150:302–308). It has long been recognized in the European literature, but largely neglected in American psychiatry except as a subtype of OCD. Also called "dysmorphophobia."

body jerk Normal movement(s) (not epileptic activity) occurring during the night at times of arousal, on falling asleep, or during periods of light sleep. Also called "hypnotic jerk"; "sleep start."

body mass index (BMI) Body weight in kilograms divided by height in meters squared (BMI = kg/m^2). BMI in the range of 25–30 is classified as overweight; BMI over 30 defines obesity (Edwards KI. Obesity, anorexia and bulimia. *Med Clin North Am* 1993;77:899–909). Recent evidence shows that BMI has strong genetic determinants, and that the direction of weight change in depression may also be genetically determined (Stunkard AJ, Fernstrom M, Price RA, Frank W, Kupfer DJ. Direction of weight change in recurrent depression. *Arch Gen Psychiatry* 1990;47:857–860).

"body stuffer" Street term for a drug dealer or user who swallows an illicit drug (usually wrapped in a condom, plastic bag, or aluminum foil) to hide it in the gastrointestinal tract to avoid detection/arrest. Packets generally contain 3–6 g of drug. The practice can be very hazardous. If a package should rupture, the smuggler will quickly absorb a very large amount of the drug, resulting in seizures, protracted coma, or death (Howell S, Ezell A. An example of cocaine tolerance in a gunshot wound fatality. *J Anal Toxicol* 1990;14:60–61; Young JD, Crapo LM. Protracted phencyclidine coma from an intestinal deposit. *Arch Intern Med* 1992;152:859–860). Also called "mule."

bolasterone (Finiject 30) Commonly abused anabolic steroid.

boldenone Commonly abused anabolic steroid.

boldenone undencyclate (Equipose) Anabolic steroid marketed primarily for use in the treatment of debilitation in horses, but commonly diverted to the underground steroid market for human use. An injectable agent formulated in sesame oil, it has a rapid onset of action, yet provides relatively stable high drug concentrations over a prolonged period. The package insert notes that at the recommended dose of 0.5 mg/lb of body weight administered every 3 weeks, overaggressive-

ness (in horses) is a potential adverse reaction that may persist for 6–8 weeks after drug administration.

bolus 1. Intravenous (IV) infusion of a drug within a few seconds. **2.** Brief (20–30 minutes) infusion of a drug relative to its elimination half-life. A multiple IV bolus results in drug accumulation as indicated by rising drug levels with each succeeding infusion.

Bolvidon See **mianserin.**

bombesin (BBS) 14-amino-acid residue peptide, originally isolated from frog skin, that produces satiety. It is found in humans, but is structurally related to gastrin-releasing peptide. It exists in at least two peripherally active forms, BBS-9 and BBS-14. When given intravenously to man, BBS stimulates gastric acid secretion and increases serum gastrin, but no changes are seen in growth hormone, prolactin, thyrotropin, luteinizing hormone, or follicle-stimulating hormone. Bombesin acts on the adrenal medulla, and sympathetic, parasympathetic, and (presumably) central nervous systems. BBS infusions have no behavioral effects in man because of the blood-brain barrier.

"bombit" Street name for methamphetamine.

bonbon sign Pressing the tongue against the cheek, giving the perception of a candy (bonbon) in the mouth. There occasionally may be repetitious movements of the tongue over the buccal lining that also push out the mouth. It is one of the manifestations of the buccal-lingual-masticatory syndrome of tardive dyskinesia.

bondage Use of ropes, cords, chains, fabric, gags, etc., to bind or constrict the body in a manner superfluous for, or irrelevant to, physiological asphyxia (e.g., tying the ankles). See **autoerotic asphyxia.**

Bondormin See **brotizolam.**

bone marrow Source of cellular components (stem cells) of the blood that proliferate and then differentiate into erythrocytes (red cells), leukocytes (white cells), and platelets. Differentiation is influenced by regulators specific to one cell line; depression of the marrow may affect the stem cells or the individual cell lines. Drugs can produce blood dyscrasias by affecting either the marrow cells or, less commonly, the circulating blood cells.

Bonferroni t procedure In analysis of variance, t procedure with alpha level adjusted by the number of multiple comparisons of group means following a significant f test. Also called Dunn multiple-comparison procedure.

Bonserin See **mianserin.**

Bonton See **lorazepam.**

Bontril See **phenmetrazine.**

"booting"   Slang term used when blood is drawn from the vein into the syringe and reinjected with an illicit drug such as cocaine or heroin.

"bopping"   Street term for use of amyl or butyl nitrite ampules.

borderline   **1.** Originally, characteristic of disorders intermediate between the neuroses and the psychoses. *Borderline,* the closely related *pseudoneurotic schizophrenia,* and other terms were used to describe patients seen as stably unstable, manifesting ego weakness, high levels of anxiety, primitive defenses, multiple symptoms, poor impulse control, and transient psychotic episodes. **2.** In DSM-IV, a type of personality disorder. The efficacy of pharmacological treatment in borderlines is now well established (Zanarini MC, Frankenburg FR, Gunderson JG. Pharmacotherapy of borderline patients. *Compr Psychiatry* 1988;29:372–378). In many instances, it is necessary to combine pharmacological treatments with psychotherapy. The nature of the borderline character raises some special psychological problems with regard to the combination of these two forms of therapy (Perry S. Combining antidepressants and psychotherapy: rationale and strategies. *J Clin Psychiatry* 1990;51:16–20).

botulinum toxin   (Oculinum) The most potent biologic neurotoxin and the first microbial protein used for the treatment of human disease (Schantz EJ, Johnson EA. Properties and use of botulinum toxin and other microbial neurotoxins in medicine. *Microb Rev* 1992;56:80–92). There are two types, A and F. Type A (BtA) is one of the most lethal biologic toxins. It is of particular interest because of its therapeutic value in the treatment of a variety of neurological and ophthalmological disorders, including strabismus, nystagmus, various dystonias, tremor, and hemifacial spasm. Preliminary reports indicate that it may be useful for the treatment of focal dystonias such as writer's or musician's cramps. In hand and limb dystonias, weakness is a desired effect, and tenderness at the injection site is noted in up to 20% of cases. The toxin is acceptable therapy for cervical dystonia. Women and thin people tend to be more prone to complications, the most common of which are swallowing difficulty, neck weakness, and pain. The symptoms are generally short-lived, but weakness can be excessive until the appropriate dose for the individual is determined. For generalized neuromuscular disorders, the toxin is indicated only for very severe localized abnormalities; otherwise, too much toxin would be required. In oromandibular dystonia, the toxin is more effective for jaw-closing than for other variants. Adductor dysphonia seems to respond to the toxin; so might selected cases of abductor dysphonia, but there is risk of local paralysis and airway obstruction. For both forms of spasmodic dysphonia, severity of dysphagia may sometimes warrant discontinuation of treatment. Successful use of botulinum toxin in a case of severe mixed tardive dyskinesia and dystonia has been reported (Stip E, Faughan M, Desjardin I. Botulinum toxin in a case of severe tardive dyskinesia mixed with dystonia. *Br J Psychiatry* 1992;161:867–868). Botulinum toxin type F has proved effective in patients with torticollis who have become resistant to BtA and who have antitoxin antibodies (Ludlow CL, Hallett M, Rhew K, et al. Therapeutic use of type F botulinum toxin. *N Engl J Med* 1992;326:349–350). Analysis of 157 patients who received at least five separate treatments with repeated injections over an 8-year period showed that on the same total dose per treatment session, duration of benefit increased and the number of complications decreased (Jenkovic J, Schwartz KS. Longitudinal experience with botulinum toxin injections for treatment of blepharospasm and cervical dystonia. *Neurology* 1993;43:834–836).

bowel obsession   Variant of obsessive-compulsive disorder characterized by excessive preoccupation with sudden loss of bowel control. It also occurs in agoraphobia without panic and social phobia. Case reports document successful treatment with clomipramine, doxepin, imipramine, nortriptyline, benzodiazepines, and behavioral techniques.

box and whisker plot   Graph that displays both frequencies and distribution of observation. Also called "box plot."

"boxer's brain"   See **dementia pugilistica.**

box plot   See **box and whisker plot.**

"boy"   Street name for heroin.

bradykinesia   Extrapyramidal disorder characterized by diminution in the velocity of normal movements and paucity of movements; inability to initiate and conduct movement at a normal speed associated with a sense of weakness or fatigue. It is a cardinal feature of parkinson syndromes (e.g., the "masked facies" of Parkinson's disease) that represents decreased nigrostriatal dopaminergic activity. It should be distinguished from drug-induced akinesia. The bradykinetic patient is slowed, less expressive, and mask-like; blinks infrequently; and turns the whole body rather than eyes and head separately. Pharmacological agents that have been used to treat bradykinesia, with varying degrees of success, include tricyclic antidepressants (e.g., protriptyline, nortriptyline), dopaminergic agents (e.g., levodopa/carbidopa, amantadine, bromocriptine, pergolide), and psychostimulants (methylphenidate and pemoline).

bradykinin Peptide with a wide spectrum of proinflammatory actions. It activates nociceptive afferent nerves, increases vascular permeability, promotes vasodilation, and induces positive chemotaxis of leukocytes. Bradykinin is liberated by the enzymatic cleavage of its precursor, kininogen, by the enzyme kallikrein.

bradyphrenia See **dementia, subcortical** (preferred term).

brain derived neurotrophic factor (BDNF) Naturally occurring member of the neurotrophin growth factor family, discovered in 1991, that can preferentially stimulate growth of dopaminergic cells of the substantia nigra that are destroyed in Parkinson's disease. The discovery is expected to result in development of new drugs to treat Parkinson's disease. BDNF has a different neuronal specificity to nerve growth factor, interacting with the central rather than peripheral projections of sensory neurons.

brain electrical activity mapping (BEAM) Computerized spatial and temporal extension of conventional electroencephalography capable of demonstrating characteristic findings of abnormal electrophysiology in schizophrenia, learning disabilities, and a variety of disorders seen in conjunction with psychostimulant and hallucinogen abuse. Preliminary BEAM studies indicate significant differences between the electrical activity maps of patients with dementia of the Alzheimer's type and normal control subjects or patients with vascular dementia. See **brain imaging.**

brain function Inner workings of the brain; functions the brain performs. It should not be confused with brain structure.

brain imaging Radiological techniques that assess in vivo structural and functional neuroanatomy, including x-ray computed tomography (CT), magnetic resonance imaging (MRI), MRI spectroscopy (MRS), regional cerebral blood flow (rCBF), positron emission tomography (PET), single photon emission computed tomography (SPECT), magnetoencephalography, and brain electrical activity mapping (BEAM).

brain metabolism Process by which the brain synthesizes and degrades various chemicals, and alteration of its cells for repair, energy control, and function.

brain organization Association among various brain areas as they interact to receive, process, and integrate the internal and external experiences of the individual.

brainstem auditory-evoked response (BAER) Sensitive, noninvasive measure of nerve impulse transmission stimulated in the ear (auditory clicks delivered through head phones) and traveling through the brain stem to the auditory cortex in the temporal lobe. As the impulses course through auditory nerve and brain stem, wave forms measured across the scalp are generated. The waves correspond roughly to known synaptic areas of hearing and can localize lesions along the lateral tracts in the brain stem. BAER characteristics are not altered by therapeutic or toxic doses of neuroleptics, or significantly affected by cognitive effects or levels of arousals including anesthesia (differentiating them from event-related potentials) (Chiappa KH, Gladstone KJ, Young RR. Brain stem auditory responses. Studies of waveform variations in 50 normal human subjects. *Arch Neurol* 1979;36:81–87). It has been used as a probe in autism with contradictory results. See **brainstem-evoked potential; brainstem evoked-response audiometry; somatosensory evoked potential.**

brainstem-evoked potential (BSEP) Exogenous evoked-response potential (ERP) that measures electrical transmission of impulses traveling through the brain stem. A stimulus is generated in a peripheral nerve (arm, leg, face, or ear), and the evoked response is measured at various points along the known route of transmission (near field) and over the cortex (far field). The most commonly used BSEP is the brain stem auditory evoked response (BAER). Another evoked response that can yield information on brain stem function is the somatosensory evoked potential. In general, evoked responses are affected by trauma, pressure, and ischemia, but resist the effects of drugs and toxins. Therefore, these tests are helpful in evaluating patients on therapeutic doses of neuroleptic and most sedative hypnotic medications. See **brainstem auditory-evoked response; somatosensory evoked potential.**

brainstem-evoked response audiometry Method of measuring high-frequency hearing when a person is asleep, sedated, or uncooperative by analysis of the early wave forms of the brainstem auditory-evoked response. It may be useful in a mentally handicapped person unable to cooperate with other forms of hearing testing. It involves small electrodes being placed on the forehead, on the scalp, and behind each ear. A headphone is held against the ear, and a clicking noise is delivered through it. This generates tiny electrical potentials in the nerve of the ear and the pathway to the brain that are picked up by the electrodes and processed on a computer to give a visual display. The information on hearing is limited to high frequencies and is not always reliable. Response also changes with age. See **brainstem auditory-evoked potential.**

brain stimulation reward Experimental procedure whereby an animal learns to receive brief, low-intensity electrical stimuli to subcortical regions of the brain that elicit a reward.

brain stress test One of a group of tests developed for imaging the brain in an active state because disease is manifested most provocatively during brain activation. There are three classes: cognitive, motoric, and pharmacological; the latter has been most thoroughly studied.

brand name drug Trademark or brand name selected by the company marketing the product. Trademark selection involves extensive research to avoid confusion with existing trademarks and generic names for other products. Emphasis is on development of a distinctive trademark that will be easily written and remembered by physicians. Frequently, the trademark must be capable of being registered in most countries of the world. The process involves computer searching of registered trademarks, computer analysis of the structural and phonetic composition of the proposed trademark in a number of languages, and extensive market research and analysis by panels of physicians, pharmacists, and other health practitioners. If a newly proposed trademark survives this scrutiny, it is submitted for registration as a trademark in many countries. In the United States, the Patent and Trademark Office employs specially trained attorneys who examine the proposed trademark to ensure that it is free from possible confusion with other registered trademarks. If the trademark survives that examination, it is published in the office's Official Gazette for opposition by any interested party. If it survives these steps, it becomes a registered trademark entitled to certain legal protections. In the United States, the process could take over a year (Beary JF. Confusion about drug names. *N Engl J Med* 1991;325:588–589).

Brantur See **minaprine.**

breakthrough anxiety See **anxiety, breakthrough.**

bretazenil (RO 16-6028) Partial benzodiazepine agonist that is a v receptor ligand. It is a high-potency benzodiazepine with a rapid onset of action (first effects are experienced a few minutes after oral administration) and short mean elimination half-life of 2–4 hours. Placebo-controlled, double-blind studies indicate that it is effective in suppressing panic attacks with beneficial effects on anticipatory anxiety and phobic avoidance.

Brevibloc See **esmolol.**

Brevital See **methohexital.**

"brick" Street name for a cannabinol.

"bridling" Type of perioral dyskinesia, seen in patients with tardive dyskinesia, characterized by retraction of one or both corners of the mouth.

brief depression See **depression, brief.**

brief reactive psychosis See **psychosis, brief reactive.**

brief stimulus therapy (BST) Form of mild electroshock therapy.

bright light therapy See **phototherapy.**

British National Formulary (BNF) Concise, basic drug prescribing guide produced by a "Joint Formulary Committee" set up by the British Medical Association and the Pharmaceutical Society of Great Britain for use by British physicians.

Brocadisipal See **orphenadrine.**

brofaromine (CGP 11 305 A) (Consonar) (BRO) Putative antidepressant that is a selective and reversible inhibitor of monoamine oxidase-A (RIMA). It is less liable to potentiate pressor responses to tyramine in man compared to classic monoamine oxidase inhibitors. It is also less likely to interact with sympathomimetic amines in over-the-counter medications. It may be useful in the treatment of social phobias. Compared to tricyclic antidepressants, BRO has the advantage of not causing anticholinergic side effects. Among its side effects are middle or late insomnia, or superficial sleep (Haffmans J, Knegtering R. The selective reversible monoamine oxidase-A inhibitor brofaromine and sleep. *J Clin Psychopharmacol* 1993;13:291–292). Early side effects that subside quickly are nausea, dizziness, dry mouth, and feeling cold. In some patients nausea can be alleviated by taking BRO with food. Double-blind studies in patients with bulimia nervosa indicate significant reduction in intake of nonbinge meals and significant weight loss compared to placebo. BRO has been found effective and safe in the treatment of depressed geriatric patients. Double-blind studies also indicate that it is effective for panic disorder. Clinical trials in Europe indicate it is a well tolerated, effective treatment for excessive daytime sleepiness and REM sleep–associated symptoms in narcolepsy.

brofaromine + lithium Co-administration in patients nonresponsive to brofaromine may result in therapeutic response with no serious adverse effects (Nolan WA, Haffmans J, Bouvy PF, Duivenvoorden HJ. Monoamine oxidase inhibitors in resistant major depression. A double-blind comparison of brofaromine and tranylcypromine in patients resistant to tricyclic antidepressants. *J Affective Disord* 1993;28:189–197).

brofaromine + maprotiline Brofaromine augments therapeutic response in patients refractory to maprotiline without serious drug-drug interactions.

brofaromine + phenylephrine Administration of phenylephrine (PE; Neo-Synephrine) to patients taking 75 mg brofaromine twice daily caused no clinically relevant increases in blood pressure before or during brofaromine treatment (Gleiter CH, Muhlbauer B, Gradin-Frimmer G, et al. Administration of sympathomimetic drugs with the selective MAO-A inhibitor brofaromine: effect on blood pressure. *Drug Invest* 1992;4:149–154).

brofaromine + phenylpropanolamine The slow-release formulation (75 mg) of phenylpropanolamine (PPA) does not cause a clinically relevant increase in blood pressure before or during brofaromine therapy, whereas rapid-release PPA (25–75 mg) may cause a significant pressor response that may still be evident after 3 days. Rapid-release PPA should be avoided during brofaromine therapy (Gleiter CH, Muhlbauer B, Gradin- Frimmer G, et al. Administration of sympathomimetic drugs with the selective MAO-A inhibitor brofaromine: effect on blood pressure. *Drug Invest* 1992;4:149–154).

bromazepam (Lectopam; Lenitin; Lexotan; Lexotanil) 1,4 benzodiazepine marketed in Europe for its anticonvulsant properties. It is oxidatively metabolized and has a long elimination half-life.

bromazepam + clomipramine In outpatients with major depressive disorder or dysthymic disorder, co-administration was effective and well tolerated (Cottraux J, Riant N. Alpidem versus bromazepam in depressed outpatients treated with clomipramine. A controlled comparison. *Clin Neuropharmacol* 1992;15[suppl 1/B]:521B).

bromazepam + fluvoxamine Bromazepam plasma concentrations increased by 2.4 times after multiple doses of fluvoxamine (Van Harten J, Holland RL, Wesnes K, et al. Kinetic and dynamic interaction study between fluvoxamine and benzodiazepines. Poster presented at the Second Jerusalem Conference on Pharmaceutical Sciences and Clinical Pharmacology, Jerusalem, May 24–29, 1992).

bromerguride First 8 alpha-aminoergoline derivative with central dopamine antagonistic properties in a number of neuropharmacological and neurobiochemical tests. It is derived from lisuride by one-step bromination. In an open clinical trial, it had antipsychotic activity in schizophrenic patients. Positive symptoms were decreased within 3 days of treatment. Negative symptoms improved when they were related to the presence of positive symptoms; bromerguride was less active in influencing predominant negative symptoms. It does not cause extrapyramidal reactions or elevation of prolactin levels. Bromerguride labeled with radioactive isotope bromine 76 has been successfully used in primates and humans for positron emission tomography (PET) studies (Loschmann PA, Horowski R, Wachtel H. Bromerguride—an ergoline derivative with atypical neuroleptic properties. *Clin Neuropharm* 1992;15:[suppl 1, Pt A]:263A–264A).

Bromidol See **bromperidol.**

bromism Intoxication resulting from the accumulation of bromide. It may be manifested by mental dulling; memory disturbances; skin lesions; weakness; tremor of the hand, face, and tongue; ataxia; fetid breath; coated tongue; delirium; hallucinations that may last for weeks; schizophreniform psychosis; or pseudoepilepsy. Once common, bromism is seen most often today in patients who self-administer bromide-containing over-the-counter preparations.

bromocriptine (Parlodel) Ergot alkaloid structurally related to dopamine (DA). It has a biphasic effect that depends on the dose. In low doses, bromocriptine may preferentially activate DA presynaptic receptors and thereby act as an antagonist; at high doses, it mimics the action of dopamine, acting directly at the postsynaptic receptor sites. It has high affinity for the D_2D_A receptor. Its agonistic actions on the D_2 receptor appear to depend on stimulation of D_1D_A receptors. In addition, there is evidence that bromocriptine might be a partial agonist or mixed agonist-antagonist at the D_2 presynaptic receptor. Since bromocriptine has no effect on D_1 receptors, availability of presynaptic DA or independent stimulation of the D_1 receptor by other pharmacological agents is required for bromocriptine to produce its behavioral effects (Markou A, Koob GF. Bromocriptine reverses the elevation in intracranial self-stimulation thresholds observed in a rat model of cocaine withdrawal. *Neuropsychopharmacology* 1992;7:213–224). Bromocriptine can only be given orally. Absorption begins in 20–40 minutes, with peak blood levels at 1–2 hours; half-life is about 7 hours. Over 90% undergoes first-pass hepatic metabolism. In patients with compromised mental status and/or dysphagia, it is administered by means of a nasogastric tube, with some risk of aspiration. Bromocriptine is presently used in the treatment of amenorrhea, galactorrhea, and acromegaly, and in the prevention of physiologic lactation and Parkinson's disease. Its most significant side effect is orthostatic hypotension, although it may also cause nausea, vomiting, and hallucinations. Adverse effects can be minimized by slow introduction over several weeks. Like other dopamine agonists, it is indicated for Parkinson's disease patients who have not responded optimally to levodopa drugs or who have developed "on-off" fluctuations or moderate to severe drug-induced dyskinesia refractory to adjustments of levodopa dosage and timing. In Parkinson's disease patients, the most common side effects of bromocriptine are nausea, vomiting, dyspepsia, hypotension, hallucinations, psychosis, and dyskinesias. Long-term therapy can be associated with cramps and pains in the legs, often at night, with or without claudication. Generally, these side effects subside after bromocriptine is discontinued. Bromocriptine can cause a variety of psychiatric complications (nightmares, wanderings, confusion, delusions, and sometimes aggressive psychosis) that can be difficult to manage and that persist for days after dosage reduction or discontinuation. Parkinson patients who have psychotic symptoms on levodopa drugs are very likely to be worse on bromocriptine. Bromocriptine is often used for the treatment of neuroleptic malignant syndrome (NMS) in doses of 5–10 mg three times a day. Some patients have been given up to 60 mg/day. There may be rapid improvement within a few hours (3+), but response is variable. To date, bromocriptine has not exacerbated any underlying psychosis in NMS patients. It has not been proven effective in the treatment of tardive dyskinesia. It may be used for maintenance of cocaine abstinence (Sitland-Marken PA, Wells BV, Froemming JH, et al. Psychiatric applications of bromocriptine therapy. *J Clin Psychiatry* 1990; 51:68–82) and has been used with limited success for treatment of cocaine withdrawal (Giannini AJ, Folts DJ, Feather JN, Sullivan BS. Bromocriptine and amantadine in cocaine detoxification. *Brain Res* 1989;29:11–16). Although bromocriptine is believed to have almost no abuse potential in humans (Gawin FH. Chronic neuropharmacology of cocaine: progress in pharmacotherapy. *J Clin Psychiatry* 1988;49[2 suppl]:12), a case of abuse has been reported (Ross RG, Ward NG. Bromocriptine abuse. *Biol Psychiatry* 1992;31:404–406). Bromocriptine has been used to treat attention-deficit disorder in chemically dependent patients (Cavanaugh R, Clifford JS, Gregory WL. The use of bromocriptine for the treatment of attention deficit disorder in two chemically dependent patients. *J Psychoactive Drugs* 1989; 21:217–220). Controlled studies in depressed patients refractory to standard antidepressant therapy indicate that bromocriptine has antidepressant efficacy comparable to that of standard tricyclic antidepressants (Wells BG,

Marken PA. Bromocriptine in the treatment of depression. *Drug Intell Clin Pharm* 1989;23: 601–602). Pregnancy risk category C.

bromocriptine + alcohol To avoid severe side effects due to measured alcohol intolerance, bromocriptine-treated patients should not drink alcohol .

bromocriptine + antihypertensive Bromocriptine can cause hypotension and may potentiate antihypertensive drugs. To prevent hypotension, reduction of antihypertensive dosage may be warranted if both drugs are prescribed.

bromocriptine + clozapine Co-administration in the treatment of co-morbid psychosis in patients with Parkinson's disease has produced clearing of psychotic illness, with no serious adverse interactions or worsening of parkinsonism (Wolk SI, Douglas CJ. Clozapine treatment of psychosis in Parkinson's disease: a report of five consecutive cases. *J Clin Psychiatry* 1992;53:373–376).

bromocriptine + dantrolene Co-administration is often used for the treatment of neuroleptic malignant syndrome without serious adverse interactions.

bromocriptine + fluoxetine No adverse interactions in depressed parkinson patients have been reported (Lauterbach EC. Dopaminergic hallucinosis with fluoxetine in Parkinsons disease. *Am J Psychiatry* 1993;150:1750).

bromocriptine growth hormone challenge test (BGHT) Test used as an index of D_2 receptor activity within the central nervous system and to adjust the dose of antipsychotic drugs for maximum therapeutic effect.

bromocriptine + haloperidol Double-blind crossover studies indicate that bromocriptine enhances therapeutic response to haloperidol in chronic schizophrenia.

bromocriptine + imipramine Co-administration has been used effectively to augment antidepressant response to imipramine. Side effects may include nausea, dizziness, and headache (Waerens J, Gerlach J. Bromocriptine and imipramine in endogenous depression. A double-blind controlled trial in outpatients. *J Affect Disord* 1981;3:193–202).

bromocriptine + monoamine oxidase inhibitor (MAOI) Bromocriptine may be used safely with monoamine oxidase type A inhibitors. Although their strength is less than that occurring with optimal doses of levodopa, substantial improvement in the disabilities of Parkinson's disease may occur.

bromocriptine + neuroleptic Adjunctive, low-dose bromocriptine has been reported to improve psychotic symptoms in neuroleptic-resistant schizophrenia without producing adverse drug-drug interactions. It has been co-administered with chlorpromazine, flupen-thixol, fluphenazine, and haloperidol (Wolf M-A, Diener J-M, Lajeunnesse C, et al. Low-dose bromocriptine in neuroleptic-resistant schizophrenia. A pilot study. *Biol Psychiatry* 1992;31:1166–1168).

4-bromo-2,5-dimethoxy-amphetamine (DOB) Methamphetamine analog designer drug with potent hallucinogenic and sympathomimetic properties. It is relatively long-acting, with symptoms beginning 3–4 hours after ingestion and taking up to 24 hours to resolve. It has been sold impregnated in blotter paper, some-times as lysergic acid diethylamide (LSD). Substance abusers use it as a hallucinogen. Also called "bromo-DMA."

bromo-DMA See **4-bromo-2,5-dimethoxy-amphe-tamine.**

bromperidol (Azurene; Bromidol; Consilium; Impromen; Tesoprel) (BRP) Potent buty-rophenone derivative neuroleptic in which the chlorine halogen of haloperidol (HAL) is replaced by the halogen bromine. It has rela-tively selective binding affinity for dopamine D_2, as compared with dopamine D_1, serotonin S_2, histamine H_1, and adrenergic alpha$_1$ bind-ing sites in the brain (Leysen JE, Janssen PAJ. Specificity of ligands used in psychiatric re-search. *In* Sen AK, Lee T [eds], *Receptors and Ligands in Psychiatry.* Cambridge, UK: Cam-bridge University Press, 1988, pp 526–543). BRP has a longer half-life (30+ hours) than HAL and can be administered in a single daily dose. It has a slight sedative effect. Clinical trials indicate that BRP has a specific action against delusions and hallucinations while causing fewer extrapyramidal and other side effects (e.g., psychomotor inhibition) than HAL. Its major metabolite is reduced brom-peridol (Someya T, Inaba T, Tyndale RF, Tang SW, Takahashi S. Conversion of bromperidol to reduced bromperidol in human liver. *Neu-ropsychopharmacology* 1991;5:177–182).

bromperidol decanoate Long-acting injectable formulation of bromperidol. It has been shown to be effective and reasonably safe in the treatment of schizophrenia (McLaren S, Cookson JC, Silverstone T. Positive and nega-tive symptoms, depression and social disability in chronic schizophrenia: a comparative trial of bromperidol and fluphenazine decanoates. *Int Clin Psychopharmacol* 1992;7:67–72).

"Brompton's cocktail" Mixture of heroin, co-caine, ethanol, and a phenothiazine neurolep-tic used for the treatment of severe pain.

brotizolam (Bondormin; Dormex; Indormyl; Ladormin; Ladorum Landormin; Lenderm; Lendorm; Lendormin; Lenormin; Sintonal) Thienodiazepine with pharmacological effects comparable to the benzodiazepines. It is me-tabolized by hepatic microsomal oxidation. Although it is considered a benzodiazepine from a clinical standpoint, the 26th Expert Committee on Drug Dependence of the World Health Organization concluded that it does not need to be controlled. It is currently (1994) the only thienodiazepine marketed anywhere in the world.

"brown" Street name for heroin.

"brownie" Street name for dextroamphet-amine.

"brown sugar" Street name for heroin.

bruxism Teeth clenching with protrusive or lat-eral jaw movements.

bucco-lingual-masticatory syndrome (BLM) Most common form of tardive dyskinesia. See **tardive dyskinesia.**

bufotenin (5-hydroxy-N,N-dimethyltryptamine) Methylated indolamine serotonin analog that produces hallucinogenic effects similar to those seen following lysergic acid diethyla-mide (LSD) or mescaline administration. It is metabolized mainly through oxidative deami-nation by monoamine oxidase (Karkkainen J, Raisanen M. Nialamide, an MAO inhibitor, increases urinary excretion of endogenously produced bufotenin in man. *Biol Psychiatry* 1992;32:1042–1048).

bug, cocaine See **cocaine bug.**

bulimarexic Bulimia nervosa patient who binge-eats and purges.

bulimia Eating disorder that may be either a symptom or a syndrome. It is manifested by insatiable hunger resulting in compulsive or binge eating. Bulimics lose control over eating behavior and consume large quantities of calorie-rich food. To reduce caloric intake, they purge by self-induced vomiting, exces-sively restricted dieting, or prolonged periods of fasting. Bulimics have a propensity to abuse alcohol and psychoactive drugs (most com-monly marijuana and stimulants). They also abuse laxatives, diuretics, and diet pills to counteract the effects of binge eating. Laxa-tive abuse can cause severe medical problems, notably electrolyte disturbances (e.g., hy-pokalemia). Diuretic abuse can also lead to alterations in electrolytes and dehydration. See **bulimia nervosa; bulimia/diuretic misuse.**

bulimia/diabetes An unknown number of bu-limics also are diabetic. Their abnormal eating habits can cause their blood glucose levels to fluctuate considerably. Their consumption of excessive quantities of high-calorie foods and simple carbohydrates (e.g., cookies and candy) can cause acute hyperglycemia. If they do not adjust insulin in response to increased caloric intake—and many do not—diabetic ketoacidosis may occur. Because insulin in-creases glucose metabolism and causes weight gain, some diabetic bulimics induce glycosuria by intentional insulin overdosing. Bulimic diabetics who purge risk hypoglycemia because of a relative excess of insulin. Clinical experience substantiates that long-term vascular problems may occur secondary to abnormal eating and purging habits (Hillard JR, Hillard PJA. Bulimia, anorexia nervosa and diabetes. Deadly combinations. *Psychiatr Clin North Am* 1984;7:367–379).

bulimia/diuretic misuse Among the clinical signs and symptoms of bulimia is diuretic abuse. Misused prescription drugs include (a) loop diuretics, either ethacrynic acid (Edecrin) or furosemide (Lasix); (b) potassium-sparing diuretics, either spironolactone (Aldactone) or triamterene (Dyrenium); and (c) thiazides—chlorothiazide (Diuril) or hydrochlorothiazide (Hydro Diuril). Loop diuretic misuse can cause secondary problems: hyponatremia, hypercalcuria, hypovolemia, and hypokalemic alkalosis and low serum magnesium levels. Misused/abused over-the-counter diuretics (e.g., ammonium chloride) may cause transient kidney function impairment, low serum calcium and potassium levels, hyperglycemia, metabolic acidosis, and other manifestations of ammonium chloride toxicity.

bulimia nervosa Eating disorder of unknown etiology, common in women, that is characterized by bingeing and purging, disturbances of mood, and neuroendocrine abnormalities. Bulimia occurring in males has received relatively little attention in the literature. Bulimic patients have diminished caloric requirements and reduced metabolic rate. Bulimic women have alterations of neurotransmitter systems known to contribute to modulation of feeding, mood, and neuroendocrine function. Bulimics have increased cerebrospinal fluid concentrations of peptide YY (PYY), a potent stimulant of feeding in experimental animals; increased PYY activity may contribute to patients' drive to binge. Bulimia nervosa is associated with excessive levels of the brain hormone vasopressin, which is believed to affect thirst, blood pressure, learning, and memory. Bulimia may be punctuated by sudden decisions to binge and purge, with little regard for the considerable physical risk incurred or for the inevitable dysphoria afterwards. There is a high prevalence of impulsive behavior in bulimia nervosa (Fahy T, Eisler I. Impulsivity and eating disorders. *Br J Psychiatry* 1993;162:193–197). Bulimic patients report binge eating 2–20 times per week; half binge daily, and a third binge multiple times a day. Approximately a third report using laxatives. Each binge may be followed by depressed mood,

self-criticism, and often self-induced vomiting. Patients may show dental enamel erosions, abrasions, and scars on knuckles from induced vomiting (Russell's sign). Also observed secondary to induced vomiting are enlarged parotid glands, amenorrhea, hypokalemia, and esophageal irritation with mucosal tears. Chronic ipecac (emetine) use may result in cardiomyopathy; cardiac failure due to ipecac intoxication is a serious consequence. Vomiting or use of diuretics and laxatives can cause hypokalemia alkalosis and metabolic acidosis, dehydration, increased potassium excretion, weakness, lethargy, acute dilatation of the stomach (rare), and at times, cardiac arrhythmias that can lead to cardiac arrest, all made even worse by fasting. A subpopulation of patients engages in regular binge eating without purging. A minority of patients (one-third) have co-existent anorexia nervosa (anorexia nervosa—bulimia variant) and present with low body weight and other features of anorexia nervosa such as fear of fatness, vigorous exercising, and amenorrhea. They have a worse prognosis than those with bulimia nervosa alone. Typically, all types of bulimic patients have a history of numerous strict or fad diets, punctuated by recurrent episodes of binge eating and persistent overconcern with body shape and weight. Major depressive disorders and alcohol and drug abuse coexist in a large number of bulimic patients and their first-degree family members. Bulimia can be a symptom in a variety of medical disorders, or a component of the anorexia nervosa syndrome. It is also encountered alone as a separate syndrome in which the patient's weight is comparatively normal. There is no substantive evidence to support the hypothesis that childhood sexual abuse is a risk factor for bulimia nervosa. See **cholecystokinin; eating disorder/pregnancy.**

bulimia nervosa, multisymptomatic Disorder characterized by a disturbed eating pattern and problems in impulse control resulting in drug abuse, alcohol abuse, self-mutilation, kleptomania, and/or sexual disinhibition. There also may be symptoms of obsessive-compulsive disorder. Manipulation of food is associated to a varying degree with alcohol and drug abuse.

bulimia nervosa/pharmacotherapy Controlled studies have demonstrated the efficacy of cognitive, behavioral, and psychopharmacological treatments in alleviating bulimic symptoms in the short term. Antidepressants used include tricyclics (TCAs—imipramine, desipramine), monoamine oxidase inhibitors (MAOIs—phenelzine, isocarboxazid), serotonin uptake inhibitors (fluoxetine), and trazodone. Long-term outcome studies, however, show a high relapse rate. TCA and MAOI doses used to treat bulimia nervosa are generally the same as those used to treat mood disorders, but higher fluoxetine doses (60 mg/day) seem more effective than lower doses (20 mg/day). Carbamazepine and lithium have been less effective than TCAs and MAOIs; their adjunctive use in eating disorders should rest on consideration of other co-morbid conditions. Several medication trials are sometimes required to establish the proper medication for a given patient. According to the American Psychiatric Association Practice Guidelines for Eating Disorders, antidepressants may reduce symptoms of binge eating and purging independent of the presence of depression. They should not constitute the entire treatment, but may be helpful for patients with significant symptoms of depression, anxiety, obsessions, or certain impulse disorder symptoms, and for patients who have failed previous attempts at appropriate psychosocial therapy. If bulimic symptoms do not respond to medication, it is important to determine if the patient took the medication shortly before vomiting. Medication serum levels should be obtained to determine if presumably effective levels have been achieved (American Psychiatric Association Practice Guideline for Eating Disorders. *Am J Psychiatry* 1993;150:207–228).

bulimia, normal-weight Disturbed appetite, mood, and neuroendocrine function often responsive to antidepressants. See **bulimia.**

"bulking out" Street term used by weight lifters and body builders to describe the expansion in muscle size induced by androgenic/anabolic steroids.

"bullet" Street name for a central nervous system depressant or volatile nitrite (e.g., amyl nitrite sold in "head shops," pornography stores, and novelty shops, and through mail order houses).

Bunil See **melperone.**

Buprenex See **buprenorphine.**

buprenorphine (Buprenex; Temgesic) Analgesic currently approved by the Food and Drug Administration (FDA) for moderate to severe pain. It is approximately 30 times more potent than morphine and interacts primarily with the mu-receptor. It has dual action as a partial opioid agonist, or mixed agonist-antagonist, with a biphasic dose-response curve that limits agonist effects, making it remarkably safe and free from toxicity. It has been reported to have antidepressant properties and has produced marked benefit for at least some treatment-refractory depressives. Since 1978, research data have suggested that 1–32 mg/day may be

effective therapy for heroin addiction, because heroin's high is antagonized by buprenorphine; 8 mg/day can be as effective as 60 mg/day of methadone. A clinically important consequence of its antagonist properties appears to be that, when buprenorphine use is abruptly terminated, the withdrawal syndrome is relatively mild and brief compared with withdrawal from methadone. It is also more difficult to overdose with buprenorphine than with methadone, because at higher doses its antagonistic effects limit the opiate effects of sedation, respiratory depression, and hypotension (Johnson RE, Jaffe JH, Fudala PJ. Controlled trial of buprenorphine treatment for opioid dependence. *JAMA* 1992;267:2750–2755; Resnick RB, Galanter M, Pycha C, et al. Buprenorphine: an alternative to methadone for heroin dependence treatment. *Psychopharm Bull* 1992;28:109–113). Preliminary human studies indicate that buprenorphine treatment may be associated with significantly less cocaine abuse than treatment with methadone maintenance is. This is important, because combined opioid and cocaine dependence is a major clinical problem; up to 70% of heroin addicts are also cocaine-dependent, and more than half continue to use cocaine during methadone maintenance. This combined addiction has been associated with the spread of acquired immunodeficiency syndrome (AIDS) through needle sharing and the combined immunosuppressive effects of both drugs. Physical dependence on buprenorphine is less severe than dependence on morphine, even with chronic use. Buprenorphine does have abuse potential: substance abusers may intravenously inject sublingual tablets or snort crushed tablets like snuff (San L, Cami J, Fernandez T, et al. Assessment and management of opioid withdrawal symptoms in buprenorphine-dependent subjects. *Br J Addict* 1992;87:55–62). Abuse among opioid addicts who spontaneously switched from heroin to intravenous buprenorphine has been increasingly reported because it is an unadulterated, easily available drug that produces subjective effects very close to those of intravenously administered heroin (Torrens M, San L, Cami J. Buprenorphine versus heroin dependence: comparison of toxicologic and psychopathologic characteristics. *Am J Psychiatry* 1993;150:822–824). Schedule V; pregnancy risk category C. See **buprenorphine + cocaine.**

buprenorphine + amitriptyline In normal subjects, sublingual buprenorphine (0.4 mg) and oral amitriptyline (50 mg) mildly impaired performance on a number of psychomotor tests. The combination can be used with reasonable safety (Saarialho-Kere U, Mattila MJ, Paloheimo M, Seppala T. Psychomotor, respiratory and neuroendocrinological effects of buprenorphine and amitriptyline in healthy volunteers. *Eur J Clin Pharmacol* 1987;33:139–146).

buprenorphine + cocaine Sublingual buprenorphine maintenance (12–16 mg/day) suppresses illicit opioid use and attenuates cocaine use. Buprenorphine has no significant effects on cocaine euphoria (Schottenfeld RS, Pakes J, Ziedonis D, Kosten TR. Buprenorphine: dose-related effects on cocaine and opioid use in cocaine-abusing opioid-dependent humans. *Biol Psychiatry* 1993;34:66–74). In a study of acute co-administration effects, the "high" from a relatively low dose of buprenorphine was more intense and longer-lasting than that from cocaine, and subjects preferred the combination of the two drugs (Manelli P, Janiri L, Tempesta E, Jones RT. Prediction in drug abuse: cocaine interactions with alcohol and buprenorphine. *Br J Psychiatry* 1993;163[suppl 21]:39–45).

bupropion (Amfebutamone; Amfetamone; Wellbutrin) (BUP) Chemically unique antidepressant of the propiophenone class and the first monocyclic aminoketone to be used clinically. Structurally, it is similar to diethylpropion and amphetamines, both of which have prominent dopaminergic activity. It is extensively metabolized to pharmacologically active metabolites (hydroxybupropion, threohydrobupropion, ethrohydrobupropion) with half-lives longer than 24 hours, monitoring of which should continue for several days after BUP is discontinued. Steady-state concentration of metabolites may be 10–100 times that of BUP. Its pharmacological and clinical side effect profile differs from such profiles of the tricyclic antidepressants. It does not block norepinephrine or serotonin uptake or inhibit monoamine oxidase, but may affect dopamine. BUP may benefit patients refractory to serotonin uptake inhibitors. It has mild psychostimulant properties and, because it inhibits dopamine reuptake, has on rare occasions evoked extrapyramidal effects. BUP has no significant anticholinergic activity. Its cardiovascular profile may make it useful in the treatment of depressed patients with pre-existing cardiovascular disease. Some clinical trials have shown that BUP can be a reasonably tolerated antidepressant in depressed octogenarians and an effective treatment for adolescent depression. Because of its dopamine effects, BUP appears to have added utility in disorders with a known dopamine impairment in association with depression (Parkinson's disease, cocaine withdrawal, attention-deficit disorder). Prelimi-

nary clinical trials indicate that it may be an effective treatment for chronic fatigue syndrome, even in patients unresponsive to other antidepressants (Goodnick PJ, Sandoval R, Brickman A, Klimas NG. Bupropion treatment of fluoxetine-resistant chronic fatigue syndrome. *Biol Psychiatry* 1992;32:834–838). BUP may be ineffective in illnesses that typically are unresponsive to tricyclic antidepressants. It is not effective in panic disorder. When given in doses below 450 mg/day, seizure frequency is approximately 4/1000 (0.4%); risk increases tenfold as doses increase to 450–600 mg/day. High plasma levels of its metabolites, especially hydroxybupropion, are associated with poor response, cognitive and extrapyramidal toxicity, and seizures. BUP does not appear to induce sedation and psychomotor retardation when taken with alcohol. Like all effective antidepressants, it may provoke mania. Caution in the concurrent use of BUP and dopamine agonists, even at the lowest doses, is advisable (Settle EC, Jr. Bupropion: update 1993. *Int Drug Ther Newsl* 1993;28:29–36). Pregnancy risk category B. See **bupropion/overdose; bupropion/seizures.**

bupropion + alcohol A study showed that alcohol plus a single 100-mg dose of bupropion (BUP) did not influence time of peak BUP level or elimination half-life. Intake of 40 ml of alcohol 3.5 hours after BUP (100 mg) or placebo showed no influence of BUP on alcohol kinetics. BUP (100 mg) plus 32 ml of alcohol blocked impairment in auditory vigilance produced by alcohol alone (Posner J, Bye A, Peck AW, Whitman P. Alcohol and bupropion pharmacokinetics in healthy male volunteers. *Eur J Pharmacol* 1984;26:627–630; Hamilton KJ, Bush MS, Peck AW. The effect of bupropion, a new antidepressant drug, and alcohol and their interaction in man. *Eur J Clin Pharmacol* 1984;27:75–80).

bupropion + amantadine Bupropion (BUP) inhibits dopamine reuptake; amantadine facilitates release of presynaptic dopamine. Co-administration may cause dopaminergic overdrive, resulting in delirium. Caution during concurrent use of BUP and dopamine agonists, even at the lowest doses, is advisable (Liberzon I, Dequardo JR, Silk KR. Bupropion and delirium. *Am J Psychiatry* 1990;147:1659–1690).

bupropion/breast milk Little is known about the effects of bupropion in breast-fed infants. It is secreted in breast milk in concentrations much higher than in maternal plasma. Its two metabolites are also excreted in milk; however, bupropion and its metabolites were not detected in a single plasma sample obtained from an infant (Briggs GG, Samson JH, Ambrose PJ, Schroeder DH. Excretion of bupropion in breast milk. *Ann Pharmacother* 1993;27: 431–433).

bupropion + carbamazepine Some patients receiving carbamazepine (CBZ) and bupropion (BUP) have low plasma BUP levels and high BUP metabolite (hydroxybupropion) levels. This is attributed to the effect of CBZ on the hepatic drug metabolizing system (Popli AP, Tanquary JF, Lamparella V, Masand P. Bupropion revisited: how much is too much? Presented at the 146th annual meeting of the American Psychiatric Association, San Francisco, May 1993).

bupropion + cimetidine Co-administration may require caution because cimetidine affects the hepatic drug metabolizing system, and bupropion is extensively metabolized.

bupropion/cocaine abuse In an 8-week, open study of bupropion in six cocaine-dependent, methadone-maintained patients, bupropion was well tolerated and effective in combination with psychotherapy in substantially reducing cocaine use in five patients. One patient dropped out after 2 weeks because of an episode of hypomania, possibly a side effect of bupropion (Margolin A, Kosten T, Petrakis I, et al. Bupropion reduces cocaine abuse in methadone-maintained patients. *Arch Gen Psychiatry* 1991;48:87).

bupropion + electroconvulsive therapy (ECT) Like tricyclic antidepressants, trazodone, and fluoxetine, bupropion (BUP) has been reported to prolong seizures associated with ECT. Thus, some clinicians have speculated that it might be used beneficially to assure adequate seizure length during ECT in patients with short seizures and high seizure thresholds, similar to the way in which caffeine sodium benzoate is now often used (Figiel GS, Jarvis MR. Electro-convulsive therapy in a depressed patient receiving bupropion. *J Clin Psychopharmacol* 1990;10:376). However, delirium was reported in a 75-year-old man given BUP (75 mg twice a day) after a course of ECT, suggesting that risks of concurrent use may outweigh any potential benefit (Libergon I, Deguardo JR, Silk KR. Bupropion and delirium. *Am J Psychiatry* 1990; 147:1689–1690).

bupropion + fluoxetine Fluoxetine (FLX) can augment therapeutic response to bupropion (BUP) and vice versa. Co-administration is usually well tolerated and may sometimes be effective in patients refractory to FLX. In a controlled trial, BUP treatment was associated with moderate to marked improvement in 10 of 22 patients who had not responded to a previous trial of FLX. FLX inhibits BUP metabolism, leading to a threefold and eightfold increase in plasma levels of the metabolites hydroxybupropion and threohydroxybupropion, respectively. These compounds can interact pharmacokinetically, interfering with BUP clearance and resulting in a severe extrapyramidal syndrome with ataxia, impaired psychomotor coordination, and catatonic symptoms (Preskorn SH. Selected topics on the pharmacokinetics and drug interactions of serotonin-selective reuptake inhibitors. *Curr Psychopharmacol* 1992;11:5–12). Addition of BUP to FLX-resistant obsessive-compulsive disorder patients may reduce symptoms in some patients and worsen them in others (Goodman WK, McDougle CJ, Price LH. Pharmacotherapy of obsessive compulsive disorder. *J Clin Psychiatry* 1992; 53[suppl]:29–37). The combination causes the same type of side effects seen with either drug alone. No seizures have been reported with combined therapy (Boyer WF, Feighner JP. The combined use of fluoxetine and bupropion. Presented at the 146th annual meeting of the American Psychiatric Association, San Francisco, May 1993).

bupropion + levodopa In patients receiving levodopa, bupropion should be given cautiously, using small initial doses and small gradual dose increases. Co-administration has resulted in a high incidence of adverse reactions, including nausea, vomiting, agitation, excitement, restlessness, and tremor (Watskey EJ, Salzman C. Psychotropic drug interactions. *Hosp Comm Psychiatry* 1991;42:247–256; Goetz CG, Tanner CM, Klawans HL. Bupropion in Parkinson's disease. *Neurology* 1984;34:1092–1094).

bupropion + lithium In the treatment of rapid cycling, bupropion may augment lithium or lithium and levothyroxine in patients who have not responded to carbamazepine (Haykal RF, Akiskal HS. Bupropion as a promising approach to rapid cycling bipolar II patients. *J Clin Psychiatry* 1990;51:450–455; Apter JT, Woolfolk RL. Lithium augmentation of bupropion in refractory depression. *Ann Clin Psychiatry* 1990;2:7–10). There have been reports of changes in lithium levels, and three cases of seizures (Goodnick PJ. Pharmacokinetics of second generation antidepressants: bupropion. *Psychopharmacol Bull* 1991;27:513–518).

bupropion + monoamine oxidase inhibitor (MAOI) Animal data indicate that the acute toxicity of bupropion (BUP) is enhanced by phenelzine. BUP's manufacturer advises that concurrent administration of BUP and an MAOI is contraindicated. At least 14 days should elapse between MAOI discontinuation and BUP initiation. This recommendation is made not because of any specific known problem, but because of a lack of data (Settle EC Jr. Bupropion: general side effects. *J Clin Psychiatry Monogr* 1993;11:33–39).

bupropion/overdose The manufacturer has received 86 reports of bupropion overdoses, many of which were mixed overdoses. Of the total cases, 38 involved seizures, 34 of which were in the bupropion-alone group. In no case did seizures result in status epilepticus or chronic epilepsy. Fourteen deaths have been reported, six in patients who took bupropion alone. Cardiovascular collapse was apparently responsible for some of these deaths in the bupropion-alone group. Seven cases of sinus tachycardia or "tachycardia" have been reported, four in mixed overdoses and three with bupropion alone (Gittelman DK, Kirby MG. A seizure following bupropion overdose. *J Clin Psychiatry* 1993;43:162).

bupropion + phenelzine See **bupropion + monoamine oxidase inhibitor.**

bupropion + phenobarbital Because phenobarbital may affect hepatic drug metabolizing enzyme systems, care should be exercised in co-prescribing it with bupropion.

bupropion + phenytoin Co-administration for 2 weeks resulted in delayed gastrointestinal absorption, significantly prolonged terminal elimination half-life, and delayed clearance of phenytoin (PHT) as manifested by an increase in the area under the curve in one study. This has been attributed to the inhibition of hepatic microsomal enzymes that metabolize PHT (Tekle A, Al-Khamis KI. Phenytoin-bupropion interaction: effect on plasma phenytoin concentrations in the rat. *J Pharm Pharmacol* 1990;42:799–801).

bupropion/seizures Reports of tonic-clonic seizures related to bupropion (BUP) (450 mg/day or lower) indicate that incidence is between 0.35% and 0.44%. A cumulative 2-year probability of seizures is 0.48%. There does not appear to be a higher risk based on sex, age, or body weight. Dose escalation is not consistently related to occurrence of seizures, all of which are likely to occur within 30 hours after the last dose of BUP. BUP's epileptogenic propensity is dose-related and may be mediated by the parent compound and/or its metabolites, three of which are pharmacologically active. High BUP plasma levels (i.e., above 100 ng/ml) are unnecessary for therapeutic efficacy and are more likely to cause seizures. To reduce seizure risk, BUP therapy should be initiated at a daily dose of 225 mg (75 mg three times a day) and gradually increased by 75 mg/day to a maximum of 450 mg/day. There is a relationship between seizures and predisposing factors (i.e., drug over-

dose, alcohol withdrawal, bulimia, electroencephalogram abnormalities, organic brain disease, high plasma levels of BUP or its metabolites, and concomitant therapy with drugs that lower the seizure threshold) (Davidson J. Seizures and bupropion: a review. *J Clin Psychiatry* 1989;50:256–261; Johnson JA, Lineberry CG, Ascher JA, et al. A 102-center prospective study of seizure in association with bupropion. *J Clin Psychiatry* 1991;52:450–456). Seizure following bupropion overdose has been reported (Gittelman DK, Kirby MG. A seizure following bupropion overdose. *J Clin Psychiatry* 1993;43:162). Advancing age may inhibit BUP-induced seizures; in some studies, seizure was 80% less frequent in BUP-treated patients over age 50 (Swartz CM. Advancing age may inhibit antidepressant-induced seizure. *J Clin Psychiatry* 1993;54:202). See **bupropion/overdose.**

bupropion/sexual dysfunction Although bupropion (BUP) purportedly is devoid of adverse effects on sexual function, anorgasmia has been reported. It was effectively treated with yohimbine (Pollack MH, Hammerness P. Adjunctive yohimbine for treatment in refractory depression. *Biol Psychiatry* 1993;33:220–221).

bupropion + valproate Bupropion may increase sodium valproate plasma levels (Popli AP, Tanquary JF, Lamparella V, Masand P. Bupropion revisited: how much is too much? Presented at the 146th annual meeting of the American Psychiatric Association, San Francisco, May 1993).

bupropion + yohimbine Marked and persistent improvement in mood occurred in a patient with treatment-resistant major depression when yohimbine was added to counteract anorgasmia associated with bupropion therapy (Pollack MH, Hammerness P. Adjunctive yohimbine for treatment in refractory depression. *Biol Psychiatry* 1993;33:220–221).

Burkson's fallacy Tendency for clinical studies, especially from specialist centers, to overestimate co-morbidity rates.

burnout Physical, emotional, or attitudinal exhaustion manifested by impaired performance, fatigue, insomnia, depression, enhanced susceptibility to physical illness, and misuse of alcohol or substance abuse. It is considered a stress reaction to persistent occupational performance and emotional demands.

Buronil See **melperone.**

"buscuso" Street name for coca paste.

"bush" Street name for cannabis products in the United Kingdom.

"businessman's acid" Street name for psilocybin.

"businessman's LSD" Street name for dimethyltryptamine (DPT).

"businessman's trip"   Street term for use of dimethyltryptamine (DPT).

Buspar   See **buspirone.**

Buspimen   See **buspirone.**

buspirone   (Axoren; Bespar; Buspar; Buspimen; Cespar; Dalpas; Neurosine; Tutran) Azasperone anxiolytic that bears no obvious resemblance to other anxiolytics, including benzodiazepines (BZDs). Unlike BZDs, it neither inhibits nor stimulates $_3$H-benzodiazepine binding in in-vitro receptor systems, does not facilitate gamma-aminobutyric acid (GABA) transmission, yet has effects on both serotonergic and dopamine receptors. It has a high affinity for serotonin (5-HT)$_{1A}$ receptors and moderate affinity for dopamine D_2 receptors. In conventional therapeutic doses, it is a 5-HT$_{1A}$ partial agonist; at doses higher than 100–200 mg/day it also has partial dopamine agonist effects. Metabolites include 1-pyrimidinyl-piperazine (1-PP), an alpha$_2$-receptor antagonist. Buspirone lacks the anticonvulsant and muscle relaxant properties of BZDs, and its onset of action is slow (2–4 weeks). Its side effect profile is not known to be altered by concomitant use of other medications and it does not appear to induce movement disorders. It does not impair psychomotor performance or driving skills, even when mixed with alcohol; it may even offset some impairment due to alcohol. Unlike BZDs, it is not associated with withdrawal reactions and lacks dependence/abuse potential as evidenced by studies of drug discrimination and withdrawal in animals and clinical experience with patients, especially known substance abusers. It is safe even when given in very high doses. Placebo-controlled studies indicate that buspirone is as effective as BZDs in the treatment of generalized anxiety disorder. It is effective in social phobia and post-traumatic stress disorder, but not panic disorder. It is useful for anxiety in patients with pulmonary disease, sleep apnea, and dementia because it does not cause cognitive impairment, sedation, respiratory depression, or withdrawal symptoms. There is no cross-tolerance with BZDs and other sedative-hypnotic drugs, although buspirone has been reported less effective in patients previously treated with BZDs. In comparisons with diazepam, some patients have benefitted more from buspirone, and some more from diazepam, depending on the prevalence of concomitant symptoms differently affected by the drugs. Clinical trials have shown that in doses of 120–240 mg/day of buspirone has profound anti–tardive dyskinesia (TD) effects (Neppe VM. High dose buspirone in a case of tardive dyskinesia. *Lancet* 1989;2:1458). In an open-label study, eight patients with mild to severe TD were treated for 12 weeks with buspirone (up to 180 mg/day). Improvement was observed in TD as well as neuroleptic-induced extrapyramidal side effects such as parkinsonism and akathisia (Moss LE, Neppe VM, Drevets WC. Buspirone in the treatment of tardive dyskinesia. *J Clin Psychopharmacol* 1993;13:204–209). Preliminary data indicate that buspirone (15–30 mg/day) may be useful in levodopa-induced dyskinesias. It may possess intrinsic antidepressant activity, and appears to have efficacy in major depressive disorder in comparison with placebo. Buspirone is of particular benefit as an adjunct to carbamazepine and valproate in the treatment of psychosis associated with temporal lobe injuries. It also has been used with partial success in the treatment of post-traumatic akathisia, a frequent element of the postconcussion syndrome. Buspirone (up to 60 mg/day—average 35 mg/day) alone or in combination with low doses of a neuroleptic may significantly decrease agitation associated with dementia (Sakanye KM, Camp CJ, Ford PA. Effects of buspirone on agitation associated with dementia. *Am J Geriatr Psychiatry* 1993;1:82–84). It can be effective in reducing irritability, impatience, hostility, and perceived stress in cardiac patients with no psychiatric diagnosis. It also may reduce aggressive behavior. Its antiaggressive and anti–self-injurious effects in mentally retarded subjects have been achieved often without sedation, which can compromise adaptive and intellectual capacities and thus reduce the patient's potential to benefit from training programs. It may be useful for anxiety due to protracted alcohol abstinence (Meyer R. Anxiolytics and the alcoholic patient. *J Stud Alcohol* 1986;47:269–273). Pregnancy risk category B.

buspirone + alcohol   In contrast to almost all anxiolytics and sedative-hypnotics, buspirone does not potentiate alcohol blood concentrations or enhance alcohol's cognitive and psychomotor impairment. Nevertheless, patients should be warned of potential hazards of driving or working around operating machinery (Moskowitz H, Smiley A. Effects of clinically administered buspirone and diazepam on driving related skills performance. *J Clin Psychiatry* 1982;43:45–55).

buspirone/breast milk   The extent of buspirone excretion in human milk is unknown. It should be avoided by nursing mothers.

buspirone/benzodiazepine withdrawal   Buspirone is not cross-tolerant with benzodiazepines and does not prevent benzodiazepine withdrawal symptoms (Ashton CH, Rawlins MD, Tyrer SP. A double-blind placebo-controlled study of buspirone in diazepam withdrawal in chronic benzodiazepine users. *Br J Psychiatry* 1990;157:232–238).

buspirone + carbamazepine Buspirone is of particular benefit as an adjunct to carbamazepine in the treatment of psychosis associated with temporal lobe injuries. Co-administration has been used with partial success in the treatment of post-traumatic akathisia, a frequent element of the postconcussion syndrome.

buspirone challenge test Test used as a neuroendocrine marker of depression by determining the functional activity of hypothalamic serotonin (5-HT) receptors. Subjects fast from midnight to 9 am. After two basal blood samples are taken from the antecubital vein for a baseline prolactin level determination at 8:30 am, subjects are given 60 mg of buspirone orally at 9 am. Blood samples for prolactin levels are then taken at 30, 60, 90, 120, and 180 minutes, and prolactin is measured by a fluoroimmunoassay. Response to buspirone is determined by subtracting baseline from peak prolactin concentrations (the latter value expressed as a percentage of baseline). If prolactin serum blood level rises more in patients than in controls, the buspirone test is positive and confirms responsiveness of 5-HT$_{1A}$ receptors. Buspirone stimulates prolactin release by acting on hypothalamic 5-HT receptors since this can be blocked by specific 5-HT antagonists such as methysergide and metergoline (Yatham L, Barry S, Dinan TG. Serotonin receptors, buspirone, and premenstrual syndrome. *Lancet* 1989;1:1447–1448).

buspirone + clomipramine When buspirone was added to the therapeutic regimen of 14 obsessive-compulsive disorder (OCD) patients partially responsive to at least 3 months clomipramine monotherapy, 4 (29%) had an additional 25% reduction in OCD and 3 (21%) experienced a 25% increase in symptoms. Results suggest that adjunctive buspirone therapy is not generally associated with significant further clinical improvement in OCD or depressive symptoms, but there may be a patient subgroup that benefits (Pigott TA, L'Hereux F, Hill JL, et al. A double-blind study of adjuvant buspirone hydrochloride in clomipramine-treated patients with obsessive-compulsive disorder. *J Clin Psychopharmacol* 1992; 12:11–18).

buspirone + clozapine Buspirone has been used to augment clozapine in some patients with no adverse interactions (Meltzer HY, Cola P, Way L, et al. Cost effectiveness of clozapine in neuroleptic-resistant schizophrenia. *Am J Psychiatry* 1993;150:1630–1638).

buspirone + digoxin Co-administration may cause digoxin toxicity because buspirone displaces digoxin from blood proteins. If possible, combined use should be avoided.

buspirone + electroconvulsive therapy (ECT) No interactions have been reported.

buspirone + fluoxetine Buspirone may augment response in obsessive-compulsive child and adult patients refractory or only partially responsive to fluoxetine (FLX) (Alessi N, Bos T. Buspirone augmentation of fluoxetine in a depressed child with obsessive-compulsive disorder. *Am J Psychiatry* 1991;148:1605–1606; Jenike MA, Baer L, Buttolph L. Buspirone augmentation of fluoxetine in patients with obsessive-compulsive disorder. *J Clin Psychiatry* 1991;1;13–14). In a double-blind, crossover study, 13 FLX-treated (80 mg/day for a minimum of 10 weeks) OCD patients were given adjuvant buspirone and placebo for 4 weeks each. Buspirone dosage was gradually increased over 2 weeks; all patients reached a stable dose of 60 mg/day for the final 2 weeks of active treatment. There were no significant differences between buspirone and placebo in obsessive-compulsive, depressive, or anxiety symptoms (Grady TA, Pigott TA, L Heureux F, et al. Double-blind study of adjuvant buspirone for fluoxetine-treated patients with obsessive-compulsive disorder. *Am J Psychiatry* 1993;150:819–821). Co-administration appears to have more potent antidepressant activity than either drug alone in patients with severe depression (Jacobsen FM. A possible augmentation of antidepressant response by buspirone. *J Clin Psychiatry* 1991;52:217–220; Bakish D. Fluoxetine potentiation by buspirone: three case histories. *Can J Psychiatry* 1991:36:749–750; Joffe RT, Schuller DR. An open study of buspirone augmentation of serotonin reuptake inhibitors in refractory depression. *J Clin Psychiatry* 1993;54:269–271). However, sequential use of buspirone followed by FLX may interfere with FLX antidepressant effect (Markovitz PJ, Stagno SJ, Calabrese JR. Buspirone augmentation of fluoxetine in obsessive-compulsive disorder. *Am J Psychiatry* 1990;147:798–800; Bakish D. Fluoxetine potentiation by buspirone: three case histories. *Can J Psychiatry* 1991;36:749–750). Sequential administration also may cause a serotonin syndrome, seizures, and antagonism of buspirone's anxiolytic effects (Sternbach H. Danger of MAOI therapy after fluoxetine withdrawal. *Lancet* 1988;2:850; Bodkin JA, Teicher MH. Fluoxetine may antagonize the anxiolytic action of buspirone. *J Clin Psychopharmacol* 1989;9:150). Seizure has been reported with the combination in the absence of the serotonin syndrome (Grady TA, Pigott TA, L Heureux F, et al. Seizure associated with fluoxetine and adjuvant buspirone therapy. *J*

Clin Psychopharmacol 1992;12:70–71). Simultaneous administration of low doses of buspirone (30 mg/day) after FLX discontinuation (20 mg/day) may cause euphoria, pressured speech, disinhibition and motor hyperactivity (Lebert F, Pasquier F, Goudemand M, et al. Euphoria with buspirone after fluoxetine treatment. *Am J Psychiatry* 1993;150:167). A paradoxical reaction to buspirone augmentation of FLX has been reported (Tanquary J, Masand P. Paradoxical reaction to buspirone augmentation of fluoxetine. *J Clin Psychopharmacol* 1990;10:377).

buspirone + fluvoxamine Addition of buspirone in fluvoxamine treatment-resistant depression may produce augmentation effects. The combination appears to be safe (Joffe RT, Schuller DR. An open study of buspirone augmentation of serotonin reuptake inhibitors in refractory depression. *J Clin Psychiatry* 1993;54:269–271).

buspirone + haloperidol Buspirone may increase haloperidol (HAL) serum levels by 25% or more. Clinical significance of the interaction is uncertain, but it may increase HAL's antipsychotic effects. Clinicians should be aware of a possible pharmacokinetic interaction when interpreting clinical changes following addition of buspirone to neuroleptics in general (Goff DC, Midha KK, Brotman AW, et al. An open trial of buspirone added to neuroleptics in schizophrenic patients. *J Clin Psychopharmacol* 1991;11:193–197).

buspirone + moclobemide Currently (1994) there are no data on co-administration.

buspirone + monoamine oxidase inhibitor (MAOI) Limited clinical experience is restricted to buspirone combined with phenelzine or tranylcypromine. Several patients have been treated safely and effectively; in a few the combination has produced a slight elevation of blood pressure. At this time there are no data warranting total prohibition of combined use (Gelenberg AJ. Buspirone-MAOI interaction. *Biol Ther Psychiatry Newsl* 1990;13:36).

buspirone overdose Over 4 million patients have been treated with buspirone since its introduction. Some have taken up to 3000 mg in overdose (150 times the average anxiolytic dose). Clinical symptoms of overdose include dizziness, headaches, nausea, gastrointestinal distress, hypotension, lightheadedness, and loss of consciousness. One fatality has been reported following ingestion of 450 mg of buspirone with other drugs (alprazolam, diltiazem, alcohol, cocaine); buspirone's contributory role, if any, in this case is therefore difficult to determine (Napoliello MJ, Doman-

tay AG. Buspirone: a worldwide update. *Br J Psychiatry* 1991;159:40–44).

buspirone + perphenazine Co-administration has significantly decreased agitation associated with dementia. It is possible that buspirone and perphenazine augment each other, allowing lower doses of perphenazine to be used in difficult cases (Sakanye KM, Camp CJ, Ford PA. Effects of buspirone on agitation associated with dementia. *Am J Geriatr Psychiatry* 1993,1:82–84).

buspirone + phenelzine See **buspirone + monoamine oxidase inhibitors.**

buspirone/prolactin Prolactin release from the anterior pituitary is under the inhibitory control of dopamine and the stimulatory control of serotonin (5-HT). When hypothalamic receptors are stimulated by an appropriate 5-HT agonist, serum prolactin concentration increases. Buspirone stimulates central 5-HT_{1A} receptors and releases prolactin in a dose-related manner. Extent of release is a good measure of the sensitivity of central 5-HT_{1A} receptors and can be measured by the buspirone challenge test. See **buspirone challenge test.**

buspirone/prolactin stimulation test See **buspirone challenge test.**

buspirone + tranylcypromine See **buspirone + monoamine oxidase inhibitor.**

buspirone + trazodone Co-administration has been associated with the serotonin syndrome (Goldberg RJ, Huck M. Serotonin syndrome from trazodone and buspirone. *Psychosomatics* 1992;33:235–236).

buspirone + valproate Buspirone is of particular benefit as an adjunct to valproate in the treatment of psychosis associated with temporal lobe injuries. It also has been used with partial success in the treatment of post-traumatic akathisia, a frequent element of the postconcussion syndrome.

"bust bee" Street name for phencyclidine (PCP).

butabarbital (Barbased; Butalan; Butisol; Sarisol No 2) Barbiturate sedative-hypnotic. Peak plasma concentration occurs in 3–4 hours; duration of action is 6–8 hours. The elderly are more susceptible to its central nervous system depressant effects. Dependency and withdrawal may be associated with long-term use (3 months +). Schedule III; pregnancy risk category D.

Butalan See **butabarbital.**

Butazolidin See **phenylbutazone.**

Butisol See **butabarbital.**

butorphanol (Stadol) Opioid with some agonistic actions at the K receptor. In opioid-free individuals it can produce analgesia, but produces an abstinence syndrome in the opioid-dependent because it is a weak agonist or antagonist at mu-receptors.

butotenin See **indole.**

"button" Street name for the dried protuberance from the peyote cactus. It contains mescaline, its active ingredient.

butyl nitrite Volatile substance increasingly abused. Serious abuse effects include methemoglobinemia.

butyrophenone Class of antipsychotic drugs discovered and developed by Paul Janssen, the prototype of which is haloperidol. Others include benperidol and droperidol. All have similar side effects, mainly extrapyramidal. Butyrophenones cause little hypotension, hypothermia, or other autonomic nervous system changes, and have only weak anticholinergic properties. They are potentially less sedative because they are weak histamine receptor blockers, but their noradrenaline alpha$_1$ blocking activity affords some sedative action. They have less serotonin (5-HT)$_1$ receptor blocking potency than chlorpromazine, making them less liable to cause weight gain. Butyrophenones appear to cause few adverse cardiac effects and thus are suitable for patients with concomitant physical illness. They also do not adversely interact with the majority of drugs co-prescribed with them. As a rule, they are not potentiated by alcohol. They are available in a range of formulations: intravenous, intramuscular, and oral (tablet or liquid).

butyrylcholinesterase (BChE) Plasma enzyme that hydrolyses cocaine in humans and degrades succinylcholine, a muscle-relaxant used prior to electroconvulsive therapy (ECT). Absence of the enzyme is a rare genetic abnormality responsible for the complication of prolonged apnea after ECT when succinylcholine is given. Also called "pseudocholinesterase."

"buzz bomb" Street name for the pipe used to inhale nitrous oxide from a small metal cylinder of gas.

"buzzing" Street term for emptying a can of glue or some other dissolved solid into a plastic bag, holding the bag to the nose, and inhaling.

C

"C" Street name for cocaine.

CA Cocaine Anonymous.

cabergoline Ergoline derivative, dopaminergic agonist specific for the D_2 receptor that may be a promising agent in the treatment of Parkinson's disease. Elimination half-life is about 72 hours. It is more potent and longer-acting than bromocriptine or pergolide, and its prolactin-suppressing effect is superior to that of bromocriptine. In a randomized, double-blind study in 25 Parkinson's disease patients taking stable doses of levodopa, once-daily doses of cabergoline (0.5–2.5 mg/day) were therapeutically effective without evoking serious adverse effects. Side effects noted were similar to those caused by other dopaminergic agonists (Hutton JT, Morris JL, Brewer MA. Controlled study of the antiparkinson activity and tolerability of cabergoline. *Neurology* 1993; 43:613–616).

cachexia Chronic catabolic state manifested by marked general weight loss and wasting during the course of a chronic disease or emotional disturbance. See **anorexia nervosa.**

"cactus" Street name for the hallucinogen mescaline.

"cafe coronary" Term coined by Hangen in 1963 for obstructive asphyxia caused by aspirated food. Fatal and nonfatal coronaries have been suffered by psychiatric patients being treated with high dosages of drug(s) with antidopaminergic and/or anticholinergic activity that increase risk of choking incidents. See **dysphagia; choking incident.**

caffeine Methylated xanthine that is a powerful central nervous system stimulant in either natural or synthetic form. It is the most widely used drug in the world. It is a potent psychoactive substance, the behavioral effects of which may be mediated through brain catecholamine systems. It acts on the kidney to produce diuresis, stimulates cardiac muscle, and relaxes smooth muscle. Caffeine can be ingested from brewed coffee (100 mg/6 oz), instant coffee (65 mg/6 oz), tea (40 mg/6 oz), cola-flavored beverages (25 mg/6 oz), and over-the-counter analgesics, antihistamines, stimulants, and weight-loss aids (50–200 mg/tablet). The average caffeine intake is approximately 200 mg/day. Some individuals drink 10–20 cups of coffee daily (1000–2000 mg of caffeine). Acute toxic effects of caffeine include excitement, delirium, sensory disturbances, and focal and general tonic-clonic seizures that may be refractory to anticonvulsants. Chronic ingestion of large quantities of coffee may provoke headaches and various psychophysiological symptoms. Research findings have documented that caffeine is reinforcing in man. It can produce tolerance, dependence, and an abstinence syndrome manifested by dysphoria, headache, anxiety, lethargy, insomnia, irritability, and poor concentration (Griffiths RR, Woodson PP. Caffeine dependence and reinforcement in humans and laboratory animals. *In* Lader M [ed], *The Psychopharmacology of Addiction.* New York: Oxford University Press, 1988). Excessive caffeine intake is prevalent among psychiatric patients: 22% use more than 750 mg/day, compared to 9% of the general population. It can be a panic-inducing agent in normal persons and in panic disorder patients, most likely because of its competitive antagonism of adenosine receptors. Caffeine's anxiogenic effects are well known, and there are many reports that high caffeine ingestion can induce a state indistinguishable from a generalized anxiety disorder (GAD). Patients with GAD are abnormally sensitive to caffeine (Bruce M, Scott N, Shine P, Lader M. Anxiogenic effects of caffeine in patients with anxiety disorders. *Arch Gen Psychiatry* 1992;49:867–869). Its exact mode of action as an anxiogenic substance is unclear, as it binds to adenosine and benzodiazepine receptors. About 15% of patients with eating disorders are high caffeine consumers who experience more anxiety and binge more often than those who consume less than 250 mg/day. Excessive caffeine use can result in sleep problems (delayed sleep onset and frequent awakenings). If taken before sleep, caffeine decreases total slow wave sleep. Large quantities of caffeine might precipitate mania or mixed states in those with bipolar predisposition, who therefore should avoid it. Brown "mustaches" and nostrils are considered signs of having eaten or snorted instant coffee. See **caffeine abuse; caffeinism; caffeine withdrawal.**

caffeine abuse Characterized by (a) substance abuse history; (b) affective symptoms and sleep disturbance that respond poorly to sedation; (c) persistent caffeine-seeking and caffeine-consuming behavior; (d) observable physical signs of acute caffeine intoxication; (e) little improvement despite vigorous treatment; (f) favorable response to careful restriction of caffeine (Zaslove MO, Russell RL, Ross E. Effect of caffeine intake on psychotic inpatients. *Br J Psychiatry* 1991;159:565–567). See **caffeine intoxication, acute.**

caffeine doping Defined by the International Olympic Committee (IOC) as a urine concentration above 12 μg/ml and by the National Collegiate Athletic Association (NCAA) as a urine concentration of 15 μg/ml. Because athletes use large quantities of caffeine to improve performance, the IOC and NCAA have placed limits on caffeine ingestion among athletes. It is estimated that 2 cups of strongly brewed coffee contain 200–300 mg caffeine and yield urine concentrations of 3–6 μg/ml.

caffeine + electroconvulsive therapy See **electroconvulsive therapy + caffeine.**

caffeine intoxication, acute State manifested by restlessness, muscle twitching, tremulousness, flushed face, fever, excitement, insomnia, diuresis, tachycardia, gastric distress, and vomiting. Symptoms may occur after just a few cups of coffee. At dosages greater than 1 g/day, muscle twitching, rambling flow of thought and speech, cardiac arrhythmias, periods of inexhaustability, and psychomotor agitation may occur. At dosages above 10 g/day, death may result from seizures and respiratory failure. Acute caffeine toxicity is responsible for several reported deaths annually; physical signs above may presage seizures and coma (Dreisbach RH, Robertson WO. *Handbook of Poisoning,* 12th ed. Norwalk, CT: Appleton & Lange, 1987).

caffeine + lithium See **lithium + caffeine.**

caffeinism Clinical syndrome produced by acute or chronic overuse of caffeine that is characterized mainly by dose-related central nervous system symptoms such as anxiety, sleep disturbances, mood changes, and psychophysiological complaints. It may be caused by ingestion of caffeine-containing drinks (coffee, tea, cola, cocoa), cold remedies, and some analgesics. Symptoms, which may appear with caffeine intake as low as 250 mg/day, include restlessness, excitement, insomnia, increased psychomotor activity, rambling thought and speech, and tinnitus (Greder JF. Anxiety or caffeinism: a diagnostic dilemma. *Am J Psychiatry* 1974;131:1089–1092). Many patients with caffeinism often doubt the role of caffeine in their symptoms and are willing to tolerate them to obtain its reinforcing effects. For some patients, caffeinism withdrawal effects discourage their attempts to discontinue caffeine consumption, especially when caffeine is so readily available and so quickly relieves caffeine withdrawal manifestation. See **caffeine abuse; caffeine intoxication, acute.**

caffeine/sleep Caffeine has a dose-related effect on sleep, delaying sleep onset and interfering with sleep maintenance. Intake of 300 mg (3–4 cups of regular, or 4–5 cups of instant coffee) increases number of arousals and reduces periods of rapid eye movement (REM) sleep in most people; 500 mg caffeine causes the same degree of alertness as 5 mg dextroamphetamine. Since caffeine has a half-life of 5+ hours, daytime consumption also causes insomnia and arousals. Patients who drink coffee during the day (5+ cups) may establish a cycle of coffee-induced poor sleep and resulting daytime drowsiness that they treat by drinking caffeine during the day. Over time they exhibit symptoms of caffeinism.

caffeine test Caffeine heightens taste sensitivity to quinine through an adenosinergic mechanism; sensitivity is enhanced in panic disorder (PD) patients. When PD patients are asked to separate 4 cups containing quinine from 4 cups containing water, 86% show heightened caffeine sensitivity by correctly identifying even the lowest concentration of quinine. The test may be a simple assay to identify potential panic disorder patients.

caffeine withdrawal Headache, decreased arousal, and fatigue consistently occur upon cessation of caffeine use. Other symptoms are anxiety, nausea, and craving for caffeine. Symptoms begin 12–24 hours after deprivation, peak at 20–48 hours, and last about 1 week. In one study, withdrawal symptoms reliably occurred with repeated substitutions of decaffeinated coffee in some coffee drinkers. Cessation of caffeine also has biochemical and physiological effects such as increased 3-methoxy-4-hydroxyphenylglycol (MHPG), elevated blood pressure, increased heart rate, orientation response, and decreased beta-adrenoreceptor sensitivity. Caffeine withdrawal can be severe and appears to be one reason for continued use of coffee (Hughes JR, Oliveto AH, Helzer JE, Higgins ST, Bickel WK. Should caffeine abuse, dependence or withdrawal be added to DSM-IV and ICD-10? *Am J Psychiatry* 1992;149:33–40). DSM-IV includes the following caffeine-related disorders: caffeine intoxication, caffeine-induced anxiety disorder, caffeine-induced sleep disorder, and caffeine-related disorder not otherwise specified.

Cairn's stupor Akinetic or diencephalic stupor manifested by rigidity, postural catatonia, and absence of spontaneous movement and emotion. See **mutism, akinetic.**

Calan See **verapamil.**

calcitonin gene related peptide (CGRP) 37-Amino acid peptide formed from the preprocalcitonin gene on chromosome 11. Its existence was predicted from molecular cloning studies of the calcitonin gene. The big primary ribonucleic acid (RNA) transcript produces two different peptides by alternative splicing. In thyroid C cells, the gene produces procalcitonin; in neural tissues, it produces proCGRP. CGRP can act directly as a neurotransmitter or as a trophic factor (e.g., promoting the development and growth of dopamine-containing neurons). It may also regulate the number of acetylcholine receptors at the neuromuscular junction. A study of CGRP content in brain and spinal cord in Alzheimer-type dementia (characterized by severe neuronal atrophy) found no difference from the normal in the distribution pattern. Laboratory experiences have provided so far only a partial view of the likely importance of CGRP.

calcium acetyl homotaurinate (Acamprosate) Agonist and synthetic structural analog of gamma aminobutyric acid (GABA). In controlled trials in Europe, it has been shown more effective than placebo in reducing alcohol intake in chronic alcoholic patients, suggesting that it is another possible approach to the treatment of alcoholism (Lhuintre JP, Moore N, Tran G, et al. Acamprosate appears to decrease alcohol intake in weaned alcoholics. *Alcohol Alcohol* 1990;25:613–622). Now marketed in France, especially for the prevention of alcoholism relapse, it is being studied in other European countries and Great Britain.

calcium carbimide (Temposil) Hepatic aldehyde dehydrogenase (ALDH) inhibitor that increases blood acetaldehyde levels after alcohol ingestion. It evokes sensitization to alcohol, as does disulfiram. Alcoholics treated with therapeutic doses (50 mg twice a day) experience flushing, tachycardia, tachypnea, sensations of warmth, palpitations, and shortness of breath after ingesting one or two alcoholic drinks. Onset of sensitization with carbimide is much more rapid (1 hour vs. 12 hours with disulfiram), and duration of sensitization is much shorter (24 hours vs. 21 days with disulfiram). Because of its rapid onset and short duration of action, carbimide is particularly suitable for pairing with entry into high-risk drinking situations in relapse prevention (Annis HM, Peachey JE. The use of calcium carbimide in relapse prevention counselling: results of a randomized controlled trial. *Br J Addict* 1992;87:63–72). Although alcohol-sensitizing drugs can be a powerful clinical aid in initiating a period of abstinence in alcoholic patients, reported long-term outcome results are disappointing (Institute of Medicine: *Prevention and Treatment of Alcohol Problems: Research Opportunities.* Washington, DC: Naval Academy Press, 1989). Not available in the United States.

calcium channel blocker (CCB) Any of a heterogeneous group of compounds sometimes referred to as calcium antagonists, slow channel inhibitors, or calcium modulators. They inhibit influx of calcium into a cell by receptor-operator and voltage-dependent channels, may inhibit the cal modulin myosin chain kinase system or release of calcium from the sarcoplasmic reticulum, and may modify the electrophysiological and contractile properties of the myocardium and cause vascular smooth muscle to relax. Three clinically important CCBs are available in the United States—verapamil, diltiazem, and nifedipine. They are marketed for the treatment of angina, hypertension, and other cardiovascular disorders, but also have been shown to have efficacy in some noncardiac conditions, including mania, depression, and hypertension induced by monoamine oxidase inhibitors. CCBs are orally active and readily bind to plasma protein (80–90%). First-pass hepatic metabolism is extensive for verapamil and diltiazem. Elimination half-lives of nifedipine and verapamil are 3–6 hours. Peak effect occurs within 30 minutes for nifedipine, 1–2 hours for verapamil, and 2–3 hours for diltiazem. All CCBs are rapidly absorbed. Onset of action after oral administration is usually less than 30 minutes. CCBs are generally well tolerated. Side effects are often extensions of their pharmacological properties. Adverse reactions may be categorized as cardiovascular, central nervous system, gastrointestinal, dermatological, hematological, and others. The most common side effects are due to potent vasodilatory properties and include flushing, headache, hypotension, dizziness, and lightheadedness. Peripheral edema is also a common adverse reaction. All CCBs can cause hypotension and affect cardiac rate (Dubovsky SL, Franks RD, Lifschitz M, Cohen P. Effectiveness of verapamil in the treatment of a manic patient. *Am J Psychiatry* 1982;139:502–504; El-Mallakh RS, Jaziri WA. Calcium channel blockers in affective illness: role of sodium-calcium exchange. *J Clin Psychopharmacol* 1990; 10:203–206; Jacques RM, Cox SJ. Verapamil in major [psychotic] depression. *Br J Psychiatry* 1991;158:124–125).

calcium channel blocker + carbamazepine CCBs inhibit carbamazepine (CBZ) metabolism and may lead to surprising increases in CBZ serum concentrations and some CBZ intoxication. To avoid toxicity, CCBs such as verapamil and diltiazem should not be prescribed for patients taking CBZ for bipolar disorder or epilepsy unless the CBZ dose has been lowered first. The CCB nifedipine does not affect CBZ blood levels and is less likely to produce CBZ toxicity (Ayd FJ Jr. Drug interactions that count: carbamazepine and calcium channel blockers. *Int Drug Ther Newsl* 1988;23:18).

calcium channel blocker + lithium Co-administration occasionally is used in the treatment of psychopathology and in co-morbid cardiovascular and psychiatric disorders. It may precipitate neurotoxicity manifested by nausea, weakness, tremor, ataxia, and Parkinson's disease symptoms (Price WA, Shallet JE. Lithium-verapamil toxicity in the elderly. *J Am Geriatr Soc* 1987;35:177–179).

"California sunshine" Street name for lysergic acid diethylamide (LSD).

calpain Calcium-mediated protease, activation of which has been implicated in the pathogenesis of neuron destruction following an ischemic episode.

calusterone (Methosarb) Commonly abused anabolic steroid.

Camcolit 250 See **lithium.**

Camcolit 400 See **lithium.**

camisole Canvas shirt with very long sleeves used to restrain the violently disturbed. After the shirt is securely laced, the person's arms are folded and the ends of the sleeves are fastened behind the back. Popularly called a "straightjacket."

cancer/depression See **depression/cancer.**

candidate gene Cloned human gene functionally related to a disease of interest, including genes for receptors (e.g., alpha- and beta-adrenergic receptors) and genes relevant to lactate metabolism (e.g., lactate dehydrogenase genes). Candidate genes encode for a neuroreceptor or other protein that may be involved in neurotransmission. They may play a role in the pathogenesis of schizophrenia.

"candy" Street name for barbiturates or any illicit drug (amphetamines, cocaine, lysergic acid diethylamide [LSD], pills in general).

cannabinoid Derivative or preparation from the plant *Cannabis sativa*, which contains several dozen compounds chemically related to cannabinol, including delta-9-tetrahydrocannabinol.

cannabinoid receptor (CNR) Binding site for the psychoactive component of marijuana as well as the physiological ligand anandamide (Devane WA, Hanus L, Breuer A, et al. Isolation and structure of a brain constituent that binds to the cannabinoid receptor. *Science* 1992;258:1946–1949).

"cannabis" Street name for marijuana.

cannabis dependence Psychological need for a routine pattern of cannabis use, to the point where social-occupational functioning may be impaired to some degree.

"cannabis oil" Liquid with a high tetrahydrocannabinol (THC) concentration extracted from cannabis resin.

cannabis psychosis Acute psychotic reaction, either of a manic type or schizophreniform with organic features, attributed to cannabis that subsides rapidly when the cannabis is stopped. It is reported to be common, especially in young adults and first-time users. The relationship between cannabis and psychotic conditions is complex. An acute toxic confusional state following ingestion is well documented and probably dose-dependent; thus, drug therapy for the control of disturbed behavior is usually unnecessary, except temporarily. Clinical data on the role of cannabis in the etiology of more persistent paranoid or affective disorders are sparse. That established schizophrenics use the drug is well recognized and may represent self-medication. Because of confusion about the meaning of the term and because "cannabis-induced psychosis" may obscure a diagnosis of paranoid schizophrenia, the term is best avoided (Mathers DC, Ghodse AH. Cannabis and psychotic illness. *Br J Psychiatry* 1992;161:648–653). Although many question the existence of cannabis psychosis and argue that the term should be abandoned, this does not mean there is no association between cannabis and psychosis (Thomas H. Psychiatric symptoms in cannabis users. *Br J Psychiatry* 1993;163:141–149). Also called "bhang psychosis"; "ganja psychosis"; "marijuana psychosis."

Cannabis sativa Herbaceous annual (marijuana or hemp plant) originally indigenous to India but now grown worldwide. The leaves, flowers, and seeds contain many biologically active compounds, the most important of which are the lipophilic cannabinoids, especially the psychoactive delta-9-tetrahydrocannabinol (THC). Cannabinoids are also found in two other varieties, *Cannabis indica* and *Cannabis ruderatis*. Today (1994), marijuana is more likely to be obtained from plants cultivated for their THC content (e.g., sensemilla) rather than from hemp fibers. Such preparations contain considerably more active THC. Cannabinoids are now believed to act at several specific cannabis receptors in the brain. Persistent heavy marijuana use induces significant and long-lasting deficits of short-term memory. Preparations made from the cannabis plant are known as hashish (a concentrated form of the resin containing high amounts of THC) and hashish oil (an even more concentrated form of THC). Other names for preparation of the leaves include bhang, kif, pot, and grass. When a human inhales or ingests marijuana, the liver biotransforms it into a number of metabolites. The most important active metabolite is 11-hydroxy-delta-9-THC, with effects identical to those of the parent compound. 11-Hydroxy-delta-9-THC is, in turn, converted to more polar inactive metabolites, including 11-nor-delta-9-tetrahydrocannabinol carboxylic acid (THC acid), which is excreted in urine in free and conjugated form. Although there may be no relationship between psychosis and cannabis, it has been associated with de novo psychoses and activation or relapse of pre-existing psychoses. Established psychopathology may lead to an increased intake of cannabis.

cannabis sativa/carcinogenic effect Between 1985 and 1994, there were 13 reports of cancer of the mouth and larynx among chronic marijuana smokers in Australia and the United States. Five patients had no other risk factors, and all were young. Available evidence suggests that marijuana smoking has a greater carcinogenic effect on the upper than on the lower airways (Caplan GA. Marijuana and mouth cancer. *J R Soc Med* 1991;84: 386).

Cannoc See **estazolam.**

canonical correlation analysis Advanced statistical method for examining relationships between two sets of numerical measurements made on the same set of subjects.

canonical variate analysis Statistical procedure used to isolate and assess the contribution of different factors to the variation of data.

cantharis Substance erroneously believed by many to be an aphrodisiac. It does cause the user to feel pseudosexual excitement. It has relieved priapism in some men and impotence in others. It irritates the bladder and urethra and can be toxic for both men and women. Also called "Spanish fly."

Cantor See **minaprine.**

Capgras syndrome Uncommon disorder in which the subject believes a person or persons of emotional significance has or have been replaced by imposters. There is evidence of a link between Capgras syndrome and prosopagnosia. There are reports of organic disorders associated with Capgras syndrome, including head injury, diabetes mellitus, temporal lobe epilepsy, vitamin B_{12} deficiency, hepatic encephalopathy, and dementia. Neuroimaging studies suggest that frontal lobe pathology may be important. The syndrome has been described as a feature of a number of psychotic states, but only rarely in the manic phase of a bipolar disorder (Signer SF. Capgras syndrome: the delusion of substitution. *J Clin Psychiatry* 1987;48:147–150). See **prosopagnosia.**

capillary electrophoresis See **electrophoresis.**

capillary zone electrophoresis See **electrophoresis.**

Capoten See **captopril.**

Capozide See **captopril.**

capsulotomy Psychosurgical procedure consisting of stereotactic interruption of the anterior fibers of the internal capsule (anterior capsulotomy) that is particularly effective in anxiety disorders compared to cingulotomy. However, there may be more cognitive side effects after capsulotomy, with patients showing less initiative than those who have undergone operations on other anatomical sites. Rehabilitation from capsulotomy is more prolonged than from cingulotomy. Data are accumulating that capsulotomy may be preferable for primary anxiety disorders (Boukoms AJ. The role of stereotactic cingulotomy in the treatment of intractable depression. *In* Amsterdam JD [ed], *Advances in Neuropsychiatry and Psychopharmacology, volume 2: Refractory Depression.* New York: Raven Press, 1991). See **cingulotomy.**

captopril (Acepril; Capoten; Capozide) Antihypertensive with cognitive enhancing properties that inhibit angiotensin converting enzyme (convertase), a nonspecific dipeptidyl carboxypeptidase found in various areas of the human brain and autonomic nervous system and active in the biochemical degradation of at least three neuropeptides—met-enkephalin Arg^6 Phe^7, substance P, and angiotensin I. It is a novel approach to finding drugs that may be useful therapies for Alzheimer's disease. Some studies suggest that captopril has minor antidepressant effects in patients suffering from both hypertension and unipolar recurrent depression. Its antidepressant effects are provocative, but unsubstantiated at this time (1994). Because it inhibits the proteolytic activity of human cerebrospinal fluid angiotensin convertase, its antidepressant effect may be related to increased concentrations of these and other neuropeptides in specific nuclei of the human brain.

captopril + chlorpromazine See **chlorpromazine + captopril.**

captopril + clozapine See **clozapine + captopril.**

captopril + lithium See **lithium + captopril.**

carbachol Direct-acting muscarinic acetylcholine agonist that does not penetrate the blood-brain barrier.

carbamazepine (Apo-Carbamazepine; Atretol; Convuline; Epital; Epitol; Mazepine; Sirtal; Tegretal; Tegretol; Teril) (CBZ) Iminodibenzyl tricyclic anticonvulsant developed in 1962 with particular efficacy in inhibiting abnormal temporal lobe and limbic system activity. It is the drug of choice for complex partial seizures and generalized tonic-clonic convulsive seizures. In seizure disorder patients, rectal administration of CBZ produces serum concentrations ranging from 30% to 70% of those obtained with oral administration (Olson WL. Carbamazepine suppository. *Neurology* 1990; 40:1472–1473). CBZ also has efficacy in a variety of psychiatric syndromes characterized by excitation and impulsivity, including episodic dyscontrol, mental retardation with overactivity, and hostile/violent psychoses. It is the most extensively studied antimanic alternative to lithium. Results of controlled and uncontrolled studies show that CBZ produced marked improvement in 50–70% of manic patients after 2–3 weeks. Onset of its antimanic effect occurs within 7–14 days of achieving therapeutic serum concentrations (50–150 µg/ml), and increases to a maximum over the third week (Post RM, Uhde TW, Roy-Byrne PP, et al. Correlates of antimanic responses to carbamazepine. *Psychiatry Res* 1987;21:71–83). Dose should be individually adjusted to blood levels between 4 and 12 µg/ml, titrated against clinical and side effects (Post RM. Non-lithium treatment for bipolar disorder. *J Clin Psychiatry* 1990;51[suppl 8]:9–16). Factors associated with favorable antimanic response are rapid cycling, absence of a family history of affective disorder, dysphoric mania, and no response to lithium (Post RM, Uhde TW, Roy-Byrne PP, Joffe RT. Correlates on antimanic response to carbamazepine. *Psychiatry Res* 1987;21:71–83). There is a growing body of evidence that acutely manic patients respond as well to CBZ as to lithium. However, monotherapy with either drug is not sufficient for most manic patients. Comparisons of CBZ with neuroleptics in the management of mania have shown that it has equivalent therapeutic efficacy and less neurotoxicity. Lithium plus CBZ has been shown to be therapeutically equivalent to either drug plus a neuroleptic in the treatment of mania. CBZ's acute antidepressant effects are less than its antimanic effects, producing fair or good response in about one-third of cases. Onset of action in depression is slow (up to 6 weeks) (Post RM. Time course of clinical effects of carbamazepine: implications for mechanisms of action. *J Clin Psychiatry* 1988;49[suppl]:35–46). Open trials indicate that CBZ may reduce frequency and intensity of recurrent manic and depressive episodes over extended periods. CBZ may also have therapeutic effects in the treatment of anxiety disorders, particularly panic disorder, post-traumatic stress disorder, alcohol and sedative-hypnotic withdrawal states, and behavioral dyscontrol syndromes (Keck PE Jr, McElroy SL, Friedman LM. Valproate and carbamazepine in the treatment of panic and posttraumatic stress disorders, withdrawal states, and behavioral dyscontrol syndromes. *J Clin Psychopharmacol* 1992; 12:36S–41S). CBZ has been used to treat

behavioral disturbances in overactive mentally handicapped people. CBZ is used in the treatment of trigeminal neuralgia and can be useful alone or in combination with antidepressants in the treatment of pain caused by cancer or other disorders (Kloke M, Hoffken K, Olbrich H, Schmidt CG. Antidepressants and anticonvulsants for the treatment of neuropathic pain syndromes in cancer patients. *Onkologie* 1991;14:40–43). CBZ can be crushed and poured into size-00 gelatin capsules and inserted into the rectum. Administered in this fashion, CBZ is well tolerated and well absorbed, and serum concentrations in the therapeutic range can be achieved (Storey P, Trimble M. Rectal doxepin and carbamazepine therapy in patients with cancer. *N Engl J Med* 1992;327:1318–1319). CBZ bioavailability ranges from 75% to 85%, and may vary with the formulation and manufacture of the products. Absorption of oral CBZ is rather slow, erratic, and unpredictable, and may be more rapid in chronic users. Peak plasma levels in epileptic patients occur 4–6 hours after dosing. Because CBZ induces its own metabolism, causing a drop in blood concentration (usually starting in the second week), it may take more than a month before stable serum levels are achieved. For this reason, it is necessary to initially make upward dosage adjustments and monitor serum drug concentrations frequently over a longer period until levels are stable. Serum level decline can be prevented by increasing the dosage by 2–4 mg/kg/day to a total of 14–16 mg/kg/day over the next 3 months. CBZ has a relatively narrow therapeutic range; high doses in particular can significantly influence peak plasma levels and result in dose-related adverse effects. Some of these side effects may be overcome by the slow-release formulation, where available, or by splitting the daily dosage into smaller, more frequent doses. Three to four daily doses of CBZ are preferred over twice-a-day administration to avoid transient dose-related toxicity and permit sustained anticonvulsant action. Side effects include dizziness, unsteadiness, ataxia, drowsiness, gastrointestinal disturbances/nausea, tremor, lethargy, sedation, visual disturbances, and cognitive changes. A consistent effect of CBZ has been a decrease in circulating thyroid hormones (T_4, variable changes in T_3 and TSH) without producing frank hypothyroidism or a significant effect on resting metabolic rate. Idiosyncratic reactions include hepatotoxicity, rash, Stevens-Johnson syndrome, and renal complications. CBZ also may cause hyponatremia (Yassa R, Iskandar H, Nastase C, et al. Carbamazepine and hyponatremia in patients with affective disorder. *Am J Psychiatry* 1988;145:

339–342). CBZ can cause a variety of hematological toxicities, including agranulocytosis and aplastic anemia, which may be fatal. Regular blood counts should be done in the early stages of treatment. Other disadvantages are interaction with and/or potential toxicity when combined with other anticonvulsants, some antibiotics, tricyclic antidepressants, and oral contraceptives. After prolonged treatment, abrupt CBZ withdrawal may predispose to tonic-clonic seizures. CBZ should be tapered gradually, even when used for short-term treatment, especially in patients predisposed to seizures. Pregnancy risk category C.

carbamazepine + acetaminophen Co-administration may increase risk of hepatotoxicity and decrease therapeutic effects of acetaminophen (Smith JAE, Hine ID, Beck P, Routledge PA. Paracetamol toxicity: is enzyme induction important? *Hum Toxicol* 1986;5:383–385).

carbamazepine/agranulocytosis See **carbamazepine/aplastic anemia.**

carbamazepine + alprazolam Carbamazepine (CBZ) may enhance alprazolam (ALP) metabolism, significantly lowering (>50%) plasma ALP concentration and increasing the risk of causing ALP withdrawal symptoms. CBZ may contribute to occurrence of ALP withdrawal syndrome; furthermore, continued administration of CBZ may not prevent its worsening (Arana GW, Epstein S, Molloy M, et al. Carbamazepine-induced reduction of plasma alprazolam concentrations: a clinical case report. *J Clin Psychiatry* 1988;49:448–449).

carbamazepine + amitriptyline Co-administration reduces serum amitriptyline (AMI) and nortriptyline plasma levels about 40%, undermining AMI's therapeutic efficacy unless dosage is increased and serum levels are monitored (Leinonen E, Lillsunde P, Laukkanen V, Ylitalo P. Effects of carbamazepine on serum antidepressant concentration in psychiatric patients. *J Clin Psychopharmacol* 1991;11:313–318). Following CBZ discontinuation, AMI serum level may increase unless AMI dosage is reduced.

carbamazepine/antithyroid effects Goiter and hypothyroidism have been reported infrequently in carbamazepine (CBZ)-treated patients. There is no evidence that co-prescribing CBZ and lithium increases risk of hypothyroidism. Routine thyroid hormone monitoring during CBZ therapy is not indicated. Should hypothyroidism occur, treatment is the same as that for lithium-induced hypothyroidism.

carbamazepine/aplastic anemia Carbamazepine (CBZ) can produce aplastic anemia in approximately 1 in 575,000 treated patients per year. It is most likely to occur after 2–3 months and by the end of the sixth treatment month, after which incidence drops sharply. In addition to monitoring, the clinician must be familiar with the early warning signs of this rare but serious complication. Warning signs (fever, sore throat, petechiae, or bruising) should be discussed with patients and their families during regular visits so that if they occur they can be treated without delay.

carbamazepine + barbiturate Barbiturates can markedly lower carbamazepine (CBZ) serum concentrations and impede CBZ's therapeutic efficacy.

carbamazepine + benzodiazepine Carbamazepine (CBZ) can decrease plasma levels of benzodiazepines (BZDs), reducing their efficacy. CBZ induces metabolism of clobazepam and clonazepam (Brodie MJ. Established anticonvulsants and treatment of refractory epilepsy. *Lancet* 1990;336:350–354). See **carbamazepine + alprazolam.**

carbamazepine/benzodiazepine withdrawal CBZ may be useful in the treatment of benzodiazepine withdrawal, particularly in seizure-prone patients (Rickels K, Case WG, Schweizer E. Withdrawal from benzodiazepines. *In* Hindmarch I, Beaumont G, Brandon S, Leonard BE [eds], *Benzodiazepines: Current Concepts—Biological, Clinical and Social Perspectives.* West Sussex: John Wiley & Sons, 1990.)

carbamazepine/breast milk Carbamazepine (CBZ) and its major metabolite are excreted in breast milk and can be detected in the nursing infant's plasma. Concentrations are usually low but near the therapeutic range in some infants. Although no dose-related effects have been reported, concentrations in breast milk and plasma of nursing infants have been reported to reach 60% of the maternal plasma concentration. CBZ can be used during lactation, but occasional measurements of infant plasma concentrations may be indicated, as well as close observation of the infant for jaundice and other signs of adverse idiosyncratic effects (Froescher W, Eichelbaum M, Niesen M, et al. Carbamazepine levels in breast milk. *Ther Drug Monit* 1984;6:266–271). There is a case report of cholestatic hepatitis in a newborn whose mother took CBZ throughout pregnancy and who was breastfed for 4 days prior to hospitalization (Frey B, Schubinger G, Mury JP. Transient cholestatic jaundice in a neonate associated with carbamazepine exposure during pregnancy and breastfeeding. *Eur J Pediatr* 1990;150:136–138). See **carbamazepine/pregnancy.**

carbamazepine + bupropion Some patients receiving carbamazepine (CBZ) and bupropion (BUP) have low plasma BUP levels and high

BUP metabolite (hydroxybupropion) levels. This is attributed to the effect of CBZ on the hepatic drug metabolizing system (Popli AP, Tanquary JF, Lamparella V, Masand P. Bupropion revisited: how much is too much. Presented at the 146th Annual Meeting of the American Psychiatric Association, San Francisco, May 1993).

carbamazepine + buspirone Buspirone is of particular benefit as an adjunct to carbamazepine in the treatment of psychosis associated with temporal lobe injuries. Co-administration has been used with partial success in the treatment of post-traumatic akathisia, a frequent element of the postconcussion syndrome.

carbamazepine + calcium channel blocker (CCB) CCBs inhibit carbamazepine (CBZ) metabolism and may lead to surprising increases in CBZ serum concentrations and some CBZ intoxication. To avoid toxicity, CCBs such as verapamil and diltiazem should not be prescribed for patients taking CBZ for bipolar disorder or epilepsy unless CBZ dose has been lowered first. The CCB nifedipine does not affect CBZ blood levels and is less likely to produce CBZ toxicity (Ayd FJ Jr. Drug interactions that count: carbamazepine and calcium channel blockers. *Int Drug Ther Newsl* 1988;23:18).

carbamazepine/cardiac effects Carbamazepine (CBZ) can cause a variety of cardiac conduction abnormalities, including complete heart block, intermittent sinoatrial block, both sinus and nodal bradycardia, and sick sinus syndrome. It also can secondarily cause hypotension. There are two principal forms of CBZ-induced cardiotoxicity: tachyarrhythmias occurring predominantly in young, healthy patients with elevated serum CBZ concentrations following intentional overdosage; and bradyarrhythmias and atrioventricular conduction abnormalities occurring in older patients, usually with therapeutic serum concentrations. CBZ-treated patients over age 50 should have a baseline electrocardiogram (ECG) with repeat ECGs after attainment of steady-state plasma levels. Co-administration with other compounds that affect cardiac conduction should be done cautiously. Abrupt rise in stimulation threshold causing failure of a functioning pacer was reported in a 59-year-old man. After 5 days' CBZ, he was admitted because of dizziness. ECG showed atrial and ventricular stimuli were ineffective without sensory failure. Atrial and ventricular capture occurred when ventricular and atrial pulse amplitudes were increased to 5 V. Usual causes of stimulation-threshold elevation were excluded. Plasma carbamazepine was 21 mmol/L, and the drug was continued. Two

months later, the patient received a heart transplant. Elevation of ventricular and atrial thresholds after CBZ administration accords with observations that it has class I antiarrhythmic properties (increased myocardial stimulation threshold). Attention should be paid to stimulus amplitude in patients with pacemakers before starting CBZ (Ambrosi P, Faugere G, Poggi L, Luccioni R. Carbamazepine and pacing threshold. *Lancet* 1993;342:365; Kenneback G, Bergfeldt L, Vallin H, et al. Electrophysiologic effects and clinical hazard of carbamazepine treatment for neurological disorders in patients with abnormalities of the cardiac conduction system. *Am Heart J* 1991; 121:1421–1429).

carbamazepine/children Carbamazepine (CBZ) has become a major antiepileptic drug in children as well as adults that is reported to have cognitive and behavioral advantages over other antiepileptic drugs. It is effective for the treatment of partial and generalized convulsive seizures in children. The pharmacokinetic profile in children is similar to that in adults, but half-life in long-term pediatric therapy is between 6 and 12 hours, compared with 15 hours in adults. Most common adverse effects are neurological and dose-related, and occur in up to 50% of patients, usually on dosage initiation or elevation. Most side effects dissipate over time and require no alteration in dosage. Idiosyncratic effects include hypersensitivity and hepatic and hematological reactions. Benign leucopenia occurs in 10–12% of adults and children and appears unrelated to aplastic anemia (Seetharam MN, Pellock JM. Risk-benefit assessment of carbamazepine in children. *Drug Safety* 1991;6:148–158).

carbamazepine/children, conduct disorder In 10 nonpsychotic children (ages 5–11) with long histories of highly aggressive, explosive behavior, carbamazepine (CBZ), 200–800 mg/day in divided doses, produced clinically significant symptom reduction. Four of five lithium-refractory children responded. Side effects were not serious and were eliminated or reduced with dosage adjustment (Kafantaris V, Campbell M, Padron-Gayol MV, et al. Carbamazepine in hospitalized aggressive conduct disorder children: an open pilot study. *Psychopharmacol Bull* 1992;28:193–199).

carbamazepine + chlorpromazine Carbamazepine induces microsomal enzymes, which decrease steady-state plasma concentration and increase hepatic clearance of chlorpromazine. Variable clinical results range from improvement to deterioration.

carbamazepine + chlorprothixene Co-administration increases carbamazepine concentration in blood plasma and brain, and decreases concentration of the 10,11-epoxide metabolites in these areas.

carbamazepine + cimetidine Co-administration results in increased carbamazepine (CBZ) serum concentration and possible toxicity due to its decreased clearance secondary to decreased epoxidation and autoinduction. When CBZ plasma levels are at steady state, the effect is minimal (Dalton MJ, Powell JR, Messenheimer JA Jr, Clark J. Cimetidine and carbamazepine: a complex drug interaction. *Epilepsia* 1986;27:553–558). To compensate for increased CBZ plasma level, CBZ dose should be reduced when co-administered with cimetidine. CBZ dose must be readjusted when cimetidine is discontinued.

carbamazepine + clobazam Addition of clobazam (CLB) to carbamazepine (CBZ) increases CBZ metabolism approximately 1.5 times, probably by inducing its epoxidation. CBZ induces CLB metabolism, decreasing its plasma level and interfering in its therapeutic efficacy (Levy RH, Lane EA, Guyot M, Brachet-Liermain A, Cenraud B, Loiseau P. Analysis of parent drug-metabolite relationship in the presence of an inducer: application to the carbamazepine-clobazam interaction in normal man. *Drug Metab Dispos* 1983;11:286–292). CLB has been reported to have no significant effect on the blood level/dose ratio (LDR) of CBZ. However, CBZ significantly decreases the LDR of the metabolite of CLB, N-desmethylclobazam (NCLB), thereby increasing the NCLB/CLB ratio (Sennome S, Mesdjian E. Interactions between clobazam and standard antiepileptic drugs in patients with epilepsy. *Ther Drug Monit* 1992;14:269–274).

carbamazepine + clomipramine Co-administration has improved treatment-resistant depression. Addition of carbamazepine (CBZ) to clomipramine (CMI) monotherapy produced a marked drop in CMI and desmethylclomipramine plasma levels (De la Fuente JM, Mendlewicz J. Carbamazepine addition in tricyclic antidepressant-resistant unipolar depression. *Biol Psychiatry* 1992;32:369–374). Co-administration also may increase clomipramine plasma levels (Gerson GR, Jones RB, Luscombe DK. Studies on the concomitant use of carbamazepine and clomipramine for the relief of post-herpetic neuralgia. *Postgrad Med J* 1977;53[suppl 4]:104–109).

carbamazepine + clonazepam Carbamazepine induces clonazepam metabolism, decreasing its plasma level and interfering in its therapeutic efficacy (Lai AA, Levy RH, Cutler RE. Time-course of interaction between carbamazepine and clonazepam in normal man. *Clin Pharmacol Ther* 1978;24:316–323). Co-adminis-

tration in absence seizure patients may induce absence status. See **absence status.**

carbamazepine + clozapine Co-administration is inadvisable for the following reasons. (a) Carbamazepine (CBZ), secondary to its effect on cytochrome P450 enzymes, may increase clozapine (CLOZ) clearance and interfere with its therapeutic effectiveness. After CBZ is discontinued, CLOZ plasma levels may rise within 2 weeks to levels well above the suggested therapeutic level of 1.1 mmol/L (0.35 mg/L) (Raitasuo V, Lehtovarra R, Huttunen MO. Carbamazepine and plasma levels of clozapine. *Am J Psychiatry* 1993:150:169). (b) Both drugs can cause agranulocytosis and aplastic anemia, and co-prescription may increase risk of adverse hematologic reactions.

carbamazepine + corticosteroid Carbamazepine induces corticosteroid metabolism and decreases the plasma level of corticosteroids (Brodie MJ. Established anticonvulsants and treatment of refractory epilepsy. *Lancet* 1990; 336:350–354).

carbamazepine CR (Tegretol CR; Tegretol Retard) Controlled release carbamazepine. Available in 200- and 400-mg tablets for dosage flexibility and twice-a-day dosing.

carbamazepine + danazol Carbamazepine inhibits danazol metabolism, with resultant neurotoxicity (Brodie MJ. Established anticonvulsants and treatment of refractory epilepsy. *Lancet* 1990;336:350–354).

carbamazepine/depression Carbamazepine (CBZ) is less effective in the treatment of depression than in the treatment of acute mania (Post RM. Non-lithium treatment for bipolar disorder. *J Clin Psychiatry* 1990; 51[suppl]:9–16). CBZ produces fair or good response in about one-third of cases of depression. Antidepressant action is slow, taking 6 weeks to reach its peak (Post RM. Time course of clinical effects of carbamazepine: implications for mechanisms of action. *J Clin Psychiatry* 1988;49[suppl]:35–46). Predictors of a positive response include more severely depressed, rapid cycling, more previous hospitalizations, fewer lifetime weeks of depression, bipolar depressions more than unipolar, positive response to sleep deprivation, higher cerebrospinal fluid (CSF) opiate-binding activity, and lower CSF levels of cyclic guanosine monophosphate (Ballenger JC. The clinical use of carbamazepine in affective disorders. *J Clin Psychiatry* 1988;49[suppl]:13–19).

carbamazepine + desipramine Although carbamazepine (CBZ) may lower parent desipramine (DMI) serum levels, co-administration may cause cardiac complaints, possibly because of the highly increased serum level of DMI's hydroxy metabolite, which is thought to be cardiotoxic. Increased hydroxylation rate could result from CBZ induction of desipramine-hydroxylating cytochrome P450 enzymes (Baldessarini RJ, Teicher MH, Cassidy JW. Anticonvulsant cotreatment may increase toxic metabolites of antidepressants and other psychotropic drugs. *J Clin Psychopharmacol* 1988;8:381–382).

carbamazepine/dexamethasone suppression test (DST) Carbamazepine (CBZ) significantly elevates postdexamethasone plasma cortisol values regardless of diagnosis or clinical state; thus, the DST should not be used to monitor CBZ-treated patients (Rubinow DR, Post RM, Gold PW, Uhde TW. Neuroendocrine and peptide effects of carbamazepine: clinical and mechanistic implications. *Psychopharmacol Bull* 1984;20:590–594).

carbamazepine + dextropropoxyphene Co-administration may increase carbamazepine (CBZ) levels, resulting in serious adverse effects (drowsiness, dizziness, nausea, vomiting, headache, ataxia and blurred vision) (Yu YL, Huang CY, Chin D, Woo E, Chang CM. Interaction between carbamazepine and dextropropoxyphene. *Postgrad Med J* 1986;62:231–233). CBZ dose should be reduced when it is co-administered with dextropropoxyphene and readjusted when the latter is discontinued.

carbamazepine + digoxin Carbamazepine (CBZ) can cause cardiac conduction disturbances and bradycardia and may have additive cardiotoxicity combined with digoxin. Co-administration also may result in high CBZ levels, subtherapeutic digoxin levels, confusion, ataxia, asterixis, and dyspnea. Decreasing CBZ dosage results in return to therapeutic digoxin levels and clinical improvement (Ketter TA, Post RM, Worthington K. Principles of clinically important drug interactions with carbamazepine. Part II. *J Clin Psychopharmacol* 1991; 11:306–313).

carbamazepine + diltiazem Diltiazem inhibits the P450 cytochrome oxidases located within the hepatic microsomal enzyme systems that metabolize carbamazepine (CBZ) and significantly increases its total blood levels, producing signs and symptoms of CBZ toxicity (ataxia, poor coordination, and blurred vision) (Brodie MJ, Macphie GJA. Carbamazepine neurotoxicity precipitated by diltiazem. *Br Med J* 1986;292:1170–1171). CBZ blood level can drop as much as 54% after diltiazem discontinuation (Gadde K, Calabrese JR. Diltiazem effect on carbamazepine levels in manic depression. *J Clin Psychopharmacol* 1990;10:378–379; Shaughnessy AF, Mosley MR. Elevated carbamazepine levels associated with diltiazem use. *Neurology* 1992;42:937–938). In a 60-year-old woman taking CBZ (600 mg/day) for 10 years for epilepsy, diltiazem (45 mg/day) was added for hypertension and increased after 39 days to 135 mg/day, at which time CBZ was decreased to 400 mg/day. Three days later, central nervous system symptoms began, and diltiazem was withdrawn. One week later, the patient suffered an epileptic seizure. Plasma CBZ levels peaked while the patient was taking the highest dose of diltiazem; after diltiazem withdrawal, CBZ concentration was reduced, inducing the seizure. Careful monitoring of CBZ blood levels is recommended to prevent effects associated with this combination (Maoz E, Grossman E, Thaler M, Rosenthal T. Carbamazepine neurotoxic reaction after administration of diltiazem. *Arch Intern Med* 1992;152:2503–2504).

carbamazepine + disulfiram Carbamazepine does not appear to interact with disulfiram (Krag B, Dam M, Helle A, Christensen JM. Influence of disulfiram on the serum concentrations of carbamazepine in patients with epilepsy. *Acta Neurol Scand* 1981;63:395).

carbamazepine + divalproex Co-administration may result in sustained prophylaxis for bipolar disorder in patients who have had an inadequate response to either anticonvulsant alone (Ketter TA, Pazzaglia PJ, Post RM. Synergy of carbamazepine and valproic acid in affective illness: case report and review of literature. *J Clin Psychopharmacol* 1992;12:276–281; Keck PE Jr, McElroy SL, Vuckovic A, Freidman LM. Combined valproate and carbamazepine treatment of bipolar disorder. *J Neuropsychiatry Clin Neurosci* 1992;4:319–322; Schaff MR, Fawcett J, Zajecka JM. Divalproex sodium in the treatment of refractory depressive disorders. *J Clin Psychiatry* 1993;54:380–384).

carbamazepine + doxacurium Carbamazepine shortens recovery time from neuromuscular blockade induced by doxacurium (Ornstein E, Matteo RS, Halevy JD, et al. Accelerated recovery from doxacurium in carbamazepine treated patients. *Anesthesiology* 1989;71:A785).

carbamazepine + doxepin Carbamazepine (CBZ) decreases doxepin serum concentration (Leinonen E, Lillsunde P, Laukkanen V, Ylitalo P. Effects of carbamazepine on serum antidepressant concentration in psychiatric patients. *J Clin Psychopharmacol* 1991;11:313–318). If doxepin levels are monitored, the combination can be used for pain caused by cancer or other disorders. Doxepin (50 mg) doxepin plus CBZ (800 mg) produces serum concentrations in the therapeutic range (Storey P, Trimble M. Rectal doxepin and carbamazepine therapy in patients with cancer. *N Engl J Med* 1992;327:1318–1319).

carbamazepine + doxycycline Carbamazepine decreases doxycycline plasma levels.

carbamazepine + electroconvulsive therapy (ECT) Carbamazepine (CBZ) may interact with pre-ECT anesthetic(s) and may prevent seizure induction. Many experts advise stopping CBZ during ECT therapy (Roberts MA, Attah JR. Carbamazepine and ECT. *Br J Psychiatry* 1988;153:418).

carbamazepine epoxide (CBZE) Active metabolite of carbamazepine. Half-life ranges from 10 to 20 hours. Some investigators think it is responsible for additional neurotoxicity, which may well be the case in children, especially in those also being treated with valproic acid. See **carbamazepine + valproic acid.**

carbamazepine + erythromycin Erythromycin increases plasma carbamazepine (CBZ) levels, resulting in neurotoxicity that can be accompanied by hyponatremia. Erythromycin inhibits epoxide formation as it decreases plasma CBZ-E and increases plasma CBZ/CBZ-E ratio (Wong YY, Ludden TM, Bell RD. Effect of erythromycin on carbamazepine kinetics. *Clin Pharmacol Ther* 1983;33:460–464; Jaster P, Abbas D. Erythromycin-carbamazepine interaction. *Neurology* 1986;36:594–595). To compensate for erythromycin-increased CBZ plasma level, CBZ dose should be reduced during co-administration and readjusted when erythromycin is discontinued.

carbamazepine + ethosuximide Carbamazepine increases ethosuximide clearance, reducing its plasma level and interfering with its therapeutic efficacy (Brodie MJ. Established anticonvulsants and treatment of refractory epilepsy. *Lancet* 1990;336:350–354).

carbamazepine + felbamate Co-administration increases carbamazepine (CBZ) clearance and decreases CBZ plasma concentration by 28%. If the CBZ pharmacodynamic effect is linear, 20% reduction of CBZ level would be associated with a 20% increase in seizure frequency. Patients treated with the combination may need increased CBZ dosage (Fuerst RH, Graves NM, Leppik IE, et al. A preliminary report on alteration of carbamazepine and phenytoin metabolism by felbamate. *Drug Intell Clin Pharm* 1986;20:465–466; Fuerst RH, Graves NM, Leppik IE, et al. Felbamate increases phenytoin but decreases carbamazepine concentrations. *Epilepsia* 1988;29:488–491). Interaction between felbamate and CBZ may not be as important as that between felbamate and other anticonvulsants because concentration of CBZ's active epoxide metabolite rises in parallel with the fall in the concentration of the parent drug (Albani F. Theodore WH, Washington P, et al. Effect of felbamate on plasma levels of carbamazepine and its metabolite. *Epilepsia* 1991;32:130–132). CBZ induces felbamate metabolism, resulting in lower-than-expected steady-state concentrations (Wagner ML, Leppik IE, Graves NM, et al. Felbamate serum concentrations: effect of valproate, carbamazepine, phenytoin and phenobarbital. *Epilepsia* 1990;31:642).

carbamazepine + felodipine Repeated co-administration significantly reduced felodipine maximum plasma concentration and area under the concentration-time curve (Zaccara G, Gangemi PF, Bendoni L, et al. Influence of single repeated doses of oxcarbamazepine on the pharmacokinetic profile of felodipine. *Ther Drug Monit* 1993;15:39–42).

carbamazepine + fluoxetine There are mixed data on the effect of fluoxetine (FLX) on carbamazepine (CBZ) plasma levels. Co-administration should be cautious, with frequent monitoring of CBZ levels. FLX inhibits CBZ metabolism, possibly resulting in clinically important interaction effects. There have been a few reports that addition of FLX to CBZ resulted in increased plasma levels of CBZ (27%) and its active metabolite, 10,11-epoxide (31%), increasing the risk of neurotoxicity and/or cardiotoxicity (Grimsley SR, Jann MW, Carter G, et al. Increased carbamazepine plasma concentrations after fluoxetine co-administration. *Clin Pharmacol Ther* 1991;50: 10–15; Pearson HT. Interaction of fluoxetine with carbamazepine. *J Clin Psychiatry* 1990;51: 126). Interactions may be due to FLX inhibition of CYP3A, which metabolizes CBZ (Pirmohamed M, Kitteringham N, Breckenridge A, Park BK. The effect of enzyme induction on the cytochrome P450-mediated bioactivation of carbamazepine by mouse liver microsomes. *Biochem Pharmacol* 1992;44:2307–2314). Addition of FLX to CBZ may cause parkinsonism. Clinical observations and neuroscientific and pharmacological data suggest that any drug that potentiates 5-HT effects, presumably by inhibiting dopaminergic nigrostriatal projections, may precipitate parkinsonism, especially when combined with neuroleptics or other 5-HT–enhancing drugs or when used in patients with subclinical or mild parkinsonism (Gernaat HBPE, van de Woude J, Touw DJ. Fluoxetine and parkinsonism in patients taking carbamazepine. *Am J Psychiatry* 1991;148; 1604–1605; Touw DJ, Gernaat HBPE, van der Woude J. Parkinsonisme na toevoeging van fluoxetine aan de behandeling met neuroleptica of carbamazepine. *Ned Tijdschr Geneeskd* 1992;136:332–333). A toxic serotonin syndrome was reported in an affective disorder patient treated with CBZ (200 mg/day) who had FLX (20 mg/day) added for 14 days. She also had leukopenia and thrombocytopenia. Following FLX discontinuation, all symptoms of toxicity subsided after 72 hours (Dursun

SM, Mathew VM, Reveley MA. Toxic serotonin syndrome after fluoxetine plus carbamazepine. *Lancet* 1993;342:442–443). CBZ plasma concentrations should be monitored closely for up to 3–5 weeks in any patient who has FLX added to the drug regimen. No apparent interaction occurred when FLX was added to a stable CBZ regimen in patients with epilepsy. There were no significant changes in steady-state CBZ or its metabolites during its co-administration with fluoxetine, nor were there any changes in seizure frequency, possibly because of FLX and CBZ metabolism by different hepatic isoenzymes (Spina E, Avenoso A, Pollicino AM, et al. Carbamazepine co-administration with fluoxetine or fluvoxamine. *Ther Drug Monit* 1993; 15:247–250).

carbamazepine + fluphenazine Carbamazepine's microsomal enzyme-inducing action decreases fluphenazine steady-state plasma concentration by approximately 50% and increases its hepatic clearance; clinical results range from improvement to deterioration (Jann MW, Fidone GS, Hernandez JM, Amrung JE, Davis CM. Clinical implications of increased antipsychotic plasma concentrations upon anticonvulsant cessation. *Psychiatry Res* 1989;28:153–159).

carbamazepine + fluvoxamine Co-administration may result in increased carbamazepine (CBZ) plasma concentration with resultant toxicity (Fritze J, Unsorg B, Lanczik M. Interaction between carbamazepine and fluvoxamine. *Acta Psychiatr Scand* 1991;84:583–584). Fluvoxamine (250 mg/day) plus CBZ (60 mg/day) significantly reduced obsessive-compulsive symptoms without adverse effects in a 26-year-old woman with a history of tonic-clonic seizures induced by combined levomepromazine-fluvoxamine treatment (Grinshpoon A, Berg Y, Mozes T, et al. Seizures induced by combined levomepromazine-fluvoxamine treatment. *Int Clin Psychopharmacol* 1993;8:61–62). No apparent interaction occurred when fluvoxamine was added to a stable CBZ regimen in patients with epilepsy. There were no significant changes in steady-state CBZ or its metabolites, nor were there any changes in seizure frequency, possibly because of the drugs' metabolism by different hepatic isoenzymes (Spina E, Avenoso A, Pollicino AM, et al. Carbamazepine co-administration with fluoxetine or fluvoxamine. *Ther Drug Monit* 1993;15:247–250).

carbamazepine + gemfibrozil Co-administration can increase carbamazepine plasma levels (Denio L, Drake ME, Pakalnis A. Gemfibrozil-carbamazepine interaction in epileptic patients [AES abstract]. *Epilepsia* 1988;29:654).

carbamazepine + haloperidol Carbamazepine (CBZ) powerfully induces hepatic microsomal enzymes over several weeks and increases metabolism of many drugs. It may lower haloperidol (HAL) plasma levels up to 60%, with variable clinical impact: some patients improve and have fewer extrapyramidal symptoms; others deteriorate (Arana GW, Goff DC, Friedman H, et al. Does carbamazepine-induced reduction of plasma haloperidol levels worsen psychotic symptoms? *Am J Psychiatry* 1986;143:650–651). Double-blind crossover studies indicate that adjunctive CBZ can enhance therapeutic response to HAL in chronic schizophrenia. Neurotoxicity is rare. Two cases of delirium have been reported (Kanter GL, Yerevanian BI, Ciccone JR. Case report of a possible interaction between neuroleptics and carbamazepine. *Am J Psychiatry* 1984;141:1101–1102; Yerevanian BI, Hodgman CH. A haloperidol-carbamazepine interaction in a patient with rapid-cycling bipolar disorder. *Am J Psychiatry* 1985;142:785–786). Neuroleptic malignant syndrome (NMS) developed in a 29-year-old woman with bipolar disorder 8 hours after treatment with HAL (10 mg) and CBZ (100 mg). It was treated successfully with oral nifedipine (60 mg/day) (Hermesh H, Molcho A, Aizenburg D, Munitz H. The calcium antagonist nifedipine in recurrent neuroleptic malignant syndrome. *Clin Neuropharmacol* 1988;11:552–555). Patients whose hepatic enzymes have been induced by such factors as cigarette smoking or alcohol use may not show an additional increase in hepatic clearance of HAL when CBZ is added. This may explain why HAL levels do not fall in some patients begun on CBZ, but fall sharply in others (Belknap SM, Nelson JE. Drug interactions in psychiatry. *In* Musa MN [ed], *Pharmacokinetics and Therapeutic Monitoring of Psychiatric Drugs*. Springfield, IL: Charles C Thomas, 1993, pp 57–112).

carbamazepine/hypersensitivity reactions Rashes occur in at least 5% of carbamazepine (CBZ)-treated patients. Ranging from innocent and photosensitive to life-threatening, reactions include dermatitis, maculopapular, erythema multiforme, Stevens-Johnson syndrome, Lyell's disease, and toxic epidermal necrolysis. They are very rare, accounting for less than 10% of all skin reactions to CBZ. They appear in most cases 8–12 days after initiation of therapy.

carbamazepine/hyponatremia Hyponatremia and water retention are documented side effects of carbamazepine (CBZ). Rare in children, they seem to be related to CBZ serum concentration and the patient's age. Reported frequency is 6–31%. Mild hyponatremia is usually symptomless, but if serum sodium falls below 120 mmol/L, there may be confusion, peripheral edema, and seizures. Probable mechanisms are a hypothalamic effect on osmoreceptors mediated via antidiuretic hormone, and direct action on the renal tubules. Evidence for the latter is the reversibility of CBZ's antidiuretic effect by demeclocycline, which is known to antagonize renal antidiuretic hormone receptors. Since several hyponatremia symptoms (e.g., dizziness, headache, drowsiness, and nausea) may mimic known CBZ side effects, hyponatremia should be considered when such symptoms are reported by a CBZ-treated patient.

carbamazepine + imipramine Co-administration significantly lowers desipramine (imipramine's metabolite) mean plasma levels and summed imipramine and desipramine plasma levels. This is attributed to carbamazepine induction of hepatic hydroxylase enzymes (Brown CS, Wells BG, Cold JA. Possible influence of carbamazepine on plasma imipramine concentrations in children with attention deficit hyperactivity disorder. *J Clin Psychopharmacol* 1990;10:359–362).

carbamazepine + isoniazid Isoniazid inhibits carbamazepine (CBZ) metabolism, possibly resulting in elevated CBZ plasma levels and toxicity (Block H. Carbamazepine-isoniazid interactions. *Pediatrics* 1982;69:494–495).

carbamazepine + lamotrigine Lamotrigine increases serum concentration of carbamazepine (CBZ) epoxide, an active metabolite of CBZ, thereby causing adverse effects such as dizziness and diplopia (Warner T, Patsalos PN, Prevett M, et al. Lamotrigine-induced carbamazepine toxicity: an interaction with carbamazepine-10,11-epoxide. *Epilepsy Res* 1992;11:147–150). CBZ, by inducing liver enzymes, can halve lamotrigine's half-life.

carbamazepine/leucopenia Benign leucopenia occurs in about 10–12% of adults treated with carbamazepine (CBZ). It almost always reverts to a normal white blood cell count after CBZ is discontinued. It rarely progresses to agranulocytosis or aplastic anemia.

carbamazepine + lithium Carbamazepine (CBZ) and lithium have additive or synergistic therapeutic effects in treatment-refractory bipolar illness, particularly in patients unresponsive to either drug alone. Co-administration has been found safe and effective in rapid-cycling bipolar patients. If the combination is used, CBZ levels should be 8–12 µg/ml (DiCostanzo E, Schifano F. Lithium alone or in combination for the treatment of rapid-cycling bipolar affective disorder. *Acta Psychiatr Scand* 1991;83: 456–459). Addition of lithium to depressed patients nonresponsive to CBZ monotherapy produced rapid improvement (4 days) in half of a studied group. Thirteen patients were "bipolar depressives," 8 of whom were also rapid cyclers (Kramlinger KG, Post RM. The addition of lithium to carbamazepine, antidepressant efficacy in treatment-resistant depression. *Arch Gen Psychiatry* 1989;46:794–800). However, some patients either do not respond or show loss of efficacy via development of tolerance during long-term prophylaxis (Post RM, Pazzaglia PJ, Ketter TA, George MS, Marangell L. Carbamazepine and nimodipine in refractory bipolar illness: efficacy and mechanisms. *Neuropsychopharmacology* 1993;9: 17S). Lithium is excreted by the kidney with no hepatic metabolism. Thus, pharmacokinetic interactions do not occur, although there are several pharmacodynamic interactions. Each drug may elevate the other's serum level, leading to neurotoxicity, even when blood levels of both are in the therapeutic range (Baciewicz AM. Carbamazepine drug interactions. *Ther Drug Monit* 1986;8:305–317). Toxicity can be manifested by generalized truncal tremor, ataxia, horizontal nystagmus, hyperreflexia, and muscle fasciculation, all of which usually abate within 3–7 days after CBZ discontinuation (Shukla S, Godwin CD, Long LE, Miller MG. Lithium-carbamazepine neurotoxicity and risk factors. *Am J Psychiatry* 1984; 141:1604–1606). The reactions appear to be, at least in part, associated with pre-existing central nervous system abnormalities and/or rapid, large dosage increases of the drugs (Ballenger JC. The clinical use of carbamazepine in affective disorders. *J Clin Psychiatry* 1988;49[suppl]:13–19). Patients must be monitored for signs and symptoms of neurotoxicity, serum levels of each drug must be monitored, and CBZ dose may need to be decreased. Lithium's diuretic effect overrides CBZ's antidiuretic effect. CBZ does not reverse lithium-induced diabetes insipidus. Lithium may attenuate CBZ-induced hyponatremia, but its potential to do so has not been unequivocally demonstrated (Vieweg V, Glick JL, Herring S, et al. Absence of carbamazepine-induced hyponatremia among patients also given lithium. *Am J Psychiatry* 1987; 144:943–947; Kramlinger KG, Post RM. Addition of lithium carbonate to carbamazepine: hematological and thyroid effects. *Am J Psychiatry* 1990;147:615–620).

carbamazepine + lithium/hematological effects Lithium may reverse carbamazepine (CBZ)-induced leucopenia; however, leucopenia secondary to CBZ despite concurrent lithium treatment has been reported. There is no evidence that lithium alters the course of CBZ-induced severe bone marrow depression

(Klein EM. Lithium and carbamazepine therapy in a patient with manic depressive illness: clinical effects, interactions and side effects. *Isr J Psychiatry Relat Sci* 1987;24:295–298). Neither lithium dose nor plasma level is significantly correlated with degree of change in the total white blood cell or neutrophil count.

carbamazepine + lithium/thyroid effects Co-administration produces additive antithyroidal effects, resulting in greater decreases in thyroxine and free thyroxine than with carbamazepine (CBZ) alone. Addition of lithium to CBZ can be associated with emergence of a modestly higher thyrotropin level. Regular monitoring of thyroid function during combined therapy is advisable (Kramlinger KG, Post RM. Addition of lithium carbonate to carbamazepine: hematological and thyroid effects. *Am J Psychiatry* 1990;147:615–620).

carbamazepine + loxapine Co-administration may enhance the central nervous system depressant effects of carbamazepine (CBZ), lower seizure threshold, and decrease CBZ's anticonvulsant effects. Dosage adjustments may be necessary to control seizures. Anticholinergic effects may be potentiated, leading to confusion and delirium.

carbamazepine + maprotiline Co-administration may enhance the central nervous system depressant effects of carbamazepine (CBZ), lower seizure threshold, and decrease CBZ's anticonvulsant effects. Dosage adjustments may be necessary to control seizures. In some patients anticholinergic effects may be potentiated, leading to confusion and delirium.

carbamazepine + metoclopramide Co-administration of therapeutic doses may cause acute neurotoxicity (Saudyk R. Carbamazepine and metoclopramide interaction: possible neurotoxicity. *Br Med J* 1984;288:830).

carbamazepine + methadone Addition of carbamazepine during methadone maintenance results in mild opiate withdrawal symptoms and a 60% decrease in plasma methadone trough levels (Bell J, Seres V, Bowron P, et al. The use of serum methadone levels in patients receiving methadone maintenance. *Clin Pharmacol Ther* 1988;43:623–629).

carbamazepine + methylprednisolone Carbamazepine increases methylprednisolone metabolism.

carbamazepine + mianserin Carbamazepine decreases mianserin serum concentration and may interfere with its therapeutic efficacy. Mianserin dosage may have to be increased, and its serum levels may have to be carefully monitored (Leinonen E, Lillsunde P, Laukkanen V, Ylitalo P. Effects of carbamazepine on serum antidepressant concentration in psychiatric patients. *J Clin Psychopharmacol* 1991; 11:313–318).

carbamazepine + moclobemide Co-administration in three patients for at least 4 weeks produced no adverse interactions (Amrein R, Guntert TW, Dingemanse J, et al. Interactions of moclobemide with concomitantly administered medication: evidence from pharmacological and clinical studies. *Psychopharmacology* 1992;106:S24–S31).

carbamazepine + molindone Co-administration may enhance the central nervous system depressant effects of carbamazepine (CBZ), lower seizure threshold, and decrease CBZ's anticonvulsant effects. Dosage adjustments may be necessary to control seizures. In some patients anticholinergic effects may be potentiated, leading to confusion and delirium.

carbamazepine + monoamine oxidase inhibitor (MAOI) With the exception of isoniazid, MAOIs and carbamazepine (CBZ) may be used together when required to maximize antidepressant effects. Isoniazid inhibits CBZ metabolism and substantially increases blood levels, producing toxicity manifested by disorientation, extreme drowsiness, and aggression. An interval of 14 days is recommended between discontinuation of isoniazid and initiation of CBZ, or vice versa (Wright JM, Stokes EF, Sweeney VP. Isoniazid-induced carbamazepine toxicity and vice versa. *N Engl J Med* 1982;18:1325–1327). Several reports suggest that MAOIs do not alter CBZ plasma levels. However, four patients taking phenelzine required a mean daily dose of 450 mg of CBZ (300–700 mg/day) to attain CBZ levels of 8.6–10.9 µg/ml, whereas five patients taking tranylcypromine required a mean daily dose of CBZ of 1040 mg (800–1600 mg/daily) to produce CBZ plasma levels of 8.0–11.1 µg/ml. Thus, tranylcypromine patients needed a dose 2.3 times higher to reach similar levels (Barklage NE, Jefferson JW, Margolis D. Do monoamine oxidase inhibitors alter carbamazepine blood levels? *J Clin Psychiatry* 1992;53:258).

carbamazepine + neuroleptic Carbamazepine (CBZ), a potent inducer of hepatic microsomal enzymes, may cause a significant (50% or more) decrease in the level of co-administered neuroleptics (Fast DK, Jones BD, Kusalic M, Erickson M. Effect of carbamazepine on neuroleptic plasma level and efficacy. *Am J Psychiatry* 1986;143:117–118; Jann M, Ereshefsky L, Sakalad S. Effects of carbamazepine on plasma haloperidol levels. *J Clin Psychopharmacol* 1985; 5:106–109). This can result in loss of efficacy in neuroleptic-responsive patients. Neuroleptic plasma levels should be checked if patients fail to respond to standard doses during combined therapy with CBZ. Also, abrupt CBZ discontinuation can markedly increase neuroleptic plasma levels, possibly resulting in serious side effects. In patients with affective and schizoaffective disorders, combined use is more likely to cause hyponatremia than CBZ alone. See **carbamazepine + haloperidol.**

carbamazepine neurotoxicity Drowsiness followed by incoordination and vertigo. Symptoms are nearly always transient. They are most frequent during treatment initiation or after dosage increase and usually subside spontaneously or after minor dose alterations. Risk can be minimized by gradual dosage increments over 10–14 days, since neurotoxicity is presumed to be related to serum carbamazepine concentrations.

carbamazepine + nicotinamide Nicotinamide can increase plasma carbamazepine (CBZ) levels and may cause CBZ toxicity (Bourgeois BF, Dodson WE, Ferrendelli JA. Interactions between primidone, carbamazepine and nicotinamide. *Neurology* 1982;32:1122–1126).

carbamazepine + nifedipine Co-administration may precipitate carbamazepine toxicity (Brodie MJ, Macphee GJA. Carbamazepine neurotoxicity precipitated by diltiazem. *Br Med J* 1986;292:1180).

carbamazepine + nimodipine Preliminary data indicate that nimodipine does not substantially influence carbamazepine pharmacokinetics (Ketter TA, Post RM, Worthington K. Principles of clinically important drug interactions with carbamazepine. Part II. *J Clin Psychopharmacol* 1991;11:306–313). Co-administration has been shown to be efficacious in a subgroup of patients with ultra-ultra rapid (ultradian) cycling (Post RM, Pazzaglia PJ, Ketter TA, George MS, Marangell L. Carbamazepine and nimodipine in refractory bipolar illness: efficacy and mechanisms. *Neuropsychopharmacology* 1993;9:17S). Co-administration may decrease plasma nimodipine concentrations, making increased doses necessary to achieve adequate therapeutic levels (Tartara A, Galimberti CA, Manni R, et al. Differential effects of valproic acid and enzyme-inducing anticonvulsants on nimodipine pharmacokinetics in epileptic patients. *Br J Clin Pharmacol* 1991;32:335–340).

carbamazepine + nortriptyline Carbamazepine (CBZ) may enhance hepatic hydroxylation of nortriptyline, producing relatively low levels of the parent compound and elevated ratios of the metabolite 10-hydroxynortriptyline to nortriptyline (Baldessarini RJ, Teicher MH, Cassidy JW. Anticonvulsant cotreatment may increase metabolites of antidepressants and other psychotropic drugs. *J Clin Psychopharmacol* 1988;8:381–382). In another study, CBZ reduced nortriptyline concentrations by 67% (Brosen K, Kragh-Sorensen P. Concomitant intake of nortriptyline and carbamazepine. *Ther Drug Monit* 1993;15:258–260).

carbamazepine/ocular effects Diplopia, accommodation disturbance, nystagmus, impairment of saccadic eye movements, opthalmologia, oculogyric crisis, blurred vision, mychriasis, cycloplegia, visual hallucinations, pigmented retinopathy, and papilledema have been reported. Ordinarily they are mild and often self-limiting, particularly if carbamazepine dosage is reduced or discontinued. In most cases they can be avoided with careful dose titration and monitoring. Some data suggest that incidence increases with polypharmacy (Remler BF, Leigh J, Osorio I, et al. The characteristics and mechanisms of visual disturbance associated with anticonvulsant therapy. *Neurology* 1990;40:791–796; Fraunfelder FT, Meyer SM [eds]: *Drug-Induced Ocular Side Effects and Drug Interactions.* Philadelphia: Lea & Febiger, 1989; Goldman MJ, Schultz-Ross RA. Adverse ocular effects of anticonvulsants. *Psychosomatics* 1993;34:154–158).

carbamazepine + oral contraceptive Because carbamazepine (CBZ) induces metabolism of oral contraceptives, their effectiveness may be reduced with co-administration. Birth control failure may occur unless a higher dose formulation of the contraceptive is prescribed (estrogen dose of 50–100 μg) (Mattson RH, Cramer JA, Darney PD, Naftolin F. Use of oral contraceptives by women with epilepsy. *JAMA* 1986;256:238–240). See **carbamazepine/teratogenesis.**

carbamazepine + other drugs Awareness of carbamazepine (CBZ) drug interactions is essential for the safe and effective treatment of patients requiring medication combinations. CBZ induces metabolism of many drugs, undermining their efficacy, and other drugs can inhibit CBZ metabolism, increasing risk of CBZ toxicity. Monitoring CBZ plasma levels and adjusting CBZ dose usually alleviates interaction problems.

carbamazepine overdose Data from 33 patients treated for overdose (1.6–45 g), with 51% of cases involving other drugs, indicates the following symptoms: diminished consciousness, mydriasis, abnormal muscle tone, tendon reflexes, ataxia, nystagmus, and opthalmoplagia. Seizures occurred in 24%. Hyponatremia occurred in 12%, and there was transient evidence of hepatic dysfunction in 50%. Incidences of hyperglycemia and hypokalemia were related to higher drug levels. Management was largely supportive: avoidance of drug interactions, large doses of activated charcoal, airway management, and correction of electrolyte disturbances (Seymour JF. Carbamazepine overdose: features of 33 cases. *Drug Safety* 1993;8:81–88). Flumazenil has been reported effective in cases of carbamazepine poisoning (Martens F, Koppel C, Ibe K, et al. Clinical experience with the benzodiazepine antagonist flumazenil in suspected benzodiazepine or ethanol poisoning. *J Clin Toxicol* 1990;28:341–356; O'Sullivan GF, Wade DN. Flumazenil in the management of acute overdosage with benzodiazepines and other agents. *Clin Pharmacol Ther* 1987;42:254).

carbamazepine overdose/children In a study of 82 pediatric patients (ages 1–17) with carbamazepine (CBZ) poisoning, serum CBZ level was related to depth of coma, convulsions, hypotension, and need for mechanical ventilation. In 10 patients in deep coma, mean serum level was 213 mmol/L; in 4 of the 10, large doses of inotropic agents were required; 1 patient was treated with plasmapheresis; and 2 died. In 27 patients with moderate coma, mean CBZ serum level was 112 mmol/L; 2 of the 27 had convulsions. In 45 patients with normal or mildly depressed consciousness, mean CBZ serum level was 73 mmol/L (Tibbals J. Acute toxic reaction to carbamazepine: clinical effects and serum concentrations. *J Pediatr* 1992;121:295–299).

carbamazepine + oxiracetam Carbamazepine influences the half-life of oxiracetam, necessitating its more frequent administration. No adverse interactions have been reported.

carbamazepine + pancuronium Carbamazepine decreases response to pancuronium and shortens recovery time from it (Desai P, Hewitt PB, Jones RM. Influence of anticonvulsant therapy on doxacurium and pancuronium-induced paralysis. *Anesthesiology* 1989;71:A784).

carbamazepine + paroxetine Co-administration in well controlled epileptics was well tolerated in a single-blind, placebo-controlled study. No seizures or clinically relevant changes in carbamazepine plasma concentrations occurred (Mikkelsen M, Anderson BB, Dam M, et al. Paroxetine: no interaction with anti-epileptic drugs. *Psychopharmacology* 1991;103:B13).

carbamazepine + perphenazine Carbamazepine can substantially reduce perphenazine plasma levels, making it difficult to achieve effective antipsychotic drug levels (Nelson JC. Combined treatment strategies in psychiatry. *J Clin Psychiatry* 1993;54[suppl 9]:42–49).

carbamazepine + phenobarbital Phenobarbital can adversely affect carbamazepine (CBZ) metabolism, doubling CBZ epoxide plasma levels. When drugs that stimulate epoxide formation are co-administered with CBZ, serum levels may remain relatively normal, but intoxi-

cation can occur from high metabolite concentrations.

carbamazepine + phenytoin Each drug may lower the other's plasma level, resulting in reduced therapeutic efficacy. Through induction of hepatic microsomal enzymes, each may decrease the other's steady-state concentrations (Hansen J, Siersbaek-Nielsen K, Skovsted L. Carbamazepine-induced acceleration of diphenylhydantoin and warfarin metabolism in man. *Clin Pharmacol Ther* 1971;12:539–543; Zielinski JJ, Haidukewych D, Lehata BJ. Carbamazepine-phenytoin interaction: elevation of plasma phenytoin concentrations due to carbamazepine comedication. *Ther Drug Monit* 1983;7:51–53). Altered mental status occurred in a patient treated with phenytoin (450 mg/day) and carbamazepine (600 mg/day) (Browne TR, Feldman RG, Mikati MA, et al. Nineteen-year-old man with altered mental status. *J Clin Pharmacol* 1992;32:511–519).

carbamazepine + pimozide Co-administration may enhance the central nervous system depressant effects of carbamazepine (CBZ), lower seizure threshold, and decrease the anticonvulsant effects of CBZ. Dosage adjustments may be necessary to control seizures. In some patients, anticholinergic effects may be potentiated, leading to confusion and delirium.

carbamazepine + prednisolone Because it is a powerful inducer of hepatic microsomal enzymes, carbamazepine increases metabolism of prednisolone.

carbamazepine/pregnancy Some investigators have found that carbamazepine (CBZ) serum levels remain constant during pregnancy; others have noted that dose increases of 25% or higher may be needed because of altered gastrointestinal, hepatic, and renal functioning. CBZ freely crosses the placenta. Cord serum concentrations are approximately equal to those in maternal serum. Minor craniofacial defects, fingernail hypoplasia, and developmental delay have been associated with CBZ alone or in combination with other medications. When it is essential to prescribe CBZ during pregnancy, serum concentrations should be monitored closely, since adverse fetal effects have been associated with high blood concentrations (Miller LJ. Clinical strategies for the use of psychotropic drugs during pregnancy. *Psychiatr Med* 1991;9:275–298). CBZ is virtually undetectable within 2 weeks of birth. See **carbamazepine/breast milk; carbamazepine/teratogenesis.**

carbamazepine/pregnancy test Carbamazepine (CBZ) may interfere with some pregnancy tests that ordinarily are about 98% reliable. Inconclusive and false-negative results have been reported in some women taking CBZ (Lindhout D, Meinardi M. False-negative pregnancy test in women taking carbamazepine. *Lancet* 1982;2:505). See **carbamazepine + oral contraceptive.**

carbamazepine + primidone Co-administration may lower carbamazepine (CBZ) plasma level and reduce therapeutic efficacy. CBZ may decrease metabolism of primidone to its metabolites; increased primidone levels have been reported (Pippenger CE. Clinically significant carbamazepine drug interactions: an overview. *Epilepsia* 1987;28:S71–S76).

carbamazepine + ranitidine Ranitidine does not inhibit the hepatic microsomal enzyme oxidase system and hence does not alter the levels of hepatically metabolized anticonvulsants, such as carbamazepine (Webster LK, Mihaly GW, Jones DB, et al. Effect of cimetidine and ranitidine on carbamazepine and sodium valproate pharmacokinetics. *Eur J Clin Pharmacol* 1984;27:341–343).

carbamazepine/systemic lupus erythematosus (SLE) Carbamazepine (CBZ)-induced SLE has been reported frequently since 1966. All patients suffered from neurological diseases, in most cases epileptic disorders, and usually had been treated with CBZ for 1 year or longer. Antihistone antibodies, which are more often found in drug-induced SLE (90%) than in idiopathic SLE (30%–70%), are found in patients with CBZ-induced SLE, strongly suggesting that the SLE is due to CBZ (Schmist ST, Welcker M, Greil W, Schattenkirchner M. Carbamazepine-induced systemic lupus erythematosus. *Br J Psychiatry* 1992;161:560–561).

carbamazepine/teratogenesis Carbamazepine (CBZ) was suggested as the drug of choice for epileptic women of child-bearing potential. Since 1989, anecdotal reports have indicated that CBZ is a minor teratogen. Despite concerns, the case against CBZ remains to be proven by large, prospective, multicenter investigations based on pregnancy registers. CBZ treatment should not preclude a woman from childbearing. More than 90% of such pregnancies are uneventful and result in a healthy baby (Anon. Teratogenesis with carbamazepine. *Lancet* 1991;337:1316–1317; Rosa FW. Spina bifida in infants of women treated with carbamazepine during pregnancy. *N Engl J Med* 1991;324:674–677).

carbamazepine + terfenadine Co-administration caused confusion, disorientation, visual hallucinations, nausea, and ataxia soon after beginning treatment with terfenadine (Seldane) 60 mg twice a day. Free carbamazepine blood concentration was nearly 3 times higher than the upper limit of the therapeutic range.

Symptoms remitted following discontinuation of terfenadine (Hirschfeld S, Jarosinski P. Drug interaction of terfenadine and carbamazepine. *Ann Intern Med* 1993;188:907–908).

carbamazepine + theophylline Co-administration may decrease theophylline blood levels and cause some interference with its therapeutic effects (Mitchell EA, Dower JC, Green RJ. Interaction between carbamazepine and theophylline. *N Z Med J* 1986;99:69–70).

carbamazepine + thioridazine Co-administration produces no significant changes in steady state plasma levels of either carbamazepine or its metabolite, 10,11-epoxide.

carbamazepine + thiothixene Carbamazepine increases thiothixene clearance, decreasing steady-state plasma levels and possibly interfering with therapeutic efficacy (Ereshefsky L, Jann MW, Saklad SR, Davis CM. Bioavailability of psychotropic drugs: historical perspective and pharmacokinetic overview. *J Clin Psychiatry* 1986;47[suppl]:6–15).

carbamazepine + thyroxine Use of carbamazepine in thyroxine-substituted hypothyroid children requires an increased dose of thyroxine to maintain a euthyroid state.

carbamazepine + tricyclic antidepressant (TCA) Carbamazepine (CBZ) induces metabolism of TCAs, resulting in lower plasma levels and possible depressive relapse (Preskorn SH, Burke MJ, Fast GA. Therapeutic drug monitoring: principles and practice. *Psychiatr Clin North Am* 1993;16:611–645). If patients fail to respond to standard TCA doses or develop adverse effects, CBZ, TCA, and TCA metabolite levels should be checked (De la Fuente JM. Carbamazepine-induced low plasma levels of tricyclic antidepressants. *J Clin Psychopharmacol* 1992;12:67–68).

carbamazepine + valproate Valproate inhibits metabolism of carbamazepine (CBZ), increasing its blood concentration. Conversely, CBZ increases metabolism of valproate, decreasing its blood level over 60%, so that quite high doses may be needed to obtain therapeutic serum levels (Jann MW, Fidone GS, Israel MK, et al. Increased valproate serum concentrations upon carbamazepine cessation. *Epilepsia* 1988;29:578–581; Keck PE, Jr, McElroy SL, Vuckovic A, et al. Combined valproate and carbamazepine treatment of bipolar disorder. *J Neuropsychiatry Clin Neurosci* 1991;4:319–322). Both drugs compete for protein binding sites; when they are administered together, the concentration of the free fraction (bioactive component) of the drug may increase. Thus, dosages previously tolerated with a single agent may result in enhanced central nervous system effects and even toxicity when co-administered. Adding valproate to ongoing

CBZ therapy can result in a decrease in CBZ concentration and increase the CBZ metabolite 10,11-epoxide, while CBZ in turn may induce oxidation of valproate through a microsomal P450-mediated process. Acute psychosis occurred in a patient on long-term valproate therapy following addition of CBZ, even though CBZ levels were "nontoxic" (McKee RJW, Larkin JG, Brodie MJ. Acute psychosis with carbamazepine and sodium valproate. *Lancet* 1987;1:167). Co-administration requires monitoring of drug serum levels and awareness of clinical signs and symptoms of toxicity. Data indicate that co-administration is safe for bipolar and schizoaffective patients, but more effective in the former. Bipolar patients refractory to carbamazepine or valproate alone are likely to respond, suggesting a possible synergistic effect (Token M, Castillo JM, Pope HG, Jr. Concurrent use of valproate and carbamazepine in bipolar disorder. Presented at the 146th Annual Meeting of the American Psychiatric Association, San Francisco, May 1993).

carbamazepine + valproic acid Co-administration has been used in epileptic patients without problems. It also may result in sustained prophylactic response in bipolar patients inadequately responsive to CBZ or valproic acid (VPA) alone (Ketter TA, Pazzaglia PJ, Post RM. Synergy of carbamazepine and valproic acid in affective illness: case report and review of literature. *J Clin Psychopharmacol* 1992;12:276–281; Keck PE Jr, McElroy SL, Vuckovic A, Friedman LM. Combined valproate and carbamazepine treatment of bipolar disorder. *J Neuropsychiatry Clin Neurosci* 1992;4:319–322). Although not an enzyme inducer, VPA inhibits carbamazepine (CBZ) metabolism and displaces it from plasma proteins, increasing the free CBZ fraction that is active and available to be metabolized. Depending on which effect predominates, total CBZ level can rise, fall, or not change. VPA inhibits epoxide hydrolase, increasing the plasma level of CBZ-epoxide (CBZ-E), at times without altering total plasma CBZ level (Sovner R. A clinically significant interaction between carbamazepine and valproic acid. *J Clin Psychopharmacol* 1988;8:448–449). Because of their complex pharmacokinetics, it may be useful to monitor plasma levels of both CBZ and VPA during combined therapy. VPA serum concentrations have been reported to increase in some patients following CBZ discontinuation (Jann MW, Fidone GS, Israel MK, Bonadero P. Increased valproate serum concentrations upon carbamazepine cessation. *Epilepsia* 1988;29:578–581). The combination should probably be avoided in pregnancy because of the possibility of increased risk of congenital malformations.

carbamazepine + verapamil Co-administration may result in elevated carbamazepine (CBZ) plasma levels and sometimes CBZ toxicity. To compensate for increased CBZ plasma level, CBZ dose should be reduced or nifedipine should be used as an alternative to verapamil (Macphee GJA, McInnes GT, Thompson GG, Brodie M. Verapamil potentiates carbamazepine neurotoxicity: a clinically important inhibitory interaction. *Lancet* 1986;1:700–703; Price WA, DiMarzio LR. Verapamil-carbamazepine neurotoxicity. *J Clin Psychiatry* 1988;49:80). CBZ dosage should be readjusted when verapamil is discontinued.

carbamazepine + vigabatrin No significant changes in carbamazepine (CBZ) plasma levels have been reported. Two patients developed acute encephalopathy after vigabatrin was added to CBZ. Both had stupor and slowed electroencephalographic background activity, dysphoria, and irritability. One developed a novel type of seizure, the other, myoclonic status epilepticus. In the first case serum CBZ was slightly raised, but clinical symptoms could not be related to intoxication with CBZ or its epoxide. It is unknown whether an interaction between vigabatrin and CBZ caused acute encephalopathy, which has been reported with vigabatrin monotherapy (Salke-Kellerman A, Baier H, Rambeck B, Boenigk HE, Wolf P. Acute encephalopathy with vigabatrin. *Lancet* 1993;342:185).

carbamazepine + viloxazine Co-administration may increase serum carbamazepine (CBZ) levels up to 50%, but only slightly increase its epoxide levels. There may be symptoms of CBZ intoxication (fatigue, dizziness, ataxia). Viloxazine discontinuation produces symptom remission and return of serum CBZ level to initial value (Pisani F, Fazio A, Oteri G, et al. Elevation of plasma carbamazepine and carbamazepine 10,11-epoxide levels by viloxazine in epileptic patients. *Acta Pharmacol* 1986;59[suppl 5/II]:109; Pisani F, Fazio A, Oteri G, et al. Carbamazepine-viloxazine interaction in patients with epilepsy. *J Neurol Neurosurg Psychiatry* 1986;49:1142–1145).

carbamazepine + warfarin Carbamazepine (CBZ), a powerful inducer of hepatic microsomal enzymes, can decrease warfarin's effectiveness; dosage adjustments based on monitoring of prothrombin time may be necessary during and after CBZ (Hansen J, Siersbaek-Nielsen K, Skovsted L. Carbamazepine-induced acceleration of diphenylhydantoin and warfarin metabolism in man. *Clin Pharmacol Ther* 1971;12:539–543).

carbamazepine + zopiclone Although co-administration reduces plasma concentrations of each drug, it also produces clear additive impairment of psychomotor performance (Kuitunen T, Mattila MJ, Seppala T, et al. Actions of zopiclone and carbamazepine, alone and in combination, on human skilled performance in laboratory and clinical tests. *Br J Clin Pharmacol* 1990;30:453–461).

carbidopa (Lodosyn) Peripheral aromatic amino acid decarboxylase inhibitor that inhibits hepatic enzymes but does not enter the brain. When co-administered with levodopa, it increases brain catecholamine levels, potentiating and increasing levodopa's duration of effect in parkinson patients. With co-administration, the effective dose of levodopa can be reduced significantly and its peripheral side effects are largely eliminated, but abnormal involuntary movements tend to develop earlier and in more severe form.

carbidopa/levodopa See **levodopa/carbidopa.**

carbimide See **calcium carbimide.**

Carbolith See **lithium.**

carbon dioxide (CO$_2$) challenge test Double-breath inhalation of high-dose (5–30%) CO$_2$ to assess sensitivity. See **carbon dioxide/panic disorder.**

carbon dioxide/panic disorder Panic disorder (PD) and social phobia patients are reported to be hypersensitive to the anxiogenic effects of inhaled carbon dioxide (CO$_2$). Inhalations of 5% and 30% are frequently used as provocation techniques for experimental induction of panic attacks in PD patients with or without agoraphobia. Of numerous agents capable of inducing panic, CO$_2$ offers significant advantages. It is easily administered, well tolerated, and one of the most reliable panicogens. Various concentrations induce more anxiety and panic attacks in patients than in comparison subjects, suggesting that respiratory disturbance is a key component in the pathophysiology of panic. However, studies indicate that its specific panicogenic effect in panic patients goes beyond simple breathlessness (Papp LA, Klein DF, Martinez J, et al. Diagnostic and substance specificity of carbon-dioxide-induced panic. *Am J Psychiatry* 1993;150:250–257).

carcinoid syndrome Disease due to a 5-hydroxytryptamine secreting tumor usually located in the gastrointestinal tract.

Cardizem See **diltiazem.**

caroxazone Selective, reversible inhibitor of monoamine oxidase-B being investigated as an antidepressant.

carphenazine (Proketazine) Piperazine phenothiazine no longer marketed in the United States.

carrier One who is heterozygous for a normal gene and an abnormal gene that is not ex-

pressed phenotypically, though it may be detectable.

carrier trait See **trait, carrier.**

carryover effect Influence of treatments administered before the trial period on results of any other treatments administered during the trial. Before a trial is started, a washout period for previously administered treatment may be needed to ensure absence of carryover effects. They also can be minimized by delaying the second treatment administration, thereby allowing effects of one drug to dissipate before administering the other. Carryover effects can complicate interpretation and analysis when a subsequent treatment's apparent activity is actually due to the previous treatment. They also can weaken the scientific and statistical basis for choosing a crossover design. See **washout.**

"cartwheel" Street name for (a) amphetamines; (b) Dexedrine.

case-control study Observational study in which characteristics of people with a disease or with a particular condition (the *case* patients) are compared with individuals in whom the condition or disease is absent (the *control* subjects). Case patients and control subjects are compared with respect to existing or past attributes or exposures thought to be relevant to development of the condition or disease under study (Schesselman JJ. *Case Control Studies.* New York: Oxford University Press, 1982). Case-control studies are used extensively to study adverse drug reactions and, occasionally, beneficial drug effects. They can be used to study multiple exposures and uncommon diseases. They require few subjects and are logistically easy, fast, and inexpensive. Disadvantages are difficulty in selection of control subjects, possibly biased exposure data, and inability to assess incidence. Also called "retrospective study."

case history study Study based on reports from a series of cases.

case index Person in a family or group who is the subject of investigation.

case management Identification, coordination, and monitoring of services for patients with severe illness. Focus is on integrating and mobilizing resources to meet individual patient needs. In clinical case management, a highly skilled psychiatric professional is directly concerned with all aspects of the patient's physical and social environment. Clinical case managers arrange access to appropriate services and provide a range of interventions (intermittent psychotherapy, training in community living skills, psychoeducation of patient and family, and support during crises).

case report Report on a single or very small number of patients. In pharmacoepidemiology, it describes exposure to a drug followed by an unusual, usually adverse, outcome. Case reports are useful for generating hypotheses, but cannot be used for hypothesis testing.

case series Reports examining clinical outcomes of a collection of patients, all of whom had a single exposure. No attempt is made to verify specific hypotheses or compare results with another group of cases. Case series also examine antecedent exposures of patients with a common disease. No control group is present. Case series can provide descriptive data on disease characteristics, but cannot be used for hypothesis testing because there are no control groups. Also called "longitudinal observational study."

case series study Descriptive account of interesting or intriguing characteristics observed in a group of subjects.

catalase system Pathway of alcohol metabolism involving use of hydrogen peroxide.

catalepsy Trance-like state with generalized unresponsiveness in which muscles are held rigid for a long period and the person's limbs will remain in any position in which they are placed. It is characteristic of catatonic schizophrenia and some forms of hysteria, and may occur in patients with affective disturbances, both psychotic and nonpsychotic. Treatment with neuroleptics or electroconvulsive therapy is effective. Also called "flexibilitas cerea"; "waxy flexibility."

catalyst Substance that increases the rate of a chemical reaction without itself undergoing chemical transformation. Enzymes are biological catalysts that increase the rate of reactions in living tissue.

catamnesis Medical history of a patient following a given illness. Also called "follow-up history."

catamnestic study Study based on the past history of a case or cases.

cataplexy Transient, sudden loss of skeletal muscle tone that is one of the distinct features of narcolepsy. It may consist of buckling knees, sagging head, or complete collapse without loss of consciousness. Episodes can result in injury to the patient. It should not be confused with the trance-like state called "catalepsy." Primary treatment is with medications that suppress rapid eye movement (REM) sleep, including tricyclic antidepressants (e.g., imipramine, protriptyline), monoamineoxidase inhibitors (e.g., phenelzine, tranylcypromine), amphetamines, and methylphenidate. Clomipramine is considered a superior treatment (Douglass AB, Hays P, Pazderka F, Russell JM. Florid refractory

schizophrenias that turn out to be treatable variants of HLA-associated narcolepsy. *J Nerv Ment Dis* 1991;179:12–17).

Catapres See **clonidine**.

Catapres-TTS See **clonidine skin patch**.

catatonia Syndrome secondary to medical and/or neurological disorders characterized by (a) stupor associated with either marked rigidity or flexibility of the musculature; or (b) overactivity in conjunction with various manifestations of stereotypy. Often erroneously considered a manifestation only of schizophrenia, it is often seen in mania, depression, infections, endocrinopathy, and drug toxicity. In a study comparing computerized tomography (CT) scans of five catatonic patients with scans of five non-catatonic patients, all catatonic patients showed atrophy of the brainstem and cerebellar vermis (Joseph AB, Anderson WH, O'Leary DH. Brain stem and vermis atrophy in catatonia. *Am J Psychiatry* 1985;142:352–354). Every case of catatonia or catalepsy should have a full neurological and general medical investigation, including neuroimaging and electroencephalogram (EEG) examinations. Electroconvulsive therapy (ECT) has been known to be an effective treatment for catatonia since 1938, and was endorsed by an American Psychiatric Association task force as an effective treatment for catatonic subtypes of schizophrenia (American Psychiatric Association Task Force on Electroconvulsive Therapy: *The Practice of Electroconvulsive Therapy: Recommendations for Treatment, Training, and Privileging*. Washington, DC: APA, 1990). Although the Task Force listed catatonia secondary to medical conditions as an indication for ECT, caution is warranted; medical and/or neurological disorders underlying catatonia should be treated as aggressively as possible, and ECT should be used only when symptoms are refractory to psychopharmacological interventions or are more life-threatening than the underlying medical/neurological disorder. However, in patients with malignant catatonia in whom the catatonic process produces severe and life-threatening medical/neurological complications, ECT should be considered a first-line therapy (Rummans TA. Medical indications for electroconvulsive therapy. *Psychiatr Ann* 1993;23:27–32). Lorazepam, clonazepam, and diazepam induce temporary remission of catatonic symptoms. Benzodiazepine treatment is usually considered diagnostic because symptoms return as the drug's therapeutic effects wane. Neuroleptic malignant syndrome should be considered in the differential diagnosis of any case of acute catatonia (Levenson JL. Neuroleptic malignant syndrome. *Am J Psychiatry* 1985;142:1137–

1145; White DAC, Robins AH. Catatonia: harbinger of the neuroleptic malignant syndrome. *Br J Psychiatry* 1991;158:419–421).

catatonia, deadly See **catatonia, lethal.**

catatonia, hyperthermic See **catatonia, lethal.**

catatonia, lethal Term coined by Stauder (1934) for a rare, often fatal psychiatric disorder manifested by psychosis, agitation, high blood pressure, hyperpyrexia (temperatures up to 108° F), delirium, tremulousness, tachycardia, diaphoresis, and catatonic rigidity. It may develop during a variety of organic and functional illnesses. It can be conceptualized as an exhaustion syndrome, caused and maintained by relentless psychomotor excitement lasting days to weeks, that progresses to cachexia, organic-like delirium, convulsions, and coma (Stauder KH. Die todliche Katatonie. *Arch Psychiatr Nervenkr* 1934;102:614–634; Pearlman CA. Neuroleptic malignant syndrome: a review of the literature. *J Clin Psychopharmacol* 1986;6:257–273). Since 1960, over 300 cases have been reported. Lethal catatonia should be included in the differential diagnosis of high fevers. Electroconvulsive therapy may be the treatment of choice for functional lethal catatonia. Organic lethal catatonia responds to treatment of the underlying disorders (e.g., cerebral thrombosis, hyperthyroidism, or sedative-hypnotic withdrawal). Neuroleptics are not helpful and may make lethal catatonia worse. Also called "deadly catatonia"; "hyperthermic catatonia."

catatonia, neuroleptic-induced Orally or intramuscularly administered neuroleptics, especially high-potency ones, may cause a syndrome strikingly similar to catatonic stupor. It may develop during intramuscular neuroleptic therapy for acute catatonic schizophrenia as well as during rapid neuroleptization with an intramuscularly administered neuroleptic for other types of schizophrenic and nonschizophrenic psychosis, thereby posing a serious diagnostic and management dilemma. Symptoms include withdrawal, mutism, and a variety of neuromuscular and extrapyramidal symptoms (e.g., bizarre posturing, rigidity, immobility, and catalepsy). They may be quickly followed by life-threatening pulmonary and/or cardiovascular complications and dehydration that may be resistant to intensive medical therapy. Extrapyramidal symptoms in patients with neuroleptic-induced catatonia generally are refractory to even massive doses of antiparkinson medications. Catatonia as a side effect of neuroleptics is now seen more often than catatonic schizophrenia. Because catatonic schizophrenia is relatively uncommon and because neuroleptic-induced catato-

nia may be life-threatening, the drug should be presumed responsible for catatonic symptoms that appear or worsen shortly after initiation of neuroleptic therapy. To avert potential pathological sequelae, the neuroleptic should be discontinued immediately. Although catatonic symptoms may persist because of the long elimination half-life of many neuroleptics, symptoms usually resolve within several days to a few weeks. However, progressive medical complications may develop that may be irreversible or fatal despite intensive treatment.

catatonic behavior Marked motor activity, apparently purposeless and not influenced by external stimuli.

catatonic negativism Apparently motiveless resistance to instructions or attempts to be moved. When passive, the person may resist any effort to be moved; when active, he or she may do the opposite of what is asked (firmly clench jaws when asked to open mouth).

catatonic posturing Voluntary assumption of an inappropriate or bizarre posture, usually held for a long period.

catatonic rigidity Maintenance of a rigid posture against all efforts to be moved.

catatonic stupor Marked decrease in reactivity to the environment and reduction in spontaneous movements and activity, sometimes to the point of appearing to be unaware of one's surroundings.

catatonic waxy flexibility See **catalepsy.**

"catatonos raptus" See **delirium acutum** (preferred term).

Catatrol See **viloxazine.**

cat box DNA sequence that regulates transcription of eukaryotic genes, frequently with some tissue specificity. It is located about 70–80 bases upstream from the start of the transcription.

catchment area Geographic region (well- or ill-defined) in which clients of a particular health facility reside.

catecholamine Any organic compound containing a catechol nucleus (a benzene ring with two adjacent hydroxyl substituents) and an amine group. Catecholamines are formed in adrenal chromaffin cells, sympathetic nerves, sympathetic ganglia, and central neurons from their amino acid precursor tyrosine by a sequence of enzymatic steps. The biosynthetic pathway for their formation is tyrosine to dopa to dopamine and then to norepinephrine and epinephrine, depending on availability of phenylethalanine-N-methyl transferase and dopamine-beta-hydroxylase. Some are neurotransmitters that exert important effects on peripheral and central nervous system activity (e.g., norepinephrine [noradrenaline], epinephrine [adrenaline], and dopamine). In practice, the term means dopamine and its metabolic products, norepinephrine, and epinephrine. See **biogenic amine.**

catecholamine hypothesis of depression Postulation that some, if not all, depressions are associated with an absolute or relative deficiency of catecholamines, particularly norepinephrine (NE), at functionally important adrenergic receptor sites in the brain. This hypothesis is based on indirect pharmacological evidence from studies of drug effects on catecholamines, especially NE, and on affective states. Drugs that deplete and inactivate NE centrally produce sedation or depression, whereas drugs that increase or potentiate brain NE are associated with behavioral stimulation or excitation, and generally have antidepressant effects in man (Bunney WE, Davis JM. Norepinephrine in depressive reactions. *Arch Gen Psychiatry* 1965;13:1160–1162; Schildkraut JJ. The catecholamine hypothesis of affective disorders: a review of supporting evidence. *Am J Psychiatry* 1965;122:509–514). The hypothesis stimulated an entire generation of investigations in biological psychiatry.

catecholestrogen 2- and 4-hydroxylated metabolites of estrone and estradiol. Although they have been known and studied for over 40 years, their functional roles remain elusive. Their formation represents a major route of estrogen metabolism in various tissues, including the brain, where they are of particular interest to neuroendocrinologists because they interact with the catecholaminergic system. Recent findings that they exert behavioral effects indicate they may not be merely inactive metabolites. Main route of catecholestrogen degradation is by catechol-O-methyltransferase (COMT).

catechol-O-methyltransferase (COMT) Enzyme that plays a major role in the metabolism of endogenous circulating and administered catecholamines. It methylates dopamine to 3-O-methyltyramine. COMT and monoamine oxidase are the two principal enzymes involved in the metabolism of dopamine.

categorical data Counted measures, always given in whole numbers.

categorical observation Variable whose values are categories that are qualitatively different (e.g., pregnant vs. nonpregnant).

catharsis Relief due to release of pent-up emotions. It occurs when a patient releases feelings (anger, affection, sorrow, grief) about past or present material that have previously been difficult or impossible to discharge (Bloch S, Crouch E. *Therapeutic Factors in Group Psychotherapy.* Oxford: Oxford University Press, 1985).

caudate nucleus Part of the corpus striatum, which is a part of the basal ganglia.

causalgia Particularly intense, diffuse burning sensation of the skin along the distribution of a peripheral nerve following partial damage to peripheral nerve trunks. It is accompanied by cutaneous changes, including swelling, redness, and temperature changes.

cause-specific mortality rate Mortality rate from a specific disease.

"CD" Street name for glutethimide.

CD4 cell T helper lymphocyte, a subset of lymphocytes identified by their differential functions and specific cell-surface markers. Decreased number and steady-state decline of CD4 cells predicts the development of clinical acquired immunodeficiency syndrome (AIDS) in human immunodeficiency virus (HIV)-seropositive individuals. Biologically significant alterations in lymphocyte subsets (T cells, T cell subsets, and B cells) may occur without changes in the total number of circulating lymphocytes. There are no relationships between depressive disorders or depressive symptoms and counts of CD4 cells in HIV-positive homosexual men.

cDNA library Clones containing a single independent DNA molecule.

Celance See **pergolide.**

cell **1.** Smallest component of life; a complex collection of molecules bounded by a membrane. **2.** Category of counts or values in a contingency table.

Celontin See **methsuximide.**

censored observation Incomplete observation in a study that occurs when a subject drops out before an experiment ends (right censor), enters after it begins (left censor), or both.

centimorgan (cM) Genetic "distance" at which likelihood that two genes will be separated in meiosis equals 50%, which would occur by random chance. See **linkage; linkage map.**

central anticholinergic syndrome (CAS) Toxic disorder that occurs in patients receiving a high dose of a single anticholinergic medication or a combination of two or more medications with antimuscarinic actions. Symptoms include temperature elevation, dry flushed skin, dry mouth, blurred vision, dilated and nonreactive pupils, constipation, decreased bowel sounds, rapid heart rate, urinary retention, flushed face, and confusion. Severe cases may be manifested by seizures, hyper-reflexia, fever, slurred speech, and ataxia. CAS occurs often in elderly patients and those who have just undergone operations who take one or more (usually the latter) drugs with anticholinergic properties, such as scopolamine, atropine, cyclopentolate, antihistamines (e.g., diphenhydramine, hydroxyzine, chlorpheniramine, promethazine), antiparkinson drugs (e.g., benztropine, biperiden, trihexyphenidyl), tricyclic antidepressants (e.g., amitriptyline, nortriptyline, imipramine, clomipramine, doxepin), and neuroleptics (e.g., chlorpromazine, thioridazine, mesoridazine). CAS may superficially mimic neuroleptic malignant syndrome (NMS); however, in NMS, there is diaphoresis, rigidity, and no dry mouth or change in pupillary function.

central excitatory syndrome See **serotonin syndrome.**

central limit theorem Principle that the distribution of means is approximately normal if the sample size is large enough, regardless of the underlying distribution of original measurements.

central nervous system (CNS) See **nervous system, central.**

central nervous system (CNS) depressant Substance that produces depression of CNS function, including alcohol, inhalation agents (anesthetics), some sedative-hypnotic drugs (barbiturates, nonbarbiturates [e.g., antihistamines, glutethimide, chloral hydrate, benzodiazepines]), some neuroleptics (e.g., phenothiazines), and some antidepressants (e.g., tricyclics). These nonspecific depressants share the ability to depress excitable tissue at all levels of the CNS by stabilizing neuronal membranes, which leads to a decrease in the amount of transmitter released by the nerve impulse and a general depression of postsynaptic responsiveness and ion movement. Effects are dose-related and depend on formulation (particle size) and route of administration. CNS depressants have additive effects when taken together.

central nervous system (CNS) depressant + amoxapine Combined use increases CNS depression beyond that caused by either drug alone.

central nervous system (CNS) depressant + antihistamine Co-administration may cause drowsiness and impaired attention, resulting in accidents and/or falls.

central nervous system (CNS) depressant + diphenhydramine Co-administration may produce moderate to severe sedation or induce drowsiness and various degrees of sleep.

central nervous system (CNS) depressant/intoxication Manifestations range from varying degrees of sedation to coma. Treatment varies according to type of CNS depressant. In every case, treatment should basically consist of emesis, lavage, and supportive care. The treating physician should always be on the alert for concomitant ingestions.

central nervous system (CNS) depressant + nalbuphine Phenothiazines and other tranquilizers, sedative-hypnotics, alcohol, and other CNS depressants produce additive effects when co-administered with nalbuphine. If combined therapy is contemplated, dosage of one or both agents should be reduced.

central nervous system (CNS) depressant + orphenadrine Co-administration may produce additive CNS depressant effects and may necessitate reduction of the dosage of both drugs.

central nervous system (CNS) depressant + thioridazine Thioridazine + alcohol, anesthetics, barbiturates, narcotics, or other CNS depressants increases CNS depression.

central nervous system (CNS) infusion Drug delivery system using an implantable pump connected to a Silastic intraventricular catheter. It offers numerous potential advantages for drug delivery to the brain and may be a treatment for dementia. Risks are related to the surgery associated with implantation and to the possibility of increased neurotoxicity of centrally administered drugs.

central nervous system (CNS) stimulant Drug that produces widespread, dose-dependent excitation leading ultimately to convulsions. The drugs are classified on the basis of their mechanism of action and their presumed major action at different levels of the neuraxis. Methylxanthines, cocaine, amphetamine, methamphetamine, ephedrine, mephentermine, methylphenidate, phenmetrazine, and pipradol are classified as corticostimulants; pentetrazol, picrotoxin, and bemegride are brainstem stimulants; strychnine is a spinal cord stimulant.

central nervous system (CNS) stimulant + amantadine Co-administration may result in additive stimulation and should be used with caution.

central pontine myelinolysis (CPM) Selective loss of myelin involving the center of the basal pons and other extrapontine areas of the brain where gray and white matter intermix. It accompanies many chronic debilitating diseases and is most often seen in malnourished alcoholics. Symptoms of the fulminant state include dysarthria, impaired swallowing, pseudobulbar signs, quadriparesis, and quadriplegia. Although early experience suggested an invariably poor outcome, recovery has been documented in patients who clinically seemed to show dissociation at the pontine level: brisk reflexes, extensor plantars, quadriparesis leading to quadriplegia, and dysarthria, giving a "locked-in" appearance. Symptom severity seems to vary with lesion size. Hemiparesis, spastic weakness of the arms, and oculomotor abnormalities are noted in milder cases, whereas small lesions in the mid-pons give rise to few clinical symptoms. Confusion or stupor are often present (McColl P, Kelly C. A misleading case of central pontine myelinolysis. Risk factors for psychiatric patients. *Br J Psychiatry* 1992;160:550–552). CPM has been attributed to too-rapid correction of hyponatremia (serum sodium level below 135 mEq/L) in a number of cases, but major ambiguities include whether severity and/or chronicity of hyponatremia prior to correction contribute to demyelinization and what constitutes a safe correction rate for different degrees of hyponatremia. Severe hyponatremia (serum sodium level below 120 mEq/L) may lead to severe neurological damage or death. Long-term psychiatric symptoms due to CPM include personality change, inappropriate affect, and/or delusions not present prior to CPM development (Muller RJ, Donner TW. Correction rate of severe hyponatremia and central pontine myelinolysis. *Am J Psychiatry* 1992;149:715–716). Also called "osmotic demyelination syndrome." See **hyponatremia.**

Centrax See **prazepam.**

centromere Constricted portion of the chromosome separating its two arms.

centrophenoxine Psychotropic agent synthesized in 1959 as the p-chlorphenoxyacetic acid ester of dimethylaminoethanol, a precursor of acetylcholine. It has been claimed to produce changes in neuronal lipopigment. It has been advocated for the treatment of various forms of dementia, stroke, and head injuries, although the clinical literature is sparse and inconclusive.

cerebellum Brain mass located above the pons and medulla and beneath the posterior portion of the cerebrum.

cerebral blood flow (CBF) study Measurement of regional cerebral blood flow, which is intimately associated with local neuronal activity in the brain. Done since 1948, primarily in schizophrenic patients, the studies have been used to investigate physiological dysfunction in the central nervous system. Techniques used are rapid and noninvasive, but their use is limited by poor spatial resolution. See **regional cerebral blood flow.**

cerebral concussion Reversible or irreversible disruption of neural function by trauma occurring in a diffuse, symmetrical manner throughout the brain.

cerebral electrostimulation See **electrosleep.**

cerebral electrotherapy (CET) See **electrosleep.**

cerebral insufficiency Putative state in the elderly characterized by difficulties of concentration and of memory; absentmindedness; confusion; lack of energy; tiredness; decreased physical performance; depressive mood; anxiety; dizziness; tinnitus; and headache. The symptoms, said to be relieved by ginkgo treatment, have been associated with impaired cerebral circulation; sometimes they are thought to be early indications of dementia, of either degenerative or multiple infarct type but often no explanation can be found.

cerebral laterality Functional specialization of the nervous system that is found to a different degree on one side or the other of the neuraxis. Lateralization of the human brain is a normal condition. In general, female brains are theorized to be less asymmetric and lateralized than male brains. In turn, male brains may be a variation on female brains that have been modified and lateralized more than normal under the influence of male hormones. This theory of lateralization has been used to explain and predict various phenomena, including differences in male and female psychology and neuropsychological functioning, and the observation that paraphilias are more likely to occur in males than females. Cerebral laterality is not synonymous with dominance, asymmetry, or handedness.

cerebral palsy Congenital disorder consisting of bilateral, symmetrical atrophy of the nerve cells and gliosis, mainly of the pyramidal tracts, resulting in weakness and spasticity of the lower limbs. It may also be manifested by involuntary movements, ataxia, and some degree of mental deficiency.

cerebromalacia Change (lesion) in white matter of the brain associated with aging and believed to be associated with increased water content in the tissue due to cerebrovascular disease. It can be demonstrated by imaging technologies such as computed tomography (CT) and magnetic resonance imaging (MRI).

cerebrovascular accident See **stroke** (preferred term).

Cerepax See **temazepam.**

Cerespan See **papaverine.**

Ceretec See **technetium-99m hexamethylpropyleneamine.**

cervical dystonia See **dystonia, cervical.**

Cesamet See **nabilone.**

Cespar See **buspirone.**

Cetrane See **quazepam.**

C-fos Immediate early gene that serves as a transcription factor for the expression of other genes. It is the prototypical member of a class of oncogenes. It encodes a 55,000 molecular weight phosphoprotein FOS, which is thought to assist in the regulation of "target genes" containing an AP-I binding site. C-fos is also involved in actions of central nervous system drugs. See **oncogene.**

CGS-20625 Pyrazolopyridine that is a potent and selective agonist for the central benzodiazepine receptor complex. Its profile indicates partial agonist or mixed agonist/antagonist properties, and it is predicted to have high anxiolytic potency with minimal sedation and alcohol potentiating liability. In a phase I, double-blind, dose-finding study with pharmacodynamic and pharmacokinetic evaluations in healthy male volunteers, it was "typically" anxiolytic with central nervous system effects similar to those of diazepam and estazolam. Study results suggest that doses of 40–80 mg would have long-lasting clinical anxiolytic effects.

chance agreement Measure of the proportion of times two or more raters would agree by chance in their measurement or assessment of a phenomenon.

character spectrum disorder (CSD) Subdivision of "characterological depression," a form of personality disorder unresponsive to medication and more common in women. Patients have normal rapid eye movement (REM) latencies, more intermittent dysphoria, positive family histories of alcoholism, developmental history characterized by parental separation or divorce, and a dependent, histrionic, or sociopathic personality. They should be evaluated for histories of childhood sexual abuse. CSD overlaps to some extent with depression spectrum disorder and neurotic depression.

"charas" Street name for the cannabinols.

Charcot's disease See **amyotrophic lateral sclerosis.**

"chasing ghosts" Street term for transient compulsive foraging behavior associated with crack cocaine use. See **compulsive foraging behavior.**

"chasing the dragon" Street term for inhalation of sublimated heroin after treating it on tinfoil. In the United Kingdom, chasing was a route of initiation to heroin secondary to injection and snorting until the mid-1970s. By 1979, there were as many initiations by chasing as by injection. By 1981, over half the heroin initiations were by chasing; by 1985, more than three-fourths; and since 1988, an estimated 94% have been by chasing. Chasing could alter the importance of heroin use in human immunodeficiency virus (HIV) transmission.

"cheap cocaine" Street name for phencyclidine (PCP).

"checker" Obsessive-compulsive disorder patient obsessed with doubt (usually fear of harming or offending others) or a need for symmetry. Checkers fear they have not turned off the stove or locked the door, or that a bump in the road was a body. They check repetitively, which often contributes to even greater doubt.

"cheese reaction" See **monoamine oxidase inhibitor/"cheese reaction."**

chelating agent Compound that sequesters a metallic ion, thereby inactivating it.

chemical dependence Generic term for psychological or physical dependency, or both, on an exogenous substance. Like alcohol dependence, it is a chronic behavior disorder with genetic, psychosocial, and environmental factors influencing development and manifestations. Often progressive and fatal, it is characterized by continuous or periodic (a) impaired control over drug use/drinking; (b) preoccupation with the drug/alcohol; (c) continued drug/alcohol use despite adverse consequences; and (d) distortions in thinking, most notably denial.

chemoarchitecture of the central nervous system Complex distribution of various endogenous neuroactive compounds and receptors within the brain and spinal cord.

chemoreceptor Receptor, usually peripheral, that is selectively excited by chemical agents (e.g., olfactory and gustatory receptors for smell and taste).

chemoreceptor trigger zone Zone in the area postrema in the floor of the fourth ventricle of the brain that contains receptors for dopamine, histamine, and acetylcholine, inhibition of which partly accounts for the antiemetic properties of prochlorperazine (dopamine blockade), diphenhydramine (histamine blockade), and scopolamine (acetylcholine blockade), respectively.

chemotherapy Use of a chemical to treat or limit further progress of a clinically recognizable disease.

"chewing-spitting syndrome" Variant of bulimia nervosa in which the patient eats very slowly, lets food melt in the mouth, and then spits it out (Vandereycken W, Meermann R. *Anorexia Nervosa: A Clinician's Guide to Treatment.* Berlin-New York: Walter de Gruyter, 1984).

Cheyne-Stokes respiration Breathing pattern characterized by regular "crescendo-decrescendo" fluctuations in respiratory rate and tidal volume. Cheyne-Stokes respiration during sleep can give rise to the symptoms of sleep apnea.

chiasma Point where a crossover between paternal and maternal chromatids has occurred during meiosis.

child abuse Physical abuse and neglect (often chronic) of children, usually infants, toddlers, or preschoolers. They may present with minor or major injuries with explanations that often do not fit the injury. Injuries are usually characteristic and identifiable to well trained professional workers. Handicapped children have been found to be over-represented among abused children; some children may suffer severe brain damage and be permanently mentally handicapped, often with other associated disabilities such as spasticity, epilepsy, or blindness. Abuse may be due to abnormal behavior from the handicapped child that interferes with attachment, or the parents' reaction to the knowledge that the child is handicapped.

childhood anxiety disorder DSM-IV includes three applied to children: separation anxiety disorders, overanxious disorder, and avoidant disorder; and five applied to both children and adults: phobic disorder, panic disorder, generalized anxiety disorder, obsessive-compulsive disorder, and post-traumatic stress disorder.

child molester See **child sexual abuse; pedophile.**

child molester, preferential See **pedophile, preferential.**

child molester, situational See **pedophile, situational.**

child neglect Failure to provide needed, age-appropriate care (National Center on Child Abuse and Neglect. National Child Abuse and Neglect Data System—Working Paper 1: 1990 Summary Data Component. Washington, DC: US Dept. of Health and Human Services, 1992. Publication ACF 92-30361).

child physical abuse Acts that cause or could have caused physical injury to a child (National Center on Child Abuse and Neglect. National Child Abuse and Neglect Data System—Working Paper 1: 1990 Summary Data Component. Washington, DC: US Dept. of Health and Human Services, 1992. Publication ACF 92-30361).

child psychological (emotional) abuse Acts or omissions that caused or could have caused conduct, cognitive, affective, or other mental disorders (National Center on Child Abuse and Neglect. National Child Abuse and Neglect Data System—Working Paper 1: 1990 Summary Data Component. Washington, DC: US Dept. of Health and Human Services, 1992. Publication ACF 92-30361).

child sexual abuse (CSA) Involvement of dependent, developmentally immature children and adolescents in sexual activities they do not fully comprehend, are unable to give informed consent to, and that violate the social taboos of family roles (Schecter MD, Roberge L. Sexual exploitation. *In* Helfer RE, Kempe Ch [eds], *Child Abuse and Neglect: The Family and the Community.* Cambridge, MA: Ballinger, 1976, pp 127–142). CSA may include acts from fondling to intercourse; intercourse between similarly aged adolescents just below the legal age of consent; sadistic sexual assaults by adults on infants; single incidents perpetrated by strangers; and frequent contacts over many years by family members or well known family friends. It also may involve exploitation such as involvement of a child in sexual activity to provide financial benefit to the perpetrator, including contacts for sexual purposes, prostitution, and/or pornography (National Center on Child Abuse and Neglect). CSA is considered a common and previously underestimated problem in modern society. Accurate estimation of prevalence rates and outcome is made difficult by under-reporting, different diagnostic criteria, and reluctance of victims to reveal information, even in "therapeutic settings." Depression is the symptom most commonly reported among adults who were sexually abused as children. Others are anxiety, tension, and sleeping difficulties. An association between eating disorders and a history of child sexual abuse has also been found (National Child Abuse and Neglect Data System—Working Paper 1: 1990 Summary Data Component. Washington, DC: US Dept. of Health and Human Services, 1992. Publication ACF 92-30361).

child sexual abuse, types (a) *Noncontact*: exposure, spying, indecent suggestion, pornography; (b) *Nongenital contact*: touching of breasts or buttocks, inappropriate kissing, attacks with an obvious sexual motive that stopped before any sexual behavior occurred; (c) *Genital contact, child*: touching of the child's genital area, either clothed or unclothed; (d) *Genital contact, abuser*: forcing or persuading the child to touch the abuser's genital area; (e) *Attempted intercourse*: attempts involving immobilization of the child and attempted removal of clothing; and (f) *intercourse*: any act involving penile penetration of the genital or anal area, whether or not ejaculation takes place (Anderson J, Martin J, Mullen P, et al. Prevalence of childhood sexual abuse experiences in a community sample of women. *J Am Acad Child Adolesc Psychiatry* 1993;32:911–919).

chimera Individual composed of cells derived from different zygotes. In human genetics it refers to blood group chimerism, a phenomenon in which dizygotic twins exchange hematopoietic stem cells in utero and continue to form blood cells of both types; or to "whole-body" chimerism, in which two separate zygotes are fused into one individual.

"China white" Street name for (a) designer drugs with opiate effects; (b) potent heroin preparations; (c) 3-methylfentanyl.

"chipper" Individual who reputedly takes drugs regularly but continues to function in the community. Chippers are a subgroup of drug users who do not belong to established categories. Also called "controlled user."

"chira" Street name for hashish.

chi-squared Statistical technique in which variables are categorized to determine whether score distribution is due to chance or to experimental factors.

chi-squared distribution Distribution used to analyze counts in frequency tables. Sum of squares of n independent random variables, each with the standard normal distribution, is called chi-squared distribution with n degrees of freedom.

chi-squared test (x^2) Statistical test based on comparison of a test statistic to a chi-squared distribution. The Pearson chi-squared test is probably the best known.

chloral hydrate (Noctec; Novo-Chlorhydrate) Piperidinedione sedative/hypnotic with a short elimination half-life (6–8 hours). It is metabolized by the alcohol dehydrogenase (ADH) enzyme system in the liver to form the metabolite trichloroethanol, also an active sedative/hypnotic. The metabolite has a half-life of approximately 8 hours. Chloral hydrate is available as a liquid or in capsules containing the liquid. Side effects are rare but can include drowsiness, dizziness, unsteadiness, dry mouth, stomach irritation, excessive bloating and flatus, and excitement. It is suitable for children and the elderly because it is unlikely to have side effects such as confusion. Tolerance and dependence may develop, and sudden withdrawal after long-term use may cause an abstinence syndrome similar to that of barbiturates, though generally less intense. Discontinuation should be gradual. Schedule IV; pregnancy risk category C.

chloral hydrate + clozapine No significant adverse interactions between therapeutic doses have been reported.

chloral hydrate + fluoxetine Co-administration causes moderate, prolonged drowsiness, possibly due to fluoxetine interference with the metabolic degradation of chloral hydrate or to fluoxetine displacement of chloral hydrate from its binding sites (Devarajan S. Interactions of fluoxetine and chloral hydrate. *Can J Psychiatry* 1992;37:590–591).

chloral hydrate + fluvoxamine Chloral hydrate (500–1500 mg) has been prescribed for insomnia in fluvoxamine-treated patients without adverse effects (Mallya GK, White K, Waternaux C, et al. Short- and long-term treatment of obsessive-compulsive disorders with fluvoxamine. *Ann Clin Psychiatry* 1992;4:77–80).

chloral hydrate + furosemide Chloral hydrate affects the hepatic drug-metabolizing system and thus may interfere with a number of other drugs metabolized in the liver. When co-prescribed with the diuretic furosemide, it may cause a syndrome of sympathetic instability.

chloral hydrate intoxication Basic treatment of acute intoxication with all central nervous system depressants is similar to that of barbiturate intoxication. Unabsorbed drug should be removed by lavage or catharsis, respiratory and cardiovascular systems should be stabilized, and drug elimination should be expedited by whatever techniques are feasible for each drug. For chloral hydrate overdose, forced diuresis is of limited benefit. Hemodialysis is more effective and should be used with the same indications as barbiturate overdose. Lipid dialysis increases elimination rate.

chloral hydrate + phenytoin Co-administration can significantly reduce (up to 70%) phenytoin levels.

chloral hydrate + warfarin Co-administration may displace warfarin from its plasma protein binding sites, resulting in increased anticoagulation effects and risk of bleeding.

chlordehydromethyltestosterone Commonly abused anabolic steroid.

chlordesipramine One of the metabolites of clomipramine.

chlordiazepoxide (A-Poxide; Clipoxide; Librium; Libritabs; Servium; SK-Lygen) The first benzodiazepine (BZD) anxiolytic, available since 1960. It is a 1,4-benzodiazepine metabolized by hepatic microsomal oxidation. It is moderately long-acting and well absorbed orally; blood concentrations peak in several hours. Main metabolites (desmethylchlordiazepoxide, demoxepam, and desmethyldiazepam) are pharmacologically active. Half-life varies from 6 to 30 hours. N-desmethyldiazepam (DMDZ), a very long-lasting metabolite, accumulates to high levels after a week. Chlordiazepoxide does not need to be given more than twice daily. Like some other benzodiazepines, it may paradoxically increase irritability and hostility, producing the so-called "Librium rage." Pregnancy risk category D, Schedule IV.

chlordiazepoxide + alcohol Acute alcohol ingestion, even in chronic users, reduces chlordiazepoxide elimination and increases its plasma level (Desmond PV, Patwardhan RV, Schenker S, Hoyumpa AM. Short-term ethanol administration impairs the elimination of chlordiazepoxide [Librium] in man. *Eur J Clin Pharmacol* 1980;18:275–278).

chlordiazepoxide + amitriptyline (Limbitrol) Combination of a benzodiazepine (chlordiazepoxide) and a tricyclic antidepressant (amitriptyline) marketed for the relief of moderate to severe depression associated with moderate to severe anxiety. Both components act on the central nervous system. Adverse reactions are those associated with use of either component alone. Most frequently reported are drowsiness, dry mouth, constipation, blurred vision, dizziness, and bloating.

chlordiazepoxide + amitriptyline/pregnancy
Safe use during pregnancy and lactation has not been established because of the chlordiazepoxide component. According to the manufacturer: "An increased risk of congenital malformations associated with the use of minor tranquilizers (chlordiazepoxide, diazepam, and meprobamate) during the first trimester of pregnancy has been suggested in several studies. Because the use of these drugs is rarely a matter of urgency, their use during this period should almost always be avoided. The possibility that a woman of childbearing potential may be pregnant at the time of institution of therapy should be considered. Patients should be advised that if they become pregnant during therapy or intend to become pregnant they should communicate with their physicians about the desirability of discontinuing the drug." (*Physician's Desk Reference* 1993, pp 2020–2023).

chlordiazepoxide + cimetidine Combined use inhibits chlordiazepoxide hydroxylation, increasing its plasma concentration.

chlordiazepoxide overdose Overdose with chlordiazepoxide alone usually does not cause life-threatening intoxication in physically healthy patients. Management consists of eliminating unabsorbed drug from the gastrointestinal tract and supporting the patient until he or she awakens. Judicious use of flumazenil can quickly reverse chlordiazepoxide intoxication. See **flumazenil.**

chlorimipramine See **clomipramine.**

chlormethiazole (Heminevrin) Sedative/hypnotic with anticonvulsant activity. Onset of action is rapid, but duration of action is shorter than long-acting benzodiazepines. Action on the gamma aminobutyric acid (GABA)$_A$ receptor site, similar to that of barbiturates, has been demonstrated. Half-life is short (1–4 hours). It does not accumulate and is well tolerated. Although it has some hypnotic effect, it does not produce undue sedation in normal doses. It is relatively free of hangover effects and thus has been recommended for use in the elderly. It has improved the behavior of patients with various types of dementia at doses not causing disturbing somnolence or other significant side effects. Short-term administration (7–10 days) is advisable

to minimize risk of tolerance, dependence, and withdrawal symptoms on abrupt discontinuation. Like all central nervous system sedative/hypnotics, chlormethiazole should not be discontinued abruptly. It has been used for alcohol and narcotic withdrawal in Great Britain and Europe, but there may be risk of dependence, especially with high doses. Not available in the United States.

chlorpheniramine (Teldrin) Antihistamine with anticholinergic properties often prescribed as a sedative or antianxiety agent. It may cause anticholinergic delirium, especially in the elderly.

Chlorpromanyl See **chlorpromazine**

chlorpromazine (Chlorpromanyl; Largactil; Novo-Chlorpromazine; Ormazine; Promaz; Prozil; Sonazine; Taroctyl; Thorazine; Thor-Prom) (CPZ) Aliphatic phenothiazine neuroleptic used primarily as an antipsychotic agent and in the treatment of nausea and vomiting. Synthesized in 1950 and first used in psychiatry in 1952, this prototypical antipsychotic agent was one of the most widely used drugs in psychiatry. Antipsychotic efficacy and some side effects (e.g., extrapyramidal reactions) are attributed to central dopamine receptor blockade. Crystallographic data demonstrating that CPZ's molecular configuration is similar to that of dopamine could explain CPZ's ability to block dopamine receptors. Following oral administration, CPZ is well absorbed and metabolized by the liver, with peak plasma concentrations occurring in 1–3 hours. Elimination half-life is 8–17 hours. CPZ is metabolized by sulphoxidation, hydroxylation, N-oxidation, and demethylation, these often succeeding each other. Nearly 100 of an estimated 150 metabolites have been detected in blood or urine. Eventually, metabolites of low lipophilicity are produced, or conjugates are formed and excreted renally. Metabolites such as the sulfoxide have little pharmacological activity, whereas the hydroxyl derivatives are more pharmacologically active. Poor responders to CPZ have high levels of the sulfoxide metabolite, whereas responders have high levels of CPZ or its unconjugated hydroxy metabolites. CPZ is strongly protein-bound and preferentially accumulates in the brain with a brain/plasma ratio of about 5:1. After treatment termination, excretion of drug or one of its metabolites may continue for several months. CPZ may cause a variety of anticholinergic effects, orthostatic hypotension, reflex tachycardia, delayed ejaculation, galactorrhea, decreased libido, weight gain, and early- and late-onset extrapyramidal reactions. Uncommon adverse effects include cholestatic jaundice, photosensitivity, lens and corneal opacities, and agranulocytosis. Pregnancy risk category C.

chlorpromazine + benztropine Benztropine is sometimes co-prescribed with chlorpromazine to treat or prevent acute early onset extrapyramidal reactions. The regimen may reverse some of chlorpromazine's therapeutic effects or cause additive anticholinergic toxicity (Singh MM, Smith JM. Reversal of some therapeutic effects of an antipsychotic agent by an antiparkinsonian drug. *J Nerv Ment Dis* 1973; 50:157).

chlorpromazine + captopril A patient tolerant of higher doses of each drug alone developed supine hypotension with postural syncope when treated with lower doses of both drugs simultaneously. The interaction recurred on rechallenge with low-dose captopril (6.25 mg twice a day) (White WB. Hypotension with postural syncope secondary to the combination of chlorpromazine and captopril. *Arch Int Med* 1986;146:1833–1834).

chlorpromazine + carbamazepine Carbamazepine induces microsomal enzymes, which decrease steady-state plasma concentration and increase hepatic clearance of chlorpromazine. Variable clinical results range from improvement to deterioration.

chlorpromazine + cimetidine Cimetidine reduces chlorpromazine (CPZ) steady state plasma concentration and thus may impair its therapeutic effects (Howes CA, Pullar T, Sourindhrin I, et al. Reduced steady-state concentrations of chlorpromazine and indomethacin in patients receiving cimetidine. *Eur J Clin Pharmacol* 1983;24:99–102). There may be an adverse interaction manifested by excessive sedation and deterioration in performance levels, necessitating reduction in CPZ dosage (Byrne A, O'Shea B. Adverse interaction between cimetidine and chlorpromazine in two cases of chronic schizophrenia. *Br J Psychiatry* 1989;155:413–415).

chlorpromazine/cornea Chlorpromazine (CPZ) can produce corneal and conjunctival changes. Corneal changes fall into two categories: lenticular and epithelial. Fine white and light brown granular deposits on the endothelium and in the stroma, limited to the exposed portion of the cornea, are found in association with the lenticular changes produced with prolonged therapy. They appear to be related to total dosage (usual threshold for their appearance is around 1000 g), and intensity progresses with larger total dosage. Although lesions may improve after CPZ cessation, there have been no reports of their complete disappearance. Epithelial keratopathy differs from deep corneal changes in that it is not necessarily associated with lens

changes, is related to high daily CPZ dosage, and can appear within a period of months. It is characterized by faint, diffuse opacification of the entire exposed portion of the epithelium with linear and curvilinear brownish and white opacifications radiating from a horizontal line just below the optic axis. Almost identical to chloroquine keratopathy, it is known to be at least partially reversible.

chlorpromazine equivalent Antipsychotic dosage considered equivalent to 100 mg of chlorpromazine (CPZ). The following formula is frequently used: 100 mg CPZ = 100 mg of thioridazine = 5 mg of trifluoperazine = 2.5 mg of haloperidol = 2 mg of pimozide. Fluphenazine decanoate (25 mg) is considered equivalent to 291.7 mg/day of CPZ. Other equivalents can be calculated by multiplying a CPZ equivalent ratio by dose and its frequency (Baldessarini RJ, Davis JM. What is the best dose of neuroleptics in schizophrenia? *Psychiatry Res* 1980;3:115–122)

chlorpromazine + fluoxetine Even small doses of fluoxetine (<10 mg) added to chlorpromazine may produce dry mouth and pronounced orthostatic hypotension.

chlorpromazine + lithium Co-administration may cause neurotoxicity manifested by confusion, disorientation, ataxia, falls, and extrapyramidal symptoms (tremors, drooling, and akathisia). Lithium lowers plasma levels of orally administered chlorpromazine, an interaction thought to be due to altered absorption and perhaps increased gut metabolism (Rivera-Calimlin L, Kerzner B, Karch FE. Effect of lithium on plasma chlorpromazine levels. *Clin Pharmacol Ther* 1978;23:451–455).

chlorpromazine + metoclopramide Co-administration may evoke severe extrapyramidal reactions. Fatal acute dystonia has been reported (Schou H, Kongstad LL. Acute dystonia with fatal outcome. A possible adverse drug reaction in the simultaneous administration of chlorpromazine and metoclopramide. *Ugeskr Laeger* 1986;148:2357–2358).

chlorpromazine + nicotine Nicotine lowers chlorpromazine (CPZ) plasma level. Unless CPZ dosage is reduced after smoking cessation, CPZ plasma level may increase markedly and result in sedation (Stimmel GL, Falloon IRH. Chlorpromazine plasma levels, adverse effects and tobacco smoking: case report. *J Clin Psychiatry* 1983;44:420–422).

chlorpromazine + orphenadrine Orphenadrine induces microsomal oxidizing enzymes that reduce chlorpromazine plasma concentration and may interfere with its therapeutic effects (Loga S, Curry S, Lader M. Interactions of orphenadrine and phenobarbitone with chlorpromazine:plasma concentration and effects in man. *Br J Clin Pharmacol* 1985;2:197–208).

chlorpromazine overdose Earliest signs are drowsiness with or without agitation and confusion. Dystonias, twitching, and convulsions occur, and the electroencephalograph contains prominent slow waves. Hypotension is often profound, and cardiac arrhythmias may supervene; hypothermia is common and may be marked. Anticholinergic effects may be intense and worsen the prognosis. Extrapyramidal reactions are usually not a problem, perhaps because they are counteracted by the anticholinergic actions of the drug.

chlorpromazine + phenobarbital Phenobarbital reduces chlorpromazine (CPZ) plasma concentration by inducing microsomal oxidizing enzymes and may interfere with CPZ's therapeutic effects (Loga S, Curry S, Lader M. Interactions of orphenadrine and phenobarbitone with chlorpromazine: plasma concentration and effects in man. *Br J Clin Pharmacol* 1985;2:197–208).

chlorpromazine + phenytoin Chlorpromazine (CPZ) may increase phenytoin levels, but generally its effects are not significant (Kuth H. Interactions between anticonvulsants and other commonly prescribed drugs. *Epilepsia* 1984; 25[suppl 2]:118–131). CPZ's inhibition of hepatic mono-oxygenase activity may reduce the rate of phenytoin metabolism, resulting in a rise in plasma phenytoin concentration with increased risk of toxicity (Aronson JK, Hardman M, Reynolds DJM. Phenytoin. *Br Med J* 1992;305:1215–1218).

chlorpromazine/pregnancy Possible withdrawal following maternal chlorpromazine (CPZ) exposure during pregnancy was reported in the neonate of a woman taking CPZ (300 mg/day) for 4 years. Shortly after birth, the newborn had cyanotic spells and tremor involving all limbs, and later had episodes of hyperthermia. There was no evidence of neonatal sepsis. After 25 days, the newborn was asymptomatic. Neurological development was normal at 1 year of age (Ben-Amitai D, Merlob P. Neonatal fever and cyanotic spells from maternal chlorpromazine. *Ann Pharmacother* 1991;25:1009–1010).

chlorpromazine + propranolol Propranolol may retard chlorpromazine (CPZ) elimination, resulting in elevation of its serum concentration and enhancement of its therapeutic effects (Greendyke RM, Kanter DR. Plasma propranolol levels and their effects on plasma thioridazine and haloperidol concentrations. *J Clin Psychopharmacol* 1987;7:178–182; Peet M, Middlemiss DN, Yates RA. Propanolol in schizophrenia: clinical and biochemical aspects of combining propranolol with chlorpro-

mazine. *Br J Psychiatry* 1981;138:112–117). Adverse cardiovascular changes have occurred in some patients when propranolol is added to CPZ (Miller FA, Rampling D. Adverse effects of combined propranolol and chlorpromazine therapy. *Am J Psychiatry* 1982;139:1189–1199).

chlorpromazine + tricyclic antidepressant (TCA) Co-administration may elevate chlorpromazine plasma levels and tricyclic antidepressant plasma concentration, causing additive anticholinergic effects and excessive sedation.

chlorpromazine + valproate Co-administration may decrease valproate blood level and necessitate quite high doses to obtain therapeutic serum levels (Ishizaki T, Chiba K, Saito M, et al. The effect of neuroleptics [haloperidol and chlorpromazine] on the pharmacokinetics of valproic acid in schizophrenic patients. *J Clin Psychopharmacol* 1984;4:254–261).

chlorpromazine + valproic acid Chlorpromazine may competitively inhibit metabolism of valproic acid, decrease its clearance, and result in valproic acid toxicity.

chlorpromazine + zolpidem Co-administration may increase sedation without altering pharmacokinetics of either drug.

chlorprothixene (Taractan; Tarasan; Truxal) Thioxanthene analog of chlorpromazine (CPZ) that is roughly equipotent to CPZ as a neuroleptic but has a faster onset of action and, like CPZ, is effective in potentiating hypnotic compounds. Antipsychotic efficacy is generally comparable to that of other neuroleptics. It is also useful in manic depressive illness and in depressed patients (Gardos G, Cole JO. A forgotten antipsychotic. *Hosp Comm Psychiatry* 1990;41:1261–1262). Pregnancy risk category C.

chlorprothixene + carbamazepine Co-administration increases carbamazepine concentration in blood plasma and brain, and decreases concentration of the 10,11-epoxide metabolites in these areas.

choice reaction time (CRT) Task that assesses cognitive processes, including alertness, power of concentration, and ability to respond rapidly (Frewer LJ, Hindmarch I. The effects of time of day, age and anxiety on a choice reaction task. *In* Hindmarch I, Aufdembrinke B, Ott H [eds], *Psychopharmacology and Reaction Time*. Chichester: Wiley, 1988). The CRT measures motor, recognition, and total reaction time in choosing and response among various alternatives.

choking incident Acute event associated with ingestion of food or drink in which the patient coughs incessantly, changes color, and cannot speak and cough effectively. It usually terminates by expulsion of solid or liquid food. Choking incidents, frequent in psychiatric patients with dysphagia, have been classified into five groups: bradykinetic, dyskinetic, fast eating syndrome, paralytic, and medical (Bazemore PH, Tonkonogy J, Ananth R. Dysphagia in psychiatric patients: clinical and videofluoroscopic. *Dysphagia* 1991;6:2–5). See **dysphagia.**

cholecystokinin (CCK) 33-amino-acid neuropeptide that co-localizes with dopamine in some mesolimbic dopamine cells. CCK exists in various forms and has a variety of peripheral and central nervous system (CNS) actions. One of the most potent excitants of dopamine cell activity, it appears to affect both presynaptic mesolimbic cell activity and postsynaptic responses to its cotransmitter, dopamine. Like other neuropeptides, it cannot cross the normal blood-brain barrier. It is secreted by the gastrointestinal tract in response to food intake and is thought to contribute to satiety. Bulimic women may have reduced CCK secretion; some may binge on large meals to provoke enough CCK secretion to become satiated. Predominant CNS forms include the octapeptide (CCK-8) and tetrapeptide (CCK-4) forms. Three forms of naturally occurring CCK have been found in the gut with varying amino acid lengths: CCK-8, CCK-33, and CCK-39. CCK receptors are classified into two subtypes, CCK-A, and CCK-B. Controlled studies indicate CCK-4 can cause dose-dependent panic symptoms. Panic disorder patients are more sensitive to the panicogenic properties of CCK-4 than control subjects with no personal or family history of mental illness or panic attacks. Preliminary evidence suggests that CCK-4 may prove to be a useful challenge test for research in the pathophysiology of this illness (Bradwejn J, Koszycki D, Bourin M. Dose ranging study of the effects of cholecystokinin in healthy volunteers. *J Psychiatr Neurosci* 1991;2:91–95).

cholecystokinin-octapeptide (CCK-8) Neuropeptide found in the central nervous system, believed to be the most prevalent form of cholecystokinin in the CNS. CCK-8 and various analogs may modulate central nervous system dopamine neurotransmission and thus have been studied as potential antipsychotic agents. CCK-8 antagonizes mu- or k-opioid receptors and may play a role in the development of heroin tolerance.

cholecystokinin (CCK)/schizophrenia Acute CCK administration improved schizophrenic symptoms in 13 of 15 clinical trials (including three double-blind studies). In a study of effects of chronic administration, 10 of 12 paranoid schizophrenic outpatients resistant to standard neuroleptic treatment improved beginning with the first week of treatment. There were no significant side effects (Nestoros JN. Chronic cholecystokinin administration to paranoid schizophrenic patients. *Neuropsychopharmacology* 1993;9:56S).

cholecystokinin-tetrapeptide (CCK-4) Neuropeptide that binds preferentially to central nervous system (CNS) CCK receptors and has profound anxiogenic effects in humans. When given intravenously, it induces panic attacks and behavior thought to reflect anxiety in panic disorder patients, and panic in 50–80% of healthy volunteers similar to attacks induced with carbon dioxide in panic patients. Panic disorder patients have significantly lower cerebrospinal fluid concentrations of cholecystokinin, which may reflect increased CNS cholecystokinin receptor sensitivity, reduced numbers of receptors, or a compensatory reduction in cholecystokinin octapeptide secondary to theoretically increased central CCK-4 activity (Bradwejn J, Koszycki D, Bourin M. Dose ranging study of the effects of cholecystokinin in healthy volunteers. *J Psychiatr Neurosci* 1991;2:91–95; Bradwejn J, Koszycki D, Shriqui C. Enhanced sensitivity to cholecyctokinen tetrapeptide in panic disorder: clinical and behavioral findings. *Arch Gen Psychiatry* 1991;48:603–610; Bradwejn J, Koszycki D, Annable L, et al. A dose-ranging study of the behavioral and cardiovascular effects of CCK-tetrapeptide in panic disorder. *Biol Psychiatry* 1992;32:903–912).

choline Naturally occurring dietary constituent, the principle source of which is phosphatidylcholine or a less pure preparation called lecithin, a precursor of acetylcholine. The brain cannot synthesize choline. It is found in many foods (e.g., liver, fish, meat, eggs) used by the body to make acetylcholine. After several days, it produces an unpleasant "fishy" body odor and dose-limiting gastrointestinal irritation. It has been used for the treatment of cognitive impairment associated with Alzheimer's disease with no significant benefit and tested with minimal results in tardive dyskinesia.

choline acetyltransferase (ChAT) Enzyme necessary for synthesis of the neurotransmitter acetylcholine; considered one of the best markers for a cholinergic neuron. Activity is severely reduced in discrete areas (e.g., nucleus basalis) of the brain in Alzheimer's disease patients.

choline alfoscerate (Gliatilin) Nootropic drug marketed outside the United States.

cholinergic Relating to nerve fibers, tracts, or pathways in which synaptic transmission is mediated by acetylcholine (e.g., parasympathetic nerve fibers and somatic motoneurons).

cholinergic-adrenergic hypothesis Postulation that mania/depression is a disease of adrenergic dominance, and depression is a disease of cholinergic dominance. It also suggests that depression results from a relative predominance of central cholinergic as compared with aminergic neurotransmission. Consistent with the hypothesis, sleep abnormalities of depression (e.g., short rapid eye movement [REM] latency, increased REM density, and short total sleep time) may result from functional predominance of central cholinergic to aminergic neurotransmission (Janowsky DS, El-Yousseff MK, Davis JM. A cholinergic-aminergic hypothesis of mania and depression. *Lancet* 1972;2:632). Human studies with physostigmine tend to support the hypothesis.

cholinergic crisis Syndrome resulting from acetylcholine accumulation at muscarinic and nicotinic receptors. Signs occur rapidly (minutes to several hours) after intoxication and may lead to death. Muscarinic effects include nausea and vomiting, myosis and headache, sialorrhea, rhinorrhea, bronchoconstriction, bradycardia and other arrhythmias, and urinary and fecal incontinence. Nicotinic effects include muscle twitching and weakness. Central nervous system effects include ataxia, convulsions, and coma.

cholinergic effect Any of the effects due to stimulation of the parasympathetic nervous system, similar to those induced by acetylcholine (e.g., hypersalivation, diarrhea, frequent urination).

cholinergic hypothesis of Alzheimer's disease Premise that Alzheimer's disease is due to disturbance in cholinergic function, based on observations that cholinergic blockade interferes with some normal memory processes and patients with Alzheimer's disease have deficits in cortical acetylcholine (ACh) and several other neurotransmitters that parallel the degree of dementia. It has led to strategies to increase brain ACh activity to treat Alzheimer's disease, including precursor loading, cholinesterase inhibition, and use of direct muscarinic ACh agonists (carbachol and bethanechol).

cholinergic nerve Any of the nerves that release acetylcholine, the neurotransmitter for parasympathetic and sympathetic preganglionic fibers and neuromuscular junction fibers.

cholinergic rapid eye movement induction test (CRIT) Administration of a cholinergic muscarinic receptor agonist (e.g., arecoline) to affective disorder patients and normal control subjects to determine if depression is associated with enhanced induction of rapid eye movement (REM) sleep by muscarinic agonists. Elapsed time from infusion of arecoline during the second non-REM period to the onset of the second REM period is measured. The test has shown that arecoline induces REM sleep in a dose-dependent fashion in patients and control subjects compared with placebo infusions. Results support the hypothesis that patients with affective disorder show a functional supersensitive induction of REM sleep in response to muscarinic receptor agonists and may be consistent with the hypothesis that functional muscarinic "up-regulation" is associated with depression (Gillin JC, Sutton L, Ruiz C, et al. The Cholinergic Rapid Eye Movement Induction Test with arecoline in depression. *Arch Gen Psychiatry* 1991;48:264–270).

cholinergic rebound Relapse and withdrawal symptoms that may occur when a drug with anticholinergic effects is discontinued abruptly.

cholinergic receptor One of two types of receptors, nicotinic and muscarinic, each of which has a selective preference for nicotinic and muscarinic drugs, respectively. See **muscarinic receptor; nicotinic receptor.**

cholinesterase Enzyme (butyrylcholinesterase or pseudocholinesterase) found in blood and various other tissues that breaks down (hydrolyzes) acetylcholine. Acetylcholinesterase or true cholinesterase plays an important role in transmission of nervous impulses by preventing build-up of acetylcholine at nerve endings.

cholinesterase inhibitor Drug (e.g., tacrine, physostigmine) that exerts modest but clinically significant cognitive effects in patients with Alzheimer's disease (Schneider LS, Olin JT, Pawluczyk S. A double-blind crossover pilot study of l-deprenyl [selegiline] combined with cholinesterase inhibitor in Alzheimer's disease. *Am J Psychiatry* 1993;150:321–323).

cholinoceptor See **cholinergic receptor.**

cholinomimetic Substance that stimulates postsynaptic muscarinic receptors and has an action similar to that of acetylcholine. The term has been proposed as a replacement for *parasympathomimetic*, which is less accurate.

chorea Continuous, randomly distributed, irregularly timed involuntary muscle jerks. Limbs, trunk, and facial features are continually disturbed by brief unpredictable movements. Walking is interrupted by lurches, stops, and starts (dancing gait). Fine manipulations with the hands, speech, and respiration are similarly disturbed. Typical chorea is unmistakable, but in some patients it resembles myoclonus and torsion dystonia.

chorea, chronic progressive See **Huntington's disease.**

choreiform movement Irrepressible, involuntary, nonrepetitive, jerky, and abrupt movement of roughly normal pattern resembling an incomplete gesture. If mild, the person may just seem clumsy and fidgety. If severe, there is almost continuous writhing movement. Movements may occur in limbs or facial muscles. In several diseases such as Huntington's chorea, movements are very characteristic; most are not associated with mental handicap. Chorea may occur, however, where any form of brain damage affects the basal ganglia of the brain (viral encephalitis, cerebral palsy, Wilson's disease, problems at birth). In these cases it is frequently associated with mental handicap.

choreoathetosis Coexistence of chorea and athetosis.

"Chris" Street name for a central nervous system stimulant.

"Christine" Street name for a central nervous system stimulant.

"Christmas tree" Street name for (a) amobarbital plus secobarbital; (b) dextroamphetamine; (c) a combination of weak and potent varieties of marijuana.

chromatic In genetics, relating to the protoplasmic cell substance called "chromatin" that stains the nuclear network and is the genetic material of the nucleus.

chromatid Two sister strands making up a chromosome and held together by the centromere. Upon centromere division, each will become a separate chromosome.

chromatin Composite material (DNA, RNA, and protein) of a chromosome.

chromatography Method of separating compounds based on their differential adherence to particles of an absorbing substance.

chromomere Minute nodules in the chromosomes of a cell nucleus forming a chain of chromatic bodies in the early stages of mitosis that are strung like beads on a fine thread. Many chromomeric nodules are thought to be too small to be visible.

chromosomal aberration Abnormality of chromosome number or structure detectable by standard cytogenetic techniques (Gardner RJM, Southerland GR. *Chromosome Abnormalities and Genetic Counseling.* New York: Oxford University Press, 1989). Abnormalities associated with various genetic disorders are valuable for localizing and isolating causative genes. They also have provided important clues to the genetic cause of behavioral disorders (Bassett AS. Chromosomal aberrations in schizophrenia. Autosomes. *Br J Psychiatry* 1992; 161:323–334).

chromosomal disorder Genetic disease in which there is a demonstrable abnormality in the individual's chromosome complement.

chromosome Carrier of genetic information consisting of long strands of DNA in a protein framework that are constant in number in each species. The normal number in humans is 46 (22 pairs of autosomes and 2 sex chromosomes, XX or XY). Chromosomes are unimaginably long, tightly coiled strands of DNA protein (deoxyribonucleic acid); genes are segments of the DNA strand that instruct individual cells to manufacture specific chemicals (e.g., genes in bone cell nuclei instruct the cell to synthesize bone proteins). Chromosomes are visible in a dividing cell as deeply staining rod-shaped or J-shaped structures.

chromosome banding Various intrachromosomal regions of varying intensities brought out by differential staining.

chromosome mapping Determining the position and order of gene loci on a chromosome, especially by analyzing the frequency of recombination between the loci.

chromosome translocation Rare occurrence in which part or nearly all of one chromosome joins or becomes part of another. All genetic material is still present in the cell, but arranged abnormally; the person (translocation carrier) is healthy and normal. This is called "balanced translocation." When the cells divide to make eggs or sperm, however, there cannot be equal division of the translocated pair of chromosomes: one cell may get most or all of the genetic material of the pair, while the other gets little or none. Translocation carriers are at high risk for having a child with abnormal chromosomes. The child has an unbalanced translocation or deletion of chromosome. Sometimes an unbalanced translocation arises as a fresh mutation, a kind of genetic accident, in which both parents have completely normal chromosomes. Translocation causes the extra chromosomal material in 3% of people with Down syndrome.

chromosome walking Narrowing the genetic distance between loci using relevant DNA markers in chromosomal areas.

chronergy Rhythmic changes in any effects of a drug, including its therapeutic and toxic effects. It depends on the chronesthesy of the target biosystem and the chronopharmacokinetics of the drug (Reinberg A, Smolensky MH. Circadian changes of drug disposition in man. *Clin Pharmacokinet* 1982;7:401–420)

chronesthesy Rhythmic changes in the susceptibility of a target biosystem to a drug. The biosystem includes molecular and membrane phenomena (e.g., receptors) and related metabolic functions. Chronesthesy involves all levels of biological organization (e.g., cells, organ-systems) including bacteria, parasites, and tumors (Tolstoi LG. A review of chronobiology and chronopharmacology. *Pharmacy Times* 1992;58:118–126).

chronic Referring to duration of an illness or therapy. The U.S. National Center for Health Statistics designates a condition as "chronic" if it exists for 3 or more months.

chronic akathisia See **akathisia, chronic.**

chronic alcoholism See **alcoholism, chronic.**

chronic brain syndrome (CBS) Irreversible diffuse disturbance of brain tissue resulting in some permanent alteration in brain function. It usually evolves slowly and as imperceptibly as the unfolding of a flower. Over time it may be manifested by dementia, delirium, stupor, or coma.

chronic Epstein-Barr virus (CEBV) See **chronic fatigue syndrome.**

chronic fatigue immune deficiency syndrome (CFIDS) See **chronic fatigue syndrome.**

chronic fatigue syndrome (CFS) Formally defined by the Centers for Disease Control (1988) as a symptom complex of extreme fatigue in combination with numerous signs of impaired immune state (e.g., fever and lymphadenopathy). Onset is after an acute, apparently viral infection. It is characterized by generalized, chronic, persistent, or relapsing fatigue, present for more than 6 months, that causes major disruption of usual daily activities. Other criteria include major symptoms (concentration/memory impairment, lymphadenopathy), or one major and three minor symptoms (myalgia, arthralgia, depression, tinnitus). About one-third of patients complain of palpitations or unsteadiness, or both. Physical signs, however, are inconsistent or absent, and routine laboratory tests yield normal results. Any psychological disturbance is likely to be a consequence, rather than an antecedent risk factor of, the syndrome. Fluoxetine (20 mg/day) improves immunologic NK cytotoxicity and cytotoxic T cell number and activation independent of fluoxetine's antidepressant effect (David A, Wessely S, Pelosi A. Chronic fatigue syndrome (ME)—signs of a new approach. *Br J Hosp Med* 1991; 45:158–163; Lloyd A, Gandevia S, Hales J. Muscle performance, voluntary activation, twitch properties and perceived effort in normal subjects and patients with chronic fatigue syndrome. *Brain* 1991;114:85–98). Also called "chronic fatigue immune deficiency syndrome (CFIDS)"; "chronic Epstein-Barr virus (CEBV)"; "myalgic encephalomyelitis"; "Royal Free disease"; "postviral fatigue syndrome." See **chronic fatigue syndrome/Centers for Disease Control case criteria.**

chronic fatigue syndrome/Centers for Disease Control case criteria Major criteria are (a) new onset of persistent or relapsing, debilitat-

ing fatigue or easy fatigability that does not resolve with bedrest and is severe enough to impair average daily activity below 50% of premorbid activity level, lasting for a period of at least 6 months; or (b) exclusion of other clinical conditions or medication effects by appropriate history, physical examination, or laboratory tests. In addition, six or more of the following must have begun at or after onset of fatigue and must be persistent or recurring: (a) mild fever or chills; (b) sore throat; (c) painful anterior or posterior cervical or axillary lymph nodes; (d) generalized muscle weakness; (e) myalgia; (f) prolonged postexertional fatigue; (g) headaches; (h) migratory arthralgia; (i) neuropsychological complaints (including photophobia, transient scotomata, forgetfulness, irritability, confusion, depression, poor concentration); (j) sleep disturbance; and (k) abrupt onset of main symptom complex. Alternatively, there must be eight or more of the symptom criteria or two or more of the following physical criteria, which must be documented on at least two occasions, at least one month apart: (a) low-grade fever (oral temperature of 37.6–38.6° C or rectal temperature of 37.8–38.8° C); (b) nonexudative pharyngitis; and (c) palpable anterior or posterior cervical or axillary lymph nodes (Holmes GP, Kaplan JE, Gantz NM, et al. Chronic fatigue syndrome: a working case definition. *Ann Intern Med* 1988;108: 387–389).

chronic pain, psychiatric aspects Depression is frequently associated with chronic pain; 30–40% of patients attending chronic pain clinics fulfill operational criteria for depression. A significant proportion have biological symptoms of depression with failure of dexamethasone to suppress cortisol secretion and reduced binding affinity of $[^3H]$-imipramine binding to platelet membranes. Antidepressants are often effective in these patients (Tyrer S. Psychiatric assessment of chronic pain. *Br J Psychiatry* 1992;160:733–741).

chronic primary major depression Unresolved major depressive episode of late onset with no evidence of pre-existing chronic minor disorder. It may be unipolar or bipolar.

chronic progressive chorea See **Huntington's disease.**

chronic secondary major depression Unremitting major depression arising secondary to physical ill health or nonaffective psychiatric disorder.

chronobiology Study of the effects of rhythms or other periods on biological processes and their responses to interventions.

chronobiotic Drug that alters biological rhythms.

chronopharmacology Study of influences of biological rhythms on the pharmacokinetics, effectiveness, and toxicology of different drugs (Marks V, English J, Aherne W, et al. Chronopharmacology. *Clin Biochem* 1985;18:154–157). There are two major subdisciplines, chronopharmacokinetics and chronopharmacodynamics.

chronopharmacodynamics Time-dependent or rhythmic changes in the therapeutic and toxic effects of a drug. Atenolol, cimetidine, diazepam, morphine, nifedipine, and prednisone are drugs with documented daily changes in their pharmacodynamics (Lemmer B, Lagreque G. Chronopharmacology and chronotherapeutics: definitions and concepts. *Chronobiol Int* 1987;4:319–329).

chronopharmacokinetics Time-dependent or rhythmic changes in a drug's absorption, distribution, metabolism, and/or excretion. Circadian rhythms in physiological functions such as blood volume, serum proteins, and liver and kidney function may alter drug pharmacokinetics so that they are not constant throughout a 24-hour period. Diazepam, nortriptyline, and propranolol are drugs with documented daily changes in their pharmacokinetics (Lemmer B, Labrecque G. Chronopharmacology and chronotherapeutics: definitions and concepts. *Chronobiol Int* 1987;4:319–329).

chronotherapy Treatment of delayed sleep phase syndrome consisting of a phase delay of approximately 3 hours on each consecutive day. This schedule must be rigorously maintained; if the subject is allowed a late night, original complaints recur.

Ciatyl See **zuclopenthixol.**

"Ciba" Street name for glutethimide.

cimetidine (Tagamet) Histamine H_2 receptor antagonist frequently used to decrease gastric acid production and treat ulcers. It may cause depression. By binding to the cytochrome P450 oxidizing system in hepatic microsomes, as well as by reducing hepatic blood flow, it reduces metabolism of certain drugs (e.g., diazepam, warfarin, chlorpromazine, clozapine).

cimetidine + adinazolam See **adinazolam + cimetidine.**

cimetidine + alprazolam See **alprazolam + cimetidine.**

cimetidine + amoxapine See **amoxapine + cimetidine.**

cimetidine + benzodiazepine See **benzodiazepine + cimetidine.**

cimetidine + bupropion See **bupropion + cimetidine.**

cimetidine + carbamazepine See **carbamazepine + cimetidine.**

cimetidine + chlordiazepoxide See **chlordiazepoxide + cimetidine.**

cimetidine + chlorpromazine See **chlorpromazine + cimetidine.**

cimetidine + clomipramine See **clomipramine + cimetidine.**

cimetidine + clorazepate See **clorazepate + cimetidine.**

cimetidine + clozapine See **clozapine + cimetidine.**

cimetidine + desipramine See **desipramine + cimetidine.**

cimetidine + diazepam See **diazepam + cimetidine.**

cimetidine + doxepin See **doxepin + cimetidine.**

cimetidine + flurazepam See **flurazepam + cimetidine.**

cimetidine + imipramine See **imipramine + cimetidine.**

cimetidine + meperidine See **meperidine + cimetidine.**

cimetidine + methadone See **methadone + cimetidine.**

cimetidine + moclobemide See **moclobemide + cimetidine.**

cimetidine + morphine See **morphine + cimetidine.**

cimetidine + neuroleptic See **neuroleptic + cimetidine.**

cimetidine + paroxetine See **paroxetine + cimetidine.**

cimetidine + phenytoin See **phenytoin + cimetidine.**

cimetidine + propranolol See **propranolol + cimetidine.**

cimetidine + sertraline See **sertraline + cimetidine.**

cimetidine + tacrine See **tacrine + cimetidine.**

cimetidine + triazolam See **triazolam + cimetidine.**

cimetidine + warfarin See **warfarin + cimetidine.**

cimetidine + zolpidem See **zolpidem + cimetidine.**

cimoxatone Selective, reversible inhibitor of monoamine oxidase (MAO)-A that has been shown to be a clinically effective antidepressant. Like other reversible selective MAO-A inhibitors, it appears to cause less potentiation of the pressor response to tyramine than irreversible MAO inhibitors (Kapfhammer HP, Hoff P, Golling H, Schmauss M. Cimoxatone and moclobemide, two new MAO-inhibitors, in the treatment of major depressive disorder. *Pharmacopsychiatry* 1986;19:247–248).

cingulate gyrus Crescent-shaped convolution of the medial surface of the cerebral hemisphere, lying immediately above the corpus callosum. It is part of "Papez's circle."

cingulotomy Form of psychosurgery in which the cingulate gyrus is removed to treat otherwise intractable depression or obsessive-compulsive disorder. It is occasionally used for the treatment of other psychiatric disorders (Jenike M, Baer L, Ballatine HT, et al. Cingulotomy for refractory obsessive-compulsive disorder: a long-term follow-up of 33 patients. *Arch Gen Psychiatry* 1991;48:548-555). See **lobotomy; tractotomy, stereotactic.**

cingulum Bilateral bundle of white nerve fibers that connect the frontal cortex, thalamic nuclei, and hippocampal formation. It is at the crossroads of the limbic system.

cinolazepam Benzodiazepine (BZD) with higher affinity for BZD receptors in the cerebellum than for those in the hippocampus and other brain tissues.

Cipramil See **citalopram.**

circadian dyschrony When the human biological clock is not synchronous with the 24-hour day. A common cause is modern technology that requires constantly shifting light-dark cycles, disrupting the sleep-wake cycle. It also can occur if the circadian system malfunctions because of certain sleep disorders, manic-depressive illness, and endocrine disorders. In the elderly, pathophysiological changes in the retina may reduce sensitivity to light and cause circadian dyschrony.

circadian phase sleep disorder There are two types: phase advance or advanced sleep phase syndrome, and phase delay or delayed sleep phase syndrome. In the former, individuals have difficulty staying up past 9 pm and awaken early in the morning. In the latter, individuals have difficulty falling asleep before 1 or 2 am. Either can be treated with appropriately timed bright light exposure. Phase advance patients should be exposed to 1–2 hours of 2500-lux light 1 hour before bedtime. Phase delay patients should be exposed to bright light as soon as they awaken in the morning. Both treatments produce corrective phase change. Oral melatonin (0.5 mg) also corrects circadian phase shifts in humans. The phase response curve is nearly opposite to that for light. Phase advance patients should be given melatonin when they awaken in the morning, or about 14 hours before onset of their (endogenous) melatonin production in the evening. Phase delay patients should be given melatonin in the afternoon, about 6 hours before onset of their endogenous melatonin production (Lewy AJ, Sack RL. Chronobiologic treatments of circadian phase disorders. Presented at the 1992 Annual Meeting of the American College of Neuropsychopharmacology, San Juan, Puerto Rico).

circadian rhythm Biological rhythm with a period of around 24 hours. They are generated by an internal clock or pacemaker in the brain that is synchronized to daily environmental time cues, most importantly the light-dark cycle. Functions that vary with circadian rhythm include body temperature, sleep and wakefulness, release of many hormones, alertness, and memory. Circadian rhythms may be classified according to whether they arise outside the organism (representing passive response to rhythmic environmental change) or within the organism (endogenous rhythms). Disturbances of circadian rhythm in depressed patients are likely to be manifested in phase variability rather than in phase advance. With respect to sleep, circadian rhythm refers to sleep/wake cycles.

circannual rhythm Near 365-day rhythm synchronized with annual rhythms in the external world.

circasemidian rhythm Biological rhythm with a period of about half a day.

circumscribed cortical atrophy See **Pick's disease.**

circumstantial-situational drug use World Health Organization classification of drug use defined as a task-specific, self-limited use that is variably patterned and differing in frequency, intensity, and duration. Drug use is motivated by the perceived need to achieve a known and anticipated drug effect to cope with a specific condition or situation.

circumstantiality Style of speaking or writing characterized by multiple, often peripheral, details and excessive clarifications, qualifications, and circumlocutions. See **viscosity, interpersonal.**

circumventricular organ (CVO) One of about a half dozen tiny areas of brain surrounding the ventricles. Most notable is the chorioid plexus, which lines the lateral ventricle, the roof of the third ventricle, and the fourth ventricle. Other CVOs include the posterior pituitary at the floor of the third ventricle, the pineal gland at the dorsal area of the third ventricle, and the subcommissural organ at the dorsal aspect of the third ventricle. Three CVOs are particularly involved in neuroendocrine regulation. The presence of CVOs in brain allows for rapid uptake at the nerve ending of neuroendocrine substances from the circulation.

cirrhosis Chronic liver disease marked by scarring of liver tissue and eventually liver failure, frequently due to chronic alcoholism.

cisapride (Alimix; Prepulsid) Primary serotonin (5-HT)$_2$ antagonist that distinguishes between 5-HT$_2$ and 5-HT$_{1C}$ receptors. Chemical structure is similar to that of metoclopramide. Lacking central dopamine receptor blocking effects, it does not cause hyperprolactinemia, dyskinesia, or other extrapyramidal symptoms occasionally seen with metoclopramide.

cis-doxepin One of the geometric isomers of the tricyclic antidepressant doxepin.

cis-N-desmethyldoxepin Metabolite of cis-doxepin.

Cisordinal See **zuclopenthixol.**

Cisordinal Acutard See **zuclopenthixol.**

cis (Z)-clopenthixol (Clopixol) See **zuclopenthixol.**

cis (Z)-flupenthixol decanoate See **flupenthixol decanoate.**

citalopram (Cipramil; Seropram) Serotonin uptake inhibitor with antidepressant efficacy. It blocks uptake of serotonin into serotonergic neurons, with little effect on noradrenaline or dopamine uptake. Pharmacokinetics are characterized by high bioavailability after oral administration and plasma half-life of 30–40 hours. It has no anticholinergic, antihistaminic, or alpha-adrenergic properties. It is considered both a mood stabilizer and an emotional stabilizer. It reduces overactivity in the hypothalamic-pituitary-adrenal axis, improves emotional disturbances in demented patients, and affects emotional bluntness, irritability, anxiety, fear-panic, and restlessness. Most commonly reported side effects include nausea, headache, and sweating. Preliminary trials suggest that citalopram may be a possible treatment for alcoholism. Studies with nondependent alcohol abusers show that it decreases number of drinking days and total amount of alcoholic drinking (Naranjo CA, Sellers EM, Sullivan JT, et al. The serotonin uptake inhibitor citalopram attenuates ethanol intake. *Clin Pharmacol Ther* 1987;41:266–274). In male nondepressed problem drinkers, 40 mg/day, but not 20 mg/day, significantly reduced the number of drinks consumed and increased the number of abstinent days. In a randomized, double-blind, crossover study in 16 healthy subjects (ages 26–29) who were heavy drinkers, citalopram (40 mg/day) for 7 days significantly decreased drinking (average, 17.5%) and increased the percentage of days abstinent. Citalopram decreased interest in, desire for, craving for, and liking of alcohol, but had no significant effects on the subjective feelings of intoxication (Naranjo, CA, Poulos CX, Bremmer KE, Lanctot KL. Citalopram decreases desirability, liking, and consumption of alcohol in alcohol-dependent drinkers. *Clin Pharmacol Ther* 1992; 51:729–739).

citalopram + alcohol In one study, no interactions were detected in healthy volunteers (Lader M, Melhuish A, Frecka G, et al. The effects of citalopram in single and repeated doses and with alcohol on physiological and psychological measures in healthy subjects. *Eur J Clin Pharmacol* 1986;31:183–190). Citalopram may decrease alcohol consumption (Naranjo CA, Poulos CX, Bremmer KE, Lanctot KL. Citalopram decreases desirability, liking, and consumption of alcohol in alcohol-dependent drinkers. *Clin Pharmacol Ther* 1992; 51:729–739).

citalopram + amitriptyline Addition of citalopram to previously initiated amitriptyline therapy has no influence on plasma amitriptyline and nortriptyline (Baumann P. Clinical pharmacokinetics of citalopram and other selective serotonergic reuptake inhibitors [SSRI]. *Int Clin Psychopharmacol* 1992;6[suppl 5]:13–20; Baettig D, Bondolfi G, Montaldi S, et al. Tricyclic antidepressant plasma levels after augmentation with citalopram. *Eur J Clin Pharmacol* 1993;44:403–405).

citalopram + clomipramine No pharmacokinetic interaction has been reported (Baumann P. Clinical pharmacokinetics of citalopram and other selective serotonergic reuptake inhibitors [SSRI]. Int Clin Psychopharmacol 1992;6[suppl 5]:13–20; Baettig D, Bondolfi G, Montaldi S, et al. Tricyclic antidepressant plasma levels after augmentation with citalopram. A case study. *Eur J Clin Pharmacol* 1993;44:403–405).

citalopram + lithium Addition of lithium may improve affective illness in citalopram nonresponders.

citalopram + maprotiline Co-administration apparently produces no pharmacokinetic interactions or adverse effects (Baettig D, Bondolfi G, Montaldi S, et al. Tricyclic antidepressant plasma levels after augmentation with citalopram. A case study. *Eur J Clin Pharmacol* 1993; 44:403–405).

citalopram + moclobemide Three cases of fatal serotonin syndrome were reported in patients who took overdoses of moclobemide and citalopram. Death occurred rapidly (3–16 hours) (Neuvonen PJ, Pohjola-Sintonen S, Tacke U, Vuori E. Five fatal cases of serotonin syndrome after moclobemide-citalopram or moclobemide-clomipramine overdoses. *Lancet* 1993; 342:1419).

citalopram/obsessive-compulsive disorder Initiation of treatment for obsessive-compulsive disorder may transiently increase obsessions (Bejerot S, Humble M. Citalopram treatment of obsessive-compulsive disorder: a pilot study of antiobsessive efficacy. *Biol Psychiatry* 1991; 29:443S).

citalopram/Parkinson's disease In contrast to fluoxetine, citalopram did not aggravate parkinsonism or tardive dyskinesia in 13 psychotic inpatients (Korsgaard S, Noring V Poolsen UJ,

Gerblack J. Effects of citalopram, a specific serotonin uptake inhibitor, in tardive dyskinesia and parkinsonism. *Clin Neuropharm* 1986;9: 52–57).

citrated calcium carbimide Substance that inhibits breakdown of acetaldehyde. It is used as an alternative to disulfiram in the treatment of alcoholism. Duration of action is shorter than that of disulfiram, but the alcohol-induced acetaldehyde syndrome usually is less intense. Available in Canada, but not in the United States.

clanging Speech in which sounds, rather than meaningful, conceptual relationships, govern word choice; it may include rhyming and punning (DSM-IV). The term is generally applied only when it is a manifestation of a pathological condition; it is not used to describe the rhyming word play of children. Clanging is observed most commonly in schizophrenia and manic episodes.

class limit Subdivision of a numerical characteristic when it is displayed in a frequency table or graph.

classic conditioning Complex learning task involving association of a conditioned and unconditioned stimulus. The conditioned stimulus always precedes the unconditioned stimulus, with only a brief interval between them.

classification Grouping together into separate classes or names (e.g., mental disorders, substance abuse disorders).

classification of mental disorders System of scientifically organizing mental disorders according to different criteria (e.g., behavioral symptoms) to yield uniform diagnoses.

clearance (Cl) Apparent volume of blood from which a drug is removed in a given unit of time. It also is conceptualized as the rate of elimination of a drug at a given concentration of that drug. It is the most important pharmacokinetic variable, ultimately determining maintenance dose and steady-state plasma level. Total body clearance determines steady-state drug concentration, regardless of volume of distribution or half-life. Clearance also is crucial in determining treatment of accidental or deliberate overdose. Clearance often encompasses both metabolism and hepatic or renal elimination. Water-soluble, non–protein-bound drugs are eliminated primarily by renal filtration. By glucuronidation, the liver makes drugs more water-soluble for easy removal from the circulation by the kidney. Compromised kidney or liver function, concomitant drugs, diet, age, and various disease states affect the body's ability to clear a drug. Because drug clearance is usually slower in the elderly, dosage changes should be made at less-frequent intervals to allow maximal steady-state accumulation.

clearance, intrinsic Clearance of a drug from an organ or organ system under conditions of unrestricted blood flow.

clenbuterol Sympathomimetic agonist with anabolic properties in animals. It achieved notoriety at the 1992 Olympics when its use by some athletes was disclosed even though no reputable scientific studies had been published showing muscle-enhancing effects in humans. Large doses may cause cardiac arrhythmias, tremor, and serious hypokalemia (Perry HM, Littlepage BNC. Misusing anabolic drugs. *Br Med J* 1992;305:1241–1242).

"clinging" See **viscosity, interpersonal.**

clinical algorithm Description of steps to be taken in patient care in specified circumstances, including observations to be made, decisions to be considered, and actions to be taken. Algorithms describe and organize the multiple factors and considerations that characterize medical diagnosis and treatment. The basic goal of clinical algorithms is to identify how these factors and considerations should be used to divide patients into subcategories that are best treated differently (i.e., those who will or will not be likely to derive significant benefit from a particular procedure or management strategy). Algorithms have been shown to result in faster learning, higher retention, and better compliance with established practice standards than prose text because they help organize thought in a visible way. Algorithms have also been used successfully for retrospective quality review (Hadorn DC, McCormick K, Diokono A. An annotated algorithm approach to clinical guideline development. *JAMA* 1992;267:3311–3314).

clinical equipoise Willingness of a community of physicians to have their patients pursue any of the treatments being tested in a randomized trial, since none of them have been clearly established as preferable.

clinical investigator See **investigator, clinical.**

clinical pharmacology Study of the effects of drugs in humans.

clinical pharmacokinetics Study of the uptake, distribution, binding, elimination, and biotransformation of drugs in humans. One aim is detection of patient subpopulations at risk of showing abnormally high or abnormally low blood concentrations when given normal doses of a drug. Genetic factors, age, and use of other drugs (e.g., phenothiazines, tobacco, alcohol) are responsible for the large interindividual variability in steady-state concentrations of many drugs, including tricyclic antidepressants.

clinical psychologist See **psychologist, clinical.**

clinical significance Relevance of a particular observation in a clinical study.

clinical test Test used in diagnosis. Included are physiological tests (e.g., blood or urine analysis), electrophysiological tests (e.g., electroencephalogram, electrocardiogram), and questionnaires (e.g., Minnesota Multiphasic Personality Inventory).

clinical trial Research activity that involves administration of a drug or other treatment regimen to patients to evaluate indications, safety, and efficacy. Meaning of the term varies widely, ranging from first use with no control treatment to a rigorously designed and executed study involving objective tests, controlled treatments, and randomization.

clinical trial, premarketing Clinical trial designed to determine such factors as indications, efficacy, and safety of a new drug. There are three phases. See **phase 1 trial; phase 2 trial; phase 3 trial.**

clinometrics Evaluation of indices (arbitrary ratings) used to evaluate, describe, or measure symptoms, physical signs, and other distinctly clinical phenomena in medicine. Clinometric indices transform qualitative "soft" data into nominal or quantitative scales used as summary measures for clinical and research activities. A well known example is the Apgar score for quantifying the condition of a newborn (Feinstein AR. *Clinometrics.* New Haven: Yale University Press, 1987).

Clinoril See **sulindac.**

Clinovir See **medroxyprogesterone.**

Clipoxide See **chlordiazepoxide.**

clobazam (Frisium; Urbanyl) (CLB) Benzodiazepine (BZD) with potent anticonvulsant activity in a variety of seizure disorders including myoclonic and complex partial seizures. Its structure (1,5-benzodiazepine) differs slightly from those of clonazepam and diazepam (1,4-benzodiazepine); biotransformation is by the oxidative reaction of N-demethylation. It is used in epilepsy, usually in addition to other anticonvulsants when seizures are difficult to control. It is introduced gradually to prevent sedation and withdrawn gradually to prevent withdrawal seizures. CLB has been shown to be effective for partial status epilepticus. It may be a useful adjuvant to other agents because of its safety profile and the fact that it can be given orally and therefore in an outpatient setting (Benavente O, Guberman A, Hogan MJ. The use of oral clobazam for partial status epilepticus. *Neurology* 1993; 43[suppl]A198). It causes less sedation and has less effect on psychomotor performance than other BZDs. Tolerance to its anticonvulsant effect develops with oral administration. As with clonazepam, only a few patients achieve worthwhile improvement in seizure control with long-term dosing. Intermittent use may reduce the likelihood of tolerance. Commonly reported side effects include depression, irritability, and tiredness (Brodie MJ. Established anticonvulsants and treatment of refractory epilepsy. *Lancet* 1990;336:350–354). CLB has been found as effective as alprazolam for panic disorder and generalized anxiety. When used for anxiety, clinical and side effects are very similar to diazepam's.

clobazam + alcohol Acute alcohol ingestion, even in chronic alcohol users, reduces elimination and increases plasma level of clobazam (Taeber K, Badian M, Brettel HF, et al. Kinetic and dynamic interaction of clobazam and alcohol. *Br J Clin Pharmacol* 1979;7:91S–97S).

clobazam + carbamazepine Addition of clobazam (CLB) to carbamazepine (CBZ) increases CBZ metabolism approximately 1.5 times, probably by inducing its epoxidation. CBZ induces CLB metabolism, decreasing its plasma level and interfering in its therapeutic efficacy (Levy RH, Lane EA, Guyot M, Brachet-Liermain A, Cenraud B, Loiseau P. Analysis of parent drug-metabolite relationship in the presence of an inducer: application to the carbamazepine-clobazam interaction in normal man. *Drug Metab Dispos* 1983;11:286–292). CLB has been reported to have no significant effect on the blood level/dose ratio (LDR) of CBZ. However, CBZ significantly decreases the LDR of the metabolite of CLB, N-desmethyl-clobazam (NCLB), thereby increasing the NCLB/CLB ratio (Sennome S, Mesdjian E. Interactions between clobazam and standard antiepileptic drugs in patients with epilepsy. *Ther Drug Monit* 1992;14:269–274).

clobazam + oxiracetam Clobazam influences the half-life of oxiracetam, necessitating its more frequent administration. No adverse interactions have been reported.

clobazam + phenobarbital Clobazam (CLB) has been reported to have no significant effect on the blood level/dose ratio (LDR) of phenobarbital (PB). However, PB significantly decreased LDR of the CLB metabolite N-desmethyl-clobazam (NCLB), thereby increasing the NCLB/CLB ratio (Sennome S, Mesduian E. Interactions between clobazam and standard antiepileptic drugs in patients with epilepsy. *Ther Drug Monit* 1992;14:269–274).

clobazam + phenytoin Clobazam (CLB) has been reported to have no significant effect on the blood level/dose ratio (LDR) of phenytoin (PHT). However, PHT significantly decreased LDR of the CLB metabolite N-desmethyl-clobazam (NCLB), thereby increasing the NCLB/CLB ratio (Sennome S, Mesdjian E. Interactions between clobazam and standard antiepileptic drugs in patients with epilepsy. *Ther Drug Monit* 1992;14:269–274).

clobazam + valproic acid   Clobazam (CLB) has been reported to have no significant effect on the blood level/dose ratio (LDR) of valproic acid (VPA). However, VPA significantly decreased LDR of the CLB metabolite N-desmethylclobazam (NCLB), thereby increasing the NCLB/CLB ratio (Sennome S, Mesdjian E. Interactions between clobazam and standard antiepileptic drugs in patients with epilepsy. *Ther Drug Monit* 1992;14:269–274).

clock, biological   See **biological clock.**

clockwise shift   Work shift that progresses from midnight to day to swing.

clofibrate   Selective inducer of microsomal enzymes and beta-oxidation mitochondrial metabolism.

clofibrate + valproate   Co-administration increases valproate clearance (Heinemeyer G, Nau H, Hildebrandt AG, Roots I. Oxidation and glucoronidation of valproic acid in male rats—influence of phenobarbital, 3-methylcholanthrene, beta-naphthofarone and clofibrate. *Biochem Pharmacol* 1985;34:133–139).

clometacin + lithium   See **lithium + clometacin.**

clomipramine   (Anafranil; Maronil) (CMI) Tertiary tricyclic antidepressant (TCA) similar in structure to imipramine (IMI) with chlorine in the 3 position. The chlorine atom conveys properties that significantly inhibit serotonin reuptake and that are present in varying degrees in other TCAs. Compared to IMI, CMI is much more potent with respect to serotonin reuptake inhibition. It is not entirely selective, however, because its metabolite, desmethylclompramine, powerfully inhibits norepinephrine reuptake. CMI is as effective as IMI in the treatment of depression and clearly superior in the treatment of obsessive-compulsive disorder (Zohar J, Insel TR. Drug treatment of obsessive-compulsive disorder. *J Affective Disord* 1987;13:193–202; Clomipramine Collaborative Study Group. Clomipramine in the treatment of patients with obsessive-compulsive disorder. *Arch Gen Psychiatry* 1991;48:730–738). Comparative trials in panic disorder patients have shown that low doses of CMI are significantly more effective than diazepam, and that low and high doses of CMI and alprazolam are effective and comparable. Some clinical evidence suggests that CMI may be effective in the treatment of pathological gambling. Therapeutic blood levels have not been established, but a reasonable maximum dose, if tolerated, is 250 mg/day. CMI's side effect profile is much like those of other TCAs. Withdrawal symptoms have been reported following abrupt discontinuation, including dizziness, nausea, vomiting, headache, malaise,

sleep disturbance, hypothermia, and irritability. Some patients also may experience a worsening of psychiatric status. In men, CMI may cause a dose-related delay or inhibition of ejaculation due to alpha-adrenergic blockade. High doses may also cause erectile impotence. Anorgasmia has been reported in women. Dosage adjustment can alleviate these sexual side effects in most instances. Also called "chlorimipramine." Pregnancy risk category C.

clomipramine/agranulocytosis   Clomipramine-induced hematologic side effects (pancytopenia and agranulocytosis) have been reported (Magni G, Urbani A, Silverstro A, Grassetto M. Clomipramine induced pancytopenia. *J Nerv Ment Dis* 1975;5:309–310; Sounami RL, Ashton CR, Lee-Potter JP. Agranulocytosis and systemic candidiasis following clomipramine therapy. *Postgrad Med J* 1976;52:472–474). A case of agranulocytosis associated with clomipramine was successfully treated with granulocyte-colony stimulating factor (G-CSF) (Hunt KA, Resnick MP. Clomipramine-induced agranulocytosis and its treatment with G-CSF. *Am J Psychiatry* 1993;150:522–523).

clomipramine + alcohol   In recently abstinent alcoholic patients, clomipramine demethylation may be inhibited, even for several weeks or months after alcohol withdrawal (Balant-Gorgia AE, Gay M, Gex-Fabry M, et al. Persistent impairment of clomipramine demethylation in recently detoxified alcoholic patients. *Ther Drug Monit* 1992;14:119–124).

clomipramine + alpidem   Co-administration had a slightly superior effect on depression and anxiety compared to clomipramine + bromazepam and was well tolerated (Cottraux J, Riant N. Alpidem versus bromazepam in depressed outpatients treated with clomipramine. A controlled comparison. *Clin Neuropharmacol* 1992;15[suppl 1/B]:521B).

clomipramine + alprazolam   Study of co-administration kinetics in 45 healthy male volunteers indicates no significant changes (Carson SW, Wright CE, Millikin SP, et al. Pharmacokinetic evaluation of the combined administration of alprazolam [ALP] and clomipramine (CMI). *Clin Pharmacol Ther* 1992;51:154).

clomipramine + anticholinergic   Co-administration increases risk of adverse anticholinergic effects. Careful dosage adjustment of clomipramine and/or the anticholinergic may be necessary to avoid toxicity.

clomipramine + barbiturate   Co-administration increases clomipramine (CMI) metabolism, resulting in lower levels of CMI and its active metabolite, desmethylchlorimipramine, and possibly interfering with CMI's therapeutic effects (Peters MD, Davis SK, Austin LS. Clomipramine: an antiobsessional tricyclic antide-pressant. *Clin Pharm* 1990;9:165–178).

clomipramine + bentazepam In a multicenter, open study in patients with major depression, clomipramine (CMI) + bentazepam (BZP) was better than CMI alone in reducing anxi-ety, with equal or better tolerability (Calcedo Ordonez A, Arosamene X, Otero Perez FJ, et al. Clomipramine/bentazepam in the treat-ment of major depressive disorders. *Hum Psy-chopharmacol* 1992;7:115–122).

clomipramine + benzodiazepine No pharmaco-kinetic interactions have been detected.

clomipramine/breast milk Clomipramine (CMI) has been detected in human milk, usually in small quantities. Because of the possibility of harm to the newborn infant, CMI therapy should be temporarily discontinued and rein-stituted if relapse occurs in the mother.

clomipramine + bromazepam In outpatients with major depressive disorder or dysthymic disorder, co-administration was effective and well tolerated (Cottraux J, Riant N. Alpidem versus bromazepam in depressed outpatients treated with clomipramine. A controlled com-parison. *Clin Neuropharmacol* 1992;15[suppl 1/B]:521B).

clomipramine + buspirone When buspirone was added to the therapeutic regimen of 14 obses-sive-compulsive disorder (OCD) patients par-tially responsive to at least 3 months' clomi-pramine (CMI) monotherapy, 4 (29%) had an additional 25% reduction in OCD and 3 (21%) experienced an increase in symptoms of 25%. Results suggest that adjunctive bus-pirone therapy is not generally associated with significant further clinical improvement in OCD or depressive symptoms, but there may be a patient subgroup that benefits (Pigott TA, L'Hereux F, Hill JL, et al. A double-blind study of adjuvant buspirone hydrochloride in clomi-pramine-treated patients with obsessive-com-pulsive disorder. *J Clin Psychopharmacol* 1992; 12:11–18).

clomipramine + carbamazepine Co-administra-tion has improved treatment-resistant depres-sion. Addition of carbamazepine to clomi-pramine (CMI) monotherapy produced a marked drop in CMI and desmethylclomi-pramine plasma levels (De la Fuente JM, Mendlewicz J. Carbamazepine addition in tri-cyclic antidepressant-resistant unipolar depres-sion. *Biol Psychiatry* 1992;32:369–374). Co-ad-ministration also may increase clomipramine plasma levels (Gerson GR, Jones RB, Lus-combe DK. Studies on the concomitant use of carbamazepine and clomipramine for the re-lief of post-herpetic neuralgia. *Postgrad Med J* 1977;53[suppl 4]:104–109).

clomipramine challenge test Pharmacological probe that measures neuroendocrine re-sponse to acute, intravenously administered clomipramine (CMI). An intravenous line is started at 8:30 am and kept patent with a slow drip of normal saline solution. Blood samples are obtained after 30, 45, and 60 minutes for determination of baseline hormone concen-trations. Immediately after the last sample, 100 ml of normal saline containing 12.5 mg of CMI is infused over 15 minutes. Additional blood samples are obtained after 30, 45, 60, 90, 120, and 150 minutes. Intravenous CMI administration minimizes interindividual dif-ferences in rate and degree of absorption seen with oral pharmacological challenges, avoids the "first-pass" effect of hepatic metabolism, and delays formation of demethylated clomi-pramine and minimizes its effect on norepi-nephrine during hormonal measurements. Depressed patients apparently have abnormal neuroendocrine responses to intravenously administered CMI (Golden RN, Ekstrom D, Brown TM, et al. Neuroendocrine effects of intravenous clomipramine in depressed pa-tients and healthy subjects. *Am J Psychiatry* 1992;149:1168–1175).

clomipramine + cimetidine Cimetidine inhibits metabolism of clomipramine (CMI), increas-ing CMI plasma level and the risk of CMI toxicity.

clomipramine + citalopram No pharmacoki-netic interaction has been reported (Bau-mann P. Clinical pharmacokinetics of citalo-pram and other selective serotonergic reuptake inhibitors [SSRI]. *Int Clin Psychophar-macol* 1992;6[suppl 5]:13-20; Baettig D, Bon-dolfi G, Montaldi S, et al. Tricyclic antidepres-sant plasma levels after augmentation with citalopram. A case study. *Eur J Clin Pharmacol* 1993;44:403–405).

clomipramine + clonazepam Adjuvant clon-azepam treatment may be associated with ad-ditional antianxiety and possible antiobsessive effects in obsessive-compulsive disorder pa-tients.

clomipramine + clonidine There is one report of successful use of clonidine to augment clomipramine in obsessive-compulsive disor-der (Lipsedge MS, Prothero W. Clonidine and clomipramine in obsessive-compulsive disor-der. *Am J Psychiatry* 1987;144:965–966). Others have reported unimpressive results (Hol-lander E, Fay M, Liebowitz MR. Clonidine and clomipramine in obsessive-compulsive disor-der. *Am J Psychiatry* 1988;145:388–389.

clomipramine + clorgyline Co-administration or sequential administration, even within 4 weeks of clorgyline discontinuation, may cause a serotonin syndrome. This occurred in two patients given a single dose of clomipramine 4 weeks after the last dose of clorgyline (Insel TR, Roy BF, Cohen RM, Murphy DL. Possible development of the serotonin syndrome in man. *Am J Psychiatry* 1982;139:954–955). See **serotonin syndrome.**

clomipramine + dextropropoxyphene Co-administration may raise the plasma concentrations of clomipramine and desmethyl-clomipramine to 3 times the level in control subjects (Luscombe DK, Jones RB. Effects of concomitantly administered drugs on plasma levels of clomipramine and desmethylclomipramine in depressive patients receiving clomipramine therapy. *Postgrad Med J* 1977;53[suppl 4]:77–78).

clomipramine + diazepam Diazepam does not appear to influence plasma levels or clinical efficacy of clomipramine (CMI) (Luscombe DK, Jones RB. Effects of concomitantly administered drugs on plasma levels of clomipramine and desmethylclomipramine in depressive patients receiving clomipramine therapy. *Postgrad Med J* 1977;53[suppl 4]:77–78). Co-administration (CMI 50–225 mg/day + diazepam 10–45 mg/day) has been used with benefit and good tolerance in phobic and obsessive-compulsive disorder (Cassano GB, Castrogiovanni P, Mauri M, et al. A multicenter controlled trial in phobic-obsessive psychoneurosis. The effect of chlorimipramine and of its combinations with haloperidol and diazepam. *Progr Neuropsychopharmacol Biol Psychiatry* 1981;5:129–138).

clomipramine + digoxin Co-administration may produce elevated serum concentrations of both drugs.

clomipramine + enalapril In two patients treated with enalapril for hypertension, addition of clomipramine (CMI) for dysthymia produced rapid improvement of depressive symptoms followed by signs of antidepressant toxicity. CMI plasma level was unusually high, and the ratio of clomipramine to its metabolite, desmethylclomipramine, also was high. This suggests that enalapril inhibits hepatic demethylation, the initial step in CMI biotransformation (Toutoungi M. Potential effect of enalapril on clomipramine metabolism. *Hum Psychopharmacol* 1992;7:147–149).

clomipramine + ethosuximide Co-administration may decrease steady-state plasma concentrations of clomipramine and its desmethyl metabolite compared with controls (Luscombe DK, Jones RB. Effects of concomitantly administered drugs on plasma levels of clomipramine and desmethylclomipramine in depressive patients receiving clomipramine therapy. *Postgrad Med J* 1977;53[suppl 4]:77–78).

clomipramine + fenfluramine Fenfluramine has been reported to potentiate the effects of clomipramine (CMI) in a few obsessive-compulsive disorder patients partially responsive to CMI. In one patient, the combination was discontinued because of marked postural hypotension (Judd FK, Chua P, Lynch C, Norman T. Fenfluramine augmentation of clomipramine treatment of obsessive compulsive disorder. *Aust N Z J Psychiatry* 1991;25:412–4; Hollander E, DeCaria CM, Schneier FR, et al. Fenfluramine augmentation of serotonin reuptake blockade antiobsessional treatment. *J Clin Psychiatry* 1990;51:119–23).

clomipramine + fluoxetine Fluoxetine (FLX) inhibits the metabolic pathways involved in tricyclic antidepressant biotransformation (Bertschy G, Vandel S, Francois T, et al. Metabolic interaction between tricyclic antidepressant and fluvoxamine and fluoxetine, a pharmacogenic approach. *Clin Neuropharmacol* 1992;15:[Suppl 1/A]:78a–79a). Co-administration was effective in adult patients with severe obsessive compulsive disorder (OCD) refractory to FLX or clomipramine (CMI alone). In other cases, adjunctive FLX produced benefits with no additional side effects (Browne M, Horn E, Jones TT. The benefits of clomipramine-fluoxetine combination in obsessive compulsive disorder. *Can J Psychiatry* 1993;38:242–243). Similar benefits have been reported in adolescents with OCD (Simeon JG, Thatte S, Wiggins D. Treatment of adolescent obsessive-compulsive disorder with a clomipramine-fluoxetine combination. *Psychopharmacol Bull* 1990;26:285–290). Combined use of these two serotonergic agents did not produce the serotonin syndrome. FLX may potentiate CMI's capacity to induce convulsions either by increasing its serum concentration or by some additive effect. Drugs with known seizure potential should be administered very cautiously in conjunction with high-dose FLX.

clomipramine + fluphenazine decanoate Addition of clomipramine (CMI) (300 mg/day) to ongoing treatment with fluphenazine decanoate (25 mg every 2 weeks) markedly improved both schizophrenic and obsessive-compulsive symptoms in a patient with a 7-year history of undifferentiated schizophrenia (Zohar J, Kaplan Z, Benjamin J. Clomipramine treatment of obsessive-compulsive symptomatology in schizophrenic patients. *J Clin Psychiatry* 1993;54:385–388).

clomipramine + fluvoxamine Fluvoxamine (FVX) inhibits clomipramine demethylation (CMI), markedly enhancing plasma levels of CMI and its metabolite, desmethylclomipramine. The increase may lead to a potentiation of the antidepressant effect in some patients, but also may cause adverse reactions. CMI also increases FVX plasma level. During co-administration, serum level monitoring of both drugs is indicated (Bertschy G, Vandel S, Vandel B, et al. Fluvoxamine-tricyclic antidepressant interaction—an accidental finding. *Eur J Clin Pharmacol* 1991;40:119–120). Co-medication appears to be well tolerated without signs of cardiotoxic or central nervous system side effects. FVX inhibitory effects on CMI metabolism disappeared within at least 1–2 weeks after FVX discontinuation (Haertter S, Wetzel H, Hammes E, Hiemke C. Inhibition of antidepressant demethylation and hydroxylation by fluvoxamine in depressed patients. *Psychopharmacology* 1993;110:302–308). A patient who had undergone cingulotomy had seizures on one occasion while taking both CMI and FVX (Jenike MA, Baer L, Ballantine HT, et al. Cingulotomy for refractory obsessive-compulsive disorder. A long-term follow-up of 33 patients. *Arch Gen Psychiatry* 1991;48:548–555).

clomipramine + haloperidol Haloperidol (HAL) may increase plasma concentration of clomipramine (CMI), augmenting its effects. CMI (75–175 mg/day) + HAL (3–7 mg/day) has been used with benefit and good tolerance in phobic and obsessive-compulsive patients (Cassano GB, Castrogiovanni P, Mauri M, et al. A multicenter controlled trial in phobic-obsessive psychoneurosis. The effect of chlorimipramine and of its combinations with haloperidol and diazepam. *Progr Neuropsychopharmacol Biol Psychiatry* 1981;5:129–138). Co-administration produced marked improvement in delusions, hallucinations, and obsessive symptoms and completely eradicated tics in a patient with Tourette's syndrome, obsessive-compulsive disorder, and schizophrenia (Escobar R, Bernardo M. Schizophrenia, obsessive-compulsive disorder, and Tourette's syndrome: a case of triple co-morbidity. *J Clin Neuropsychiatr Clin Neurosci* 1993;5:108).

clomipramine + levomepromazine Co-administration significantly increases clomipramine plasma level (Balant-Gorgia AE, Balant LP, Genet C, et al. Importance of oxidative polymorphism and levomepromazine treatment on the steady-state blood concentrations of clomipramine and its major metabolites. *Eur J Clin Pharmacol* 1986;31:449–455).

clomipramine + lithium Lithium does not augment antiobsessional response to clomipramine (CMI) (Pigott TA, Pato MT, L'Heureux F, et al. A controlled comparison of adjuvant lithium carbonate or thyroid hormone in clomipramine-treated patients with obsessive-compulsive disorder. *J Clin Psychopharmacol* 1991;11:242–248). High dose CMI +

lithium has been reported very effective in some patients with resistant endogenous depression (Hale AS, Procter AW, Bridges PK. Clomipramine, tryptophan and lithium in combination for resistant endogenous depression: seven case studies. *Br J Psychiatry* 1987; 151:213–217; Stein G, Bernadt M. Lithium augmentation therapy in tricyclic-resistant depression. A controlled trial using lithium in low and normal doses. *Br J Psychiatry* 1993;162: 634–640; Feder R. Lithium augmentation of clomipramine. *J Clin Psychiatry* 1988;49:458).

clomipramine + mebanazine Clomipramine (CMI) should not be co-administered with mebanazine or within 14 days after mebanazine discontinuation, nor should mebanazine be given to a patient already receiving CMI. Either regimen may cause hypertension, collapse, convulsions, coma, and death.

clomipramine + methylphenidate Co-administration increases the plasma level of clomipramine (CMI) and risk of CMI toxicity.

clomipramine + moclobemide The serotonin syndrome occurred in a 76-year-old woman the day after she was switched to moclobemide (300 mg/day) following several months of treatment with clomipramine (50 mg/day). After a few days, she recovered fully. She also was taking levodopa-benserazide, bromocriptine, triazolam, diflunisal, dextropropoxyphene, estradiol, and lactulose (Spigest O, Mjorndal T, Lovheim O. Serotonin syndrome caused by a moclobemide-clomipramine interaction. *Br Med J* 1993;306:248). Fatal serotonin syndrome was reported in two patients who took an overdose of moclobemide and clomipramine (Neuvonen PJ, Pohjola-Sintonen S, Tacke U, Vuori E. Five fatal cases of serotonin syndrome after moclobemide-citalopram or moclobemide-clomipramine overdoses. *Lancet* 1993;342:1419). Data from a patient who overdosed with moclobemide and clomipramine along with 20 mg of flunitrazepam and a bottle of wine suggest a possible interaction with an additive effect that may lead to serious toxicity (Myrenfors PG, Eriksson T, Sandstedt CS, Sjoeberg G. Moclobemide overdose. *J Intern Med* 1993;233:113–115).

clomipramine + monoamine oxidase inhibitor (MAOI) Co-administration may induce hyperpyrexia, muscle spasms, convulsions, coma, and death. It should be reserved for highly refractory depression.

clomipramine + morphine Co-administration increases morphine's bioavailability and degree of analgesia. Although the interaction is useful, morphine toxicity also may be increased (Ventafridda V, Ripamonti C, DeConno F, et al. Antidepressants increase bioavailability of morphine in cancer patients. *Lancet* 1987;1:1204).

clomipramine/neonate Clomipramine (CMI) or its metabolites may induce neonatal adverse effects such as respiratory distress, hypotonia, feeding difficulties, diaphoresis, and jitteriness. Symptoms are usually related to plasma level of CMI and its metabolites in the neonate; they usually disappear without specific treatment as plasma levels fall (Schimmel MS, Katz E, Shaag Y, Patuszak A, et al. Toxic neonatal effects following maternal clomipramine therapy. *Clin Toxicol* 1991;29:479–484).

clomipramine + neuroleptic Addition of clomipramine (CMI) to ongoing neuroleptic treatment in schizophrenic patients with obsessive-compulsive symptoms has been associated with specific reduction of those symptoms. CMI has been co-administered with chlorpromazine, haloperidol, and fluphenazine decanoate (Zohar J, Kaplan Z, Benjamin J. Clomipramine treatment of obsessive-compulsive symptomatology in schizophrenic patients. *J Clin Psychiatry* 1993;45:385–388).

clomipramine + nicotine Nicotine increases metabolism of clomipramine (CMI), resulting in lower levels of CMI and its active metabolite, desmethylclomipramine, and possibly interfering with CMI's therapeutic effects (Peters MD, Davis SK, Austin LS. Clomipramine: an antiobsessional tricyclic antidepressant. *Clin Pharm* 1990;9:165–178).

clomipramine + oral contraceptive Co-administration in some patients produced steady-state plasma levels of clomipramine (CMI) above the range observed in patients receiving CMI alone (Luscombe DK, Jones RB. Effects of concomitantly administered drugs on plasma levels of clomipramine and desmethylclomipramine in depressive patients receiving clomipramine therapy. *Postgrad Med J* 1977; 53[suppl 4]:77–78).

clomipramine + oxprenolol Co-administration does not appear to influence clomipramine (CMI) plasma levels or clinical efficacy (Luscombe DK, Jones RB. Effects of concomitantly administered drugs on plasma levels of clomipramine and desmethylclomipramine in depressive patients receiving clomipramine therapy. *Postgrad Med J* 1977;53[suppl 4]:77–78).

clomipramine + paracetamol Co-administration may raise the plasma concentrations of clomipramine (CMI) and desmethylclomipramine to three times higher than in controls (Luscombe DK, Jones RB. Effects of concomitantly administered drugs on plasma levels of clomipramine and desmethylclomipramine in de-

pressive patients receiving clomipramine therapy. *Postgrad Med J* 1977;53[suppl 4]:77–78).

clomipramine + phenelzine Addition of phenelzine (60 mg/day) to clomipramine (CMI) at a reduced dose of 150 mg/day resulted in almost complete disappearance of avoidance behavior and agoraphobia within 2 weeks in a patient who remained completely symptom-free for about 2 years. Low maintenance doses of the drugs produced no significant side effects (Klein E, Metz L. Differential drug response of panic and agoraphobic avoidance in a case of panic disorder. *Acta Psychiatr Scand* 1990;82:86–87). Catastrophic illness manifested by hyperpyrexia (110° F), blood pressure lability, tachycardia, renal failure, and coma occurred in a patient treated with clomipramine, phenelzine, and chlorpromazine (Stern TA, Schwartz JH, Shuster JL. Catastrophic illness associated with the combination of clomipramine, phenelzine and chlorpromazine. *Ann Clin Psychiatr* 1992;4:81–85). The serotonin syndrome, resulting from an interaction between phenelzine (which reduces serotonin metabolism within neurons) and clomipramine (which inhibits serotonin uptake at synapses), has been reported (Nierenberg DW, Semprebon M. The central nervous system serotonin syndrome. *Clin Pharmacol Ther* 1993;53:84–88). Thus, addition of clomipramine to phenelzine should be considered potentially dangerous and probably should be avoided.

clomipramine + phenobarbital Co-administration can decrease steady-state plasma concentrations of clomipramine and its desmethyl metabolite compared with such concentrations in control subjects (Luscombe DK, Jones RB. Effects of concomitantly administered drugs on plasma levels of clomipramine and desmethylclomipramine in depressive patients receiving clomipramine therapy. *Postgrad Med J* 1977;53[suppl 4]:77–78).

clomipramine + phenytoin Co-administration can decrease steady-state plasma concentrations of clomipramine and its desmethyl metabolite compared with such concentrations in control subjects (Luscombe DK, Jones RB. Effects of concomitantly administered drugs on plasma levels of clomipramine and desmethylclomipramine in depressive patients receiving clomipramine therapy. *Postgrad Med J* 1977;53[suppl 4]:77–78).

clomipramine + pimozide Pimozide (1 mg every day increased to 2 mg twice a day) may augment therapeutic response to clomipramine (CMI) in trichotillomania partially responsive or refractory to CMI alone (Stein DJ, Hollander E. Low-dose pimozide augmentation of serotonin reuptake blockers in the treatment of trichotillomania. *J Clin Psychiatry* 1992;53:123–126). See **trichotillomania.**

clomipramine/pregnancy No teratogenic effects attributable to clomipramine (CMI) have been observed in animals or offspring of the few women who took CMI during pregnancy. However, withdrawal symptoms, including jitteriness, tremor, and seizures, have been reported in neonates whose mothers took CMI until delivering. During pregnancy, CMI should be taken with caution and only when potential benefits justify potential risks to the fetus. If possible, CMI therapy should be stopped 1 month before anticipated delivery or restricted to the lowest beneficial doses. See **clomipramine/neonate.**

clomipramine + propoxyphene Elevated plasma clomipramine (CMI) levels were found in two of three patients receiving propoxyphene with paracetamol. CMI plasma levels above the range observed in patients receiving CMI alone tended to be associated with poor therapeutic response and more unwanted effects (Luscombe DK, Jones RB. Effects of concomitantly administered drugs on plasma levels of clomipramine and desmethylclomipramine in depressive patients receiving clomipramine therapy. *Postgrad Med J* 1977;53[suppl 4]:77–78).

clomipramine + propranolol Clomipramine (CMI) (150 mg/day) + propranolol (dosage unknown) was well tolerated and effective prophylaxis for 7 years in a patient with major depression and recurrent paroxysmal tachycardia (Jouvent R, Baruch P, Simon P. *Am J Psychiatry* 1986;143:1633).

clomipramine + S-adenosylmethionine Co-administration produced a toxic interaction diagnosed as a probable serotonin syndrome in an elderly patient. Symptoms consisted of increasing anxiety, agitation, and confusion, followed by verbal unresponsiveness and stupor with tachycardia (130 beats/minute), tachypnea (30 respirations/minute), diarrhea, myoclonus, generalized tremors, rigidity, hyper-reflexia, shivering, profuse diaphoresis, and dehydration. On admission, temperature was 40.5° C, which rose to 43° C. Intensive treatment resulted in complete medical recovery (Iruela LM, Minguez L, Merino J, Monedero G. Toxic interaction of S-adenosylmethionine and clomipramine. *Am J Psychiatry* 1993; 150:522).

clomipramine + sulpiride Co-administration has been reported useful in the treatment of severe depression (Masquin A. Association du Dogmatil et de l'anafranil chaus le traitement des melancolies. *Information Psychiatrique* 1972; 48:218–219).

clomipramine + sympathomimetic Co-administration increases risk of sympathomimetic effects. Careful dosage adjustment of one or both drugs may be necessary to avoid toxicity.

clomipramine + thiothixene Very rapid development of a tardive dyskinesia–like syndrome was reported. It remitted rapidly following discontinuation of clomipramine (Gersten SP. Tardive dyskinesia-like syndromes with clomipramine. *Am J Psychiatry* 1993;150:165–166).

clomipramine + thyroid drug Co-administration increases risk of cardiac arrhythmias.

clomipramine + tranylcypromine Clomipramine (CMI) should not be prescribed during tranylcypromine therapy or within 14 days after its discontinuation; nor should tranylcypromine be added to CMI therapy. Either regimen may cause hypotension, collapse, convulsions, coma, and death. Disseminated intravascular coagulation, agitated delirium, hyperpyrexia, tachycardia, and rigidity occurred in a patient when CMI was added to chronic tranylcypromine therapy (Tackley RM, Tregaskis B. Fatal disseminated intravascular coagulation following a monoamine oxidase inhibitor/tricyclic interaction. *Anesthesia* 1987;42:760–763). However, CMI plus tranylcypromine plus trifluoperazine has been used safely and effectively in some patients with treatment-resistant depression (Schmauss M, Kapfhammer HP, Meyr P, Hoff P. Combined MAO-inhibitor and tri [tetra] cyclic antidepressant treatment in therapy resistant depression. *Progr Neuropsychopharmacol Biol Psychiatry* 1988;12:523–532).

clomipramine + triiodothyronine (T3) Addition of T3 to patients partially responsive to clomipramine did not improve therapeutic response (Pigott TA, Pato MT, L'Heureux F, et al. A controlled comparison of adjuvant lithium carbonate or thyroid hormone in clomipramine-treated patients with obsessive-compulsive disorder. *J Clin Psychopharmacol* 1991;11:242–248). See **clomipramine + thyroid drug.**

clomipramine + tryptophan Co-administration augments antiobsessional response to clomipramine.

clomipramine + valproate Co-administration may have beneficial effects in the treatment of pain. In some patients, especially the elderly, co-administration may cause undesirable drowsiness.

clomipramine + warfarin Co-administration may increase plasma concentrations of both drugs, resulting in adverse effects.

clomipramine + yohimbine In a double-blind crossover placebo study, yohimbine (4 mg three times a day) significantly increased systolic blood pressure in 12 depressed patients with orthostatic hypotension induced by clomipramine. The effect was possibly due to pharmacodynamic and pharmacokinetic interactions between yohimbine and clomipramine or desmethylclomipramine (Lacomblez L, Bensimon G, Isnard F, et al. Effect of yohimbine on blood pressure in depressed patients with orthostatic hypotension induced by clomipramine. *Fundam Clin Pharmacol* 1989; 3:579).

clonazepam (Clonex; Clonopin; Klonopin; Leponex; Riootril; Rivotril) (CNP) High potency 1,4-benzodiazepine (BZD) marketed as an anticonvulsant, with an affinity for central BZD receptors exceeded only by midazolam and triazolam. It also may influence central serotonergic function. Half-life is relatively long (20–50 hours). Following oral administration, peak concentrations occur between 1 and 4 hours. Delayed absorption rate contributes to a relatively slow onset of action (2–3 hours). CNP undergoes nitroreduction to 7-aminoclonazepam, followed by acetylation to 7-acetamidoclonazepam. There are five metabolites, none of which contributes appreciably to pharmacological effects. Effective dosage is 1–6 mg/day. The long half-life allows twice- a-day dosing without interdose rebound anxiety or withdrawal. CNP is effective in the treatment of myoclonic and generalized tonic-clonic seizures. Sedation and tolerance have been reported in most studies; alternate-day administration has been used to offset these side effects in patients with refractory epilepsy. Few patients benefit greatly from long-term treatment, and nearly 50% will have an exacerbation of seizures when CNP is withdrawn, especially if there is pre-existent cerebral damage (Brodie MJ. Established anticonvulsants and treatment of refractory epilepsy. *Lancet* 1990;336:350–354). CNP has antipanic, anxiolytic, and antimanic properties and has been used in managing disturbed psychotic behavior. Although it has been used to treat mania, mania can be associated with CNP therapy (Dorevitch A. Mania associated with clonazepam. *Ann Pharmacother* 1991;25:938–939). The most effective antipanic maintenance dose has been 2–3 mg/day, although some patients require more. CNP has been used to treat behavior disorders in the mentally retarded; neurological disorders, including Gilles de la Tourette's syndrome; myoclonus; restless legs syndrome; cerebellar tremor; facial spasm; intention tremor; and neuroleptic-induced akathisia. It reduces obsessive-compulsive disorder symptoms; about 40% of clomipramine-refractory subjects have a clinically significant response to CNP. Improvement is unrelated to changes in anxiety, oc-

curs early in treatment, and is more pronounced than with other medications during the first 3 weeks of treatment (Hewlett WA, Vinogradov S, Agras WS. Clomipramine, clonazepam, and clonidine treatment of obsessive-compulsive disorder. *J Clin Psychopharmacol* 1992;12:420–430). CNP can be used for long-term treatment of social phobia patients, including many patients refractory to prior therapies (Davidson JRT, Ford SM, Smith RD, et al. Long-term treatment of social phobia with clonazepam. *J Clin Psychiatry* 1991; 52[suppl]:16–20). Sleep laboratory studies indicate that CNP (0.5 mg at bedtime) significantly improves sleep induction and maintenance with both short-term and continued use. Following abrupt discontinuation, there is moderate to marked delayed rebound insomnia. CNP should be discontinued gradually. Most frequent side effects are mild transient sedation and ataxia. Pregnancy risk category C; Schedule IV.

clonazepam/breast milk Measurable clonazepam concentrations occur in breast milk and infant plasma. Although data are scant, monitoring of infant plasma concentrations may be indicated (Soderman P, Matheson I. Clonazepam in breast milk. *Eur J Pediatr* 1987;147: 212–213).

clonazepam + carbamazepine Carbamazepine (CBZ) induces clonazepam metabolism, decreasing its plasma level and interfering in its therapeutic efficacy (Lai AA, Levy RH, Cutler RE. Time-course of interaction between carbamazepine and clonazepam in normal man. *Clin Pharmacol Ther* 1978;24:316–323). Co-administration in absence seizure patients may induce absence status. See **absence status.**

clonazepam + clozapine Except for some transient sedation, no significant adverse interactions between therapeutic doses have been reported. Clonazepam's calming effect may reduce the need for increased clozapine (CLOZ) dosage in anxiety only partially mitigated by CLOZ.

clonazepam + desipramine Ordinarily, benzodiazepines do not significantly alter tricyclic antidepressant serum levels. However, there is a report of a rather dramatic decrease in serum desipramine (DMI) concentration after addition of clonazepam (CNP). When CNP was discontinued, there was a rebound increase in DMI plasma level (Deicken RF. Clonazepam-induced reduction in serum desipramine concentration. *J Clin Psychopharmacol* 1988;8:71–73).

clonazepam + fluoxetine No serious adverse interactions have been reported. Adjuvant clonazepam (CNP) may be associated with additional antianxiety and possible antiobsessive effects when combined with fluoxetine (FLX) in the treatment of obsessive-compulsive disorder (OCD). CNP (0.5 mg twice or three times a day) added to FLX in seven OCD patients resistant to behavior therapy produced improvement of more than 20% in only one patient (Jenicke MA. Augmentation strategies for treatment-resistant obsessive compulsive disorder. *Harvard Rev Psychiatry* 1993;1:17–26).

clonazepam + haloperidol See **clonazepam + neuroleptic.**

clonazepam + isocarboxazid Co-administration is more effective in treating panic disorder than either drug alone.

clonazepam + lithium Co-administration may be effective and safe in acute mania (Gonliaev G, Licht RW, Vestergaard P. Treatment of acute mania with lithium and clonazepam or zuclopenthixol and clonazepam. *Clin Neuropharm* 1992;15[suppl 1]:210B). Combined use may result in lithium toxicity secondary to a rise in serum lithium levels.

clonazepam + neuroleptic In a double-blind crossover study of acute mania with adjunctive haloperidol, clonazepam (mean dose, 10.4 mg/day) was superior to lithium (mean dose, 1691 mg/day) in controlling motor overactivity and logorrhea. In addition, total haloperidol dose administered was lower during clonazepam treatment (Chouinard G, Young SN, Anarable L. Antimanic effect of clonazepam. *Biol Psychiatry* 1983;18:451–466). In a double-blind study of schizophrenia, clonazepam (3 mg/day) added to haloperidol produced modest improvement in Brief Psychiatric Rating Scale and Extrapyramidal Side Effects Scale scores, but no changes in specific symptoms (Altamura AC, Mauri MC, Mantero M, Brunetti M. Clonazepam/haloperidol combination therapy in schizophrenia: a double-blind study. *Acta Psychiatr Scand* 1987;76:702–706).

clonazepam + phenelzine Two cases of facial flushing have been reported. The mechanism for the interaction is unknown, but has been attributed to additive or synergistic serotonergic effects (Karagianis JL, March H. Flushing reaction associated with the interaction of phenelzine and clonazepam. *Can J Psychiatry* 1991;36:389). After taking clonazepam (0.5 mg at bedtime), a patient who had been stabilized for 9 years on phenelzine (45 mg/day) experienced severe occipital headache (Eppel AB. Interaction between clonazepam and phenelzine. *Can J Psychiatry* 1990;35:647).

clonazepam + phenytoin In an epileptic patient, phenytoin (300 mg/day) and clonazepam (CNP) (1.5 mg/day) resulted in decreased phenytoin plasma levels (from 22 to 16 µg/ml) and increase in seizures. CNP dosage was gradually reduced by 0.5 mg/week and finally discontinued; phenytoin was maintained at 375 mg/day. Signs of intoxication resolved.

clonazepam/pregnancy Available data indicate that benzodiazepines are safer during pregnancy than other anxiolytics and antidepressants. Some investigators report no serious adverse consequences of clonazepam (CNP) during pregnancy (Liebowitz MR. Discussion. *J Clin Psychiatry* 1993;54[suppl 5]:18). Use throughout pregnancy was associated with mild transient sedation (Kriel RL, Cloyd J. Clonazepam and pregnancy. *Ann Neurology* 1982;11:544). There is a case report of floppy infant syndrome attributed to CNP during pregnancy (Fisher JB, Edgren BE, Mammel MC, et al. Neonatal apnea associated with maternal clonazepam therapy: a case report. *Obstet Gynecol* 1985;66:343–355).

clonazepam/psychotic agitation Intramuscularly administered clonazepam (CNP) (2–3 mg every 30–60 minutes) in 16 patients with psychotic agitation produced tranquilization in 1.5–6 hours with no adverse effects (Benazzi F. Intramuscular clonazepam for the treatment of psychotic agitation. *Can J Psychiatry* 1991;36:697). Intramuscularly administered CNP (4–5 mg every 30–60 minutes) was even more rapidly effective (30–60 minutes) in 12 patients with acute psychotic agitation, again with no clinically significant side effects (Benazzi F, Mazzoli M, Rossi E. Benzodiazepines and acute psychotic agitation. *Can J Psychiatry* 1992;37:732–733).

clonazepam + sertraline Low-dose clonazepam has been added at bedtime for sertraline-treated patients with pressor test pretreatment insomnia. The regimen has been safe and efficacious (Kline NA, Dow BM, Brown SA, Matloff JL. Sertraline efficacy in depressed combat veterans with posttraumatic stress disorder. Presented at the 146th Annual Meeting of the American Psychiatric Association, San Francisco, May 1993).

clonazepam + valproate Co-administration may induce absence status in patients subject to absence seizures. See **absence status.**

clonazepam + zuclopenthixol Co-administration is safe and effective in acute mania (Gonliaev G, Licht RW, Vestergaard P. Treatment of acute mania with lithium and clonazepam or zuclopenthixol and clonazepam. *Clin Neuropharm* 1992;15[suppl 1]:210B).

clone Population of cells derived from a single precursor cell by repeated mitosis and all having the same genotype.

Clonex See **clonazepam.**

clonic movement See **clonus.**

clonidine (Catapres; Dixaret) Antihypertensive reported (1978) to be effective in ameliorating opioid withdrawal symptoms. It has also been used to diminish symptoms of alcohol and smoking withdrawal. By activating alpha-2 autoreceptors, it decreases abnormally high noradrenergic activity in the locus ceruleus during withdrawal. It has been combined with naltrexone to provide more rapid (abrupt) opioid withdrawal over 3–5 days. Clonidine does not relieve all opioid withdrawal symptoms; patients continue to complain of craving, insomnia, and muscle aches. It also produces major side effects (hypotension, sedation) when used in the high doses needed to control opioid withdrawal (Jaffe JH. Pharmacological agents in treatment of drug dependence. *In* Meltzer HY [ed], *Psychopharmacology, the Third Generation of Progress*. New York: Raven Press, 1987, pp 1605–1616; Senft RA. Experience with clonidine-naltrexone for rapid opiate detoxification. *J Substance Abuse Treat* 1991;8:257–259). Clonidine may be useful in the treatment of stuttering in children, generalized anxiety and possibly panic disorders, and Tourette's syndrome and attention-deficit hyperactivity disorder when first-line drugs (e.g., stimulants) are ineffective. It can be used to test the functional sensitivity of certain adrenergic systems. In young adults and panic disorder patients, a blunted growth hormone response to clonidine occurs, as well as a decrease in blood pressure and peripheral 3-methoxy-4-hydroxyphenylglycol (MHPG). Clonidine causes a decrease in cerebrospinal fluid noradrenaline in younger, but not in older, subjects (Uhde TW, Vittone BJ, Siever LJ, et al. Blunted growth hormone response to clonidine in panic disorder patients. *Biol Psychiatry* 1986;21:1081–1085; Charney DS, Heninger GR. Abnormal regulation of noradrenergic function in panic disorders: effects of clonidine in healthy subjects and panics with agoraphobia and panic disorder. *Arch Gen Psychiatry* 1986;43:1042–1054; Raskind MA, Peskind ER, Veith RC, et al. Increased plasma and cerebrospinal fluid norepinephrine in older men: differential suppression by clonidine. *J Clin Endocrinol Metab* 1988;66:438–443). There are conflicting reports of clonidine's efficacy in reducing obsessive-compulsive disorder symptoms (Kensevich JW. Successful treatment of obsessive-compulsive disorder with clonidine hydrochloride. *Am J Psychiatry* 1982;139:364–365; Hewlett WA, Vinogradov S, Agras WS. Clomipramine, clonazepam, and clonidine treatment of obsessive-compulsive disorder. *J Clin Psychopharmacol* 1992;12:420–430). Clonidine is considered obsolete for treatment of hypertension and migraine prophylaxis. Pregnancy risk category C.

clonidine/abuse In 1992, reports began to appear of clonidine's being used to boost methadone effects. Street dose reported is 0.3 mg three times a day; over time it can increase to 30 tablets/day. Symptoms due to abrupt withdrawal from clonidine include nervousness, tachycardia, headache, sweating, and rebound hypertension; many mimic patients' withdrawal from opiates or side effects from cocaine, clouding the clinical picture and complicating appropriate assessment and management.

clonidine + amphetamine Co-administration is effective in children refractory to either medication alone (Mandoki MW. Clonidine D-amphetamine combination in the treatment of children with attention deficit hyperactivity disorder. *Neuropsychopharmacology* 1993;9: 183S).

clonidine/breast milk Measurement of clonidine concentration in the plasma of a breast-fed infant and in the plasma and milk in a woman treated with oral clonidine (37.5 μg twice a day) showed that drug concentration was 0.33 ng/ml in maternal plasma, 0.60 ng/ml in milk, and undetectable in infant plasma. If daily milk consumption had been 150 ml/kg, the infant would have ingested 90 ng/kg/day of clonidine, compared to the maternal drug dosage of 320 ng/kg/day. Thus, the infant's relative dosage would have been 6.8%. No adverse effects were observed in the infant. Clonidine is considered a second-choice drug for the treatment of hypertension in nursing women (Bunjes R, Schaefer C, Holzinger D. Clonidine and breast-feeding. *Clin Pharm* 1993;12:178–179).

clonidine challenge test Clonidine stimulates hypothalamic postsynaptic alpha-2 adrenergic receptors to induce secretion of growth-hormone-releasing factor and a discrete pulse of growth hormone (GH) release over the usual low baseline levels in humans. The response is reported to be impaired in some depressed patients (Mitchell PB, Bearn JA, Corn TH, Checkley SA. Growth hormone response to clonidine after recovery in patients with endogenous depression. *Br J Psychiatry* 1988;152: 34–38). GH response to clonidine is being used as an indirect index of noradrenergic function in various pathological conditions, particularly depressive disorders. However, blunted clonidine response is not specific for depression and does not normalize when the patient recovers. It is unclear if blunted clonidine response is a marker for some aspects of depression or vulnerability. Social phobic and panic-disorder patients had similar, significantly blunted GH increments after intravenously administered clonidine (2 μg/kg) (Tancer ME, Stein MB, Uhde TW. Growth hormone response to intravenous clonidine in social phobia: comparison to patients with panic disorder and healthy volunteers. *Biol Psychiatry* 1993;34:591–595).

clonidine + clomipramine Co-administration has been reported both effective and ineffective in the treatment of obsessive-compulsive disorder (Lipsedge MS, Prothero W. Clonidine and clomipramine in obsessive-compulsive disorder. *Am J Psychiatry* 1987;144:965–966; Hollander E, Fay M, Liebowitz MR. Clonidine and clomipramine in obsessive-compulsive disorder. *Am J Psychiatry* 1988;145:388–389).

clonidine + fluoxetine Co-administration is ineffective in the treatment of obsessive compulsive disorder. Side effects, mainly excessive sedation and unsteadiness, necessitated clonidine discontinuation before the end of a 1-month trial in over 50% of patients (Jenike MA. Augmentation strategies for treatment-resistant obsessive-compulsive disorder. *Harvard Rev Psychiatry* 1993;1:17–26).

clonidine/methadone withdrawal Clonidine is more effective than placebo in alleviating signs and symptoms of methadone withdrawal, but does not substantially reduce craving, insomnia, or muscle aches. Dosage is titrated against severity of withdrawal symptoms; average is 5 µg/kg of body weight, and the average adult needs 0.3 mg/day. Initially clonidine can be sedating, and should be used carefully in outpatients because of its hypotensive actions (Kleber HD, Riordan CE, Rounsaville BJ, et al. Clonidine in outpatient detoxification from methadone maintenance. *Arch Gen Psychiatry* 1985;42:391–394). See **clonidine/abuse.**

clonidine + methylphenidate In children and adolescents with attention deficit hyperactivity disorder whose attentional capacity improved with stimulant treatment, behavioral problems improved with adjunctive clonidine (Huessy H, Cohen S, Blair C, Rood P. Clinical explorations in adult minimal brain dysfunction. *In* L Bellak [ed], *Psychiatric Aspects of Minimal Brain Dysfunction in Adults.* New York: Grune & Stratton, 1979; Hunt RD, Minderaa MD, Cohen DJ. Clonidine benefits children with attention deficit hyperactivity: report of a double-blind placebo-crossover therapeutic trial. *J Am Acad Child Adolesc Psychiatry* 1985; 24:617–629; Gammon GD. Combined medications for ADD subtypes. Presented at the 1993 Annual Meeting of the American Psychiatric Association, San Francisco, May 25, 1993). Co-administration has been shown to have a greater effect on physical aggression and verbal oppositionality than either medication alone.

clonidine + naltrexone Co-administration in opioid-dependent patients shortens the opioid withdrawal syndrome significantly without substantially increasing patient discomfort (Kleber HD, Topazian M, Gaspari J, et al. Clonidine and naltrexone in outpatient treatment of heroin withdrawal. *Am J Drug Alcohol Abuse* 1987;13:1–17). The combination can reduce methadone detoxification to 3–5 days.

clonidine + naltrexone + diazepam Co-administration has been shown to significantly reduce average opioid withdrawal time from 3.3 to 2.3 days, despite lower clonidine dosage and significantly lower diazepam dosage on the second day.

clonidine skin patch (Catapres-TTS) Clonidine formulation used in outpatient settings to suppress withdrawal symptoms, especially from cigarette smoking or benzodiazepines (BZDs). Standard approach is to use Catapres-TTS No. 2 (equivalent to 0.2 mg/day). If baseline systolic blood pressure is less than 100 mm Hg, or the patient is of small build or reports sensitivity to clonidine, a No. 1 patch can be used. Adequate blood levels are reached in 3–4 days. Tapering usually starts only after that interval to accomplish BZD discontinuation over about 2 weeks; the patch is continued for 1–2 weeks after reaching zero dose. Hypotensive effects and rapid development of tolerance to antiwithdrawal effects limit clonidine's usefulness.

clonidine withdrawal Abrupt cessation of long-term clonidine therapy may be followed by symptoms of sympathetic overactivity including insomnia, anxiety, tremor, sweating, restlessness, vivid dreams, headache, nausea, vomiting, diarrhea, abdominal pain, salivation, and hiccups. Other effects include delirium and exacerbation of pre-existing manic and schizophrenic psychoses (Paykel, ES, Felminger R, Watson JPL. Psychiatric side effects of anti-hypertensive drugs other than reserpine. *J Clin Psychopharmacol* 1982;2:14–39; Adler LE, Bell J, Kuch D, et al. Psychosis associated with clonidine withdrawal. *Am J Psychiatry* 1982;139: 110–112; Diamond BI, Borison RL, Katz R, DeVeaugh-Geiss J. Rebound withdrawal reactions due to clomipramine. *Psychopharmacol Bull* 1989;25:209–212).

cloning, molecular Process of biological purification and amplification of specific DNA fragments. Recently developed techniques have permitted the identification and sequencing of the primary structure of several receptors that may have a role in the pathophysiology of psychiatric disorders.

cloning, positional Set of techniques by which disease genes are identified through their position in the genome rather than their function. Initial stages rely on linkage analysis, which seeks to find congregations of genetic markers with the disease in question in multiple affected families. Clues about where to begin the search for linked markers may be provided by cytogenetic abnormalities. Positional cloning is one of the strategies being used to determine the molecular genetics of schizophrenia (Collins FS. Positional cloning: let's not call it reverse any more. *Nature Genetics* 1992;1:3–6).

cloning vector Plasmid or bacteriophage used to "transport" inserted DNA to produce more material or a protein product.

Clonopin See **clonazepam**.

clonus Movement characterized by involuntary alternating rapid muscle contraction and relaxation. It may occur in limbs affected by cerebral palsy when placed in a particular position or when stretched. The clonic stage of an epileptic seizure is characterized by regular jerking movements. Ankle clonus occurring when the Achilles tendon is stretched may be a sign of brain damage.

clopenthixol decanoate See **zuclopenthixol decanoate.**

Clopixol See **zuclopenthixol.**

Clopixol Acuphase See **zuclopenthixol acetate.**

Clopixol Acutard See **zuclopenthixol acetate.**

Clopixol Decanoate See **zuclopenthixol decanoate.**

clorazepate (Novoclopate; Tranxene; Tranxal; Tranxilium) Benzodiazepine (BZD) anxiolytic with a long half-life (30–100 hours) similar to that of prazepam. Liver 450 biotransformation gives rise to its primary metabolite, nordiazepam (N-desmethyldiazepam), which appears quickly in the bloodstream. Onset of action is more rapid than that of prazepam. Like all BZDs, it may produce tolerance, dependence, and withdrawal, and should be discontinued gradually. Pregnancy risk category D; schedule IV.

clorazepate + alcohol Acute alcohol ingestion, even in chronic alcohol users, reduces clorazepate elimination and increases its plasma level (von Staak M. Moosmayar A. Pharmacokinetic studies on interactions between dipotassium clorazepate and alcohol after oral administration. *Arzneimittel-Forschung* 1978;28:1187–1191).

clorazepate + antacid Antacids impair clorazepate absorption and decrease its effects.

clorazepate/breast milk Clorazepate's primary metabolite, nordiazepam, is secreted in human milk and may adversely affect the nursing neonate. Breastfeeding should be avoided.

clorazepate + cimetidine Co-administration inhibits clorazepate hydroxylation.

clorgyline (CLO) Irreversible, selective inhibitor of monoamine oxidase-A with antidepressant activity similar to that of imipramine and amitriptyline. Efficacy in unipolar and bipolar depression is superior to that of the monoamine oxidase inhibitor (MAOI) pargyline. Oral and intravenous tyramine pressor tests show no safety advantage over nonselective MAOIs. No longer available in the United States.

clorgyline + clomipramine Co-administration or sequential administration (even within four weeks of clorgyline discontinuation may cause the serotonin syndrome. It occurred in two patients given a single dose of clomipramine 4 weeks after the last dose of clorgyline (Insel TR, Roy BF, Cohen RM, Murphy DL. Possible development of the serotonin syndrome in man. *Am J Psychiatry* 1982;139:954–955). See **serotonin syndrome.**

clorgyline + lithium In treatment-refractory depression, lithium may potentiate clorgyline's antidepressant effect without adverse interactions (Potter WZ, Murphy DL, Wehr TA, et al. Clorgyline, a new treatment for patients with refractory rapid-cycling disorders. *Arch Gen Psychiatry* 1983;39:505–510). See **lithium + monoamine oxidase inhibitor (MAOI).**

clostebol Commonly abused anabolic steroid.

clouding of consciousness Condition seen in acute and chronic brain disorders, manifested by impaired orientation, perception, and attention; drowsiness; slowed reaction; and muddled thinking.

clovoxamine Serotonin uptake inhibitor antidepressant not available in the United States.

clovoxamine + alcohol There is some evidence that clovoxamine does not interact with alcohol (Stromberg C, Mattila MJ. Acute comparison of clovoxamine and mianserin, alone and in combination with ethanol, on human psychomotor performance. *Pharmacol Toxicol* 1987;60:374–379).

clovoxamine + digoxin Clovoxamine has no effect on serum levels, volume of distribution, elimination half-life, or total body clearance of digoxin (Ochs HR, Greenblatt DJ, Verburg-Ochs B, Labedski L. Chronic treatment with fluvoxamine, clovoxamine and placebo: interaction with digoxin and effects on sleep and alertness. *J Clin Pharmacol* 1989;29:91–95).

Cloxazepam See **loxapine.**

cloxazolam (Olcadil) Benzodiazepine hypnotic not available in the United States.

clozapine (Clozaril; Lepotex) (CZP, CLOZ) Atypical dibenzodiazepine antipsychotic marketed for the treatment of drug-refractory schizophrenia. It is chemically related to but pharmacologically different from the neuroleptic loxapine. It has a unique profile of activity at a variety of receptor classes (dopaminergic, serotonergic, adrenergic, histaminergic, and cholinergic). CLOZ produces greater dopamine turnover changes in the limbic system than in the corpus striatum. Quantitative autoradiographic studies clearly differentiate it from typical antipsychotics: it upregulates dopamine D_1, but not D_2, and downregulates serotonin $(5\text{-}HT)_2$ receptors; in contrast, haloperidol upregulates D_2 and has no effect on D_1 or $5\text{-}HT_2$ receptors. It also potently blocks $5\text{-}HT_{1C}$ and $5\text{-}HT_3$. It has been shown to exhibit a relatively strong preference for the D_4 receptor, which has greater affinity for CLOZ than any other antipsychotic (Van Tol HHM, Bunzow JR, Guan HC, et al. Cloning of the gene for human D4 receptor with high affinity for the antipsychotic clozapine. *Nature* 1991;350:610–619). Unlike typical antipsychotics, CLOZ produces only slight, transient elevations in serum prolactin levels, even at moderate to high doses. It appears less likely than standard antipsychotics to cause extrapyramidal symptoms and tardive dyskinesia, thus demonstrating that antipsychotic and extrapyramidal effects can be dissociated. Candidates for CLOZ are schizophrenic patients unresponsive to adequate clinical trials (800+ mg/day chlorpromazine equivalents for at least 6 weeks) of two or more typical antipsychotics. Lack of response is indicated by persistent, moderate-to-severe delusions, hallucinations, or thought disorders. Approximately 30% of patients resistant to standard antipsychotics improve with CLOZ. Follow-up of CLOZ-responsive schizophrenic patients for 22–36 months after initial response indicates that about 50% maintain improvement. Compared to the same period before CLOZ treatment, there was a significant decrease in the number and duration of hospitalizations, and patients were living more independently and had higher rates of employment (Miller DD, Perry PJ, Cadoret R, Andreasen NC. A two and one-half year follow-up of treatment-refractory schizophrenics treated with clozapine. *Biol Psychiatry* 1992;31:85A). CLOZ can be started immediately after discontinuation of the previous typical antipsychotic. Treatment is initiated with 12.5 or 25 mg/day and increased 25 mg/day unless cardiovascular effects or excessive sedation intervene. After achieving 175 mg/day, dosages may be increased at 50-mg increments until clinical response or side effects occur. Mean effective dose is about 400 mg/day. High doses may be needed for certain patients and may increase side effects. Plasma level monitoring indicates that CLOZ has a therapeutic threshold plasma level of 350 ng/ml; response occurs in about 65% of patients above this level and only in 22% with levels below it. Average dose of 380 mg/day is needed to achieve a plasma level of 350 ng/ml (Perry P, Miller D, Arndt SV, et al. Clozapine and norclozapine concentrations and clinical

response in treatment refractory schizophrenic patients. *Am J Psychiatry* 1991;148:231–235). Plasma levels can be significantly influenced by dose, sex, smoking, weight, and age. In addition to efficacy in treatment-refractory schizophrenia, CLOZ may be more effective than typical antipsychotics in nonrefractory schizophrenia (Kahn RS, Davidson M, Siever L, et al. Serotonin function and treatment response to clozapine in schizophrenic patients. *Am J Psychiatry* 1993;150:1337–1342). CLOZ may be effective in schizoaffective patients and patients with psychotic mood disorders who are treatment-resistant or intolerant of side effects of typical antipsychotics. It reduces drug-induced psychosis without worsening Parkinson's disease symptoms in patients with Parkinson's disease, who are very sensitive to the antipsychotic and the potential extrapyramidal effects of clozapine, both of which occur at very low doses (25–100 mg/day). Bipolar disorder patients with dysphoric mania, psychosis, and chronic disability refractory to lithium, standard antipsychotics, and anticonvulsants have responded favorably to CLOZ; improvement was sustained over a 3-to 5-year follow-up (Suppes T, McElroy SL, Gilbert J, et al. Clozapine in the treatment of dysphoric mania. *Biol Psychiatry* 1992;32:270–280). CLOZ side effects at regular doses are transient sedation (39%), hypersalivation (31%), tachycardia (25%), constipation (14%), hypotension (5%), hypertension (4%), weight gain (4%), and pyrexia. Weight gain is greatest during the first 16 weeks of treatment and decreases thereafter. In many patients, better clinical response is associated with weight gain; in others it is unacceptable and results in noncompliance; in a few patients it increases health risks associated with obesity. Polyserositis (general inflammation of serous membranes with serous effusion), pericardial effusion, and pleural effusion have been reported; whether they are a direct result of CLOZ therapy is unknown (Daly JM, Goldberg RJ, Braman SS. Polyserositis associated with clozapine treatment. *Am J Psychiatry* 1992;149:1274–1275). There is a case report of priapism (Seftel A, Tejada IS, Szetela B, et al. Clozapine-associated priapism: a case report. *J Urol* 1992; 147:146–148). Most serious side effects are seizures and agranulocytosis. Pregnancy risk category B. See **clozapine/agranulocytosis.**

clozapine/agranulocytosis Compared with standard antipsychotics, clozapine (CLOZ) causes a higher incidence of agranulocytosis; cumulative incidence in the United States is approximately 1–2%. CLOZ's granulocytotoxic effects may be produced by an immune-mediated mechanism or specific gene products contained in the major histocompatibility complex (MHC) haplotypes that may be involved in mediating drug toxicity (Lieberman JA, Johns CA, Kane JM, et al. Clozapine-induced agranulocytosis: non-cross reactivity with other psychotropic drugs. *J Clin Psychiatry* 1988;49:271–277; Lieberman JA, Yunis J, Egea E, et al. HLA-B38, DQw3 and clozapine-induced agranulocytosis in Jewish patients with schizophrenia. *Arch Gen Psychiatry* 1990;47: 945–948). A specific MHC haplotype (HLA-B16, variant B39, DR4, DQw3) may be associated with susceptibility to CLOZ-induced agranulocytosis (Pfister GM, Hanson DR, Roerig JL, Landbloom R, Popkin MK. Clozapine-induced agranulocytosis in a Native American: HLA typing and further support for an immune-mediated mechanism. *J Clin Psychiatry* 1992;53:242–244). HLA typing may prove to be useful in predicting risk. Early administration of filgastrim, a granulocyte macrophage colony-stimulating factor, reduces duration of .agranulocytosis in patients with the most severe form of CLOZ-induced bone marrow suppression (Gerson SL, Gullion G, Yeh HS, Masor C. Granulocyte colony-stimulating factor for clozapine-induced agranulocytosis. *Lancet* 1992;340:1097). In patients re-exposed to CLOZ, agranulocytosis recurred more quickly the second time. Patients with a history of CLOZ-induced agranulocytosis should not be re-exposed to it (Safferman AZ, Lieberman JA, Alvir JM, et al. Rechallenge in clozapine-induced agranulocytosis. *Lancet* 1992; 339:1296–1297). There is, however, a single case report of successful CLOZ treatment after agranulocytosis induced by other neuroleptics, suggesting non–cross-reactivity between CLOZ and other neuroleptics in induction of agranulocytosis (Bauer M, Mackert A. Clozapine treatment after agranulocytosis induced by classic neuroleptics. *J Clin Psychopharmacol* 1994;14:71–73).

clozapine/akathisia Clozapine causes a much lower incidence of rigidity, bradykinesia, and coarse tremor than typical antipsychotics. Reports indicating that clozapine has a low incidence of akathisia suggest that it should be investigated as a possible treatment for tardive akathisia (Levin H, Chengappa R, Kambhampati RK, et al. Should chronic treatment-refractory akathisia be an indication for the use of clozapine in schizophrenic patients? *J Clin Psychiatry* 1992;53:248–251; Safferman AZ, Lieberman JA, Pollack S, Kane JM. Akathisia and clozapine treatment. *J Clin Psychopharmacol* 1993;13:286–287; Friedman JH. Akathisia with clozapine. *Biol Psychiatry* 1993;33:852–853).

clozapine + anticholinergic Co-administration can cause moderate to severe anticholinergic toxicity.

clozapine + antihypertensive Co-administration may enhance the pharmacological effect of antihypertensives.

clozapine + atenolol Atenolol has been used successfully to counteract clozapine-induced tachycardia with no adverse interactions.

clozapine + benzodiazepine Co-administration can produce severe sedation, hypersalivation, hypotension, toxic delirium, collapse, loss of consciousness, and respiratory arrest. Symptoms usually occur within 1–2 days of starting high doses of clozapine (CLOZ) in patients taking long-acting benzodiazepines (BZDs) (Grohmann R, Ruther E, Sassim N, Schmidt LG. Adverse effects of clozapine. *Psychopharmacology* 1989;99[suppl]:S101–S104; Cobb CD, Anderson CB, Seidel DR. Possible interaction between clozapine and lorazepam. *Am J Psychiatry* 1991;148:1606–1607; Friedman LJ, Tabb SE, Sanchez CJ. Clozapine—a novel antipsychotic agent. *N Engl J Med* 1991;325:518). Although such reactions are rare, BZDs should be used cautiously when initiating CLOZ treatment. Whether BZDs increase frequency of respiratory arrest or sudden death due to other causes in CLOZ-treated patients, and whether risk is greater than with other drugs, is unclear. BZDs are sometimes needed to treat anxiety when initiating CLOZ in neuroleptic-free patients. Naber et al. report no additional adverse effects of the combination of BZDs and CLOZ (Naber D, Holzbach R, Perro C, et al. Clinical management of clozapine patients in relation to efficacy and side effects. *Br J Psychiatry* 1992;160[suppl 17]:54–59). Some therapists co-prescribe BZDs to treat agitation, anxiety, seizure disorder, or refractory psychotic symptoms in CLOZ-treated patients. In eight treatment-refractory patients, CLOZ (mean daily dose 860.50 mg) plus lorazepam (3.88 mg/day) or clonazepam (1.5 mg/day), for a mean duration of 15.44 months, produced significant improvement without serious respiratory depression or arrest. Results suggest that CLOZ-BZD therapy, when carefully monitored, may be safe and clinically effective for some patients (Grace JJ, Priest B, Yadav M. Long-term clozapine and benzodiazepines: eight case reviews. Presented at the 146th Annual Meeting of the American Psychiatric Association, San Francisco, May 1993). Clinicians need to compare the risk/benefit ratio of combining a BZD and CLOZ with the disadvantages of continued use of typical neuroleptic drugs. When the combination is first given, it may be desirable to have the patient hospitalized or observed in an outpatient setting for 2–4 hours (Meltzer HY. New drugs for the treatment of schizophrenia. *Psychiatr Clin North Am* 1993;16:365–385). See **clozapine + diazepam.**

clozapine + benztropine Benztropine has been used to successfully counteract clozapine-induced hypersalivation with no serious adverse interactions.

clozapine/breast milk Clozapine may be excreted in breast milk and may cause sedation, decreased sucking, restlessness or irritability, seizures, and cardiovascular instability in the nursing neonate. Clozapine-treated women should not nurse.

clozapine + bromocriptine Co-administration in the treatment of co-morbid psychosis in patients with Parkinson's disease produced clearing of psychotic illness, with no serious adverse interactions or worsening of parkinsonism (Wolk SI, Douglas CJ. Clozapine treatment of psychosis in Parkinson's disease: a report of five consecutive cases. *J Clin Psychiatry* 1992;53:373–376).

clozapine + buspirone Buspirone has been used to augment clozapine in some patients with no adverse interactions (Meltzer HY, Cola P, Way L, et al. Cost effectiveness of clozapine in neuroleptic-resistant schizophrenia. *Am J Psychiatry* 1993;150:1630–1638).

clozapine + captopril Either drug alone may cause agranulocytosis; co-administration increases risk.

clozapine + carbamazepine Co-administration is inadvisable for the following reasons. (a) Carbamazepine (CBZ), secondary to its effect on cytochrome P450 enzymes, may increase clozapine (CLOZ) clearance and interfere with its therapeutic effectiveness. After CBZ is discontinued, CLOZ plasma levels may rise within 2 weeks to levels well above the suggested therapeutic level of 1.1 mmol/L (0.35 mg/L) (Raitasuo V, Lehtovarra R, Huttunen MO. Carbamazepine and plasma levels of clozapine. *Am J Psychiatry* 1993;150:169). (b) Both drugs can cause agranulocytosis and aplastic anemia, and co-prescription may increase risk of adverse hematological reactions.

clozapine + chloral hydrate No significant adverse interactions between therapeutic doses have been reported.

clozapine + cimetidine Chronic cimetidine cotreatment with clozapine (CLOZ) may increase CLOZ serum levels and cause toxicity manifested by marked diaphoresis, dizziness, vomiting, generalized weakness, and postural hypotension, which resolves after cimetidine is discontinued. This pharmacokinetic interaction is attributed to inhibition of hepatic metabolism of CLOZ secondary to the effects of cimetidine on cytochrome P450 oxidative enzymes (Symanski S, Lieberman JA, Picou D, et al. A case report of cimetidine-induced clozapine toxicity. *J Clin Psychiatry* 1991;52:21–22).

clozapine + clonazepam Except for some transient sedation, no significant adverse interactions between therapeutic doses have been reported. Clonazepam's calming effect may reduce the need for increased clozapine (CLOZ) dosage in anxiety only partially mitigated by CLOZ.

clozapine + diazepam Co-administration can cause collapse with loss of consciousness, no visible respiration, and no measurable blood pressure. Symptoms are rare and promptly respond to appropriate therapy (Sassim N, Grohmann R. Adverse drug reactions with clozapine and simultaneous application of benzodiazepines. *Pharmacopsychiatry* 1988;21:306–307). See **clozapine + benzodiazepine.**

clozapine + diphenhydramine No significant adverse interactions between therapeutic doses have been reported.

clozapine + divalproex Priapism has been reported with co-administration for about 5 weeks. Attempts to renew treatment resulted in recurrence of priapism (Seftel AD, Saenzde Tejada I, Szetela B, et al. Clozapine-associated priapism: a case report. *J Urol* 1992;147:146–148). Whether priapism was due to the combination is uncertain since priapism has been reported with clozapine monotherapy (Ziegler J, Behar D. Clozapine-induced priapism. *Am J Psychiatry* 1992;149:272–273).

clozapine + electroconvulsive therapy (ECT) Clozapine (CLOZ) is associated with increased seizure risk as daily dosage increases (Haller E, Binder RL. Clozapine and seizures. *Am J Psychiatry* 1990;147:1069–1071). Spontaneous seizures following one ECT treatment was reported in a patient receiving CLOZ (800 mg/day), propranolol (60 mg/day), and diazepam (20 mg/day). CLOZ and propranolol were tapered over 14 days and stopped 4 days before ECT administration; diazepam was reduced to 5 mg/day 72 hours before ECT. It is unclear whether CLOZ contributed to seizures in this case. A 1-in-500 incidence of tardive seizure phenomenon following ECT has been reported (Fink M. CNS sequelae: risks of therapy and their prophylaxis. *In* Shagass C, Friedhoff A [eds], *Psychopathology and Brain Dysfunction.* New York: Raven Press, 1977). Relatively rapid tapering of long-term diazepam treatment also may have been a factor. It is recommended that 7–10 days should elapse between clozapine discontinuation and ECT administration (Masiar SJ, Johns CA. ECT following clozapine. *Br J Psychiatry* 1991;158:135).

clozapine/fever Drug fever has been reported with clozapine. Generally, it is transient and mild, seldom exceeding 101° F (38.3° C). Severe diarrhea with spiking fever requiring transfer to intermediate care was reported in connection with too-low doses (Patterson BD, Jennings JL. Spiking fever and profuse diarrhea with clozapine treatment. *Am J Psychiatry* 1993;150:1126).

clozapine + fluoxetine Co-administration may be useful in the treatment of schizophrenia (Cassady SL, Thaker GK. Addition of fluoxetine to clozapine. *Am J Psychiatry* 1992;149:1274). Obsessive-compulsive symptoms have developed during clozapine (CLOZ) treatment of chronic schizophrenia (Patil VJ. Development of transient obsessive-compulsive symptoms during treatment with clozapine. *Am J Psychiatry* 1992;149:272). In some patients symptoms did not resolve spontaneously, but responded to fluoxetine (FLX) (20–40 mg/day) with no compromise of CLOZ effectiveness (Patel B, Tandon R. Development of obsessive-compulsive symptoms during clozapine treatment. *Am J Psychiatry* 1993;150:836). FLX may potentiate CLOZ's capacity to induce convulsions either by increasing its serum concentration or by some additive effect. Drugs with known seizure potential should be administered very cautiously in conjunction with high-dose FLX. Co-administration also may result in CLOZ toxicity associated with elevated plasma levels.

clozapine/hyponatremia Acute hyponatremia (sodium 113 mmol/L) was reported in a 39-year-old woman with schizophrenia who received clozapine (350 mg/day) for 7 weeks. It reverted to normal after clozapine was stopped and fluid was restricted (Ogilvie AD, Croy MF. Clozapine and hyponatremia. *Lancet* 1992;340:672).

clozapine/hypersalivation Distressing and potentially hazardous excessive salivation occurs in about one-third of clozapine-treated patients. Dosage reduction or treatment with an anticholinergic drug may help. Amitriptyline (75–100 mg/day) added to clozapine (400–600 mg/day) may produce marked sustained improvement without exacerbating psychotic symptoms (Copp PJ, Lansent R, Tennent TG. Amitriptyline in clozapine-induced sialorrhea. *Br J Psychiatry* 1991;159:166). Clonidine, which causes dry mouth by suppressing sympathomimetic sialagogic mechanisms, also may be helpful. Usually, one patch containing 0.1 mg or 0.2 mg per week is sufficient (Grabowski J. Clonidine treatment of clozapine-induced hypersalivation. *J Clin Psychopharmacol* 1992;12:69–70).

clozapine + levodopa/carbidopa Some psychotic parkinsonism patients tolerate and respond well to co-administration; in others it may produce mild to marked orthostatic hypotension and obtunded sensorium (Wolk SI, Douglas CJ. Clozapine treatment of psychosis in Parkinson's disease: a report of five consecutive cases. *J Clin Psychiatry* 1992;53:373–376).

clozapine + lithium Co-administration may be effective in bipolar disorder unresponsive to lithium or anticonvulsants alone. However, neurotoxicity, neuroleptic malignant syndrome, seizures, confusional states, and dyskinesias have been reported (Blake LM, Marks RC, Luchins DJ. Reversible neurological symptoms with clozapine and lithium. *J Clin Psychopharmacol* 1992;12:297–298; Pope H, Cole J, Choras P, Fulwiller C. Apparent neuroleptic malignant syndrome with clozapine and lithium. *J Nerv Men Dis* 1986;174:493–494). The first fatal case of agranulocytosis in the United States occurred with CLOZ + lithium. Death occurred in association with lithium tapering and discontinuation, suggesting that lithium withdrawal may have played a role (Gerson SL, Lieberman JA, Friedenberg WR, et al. Polypharmacy in fatal clozapine-associated agranulocytosis. *Lancet* 1991;338:262–263). A nonfatal case of CLOZ-induced agranulocytosis during lithium treatment was reported in a 53-year-old schizoaffective woman of Ashkenazi origin. She was treated with granulocyte-macrophage colony-stimulating factor, 300 mg administered subcutaneously over 3 days without improvement. She was then treated with interleukin-3 (300 mg/day subcutaneously for another 16 days). Agranulocytosis lasted 27 days until complete recovery. Based on these two cases, criteria for CLOZ discontinuation (white blood cell count [WBC] <3000/mm^3 or granulocyte count >1500/mm^3) are insufficient for detecting agranulocytosis in the presence of lithium. Consistent tendency of the WBC to decrease from baseline levels is a better indicator for CLOZ discontinuation (Valevski A, Modai I, Lahav M, Weizman A. Clozapine-lithium combined treatment and agranulocytosis. *Int Clin Psychopharmacol* 1993;8:63–65). Reports of adverse interactions suggest that lithium should be used with CLOZ only if manic symptoms are not adequately controlled with CLOZ.

clozapine + lorazepam Addition of low-dose lorazepam (LOR) (1 mg orally or intramuscularly, or 2 mg intramuscularly) to clozapine (CLOZ) (100–200 mg/day) produced marked sedation, excessive sialorrhea, ataxia, and unresponsiveness to verbal stimuli, suggesting a clinically significant, synergistic, pharmacodynamic interaction. Benzodiazepines should be used cautiously when initiating CLOZ (Cobb CD, Anderson CB, Seidel DR. Possible interaction between clozapine and lorazepam. *Am J Psychiatry* 1991;148:1606–1607). There are reports, however, of response to combined treatment, deterioration after LOR withdrawal, and improvement with LOR resumption (Konafsky D, Lindenmayer J-P. Relapse following lorazepam withdrawal. *Am J Psychiatry* 1993;150:348–349). See **clozapine + benzodiazepine.**

clozapine + methylphenidate Methylphenidate up to 80 mg/day has been used with therapeutic doses of clozapine (CLOZ) to alleviate CLOZ-induced sedation with no adverse interactions or aggravation of psychosis.

clozapine/myoclonic jerks, drop attacks Myoclonic jerks and drop attacks have occurred in clozapine-treated patients and have been noted to precede grand mal seizures. Various types of clozapine-induced seizures (myoclonic, atonic, and grand mal seizures) may occur in the same patient (Berman I, Salma A, DuRand CJ, Green AI. Clozapine-induced myoclonic jerks and drop attacks. *J Clin Psychiatry* 1992;53:329–330; Gouzoulis E, Ozdaglar A, Kasper J. Myoclonic seizures followed by grand mal seizures during clozapine treatment. *Am J Psychiatry* 1993;150:1128). See **clozapine/seizures.**

clozapine/neuroleptic malignant syndrome Clozapine monotherapy has been reported to cause neuroleptic malignant syndrome (NMS). Lithium co-administration may increase the likelihood of NMS (Das Gupta K, Young A. Clozapine-induced neuroleptic malignant syndrome. *J Clin Psychiatry* 1991;52: 105–107; Anderson E, Powers P. Neuroleptic malignant syndrome associated with clozapine use. *J Clin Psychiatry* 1991;52:102–104; Miller D, Sharafuddin MJA, Kathol RG. A case of clozapine-induced neuroleptic malignant syndrome. *J Clin Psychiatry* 1991;52:99–101).

clozapine + nicotine Nicotine reduces the average plasma level of clozapine (CLOZ) in smokers compared to nonsmokers. Patients should be monitored closely after smoking cessation, since this may increase CLOZ serum level and side effects (Haring C, Fleischhacker W, Schett P, et al. Influence of patient-related variables on clozapine plasma levels. *Am J Psychiatry* 1990;147:1471–1475).

clozapine + nortriptyline Co-administration can be effective and safe for depression occurring during clozapine treatment for chronic schizophrenia.

clozapine-N-oxide (NOX) Metabolite of clozapine.

clozapine overdose In 150 acute overdoses, most frequent symptoms were impaired vigilance and tachycardia. Major complications were aspiration pneumonia associated with coma, electrocardiographic changes, hypotension leading to renal failure, and seizure. The most common cause of mortality has been aspiration pneumonia (Le Blaye I, Donatini B, Hall M, et al. Acute overdosage with clozapine: review of the available clinical experience. *Pharm Med* 1992;6:169–178).

clozapine/Parkinson's disease Over 100 patients with idiopathic Parkinson's disease (PD) have been treated with clozapine for psychosis or relief of tremor or akathisia. Some have responded to low doses (25–75 mg/day); others have required 75–250 mg/day. Those treated with 25–150 mg/day improved, usually within a week, with a reduction in hallucinations and delusions without any worsening of PD. Higher doses, however, were associated with more adverse effects: sedation, worsening of orthostatic hypotension, hypersalivation, and delirium. Some patients responded to 25–37 mg/day with no ill effects during an 8-month treatment program and upon withdrawal of clozapine (Ostergaard K, Dupont E. Clozapine treatment of drug induced psychotic symptoms in later stages of Parkinson's disease. *Acta Neurol Scand* 1988;78:349–350; Friedman JH, Lannon MC, Caley C. Clozapine for movement disorder patients: a retrospective analysis of 38 patients. *Ann Neurol* 1992;32:277; Wolters EC, Hurwitz RE, Mak E, et al. Clozapine in the treatment of parkinsonian patients with dopaminergic psychosis. *Neurology* 1990; 40:832–834; Bernardi F, Del Zompa M. Clozapine in the management of psychosis in idiopathic Parkinson's disease. *Neurology* 1990;40: 1151). Resting tremor in PD patients may respond to low doses (12.5 mg/day) of clozapine. In some patients, clozapine dosage has had to be raised to a maximum of 37.5 mg/day. In other patients, titration of the clozapine dosage to 75 mg/day has been effective; a high percentage have experienced sedation but no worsening of PD symptoms. Small clozapine doses may be an effective alternative in the treatment of parkinsonian tremors unresponsive to conventional agents (Friedman JH, Lannon MC. Clozapine treatment of tremor in Parkinson's disease. *Mov Disord* 1990;5:225–229; Pakkenberg H, Pakkenberg B. Clozapine in the treatment of tremor. *Acta Neurol Scand* 1986;73:295–297; Jones KM, Stoukides CA. Clozapine in treatment of Parkinson's disease. *Ann Pharmacother* 1992;26: 1386–1387; Scholz E, Dichgens J. Treatment of drug induced exogenous psychosis in parkinsonism with clozapine and fluperlapine.

Eur Arch Psychiatry Neurol Sci 1985;235:60–64; Bear J, Lawson W, Burns S, Tarke U. Clozapine in idiopathic parkinsons. *Biol Psychiatry* 1989;25:163A; Roberts HE, Dean RC, Stoudemire A. A clozapine treatment of psychosis in Parkinson's disease. *J Neuropsychiatry Clin Neurosci* 1989;1:190–192; Pfeiffer RF, Kang J, Graber B, et al. Clozapine for psychosis in Parkinson's disease. *Mov Disord* 1990;5:239–242; Kahn N, Freeman A, Juncos JL, et al. Clozapine is beneficial for psychosis in Parkinson's disease. *Neurology* 1991;41:1699–1700; Melamed E, Achiron A, Sharpiro A, Davidovicz S. Persistent and progressive parkinsonism after discontinuation of chronic neuroleptic therapy: an additional tardive syndrome? *Clin Neuropharmacol* 1991;14:273–278; Factor SA, Brown DB. Clozapine prevents recurrence of psychosis in parkinson's disease. *Mov Disord* 1992;7:125–131; Gershanik O, Garcia S, Papa S. Scipioni O. Analysis of the mechanism of action of clozapine in Parkinson's disease. *Mov Disord* 1992;7:101; Lew MF, Waters C. Treatment of parkinsonism with psychosis using clozapine. *Mov Disord* 1992;7:100; Linazasaro G, Suarez JA. Clozapine in Parkinson's disease: three years experience. *Mov Disord* 1992;7:100; Rosenthal SH, Fenton ML, Harnett DS. Clozapine for the treatment of levodopa-induced psychosis in Parkinson's disease. *Gen Hosp Psychiatry* 1992;14:285–286; Linazasaro G, Marti Masso JF, Suarez JA. Nocturnal akathisia in Parkinson's disease: treatment with clozapine. *Mov Disord* 1993;8:171–174).

clozapine + perazine Agranulocytosis has been reported (Grohmann R, Schmidt LG, Spiess-Kiefer C, Ruther E. Agranulocytosis and significant leukopenia with neuroleptic drugs. Results from the AMUP program. *Psychopharmacology* 1989;[suppl]:109s–112s).

clozapine + pergolide Co-administration in the treatment of co-morbid psychosis in patients with Parkinson's disease produced clearing of psychotic illness, with no serious adverse interactions or worsening of parkinsonism (Wolk SI, Douglas CJ. Clozapine treatment of psychosis in Parkinson's disease: a report of five consecutive cases. *J Clin Psychiatry* 1992;53:373–376).

clozapine + phenytoin Addition of phenytoin to clozapine (CLOZ) may increase CLOZ clearance by inducing hepatic cytochrome P450 oxidase enzymes, significantly decrease (65–85%) CLOZ steady-state plasma concentrations, and produce clinical deterioration requiring increased CLOZ dosage (Miller DD. Effect of phenytoin on plasma clozapine concentrations in two patients. *J Clin Psychiatry* 1991;52:23–25).

clozapine/polydipsia Case reports describing improvement in polydipsia with clozapine treatment indicate that it could be the first definitive treatment for the disorder. Longitudinal studies are needed (Verghese C, DeLeon J, Simpson GM. Neuroendocrine factors influencing polydipsia in psychiatric patients: an hypothesis. *Neuropsychopharmacology* 1993;9:157–166; Spears NM, Leadbetter RA, Shutty MS. Influence of clozapine on water dysregulation. *Am J Psychiatry* 1993;150:1430–1431).

clozapine/pregnancy As of 1993, at least 15 women were known to have been exposed to clozapine during gestation with no known adverse sequelae in their newborns (Lieberman J, Safferman AZ. Clinical profile of clozapine: adverse reactions and agranulocytosis. *In* Lapierre Y, Jones B [eds], *Clozapine in Treatment Resistant Schizophrenia: A Scientific Update.* London: Royal Society of Medicine, 1992; Waldman MD, Safferman AZ. Pregnancy and clozapine. *Am J Psychiatry* 1993;150:169).

clozapine/priapism Clozapine should be added to the list of antipsychotic agents that may cause priapism. Despite prompt intervention, impotence may still be a consequence (Ziegler J, Behar D. Clozapine-induced priapism. *Am J Psychiatry* 1992;149:272–273; Rosen S, Hanno P. Clozapine-induced priapism. *J Urol* 1992;148:876–877).

clozapine + ranitidine Co-administration is well tolerated, with no effect on clozapine (CLOZ) plasma level. Ranitidine may be more effective than cimetidine in alleviating CLOZ-induced nausea and dyspepsia.

clozapine reinitiation In patients who have had even a brief interval (2 days or more) off clozapine (CLOZ), treatment should be restarted with half a 25-mg tablet (12.5 mg) once or twice daily. If it is well tolerated, it may be feasible to titrate to the therapeutic dose more rapidly than recommended for initial therapy. However, a patient who previously experienced respiratory or cardiac arrest with initial dosing (but then was titrated successfully to a therapeutic level) should be retitrated with extreme caution even after only 24 hours' discontinuation. Patients and caregivers should be cautioned about interrupting CLOZ treatment and advised that interruptions of 2 or more days should prompt them to contact their physician for dosing instructions before restarting the drug.

clozapine + rifampin Rifampin may hasten clozapine elimination, lower its steady-state concentration, and possibly interfere with its therapeutic efficacy.

clozapine/seizures That clozapine (CLOZ) may induce seizures is substantiated by reports of CLOZ-induced generalized convulsions. Epileptics with a history of seizures of any type, or patients with organic brain disease, may be at greater risk for exacerbation of an underlying seizure disorder. Seizure history, however, is not an absolute contraindication for CLOZ use. Seizure incidence is 1–2% with dosages less than 300 mg/day, 4% with 300–600 mg/day, and 5% with 600–900 mg/day. Myoclonic epilepsy has been reported in patients receiving doses above 600 mg/day. Thus, seizures seem to be dose-related (Povison UJ, Noring U, Fog R, et al. Tolerability and therapeutic effect of clozapine. *Acta Psychiatr Scand* 1985; 71:176–185; Lindstrom LH. The effect of long-term treatment with clozapine in schizophrenia: a retrospective study in 96 patients treated with clozapine for up to 13 years. *Acta Psychiatr Scand* 1988;77:524–539; Haller E, Binder RL. Clozapine and seizures. *Am J Psychiatry* 1990; 147:1069–1071; Thompson AE, O'Grady JC, Walls TJ. Clozapine-related seizures. *Psychol Bull* 1992;16:515–516). See **clozapine/myoclonic jerks and drop attacks.**

clozapine syndrome Disorder of drive, mood, and hedonic functioning induced by clozapine.

clozapine/tardive dyskinesia Tardive dyskinesia may not respond to clozapine unless relatively high doses are given for at least several months (Liberman JA, Saltz BL, Johns Ca, et al. The effects of clozapine on tardive dyskinesia. *Br J Psychiatry* 1991:158:503–510).

clozapine + trazodone No significant adverse interactions between therapeutic doses have been reported.

clozapine + tricyclic antidepressant (TCA) Co-administration may increase incidence of delirium, possibly because of additive central cholinergic activity. Agranulocytosis has been reported (Grohmans R, Schmidt LG, Spieb-Kiefer C, Ruther E. Agranulocytosis and significant leukopenia with neuroleptic drugs. Results from the AMUP program. *Psychopharmacology* 1989;99:109–112).

clozapine + trifluoperazine Agranulocytosis has been reported (Adams CE, Riccio M, McCarthy D, et al. Agranulocytosis induced by clozapine with the early addition of trifluoperazine: a case report. *Int Clin Psychopharmacol* 1990;5: 287–290).

clozapine + valproate Some manic, mixed manic, or schizoaffective patients with manic symptoms, particularly those unresponsive to lithium or anticonvulsants alone, may respond to co-administration with no adverse interactions. It also has been used to decrease risk of clozapine-induced seizures. No data are available on valproate effects on clozapine plasma levels (Meltzer HY. New drugs for the treat-

ment of schizophrenia. *Psychiatr Clin North Am* 1993;16:365–385).

clozapine + valproic acid Co-administration is used to decrease risk of clozapine-induced seizures.

clozapine withdrawal dyskinesia Clozapine cannot induce tardive dyskinesia (TD) and may have therapeutic effects in TD; however, there is a case report of a patient with severe TD/dystonia who developed severe rebound dyskinesia after clozapine therapy was stopped abruptly after 1 month. Rebound dyskinesia resolved when clozapine was reinstituted (Votolato NA, Smith SL, Olson SC, Martin DJ. Rebound dyskinesia on the abrupt discontinuation of clozapine in a patient with tardive dyskinesia. Presented at the ASHP Midyear Clinical Meeting 1993).

clozapine withdrawal syndrome (Meltzer E. Clozapine withdrawal syndrome. *Psychiatric Bull* 1993;17:626)

Clozaril See **clozapine.**

cluster Computer-assisted pulse analysis program to assess total hormone secretion.

cluster analysis Set of statistical methods used to group variables or observations into strongly interrelated subgroups.

cluster headache See **headache, cluster.**

cluster random sample See **sample, cluster random.**

cluttering Disorder of speech fluency in which rate and rhythm of speech are affected and speech intelligibility is impaired. There are alternating pauses and bursts of speech that produce groups of words unrelated to the grammatical structure of the sentence (DSM-IV). Severity ranges from somewhat annoying but generally intelligible speech to virtually unintelligible speech. Cluttering is distinct from stuttering, which is characterized by irregular repetition of syllables, words, or phrases; hesitation and interruptions in the flow of speech; and accompanying facial grimaces. Stutterers are aware of their difficulties; clutterers usually are not. Stuttering prevalence in the general population is 1%; cluttering is much rarer, but prevalence is not established. Both may occur in members of the same family or in the same person; frequency of concordance is unknown (Weiss DA. *Cluttering.* Englewood Cliffs, NJ: Prentice-Hall, 1964).

C_{max} See **maximum plasma concentration.**

"coast to coast" Street name for central nervous system stimulants.

co-beneldopa (Madopar) Generic for a fixed dose combination of levodopa + benserazide used in the treatment of parkinsonism. Marketed in England. Also called "co-dieldopa." See **benserazide; levodopa.**

coca paste Cocaine preparation made by adding sulfuric acid, kerosene or gasoline to macerated coca leaves. The dry paste contains 40–90% cocaine sulfate, coca alkaloids, alkalis, and other by-products or contaminants. Used almost exclusively in South America, it is smoked, often mixed with marijuana or tobacco (Parper JA, Van Thiel DH. Respiratory complications of cocaine abuse. *In* Galantur M [ed], *Recent Developments in Alcoholism, volume 10: Alcohol and Cocaine: Similarities and Differences.* New York: Plenum Press, 1993, pp 363–377). Also called "basuco."

cocaethylene Ethyl ester of benzoylecgonine found in blood and urine of users of cocaine (COC) and alcohol, but not when only COC is used. In the presence of COC and alcohol, the liver metabolizes COC to its ethyl homolog, cocaethylene, which is equipotent to COC in inhibition of ligand binding to dopamine transporters, inhibition of dopamine reuptake, and ability to increase extracellular dopamine. It is reinforcing in animals. In humans, it provides the same feelings of euphoria and well-being as COC, only more intensely and for longer periods, which may explain why COC-dependent individuals frequently use alcohol in combination with COC. Cocaethylene is more lethal than COC (Sands BF, Cirualo DA. Cocaine drug-drug interactions. *J Clin Psychopharmacol* 1992;12:49–55). See **cocaine + alcohol.**

cocaine (COC) Alkaloid extracted from leaves of the plant *Erythroxylon coca*, native to South America. It has considerable influence on monoaminergic neurotransmission in the brain. Once absorbed, it is rapidly broken down by esterases (including cholinesterases) released simultaneously with dopamine in the brain. It has considerable influence on monoaminergic neurotransmission in the brain. It binds with high affinity to dopamine, norepinephrine, and serotonin uptake sites, preventing their reuptake from the synaptic cleft and leading to their increased concentration in the synapse (Ritz MC, Cone EJ, Kuhar MJ. Cocaine inhibition of ligand binding at dopamine, norepinephrine and serotonin transporters: a structure-activity study. *Life Sci* 1990;46:635–645). Chronic COC use may lead to a "serotonin-deficit" form of serotonin dysregulation (Galloway MP. Regulation of dopamine and serotonin synthesis by acute administration of cocaine. *Synapse* 1990;6:63–72). Principal human metabolites are benzoylecgonine and ecgonine methyl ester, which are excreted in urine, where they can be detected for at least 24 hours after COC use. COC is a potent sympathomimetic agent that potentiates actions of catecholamines in the autonomic nervous system. It is also a central nervous system stimulant, causing garrulousness, restlessness, excitement, feelings of increased muscular strength, enhanced alertness and sensory experience, elevated feelings of self-esteem and confidence, and euphoria. In animals and man it is a powerfully addictive euphoriant. When it is freely available, animals will self-administer COC until stopped by a seizure, then repeat the process until supplies are exhausted. Euphoria of acute administration is attributable to COC dopamine reuptake blocking. In clinical trials, drugs that modulate dopamine function (e.g., bromocriptine, carbamazepine, amantadine, flupenthixol, desipramine) have met with limited or equivocal success in the alleviation of COC craving. Chronic cocaine abuse produces a dopamine deficit manifested by (a) high prolactin levels that may persist for a month after COC discontinuation; (b) marked decrease in dopamine D_2 receptors (revealed by positron emission tomography [PET] studies) that may last at least 2 weeks; (c) mild parkinsonian tremors during cocaine withdrawal; and (d) anhedonia during COC abstinence. With sudden cessation of COC use, there is a relative decrease in postsynaptic dopamine availability. Neuroleptic malignant syndrome has been reported in association with COC abuse. In seven patients, respiratory failure and death ensued within hours (Kosten TR, Kleber HD. Rapid death during cocaine abuse. A variant of neuroleptic malignant syndrome. *Am J Drug Alcohol Abuse* 1988; 14:335–346). COC has local anesthetic and ischemic actions. Any site of repeated application is likely to be damaged (e.g., nosebleed, abscesses, asthma). See **cocaine binging.**

cocaine abuse In humans, compulsive cocaine (COC) use occurs even when tolerance to euphorigenic actions has developed. There are distinct phases in the COC abuse cycle, including euphoria, crash, and craving, based on clinical symptoms and length of drug-free interval. Mood and motivation are lowered in the intervals between episodes of taking COC, but improve briefly during bouts of drug-taking, creating a vicious cycle with higher and higher doses needed to achieve any temporary relief. Such repeated use depresses dopamine synthesis; in time, toxic dopamine metabolites kill cells in the midbrain, and regulation of D_2 receptors in forebrain terminal fields is disrupted (Gawin F, Ellinwood EH. Cocaine and other stimulants: actions, abuse and treatment. *N Engl J Med* 1988;318: 1173–1182). There is no evidence that such toxic effects are reversible.

cocaine abuse/extrapyramidal susceptibility Cocaine (COC) abusers frequently have symptoms for which a neuroleptic may be indicated. COC abuse is associated with marked susceptibility to development of an acute neuroleptic-induced dystonic reaction.

cocaine/administration methods Cocaine (COC) is self-administered by snorting or sniffing, freebase smoking, and intravenous injection. See **cocaine adverse effects/intravenous use; cocaine adverse effects/nasal use; cocaine adverse effects/smoking.**

cocaine adverse effects/intravenous use Bloodborne elements secondary to nonsterile needle use include human immunodeficiency virus (HIV), hepatitis A and B and delta agent, and non-A and non-B infections. Inadvertent arterial injection can cause intense vasoconstriction with resultant gangrene. Contamination with cocaine adulterants (e.g., local anesthetics, sugar, toxins) can produce complications. Inert compounds (e.g., talc, cornstarch) may produce pulmonary vascular fibrosis and thrombi, resulting in pulmonary hypertension. Pulmonary parenchymal disease with atelectasis and granuloma formation are seen alone or together with granulomas in the brain, liver, and spleen (Taylor WA, Slaby AE. Acute treatment of alcohol and cocaine emergencies. *In* Galanter M [ed], *Recent Developments in Alcoholism, volume 10: Alcohol and Cocaine: Similarities and Differences.* New York: Plenum Press, 1992, pp 179–191).

cocaine adverse effects/nasal use Snorting can cause intense vasoconstriction that may result in inflammation and ulceration of the nasal septum, culminating in some patients in perforations that may require surgical correction. Rhinitis, sinusitis, ethmoiditis, and nasal bleeding also may occur (Taylor WA, Slaby AE. Acute treatment of alcohol and cocaine emergencies. *In* Galanter M [ed], *Recent Developments in Alcoholism, volume 10: Alcohol and Cocaine: Similarities and Differences.* New York: Plenum Press, 1992, pp 179–191).

cocaine adverse effects/smoking Freebase and crack users smoking cocaine (COC) may show evidence of obstructive airway disease, hoarseness, and bronchitis. Pneumomediastinum and pneumopericardium can result from COC inhalation (Taylor WA, Slaby AE. Acute treatment of alcohol and cocaine emergencies. *In* Galanter M [ed], *Recent Developments in Alcoholism, volume 10: Alcohol and Cocaine: Similarities and Differences.* New York: Plenum Press, 1992, pp 179–191).

cocaine + alcohol Alcohol is often coabused with cocaine. A national U.S. survey in 1990 found that over 90% of all cocaine abusers used alcohol and cocaine concomitantly during the month preceding the interview, and 75% reported using each of these substances at the same time on at least one occasion during the previous month (Grant BF, Harford TC. Concurrent and simultaneous use of alcohol with cocaine: results of a national survey. *Drug Alcohol Dep* 1990;25:97–104). In a study of acute effects of co-administration, subjective perception of intoxication "high" was significantly more pronounced after both drugs than after alcohol alone (Manelli P, Janiri L, Tempesta E, Jones RT. Prediction in drug abuse: cocaine interactions with alcohol and buprenorphine. *Br J Psychiatry* 1993; 163[suppl 2]:39–45). The enhanced and prolonged euphoria from alcohol and cocaine reported in most users was confirmed by subjective and electroencephalogram (EEG) data in this study (Farre M, Llorenti M, Ugena B, et al. Interaction of cocaine with ethanol: a pilot study in humans. *In Abstracts, 1990.* Richmond: Committee on Problems of Drug Dependence, 1990). Combining cocaine and alcohol enhances cocaine-induced hepatotoxicity (Boyer CS, Petersen DR. Potentiation of cocaine mediated hepatotoxicity by acute and chronic alcohol. *Alcohol Clin Exp Res* 1990;14: 28–31). It also produces neuroactive compounds in the body, including an active metabolite, cocaethylene. Co-administration in rats produces neurobiological changes resulting in enhanced anxiogenic responses to cocaine during the withdrawal period. Thus, polyabuse of alcohol and cocaine over long periods may exacerbate anxiety-related symptoms associated with cocaine abuse, further promoting abuse of anxiolytic drugs, which themselves are known to produce dependence (Prather PL, Lal H. Protracted withdrawal: sensitization of the anxiogenic response to cocaine in rats concurrently treated with ethanol. *Neuropsychopharmacology* 1992;6:23–29). Relatively little is known about combined use effects on the cardiovascular system; it does increase heart rate significantly more than predicted by an effect-addition model of drug interaction. In a study of overdose deaths, persons with underlying coronary artery disease had an approximately 18-fold increased risk of sudden death when alcohol and cocaine were used together compared with cocaine alone (Rose S, Hearn WL, Hince GW, et al. Cocaine and coca ethylene concentration in human post-mortem cerebral cortex. *Soc Neurosci Abstr* 1990;16:14). See **cocaethylene.**

Cocaine Anonymous (CA) Self-help group for cocaine addicts similar in many respects to Alcoholics Anonymous.

cocaine baby Child exposed to cocaine in utero. Those who survive may have permanent neurological damage, including visual impairments, mental retardation, symptoms of stroke, and impaired ability to learn to function (Gold MS. Cocaine (+crack): clinical aspects. *In* Lowenson JH, Ring P, Millman RB [eds], Langrod JG [assoc ed], *Substance Abuse. A Comprehensive Textbook*, 2nd ed. Baltimore: Williams & Wilkins, 1992; pp 205–221). See **cocaine/neonate, cocaine/pregnancy.**

cocaine binging Use of more than 4 g/day for 2 or more days, during which abusers become unable to stop using until cocaine (COC) supply is exhausted. Up to 15–25 intravenous injections in a single day are not uncommon, with boluses readministered as often as every 10 minutes as users attempt to recreate the rush of COC euphoria. Those injecting every 10–15 minutes may leave the needle in their vein and top it up every few minutes. Abusers average 1–3 binges/week, lasting from 8 to 24 hours. During binges, they have no interest in sex, nourishment, sleep, safety, survival, money, morality, loved ones, or responsibility. After binging, abusers may go 1/2 day to 5 days with no COC use. Shortly after cessation of binging, COC withdrawal syndrome begins. See **cocaine withdrawal.**

"cocaine blues" Street term for a moderate to severe depressed state that sometimes follows withdrawal from cocaine.

cocaine/breast milk Cocaine (COC) is found in human breast milk for hours, disappearing at a rate of only 4–5% in 2 hours. Infants appear highly susceptible to effects of COC exposure during breast feeding. COC intoxication with seizures have been reported in breastfed neonates. There also is a report of toxicity in an infant who nursed after the mother used topical COC powder as an anesthetic for nipple soreness. Breast feeding should be avoided by nursing women using COC (Young SL, Vosper HJ, Phillips SA. Cocaine: its effects on maternal and child health. *Pharmacotherapy* 1992;12:2–17).

cocaine + buprenorphine Sublingual buprenorphine maintenance (12–16 mg/day) suppresses illicit opioid use and attenuates cocaine use. It has no significant effects on cocaine euphoria (Schottenfeld RS, Pakes J, Ziedonis D, Kosten TR. Buprenorphine: dose-related effects on cocaine and opioid use in cocaine-abusing opioid-dependent humans. *Biol Psychiatry* 1993;34:66–74). In a study of acute co-administration effects, the "high" from a relatively low dose of buprenorphine was more intense and longer-lasting than that from cocaine, and subjects preferred the combination of the two drugs (Manelli P, Janiri L, Tempesta E, Jones RT. Prediction in drug abuse: cocaine interactions with alcohol and buprenorphine. *Br J Psychiatry* 1993;163[suppl 21]:39–45).

cocaine bug Common, unpleasant, tactile paraesthesia that may appear during withdrawal from cocaine. Sensations are described as itching, biting, crawling, or sticking due to an insect. Also called "Magnan's sign."

cocaine/cardiovascular effects Intense peripheral vasoconstriction, increased heart rate, increased myocardial oxygen demand, and hypertension believed to be due to the interaction of catecholamine and other vasoconstrictive substances on receptor sites leading to release and reuptake blockade of norepinephrine and dopamine. Effects are dose-related and may be complicated by concomitant use of other drugs (e.g., opiates, alcohol, barbiturates, and amphetamines) (Taylor WA, Slaby AE. Acute treatment of alcohol and cocaine emergencies. *In* Lowenson JH, Ring P, Millman RB [eds], Langrod JG [assoc ed], *Substance Abuse. A Comprehensive Textbook*, 2nd ed. Baltimore: Williams & Wilkins, 1992; pp 179–191).

cocaine/choreoathetoid movements Abnormal movements associated with cocaine use are rare (1 in 100+ cases). These include chorea, tics, dystonia, operoclonus, and bruxism. They tend to occur in young abusers (ages 21–29) during acute intoxication or the next 24 hours. They are self-limiting and of short duration (3–5 days). They may be due to increased basal ganglia dopamine secondary to reuptake blockade, or to basal ganglia ischemia induced by cocaine vasoconstriction (Daras M, Koppel BS, Atos-Radgion E, Tuchman AJ. Cocaine-induced choreoathetoid movements. *Neurology* 1993;43[suppl]:A309).

cocaine/cornea Infectious keratitis and corneal epithelial defects have occurred in crack cocaine users (Sachs R. Corneal complications associated with the use of crack cocaine. *Ophthalmology* 1993;100:187–191).

cocaine craving, cue-precipitated After cocaine (COC) withdrawal symptoms subside, exposure to a stimulus associated with previous use can provoke craving and further use. Cues include mood; availability of COC; and/or proximity of other users, pipes, or other paraphernalia. They may produce a powerful sensation of stimulation similar to a COC high (Allen DF, Jekel JF. *Crack: The Broken Promise.* London: Macmillan Press, 1991). If not reacted to or followed by COC use, cues gradually lose their effect by the process of extinction (Powell J, Gray JA, Bradley BP, et al. The effects of exposure to drug-related cues in detoxified opiate addicts: a theoretical review and some new data. *Addict Behav* 1990;15:339–

354; Strang J, Johns A, Caan W. Cocaine in the UK—1991. *Br J Psychiatry* 1993;162:1–13).

cocaine dependence Syndrome manifested by such symptoms as hypertension, sweating, central nervous system excitation, overestimation of physical and mental capacities, and pleasurable illusions and hallucinations. Dependence can occur without the clear physiological withdrawal symptoms found with alcohol, benzodiazepines, and opiates. Thoughts about obtaining and using cocaine seem to be linked more closely with repeating and sustaining euphoric effects than perceived need to relieve withdrawal symptoms. However, users do describe a withdrawal syndrome that has been observed in clinical settings.

cocaine + desipramine Desipramine (DMI) may reduce use and craving for cocaine (COC), as well as frequency, intensity, and duration of COC binges. Patients maintained on DMI report both a reduction in desire or need to use COC beyond the several days of abstinence between binges and a reduced desire to prolong their binges. Although DMI may not alter a COC "high," it attenuates desire for COC (Kosten TR, Morgan CH, Falcione J, Schottenfeld RS. Pharmacotherapy for cocaine-abusing methadone maintained patients using amantadine or desipramine. *Arch Gen Psychiatry* 1992;49:894–898; Ardnt I, Dorozynsky L, Woody G, et al. Desipramine treatment of cocaine dependence in methadone maintenanced patients. *Arch Gen Psychiatry* 1992;49:888–893). Combined use has not produced serious cardiotoxic effects (Kosten T, Garvin FH, Silverman DG, et al. Intravenous cocaine challenges during desipramine maintenance. *Neuropsychopharmacology* 1992;7:169–176).

cocaine euphoria Up to 80% of regular high-dose cocaine users may show acute effects of disinhibition, euphoria, impaired judgment, grandiosity, impulsiveness, hypersexuality, compulsively repeated actions, and marked psychomotor agitation with decreased fatigue. The state is clinically similar to hypomanic or manic episodes, but often subsides within 30 minutes (Gawin F, Ellinwood EH. Cocaine and other stimulants: actions, abuse and treatment. *N Engl J Med* 1988;318:1173–1182; Strang J, Johns A, Caan W. Cocaine in the UK—1991. *Br J Psychiatry* 1993;162:1–13).

cocaine gene Gene for the rat brain protein on which cocaine acts to produce its euphoric and addictive effects, cloned in 1991. The protein, located at nerve endings of brain cells, pumps dopamine back into the nerve terminals from which it was released. Cocaine binds to the pump and clogs it, flooding with dopamine the narrow space between sending and receiving brain cells and causing the euphoric "rush." The gene that makes the protein is called the "dopamine transporter" (Shimada S, Kitayama S, Lin C, et al. Cloning and expression of a cocaine-sensitive dopamine transporter complimentary DNA. *Science* 1991;254:576–578).

cocaine hallucinosis With continued cocaine use, euphoric stimulation becomes dysphoria. Hallucinations can appear in several modalities: voices may be heard, lights sparkle at the edge of the field of vision ("snow lights"), and insects may be felt under the skin ("cocaine bugs") (Strang J, Johns A, Caan W. Cocaine in the UK—1991. *Br J Psychiatry* 1993;162:1–13). See **"cocaine bug"; "snow light."**

cocaine + methadone Methadone may increase or prolong cocaine euphoria ("speedball" effects) or attenuate the anxiety and dysphoria associated with cocaine use (Schottenfeld RS, Pakes J, Ziedonis D, Kosten TR. Buprenorphine: dose-related effects on cocaine and opioid use in cocaine-abusing opioid-dependent humans. *Biol Psychiatry* 1993;34:66–74).

cocaine + monoamine oxidase inhibitor (MAOI) Recreational drug use, especially cocaine use, increases risk of hypertensive crises during or within several weeks of discontinuation of MAOI therapy (Devabhaktuni RV, Jampala VC. Using street drugs while on MAOI therapy. *J Clin Psychopharmacol* 1987;7:60–61).

cocaine/neonate Neonatal complications associated with maternal cocaine (COC) use include congenital malformations, decreased fetal growth, seizures, cerebral infarction and hemorrhage, auditory system deficits, sudden infant death syndrome, cardiac arrhythmias, necrotizing enterocolitis, and behavioral changes. Developmental delay continues throughout the first year of life (Young SL, Vosper HJ, Phillips SA. Cocaine: its effects on maternal and child health. *Pharmacotherapy* 1992;12:2–17). In one study of 137 children exposed to COC in utero, 21 were premature and 2 died of sudden infant death syndrome (Weathers WT, Crane MM, Sauvain KJ, Blackhurst DW. Cocaine use in women from a defined population: prevalence at delivery and effects on growth in infants. *Pediatrics* 1993;91:350–354). A retrospective study of 70 children exposed to cocaine in utero showed significant neurodevelopmental abnormalities, including language delay in 94% and extremely high frequency of autism (11.4%); the high rate of autistic disorders, which is not known to occur in children exposed to alcohol or opiates alone, suggests specific cocaine effects (Davis E, Fennoy I, Laraque D, et al. Autism and developmental abnormalities in children with perinatal cocaine exposure. *J Natl Med Assoc* 1992;84:315–319). Neurobehavioral assessments of 56 neonates exposed to cocaine prenatally disclosed significantly depressed performances on the habituation cluster, but not on other neurobehavioral assessment clusters (Mayes LC, Granger RH, Frank MA, et al. Neurobehavioral profiles of neonates exposed to cocaine prenatally. *Pediatrics* 1993;91:778–783). See **cocaine/pregnancy.**

cocaine overdose Manifestations include euphoria, disorientation, behavioral changes, mydriasis, acute toxic psychosis, and coma that can be misconstrued as a primary psychiatric illness. There may be acute cardiac events, vascular ruptures, excited delirium, agitation, hyperthermia, seizures, blood glucose abnormalities, and a myriad of other signs and symptoms. Chronic COC abuse is associated with left ventricular hypertrophy. Infection is a common fatal complication of intravenous use. Use of noninjected COC is also associated with human immunodeficiency virus (HIV) exposure, particularly through exchange of sex for drugs. COC use has been associated with fatal accidents, suicides, and homicides. With the exception of alcohol, no other drug of abuse is so closely linked to violent, premature death. Overdose death usually occurs very rapidly, with respiratory collapse often preceded by excited delirium or dysphoria, hyperthermia, grand mal seizures, or malignant arrhythmias (Wetli CW, Fishbain DA. Cocaine-induced psychosis and sudden death in recreational cocaine users. *J Forens Sci* 1985;30:873–880). Although vascular, respiratory, thermoregulatory, and cardiac dysfunctions are frequently associated with COC overdose, the physiological and biochemical sequelae of administration of amounts that result in death are not well understood.

cocaine/pregnancy Male cocaine (COC) use has been linked to abnormal development of offspring. Recent research suggests that sperm may act as a vector to transport COC into an ovum. Maternal COC use during pregnancy may increase incidence of premature delivery, low birth weight, shorter length, smaller head circumference, smallness for gestational age, and abruption of the placenta that may result in fetal death. Infants' neurobehavioral characteristics commonly include sleep pattern disturbances, tremor, motor hyperactivity, feeding difficulties, hypotonia, vomiting, sneezing, a high-pitched cry, and tachypnea. COC effects can also include autism, suspected retardation, or other nervous system deficits. The neuroteratology of COC results from its rapid transit across the placenta and fetal blood-brain barriers, as well as abrupt increases in maternal blood pressure and placental vasoconstriction, and increased uterine

contractibility in response to increased levels of norepinephrine. Brain imaging studies in COC newborns have revealed ischemic cerebral lesions that, when large, may lead to clinical manifestations (Volpe JJ. Effect of cocaine use on the fetus. *N Engl J Med* 1992; 327:399–407; Dixon SD, Bejar R. Echoencephalographic findings in neonates associated with maternal cocaine and methamphetamine use: incidence and clinical correlates. *J Pediatr* 1989;115:770–778; Handler A, Kistin N, Davis F, Ferre C. Cocaine use during pregnancy: perinatal outcomes. *Am J Epidemiol* 1991;133:818–825; Gratacos E, Torres PJ, Antolin E. Use of cocaine during pregnancy. *N Engl J Med* 1993;329:667). Acute COC withdrawal symptoms are usually mild to absent in infants. Long- term effects on intelligence and school behavior are not yet known (Corwin MJ, Lester BM, Sepkoski C, et al. Effects of in utero cocaine exposure on newborn acoustical cry characteristics. *Pediatrics* 1992;89:1199–1203). A 2-year follow-up of infants exposed to COC and cannabis and/or alcohol found that by 1 year of age, they had caught up in mean length and weight compared to control subjects (Chasnoff IJ, Griffith DR, Freier C, Murray J. Cocaine/polydrug use in pregnancy: two-year follow-up. *Pediatrics* 1992;89:284–289). A meta-analysis to examine fetal effects of COC use during pregnancy indicated that it was associated with very few fetal adverse effects. Results, however, depended on the type of comparison conducted. When infants exposed to COC were compared to middle-class nonusers, COC groups were often different from control groups. When compared to infants exposed in utero to other drugs of abuse, but not COC, most differences were eliminated (Koren G, Graham K. Cocaine in pregnancy: analysis of fetal risk. *Vet Hum Toxicol* 1992;34:263–264). See **cocaine/neonate.**

cocaine psychosis Toxic reaction induced by chronic cocaine (COC) use characterized by paranoid (persecutory) delusions and hallucinations. The most common paranoid delusion centers on being followed or sought by law enforcement agents. Most common hallucinations are auditory, but visual, tactile, and olfactory hallucinations may occur; they are typically focused on activities related to illicit drug abuse and usually consistent with the delusional system. Subjects lack insight and may become violent. Hypomanic symptoms with irritability, impaired concentration, pressured speech, disorganized thoughts, and grandiosity also can occur. Depressive symptoms, especially during the withdrawal stage and/or early abstinence stage, are common (Taylor WA, Slaby AE. Acute treatment of alcohol and cocaine emergencies. *In* Galanter M [ed], *Recent Developments in Alcoholism, volume 10: Alcohol and Cocaine: Similarities and Differences.* New York: Plenum Press, 1992, pp 179–191). Behavioral stereotypies are noted in about 40% of individuals with COC psychosis; others develop cataleptic-like behavior, depression, social withdrawal, and abnormal involuntary movements. COC psychosis is more likely to be induced by inhalation or intravenous intake than by oral or intranasal administration. Often, the first psychotic episode follows change from the intranasal to the intravenous or inhalation route of administration. Amount of COC used is a stronger predictor of development of psychosis than duration of use; however, with continued use, psychotic episodes occur with increasing frequency and onset is more rapid, even though in many cases COC dose remains stable or decreases. This may be due to kindling or behavioral sensitization (Hall WC, Talbert RL, Ershefsky L. Cocaine abuse and its treatment. *Pharmacotherapy* 1990;10:47–63). Psychosis is usually transient (24 hours), but may be prolonged after long binges or if there is pre-existing functional psychiatric illness (Gawin F, Ellinwood EH. Cocaine abuse treatment: open pilot trial with desipramine and lithium carbonate. *Arch Gen Psychiatry* 1990;41:903–909). Risk appears to be higher in males. COC psychosis and that resulting from amphetamine are very similar (Fischman MW. The behavioral pharmacology of cocaine in humans. *In* Grabowski J [ed], *Cocaine: Pharmacology, Effects and Treatment of Abuse, NIDA Research Monograph 50.* Washington, DC: Department of Health and Human Services, 1984, pp 72–91; Angrist B. Cocaine and prior stimulant epidemics. *In* Volkow ND, Swann AC [eds], *Cocaine in the Brain.* London: Rutgers University Press, 1990, pp 7–24).

cocaine run Consumption of all available cocaine (COC) and all that the user can readily acquire. Between "runs" there may be a period of spontaneous detoxification accompanied by fatigue, exhaustion, depression, and episodes of craving ("crash"). See **cocaine binging.**

cocaine/seizures "Kindled" seizures are often associated with cocaine (COC) intoxication. Proposed mechanisms include hyperpyrexia, neurohumoral imbalances, and cerebral ischemia secondary to vasoconstriction. Risk escalates with repeated COC use because of increased central nervous system sensitization (Post RM. Clinical implications of a cocaine-kindling model of psychosis. *Clin Neuropharmacol* 1977;2:25–42). Seizures are prevalent in adolescents who are frequent (25–100 times)

COC users. Occurrence of seizures is or may be significantly higher in adolescents who smoke crack than in those who snort COC (Schwartz RH. Seizures associated with smoking "crack." A survey of adolescent "crack" smokers. *West J Med* 1989;150:213). Infants and young children are also susceptible to COC-induced seizures.

cocaine "snorting" Cocaine (COC) is frequently snorted (insufflation) or "tooted" in "lines" or "rails" about 1 ½ inches long and 1/8 inches thick. Powdered COC is poured onto a hard surface (mirror, glass, slab of marble) and arranged into lines with a razor blade, knife, or credit card. One line is snorted into each nostril via a rolled bill, straw, miniature "coke spoon," or specially grown fingernail.

cocaine/street names base (freebase), big flake, blow, C, candy, coke, crack, death hit (with strychnine), dust, flake, freebase, girl, girls and boys (with heroin), gold dust, happy dust, joy powder, lady, liquid lady (with alcohol), nose candy, nose powder, paradise, Persian heroin (freebase with high-purity heroin) pier, rock, rock candy, she, sleigh ride, snow, speedball (with heroin), sugar, toot, white lady, zoom.

cocaine/suicide Studies have shown that chronic cocaine (COC) users experience intense suicidal ideation, particularly in the withdrawal phase, that can last for several days immediately after a COC binge. Young COC abusers often commit suicide; 30% of those under age 30 who committed suicide in the San Diego Suicide Study (conducted in the early 1980s) had histories of COC use. In 1986, 7% of all COC-positive deaths in New York City were suicides (Tardiff K, Gross EM, Wu J, et al. Cocaine positive fatalities. *J Forensic Sci* 1989;34:53–63). After crack COC became widely available in New York City, autopsy determination of the prevalence of COC metabolites in persons who committed suicide in 1985 showed that one of every five subjects had used COC within days of death. In addition, alcohol was detected in one-half of all COC users at autopsy (Marzule PM, Tardiff K, Leon AC, et al. Prevalence of cocaine use among residents of New York City who committed suicide during a one-year period. *Am J Psychiatry* 1992;149:371–375).

cocaine/toxicity Manifestations include agitation, dilated pupils, tachycardia, hypertension, hallucinations, hypertonia, hyper-reflexia, hyperactivity, irritability, hyperthermia, arrhythmia, vasoconstriction, headaches, seizures, vertigo, tinnitus, and partial sensory loss. In severe cases convulsions, coma and metabolic acidosis may develop. Treatment with intravenously administered diazepam may be all that is necessary; intravenously administered propranolol may be warranted in severe cases. Acute effects of cocaine (COC) are dose-related, but clinical presentation also depends on the pattern and route of use and whether other drugs or alcohol have been used. COC's toxic effects are probably a result of its interference with noradrenaline and serotonin reuptake.

cocaine/violence In the early phase of cocaine (COC) intoxication, euphoria can quickly turn to irritability, agitation, suspiciousness, and violence, especially with crack or intravenous COC use. In a COC binge, suspiciousness may turn to paranoid delusional thinking and violence. Heavy COC use has caused manic-like delirium with severe violence. Craving for COC also may result in violence, as the addict desperately seeks more COC or the money to purchase it.

cocaine withdrawal Descriptions obtained from outpatients divide course of cocaine (COC) withdrawal into several phases: (a) "Crash" lasting up to 4 days and including symptoms of agitation and anorexia, followed by fatigue, exhaustion, depression, hyperphagia, hypersomnia, and diminished craving. (b) Withdrawal following the first 4-day period and lasting up to 10 weeks. In this phase, mood and sleep normalize but powerful COC cravings may still arise, especially in response to stimuli associated with COC use. There is a great danger of relapse during this period. (c) Extinction. Manifestations of the phases partly reflect the interplay of neurotransmitter depletion and learned responses. Treatment is essential to alleviate discomfort and psychological pain and to prevent relapse (Koob GF, Bloom FE. Cellular and molecular mechanisms of drug dependence. *Science* 1988;242:715–723). During the initial withdrawal phase, bromocriptine has been recommended to reduce craving; during the second phase, desipramine therapy has been recommended. However, efficacy is not overwhelming. Other drugs used without much solid evidence for efficacy include imipramine, trazodone, phenelzine, fluoxetine, sertraline, bupropion, lithium, neuroleptics (chlorpromazine, fluphenazine), mazindol, carbamazepine, buprenorphine, levodopa, and tyrosine. Some investigators have observed a nonphasic gradual decline of depression and craving in hospitalized COC addicts. Amantadine is probably as effective as bromocriptine and is perhaps less toxic, but its effectiveness in maintaining short-term abstinence may decrease with time (Thompson DF. Amantadine in the treatment of cocaine withdrawal. *Ann Pharmacother* 1992;26:933–935).

cocainism See **cocaine dependence.**

co-careldopa (Sinemet) Fixed combination of levodopa + carbidopa used in the treatment of parkinsonism. See **levodopa/carbidopa.**

cocktail, lytic See **lytic cocktail.**

COC-LOG Longitudinal database used to assess cocaine (COC)-associated emergency department patient visits in one particular emergency department. Data show that COC toxicity remained relatively constant over a 4-year period. Majority of use was through smoking crack; major differences in toxicity were not seen between this route and intravenous use. There was a relatively low prevalence of severe cardiac toxicity and deaths. In the first 3 years after emergency department discharge, deaths occurred almost twice as frequently as in age-, race-, and sex-matched controls. Urine drug testing of pregnant patients suggested that documentation of recent COC use by history alone underestimates prevalence by approximately 4 times (Watson WA. Longitudinal assessment of cocaine toxicity in emergency department patients. *J Pharm Pract* 1993;6:74–82).

cocooning Clinical sign of depression in geriatric patients manifested by requests that curtains be drawn between patient beds, keeping TV and radio turned off, wrapping up in a sheet or blanket, psychomotor retardation, depressed facies, hesitant speech, and slow response to verbal stimulation (Baker FM, Miller CL. "Cocooning": a clinical sign of depression in geriatric patients. *Hosp Comm Psychiatry* 1991;42:845–846).

"code" Simplified set of symbols (alpha and/or numeric) substituted for more complex descriptions of medical signs, symptoms, procedures, and diagnoses. Simple codes may be a few numbers that relate to a single word or phrase. Numbers themselves need have no meaning or relationship to any other numbers in the system. This type of coding allows for more rapid data input and uses little computer space. More sophisticated codes use a hierarchial structure in which numbers have intrinsic meaning for output as well as input (Westland MM. Coding: the mortar in the bricks of data analysis. *Drug Information J* 1991; 25:197–200).

codeine Drug, usually made from morphine, used as an analgesic or antitussive. Use may be associated with dependence, but addiction is less likely than with morphine. Also called "diamorphine."

codeine + monoamine oxidase inhibitor (MAOI) See **monoamine oxidase inhibitor + codeine.**

co-dependence Characteristic symptoms occurring in persons who live with a chemically dependent person (e.g., external referencing, caretaking, self-centeredness, control issues, dishonesty, frozen feelings, perfectionism, and fear). Co-dependence has generally replaced the concept of "enabling" and focuses attention on the suffering of those who live or have lived with a chemically dependent person.

co-dergocrine See **dihydroergotoxine.**

co-dieldopa See **co-beneldopa.**

codominance Expression of both alleles in the heterozygote.

codominant inheritance Genetic condition in which a heterozygote is phenotypically distinguishable from the homozygote.

codon Triplet of three bases in a DNA or RNA molecule that encodes a specific single amino acid according to the genetic code.

codon, nonsense Triplet of three adjacent bases of a DNA or RNA molecule that does not conform to the norm.

coefficient of correlation Degree of relationship between two sets of paired measurements. Coefficients are positive or negative depending on whether paired measures vary in the same or in opposite directions. They can be computed in a variety of ways. The most common assumes a straight-line relationship between the instruments (the product-moment method), and is referred to as r. Statistically significant correlation does not necessarily imply a cause and effect relationship. Also called "correlation coefficient."

coefficient of determination Square of the correlation coefficient. It is interpreted as the amount of variance in one variable that is accounted for by knowing the second variable.

coefficient of variation Standard deviation as a percentage of the mean. The standard deviation is divided by the mean, then multiplied 100 times to convert to a percentage. Coefficients of variation are independent of the units of observation and are useful when interest is on the size of variation relative to the size of observation. They are meaningful only if the variable is measured on a ratio scale.

cofactor Compound or ion that facilitates an enzyme-catalyzed reaction without being directly involved in it.

Cogentin See **benztropine.**

Cognex See **tacrine.**

cognition Intellectual functions including perceiving, remembering, imagining, conceiving, understanding, judging, and reasoning. See **cognitive deficit; cognitive skills.**

cognitive activator See **nootropic drug.**

cognitive behavior therapy Combination of behavioral and cognitive procedures used to change patients' behaviors, attitudes, and cognitive distortions such as low self-esteem (Fairburn CG, Jones R, Peveler RC, et al. Psychotherapy and bulimia nervosa. Longer-term effects of interpersonal psychotherapy, behavior therapy, and cognitive behavior therapy. *Arch Gen Psychiatry* 1993;50:419–428).

cognitive deficit Impairment in cognitive functions that has a variety of causes. For example, drug and alcohol abuse may cause persisting cognitive impairment because of the combined influences of direct action on the brain, indirect effects of drug use (lifestyle), disruption of organ-system integrity (liver, pancreas, heart), and infection.

cognitive enhancer See **nootropic drug.**

cognitive impairment disorder See **organic mental disorder.**

cognitive laboratory (COGLAB) Collection of test batteries administered by a microcomputer that can be finished in about 40 minutes by a normal college student and in 40–60 minutes by a patient with chronic schizophrenia (Spaulding W, Garbin CP, Crinean WJ. The logical and psychometric prerequisites for cognitive therapy of schizophrenia. *Br J Psychiatry* 1989;155:[Suppl 5]:69–73).

cognitive performance Higher brain functions (e.g., memory, image, and sound recognition; thinking; reasoning; judgment; fine and/or complex motor skills; acting on nontangible stimuli).

cognitive science Study of conscious experience. It encompasses phenomena ranging from introspection to mechanisms underlying sensory information processing.

cognitive side effects Drug-related cognitive deficits. They may be subtle; the patient is often unaware of them and is unlikely to spontaneously complain of them. Effects of benzodiazepines (BZDs) on memory are among the frequent cognitive side effects of these drugs. BZDs often impair the recall or utilization of information acquired before the drug was taken. Among the elderly, there is a statistically significant association of sedative-hypnotic drug use with cognitive impairment. See **cognitive toxicity/drug induced.**

cognitive skills Skills needed to carry out activities involved in intellectual function (e.g., perceiving, remembering, imagining, conceiving, understanding, judging, and reasoning). They are acquired during human development in a fairly predictable sequence. Mentally handicapped individuals seem to have a cognitive deficit or disability because their cognitive skills are poorly developed.

cognitive test Test that measures the higher functions of the brain (memory, language, speech, and arithmetic skills, decide and react, continuous performance, IQ).

cognitive theory Theory, developed by Aaron Beck in 1969, that thinking and meanings affect feelings and behavior; that cognitive activity can be monitored and altered; and that behavior change can occur through cognitive change (Dobson KS [ed]: *Handbook of Cognitive-Behavioral Therapies.* New York: Guilford Press, 1988). Cognitive theory forms the theoretical basis for cognitive therapy.

cognitive therapy Treatment pioneered by Aaron Beck, Dan Meichenbaum, and Michael Mahoney that shares some aspects of Albert Ellis's rational emotive therapy. It was originally formulated as a standardized, brief (15–20 sessions) form of psychotherapy for depression characterized by highly specific learning experiences. It was later developed for the treatment of anxiety and substance abuse and eating disorders, and was extended to provide a model for long-term psychotherapy as well. Each session consists of choosing the problem focus, cognitive work, assignment of homework, and a summary. Cognitive work entails gathering background details, identifying automatic thoughts and cognitive errors, proposing experiments, challenging cognitions or schemas, or generating alternative ways to view a problem (Schuyler D. *A Practical Guide to Cognitive Therapy.* New York: WW Norton, 1991). For example, in the treatment of depression, each persistent negative construct that accompanies depressed affect (e.g., I am a bad person; nobody likes me; I am going to fail) is identified, its frequency and circumstances are noted, and it is posed as a specific testable hypothesis to which rules of reason are applied and for which evidence is gathered from everyday events. To initially orient and involve patients, they may be assigned concrete reading material on coping with depression and written self-reports (e.g., a weekly activity schedule to chart tangible behaviors, a mastery and pleasure schedule to rank degree of gratification and accomplishment) (Young JE, Beck AT. Cognitive therapy: clinical applications. *In* Rush AJ [ed], *Short-Term Psychotherapies for Depression.* New York: Guilford Press, 1982).

cognitive toxicity/drug-induced Drugs that may induce cognitive toxicity include (a) psychotropics (tricyclic antidepressants, neuroleptics, benzodiazepines, lithium, psychostimulants, bromides, glutethimide, and meprobromate); (b) anticholinergic agents (e.g., anticholinergic antiparkinsonian drugs); (c) antihypertensives (methyldopa, propranolol, clonidine, diuretics); (d) anticonvulsants (barbiturates, phenytoin, ethosuximide); (e) anti-histamines; (f) narcotic analgesics; (g) antiparkinson agents (L-dopa, bromocriptine, pergolide); and (h) cardiovascular agents (digitalis, quinidine, procainamide).

cogwheel phenomenon Rhythmical, repetitive interruption of passive movement of a limb about a joint. Active cogwheel phenomena are repetitive interruptions to movement carried out by the patient.

cogwheel rigidity Form of cogwheel phenomenon assumed to be pathognomic of parkinsonism.

coherence Measure of linear correlation in the frequency domain between two signals. It is interpreted as the degree of coupling between two signals. Coherence of the electroencephalographic signal recorded from electrodes over different brain regions is assumed to index anatomical or functional coupling between the brain regions under the electrodes (Nagase Y, Okubo Y, Matsuura M, et al. EEG coherence in unmedicated schizophrenic patients: topographical study of predominantly never medicated cases. *Biol Psychiatry* 1992;32:1028–1034).

coherence with existing information See **biological plausibility.**

cohesiveness In group therapy, feeling of togetherness or esprit de corps experienced by group members. The patient feels accepted and no longer isolated from others (Bloch S, Crouch E. *Therapeutic Factors in Group Psychotherapy.* Oxford: Oxford University Press, 1985).

cohort Designated group of persons in a study who are followed over time.

cohort analysis Tabulation and analysis of morbidity or mortality rates in a specific group of patients (cohort) identified at a particular period and studied as they pass through different stages during their lifetime.

cohort analytic study Prospective investigation of factors that might cause a disorder in which a cohort free of the disorder but exposed to its putative cause is compared with a cohort also free of the disorder but not exposed to the putative cause. Both cohorts are followed to compare incidence of the disorder (Anon. Glossary of methodologic terms. *JAMA* 1992;268:43–44).

cohort effect Shared temporal experience, usually the year or decade of birth, that is associated with different rates of illness throughout life.

cohort study Observational study of a group of people with a specified characteristic or disorder who are followed-up over a period to detect new events. Distinguishing factors are (a) groups to be studied (cohorts) are defined in terms of characteristics evident prior to appearance of disorder being investigated; (b) cohorts are observed over a period to determine the frequency of the disorder among them. Cohort studies generally identify and compare exposed patients with unexposed patients or with patients who receive a different exposure. The major difference between cohort and case-control studies is the basis on which patients are recruited into the study. Cohort studies have the major advantage of being free of the major problem that plagues case-control studies: the difficult process of selecting a healthy control group. Cohort studies are performed by following a group of patients exposed to a drug and comparing their experience to that of an unexposed control group, or to patients exposed to another drug of the same class. Advantages of cohort studies are ability to study multiple outcomes and uncommon exposures, reduced chance of selection bias and biased exposure data, and ability to assess incidence. Disadvantages are possibly biased outcome data, expense (may take years to complete), lack of suitability for rare diseases, ability to study only a few exposures, and loss of subjects. Cohort studies are usually prospective, but may be retrospective.

"coke"   Street name for cocaine.

"coke bug"   Street name for the tactile hallucination that live insects are crawling on the skin, which is common with cocaine use.

"cokehead"   Street name for a person who uses cocaine despite its adverse effects.

"cold turkey"   Abrupt discontinuation of a drug on which a person is physically dependent without using any drug therapy to alleviate withdrawal symptoms. Originally the term referred to the goose flesh that typically occurs during severe opiate withdrawal. See **detoxification.**

colony-stimulating factor   (CSF) One of a group of molecules that can stimulate hemopoiesis in vitro. With the advent of recombinant DNA technology and gene cloning, sufficient amounts of pure material have been synthesized to allow development for clinical use. Two molecules, granulocyte colony-stimulating factor (G-CSF) and granulocyte-macrophage colony-stimulating factor (GM-CSF), are commercially available. GM-CSF molecules are (a) malgramostim (Leucomax); and (b) sargramostim (Leukine and Prokine). G-CSF molecules are (a) filgrastim (Neupogen); and (b) lenograstim (Neutrogin). CSFs reduce duration of severe neutropenia by enabling harvest of progenitor cells from peripheral blood. They may be of value in the treatment of aplastic anemia, myelodysplasia, and acquired immunodeficiency syndrome (AIDS);

indications are likely to increase (Steward WP. Granulocyte and granulocyte-macrophage colony-stimulating factors. *Lancet* 1993;342: 153–157).

color perfusion imaging   X-ray computed tomography (CT) combined with an injected contrast agent to create a quantifiable map of tissue perfusion displayed by means of a color scale. Spatial resolution is greater than with single photon or positron emission tomography (PET). It is more readily quantifiable than single photon emission tomography, since no scatter or attenuation corrections are required. The technique depends on a CT system with low levels of photon noise. It is potentially applicable to many CT systems already installed and it may be useful in both clinical diagnosis and research (Miles KA, Hayball M, Dixon AK. Colour perfusion imaging: a new application of computed tomography. *Lancet* 1991;337:643–645).

coma   Most profound degree of stupor, manifested by total loss of consciousness and voluntary activity. It may be caused by ingestion of toxic substances, trauma, or disease.

comagram   Addition to the techniques of monitoring electrophysiological changes in the brain during loss of consciousness.

coma vigil   See **akinetic mutism.**

combination   In genetics, hereditary variations that represent effects of hybridization and that occur in cross-bred products originating from union of two individuals with unlike hereditary equipment.

combination drug   See **fixed combination drug.**

command hallucination   See **hallucination, command.**

commingling analysis   Form of segregation analysis that looks for differences in distributions in a population.

communication disorder   Form of speech or writing that impairs communication because of aberrancy of terms, content, or form but not because of failure to follow semantic or syntactic rules. Examples include pressure of speech, tangentiality, echolalia, loose associations, flight of ideas, and perseveration.

community genetics   See **genetics, community.**

community psychiatry   Psychiatry practiced in the community, often in the context of a community mental health center (CMHC), although inpatient facilities are still an important component of most services. Community psychiatry may be more stressful and demanding than in-hospital based psychiatry because of absence of some of the support and backing commonly available in the hospital setting. It is most suitable for clinically experienced psychiatrists with a special interest in developing services and who particularly enjoy working closely with patients in the community.

co-morbidity Term coined by Feinstein (1970) to describe the phenomenon of overlap of disorders in one patient. In psychiatry, co-morbidity refers to occurrence within a defined period of time (e.g., lifetime, 6 months) of two or more mental disorders that have distinct etiologies (e.g., schizophrenia and toxic delirium or anxiety and depression). There is a marked tendency for substance abuse and schizophrenia to occur together, for depression to occur with borderline personality or anxiety disorders, and for post-traumatic stress disorder to occur with depression, anxiety, and multiple personality disorder (Maser JD, Cloninger CR, eds. *Co-Morbidity of Mood and Anxiety Disorders*. Washington, DC: American Psychiatric Press, 1990; Spiegel D. Multiple personality as a post-traumatic stress disorder. *Psychiatr Clin North Am* 1984;7:101–110). Co-morbidity complicates treatment, often leading to increased hospitalization and treatment cost, decreased compliance, and poor response (McLellan AT, Luborsky L, Woody GE, et al. Predicting response to alcohol and drug abuse treatments: role of psychiatric severity. *Arch Gen Psychiatry* 1983;40:620–625).

comparative trial Study in which a new drug is compared for therapeutic efficacy with a placebo or a known effective drug for the same clinical symptoms or disorder. It is the most common therapeutic experiment.

comparison group See **control group.**

compartment Hypothetical space, not necessarily corresponding to an organ or organ system, in which a drug or neurotransmitter has different kinetic characteristics. There are two principal compartments: central (brain) and peripheral (other body tissues). The majority of psychoactive drugs enter the central compartment first and from there are distributed to peripheral compartments.

compassionate use investigational new drug (IND) Protocol less formal than treatment IND in which experimental unapproved drugs or uses of a marketed drug are made available to patients outside the traditional IND framework. The drug may be a true experimental compound or a substance that has been studied or marketed abroad but lacks any U.S. experience.

Compazine See **prochlorperazine.**

compensatory hydrocephalus See **hydrocephalus.**

compensatory tracking task Interactive test of psychomotor function in which subjects use a joystick to keep a moving cursor aligned with a moving target while responding to visual stimuli (white lights) presented in the peripheral field of vision. The response approximates divided attention required in driving (Hindmarch I, Subhan Z, Stoker MJ. The effects of zimeldine and amitriptyline on car driving and psychomotor performance. *Acta Psychiatr Scand* 1983;68:141–146). Main response measure (RMS) error is calculated as the root mean square deviation of the joystick tracking the fixed program, with a lower score indicating more accurate tracking. Responses to the peripheral stimuli are made by the subject pressing the keyboard space bar.

competitive displacement Phenomenon that occurs when two drugs capable of binding to the same sites on the protein molecule are co-prescribed. When two drugs that extensively bind to plasma proteins (e.g., warfarin and chloral hydrate or phenytoin and warfarin) are co-prescribed, fewer binding sites are available for warfarin, thereby increasing the amount of free warfarin and the risk of bleeding.

competitive inhibition Inhibition of an enzyme or receptor that depends on the relative concentration of the inhibitor, substrate, or agonist.

complementary DNA (cDNA) DNA copy of messenger RNA (mRNA). cDNA is generated from mRNA by the enzyme reverse transcriptase encoded in the genomes of retroviruses. These viruses contain an RNA genome that is converted to DNA during a phase of their life cycle. The commercially available enzyme has a variety of laboratory uses; most common is generation of cDNA for cloning purposes. The procedure is one of the steps leading to a cDNA library.

complementary event Event opposite the event being investigated.

completion rate Percentage of subjects in a survey or study on whom complete data are available for analysis.

complex partial seizure See **seizure, complex partial.**

complex segregation analysis See **segregation analysis.**

compliance Extent to which behavior (taking medication, following diets, changing lifestyle) coincides with medical or health advice (Haynes RB. Introduction. *In* Haynes RB, Taylor DW, Sackett DL [eds], *Compliance in Health Care*. Baltimore: Johns Hopkins University Press, 1979, pp 1–7). In general, one-third of patients comply, one-third sometimes comply, and one-third do not comply (Porter AMW. Drug defaulting in a general practice. *Br Med J* 1969;1:218–222). Compliance is not associated with age, sex, marital state, race, or other demographic characteristics. It may be increased by physician characteristics of enthusiasm, permissiveness, age, experience, time spent with the patient, and short waiting time. Studies have shown that only three disease factors are determinants of compliance. (a) Psychiatric patients, especially those with schizophrenia, paranoia, or personality disorders, are generally low compliers. (b) When more symptoms are reported by patients, compliance rate is lower. This finding does not support the assumption that increasing severity of symptoms encourages compliance, but instead suggests that as people notice more symptoms they begin to give up on treatment. In addition, patients with symptomatic illness such as rheumatoid arthritis become less compliant. (c) The degree of disability produced by the disease positively influences compliance; increased compliance could be the result of disease severity or increased supervision due to disability (Haynes RB. Determinants of compliance: the disease and the mechanics of treatment. *In* Haynes RB, Taylor DW, Sackett DL [eds], *Compliance in Health Care.* Baltimore: Johns Hopkins University Press, 1979, pp 49–62). Compliance also may be influenced by duration of therapy, number of times a day a drug must be taken, time of day it must be taken, and cost. Behavioral strategies (e.g., reminders, special medication containers) improve compliance (Hussar DA. Improving patient compliance—the role of the pharmacist. *In* Improving Compliance: Proceedings of a Symposium in Washington, DC, November 1, 1984, by the National Pharmaceutical Council, Reston, VA, 1985).

compliance measurement Compliance can be measured directly and/or indirectly. Direct methods, which are less subject to bias, generally involve detection of a chemical in a body fluid (e.g., determination of plasma levels of the medication or a metabolite, or a marker). Indirect methods include therapeutic or preventive outcome measurements, impression of the physician or predictability, patient interview, prescription filling dates, and pill counts. Each method has inherent advantages and disadvantages.

compliance measurement/electronic Prescription vial containing a microprocessor recording device in the lid that identifies the date and time the vial is opened. Although it does not verify that drug was consumed, it provides an accurate record of when the vial was opened, supposedly for the purpose of taking the medicine. It should be able to identify those who falsely claim they are taking medicine as prescribed (Morris LS, Schulz RM. Patient compliance—an overview. *J Clin Pharm*

Ther 1992;17:283–295). A clear relationship has been established between adherence to the prescribed regimen, as determined by electronic monitoring, and clinical outcome (Cramer JA, Mattson RH, Prevey ML, et al. How often is medication taken as prescribed? *JAMA* 1989;261:3273–3277). Although not a panacea, electronic monitoring improves clinicians' and researchers' understanding of how patients take prescribed medication.

complementarity of interaction Probability that an interaction does not occur, which is obtained by subtraction from the unity.

comprehensive drug screen Service offered by many laboratories and used by physicians when a patient's drug abuse habit is unknown. Some laboratories usually perform the most inexpensive procedure, thin-layer chromatography (TLC); however, many results are negative because of TLC's low sensitivity and not because a drug or its metabolite is not present in the sample. Different laboratories may mean different things by "comprehensive drug testing." Unless physicians are familiar with the laboratory procedures and technical language, they will be less effective in diagnosing symptoms caused by drug use.

comprehensive psychometric evaluation Evaluation with four goals: (a) to acquire objective and quantitative information about current cognitive, emotional, and social functioning; (b) to facilitate understanding of the idiosyncratic and causal interrelationships among these three spheres of functioning; (c) to elucidate etiology of a substance use disorder with respect to its origin and relative contribution of cognitive, emotional, or social disturbances; and (d) to accrue information that identifies treatment needs of the patient.

compulsion Repetitive, seemingly purposeful behaviors performed according to certain rules or in a stereotyped fashion (DSM-IV). The behavior is not an end in itself, but is designed to produce or prevent some future event or situation. However, either the activity is not connected in a realistic way with what it is designed to produce or prevent, or it may be clearly excessive. The act is performed with a sense of subjective compulsion coupled with desire to resist the compulsion (at least initially). The individual generally recognizes the senselessness of the behavior (this may not be true for young children) and does not derive pleasure from carrying out the activity, although it provides a release of tension. See **obsessive-compulsive disorder.**

compulsive drug use Drug use characterized by high frequency and high intensity levels varying in duration, usually producing some degree of psychological dependence. Dependence is such that the individual cannot at will stop such use without experiencing physical discomfort or psychological disruption.

compulsive facial picking See **impulse control disorder.**

compulsive foraging behavior In crack cocaine (COC) users, compulsive searching for drug pieces the user believes may have been accidentally dropped or misplaced where the user has been smoking crack. The user may repeatedly inspect pockets, clothes, shoes and socks, the floor, carpet, furniture, or the route taken to the place in which drug use occurs. Anything resembling crack (pebbles, candle wax, food crumbs, plaster, bits of drywall, paint chips) is carefully examined. Although users usually know the search will be in vain, they describe varying degrees of inability to resist the urge to search. The compulsive quality of the foraging behavior is associated with intense craving for COC. Onset of the behavior is usually associated with exhaustion of the user's COC supply, but may occur between "hits." Mean length of time spent foraging is 90 minutes (Rosse RB, Fay-McCarthy M, Collins JP Jr, et al. Transient compulsive foraging behavior associated with crack cocaine use. *Am J Psychiatry* 1993;150:155–156; Brady KT, Lydiard RB, Malcolm R, et al. Cocaine-induced psychosis. *J Clin Psychiatry* 1991;52:509–512). Street terms include "chasing ghosts," "geeking," and "punding."

compulsive personality Lifelong pattern of perfectionism and inflexibility associated with overconscientious and constricted emotions (DSM-IV). The concept derives from early descriptions of anal character, believed to stem from fixation at the anal stage of development leading to the triad of obstinacy, parsimony, and orderliness (Kline P. Obsessional traits, obsessional symptoms and anal eroticism. *Br J Med Psychol* 1968;41:299–305).

compulsive sexual behavior (CSB) Periods of intense involvement in sexual activity that may occur in men or women. Some may be short-lived or may reflect normal developmental processes, but sexual obsessions and compulsions may also interfere with daily functioning or be accompanied by a variety of medical problems. CSB is characterized by behavior driven by anxiety-reduction mechanisms rather than by sexual desire. Obsessive thoughts and compulsive behaviors reduce anxiety and distress, but create a self-perpetuating cycle. Sexual activity provides temporary relief, followed by further distress. Those engaging in CSB put themselves and others at risk for sexually transmitted diseases, illnesses, and injuries; often experience moral, social, and legal sanctions; and endure great emotional suffering. People with CSB may experience motor tension (trembling, shakiness, headaches, muscle aches, inability to relax, fatigue), autonomic hyperactivity (shortness of breath, tachycardia, sweating, dry mouth, dizziness, nausea, diarrhea, frequent urination, trouble swallowing) or hypervigilance ("on edge," easily startled, difficulty concentrating, insomnia, irritability). There is high co-morbidity of CSB with anxiety disorders, depression, and alcohol and drug dependence. The many manifestations of CSB can be subsumed under two basic types: paraphilic and nonparaphilic CSB (Coleman E. Is your patient suffering from compulsive sexual behavior? *Psychiatr Ann* 1992;22:320–325). Also called "erotomania," "hyperaesthesia," "hypereroticism," "hyperlibido," "hyperphilia," "hypersexuality," "nymphomania," "perversion," "satyriasis," "sexual addiction." See **compulsive sexual behavior, nonparaphilic; compulsive sexual behavior, paraphilic.**

compulsive sexual behavior, nonparaphilic Conventional and normative sexual behavior taken to a compulsive extreme. There are five subtypes: compulsive cruising and multiple partners, compulsive fixation on an unattainable partner, compulsive autoeroticism, compulsive multiple love relationships, and compulsive sexuality in a relationship (Coleman E. Is your patient suffering from compulsive sexual behavior? *Psychiatr Ann* 1992;22:320–325).

compulsive sexual behavior, paraphilic Unconventional sexual behaviors that are compulsive and devoid of love and intimacy. Eight of the most common paraphilias are described in DSM-IV (pedophilia, exhibitionism, voyeurism, sexual masochism, sexual sadism, transvestic fetishism, and frotteurism) (Coleman E. Is your patient suffering from compulsive sexual behavior? *Psychiatr Ann* 1992;22:320–325).

compulsive water drinking See **polydipsia, psychogenic** (preferred term).

computed electroencephalography topography (CET) Procedure in which a topographic map is formed by (a) recording the electroencephalogram (EEG) or evoked potential at 16 or more scalp locations; and (b) quantitating the amount of activity at each EEG frequency (delta, theta, etc.) by spectral analysis or measuring the evoked potential amplitude at a specific latency after the stimulus. CET advantages include (a) relative inexpensiveness; (b) it does not involve radioisotope administration; (c) it can be repeated without additional risk any number of times; and (d) it resolves periods as short as 1–2 seconds for EEG and 1–4 ms for evoked potentials.

computed tomography (CT) Radiographic technique for producing cross-sectional images in which a narrow x-ray beam is used to scan a tissue from multiple positrons. Detectors on the other side of the tissue, directly opposite the origin of the x-ray beam, measure the amount of beam transmitted through the tissue from each direction. A computer then determines the linear attenuation coefficient for each point in the tissue or the degree to which each point attenuated the x-ray beam. These values can then be displayed as a gray scale "anatomical" image. CT images are a graphic representation of the linear attenuation coefficients throughout a tissue slice. Tissue contrast (ability to tell one tissue from another, whether it is normal or abnormal) is therefore due to a difference in linear coefficients. Since its inception in 1973, CT has become an invaluable diagnostic and research tool, particularly in psychiatry, neurology, and neurosurgery. It is used in differentiating "functional" and "organic" psychiatric disorders; it is particularly helpful in diagnosing potentially treatable organic disorders. It could be valuable in the field of mental handicap. CT advantages include (a) less costly than magnetic resonance imaging (MRI); (b) better access; (c) it shows intracerebral bleeding (e.g., subdural hematoma, subarachnoid hemorrhage); (d) it is a good, quick screen; and (e) it provides good visualization of bony structures and calcified lesions (e.g., meningioma).

computed tomography (CT)/dementia In dementia, CT was originally used for exclusion purposes—to rule out intracranial disorders to which the dementia syndrome might be secondary. Later, attention turned to using CT to evaluate cerebral atrophy as a diagnostic step in the diagnosis of Alzheimer's disease and other causes of primary cerebral atrophy. Because of the noninvasiveness of the technique, the atrophy associated with "normal" aging can be documented, and cerebral changes associated with functional disorders in the elderly can be uncovered (Jacoby R, Levy R. Computed tomography in the elderly: 2—senile dementia, 3—affective disorder. *Br J Psychiatry* 1980;136:256–275). CT is not limited as a diagnostic tool in the study of dementia. It still has something to offer. Yet, more and more physicians are resorting to magnetic resonance and functional imaging. If CT is to remain a useful research investigation, it will need to be applied to new disorders in new ways (Burns A. Brain imaging. Computed tomography in Alzheimer's disease. *Lancet* 1993;341:601).

computed tomography (CT)/schizophrenia CT abnormalities in chronic schizophrenia include enlargement of the lateral ventricle, cortical atrophy as reflected by increased sulcal markings, third ventricle enlargement, cerebellar vermian atrophy, and reversed cerebral asymmetries. Of these, ventricular enlargement, cortical atrophy and third ventricle enlargement are the most robust findings (Sharif A, Getwirtz G, Igbal N. Brain imaging in schizophrenia: a review. *Psychiatr Ann* 1993,23:123–134).

computerized axial tomography (CAT) Technique for imaging anatomical structures using x-ray. It is used to detect and study anatomical abnormalities such as strokes, tumor, and atrophy of the brain.

computerized electroencephalogram (CEEG) See **brain electrical activity mapping.**

computerized tomography See **computed tomography.**

concentration-controlled trial (CCT) Study design in which subjects are assigned to predetermined levels of average plasma drug concentration. These target concentrations are achieved (within reasonable ranges) by an individualized pharmacokinetically controlled dosing scheme. In addition to safety concerns, which strongly suggest use of CCTs for drugs with narrow therapeutic windows, sample size considerations favor CCT use in many situations. Smaller sample sizes are possible with CCTs, which are designed to minimize the interindividual pharmacokinetic variability within comparison groups and consequently decrease the variability in clinical response within these groups. CCTs can be used to increase efficiency of the drug development process. It is proposed that in phase II of drug development, a randomized concentration-controlled trial (RCCT) be undertaken that incorporates an exit rule (for ethical reasons) that involves concentration-titration procedures. Such an integrated design (referred to as the "randomized concentration-controlled design," or "RCCTD") would facilitate valid assessment of efficacy early in drug development (Sanathanan LP, Peck CC. The randomized concentration-controlled trial: an evaluation of its sample size efficiency. *Control Clin Trials* 1991;12:780–794; Sanathanan LP, Peck C, Temple R, et al. Randomization, PK-controlled dosing, and titration: an integrated approach for designing clinical trials. *Drug Inform J* 1991;25:425–431).

concentration-time curve Curve of serum or plasma concentration versus time after administration (oral or parenteral) of a single dose of drug.

conceptual disorganization   Disorganized thinking characterized by disruption of goal-directed sequencing (e.g., circumstantiality, tangentiality, loose associations, non sequiturs, gross illogicality, or thought block). It is a positive symptom of schizophrenia.

Concillium   See **benperidol.**

concordance   In genetics, similarity in a twin pair with respect to presence or absence of a disease or trait. Study of resemblance between twins for all-or-none characteristics involves comparing the number of pairs that are concordant, where both members are affected (+ +), with the number of pairs that are discordant, where only one member is affected (+ −). Concordance rates indicate the percentage of twin pairs in a study that are similar on a given dimension. Higher concordance rates in monozygotic than in dizygotic twin pairs give a preliminary indication of a genetic factor that can be further explored by studying monozygotic twins reared apart. Twin studies in schizophrenia, manic-depressive psychosis, and other psychiatric conditions exemplify this method and extend it by introducing further categories of blood relatives, resulting in a twin-family method.

Concordin   See **protriptyline.**

concurrent control   Control subject assigned to a placebo or control condition during the same period that an experimental treatment or procedure is being evaluated.

concurrent drug use   Use of two or more drugs during the same period by the same individual, but not necessarily simultaneously or consecutively.

concurrent validity   Correlation of a measure with outside criteria in the present. It is also popular in the presentation of a psychometric test. Also called "convergent validity."

concussion   Immediate and transient impairment of brain function resulting from a head injury. Usually, an alteration of consciousness is involved.

conditional probability   Probability of event A, given that another event, B, has occurred.

confabulation   Inventing of tales and readiness to produce fluent answers to any question without regard to facts.

confidence bands   Dashed lines on each side of a regression line or curve that have a given probability of containing the line or curve in the population.

confidence interval   Measurement of the range of values within which the true population value probably lies. The specified probability is called the "confidence level," and the endpoints of the confidence interval are called "confidence limits."

confidence level   See **confidence interval.**

confidence limit   See **confidence interval.**

confirmation bias   Form of selective perception in which a person seeks data supporting his or her hypothesis and rejects data that do not.

confirmation of electroencephalogram (EEG)   Reading and interpretation of the clinically relevant findings in an EEG by an expert physician.

confounder   Nuisance variable (i.e., variable other than the risk factor and outcome under study) that may lead to incorrect data interpretations. It is related independently to both the risk factor and the outcome variable and may create an apparent association or mask a real one. To be a confounder, a variable must be a determinant of the outcome variable under study and unequally distributed among the exposed and the unexposed study subjects. Age could confound a study of the effect of a toxin on longevity if subjects exposed to the toxin are older than those not exposed (Anon. Glossary of methodologic terms. *JAMA* 1992;268:43–44).

confounding variable   See **confounder.**

confrontational psychotherapy   See **psychotherapy, confrontational.**

confusion   Impaired intellectual function and disorientation to time and place associated with a normal state of arousal. There also may be impaired recognition of others. It may be due to organic or psychic causes.

confusion, drug-induced/elderly   A number of drugs may cause the acute confusional state of delirium or mimic the more chronic cognitive decline of dementia, particularly in the elderly: benzodiazepines (BZDs), antidepressants, neuroleptics, anticholinergics, antihypertensives, digoxin, phenytoin, nonsteroidal anti-inflammatory drugs (NSAIDs), corticosteroids, barbiturates, alcohol, metoclopramide, narcotics, carbidopa, bromocriptine, H_2 blockers. BZDs can cause sedation, memory loss, and reduced energy level, which can be mistaken for dementia or even normal aging. Anticholinergic drugs (e.g., neuroleptics, tricyclic antidepressants, antihistamines, antispasmodics, antidiarrheals, antiparkinson drugs) may cause memory loss and confusion. Although antidepressant-induced confusion has been attributed to anticholinergic effects, it also has been reported with the least anticholinergic antidepressants, desipramine and trazodone. Neuroleptics given for behavioral consequences of delirium or dementia may worsen confusion because of their sedative or anticholinergic properties (Harper CM, Newton PA, Walsh JR. Drug-induced illness in the elderly. *Postgrad Med* 1989;86:245–256).

congenital   Present at birth. Heritability is not implied, however.

congenital abnormality Abnormality present at birth that may have genetic or environmental etiology. Genetic abnormality depends on chromosomes from parents together with breaks and realignments occurring at fertilization. Maternal aging increases risk of abnormalities in genes. Environmental factors interfere with embryonic development at a precise stage of organogenesis. Drugs such as thalidomide, x-rays, and infections such as maternal rubella are examples of environmental causes of congenital abnormalities. Antenatal screening is concerned with detection of central nervous system malformations and abnormalities of chromosomal origin.

congruent Concordant with what is generally considered proper, reasonable, or appropriate. Mood congruent symptoms and behavior are consistent with the patient's expressed or prevailing mood.

conjugating enzyme Drug-metabolizing enzyme that is genetically mediated. Phenotypical expression can also be induced by various environmental factors. Also called "transferase."

conjugation Chemical process that usually takes place in the liver during drug metabolism. It consists of combining the drug with glucuronic acid or sulfuric acid to form a more water-soluble compound for excretion. Conjugation is the second major step for metabolism of most psychotropic drugs. More rapid than oxidation, it results in shorter elimination half-life.

consanguinity Relationship by descent from the same ancestor. Two individuals are considered to be consanguine if they have at least one common ancestor no more remote than a great-great-grandparent. Offspring of consanguineous parents are inbred.

consecutive drug use Use of one drug followed by use of another, rather than simultaneous use.

consecutive sample Study sample in which all eligible subjects are selected on a strict "first-come, first-chosen" basis (Anon. Glossary of methodological terms. *JAMA* 1992;268:43–44).

consent, informed See **informed consent.**

conservative In statistics, quality of a test that reduces the chances of a type I error. See **error, alpha.**

Consilium See **bromperidol.**

consistency In statistics, an estimator is said to be consistent if the probability of it yielding estimates close to the true value approaches one as the sample size grows larger. Also called "internal validity."

consistency of association Consistency of a statistical relationship or association between a factor and a disease; across all strata the association remains the same.

consistency of results Degree to which results of a body of studies yield similar or discrepant data. In meta-analysis, findings of a group of studies are converted to similar units and charted in graphs or tables. In this way, discrepancies across studies become readily apparent. Consistency across studies can also be examined by various statistical indices. See **meta-analysis.**

Consonar See **brofaromine.**

constant observation (CO) Management option for patients needing intensive psychiatric nursing supervision because of an illness placing them at risk for harming themselves or others. CO is frequently used to manage the hospitalized suicidal patient. Also called "one-to-one management." See **neurological "watch."**

constant routine Chronobiological test of the endogenous pacemaker that involves a 36-hour baseline monitoring period, followed by a 40-hour waking episode of monitoring with the individual on a constant routine of food intake, position, activity, and light exposure.

construct In genetics, recombinant DNA molecule engineered to contain a variety of features for use in molecular cloning experiments. The large majority of recombinant constructs are generated from bacterial plasmid molecules.

construct validity Extent to which a test measures a defined concept or construct, as determined by a correlation coefficient. Establishing construct validity requires demonstration that the instrument is truly isolating and measuring the phenomenon of interest and nothing else. It also requires that the instrument should accurately reflect the basic nature of the behavior or disorder. See **content validity; face validity.**

consultation-liaison psychiatry See **psychiatry, consultation- liaison.**

contact paraphilias See **paraphilias, contact.**

content validity Extent to which items of a test adequately cover all facets or aspects of the domain of interest. The content of a scale (the item selection) is important. A first principle for establishing content validity is suitable representation from different facets of a construct. A second principle is inclusion of a relatively large number of items, since this helps to cancel out random error variance and thereby improves reliability. See **construct validity; face validity.**

context-dependent memory See **memory, context-dependent.**

contiguous gene syndrome Small chromosomal deletion involving several genes related only in that they lie next to one another.

contingency table Table used to display counts or frequencies for two or more nominal or quantitative variables.

contingent negative variation (CNV) Event-related potential that develops during a simple experimental situation in which stimuli and responses are serially organized. In depressed patients, CNV studies indicate abnormalities in both amplitude (too high or too low) and duration. Patients with high CNV amplitude respond better to serotonin uptake inhibitors than those with low CNV amplitude. Thus, CNV may be useful in the selection of antidepressant therapy.

continuance data Data that may take on any value within an interval and can be expressed in decimals.

continuation antidepressant drug therapy Continued administration of an antidepressant drug after disappearance of acute symptoms to maintain improvement gained. It is designed to prevent relapse and convert treatment response into remission. Continuation therapy ends when the patient meets criteria for recovery (i.e., after 4–6 months of sustained euthymia). There is considerable variability among clinicians in dosage strategies. Some routinely continue the full therapeutic dose for several months after initial control of symptoms. Others cut the therapeutic dose, usually by half or a third, and maintain the patient at this level for a number of months. Some rapidly reduce dosage following remission for the purpose of quickly discontinuing medication. Others gradually reduce dosage over 3–6 months. In some patients, especially those with a history of recurrent depression, continuation therapy should be followed by indefinite maintenance (prophylactic) antidepressant therapy. This is particularly true for those who had a depressive episode in the previous 2–3 years. Also called "stabilization therapy." See **maintenance antidepressant drug therapy**

continuation electroconvulsive therapy (ECT) ECT for patients with a history of recurring affective illness responsive to ECT and for whom pharmacotherapy alone has been ineffective in preventing early relapse or which cannot be safely administered for such a purpose.

continuity correction Adaptation to a test statistic when a continuous probability distribution is used to estimate a discrete probability distribution (e.g., using the chi-squared distribution for analyzing contingency tables).

continuous performance task (CPT) Visual vigilance task that involves monitoring a series of briefly presented stimuli (usually numbers or letters) that appear one at a time at a rapid serial rate and signaling by a button press each time a predesignated target stimulus is presented. Abnormally low CPT target detection rate characterizes 40–50% of all schizophrenic patients. Poor CPT performers are more likely to have a family history of schizophrenia than schizophrenic patients who are good CPT performers.

continuous positive airway pressure (CPAP) Standard treatment for obstructive sleep apnea. Administered through a nasal mask, it acts as a pneumatic splint maintaining the patency of the upper airways during sleep, thereby preventing occlusion of the airway and obstructive sleep apnea. Nasal CPAP is well-tolerated and compliance is good. CPAP can reverse both obstructive sleep apnea and Cheyne-Stokes respiration (Bradley TD, Shapiro CM. Unexpected presentations of sleep apnoea: use of CPAP in treatment. *Br Med J* 1993;306:1260–1262).

continuous scale Scale used to measure a numerical characteristic with values that occur on a continuum (e.g., age).

control **1.** Process of keeping relevant conditions of an experiment constant. **2.** Causing an independent variable to vary in a specified and known manner. **3.** Using a spontaneously occurring and discoverable fact as a check or standard of comparison to evaluate facts obtained after manipulation of the independent variable.

control group Group of subjects matched as closely as possible to an experimental group of subjects on all relevant aspects and exposed to the same treatments except for the independent variable under investigation. Also called "comparison group."

control, historical In clinical trials, previously collected observations on patients used as the control values against which the treatment is compared.

control, internal Control under the supervision of the investigator.

control, matched Control selected to be similar to subjects in the study group. Characteristics that can be matched include sex, age, and race.

control for In study design or analysis, taking into consideration a confounding variable.

controlled-release dosage form Drug delivery method designed to provide a more consistent pharmacological effect by reducing dosing frequency and maintaining more uniform plasma concentrations. It makes drug therapy more convenient for patients and may enhance compliance with the treatment regimen.

controlled substance categories According to the U.S. Controlled Substance Act of 1970, drugs are categorized according to their potential for abuse. The greater the potential, the more severe the limitations on their prescription. **Category I** (C I) drugs have high abuse potential and no accepted medical use (e.g., heroin, marijuana, LSD). **Category II** (C II) indicates high abuse potential; use may lead to severe physical or psychological dependence (e.g., barbiturates, amphetamines, cocaine, codeine, fentanyl, opioids, methadone). Prescriptions must be written in ink or typewritten and signed by the practitioner. Verbal prescriptions must be confirmed in writing within 72 hours and may be given only in a genuine emergency. No renewals are permitted. **Category III** (C III) indicates some abuse potential; use may lead to low-to-moderate physical dependence or high psychological dependence (e.g., nonbarbiturate sedatives, nonamphetamine stimulants, limited amounts of certain opiates, anabolic steroids). Prescriptions may be oral or written. Up to five renewals are permitted within 6 months. **Category IV** (C IV) indicates low abuse potential; use may lead to limited physical or psychological dependence (e.g., some sedative hypnotics [benzodiazepines, meprobamate, methohexital, phenobarbital], anxiolytics, nonopiate analgesics, central nervous system stimulants [diethylpropion and pemoline]). Prescriptions may be oral or written. Up to five renewals are permitted within 6 months. **Category V** (C V) drugs are subject to state and local regulation. Abuse potential is low; a prescription may not be required. Purchasers must be at least 18 years of age and furnish suitable identification. Sales must be recorded by the dispensing pharmacist.

controlled trial Experimental study in which an intervention is applied to one group of subjects and the outcome is compared with that in a similar group (control subjects) not receiving the intervention.

controlled user See **"chipper."**

convenience sample Study subjects selected at the convenience of the investigator or because they were available at a convenient time or place (Anon. Glossary of methodologic terms. *JAMA* 1992;268:43–44).

conventional electroencephalogram (EEG) EEG obtained via a multiple-lead EEG machine that amplifies the brain's electrical activity and passively outputs it to a magnetically driven ink writing system.

conventional evoked potential Evoked potential recorded by using amplifiers and an averager. It is passively presented on a display screen and/or writing unit. No analysis is done of the waveform, and the user manually makes clinically relevant measurements and interprets the signal.

convergent validity See **concurrent validity.**

conversion disorder See **dissociative disorder.**

conversion symptom Loss or alteration of physical functioning that suggests a physical disorder, but is actually a direct expression of a psychological conflict or need. Disturbance is not under voluntary control and is not explained by any physical disorder (DSM-IV). Conversion symptoms are observed in conversion disorder and may occur in schizophrenia.

Convulex See **valproic acid.**

Convuline See **carbamazepine.**

convulsion, febrile Common form of epileptic seizure disorder, occurring in 3–4% of all healthy children ages 6 months to 5 years; the majority of attacks occur between ages 6 months and 2 years. Seizures are often of the generalized tonic-clonic type. Attacks are triggered by a febrile disease; sudden, steep rise in temperature often precipitates the seizure.

convulsive status epilepticus See **status epilepticus, convulsive.**

"cook up" Street term for preparing free-base cocaine or heroin.

"copilot" Street name for central nervous system stimulants.

coprolalia Compulsive utterance of obscene words and phrases. It is often seen in Gilles de la Tourette's syndrome.

coprolalia, mental Thinking about obscene words. It sometimes is associated with Gilles de la Tourette's syndrome.

Cordarone See **amiodarone.**

Cordilox See **verapamil.**

core sleep See **sleep, core.**

Corgard See **nadolol.**

corpus striatum Part of the basal ganglia containing the caudate nucleus and the putamen.

corrected chi-squared test Chi-squared test for a 2×2 table that uses Yates' correction, making it more conservative.

correlation Extent to which two measures vary together or a measure of the strength of the relationship between two variables. It is a specific way to measure association. It is usually expressed by a coefficient that varies between +1 (perfect agreement) and –1 (perfect inverse relationship). A correlation coefficient of 0.0 would mean a perfect random relationship. The correlation coefficient signifies the degree to which knowledge of one score or variable can predict the score on the other variable. High correlation between two variables does not necessarily indicate a causal relationship between them: the correlation may follow because each of the variables is highly related to a third, yet unmeasured factor.

correlation coefficient See **coefficient of correlation.**

correlation, inverse Correlation between two variables in which increasing values of one variable are related to decreasing values of the other. Also called "negative correlation."

correlation, positive Correlation between variables in which great strength or quantity in one is associated with great strength or quantity in the other. Highest possible correlation is 1.

correspondence Relationship of two variables such that every individual score of one variable is paired with a score of the other.

corticosteroid Steroid hormone secreted by the adrenal gland (e.g., cortisol, corticosterone) and serving an anti-inflammatory and energy-conserving function. Corticosteroids may cause depression in susceptible patients.

corticosteroid + carbamazepine See **carbamazepine + corticosteroid.**

corticosterone See **corticosteroid.**

corticotropin-releasing factor (CRF) 41-Amino acid hypothalamic peptide, discovered in 1981, that is the major physiological regulator of the pituitary-adrenal axis. It controls release of hormone (ACTH) from the pituitary and other pro-opiomelanocortin-derived peptides of the anterior pituitary. There is considerable evidence that CRF is also a neurotransmitter in extrahypothalamic brain areas. It apparently mediates neuroendocrine, autonomic, and behavioral responses to stress. There is evidence that CRF-containing neurons play a role in the pathophysiology of anxiety disorders. Released following stress, CRF alters endocrine, gastrointestinal, cardiovascular, and immune function. It also appears to have a direct neurotropic action in the central nervous system (CNS). Several studies have shown increased CNS concentrations of CRF in patients with major depression, who often present with hypothalamic-pituitary-adrenocorticotropic dysfunction; CRF hypersecretion may underlie some of these changes.

corticotropin-releasing hormone (CRH) Hypothalamic peptide that plays an important role in mediating the action of endocrine, autonomic, and behavioral systems, associated with the stress response. These actions involve important interactions with other brain neurochemical systems. It has not been possible to directly assess CRH function in humans. Depressed patients have blunted responses to exogenous CRH, and normal to high concen-

trations of CRH immunoreactivity in single morning samples of lumbar cerebrospinal fluid, suggesting that depression may be associated with hypersecretion of CRH. It has also been postulated that central nervous system insufficiency of CRH may have a pathophysiologic role in certain depressive syndromes. In animals, CRH attenuates the benzodiazepine withdrawal syndrome, presumably through suppression of CRH rebound elevation in the brain (Kalogeras KT, Glowa JR, Smith MA, et al. Hypothalamic-pituitary-adrenal axis responses to benzodiazepine withdrawal: potential role of CRH in the withdrawal syndrome. *Neuropsychopharmacology* 1993;9:76S).

cortisol See **corticosteroid.**

Corynine See **yohimbine.**

cosmid Cloning vector used by molecular geneticists to package a chosen DNA strand into an ineffective virus particle.

"cosmos" Street name for phencyclidine (PCP).

cost-benefit analysis Systematic study of the ratio of negative (clinical, social, economic) factors to positive results of an intervention. Also called "cost-utility analysis."

cost-effectiveness analysis Technique that compares health effects of a treatment strategy (drugs, diagnostic tests, therapies) with resources that must be invested to adopt the strategy. In the case of therapeutics, direct and side effects of medication are quantified (e.g., years of life saved, days of morbidity averted, enhanced quality of life) and compared with costs of therapy, costs associated with clinical results, and costs induced by maltreatment or adverse reactions. These techniques are being used by pharmaceutical manufacturers and clinical researchers when evaluating new drugs. Credible results of cost-effectiveness analyses assist physicians in considering new types of treatment and in choosing between the new drug in the formulary and the tried-and-true approach.

cost-utility analysis See **cost-benefit analysis.**

Cotard's delusion Nihilistic belief that "nothing exists any longer" or "I am dead." Severity may vary from a belief by the patient that he is losing his powers of intellect and of feeling to denial of his own existence and that of the cosmos. It has been described most commonly in psychotic depression and schizophrenia, but can be elicited by organic brain disease. The most effective documented treatment is electroconvulsive therapy (Enoch MO, Tretowan WM. *Uncommon Psychiatric Syndromes*, 2nd ed. Bristol: Wright, 1979, pp 116–133).

cotinine Major metabolite of nicotine that has on average a half-life of 19 hours (Benowitz NL, Kuyt F, Jacob III P, et al. Cotinine disposition and effects. *Clin Pharmacol Ther* 1983;34: 604–611).

Cotwin control method Attempt to discriminate causal from noncausal relationships between a putative risk factor and a disorder or trait by comparing rates for the disorder in monozygotic and dizygotic twin pairs discordant for exposure to the risk factor (Cederlof R, Firberg L, Lundman T. The interactions of smoking, environment and heredity and their implications for disease etiology: a report of epidemiological studies on the Swedish twin registries. *Acta Med Scand* 1977;[suppl 612]:1–128).

counseling, genetic See **genetic counseling.**

counterbalanced design Counterbalanced order of presentation of independent variables in an experiment. One independent variable, condition A, is followed by a second independent variable, condition B. The second group is randomly allocated to receive condition B first, followed by condition A. There are many variations of the design. For example, in patients studied in four periods, the first group can be assigned the two conditions A and B in the order ABBA, and the second group can be assigned BAAB. Patients must be randomly assigned to the various conditions, and the conditions must be balanced in order of presentation in some reasonable way.

Coumadin See **warfarin.**

coumarin Coumadin.

counts See **frequency.**

co-variance 1. Variable that is possibly predictive of the outcome under study. 2. Tendency of a change in one variable to be accompanied by change in another.

co-variate Potentially confounding variable controlled for in analysis of co-variance or logistic regression.

Cox proportional-hazards model Method of survival analysis similar to multiple regression, but differing in that it predicts a dichotomous variable, taking into account a number of covariates as well as data on length of time subjects remained in a trial (i.e., censored data).

Cox regression Statistical method used when outcome is censored. Regression coefficients are interpreted as adjusted relative risk or odds ratios.

"crack" Crystalline, prepackaged combination of cocaine (COC) hydrochloride and baking soda or COC base that is heated in a crack pipe (often making a crackling sound) and then inhaled. Crack can be over 90% pure if extracted with ether or only 30% pure if prepared in a home microwave with baking soda. It is immediately and completely absorbed when smoked, delivering a highly po-

tent dose directly to the brain through the lungs. Smoking and injection are the fastest routes to the brain; smoking is much more dangerous than snorting the hydrochloride form. Neurochemical changes produced by crack contribute to personality changes and psychiatric disorders in the user: symptoms of depression, irritability, social withdrawal, and paranoia. Crack dependence seems to be more resistant to chemical dependency treatment than cocaine dependence by the intramuscular route. It has been considered responsible for the increased incidence of toxic reactions associated with COC use because of its relative purity, potency, and nearly immediate onset of action. Single photon emission computed tomography (SPECT) studies have shown a high frequency of focal perfusion abnormalities involving inferoparietal, temporal, and anterofrontal cortices and basal ganglia in crack users. Smooth pursuit eye movement (SPEM) studies have also revealed neuropsychological deficits in crack users (Rosse RB, Risher-Flowers D, Peace T, Deutsch SI. Evidence of impaired smooth pursuit eye movement performance in crack cocaine users. *Biol Psychiatry* 1992;31:1238–1240). Also called "rock."

"crack" baby Crack crosses the placental barrier, resulting in a number of immediate and delayed effects on the fetus and neonate. Effects in neonates include jitteriness, tremors, irritability, overexcitability, increased sensitivity to the mildest environmental stimulation, crying, and disturbed sleep. Calming such a child is very difficult. In the United States, there are an estimated 100,000 addicted or "crack" babies born each year, according to the U.S. National Drug Control Strategy report in 1990. See **cocaine baby.**

"crack" lung Damage to the lung(s) along with varying degrees of impaired pulmonary function that occur in chronic crack abusers (7 years+). Precise cause has not been determined. Some clinicians think it may be comparable to tobacco-induced pulmonary pathology. It is manifested by severe chest pains, respiratory symptoms, and hyperpyrexia suggesting pneumonia, but chest radiographs do not confirm this, and standard treatments for pneumonia are ineffective. Therapy with anti-inflammatory drugs may be effective.

"crack"/sexual behavior Because of its association with risky sexual behaviors, crack use may play an important role in acquisition and transmission of human immunodeficiency virus (HIV) infection. Data collected from 3,927 persons at least 18 years of age with acquired immunodeficiency syndrome (AIDS) or HIV infection between June 1, 1990, and January

31, 1993 provided detailed information on drug use and sexual activities within the past 5 years. Men who used crack but did not inject drugs were more likely to have a history of syphilis or any sexually transmitted disease (STD) than all other men. Of 672 men who used crack, regardless of injecting drug use, 189 (28%) had used crack in a crackhouse; 73 of the 189 (39%) reported having had sex in a crackhouse. The 221 women who used crack, whether or not they also injected drugs, were more likely to have a history of syphilis, gonorrhea, pelvic inflammatory disease, or any STD, and to have received money for sex more than any other women. Crack users who had been aware of their HIV infection for at least 5 years exchanged money or drugs for sex in the same proportions as crack users aware of their infection for less than 5 years. These results indicate that HIV-infected crack users continue high-risk sexual behaviors and may contribute substantially to the continuing transmission of HIV (Diaz T, Chu SY. Crack cocaine use and sexual behavior among people with AIDS. *JAMA* 1993;269:2845–2846).

[^{11}C] raclopride   Selective ligand for dopamine D_2 receptors used in positron emission tomography (PET). See **raclopride.**

"crank"   Street name for (a) methamphetamine; (b) homemade stimulant drug.

"crash"   Street term for an extreme state of exhaustion lasting from 9 hours to 4 days immediately following a cocaine (COC) binge. Manifestations include intense COC craving, lethargy, extreme dysphoria or depression, suicidal ideation, agitation, and anxiety. Within 1–4 hours, COC craving is replaced by desire to sleep. Sedatives, opiates, anxiolytics, or alcohol may be taken to induce sleep. Prolonged sleep may be punctuated by massive eating episodes. Hypersomnolence can last several days (1–5), followed by mood normalization. Clinical recovery is in part accomplished by sleep, nutrition, and replacement of neurotransmitters depleted by the prior binge. Crash symptoms resemble neurovegetative symptoms in major depression; therefore, assessments for psychiatric disorders or severity of chronic abstinence symptoms should be delayed until crash symptoms have abated. Generally, sleep normalization and 1–3 days of confirmed abstinence assure that acute post-use symptoms have ended.

Creutzfeldt-Jakob disease   (CJD) Spongiform encephalopathy or transmissible dementia in which there is a characteristic vascular, spongy appearance of the brain at postmortem examination. A typical case of CJD is that of a presenile dementia in the absence of a family history, occurring in the sixth decade of life and progressing rapidly to death within a year. It is usually accompanied by a number of neurological symptoms (e.g., hemiparesis, hemianopia, dysarthria, ataxia, parkinsonism). Initial depressive symptoms, epileptic seizures, and delirium also occur. Women are more often affected than men (ratio of 3:2). Patients classically exhibit myoclonus and have a characteristic electroencephalogram (EEG) showing periodic triphasic discharges at 1–2 Hz. Relative to other causes of presenile dementia, CJD cases tend to show early visual disturbances and a variety of motor symptoms. There is no treatment to prevent or retard development of CJD, despite occasional reports of response to amantadine.

crisis intervention   Approach based on crisis theory, which originated in the work of sociologists at the beginning of the 20th century. It was developed in the psychiatric field by Lindemann, who used it to understand and assist survivors of the Coconut Grove nightclub fire in Boston. Twenty years later, Gerald Caplan, a psychoanalyst, proposed that "a crisis occurs when an individual, faced with an obstacle to important life goals, finds that it is, for the time being, unsurmountable to the utilization of customary problem solving methods." When stress exceeds the capacity of usual coping mechanisms, a crisis ensues. Crisis intervention provides the opportunity to learn and improve coping strategies. Psychiatric emergencies can be dealt with by crisis intervention to reduce hospital admissions, length of stay, and cost.

"crisscross"   Street name for a central nervous system stimulant.

criterion-related   validity   Determination of whether an instrument co-varies with another, better established measure of the same construct or, more broadly, with outside variables to which it is expected to be related (concurrent validity). It involves a relationship between test scores and outside criteria.

criterion standard   Method with established or widely accepted accuracy for determining a diagnosis that provides a standard to which a new screening or diagnostic test can be compared. It need not be a single or simple procedure; it could include patient follow-up to observe evolution of their conditions, or consensus of an expert panel of clinicians (as is frequently used in the study of psychiatric conditions). It can also be used in studies of quality of care to indicate a level of performance, agreed to by experts or peers, to which the performance of individual practitioners or institutions can be compared (Anon. Glossary of methodological terms. *JAMA* 1992;268:43–44). Also called "gold standard."

criterion variable Something to be predicted.

criterion variance Different judges using different criteria or concepts to interpret the same data base.

critical flicker fusion (CFF) Test in which subjects are required to discriminate flicker fusion in a set of four light-emitting diodes held in foveal fixation at 1 meter. Individual thresholds are determined by the psychophysical method of limits on three ascending and three descending scales. CFF frequency (CFFF) threshold is widely accepted as a physiological measure of central nervous system activation. It allows accurate prediction of mental alertness and cognitive potential. (Hindmarch I. Critical flicker fusion frequency CFFF: the effects of psychotropic compounds. *Pharmacopsychiatria* 1982;15[suppl 1]:44–48; Parrott AC. Critical flicker fusion thresholds and their relationship to other measures of alertness. *Pharmacopsychiatria* 1982;15:39–44).

critical flicker fusion frequency (CFFF) See **critical flicker fusion.**

critical ratio Ratio of central tendency to a measure of variability, for example: the z or t score used in statistical tests.

critical region Set of values in which a test statistic must occur in order for the null hypothesis to be rejected.

critical value Value that a test statistic must exceed (in an absolute value sense) in order for the null hypothesis to be rejected.

cross-addiction Abuse of or loss of control over use of one abused substance is generally associated with abuse of or loss of control over all other intoxicating substances the person uses.

cross-cultural study Study in which populations from different cultures are compared.

cross-dependence Ability of one drug to suppress the manifestations of physical dependence produced by another and to maintain the physically dependent state (e.g., one barbiturate can substitute for another in reversing the barbiturate withdrawal syndrome, or one benzodiazepine can relieve abstinence symptoms that follow discontinuation of another). If an individual is physically dependent upon and is being withdrawn from a given narcotic, the administration of another narcotic of the same pharmacological class prevents appearance of an abstinence syndrome. This is also true for all types of central nervous system depressants.

Cross National Panic Study, Phase I First phase of a study to determine alprazolam efficacy in the treatment of panic disorder. It included seven centers in Canada, the United States, and Australia, enrolling 526 patients randomly assigned to either alprazolam or placebo. Clinical status was assessed weekly with patient diaries and other measures; 481 patients completed 3 weeks of treatment. Study outcome documented alprazolam efficacy in the short-term treatment of panic disorder.

Cross National Panic Study, Phase II Second phase of a study to determine alprazolam efficacy in the treatment of panic disorder. This phase compared alprazolam with imipramine. It included 12 sites in Europe, South America, and the United States, enrolling 1122 patients, of whom 1010 completed 3 weeks and 812 completed 8 weeks. There was greater patient acceptance and earlier efficacy in the alprazolam group, with reduction in panic attacks and other anxiety measures by week 2. By the end of the study, results were equivalent for both alprazolam and imipramine.

crossover Exchange of genetic material between homologous chromosomes. When a cell divides, it makes a copy of its entire set of paired chromosomes to provide daughter cells with a full complement of paired chromosomes. During duplication, a segment of the paternal chromosomes may cross-over and replace the same segment in the maternal chromosome; daughter cells thus end up with paired copies of the paternal segment. Ordinarily, crossover is of little consequence, since paternal genes that crossed are just as healthy as the maternal genes they replaced. If a chromosome carries an abnormality, however, crossover can be a disaster.

crossover design Study in which the same group of patients is treated at different times with all possible study treatments. After completing the first course of treatment, subjects are switched to another. The design maximizes data gained from each patient. Standard assumptions in crossover studies are that the disease is stable over the time of the study, effects of tested medication cease soon after it is discontinued, and there is no reason to believe that treatments interact with each other. Three components of crossover designs require consideration: number of treatment periods, types of treatment sequences, and number of patients for each sequence. Rules often used to strengthen the scientific and clinical validity of a crossover study are (a) treatment switch after a specified length of time; and (b) treatment switch dependent on the clinical characteristics of the patient. Since patients must receive at least two treatments to provide a complete data point, dropout rates can be high, greatly weakening the study.

"crossroads" Street name for amphetamines.

cross-sectional design Observational study in which frequency of disease, risk factors, or other characteristics in a defined population are surveyed at one particular time. Cross-sectional studies can assess prevalence, are easy to do, and can generate hypotheses. They cannot be used to evaluate timing of exposure. Also called "point prevalence study."

cross-tolerance State in which tolerance originally produced by long-term administration of one drug has the effect of causing tolerance to another drug of the same or different chemical type that has not been administered previously (e.g., tolerance to alcohol is accomplished by cross-tolerance to volatile anesthetics, barbiturates, or benzodiazepines). It occurs because of action at the same receptor site. Complete cross-tolerance seldom exists between two given narcotic analgesics, because each agent may not stimulate identical subpopulations of opioid receptors.

"crosstop" Street term for a type of illicit amphetamine (1 mg amphetamine plus some caffeine and ephedrine).

cross-validation Method of determining validity of a technique or research procedure by administering it to a second group to see if results coincide with findings obtained from the original administration.

crude rate Rate for an entire population that is not specific or adjusted for any given subset of the population.

"crystal" Street name for (a) intravenous methamphetamine; (b) phencyclidine (PCP).

Css$_{ave}$ Average infant serum concentration estimated by the equation: Css$_{ave}$ = F × infant dosage/Cl. F is the bioavailability fraction; Cl is the infant's drug clearance.

"cube" Street name for lysergic acid diethylamide (LSD).

"cube head" Street term for an habitual user of lysergic acid diethylamide (LSD).

cue On a rating scale, any of the responses that are available to the rater (e.g., "not at all," "a little," "severe"). Scale length is described in terms of the number of cues (e.g., a scale with three responses for each item is a three-point scale).

cue exposure Presentation of relevant drug-associated stimuli (paraphernalia, films of individuals' drinking or self-administering drugs) to drug abusers, with measurement of subjective, autonomic, and other responses to these stimuli.

cultural inheritance Environmental transmission resulting from parents actively or passively teaching their children customs or preferences.

cumulative 1. Constituting that which has been successively put together or summed as each new quantity is added. 2. Representing a distribution in which the sum of all elements is taken from the beginning to a certain point by adding each figure successively to the next until all the cases in the distribution have been represented.

cumulative benzodiazepine exposure (CBE) Measure of benzodiazepine (BZD) intake within a specified period that can be used as part of an operational definition of BZD abuse. It is calculated as: CBE = (daily dose) × (duration of use). Thus, in a patient taking diazepam 10 mg/day for 1 year, CBE = 10 × 365 = 3,650 mg.

cumulative frequency In a frequency table, the percentage of observations that occur at a given value plus all lower values.

cumulative meta-analysis See **meta-analysis, cumulative.**

curare Generic for various South American arrow poisons (e.g., tubocurarine, alcuronium, pancuronium, gallamine, atracurium, decamethonium, succinylcholine) that are neuromuscular blocking agents. They are used mainly as an adjuvant in surgical anesthesia to obtain relaxation of skeletal muscle. Before electroconvulsive therapy (ECT), a short-acting barbiturate and a neuromuscular-blocking agent (most often succinylcholine because of the short duration of its effects) may be used to prevent trauma during ECT. See **succinylcholine.**

Curetin See **doxepin.**

current procedural terminology (CPT) Listing of descriptive terms and identifying codes for reporting medical services and procedures performed by physicians, published by the American Medical Association. Its purpose is to provide a uniform language that accurately describes medical, surgical, and diagnostic services for effective communication among physicians and third party payers.

curvilinear relationship Relationship in which X and Y co-vary, but not in constant increments (i.e., there is not a linear relationship).

Cuvalit See **lisuride.**

C-value paradox Lack of correlation between the amount of DNA in a haploid genome and the biological complexity of the organism.

cyclandelate (Cyclospasmol) Cerebral vasodilator; one of many drugs unsuccessfully used to treat Alzheimer's disease.

cyclazocine Structural analog of pentazocine with a qualitatively similar profile. It is a narcotic antagonist that blocks the effects of morphine and heroin. It also has dysphoric effects of its own.

cycle Characteristic of an event exhibiting rhythmic fluctuations. One cycle is defined as the activity from one maximum (or minimum) to the next.

cycle length In affective disorder, period from the beginning of one episode of illness to the beginning of the next. Duration of episodes tends to be relatively constant in a given individual. Cycle length decreases (i.e., episodes occur more frequently) with an increase in the number of episodes of affective illness, whether mania or depression. There is a relationship between age of onset and frequency of relapse, with later age of onset associated with increased frequency of relapse.

cyclic adenosine monophosphate (cAMP) Postsynaptic second messenger produced by adenylate cyclase that is often associated with biogenic amine receptors. It activates protein kinase when an antagonist binds to a specific receptor on the enzyme.

cyclic antidepressant See **antidepressant, cyclic.**

"cycling" Street term for daily use of anabolic steroids for 6–8 weeks, followed by steroid discontinuation. Cycling is practiced for two purposes: (a) to avoid detection; and (b) to avoid adverse effects on pituitary and gonadal functions.

cyclobenzaprine (Flexeril) Widely prescribed muscle relaxant with potent anticholinergic properties that is a close analog of the tricyclic antidepressant amitriptyline. It decreases reuptake of norepinephrine. It has a long half-life (1–3 days) and it may persist in the brain following its disappearance from plasma. It has been used successfully in the treatment of fibromyalgia, a condition related to chronic fatigue syndrome (Goodnick PJ, Sandoval R. Psychotropic treatment of chronic fatigue syndrome and related disorders. *J Clin Psychiatry* 1993;54:13–20). It has been reported to induce psychosis, mania, and, in the elderly, delirium (Beeber AR, Manring JM. Psychosis following cyclobenzaprine use. *J Clin Psychiatry* 1983;44:151–152; Harsch HH. Mania in two patients following cyclobenzaprine. *Psychosomatics* 1984;25:791–793; Engel PA, Chapron D. Cyclobenzaprine-induced delirium in two octogenarians. *J Clin Psychiatry* 1993;54:39).

cyclobenzaprine + fluoxetine Fluoxetine inhibits hepatic metabolism of cyclobenzaprine, producing elevated cyclobenzaprine plasma levels and side effects consistent with cyclobenzaprine toxicity.

cycloid Personality characterized by alternating states of increased psychic and motor activity, usually with feelings of well-being, and of diminution of the same factors. Cycloid and cyclothymia are regarded by many as synonymous, although the latter generally refers to personality problems that are more than cycloid and less than manic-depressive reactions.

cyclopyrrolone Compound with a chemical structure different from those of traditional benzodiazepine anxiolytics and hypnotics (e.g., zopiclone).

Cyclospasmol See **cyclandelate.**

cyclosporine Powerful immunosuppressant that acts on T-lymphocytes and inhibits production of lymphokines, resulting in depression of cell-mediated immune response. It is given orally or intravenously for prophylaxis of graft rejection in organ and tissue transplantation. Adverse effects include nephrotoxicity, hypertension, and central nervous system disturbances. Careful monitoring of blood concentrations is important to minimize toxicity.

cyclosporine + nortriptyline See **nortriptyline + cyclosporine.**

cyclothymia Mild fluctuations of the manic-depressive type that resemble normal mood shifts. The role of medication in treating milder mood disorders is beginning to be explored. Valproate may be an effective treatment at significantly lower doses and blood levels than those required for mood stabilization in bipolar II disorder (Jacobsen FM. Low-dose valproate: a new treatment for cyclothymia, mild rapid cycling disorders, and premenstrual syndrome. *J Clin Psychiatry* 1993; 54:229–234).

Cylert See **pemoline.**

Cynomel See **liothyronine.**

Cyperon See **penfluridol.**

cyproheptadine (4-amino-3-p-chlorphenylbutyric acid) (Periactin) Nonselective serotonin (5-HT) receptor antagonist that binds avidly to the 5-HT_2 receptor concentrated in the frontal cortex. It is an anticholinergic, sedative antihistamine that may have antidepressant effects. In drug-free, unipolar, treatment-resistant depressed patients, it produced transient improvement; depressive symptoms returned within 2 weeks after its discontinuation. It has appetite-stimulating properties in some patients and has been used in the treatment of anorexia nervosa. Like other 5-HT antagonists, it may be useful in the treatment of tardive dyskinesia, and it may confer "atypical" characteristics to treatment with typical antipsychotic drugs. It may exacerbate some positive symptoms in some patients with chronic schizophrenia (Silver H, Blacker M, Weller MPI, et al. Treatment of chronic schizophrenia with cyproheptadine. A double-blind, placebo-controlled study. *Biol Psychiatry* 1991; 30:523–525). Cyproheptadine has been reported effective for some cases of anorgasmia induced by tricyclic antidepressants, monoamine oxidase inhibitors, and serotonin uptake inhibitors, although there may be recurrence of depressive symptoms after addition of cyproheptadine. Capacity to achieve orgasm can be restored with oral cyproheptadine (4–8 mg) taken 1–2 hours before anticipated sexual activity; efficacy may be due to blockade of serotonin receptors.

cyproheptadine + fluoxetine Cyproheptadine may reverse fluoxetine (FLX)-induced anorgasmia, but may also reverse FLX's antidepressant activity (Feder R. Reversal of antidepressant activity of fluoxetine by cyproheptadine in three patients. *J Clin Psychiatry* 1991;52:163–164; Goldbloom DS, Kennedy SH. Adverse interaction of fluoxetine and cyproheptadine in two patients with bulimia nervosa. *J Clin Psychiatry* 1991;52:261–262).

cyproheptadine + haloperidol Double-blind crossover studies indicate that cyproheptadine can enhance therapeutic response to haloperidol in chronic schizophrenia. It also may significantly reduce extrapyramidal symptoms. It did not reduce plasma prolactin level, but did decrease plasma cortisol level (Shick LH, Hak KJ, Moon LY, et al. Cyproheptadine augmentation of haloperidol in the chronic schizophrenic patient: a double-blind placebo-controlled study. *Neuropsychopharmacology* 1993; 9:55S).

cyproheptadine + imipramine Cyproheptadine has been used successfully to treat imipramine-induced anorgasmia (Steele TE, Howell EF. Cyproheptadine for imipramine-induced anorgasmia. *J Clin Psychopharmacol* 1986;6:326–327).

cyproheptadine + phenelzine Addition of cyproheptadine to the therapeutic regimen of a depressed patient responsive to phenelzine caused rapid recurrence (a few hours to four days) of depressive symptoms (Zubieta JK, Demitrack MA. Depression after cyproheptadine: MAO treatment. *Biol Psychiatry* 1992;31: 1177–1178).

cyproheptadine overdose Overdosage has resulted in short-lived generalized chorea. Myoclonic jerks persisted after chorea subsided; other, more common clinical features of anticholinergic toxicity (tachycardia, dry skin and mucous membranes, hallucinations) resolved with intravenously administered physostigmine (Samie MR, Ashton AK. Choreoathetosis induced by cyproheptadine. *Mov Disord* 1989; 4:81–84).

cyproterone (Androcur) Antiandrogenic drug believed to prevent the effect of endogenously produced and exogenously administered androgens at the target organs by means of competitive inhibition. It is used in the treatment of antisocial sexual behavior. In men, it reduces sexual drive and potency and leads to inhibition of gonadal function. These changes are reversible following discontinuation of therapy. Over the course of several weeks, cyproterone gradually impairs spermatogenesis. It occasionally leads to gynecomastia in men, sometimes combined with breast tenderness, that usually regresses after dosage reduction or discontinuation. In an elderly man, 50 mg/day produced inactivity, immobility, and falling that disappeared following discontinuation of the drug (Byrne A, Brunet B, McGann P. Cyproterone acetate therapy and aggression. *Br J Psychiatry* 1992;160:282–283). Individual dose is determined by response. Generally, treatment is started with 50 mg twice a day. Dosage increments to 100 mg 2 or 3 times/day for a short period is sometimes necessary. Treatment should be discontinued gradually.

cyproterone acetate See **cyproterone.**

Cytadren See **aminoglutethimide.**

cytochrome One of a family of hepatic microsomal drug-metabolizing enzymes. Two, P450IID6 and P450IIIA4, are thought to be responsible for the biotransformation of more than 90% of drugs used in clinical practice that are metabolized by the liver.

cytochrome 2D6 (CYP2D6) Hepatic enzyme responsible for poor metabolism of about 30 drugs, especially neuroleptics, tricyclic antidepressants, and antiarrhythmics. Individuals with the enzyme may need higher doses of these drugs to achieve a therapeutic effect (Brosen K, Gram LF. Clinical significance of the sparteine/debrisoquine oxidation polymorphism. *Eur J Clin Pharmacol* 1989;36:537–547).

cytochrome 2D6A (CYP2D6A) Mutant allele of CYP2D6 that gives rise to CYP2D6 polymorphism (Daly AK, Armstrong M, Monkman SC, et al. Genetic and metabolic criteria for the assignment of debrisoquine 4-hydroxylation [cytochrome P4502D6] phenotypes. *Pharmacogen* 1991;1:33–41).

cytochrome 2D6B (CYP2D6B) Mutant allele of CYP2D6 that gives rise to CYP2D6 polymorphism (Daly AK, Armstrong M, Monkman SC, et al. Genetic and metabolic criteria for the assignment of debrisoquine 4-hydroxylation [cytochrome P4502D6] phenotypes. *Pharmacogen* 1991;1:33–41).

cytochrome 2D6D (CYP2D6D) Mutant allele of CYP2D6 that gives rise to CYP2D6 polymorphism (Daly AK, Armstrong M, Monkman SC, et al. Genetic and metabolic criteria for the assignment of debrisoquine 4-hydroxylation [cytochrome P4502D6] phenotypes. *Pharmacogen* 1991;1:33–41).

cytochrome 2D6E (CYP2D6E) Mutant allele of CYP2D6 that gives rise to CYP2D6 polymorphism (Daly AK, Armstrong M, Monkman SC, et al. Genetic and metabolic criteria for the assignment of debrisoquine 4-hydroxylation [cytochrome P4502D6] phenotypes. *Pharmacogen* 1991;1:33–41).

cytochrome P450 Family of drug-metabolizing isoenzymes, localized in lipophilic membranes of the endoplasmic reticulum of the liver and other tissues. The enzymes are under genetic control (*P* for pigment, *450* for the maximum wave length absorption when exposed to carbon monoxide) and are required for microsomal drug oxidation. There are at least 19 human forms of P450, each with a distinct, although overlapping, substrate specificity (Kimura S, Umeno M, Skoda RC, et al. *Am J Hum Genet* 1989;45:889–905). On repeated administration, some substrates induce P450 by enhancing its rate of synthesis or reducing its rate of degradation, accelerating metabolism, and usually decreasing the pharmacological action of the inducer and co-administered drugs. Other drug substrates may inhibit P450 activity (e.g., macrolide antibiotics such as erythromycin, some barbiturates such as secobarbital, alcohol, and cimetidine). At least 10 families of P450 genes are known to constitute the P450 gene superfamily. CYP1A2, CYP2A6, CYP2B6, CYP2C, CYP2D6, and CYP3A have all been shown to metabolize clinically important drugs. CPY2D6 has been most studied and appears to be the most important to individualizing therapy thus far. Its activity can be assessed by measuring the hydroxylation capacity of some test drugs such as debrisoquine or dextromorphan. CYP2D6 metabolizes tricyclic antidepressants (TCAs), some beta-blockers, codeine by activation to morphine, some neuroleptics, anticonvulsants (e.g., carbamazepine, valproic acid), and some antiarrhythmics. About 6–10% of the U.S. population is deficient in this enzyme and fail to metabolize drugs via this pathway at a normal rate; the remainder of the population are extensive metabolizers (Cholerton S, Daly AK, Idle JR. The role of individual cytochromes P450 in drug metabolism and clinical response. *Trends Pharmacol Sci* 1992;13:434–439; Sindrup SH, Brosen K, Bjerring P, et al. Codeine increases pain thresholds to copper vapor laser stimuli in extensive but not poor metabolizers of sparteine. *Clin Pharmacol Ther* 1991;49:686–693). Individuals with normal enzyme activity slowly metabolize drugs that are substrates for it if they take other drugs that inhibit CYP2D6. Inhibition of CYP2D6 by fluoxetine increases TCA levels when fluoxetine is added to TCA drug regimens (Bergstrom RF, Peyton AL, Lemberger L. Quantification and mechanism of the fluoxetine and tricyclic

antidepressant interaction. *Clin Pharmacol Ther* 1992;51:239–248; Reidenberg MM. Clinical pharmacology. *JAMA* 1993;270:192–194).

cytochrome P450DBL (dbl) Hepatic enzyme that, in addition to the prototype substrate dextromethorphan (DM), metabolizes over 30 other drugs, including beta-blockers, tricyclic antidepressants, and neuroleptics.

cytochrome P450IIIA4 One of many cytochrome P450 hepatic enzymes that metabolizes drugs (e.g., nifedipine, some benzodiazepines, quinidine).

cytochrome P450$_{MP}$ (CYP$_{MP}$) Enzyme involved in the hydroxylation of S-mephenytoin.

cytogenetic map Map showing the location of genes on a chromosome when examined microscopically. Each chromosome has a unique appearance due to differentially staining regions (bands), each containing 1 to 5 million base pairs. Maps are at very low resolution, but help identify specific chromosomes and chromosomal regions. A karyotype, for example, is a visual representation of an individual's chromosomes that may reveal deletions, rearrangements, translocations, and other abnormalities. It is possible to localize DNA segments of interest to chromosomal regions of a cytogenetic map using sophisticated fluorescent microscopy methods.

cytogenetics Study of heredity at the microscopic level. It deals with chromosomes that carry DNA, arrangement of chromosomes, genes on the chromosomes, chemical structure of genes, and effects of abnormalities of genes and chromosomes.

cytokine Nonantibody protein that, on contact with a specific antigen, is released by certain cell populations. Cytokines act as intercellular mediators in the generation of immune response. They exert marked effects on both the hypothalamic-pituitary-adrenal and the hypothalamic-pituitary-gonadal axes, and suggest that alterations in endocrine functions that occur during stimulation of the immune system may be at least partly modulated through increased levels of interleukins. Cytokines contribute to cell growth and differentiation.

Cytomel See **liothyronine.**

cytoplasm Fluid and structures within a cell wall and surrounding the cell nucleus.

cytoskeleton Complex of proteins that make up the scaffolding of a cell. They may be used for motility of the cell or internal molecules.

cytotoxic T cell T cell that, upon activation by a specific antigen, targets and attacks the cells bearing that type of antigen. Also called "killer T cell."

D

"D" Street name for lysergic acid diethylamide (LSD).

Dale's law Principle that each neuron utilizes only one transmitter, although it is now known that more than one neurotransmitter may be contained in and released by a single neuron.

Dalmane See **flurazepam.**

Daloxin See **loxapine.**

Dalpas See **buspirone.**

DAMGO (Tyr-D-Ala-Gly-N-methyl-Phe-Gly-ol) Selective mu-opioid agonist that produces analgesia when injected into the cerebral ventricles. See **mu receptor.**

D-amphetamine See **dextroamphetamine.**

danazol (Danocrine) Gonadotropin-releasing hormone agonist. It is a synthetic androgen used in the treatment of endometriosis. It has also been used in premenstrual syndrome (PMS) and rapid-cycling manic-depressive illness.

danazol + carbamazepine See **carbamazepine + danazol.**

dangerousness Risk of inflicting serious violence on others, or causing serious psychological or physical harm or damaging property. It is not a constant quality, but subject to change according to the person's mental state and relationships with others. The best predictors of dangerousness among the psychiatrically ill are the same factors that predict dangerousness among those not mentally disordered. The poorest predictors of dangerousness among the mentally ill are factors such as diagnosis, severity of mental disorder, and personality traits.

danitracen Serotonin antagonist antidepressant. Not available in the United States.

Danocrine See **danazol.**

Dantrium See **dantrolene.**

dantrolene (Dantrium) Hydantoin derivative, long-acting peripheral muscle relaxant that may affect the release of calcium ions from muscle sarcoplasmic reticulum. It is the drug of first choice for treating malignant hyperthermia (MH) and is often used in the treatment of neuroleptic malignant syndrome (NMS). Use in patients with suspected NMS was originally based on success in the treatment of MH. It may be administered orally or intravenously; the latter route is preferable for uncooperative patients or to quickly counteract thermogenesis and muscular rigidity. Intravenous dosage is usually 50 mg every 12 hours for up to seven doses; it should be discontinued as soon as the patient can take drugs orally. Dantrolene is not recommended as a primary treatment for suspected NMS or for severe extrapyramidal symptoms. It is probably best used in NMS cases when oral bromocriptine cannot be given because of rigidity. Experts also recommend that dantrolene be considered adjunctive treatment when dopamine agonists are not rapidly effective in NMS. It should be used for as short a period as possible, and liver enzymes should be monitored. These recommendations are based in part on the fact that dantrolene-caused hepatotoxicity is often seen at dosages of over 300 mg/day and in patients treated for more than 60 days. Other side effects include drowsiness, dizziness, weakness, fatigue, and diarrhea.

dantrolene + bromocriptine Co-administration is often used for the treatment of neuroleptic malignant syndrome without serious adverse interactions.

Dapex See **phentermine.**

dapiprazole An experimental atypical neuroleptic undergoing clinical evaluations.

dapoxetine (LY210448) Selective serotonin uptake inhibitor in the early stages of investigation as an antidepressant. In animals it has very little affinity for muscarinic receptors, histamine H_1 receptors, serotonin receptors, dopamine receptors, opioid receptors, and alpha-adrenergic receptors in vivo.

DARE Acronym used in patient education about crack cocaine ("do you DARE smoke crack?"). D = for risk of Dependency, A = Abuse following recreational use, R = Recreational use following experimental use, and E = Experimental use may lead to a sequence in crack-smoking behavior with severe and negative consequences.

Darvocet See **propoxyphene.**

Darvon See **propoxyphene.**

data-set Raw data gathered by investigators.

data sheet Drug information prepared by pharmaceutical manufacturers to comply with requirements of the U.K. Medicines Act 1968, and follow requirements stipulated by the Medicines (Data Sheet) Regulations 1972. It is comparable to the U.S. package insert enclosed with each drug package for use by the medical profession. Data sheets are updated regularly and cover *presentation* (appearance of the formulation and how much drug it contains); *uses* (indications); *dosage and administration* (dose recommendations for adults and children, circumstances in which reduced doses are warranted, method and site of administration); *contraindications, warnings, etc.*

(safety data, contraindications, precautions, use in pregnancy, drug interactions, side effects, overdose management); *pharmaceutical precautions* (special storage conditions); *legal category* (whether the drug is a prescription-only medicine [POM] or can be bought from pharmacies [P]); *package quantities* (unit doses per pack); and *product license number.*

Datolan   See **zopiclone.**

Datovane   See **zopiclone.**

Datril   See **acetaminophen.**

dawn simulation light therapy   Effective treatment for winter depression consisting of exposure to a dim light that gradually increases in illuminance to a peak of only 100–500 lux before patients awaken (Avery DH, Bolte MA, Dager SR, et al. Dawn simulation treatment of winter depression: a controlled study. *Am J Psychiatry* 1993;153:113–117).

Daxolin   See **loxapine.**

day center   Outpatient or aftercare unit, ordinarily with a nonmedical staff, designed to provide company for the lonely, occupation for the handicapped, and meals for those unable to prepare them.

day-hospital care   See **partial hospitalization.**

day treatment   See **partial hospitalization.**

"d-ball"   Street name for an anabolic steroid.

"d-bol"   Street name for an anabolic steroid.

DDAVP   (1-Desamino-D-arginine-8-vasopressin) Synthetic analog of the hypothalamic peptide arginine vasopressin. It has been claimed to enhance cognition in patients with progressive dementia by facilitating access to semantic memory structures that are part of long-term memory. The claim has not been verified by large-scale, placebo-controlled trials.

Deaner   See **deanol.**

deanol   (2-dimethylaminoethanol) (Deaner) Cholinergic drug tried often during the 1970s for treatment of tardive dyskinesia (TD). At present, its value in TD is questionable.

Deanxit   Combination of the antidepressant melitracen and the neuroleptic flupenthixol. Not available in the United States.

"death hit"   Street term for cocaine mixed with strychnine.

debrisoquin   See **debrisoquine.**

debrisoquine   (Declinax) (DBQ) Peripherally active monoamine oxidase inhibitor that does not cross the blood-brain barrier. It blocks peripheral, but not central, production of homovanillic acid (HVA) and 3-methoxy-4-hydroxyphenylglycol (MHPG). It has been used to suppress the peripheral contributions of HVA to plasma and thereby enhance the degree to which plasma HVA can reflect central dopamine neuronal activity. DBQ has been used extensively in pharmacogenetic

studies to assess a subject's rate of hydroxylation (i.e., slow vs. fast). It has been studied as a pharmacogenetic probe in patients treated with tricyclic antidepressants (TCAs); those who had deficient hydroxylation of DBQ also differed from the normal population in their metabolism of TCAs. At present, however, specific drugs appear to be subject to specific metabolic processes, limiting the use of pharmacokinetic phenotyping drugs such as DBQ.

debrisoquine hydroxylase   See **debrisoquine.**

"deca"   Street name for an anabolic steroid administered by intramuscular injection. It is assumed to be nandrolone decanoate (Deca-Durabolin).

Decade of the Brain   On July 25, 1989, U.S. President George Bush signed a Congressional Resolution designating the years 1990–2000 as the "Decade of the Brain" to promote research in neuroscience and improve treatment of mental disorders.

Decadron   See **dexamethasone.**

Deca-Durabolin   See **nandrolone decanoate.**

decerebrate rigidity   See **rigidity, decerebrate.**

dechallenge   Reduction of dosage or withdrawal of a drug after occurrence of a possible adverse reaction to it. Response to dechallenge can be a major factor in assessing drug causality when an adverse drug reaction (ADR) occurs.

decision analysis   Formal model for describing and analyzing a decision.

decision tree   Graphic representation of the temporal course of a clinical problem, including choices, chance events, and outcomes. It is used in decision analysis. A series of decision options are represented as branches, and subsequent possible outcomes are represented as further branches. Decisions and eventualities are presented in the order they are likely to occur. The decision tree portrays choices available to those responsible for patient care and the probabilities of each outcome that will follow the choice of a particular action or strategy in patient care. The relative worth of each outcome is preferably also described as a utility or quality of life. In contrast to an algorithm, which is a closed system, a decision tree is an open system. See **algorithm; clinical algorithm.**

declarative memory   See **memory, declarative.**

Declinax   See **debrisoquine.**

Decolone   See **nandrolone decanoate.**

"deek"   Street name for heroin.

deep sleep   See **sleep, deep.**

deep white matter hyperintensity   (DWMH) See **subcortical hyperintensity.**

Defanyl   See **amoxapine.**

defaulter   Patient who does not follow the recommended dosages of prescribed drugs.

defense mechanism (DM) Pattern of feelings, thoughts, or behaviors that are relatively involuntary and arise in response to perceptions of psychic danger. They hide or alleviate conflicts or stressors that give rise to anxiety. Some DMs (e.g., projection, splitting, acting-out) are almost invariably maladaptive. Others (e.g., suppression, denial) may be either maladaptive or adaptive, depending on severity, inflexibility, and context.

defensive medicine Any act or failure to act by a physician performed not for the benefit of the patient but solely to avoid malpractice liability or to provide a good legal defense against a possible malpractice claim.

defensive psychiatry Ordering procedures and treatments to prevent or limit liability or avoiding procedures or treatments out of fear of a malpractice charge even though the patient might benefit from the interventions. See **defensive medicine.**

deferred diagnosis Diagnosis that is temporarily delayed because of insufficient information.

deficit, cognitive See **cognitive deficit.**

deficit symptoms See **schizophrenia/deficit symptoms.**

deficit syndrome Term proposed as a substitute for negative symptoms of schizophrenia (Carpenter WT Jr., Heinrichs DW, Wagman AMI. Deficit and nondeficit forms of schizophrenia: the concept. *Am J Psychiatry* 1988;145: 578–583). The term also denotes intractability over time and in this respect concurs with some of the key attributes of the negative symptom profile described by Crow (Crow TJ. Molecular pathology of schizophrenia: more than one disease process? *Br Med J* 1980;280: 66–68; Crow TJ. Positive and negative schizophrenic symptoms and the role of dopamine: discussion, 2. *Br J Psychiatry* 1980;137:383–386). See **subcortical hyperintensity.**

defined daily dosage (DDD) Standard for grouping and defining daily dosage of the Anatomical Therapeutic Chemical Classification (ATC), accepted by the World Health Organization (WHO) Drug Utilization Research Group for international studies of drug consumption. Examples: one DDD corresponds to 300 mg of chlorpromazine, 10 mg of diazepam, 5 mg of nitrazepam, 100 mg of imipramine, 25 mg of procyclidine, or 1 g of carbamazepine.

Defton-70 See **lofepramine.**

degree of freedom Parameter in some commonly used probability distributions (e.g., chi-squared).

dehydrochlormethyltestosterone Androgenic anabolic steroid.

deinstitutionalization Discharge from the psychiatric hospital to the community, particularly of chronically mentally ill patients who otherwise would be kept hospitalized for long periods.

deja vu "Already seen"; feeling of familiarity by a person who, when perceiving something never seen before, thinks he or she has had the experience in the past. It is a common phenomenon in normal persons that may occur more often in psychiatric and epileptic patients, particularly those with temporal lobe abnormalities.

Dekinet See **biperiden.**

Delatest See **testosterone enanthate.**

Delatestryl See **testosterone enanthate.**

delayed auditory feedback (DAF) Procedure in which normal auditory feedback of speech is drowned and disturbed by a timed, delayed feedback. At the start of DAF, subjects hear a tone in their headphones and immediately begin reading a printed text into a microphone. While they are reading they hear their own voice delayed 180 ms by a digital delay chamber. Each procedure is composed of 5 minutes of DAF, preceded and followed by two 5-minute rest periods (Badian M, Appel E, Palm D, et al. Standardized mental stress in healthy volunteers induced by delayed auditory feedback. *Eur J Clin Pharmacol* 1979;16: 171–176).

delayed onset Characteristic of a syndrome that does not become clinically significant until weeks or months after the initial stressor (e.g., post-traumatic stress disorder is specified as "delayed onset" if onset of symptoms occurs at least 6 months after the trauma).

delayed reaction Psychological response to a stressor that only occurs after time has elapsed.

delayed sleep phase syndrome (DSPS) Chronic inability to fall asleep at desired bedtime and difficulty in maintaining alertness in the morning. Patients are unable to fall asleep at the desired clock time, but have little or no difficulty if bedtime is delayed 3–5 hours. Sleep duration is normal, but forced early rising is followed by drowsiness and dysphoria. Psychiatric and psychological problems, but no specific psychiatric disorder, are common. Attempts to treat the disorder by phase advance to an early bedtime are not beneficial, but a program of progressive delay in sleep-onset time results in successful rescheduling of the sleep-wake cycle. A small placebo-controlled trial of melatonin showed substantial benefits. Sleep onset and wake times were significantly advanced towards conventional times with, surprisingly, slight reduction rather than increase in total sleep duration (Dahlitz M, Alvarez B, Vignau J, et al. Delayed sleep phase syndrome response to melatonin. *Lancet* 1991; 337:1121–1124). Bright light phototherapy also has been reported to be beneficial.

deletion of chromosome   Loss of part of a chromosome. It is a type of mutation detectable as absence of particular sequences. Loss of a tiny fragment (just a few genes) may have no noticeable effect. Generally, however, deletion of a chromosome has a major effect that varies according to the chromosome affected and the site and extent of the deletion. Deletion of the long arm is written as the letter q and of the short arm as the letter p.

deliberate self-harm syndrome   Distinct syndrome of low lethality and repetitive, direct self-destructive behavior. It begins typically in adolescence and may persist for decades, resulting in great personal and social morbidity (Pattison EM, Kahan S. The deliberate self-harm syndrome. *Am J Psychiatry* 1983;140:867–872).

deliberate self-poisoning   Deliberate ingestion of more than the prescribed amount of medical substances, or ingestion of substances never intended for human consumption, regardless of whether harm was intended.

"delicate cutters"   Subgroup of repeated wrist cutters, most of whom are women particularly sensitive to loss or unable to handle certain affects. They cut their wrists to achieve relief from mounting tension and anger. To them, wrist cutting is not painful; they are seldom candidates for pharmacotherapy.

deliriogenic   Substance capable of inducing delirium. Belladonna alkaloids and synthetic drugs with anticholinergic properties are the single most important group of deliriogenics.

delirious mania   See **Bell's mania.**

deliriousness   Disturbed state of consciousness associated with disruption of thinking. Manifested behavior can vary from dull torpor to wild agitation.

delirium   Transient organic mental syndrome characterized by global impairment of cognitive functions, including memory and perception; reduced and/or fluctuating levels of consciousness; disorientation and fear; impaired capacity to shift or maintain attention; increased or decreased psychomotor activity; disordered sleep-wake cycle; a variety of affective symptoms, including blunting or flattening of affect; and behavioral changes, including agitation, withdrawal, and lack of interest (Marin RS. Differential diagnosis and classification of apathy. *Am J Psychiatry* 1990;147:22–30). Delirium is a reversible disturbance of cerebral metabolism secondary to a cerebral insult (e.g., infection or a metabolic disturbance). The cardinal feature is day-to-day, hour-to-hour, and minute-to-minute fluctua-

tion in brain dysfunction. Onset is acute, usually within 4–6 hours, although it may evolve over several days or weeks. Prescription medications are one of the most overlooked causes of delirium, especially in the elderly. Failure to diagnose and treat delirium exposes the patient to excessive risk of morbidity and mortality. Nonpsychiatric house staff and attending physicians frequently misidentify delirium as major depression or adjustment disorder. Diagnosis of delirium can be facilitated by an electroencephalogram (Kopenen H, Partanen J, Paakkonen A, et al. EEG spectral analysis in delirium. *J Neurol Neurosurg Psychiatry* 1989;52:980–985). Rapid tranquilization generally is a reliable therapeutic regimen for acute delirium. In some patients, intravenous neuroleptic therapy is preferable to oral or intramuscular routes of administration. Any psychotropic drugs given to delirious patients should be short-acting and relatively free of anticholinergic side effects. Delirium can be subdivided into an "activated" and a "somnolent" subtype, similar to Lipowski's "hyperalert-hyperactive" and "hypoalert-hypoactive" subtypes (Lipowski ZJ. Delirium in the elderly patient. *N Engl J Med* 1989;320:578–582). These subtypes may have different phenomenologies (especially hallucinations and delusions) and etiologies. Delirium often heralds severe and life-threatening medical illness; among the elderly, 15–30% will progress to stupor, coma and death (Beresen EV. Delirium in the elderly. *J Geriatr Psychiatry Neurol* 1988;1:127–143). Failure to promptly and completely evaluate the cause of delirium may hasten death and disability if the delirium is a consequence of catastrophic medical illness. Identified risk factors include aging, malnutrition, polypharmacy, anticholinergic medication, fatigue, psychological stress, and central nervous system pathology. Also called "acute brain syndrome"; "acute confusional state"; "exogenous metabolic brain disease"; "beclouded state." See **acute confusional state.**

delirium acutum   Hyperkinetic phase of the catatonic state characterized by unprovoked outbursts of running, jumping, gyrating, screaming, or even overt aggression (Johnson J. Catatonia: the tension insanity. *Br J Psychiatry* 1993;162:733–738). Also called "catatonos raptus."

delirium, anticholinergic   Delirium secondary to muscarinic blockade. Its most common cause is treatment with potent anticholinergic medications. It is particularly common in the elderly, who are often given one or more anticholinergics concomitantly. Also called "toxic psychosis."

delirium/antihistamine   Antihistamines often prescribed as sedatives or anxiolytics (e.g., diphenhydramine, hydroxyzine, chlorphen-iramine, promethazine) may cause delirium due to their anticholinergic properties.

delirium, elderly   Delirium is common in the elderly. Sepsis and congestive heart failure are the most frequent causes on admission to general medicine wards. Drug-related delirium in the elderly is frequent and unique in terms of its etiology and good prognosis.

delirium/electroconvulsive therapy (ECT)   Delirium induced by ECT may occur in patients with structural changes in the basal ganglion and white matter (subcortical hyperintensity); the latter may serve as a risk marker for development of delirium following ECT. Patients with caudate nucleus (particularly right caudate nucleus) lesions are likely to develop delirium when receiving ECT (Figiel GC, Krishnan KRR, Doraiswamy PM. Subcortical structural changes in ECT-induced delirium. *J Geriatr Psychiatry Neurol* 1990;3:172–176). Further studies with computed tomography (CT) and magnetic resonance imaging (MRI) may help determine which patients are at risk (Black JL. ECT: lessons learned about an old treatment with new technologies. *Psychiatr Ann* 1993;23:7–14).

delirium, emergence   Short-lived delirium or acute confusional state that may occur in some patients as they emerge from an epileptic state after electroconvulsive therapy or after general anesthesia. With the use of good technique, this is rare.

delirium, postoperative   Delirium usually due to a combination of metabolic imbalances, anesthetic effects, narcotics, and infections with or without fever. It is particularly common in the elderly.

delirium tremens   (DTs) Acute, sometimes lethal brain disorder precipitated by total or partial withdrawal from excessive alcohol intake manifested by confusion, disorientation, fluctuating or clouded consciousness, agitation, insomnia, fever, tremors, ataxia and sometimes convulsions, frightening illusions, delusions, and hallucinations. It usually develops in 24–96 hours and is a medical emergency. It may be accompanied by nutritional deficiencies. Preferred medications for treatment include benzodiazepines (chlordiazepoxide, diazepam, lorazepam, oxazepam) and multivitamins (particularly thiamine, B_{12}, and folic acid). Clonidine, propranolol, chloral hydrate, or barbiturates also can be used if indicated by the patient's symptoms. A similar syndrome may follow withdrawal of high doses of barbiturates and other similar sedative hypnotics.

delirium/tricyclic antidepressant (TCA)   Delirium has been reported in 1–8% of patients treated with TCAs. It is believed to be due to their sedative and anticholinergic effects, most often the latter. TCA-induced delirium symptoms are similar to delirium of other etiologies: disorientation, confusion, altered level of consciousness, memory impairment, difficulty with concentration and attention span, altered psychomotor behavior, changes in sleep patterns, and perceptual disturbances, including frank hallucinatory activity. Psychiatric changes induced by TCAs can also appear as more specific psychiatric symptoms; agitation, psychosis, affective disturbances including both mania and depression, depersonalization, and derealization have been reported. Although these symptoms can appear as part of the spectrum of delirium, they have also been reported in isolation in TCA-treated patients who do not meet diagnostic criteria for delirium. This symptom cluster may represent a discrete form of TCA-induced toxicity (Meador-Woodruff JH. Psychiatric side effects of tricyclic antidepressants. *Hosp Comm Psychiatry* 1990;41:84–86). TCA-induced delirium is more common in the elderly, but it also can occur in the young. It happens most often when TCA plasma level is high, although it has occurred in patients with therapeutic and subtherapeutic levels. A significant percentage of patients treated with TCA doses normally considered therapeutic develop cognitive or behavioral toxicity when plasma TCA level exceeds 450 ng/ml (Meador-Woodruff JH, Akil M, Wisner-Carlson R, Grunhaus L. Behavioral and cognitive toxicity related to elevated plasma tricyclic antidepressant levels. *J Clin Psychopharmacol* 1988;8:28–32).

delta activity   See **delta electroencephalogram.**

delta electroencephalogram (EEG)   EEG predominantly in the 0–4 Hz (delta activity) range in all recorded leads. Delta EEGs are usually characterized by their moderate to high amplitude and rhythmical nature. Minimum characteristics for scoring delta waves is conventionally 75 uV (peak-to-peak) amplitude and 0.5-second duration (2 Hz) or less. Delta waves are the hallmark of deep sleep. Rhythm typically increases in normal subjects with drowsiness. It has the greatest distribution in parietal and temporal cortex, with extension into the occiput. Delta-wave increases have been noted in schizophrenics and some of their offspring. Neuroleptics reduce delta waves in schizophrenics consistent with a normalization of the EEG. In normal subjects, delta increases at the occiput are often seen with neuroleptics.

delta-receptor   Opioid receptor subtype located on presynaptic dopaminergic terminals in the corpus striatum. Delta-receptors are activated by enkephalins that have a greater affinity for them than for mu-receptors, and by beta-endorphin, which has equal agonist activity at mu-8 delta-receptors. Naloxone has less antagonist activity at delta- than at mu-receptors. Delta-receptors inhibit dopamine release.

delta sleep   See **sleep, delta.**

delta-sleep-inducing-peptide   (DSIP) Peptide that has been shown to increase sleep in insomniacs and to be decreased in patients with schizophrenia.

delta-9-tetrahydrocannabinol   See **marijuana; tetrahydrocannabinol.**

delusion   Unfounded, unrealistic, idiosyncratic belief of unknown etiology that is held without supporting evidence. It may be poorly formed, well formed, or highly systematized. Delusions are a consistent feature of many neurological and psychiatric disorders. "Organic" delusions provide important clues to regional brain dysfunction. Qualitatively and quantitatively, they are inconsistent with the patient's sociocultural or religious background. They often dominate the patient's life, resulting in inappropriate and irresponsible actions. Delusions must be distinguished from confabulation, illusions, and deficit syndromes such as prosopagnosia.

delusion, bizarre   False belief involving a phenomenon that the person's culture would regard as totally implausible (DSM-IV).

delusion, Cotard's   See **Cotard's delusion.**

delusion, grandiose   Exaggerated sense of importance, power, knowledge, or identity. It may have a religious, somatic, or other theme (DSM-IV).

delusion, nihilistic   Delusion involving the theme of nonexistence of the self or part of the self, others, or the world. A somatic delusion may also be a nihilistic delusion if the emphasis is on nonexistence of the body or part of the body (DSM-IV).

delusion of poverty   Delusion that the person is, or will be, bereft of all, or virtually all, material possessions (DSM-IV).

delusion of reference   Delusion that events, objects, or other people in the person's immediate environment have a particular and unusual significance, usually of a negative or pejorative nature. It differs from an idea of reference, in which the false belief is not as firmly held as in a delusion. If the delusion of reference involves persecution, then a persecutory delusion also is present (DSM-IV).

delusion, persecutory   Delusion that a person or group is being attacked, harassed, cheated, persecuted, or conspired against. The object of persecution is usually the subject or a person, group, or institution close to the subject (DSM-IV).

delusion, primary   First-rank symptom of schizophrenia in which meaning arises inexplicably from normal perceptions (e.g., the patient takes traffic lights changing to mean that a message is being conveyed by the colors).

delusion, somatic   Delusion whose main content pertains to the functioning of one's body (e.g., the belief that one's intestines are rotting or no longer functioning). It may be a manifestation of schizophrenia or psychotic depression.

delusion, systematized   Single delusion with multiple elaborations or a group of delusions that are all related by the person to a single event or theme (DSM-IV).

delusional depression   See **depression, delusional.**

delusional infestation   See **delusional parasitosis.**

delusional jealousy   Delusion that one's sexual partner is unfaithful.

delusional memory   Involvement of memory in delusional material (Buchanan A. Delusional memories: first-rank symptoms? *Br J Psychiatry* 1991;159:472–474). The person clearly remembers experience of past events that did not occur (Wing JK, Cooper JE, Sartorius N. *The Measurement and Classification of Psychiatric Symptoms.* London: Cambridge University Press, 1974). Delusional insight occurs not as an intuition about the world or as a change in knowledge of or about the world, but in the form of a memory (Mullen PE. The mental state and states of mind. *In* Hill P, Murray R, Thorley A [eds], *Essentials of Postgraduate Psychiatry.* London: Grune & Stratton, 1986, pp 3–36).

delusional parasitosis   Type of monosymptomatic hypochondriacal psychosis characterized by the unshakable belief of being infested with parasites. It occurs most frequently in older women, but may also affect younger men. Sufferers describe in detail the activities of the parasite (e.g., burrowing or biting) and may produce "evidence" such as fragments of the skin. An acute transient form is common in stimulant abusers (cocaine, amphetamines, methylphenidate). It also may be a symptom of schizophrenia. Pimozide is now recognized as an effective treatment in some cases. Also called "delusional infestation." See **monosymptomatic hypochondriacal psychosis.**

demand characteristics   **1.** In an experimental study, the sum total of cues that communicate to the subject(s) the purpose of the experiment and the nature of the behavior expected. Cues are derived from the manner in which subjects are solicited, the manner in which they are treated by the experimenter, scuttlebutt about the experiment, experimental instructions and, most importantly, the experimental procedure itself. Subjects may confirm the investigator's hypothesis in an effort to behave appropriately rather than respond directly to the independent variables under investigation. **2.** In nonexperimental settings, the tendency of individuals to live up to what is implicitly expected of them, a factor that may play a major role in the outcome of treatment.

Demelox See **amoxapine.**

dement Individual with an absence or reduction of intellectual faculties (intellect, memory) without global impairment of consciousness as a consequence of known organic brain disease.

dementia Global impairment of cognitive function, usually progressive (as opposed to step-wise increases, as in small strokes) that interferes with normal social and occupational activities, even though the patient is fully conscious and lucid. Although dementia is defined by impairment of memory, language, and reasoning, its most troubling aspects are often behavioral disturbances and psychiatric symptoms as a result of damage to the brain. It is an etiologically nonspecific syndrome and may be caused by Alzheimer's disease, frontal lobe degenerations, stroke, basal ganglia degenerative disorders, multiple sclerosis, trauma, brain tumors, brain infection (acquired immunodeficiency syndrome [AIDS], Creutzfeldt-Jakob disease), hydrocephalus, depression, and toxic or metabolic disorders. Differential diagnosis requires clinical, laboratory, and neuroimaging investigations (Cummings, J. Treatment challenges in dementing disorders. 1992 US Psychiatric & Mental Health Congress. Session 418;1992:194). Screaming and head-banging behavior among demented patients is not only common but often refractory to conventional drug treatment; trazodone gradually increased to 300 mg/day and adjunctive L-tryptophan titrated to 2.5 g daily has been reported to be safe and effective (Greenwald BS, Marin DB, Silverman SM. Serotonergic treatment of screaming and banging in dementia. *Lancet* 1986;2:1464–1465; O'Neil M, Page N, Adkins WN, et al. Tryptophan-trazodone treatment of aggressive behavior. *Lancet* 1986;2:859–860; Wilcock GK, Stevens J, Perkins A. Trazodone/tryptophan for aggressive behavior. *Lancet* 1987;1: 929–930). See **senile dementia of the Lewy body type.**

dementia/cognitive evaluation Cognitive dysfunction in dementia may be evaluated by Mini-Mental State examination (MMS), Blessed Memory, Information & Concentration test, and the Wechsler Adult Intelligence Scale.

dementia, end-stage Progression of dementia to the point at which severe functional impairments result in life-threatening medical complications: (a) incontinence requiring catheterization with the risk of urinary infections; (b) impaired mastication and swallowing with the risk of developing aspiration pneumonia; and (c) severe weakness prohibiting walking and necessitating bed confinement with the risk of developing bed sores. Many end-stage dementia patients are in a vegetative state; others are so cognitively impaired they cannot verbalize the pain they experience. Caring for end-stage dementia patients severely taxes the emotional, psychological, and physical resources of caregivers. Hospice care provides vital palliative care for the patient's comfort and respite from the stress relatives experience caring for the patient at home.

dementia, frontal lobe type (DFT) Form of pre-senile dementia that presents with a clinical picture suggestive of progressive, selective damage to the brain's frontal region but without the pathological or chemical hallmarks of Alzheimer's disease. Relationship with Pick's disease is unclear; most patients with DFT lack the specific balloon-like cells of Pick's disease. DFT affects the white matter of the frontotemporal areas of the brain, especially the middle and superior frontal gyri. Men and women are affected to the same degree, with onset between ages 40 and 70, most often in the mid-50s. About half of affected patients have a family history of dementia (Kisely S, Tweddle D, Pugh EW. Dementia presenting with sore eyes. *Br J Psychiatry* 1992;161:120–121).

dementia/hypomania or mania Hypomania or mania, either a first episode or secondary to drugs or another medical condition, may occur in patients with various types of dementia. If a first episode, careful medical evaluation is warranted. If mania/hypomania is not due to a tumor or other intracranial lesion, treatment is guided by the same principles used for nondemented patients. If the disorder is secondary, treatment for the primary condition should precede therapy of the affective disorder. Neuroleptics may be indicated for acute manic symptoms in Alzheimer8s disease or other demented patients with bipolar disease. Lithium may also be used, especially for long-term symptom control. However, demented patients may be susceptible to lithium neurotoxicity and may develop confusion, nausea, tremor, and ataxia with low serum levels. Neurotoxicity poses the diagnostic conundrum of distinguishing a toxic confusional state from dementia. There are too few data on carbamazepine or valproic acid for hypomania or mania in demented patients to permit recommending treatment with either drug.

dementia, hysterical   See **pseudodementia.**

dementia, irreversible   Condition diagnosed only after potentially reversible causes have been excluded on the basis of the patient's history, physical examination, and laboratory tests. See **dementia, reversible.**

dementia, Lewy body   See **senile dementia of the Lewy body type.**

dementia of the Alzheimer type   (DAT, SDAT) Insidiously deteriorating psychiatric disorder progressing from minimal symptoms with limited disability to mutism, incontinence, severe memory impairment, disorientation, and complete immobility. Clinical features exhibited are determined by the duration and rate of progression of the illness. It has been studied extensively with positron emission tomography (PET) and shown to have focal metabolic decrements in the early stages, predominantly involving the parietal and temporal lobes. Metabolic involvement becomes more generalized and severe with disease progression. Diagnosis of definite DAT requires that the patient meet clinical criteria for probable DAT and have compatible biopsy or autopsy findings. Diagnostic criteria for probable DAT include progressive worsening in memory and at least one other area of cognition, absence of delirium, onset at ages 40–90, and absence of another illness capable of producing a dementia syndrome. Possible DAT is the diagnosis when there are unusual variations in the onset, presentation, or course of the illness and there is no alternative explanation for the disease; when a second disorder is present but is not thought to be responsible for the dementia; or when only a single, slowly progressive deficit is found. Clinical features that make the diagnosis of DAT unlikely include sudden onset of the dementia, presence of focal neurological findings, or occurrence of seizures or gait disturbances early in the course of the illness. Clinical experience has demonstrated that these criteria have been consistently correct in over 80% of cases (McKhann, Drachman D, Folstein M, et al. Clinical diagnosis of Alzheimer's disease: Report of the NINCDS-ADRDA Work Group under the auspices of the Dept. of Health and Human Services Task Force on Alzheimer's Disease. *Neurology* 1984;34:939–944) See **Alzheimer's disease; senile dementia of the Alzheimer type.**

dementia, multi-infarct   (MID) This dementia is related to the extent of cerebral infarction.

Its frequency increases dramatically with age, especially in those over 85. Prevalence of vascular dementia may exceed that of Alzheimer's disease (AD) in populations with high prevalence of risk factors for vascular disease (e.g., Japanese, blacks). Since the rates of both vascular dementia and AD increase substantially with age, the number of people with either condition increases, as does the rate of so-called mixed (co-existing) cases. Mixed cases of dementia are more common than generally thought, especially in the very old.

dementia, presenile   Deterioration of the brain (dementia) with onset before old age. There is generally loss of memory, concentration, and other intellectual skills. Alzheimer's disease is the most common type; people with Down syndrome are very susceptible to the condition.

dementia, primary   Dementia occurring independently of a mental disorder and not due to drug toxicity.

dementia pugilistica   Complex encephalopathy with dementia, dysarthria, ataxia, seizures, and pyramidal tract and Parkinson8s disease features that are best regarded as pseudo-parkinsonism, due to repeated brain injury in certain boxers. Patients show old petechial hemosiderin deposits in tiny lacunae and degenerative nerve cell loss and gliosis involving the cortex and basal nuclei (Mawdsley C, Ferguson FR. Neurological disease in boxers. *Lancet* 1963;2:795–801). It is manifested by slurred speech, loss of coordination, dementia, and premature death. Postmortem brain examination reveals extensive plaques of beta protein and neurofibrillary tangles similar to those found in Alzheimer's disease. Head injury is a risk factor in their development. Other neuropathological studies of boxers' brains show that gliosis and atrophy are concentrated in the medial structures of the temporal lobe concerned with memory and behavior. Neuropsychometric testing of memory and small changes in behavior patterns are more sensitive than imaging in detecting brain damage. Also called "boxer's brain"; "punch-drunk syndrome."

dementia, reversible   See **pseudodementia.**

dementia, senile   Irreversible decline in cognitive faculties, ending in death. Incidence increases with age; it occurs in 5–10% of all adults over age 65 and in 20% over age 80. It is divided into primary and secondary dementias. A common cause is Alzheimer's disease, which is more common than usual in people with Down syndrome.

dementia, subcortical   Diseases involving the caudate nucleus and thalamus as well as white matter diseases affecting tracts interconnecting subcortical structures and connecting the dorsolateral prefrontal cortex with these subcortical nuclei. Included are degenerative basal ganglia diseases such as Huntington's, Parkinson's, and Wilson's diseases; hydrocephalus; Steele-Richardson syndrome; and idiopathic basal ganglia calcification. About two-thirds of patients with Parkinson's disease may be affected by frontal subcortical dysfunction. Thus, the conditions manifesting subcortical dementia are characterized by abnormal movements, which are usually considered to be a manifestation of basal ganglia pathology. Cardinal features of subcortical dementias are cognitive slowing, memory impairment, executive-function deficits, and mood and personality changes. Neuropsychiatric alterations are also common. Personality changes are ubiquitous and consist of apathy or irritability. Depression is common, occurring in 40% of Parkinson's disease and 25% of Huntington's disease patients. Although much less common, mania has been described in Huntington's disease, idiopathic basal ganglia calcification, and Wilson's disease. Psychosis is uncommon, but occurs more often in Huntington's patients (5–20%) and in those with idiopathic basal ganglia calcification. Cognitive impairments are characterized by marked psychosocial incompetence associated with minimal memory loss and, as a rule, absence of aphasia, apraxia, or agnosia. Many subcortical dementias have an associated motor system disturbance. Speech abnormalities, including dysarthria, hypophonia, and dysprosody, are common early in subcortical diseases. Difficulties in problem solving and abnormalities of judgment and insight may occur (Dunne FJ. Subcortical dementia. *Br Med J* 1993;307: 1–2). When simple and complex reaction times are measured, patients show a disproportionate elongation of complex reaction times. Slowing also occurs in tasks that require scanning of the memory for target items and in tests that involve rapid serial addition. Memory deficits of subcortical dementia differ from those typically seen in cortical dementias such as Alzheimer's disease, in which impaired memory storage is manifested by poor recall and abnormal recognition memory. Alzheimer's disease patients are not aided by prompting, cues, or multiple-choice lists. In subcortical dementias, recognition memory is preserved and patients derive considerable benefit from cues, prompting, and multiple-choice presentations. Subcortical dementias typically spare language skills, in contrast to Alzheimer's disease, in which aphasia is common. Patients with subcortical dementia retain language abilities until the final period of the disease, when all cognitive abilities are

compromised. Bradyphrenia (slowing of cognitive functioning), considered a cardinal feature of subcortical dementia, provides a distinction between subcortical and cortical dementia (Cummings JL. *Subcortical Dementia.* Oxford: Oxford University Press, 1990). Distinguishing between them may have some therapeutic value, as subcortical dementias may be amenable to treatment with dopamine agonists and levodopa, whereas cortical dementias (e.g., Alzheimer's disease) remain incurable. Better awareness of the cognitive deficits associated with particular dementias may lead to better management. Because of similarities in the clinical features of subcortical dementia and type II schizophrenia (especially slowness, apathy, and loss of motivation), and in the pattern of neuropsychological deficits, pathology, biochemistry, and data from brain-imaging studies, it is possible that certain schizophrenic symptoms, particularly negative symptoms and disturbance of movement, may reflect subcortical pathology (Pantelis C, Barnes TRE, Nelson HE. Is the concept of frontal-subcortical dementia relevant to schizophrenia? *Br J Psychiatry* 1992;160:442–460). Also called "bradyphrenia." See **subcortical structures.**

dementia syndrome of depression   See **pseudodementia.**

Demerol   See **meperidine.**

desmethylcitalopram   Main metabolite of citalopram. Like the parent compound, it has pronounced serotonergic activity.

demography   Study of population characteristics (e.g., size, density, fertility, mortality, growth, age distribution, migration, vital statistics) and their interaction with social and economic conditions.

Demolox   See **amoxapine.**

demoxepam   Pharmacologically active metabolite of chlordiazepoxide.

denbufylline   (BRL 30892) Novel compound that has proved active in animal models of cerebral vascular insufficiency and aging, and in preliminary studies of multi-infarct dementia (Nicholson CD, Angersbach D. Denbufylline [BRL 30892]—a novel drug to alleviate the consequences of cerebral ischaemia. *In* Krieglstein J [ed], *Pharmacology of Cerebral Ischaemia.* Amsterdam: Elsevier, 1986, pp 391–396; Saletu B, Anderer P, Firschhof PK, et al. EEG mapping and psychopharmacological studies with denbufylline in SDAT and MID. *Biol Psychiatry* 1992;32:668–681).

dendrite   Projection from a nerve cell that receives information from other, nearby cells and passes it on to the cell body. The cell body analyses the information and generates bioelectrical charges in the nerve membrane that pass the information to a nerve terminal at the end of the axon, leading to release of a neurotransmitter.

denial Mechanism in which a person fails to acknowledge some aspect of external reality that would be apparent to others (DSM-IV). See **defense mechanism.**

Deniban See **amisulpride.**

density sampling Method of selecting study control subjects in which cases are sampled only from incident cases over a specific period, and in which control subjects are interviewed throughout that period.

deoxyribonucleic acid (DNA) Macromolecule composed of a linear array of deoxyribonucleotides that have three components: nitrogenous base, sugar (deoxyribose), and phosphate. Each base is linked to adjacent ones on the same strand by the sugar and phosphate groups. The bases in DNA are either purines (adenosine [A] or guanine [G]) or pyrimidines (cytosine [C] or thymidine [T]). In the Watson-Crick helical structure of double-stranded DNA, a purine base on one strand pairs with a pyrimidine base on the opposite strand (G pairs with C, and A pairs with T). The order of these bases encodes the "information" contained in DNA. Lengths of DNA are frequently discussed in thousands of base pairs (kilobase pairs [kb]) or millions of base pairs (megabase pairs [Mb]).

Depakene See **valproic acid.**

Depakine See **valproate.**

Depakote See **divalproex; valproate.**

Depakote Sprinkle Capsule Formulation of divalproex sodium that has the most favorable absorption profile compared to syrup, capsules, and tablets. It can be used to effectively avoid gastrointestinal side effects. It can be swallowed intact or sprinkled on food.

Dep Andro See **testosterone cypionate.**

Deparcol See **diethazine.**

Depas See **etizolam.**

dependence Term with several meanings, depending on context. In the early 1960s, experts considered dependence a psychic and sometimes physical state resulting from the interaction between a person and a drug that is responsible for a variety of responses, including a compulsion to take the drug continuously or episodically to experience its psychic effects and at times to avert the discomfort of its absence. In the scientific literature, *dependence* may mean (a) a behavioral syndrome that implies compulsive, out-of-control use; (b) physical dependence, or alterations in neural systems manifested in tolerance and withdrawal when the chronically administered drug is discontinued or displaced from its receptor; and (c) a specific psychiatric diagnosis that meets an agreed-on number of criteria. Dependence represents a new dynamic equilibrium of physiological functions produced by drug actions on the organism and the organism's compensatory countermechanisms. In the presence of the drug, the dependent organism functions as it did before exposure to the drug. Presence of physical dependency is not determined directly, but assessed indirectly by withdrawal symptoms after abrupt discontinuation of the drug. In the case of drugs for which an antagonist exists (e.g., benzodiazepines, opioids), withdrawal can be elicited by administering benzodiazepine receptor antagonists such as flumazenil or naloxone. With opiates, withdrawal can be precipitated by an opiate antagonist such as naloxone. Physical dependence may or may not manifest itself while therapy is continued, depending on the duration of action of the drug involved. With short-acting agents (e.g., certain opioids) there may be mild withdrawal between doses; with longer-acting agents (e.g., flurazepam), dependence becomes apparent when withdrawal signs and symptoms occur following drug discontinuation. See **addiction.**

dependence, drug See **drug dependence.**

dependence, multiple Simultaneous dependence on more than one psychoactive substance (drugs, alcohol), including the predominant practice in which the user has a hierarchy of substance use. Multiple dependency has been on the increase, whereas the drug-dependent person who is dependent on only one drug is becoming rare.

dependence, physical See **drug dependence.**

dependence, physiological See **drug dependence.**

dependence prevention program Programs to prevent dependence among drug users not yet dependent and to preclude worsened dependence among those already drug-dependent. Since most drug-dependent persons are over age 30, dependency prevention programs focus mainly on middle-aged and older groups. However, since age at first use for alcohol, cannabis, and cocaine is about 16, dependency prevention programs should be started as soon as drug use begins.

dependence-prone Having personality factors or particular psychopathology that are likely to result in dependence on sedative/hypnotics, alcohol, and/or other substances of abuse. The term implies that the person is responsible for response to a drug, rather than the drug being the cause of their response to it.

dependence, psychic Condition in which a drug produces a feeling of satisfaction and a psychic drive that requires periodic or continuous administration of the drug to produce pleasure or avoid discomfort (World Health Organization [WHO]).

dependence, psychological   See **drug dependence.**

dependence syndrome   See **drug dependence.**

dependence, therapeutic dose   Dependence on moderate therapeutic doses of a sedative/ hypnotic drug, with no tendency to increase dosage. It may not manifest itself during ongoing therapy, but becomes apparent when withdrawal symptoms emerge following dosage reduction or drug discontinuation. It occurs frequently in patients prescribed short-half-life benzodiazepines (e.g., alprazolam), but is also seen with longer-acting agents such as diazepam. Such dependence may be responsible for complaints by patients or physicians of how difficult terminating therapeutic doses can be and for continuation of sedative/ hypnotic administration for prolonged periods.

dependent drinker   **1.** One who meets DSM-IV criteria for alcohol dependence. Current criteria do not require presence of physical dependence. **2.** One who has a compulsion to drink, takes roughly the same amount each day, has increased tolerance to alcohol in the early stages, and reduced tolerance later; suffers withdrawal symptoms when alcohol is stopped, which are relieved by consuming more; in whom drinking takes precedence over other activities; and who tends to resume drinking after a period of abstinence (Royal College of General Practitioners, 1986).

dependent sample   Sample in which values in one group can be predicted from values in the other group.

depersonalization   Nonspecific syndrome in which perception or experience of the self is altered so that the subject feels personal identity is lost and that he or she, his or her body, and/or the environment is different or unreal. Other symptoms may include mood changes; difficulty in organizing, collecting, and arranging thoughts; and a feeling that the brain has been deadened. Depersonalization has been reported in temporal-lobe epilepsy and temporal lobe migraine. Significant depersonalization has been reported 30 minutes after smoking high-potency marijuana cigarettes (Mathew RJ, Wilson WH, Humphreys D, et al. Depersonalization after marijuana smoking. *Biol Psychiatry* 1993;33:431–441). Depersonalization is known to occur in children and normal adults. It is more common in women, and most often occurs in the third and fourth decades of life. It usually lasts from 2–3 years and disappears spontaneously. Also called "feeling of unreality."

depersonalization disorder   (DPD) Dissociative disorder characterized by persistent or recurrent episodes of depersonalization, sufficiently severe to cause marked distress, in the absence of other psychiatric disorders (Chee KT, Wong KE. Depersonalization syndrome—a report of nine cases. *Singapore Med J* 1990;31:331–334). Depersonalization includes altered perception or experience of the self and a feeling of detachment from one's body or mental processes "as if in a dream." The person often feels like an outside observer of his or her own activities and thoughts. Sensory anesthesia or the sensation of not being in complete control of one's actions may occur, is egodystonic and nondelusional, and may be accompanied by lack of emotions. Derealization, evidenced by altered perception and sense of reality of the external world, frequently accompanies depersonalization. Anxiety disorders, depression, and schizophrenia are frequently accompanied by symptoms of depersonalization. Organic disorders including temporal lobe epilepsy, migraine, and marijuana abuse may also produce depersonalization (Hollander E, Carrasco JL, Mullen LS, et al. Left hemispheric activation in depersonalization disorder: a case report. *Biol Psychiatry* 1992;31:1157–1162). See **dissociative disorder.**

Depixol   See **flupenthixol.**

Depixol Injection   See **flupenthixol decanoate.**

"depo"   Street name for an anabolic steroid, usually testosterone cypionate.

depolarization   Inside of a nerve cell becoming less negatively charged relative to the outside of the nerve membrane.

Depo-Provera   See **medroxyprogesterone acetate.**

Depotest   See **testosterone cypionate.**

Depo-Testosterone   See **testosterone cypionate.**

depot   Delivery of a slow-release form of medication via intramuscular injection, usually into the deltoid or gluteal muscles, occasionally subcutaneously. Active drug is steadily released from the depot or reservoir to the blood and then to the site of action, providing duration of action from 2–4 weeks.

depot neuroleptic   See **neuroleptic, depot.**

deprenyl   See **selegiline.**

deprenyl and tocopherol antioxidative therapy of parkinsonism   (DATATOP) See **alpha-tocopherol.**

"Depressed? Sig E Caps"   Mnemonic reference to DSM-IV criteria for depression. *Depressed* refers to the primary symptom (the feeling of sadness, hopelessness, or discouragement); *Sig E Caps* refers to the first letters of words describing eight other possible problem areas: sleep, interest, guilt, energy, concentration, appetite, psychomotor skills, and suicidality.

depression State of lowered mood, often accompanied by disturbances of sleep, energy, appetite, concentration, interests, and sexual drive. It is a biologically heterogeneous illness involving many neurotransmitter and receptor systems. Different subgroups have been described (e.g., endogenous/nonendogenous, primary/secondary, unipolar/bipolar, psychotic/nonpsychotic, familial pure depressive disorder/sporadic depressive disorder). Hence, it is plausible to expect patients to respond in different ways and at different rates to antidepressant pharmacotherapy. Growing evidence suggests that depression is underdiagnosed and undertreated, especially when it accompanies physical illness. Clinicians may be inclined to regard affective symptoms as understandable when associated with serious medical conditions (e.g., cancer). Furthermore, there may be reluctance to use antidepressant drugs in case they aggravate the underlying physical condition. On the other hand, there are also diagnostic pitfalls if too much emphasis is placed on symptoms such as anorexia, weight loss, and fatigue, which are important symptoms of primary depressive illness, but which can be entirely explained by physical pathology.

depression, akinetic See **depression, postpsychotic.**

depression, atypical Depressive subtype, defined differently by various researchers, that generally includes initial insomnia, overeating, hypersomnia, a variety of anxiety and phobic symptoms, and lack of clear, endogenous symptoms such as guilt, weight loss, and anhedonia. The hyperphagia and hypersomnia that define atypical depression are in marked contrast to the cardinal symptoms of anorexia and early morning awakening of typical depression. In addition, patients with atypical depression seem passive, anergic, and apathetic, which contrasts with intense anxiety about self and ruminative preoccupation with the inevitability of loss that are characteristic of melancholia. In addition to depressed mood, diagnostic criteria include markedly increased appetite, with a weight gain of at least 4.5 kg; sleeping at least 10 hours/day; prominent, severe fatigue that creates a sensation of leaden paralysis or extreme heaviness of arms or legs; and sensitivity to rejection as a trait throughout adulthood (defined as present if rejection results in depression with functional impairment, e.g., missed work or school). Another manifestation is the triad of chocolate craving, rejection sensitivity, and applause hunger; symptoms respond poorly or incompletely to tricyclic antidepressants (TCAs), but well to monoamine oxidase inhibitors (MAOIs) and possibly to serotonin uptake inhibitors. Current clinical evidence indicates that atypical depressions in general respond well to MAOIs and nonheterocyclic antidepressants, and poorly to TCAs and electroconvulsive therapy.

depression, brief Episode of depression characterized by abrupt onset, brief duration (97% last a week or less, and two-thirds last between 2 and 4 days), increased severity (70% registered as moderate or severe on the Montgomery-Asberg Depression Rating Scale), and a median interval frequency of 18 days. Episodes are reported in a substantial majority of patients without major depression. They are distinguished from major depression by their short duration and from minor depression by their severity. Suicide attempt rate is high.

depression/cancer An unexpectedly high prevalence rate of mood disorders, especially depression, has been noted in patients with various types of cancer. A series of case studies and a few prospective studies suggest that patients with pancreatic cancer have an unusually high rate of major depression, even prior to diagnosis. There is also evidence for moderately high rates of major depression in patients with breast cancer, endometrial and cervical cancer, and malignant melanoma. A sizable percentage of cancer patients who do not fulfil categorical criteria for major depression exhibit significant depressive symptoms as assessed by dimensional measures of depression (Nemeroff CB, McDaniel JS, Reed D, et al. Cancer and depression: diagnostic and biological measures. *Neuropsychopharmacology* 1993;9:40S).

depression, catecholamine hypothesis of See **catecholamine hypothesis of depression.**

depression, characterologic See **dysthymic disorder.**

depression, delusional Distinct subtype of unipolar depression that may be characterized by uncertain response to tricyclic antidepressant (TCA) treatment, but good response to electroconvulsive therapy or to a TCA plus a neuroleptic (Glassman AK, Kantor SJ, Shostak M. Depression, delusional and drug response. *Am J Psychiatry* 1975;132:716–719; Quitkin F, Rifkin A, Klein DF. Imipramine response in deluded depressive patients. *Am J Psychiatry* 1978;135:806–811).

depression/digitalis Depressive symptoms may be a manifestation of digitalis toxicity that may be alleviated by dosage reduction to a nontoxic level. Dosage reduction also would lower risk of cardiac arrhythmias. Recognition of depression secondary to digitalis toxicity and its appropriate treatment can be life-saving.

depression, disease-related Depression may occur in reaction to an illness, but also may be inherently associated with a number of physical disorders (e.g., thyroid disease, parathyroid disease, Addison's disease, Cushing's syndrome). The possibility that these causes of secondary depression may contribute to or be the cause of a patient's depression should be excluded, especially if the depression is treatment-resistant.

depression, dopamine hypothesis of See **dopamine hypothesis of depression.**

depression, double (DD) Major depression superimposed on underlying dysthymia (chronic minor depression). As many as 25% of patients with major depression have co-existing dysthymia. Double depression is increasingly recognized as a common psychiatric disorder that is less responsive to antidepressant treatment than uncomplicated major depression. On recovery from major depression, patients return to the premorbid dysthymic baseline. Relapses are twice as common for those who do not recover completely from both depressions (Klein DN, Taylor EB, Harding K, et al. Double-depression and episodic major depression: demographic clinical, familial, personality and socioenvironmental characteristics and short-term outcome. *Am J Psychiatry* 1988;145: 1226–1231).

depression, drug-induced Depression may be precipitated in susceptible patients by a number of drugs, including antihypertensives (reserpine, beta- blockers), digitalis, alpha-methyldopa, steroids, oral contraceptives, analgesics (opiates, ibuprofen, phenacetin), amantadine, levodopa, certain phenothiazines, and phenytoin. It appears that any drug that can deplete brain catecholamine may cause depression; the drugs more likely to do so are reserpine and alpha-methyldopa.

depression, drug-induced/elderly Because a number of drugs may cause depression in the elderly, assessment of depressed elderly patients should include a comprehensive personal drug history and evaluation of the possible role of medication. Drugs that may cause depression in the elderly include benzodiazepines, barbiturates, reserpine, methyldopa, cimetidine, ranitidine, beta blockers, thiazide diuretics, corticosteroids, digoxin, theophylline, metoclopramide, and alcohol. Sedative-hypnotics and antihypertensives are the drugs most commonly associated with causing depression. Both benzodiazepines and barbiturates have been implicated. Antihypertensives most often associated with depressive symptoms are reserpine, guanethidine, methyldopa, and beta blockers; thiazide diuretics used alone for hypertension also have been

implicated (Harper CM, Newton PA, Walsh JR. Drug-induced illness in the elderly. *Postgrad Med* 1989;86:245–256).

depression, endogenous Concept of depression "arising from within," in contrast to exogenous depression that is caused by external factors.

depression, exogenous Affective illness attributed to extraneous factors, as opposed to endogenous depression, which "arises from within."

depression, geriatric In his 1910 textbook of psychiatry, Kraepelin stated that depressions are disproportionately frequent in the elderly, are often followed by dementia, and differ from depressive disorders earlier in life. Depression is the most common psychiatric diagnosis in the elderly, the dominating constituent of affective disorder, and commonly associated with physical ill health. Suicide, most frequent in old age, attests to the suffering that so many old people experience with the disorder. Missed diagnosis and failure to treat effectively and energetically are still the cardinal dangers. Depression has too often been seen as a "predictable, understandable response to the losses and declines ... [in] the season of sorrow and despair" (Jones RG. Lean, slipper'd and depressed. *Br Med J* 1987; 294:505).

depression, hypokalemic Depression with psychomotor retardation may be due to hypokalemia secondary to diuretic use. If hypokalemia is severe, the patient should be admitted to an intensive care unit because low serum potassium may produce fatal cardiac arrhythmia unless appropriate medical intervention is made.

depression, indolamine hypothesis of See **indolamine hypothesis of depression.**

depression, intermittent See **dysthymic disorder.**

depression, major (MD) Unipolar mood disorder (one or more depressive episodes) in a patient who has never had a manic or unequivocal hypomanic episode (DSM-IV). MD episodes are classified as either single-episode or recurrent. MD is manifested by vegetative symptoms (anorexia, weight loss, insomnia, hypersomnia) associated with depressed mood, loss of energy and interests, anxiety, irritability, decreased libido, difficulty concentrating, and suicidal ideation. Mild MD is manifested by few, if any, symptoms in excess of those required to make the diagnosis; moderate MD by symptoms between "mild" and "severe"; and severe (either with or without psychotic features) by several symptoms in excess of those required to make the diagnosis and causing marked interference with occupational, social, and interpersonal relationships. MD is associated with a high rate of recurrence, even when psychotic cases are excluded. Highest rate is observed during the first months after recovery from an episode. Prophylactic drug treatment reduces recurrence risk, but apparently does not affect the trend toward increasing severity of subsequent episodes.

depression, major/sleep alteration In patients with an acute episode of major depression, all-night electroencephalographic (EEG) studies have shown (a) frequent nocturnal awakenings; (b) less slow-wave sleep (especially during the first non rapid eye movement [REM] period); (c) shortened (REM) latency; (d) increased REM sleep; and (e) increased density of rapid eye movement during REM sleep (Lauer CJ, Riemann D, Wiegand M, Berger M. From early to late adulthood changes in EEG sleep of depressed patients and healthy volunteers. *Biol Psychiatry* 1991;29: 979–993).

depression, minor See **dysthymic disorder.**

depression/neuropeptides The role of neuropeptides in the etiology of depression has been examined by measuring their concentrations in cerebrospinal fluid (CSF) of depressed individuals. These studies have generally found decreased CSF somatostatin concentrations and elevations in CSF corticotropin-releasing hormone (CRH). Moreover, there is a correlation between reduction of CSF somatostatin concentration and lack of dexamethasone suppression. It is not known whether decreased CSF somatostatin is due to excessive endogenous CRH secretion or whether decreased somatostatin and elevated CRH secretion reflects two independent pathways associated with depression (Post RM, Rubinow DR, Gold PW. Neuropeptides in manic-depressive illness. *In* Nemeroff CB [ed], *Neuropeptides in Psychiatric and Neurological Disorders.* Baltimore: Johns Hopkins University Press, 1988, pp 76–115).

depression, neurotic Depressed mood that is inappropriate in duration and magnitude but that remains circumscribed and reacts to both environmental and psychological events. This form of depression is qualitatively more related to normal depressive moods than to endogenous depression. See **dysthymic disorder.**

depression, obsessional Major depressive syndrome coexistent with obsessive-compulsive features. It may be especially responsive to serotonin uptake inhibitors, even after being refractory to other agents (Montgomery SA. Selectivity of antidepressants and resistant depression. *In* Amsterdam JA [ed], *Advances in Neuropsychiatry and Psychopharmacology, vol. 2: Refractory Depression.* New York: Raven Press, 1991, pp 93–104).

depression, pharmacogenic See **depression, postpsychotic.**

depression, postpartum Depression that occurs following childbirth. It lasts longer than postpartum blues and is distinguished from puerperal depressive psychosis by lesser severity and the absence of delusions and hallucinations. Incidence may be 7–24%. It can be treated with high-dose (200 µg) transdermal estrogen patch (Henderson AF, Gregiore A, Studd JWW, et al. The treatment of severe postnatal depression with oestradiol skin patches. *Lancet* 1991;388:816). See **postpartum blues; psychosis, postpartum.**

depression, postpsychotic Co-existence of several degrees of extrapyramidal side effects and dysphoric mood states in neuroleptic-treated patients. It has a propensity to occur in bipolar patients when mania is treated with excessive doses of neuroleptics and occurs in approximately 25% of schizophrenic or schizoaffective patients responsive to antipsychotic drug therapy. It may be associated with the poor outcome features of impaired role functioning, relapse, or suicide (Becker RE. Depression in schizophrenia. *Hosp Comm Psychiatry* 1988;39:1269–1275). It also may be a significant reason why schizophrenic patients refuse to take their drugs (Van Putten T. Why do schizophrenic patients refuse to take their drugs? *Arch Gen Psychiatry* 1974;31:67–72). Symptoms include depressed mood, anhedonia, low energy level, poor concentration, and pessimism. Since these symptoms may overlap with the negative symptoms of schizophrenia, differential diagnosis may be difficult. Assessment of mood may be helpful; depressed mood is often an obvious feature in postpsychotic depression, whereas blunted affect is a central aspect of negative symptoms. If the depression seems stable and the patient does not become psychotic, symptoms may be a neuroleptic side effect, such as akinesia. Administration of the full therapeutic dose of an antiparkinson drug (e.g., benztropine, 2 mg 3 times a day) will help distinguish between depression and akinesia within a few days to a week. When depression symptoms persist despite antiparkinson drug therapy, an antidepressant should be added to the neuroleptic and antiparkinson medications. It is best to start with a low antidepressant dose (e.g., imipramine 50 mg/day) and raise dosage gradually by 50-mg increments until the full therapeutic dose is reached. Because neuroleptics and antidepressants may affect each other's metabolism, resulting in elevated blood levels, monitoring of antidepressant blood levels is prudent. It also would be prudent to check the electrocardiogram in patients who may be vulnerable to cardiac conduction defects (Siris SG. Diagnosis of secondary depression in schizophrenia: implications for DSM-IV. *Schizophr Bull* 1991;17:75–98). Also called "akinetic depression"; "pharmacogenic depression."

depression, poststroke (PSD) Major or minor depression that occurs after a stroke in approximately 50% of patients. Clinical symptoms of the major depression include sadness, anxiety, tension, loss of interest and concentration, sleep disturbance with early morning awakening, loss of appetite with weight loss, difficulty concentrating and thinking, and thoughts of death. The minor depression is characterized by sadness, sleep disturbance, loss of energy, difficulty concentrating or thinking clearly, social withdrawal, loss of interest, brooding, a pessimistic attitude toward the future, irritability, and tearfulness. The severity of physical disability, including aphasia, is not typically related to severity of depressive symptoms, suggesting that mood disorders following stroke are not merely an expected grief reaction to loss of function. Furthermore, poststroke mood disorders are associated with specific lesion loci. Depression is more frequent with left-sided stroke; it has been diagnosed in 60% of patients with left anterior lesions and in 90% of those with caudate lesions. Mania may be more common after right-sided stroke (Cummings JL. The neuroanatomy of depression. *J Clin Psychiatry* 1993;54[suppl]:14–20). Accurate diagnosis is critical because depression can significantly reduce the speed and success of stroke rehabilitation outcome. Major poststroke depression remits spontaneously in 1–2 years; whereas most patients with minor depression after a stroke remain depressed 2 years later. Either form may respond to tricyclic antidepressants such as nortriptyline (Catapano F, Galderisi S. Depression and cerebral stroke. *J Clin Psychiatry* 1990;51[suppl 9]:9–12). Electroconvulsive therapy also is very effective and generally well tolerated (Currier MB, Murray GB, Welch CC. Electroconvulsive therapy for post-stroke depressed geriatric patients. *J Neuropsychiatry Clin Neurosci* 1992;4:140–144).

depression, primary Depressive syndrome occurring in a patient with no prior history of any other psychiatric illness (e.g., alcoholism, anxiety disorder, somatization disorder, schizophrenia) or concurrent medical illness that is known to result in depression.

depression, primary unipolar There are familial subtypes: depression (or depressive) spectrum disorder and familial pure depressive disorder. The former differs from familial pure depressive disorder in having more familial anxiety, somatization disorder, more divorce, more suicide attempts, and more negative life events, and in needing more time to recover from the index episode. These patients are more likely to develop alcoholism and drug abuse. Depressive spectrum disorder patients are more likely to meet symptomatic criteria for neurotic depression (Winokur G, Coryell W. Familial subtypes of unipolar depression: a prospective study of familial pure depressive disease compared to depression spectrum disease. *Biol Psychiatry* 1992;32:1012–1018). See **depression spectrum disorder; familial pure depressive disorder.**

depression, psychotic 1. Presence of neurovegetative signs of depression, delusions, hallucinations, and/or marked formal thought disorder. 2. Depression with impaired reality testing. 3. Incapacitating depression. 4. Very severe depression that may nevertheless be seen in outpatients. A review of data on psychotic depression revealed statistically significant differences between psychotic and nonpsychotic major depression. There are greater guilt feelings and psychomotor disturbance in psychotic depression; there are significant differences in patients with psychotic and nonpsychotic depression in glucocorticoid activity, dopamine beta-hydroxylase activity, levels of dopamine and serotonin metabolites, sleep measures, and ventricle-to-brain ratios. Family studies show higher rates of bipolar disorder in first-degree relatives of probands with psychotic major depression than of probands with nonpsychotic major depression. Greater morbidity and residual impairment also have been reported in patients with psychotic depression, who respond poorly to placebo and to tricyclic antidepressants (TCAs). These differences are not due to differences in severity or endogenicity. Further studies are needed to develop an optimal set of operational criteria (Schatzberg AF, Rothschild AJ. Psychotic [delusional] major depression: should it be included as a distinct syndrome in DSM-IV? *Am J Psychiatry* 1992;149:733–745). Psychotic depression may respond to TCAs or monoamine oxidase inhibitors, but response rate is low compared to nonpsychotic depressives (Chan CH, Janicak PG, Davis JM, et al. Response of psychotic and nonpsychotic depressed patients to tricyclic antidepressants. *J Clin Psychiatry* 1987;48:197–200; Janicak PG, Pandley GN, Davis JM, et al. Response of psychotic and nonpsychotic depression to phenelzine. *Am J Psychiatry* 1988;145:93–95). Amoxapine, or a combination of amitriptyline plus perphenazine, may be useful (Anton RF, Burch EA. Amoxapine versus amitriptyline combined with perphenazine in the treatment of psychotic depression. *Am J Psychiatry* 1990;147: 1203–1208). A naturalistic, 3- to 4-year follow-up study of delusional depressives showed an 87% relapse rate, with most patients experiencing at least two relapses. These results suggest that physicians should be wary of prematurely tapering medication within the first 12 months (Aronson TA, Shukla S, Gujavarty K, et al. Relapse in delusional depression—a retrospective study of the course of treatment. *Compr Psychiatry* 1988;29:12–21).

depression rating scales Clinical Global Impressions Scale; Hamilton Rating Scale for Depression; Montgomery Asberg Depression Rating Scale; Raskin Depression Scale.

depression, reactive Disorder of relatively acute onset precipitated by some external life event. It is likely to clear up quickly once the underlying situation is resolved.

depression, recurrent brief 1. Diagnostic category with a symptom pattern identical to a major depressive episode, except that the condition lasts less than 2 weeks. Prevalence in young adults is about 10%. Suicide attempts are twice as frequent in patients with recurrent brief depression as in those with major depressive disorders (Angst J, Merikangas K, Scherdegger P, Wicki W. Recurrent brief depression: a new subtype of affective disorder. *J Affect Dis* 1990;19:87–98). 2. Major depressive syndrome characterized by short duration, high recurrence, and at least four of eight DSM-IV criteria for major depressive disorder (MDD). For multiple brief depressive episodes, prevalence rate is 3.7%; for depressive episodes of at least 2 weeks' duration, it is 3.8%. Prevalence from age 20–30 is comparable to that of MDD. Lifetime treatment rates, suicide attempts, and a positive family history of treated depression characterize recurrent brief depression as a valid subgroup of depression. It is frequently associated with MDD and dysthymia.

depression, recurrent unipolar (RU) Recurring nonbipolar depression in patients who do not have a personal history of hypomania or mania, but may have a bipolar family history.

depression, secondary Depressive syndrome secondary to an antecedent illness.

depression, sexual function Depressed individuals often have abnormalities in sexual function, including loss of sexual interest, diminished ability to maintain sexual arousal or achieve orgasm during an episode of major depression, reduced sexual activity, and loss of satisfaction in usual sexual activities (Nofzinger EA, Thase ME, Reynolds CF, III, et al.

Sexual function in depressed men. Assessment by self-report, behavioral and nocturnal penile tumescence measures before and after treatment with cognitive behavior therapy. *Arch Gen Psychiatry* 1993;50:24–30).

depression/smoking An association noted in cross-sectional studies between nicotine dependence and major depression probably reflects effects of common factors that predispose to both disorders (Breslau N, Kilbey MM, Andreski P. Nicotine dependence and major depression. New evidence from a prospective investigation. *Arch Gen Psychiatry* 1993;50:31–35). The association is not causal and arises largely from familial factors that are probably genetic and predispose to both smoking and major depression (Kendler KS, Neale MC, MacLean CJ, et al. Smoking and major depression. A causal analysis. *Arch Gen Psychiatry* 1993;50:36–43).

depression spectrum disorder (DSD) Familial subtype of primary unipolar depression that occurs in a person with a family history of alcoholism and/or antisocial personality. There may be a family history of primary depression, but none of mania. DSD is manifested by a stormy personal life, particularly with marital difficulties (Winokur G, Coryell W. Familial subtypes of unipolar depression: a prospective study of familial pure depressive disease compared to depression spectrum disease. *Biol Psychiatry* 1992;32:1012–1018). See **depression, primary unipolar.**

depression, treatment-resistant Ongoing, unremitting depression despite treatment with at least two different antidepressants or an antidepressant and a course of electroconvulsive therapy (ECT) (Remick RA, Barton JS, Patterson B, et al. On so-called treatment resistant depression. Presented at the 51st Annual Meeting, Royal College of Physicians and Surgeons of Canada. Quebec City, September 1982). Some experts believe that a trial of a tricyclic antidepressant (TCA) should not be considered a failure until tri-iodothyronine (T_3) potentiation has been tried (Goodwin FK, Prange AJ, Post RM et al. Potentiation of antidepressants effects by L-triiodothyronine in tricyclic nonresponders. *Am J Psychiatry* 1982;139:34–38). Many so-called treatment-refractory patients are given trials of only one antidepressant for too short a time, some have a psychiatric illness other than an affective disorder, and some fail to take their medication as prescribed. Several studies indicate that only a minority of treatment-resistant patients are "absolute" resistors, and that the majority of "relative" resistors can be helped substantially by accurate diagnosis and appropriate treatment with non–monoamine oxidase inhibitor

(MAOI) antidepressants, MAOIs, or electro-convulsive therapy. A patient who seems treat-ment-resistant but in fact is only relatively treatment-resistant may be safely and effica-ciously treated with one or more of the follow-ing: (a) adequate trial of a drug previously prescribed inadequately (provided there is no genetic contraindication to it); (b) adequate trial of an MAOI; (c) adequate course of ECT (at least seven treatments); (d) adequate course of any of the new, second-generation antide-pressants or serotonin uptake inhibitors; (e) any of the possible combination therapies, es-pecially a TCA plus a neuroleptic or a tricyclic plus an MAOI. An adequate trial requires no less than 4 and no more than 8 weeks of treatment with the usual therapeutic doses of each single therapy or each component of the combination. Because adequate trials can pro-duce improvement in 75–80% of so-called treat-ment-resistant depressions and because other options can benefit another 10–20%, it may be that only about 5–10% are "absolutely" treat-ment-resistant. Judicious use of newer antide-pressants may reduce the number further, so that even the so-called absolute treatment-resistant derive at least partial symptom ame-lioration.

depression, treatment-resistant/reserpine   Since 1963, a few reports have described dramatic antidepressant response in tricyclic-resistant patients with parenteral administration of re-serpine. Improvement occurred in as little as 48 hours and lasted as long as 6 months (Poldinger W. Combined administration of desipramine and reserpine or tetrabenazine in depressive patients. *Psychopharmacologia* 1963;4:308–310; Haskovec L, Rysanek K. The action of reserpine in imipramine-resistant depressive patients. *Psychopharmacologia* 1967; 11:18–30; Ayd FJ Jr. Reserpine therapy for tricyclic-resistant depressions. *Int Drug Ther Newsl* 1985;20:17–18). Findings were not rep-licated in subsequent controlled studies (Am-sterdam JD [ed]. *Refractory Depression: Advances in Neuropsychiatry and Psychopharmacology*, vol. 2. New York: Raven Press, 1991).

depression, unipolar   1. Endogenous depres-sion. 2. Any depression (including neurotic depression) that is not a bipolar disorder. 3. Psychotic depression or recurrent depression.

depression, unipolar II   See **bipolar III disorder.**

depressive affect   Emotion that accompanies an uncomplicated grief reaction to bereavement. It may also be seen in depression.

depressive neurosis   See **dysthymic disorder.**

depressive personality   See **dysthymic disorder.**

depressive spectrum disorder   See **depression spectrum disorder.**

Deprexan   See **desipramine.**

Deprimil   See **lofepramine.**

Deprol   See **meprobamate + benactyzine.**

depth electrode encephalography   Currently considered the criterion standard in determin-ing the location of seizure foci. It is a diagnos-tic technique of great importance to medically refractory epileptic patients who might be candidates for surgical excision of the seizure site. Because it is a very invasive technique, alternatives such as single positron emission computed tomography (SPECT) and positron emission tomography (PET) are being used with increasing frequency. SPECT also plays a major role in location of seizure foci (Devons MD. Comparison of SPECT application in neurology and psychiatry. *J Clin Psychiatry* 1992;53[suppl 11]:13–19).

Deptran   See **doxepin.**

Depyrel   See **trazodone.**

Deracyn CT   See **adinazolam.**

Deracyn SR   See **adinazolam SR.**

derailment   Loss of goal in thinking.

Deralin   See **propranolol.**

derealization   Feeling that one's surroundings have changed.

dermatoglyphics   Study of ridged skin on the palms and soles, customarily used in investiga-tion of chromosomal and other congenital abnormalities. Dermatoglyphic analyses are either qualitative (based on the patterns formed by the dermal ridges) or quantitative (count of dermal ridges in a pattern). Der-matoglyphic fluctuating asymmetry has been used to investigate developmental disorders providing data on the role of genetics, fetal insults, and developmental anomalies of the brain in the etiology of schizophrenia (Mellor CS. Dermatoglyphic evidence of fluctuating asymmetry in schizophrenia. *Br J Psychiatry* 1992;160:467–472).

Desoxyn   See **dextroamphetamine.**

desalkylflurazepam   Major active metabolite of both quazepam and flurazepam. It probably accounts for most of the clinical activity ob-served after flurazepam use in humans. Biotransformation of desalkylflurazepam itself appears to proceed by hydroxylation, with the hydroxylated metabolite rapidly conjugated and excreted.

descriptive statistics   See **statistics, descriptive.**

descriptive study   See **study, descriptive.**

des-enkephalin-gamma-endorphin   (DE[gam-ma]E) Neuropeptide related to the enkepha-lins. It has been tested in the treatment of chronic schizophrenia with inconclusive re-sults.

desensitization   1. Behavior therapy technique involving gradual exposure to an anxiety-provoking situation, frequently used in the treatment of phobias, often in combination with antipanic drugs. At each stage the person must overcome the anxiety before proceeding to the next, more difficult, stage. **2.** Waning of a stimulated response by the receptor resulting from continuous agonist exposure. It can be viewed as two separate processes: heterologous and homologous desensitization. The former occurs when exposure of cells to a desensitizing agent leads to diminished responses to a number of different stimuli. Homologous desensitization is much more specific and involves only loss of responsiveness to the specific desensitizing agent. See **down-regulation.**

design, experimental Plan of an experiment structured to answer specific experimental questions. It usually specifies (a) choice of subjects, species, age, sex, etc.; (b) apparatus used for stimulus presentation and response recording; (c) experimental procedure; and (d) type of analysis of results.

design variable See **variable, design.**

designer drug Illegally manufactured substance with substantial similarity in either structure or effect to substances already regulated by the Controlled Substances Act (Ziporyn T. A growing industry and menace: makeshift laboratory's designer drugs. *JAMA* 1986;256:3061–3063). Designer drugs are new chemical analogs primarily of narcotics or variations of existing controlled substances with psychedelic, stimulant, or depressive effects and potential for abuse. They are usually synthesized in clandestine laboratories, where their toxicity and potency are often vastly increased. Examples include 3,4-methylenedioxyamphetamine (MDA); 3,4-methylenedioxymethamphetamine (MDMA); "Ecstasy," an amphetamine analog; 3,4-methylenedioxyethamphetamine (MDEA); 1-methyl-4-phenyl-1,2,3,6-tetrahydropyridine (MPTP); and P-DOPE, fentanyl/opiate derivatives. Many are "designed" to escape detection since they have not been classified or scheduled by the Drug Enforcement Agency (DEA).

desipramine (Deprexan; Norpramin; Pertofrane) (DMI) Relatively nonsedating tricyclic antidepressant that is a primary metabolite of imipramine, but with fewer sedative and anticholinergic effects. It blocks reuptake of norepinephrine released at central synapses. It has low affinity for muscarinic and histaminergic receptors and only moderate affinity at alpha-1 alpha-adrenergic receptors. It is very weak against alpha-2, beta-adrenergic, and dopaminergic receptors. These pharmacological properties account for its being less likely to cause sedation, dry mouth, orthostatic hypotension, and impairment of cognition, and also for its wide use in children. It produces

stimulation in some depressed patients. It is currently being investigated as a possible treatment for cocaine dependence. Pregnancy risk category C. See **desipramine/children/cardiovascular effects.**

desipramine + alcohol In recently abstinent alcoholics who smoke, there may be decreased elimination half-life and increased clearance of desipramine compared to smoking volunteers.

desipramine + alprazolam Alprazolam can raise desipramine (DMI) plasma level and increase risk of DMI toxicity.

desipramine/breast milk Desipramine (DMI) is excreted in breast milk in concentrations equal to those in maternal serum and may be hazardous to the nursing neonate (Stancer HC, Read KL. Desipramine and 2-hydroxydesipramine in human breast milk and nursing infant's serum. *Am J Psychiatry* 1986;143:1597–1600).

desipramine + carbamazepine Although carbamazepine (CBZ) may lower parent desipramine (DMI) serum levels, co-administration may cause cardiac complaints possibly due to highly increased serum level of DMI's hydroxy metabolite, which is thought to be cardiotoxic. Increased hydroxylation rate could result from CBZ induction of desipramine hydroxylating cytochrome P450 enzymes (Baldessarini RJ, Teicher MH, Cassidy JW. Anticonvulsant cotreatment may increase toxic metabolites of antidepressants and other psychotropic drugs. *J Clin Psychopharmacol* 1988;8:381–382).

desipramine/children Since the early 1980s, DMI has been used for the treatment of children with attention-deficit hyperactivity disorder; since the mid-1980s, there have been reports of its therapeutic usefulness in the treatment of Tourette's syndrome and chronic motor tics (Spencer T, Biederman J, Kerman K, et al. Desipramine treatment of children with attention-deficit hyperactivity disorder and tic disorder or Tourette's syndrome. *J Am Acad Child Adolesc Psychiatry* 1993;32:354–360).

desipramine/children/cardiovascular effects Prior to 1990, evaluations of short- and long-term desipramine (DMI) cardiovascular effects in children showed it to be well tolerated with only minor electrocardiographic changes associated with daily doses up to 5 mg/kg. Subsequent reports of sudden death sparked mounting concern over the use and side effects of DMI in children. They also provoked published commentaries from a number of experts who concurred that the scant clinical information available precludes an accurate medical explanation. All support additional systematic investigation of side effects of tricyclic drugs in children, with careful attention paid to clinical history, cardiovascular monitoring, and documentation of side effects (Pataki CS, Carlson GA, Kelly KL, et al. Side effects of methylphenidate and desipramine alone and in combination in children. *J Am Acad Child Adolesc Psychiatry* 1993;32:1065–1072).

desipramine + cimetidine   Co-administration may result in increased serum concentration of desipramine (DMI) and possibly DMI toxicity.

desipramine + clonazepam   Ordinarily, benzodiazepines do not cause significant alterations in tricyclic antidepressant serum levels. However, there is a report of a rather dramatic decrease in serum desipramine (DMI) concentration after addition of clonazepam (CNP). When CNP was discontinued, there was a rebound increase in DMI plasma level (Deicken RF. Clonazepam-induced reduction in serum desipramine concentration. *J Clin Psychopharmacol* 1988;8:71–73).

desipramine + cocaine   Desipramine (DMI) may reduce use and craving for cocaine (COC), as well as frequency, intensity, and duration of COC binges. Patients maintained on DMI report both a reduction in desire or need to use COC beyond the several days of abstinence between binges and a reduced desire to prolong their binges. Although DMI may not alter a COC "high," it attenuates desire for COC (Kosten TR, Morgan CH, Falcione J, Schottenfeld RS. Pharmacotherapy for cocaine-abusing methadone maintained patients using amantadine or desipramine. *Arch Gen Psychiatry* 1992;49:894–898; Ardnt I, Dorozynsky L, Woody G, et al. Desipramine treatment of cocaine dependence in methadone maintenance patients. *Arch Gen Psychiatry* 1992;49:888–893). Combined use has not produced serious cardiotoxic effects (Kosten T, Garvin FH, Silverman DG, et al. Intravenous cocaine challenges during desipramine maintenance. *Neuropsychopharmacology* 1992;7:169–176).

desipramine + fenfluramine   Co-administration increases desipramine levels, but does not produce additional amelioration of depressive symptoms (Price LH, Charney DS, Delgado PL, Heninger GR. Fenfluramine augmentation in tricyclic-refractory depression. *J Clin Psychopharmacol* 1990;10:312–317).

desipramine + fluoxetine   Combined use downregulates beta-adrenergic receptors more rapidly than either drug alone and may be rapidly effective in the treatment of major depression, supporting the recent hypothesis of noradrenergic-serotonergic synergism (Eisen A. Fluoxetine and desipramine: a strategy for augment-

ing antidepressant response. *Pharmacopsychiatry* 1989;22:272–273; Nelson JC, Mazure CM, Bowers MB, Jatlow PI. Augmentation of desipramine with fluoxetine. Presented at the 146th Annual Meeting of the American Psychiatric Association, San Francisco, May, 1993; Nelson JC, Mazure CM, Bowers MB, Jatlow PI. A preliminary open study of the combination of fluoxetine and desipramine for rapid treatment of major depression. *Arch Gen Psychiatry* 1991;48:303–307; Baron BM, Ogden AM, Siegel BW, et al. Rapid down regulation of beta-adrenoceptors by co-administration of desipramine and fluoxetine. *Eur J Pharmacol* 1988;154:125–134; Vaughan DA. Interaction of fluoxetine with tricyclic antidepressants. *Am J Psychiatry* 1988;145:1478; Blier P, De Montigny CA. Basis for augmentation strategies in depression. Presented at the 146th Annual Meeting of the American Psychiatric Association, San Francisco, May 1993). The combination should be given for 4 weeks for optimal results. One week after treatment begins, there is a rise in DMI plasma level, as well as a mean change in Hamilton Depression Rating Scale (HAM-D) scores (42%). After 2 weeks, mean change in the HAM-D is about 60%. DMI and hydroxydesipramine plasma levels increase, but the higher the level the less favorable the result. In one study, addition of fluoxetine (FLX) resulted in mean DMI levels 2.5 times higher than expected (Suckow RF, Roose SP, Cooper TB. Effect of fluoxetine on plasma desipramine and 2-hydroxydesipramine. *Biol Psychiatry* 1992;31:200–204). In another study, FLX caused an average 350% increase in plasma DMI by the third week in normal volunteers receiving FLX (20 mg/day) or DMI (50 mg/day). The effect persisted for more than 21 days after discontinuation and was attributed to the longer half-life of FLX (and norfluoxetine, its major metabolite) (Preskorn SH. Unpublished data). Co-prescribing FLX and DMI or switching immediately from FLX to DMI may cause potentially toxic DMI plasma levels (van Ameringen M, Mancini C. Adverse effects of switching from fluoxetine to desipramine. *Can J Psychiatry* 1992;37:278). In some patients, a trial of FLX with low-dose DMI caused excessive anticholinergic effects (Murray MJ, Hooberman D. Fluoxetine and prolonged erection. *Am J Psychiatry* 1993;150:167–168). If FLX is given with DMI, 40% of the DMI dose, calculated using 24-hour levels, should be sufficient to attain the desired target level. The combination has not caused any serious side effects; type and frequency of side effects are similar to those reported with DMI alone.

desipramine + fluoxetine + lithium Lithium augmentation may be beneficial in patients being treated with desipramine and fluoxetine for refractory depression (Fontaine R, Ontiveros A, Elie R, et al. Lithium carbonate augmentation of desipramine and fluoxetine in refractory depression. *Biol Psychiatry* 1991; 29:946–948).

desipramine + fluvoxamine Addition of fluvoxamine (100 mg/day) to desipramine (DMI) (100–150 mg/day) dramatically increased DMI plasma concentration and was associated with adverse effects including confusion, tremor, dizziness, and seizures. The interaction is attributed to fluvoxamine8s inhibition of DMI hydroxylation (Spina E, Campo GM, Avenosa A, et al. Interaction between fluvoxamine and imipramine/desipramine in four patients. *Ther Drug Monit* 1992;14:194–196).

desipramine/growth hormone (GH) stimulation test Test that indirectly assesses central noradrenergic alpha-2 receptors. It is less cumbersome and less unpleasant from the patient's point of view than the clonidine challenge test. A fasting patient has an 18-gauge cannula inserted in a forearm vein at 8:30 am. Blood for GH estimation is taken 20 minutes later. Two baseline 8-ml samples are collected at 15-minute intervals. An oral dose of desipramine (DMI) (1 mg/kg body weight) is given. Blood for further GH estimation is collected 90, 120, and 180 minutes after oral DMI administration. GH is measured by double antibody radioimmunoassay (Dinan TG, Barry S. Growth hormone responses to desipramine in endogenous and non-endogenous depression. *Br J Psychiatry* 1990;156:680–684).

desipramine + haloperidol A grand mal seizure was reported (Mahr GC, Berchou R, Balon R. A grand mal seizure associated with desipramine and haloperidol. *Can J Psychiatry* 1987;32:463–464).

desipramine + lithium Addition of lithium in desipramine-resistant patients may heighten therapeutic response; some respond within a week (rapid responders), whereas others require 1–6 weeks (slow responders) (Dallal A, Fontaine R, Ontivero A, Elie R. Lithium carbonate augmentation of desipramine in refractory depression. *Can J Psychiatry* 1990;35:608–611).

desipramine + methadone After 2 weeks of co-administration, desipramine levels increased between 73% and 169% (Maany I, Dhopesh V, Arndt IO, et al. Increase in desipramine serum levels associated with methadone treatment. *Am J Psychiatry* 1989;146:1611–1613; Kosten TR, Gawin FH, Morgan C, et al. Desipramine and its 2-hydroxy metabolite in pa-

tients taking or not taking methadone. *Am J Psychiatry* 1990;147:1379–1380).

desipramine + methylphenidate In a double-blind placebo-controlled crossover study, nausea, dry mouth, and tremor occurred in at least twice as many children on combined therapy than on any other treatment condition. Nausea/vomiting, headaches, other aches, food refusal, and feeling "tired" were significantly more frequent during combined treatment compared with methylphenidate alone or baseline. Significantly higher ventricular heart rate was found on combined therapy compared with baseline or desipramine (DMI) or methylphenidate alone. Side effects during combined therapy appeared to be similar to and no more serious than those associated with DMI alone. No side effects were severe enough to require medication discontinuation during combined treatment. It is possible that more serious side effects did not occur because some subjects never reached the desired DMI level (125–225 ng/ml). Careful monitoring is warranted for children being treated with the combination (Pataki CS, Carlson GA, Kelly KL, et al. Side effects of methylphenidate and desipramine alone and in combination in children. *J Am Acad Child Adolesc Psychiatry* 1993;32:1065–1072).

desipramine + moclobemide Co-administration may benefit treatment-resistant depressed patients without causing serious adverse reactions (Priest R. Therapy-resistant depression. *Int Clin Psychopharmacol* 1993;7:201–202). In a pharmacodynamic study involving healthy volunteers, tyramine sensitivity was measured with each drug alone and with combined treatment to determine if tricyclic antidepressants may prevent tyramine reactions by inhibiting reuptake of sympathomimetic substances by the adrenergic neuron. Desipramine treatment decreased tyramine reactivity, which was not affected by concomitant administration of moclobemide. Co-administration was well tolerated, with no adverse events (Amrein R, Guntert TW, Dingemanse J, et al. Interactions of moclobemide with concomitantly administered medication: evidence from pharmacological and clinical studies. *Psychopharmacology* 1992;106:S24–S31).

desipramine + morphine Co-administration requires caution. Desipramine (DMI) prolongs and potentiates morphine's analgesic and respiratory depression effects. Morphine increases DMI plasma concentration, which should be monitored whenever the combination is prescribed. It is possible that these clinical effects may be observed with all opioids (Hasten PD, Horn JR. *Drug Interactions*, 6th ed. Philadelphia: Lea & Febiger, 1990).

desipramine + neuroleptic　Co-administration may increase plasma levels of both drugs (Craig Nelson J, Jatlow PI. Neuroleptic effect on desipramine steady-state plasma concentrations. *Am J Psychiatry* 1980;137:1232–1234).

desipramine + ORG 3770　Addition of the alpha$_2$ antagonist ORG 3770 in depressed patients refractory to 4 weeks' treatment with desipramine (DMI) enhanced response to DMI (Checkley S, Capstick C, O'Dwyer AM, et al. Neuroendocrine studies of the mechanism of action of antidepressant treatments. *Neuropsychopharmacology* 1993;9:23S).

desipramine + paroxetine　Paroxetine (30 mg/day) causes a threefold increase in half-life and a fivefold decrease in the clearance of serum desipramine (DMI), which is metabolized by cytochrome P$_{450}$IID$_6$ (Brosen K, Graham LF, Sindroup S. Pharmacokinetics of tricyclic antidepressants and novel antidepressants: recent developments. *Clin Neuropharmacol* 1992;15:80A–81A). Co-administration may necessitate use of lower doses than usually prescribed for either drug. In an 18-year-old man with major depression partially responsive to DMI, addition of paroxetine (20 mg/day) resulted in rapid elevation of DMI level to 503 ng/ml. Depressive symptoms improved markedly, and he experienced mild anticholinergic side effects (Pittard JT. Pharmacokinetic interaction between paroxetine and tricyclic antidepressants. *Curr Affect Illness* 1993; 12:14–15).

desipramine + pergolide　Co-administration has been used to treat patients refractory to desipramine. Response is usually rapid (within 1 week), but without incremental improvement over the next month. Some patients tolerate the combination well; others develop nausea and vomiting, which may or may not respond to lowering pergolide dose (Bouckoms A, Mangini L. Pergolide: an antidepressant adjuvant for mood disorders. *Psychopharmacol Bull* 1993;29:207–211).

desipramine + propafenone　Propafenone, a relatively new class IC antiarrhythmic agent that undergoes extensive 5-hydroxylation by the hepatic cytochrome P450 isoenzyme, may dramatically elevate serum desipramine levels (Katz MR. Raised serum levels of desipramine with the antiarrhythmic propafenone. *J Clin Psychiatry* 1991;52:432–433).

desipramine + sertraline　There may be a relatively limited pharmacokinetic interaction between sertraline and tricyclic antidepressants (Lydiard RB, Anton RF, Cunningham T. Interactions between sertraline and tricyclic antidepressants. *Am J Psychiatry* 1993;150:1125–1126;

Barros J, Asnis G. An interaction of sertraline and desipramine. *Am J Psychiatry* 1993;150: 1751). Sertraline apparently has little or no effect on desipramine (DMI) plasma concentrations. Following discontinuation of sertraline, DMI approaches baseline within 1 week. This is in contrast to the interaction of fluoxetine and tricyclic antidepressants. Co-administration decreases DMI clearance 35%, modestly correlating with sertraline and desmethylsertraline levels. Sertraline and desmethylsertraline inhibit microsomal desipramine 2-hydroxylation, but this is less potent than that caused by fluoxetine and norfluoxetine (Preskorn SH, von Moltter L, Alderman J, et al. In vitro and in vivo evaluation of the potential for desipramine interaction with fluoxetine or sertraline. Presented at the 146th Annual Meeting of the American Psychiatric Association, San Francisco, May 1993). In a patient treated with DMI (steady state 152 ng/ml) 1 week after addition of sertraline (50 mg/day), DMI level rose to 203 ng/ml. One month later, when steady-state levels of sertraline had presumably been achieved, DMI level was 240 ng/ml. There were no adverse effects and the patient reported feeling better than with prior therapy. This single case indicates a relatively modest (60%) increase in steady-state plasma DMI levels following addition of sertraline. See **fluoxetine + tricyclic antidepressant.**

desmethylchlordiazepoxide　Initial, pharmacologically active metabolite of chlordiazepoxide.

desmethylclomipramine　(DCMI) Primary metabolite of clomipramine (CMI); also a norepinephrine uptake inhibitor. It is usually present at about twice the concentration of CMI in human plasma. It has high affinity for the ^{3}H-imipramine binding site, believed to be the serotonin transporter site.

desmethylclomipramine + fluvoxamine　Fluvoxamine increases desmethylclomipramine plasma concentration. This may potentiate antidepressant effects in some patients, but also may cause adverse reactions (Bertschy G, Vandel S, Vandel B, et al. Fluvoxamine-tricyclic antidepressant interaction. *Eur J Clin Pharmacol* 1991; 40:119–120).

desmethyldiazepam　(DMDZ) Pharmacologically active metabolite of the benzodiazepines (BZDs) diazepam (DZ), chlordiazepoxide, halazepam, medazepam, and pinazepam. In many parts of the world it is administered as the pure compound for the treatment of anxiety. Several BZDs (e.g., clorazepate, ketazolam, oxazolam, prazepam) effectively serve as "prodrugs" of DMDZ, being converted to it as the major active substance. Elimination half-life is very long (approximately 65 hours).

DMDZ is biotransformed mainly by the oxidative reaction of hydroxylation, yielding oxazepam as its major metabolite. Oxazepam, in turn, is rapidly conjugated and excreted; plasma concentrations of intact oxazepam are much lower than those of the parent drug following administration of DMDZ to humans (Greenblatt DJ, Harmatz JS, Shader RI. Clinical pharmacokinetics of anxiolytics and hypnotics in the elderly. Therapeutic considerations [Part I]. *Clin Pharmacokinet* 1991;21[3]: 165–177). Hydrolysis of clorazepate dipotassium also yields DMDZ. Also called "nordiazepam."

desmethylimipramine   See **desipramine.**

desmethylmaprotiline   Pharmacologically active metabolite of maprotiline.

desmethylmianserin   Pharmacologically active metabolite of mianserin.

desmethylsertraline   Selective serotonin uptake inhibitor, but at a lower potency than the parent compound sertraline. It is inactive in an animal model predictive of antidepressant activity, and its clinical relevance is unknown.

desmopressin   (DDAVP) Analog of antidiuretic hormone used as a nasal spray once a night to effectively treat nocturnal enuresis in adults and children. Discontinuation immediately results in bed-wetting. Characteristics of patients most likely to respond favorably to DDAVP include (a) increased age; (b) presence of family history of nocturnal enuresis; (c) parental observation of a deep sleep pattern in the child; and (d) unexpectedly high volume of urine in the first morning specimen (Robson WLM, Leung AKC. Intranasal desmopressin [DDAVP] in the treatment of nocturnal enuresis—a review of efficacy studies. *Today's Therapeutic Trends* 1993;11:35–42). No serious adverse reactions have been reported in adults (Norgaard JP, Pederson ED, Djurhuus JG. Diurnal antidiuretic hormone levels in enuresis. *J Urol* 1985;134:1029–1031; Rittig S, Knudsen UB, Norgaard JP, et al. Abnormal diurnal rhythm of plasma vasopressin and urinary output in patients with enuresis. *Am J Physiol* 1989;256:664–671). Hyponatremia and seizures occurred in a child given desmopressin for enuresis (Berger V, Blanchard P, Chiffolean A, et al. Hyponatremia and seizures in a child given desmopressin for enuresis. *Therapie* 1992;47:433–434).

desmopressin + imipramine   See **imipramine + desmopressin.**

Desoxyn   See **methamphetamine.**

despair   Emotional state distinguishing suicidal patients from patients who are depressed, but not suicidal. Its development has been attributed to aloneness, murderous hate, and self-contempt or, more generally, to any state that leads to inability to maintain or envision any human connections of significance (Hendin H. Psychodynamics of suicide, with particular reference to the young. *Am J Psychiatry* 1991; 148:1150–1158).

desperation   Sense of hopelessness about change combined with a sense that life is impossible without such change.

desynchronization   Loss of the controlling relationship of a rhythmic stimulus to a rhythmic response.

Desyrel   See **trazodone.**

"det"   Street name for dimethyltryptamine.

determinant   Any factor that brings about a change in a defined characteristic.

determinism   Theory that for every action there are causal mechanisms such that no other action was possible.

detoxification   Therapeutic regimen aimed at safely and effectively withdrawing an addictive substance from a person physically dependent on continued self-administration.

detoxification, therapeutic   See **therapeutic detoxification.**

devaluation   Mechanism in which the person attributes exaggeratedly negative qualities to self or others (DSM-IV).

developmental disability   (DD) Severe and chronic mental handicap and/or physical handicap (e.g., mental retardation, autism, cerebral palsy, epilepsy and related neurological impairments) present before age 22 (Bouras N. Developmental disabilities service in California. *Bull R Coll Psychiatr* 1987;11:8–10; Bouras N. Psychiatric services to adult mentally retarded and developmentally disabled persons. American Psychiatric Association Task Force, Report 30. *Psychiatr Bull* 1992;16: 125). A wide range of psychotropic medications are prescribed in the United States for children and adults with DD. Stimulants, serotonergic antidepressants, beta-blockers, clonazepam, sodium valproate, clonidine, or naltrexone are used as adjunctive therapy for challenging behaviors. Medication trials are often accompanied by behavioral interventions and monitoring by psychologists. State regulations and fear of litigation about tardive dyskinesia restrict use of long-term neuroleptics to diagnosed psychotic disorders (Brassock D. Community mental health and mental retardation services in the United States: a comparative study of resource allocation. *Am J Psychiatry* 1992;149:175–183).

developmental toxicity   Occurrence in infants and children of unforeseen toxicity related to critical phases in organ development associated with drugs that appeared safe for adults (e.g., tetracycline, which is benign for most developmental toxicity 207 dexamethasone suppression test/children

adults, alters progression of mineral deposition in tooth development, leading to discoloration and abnormal growth). There is a concern that new drugs will produce toxicities not apparent from adult testing. There is a need, therefore, for (a) careful testing in realistic young animal models; (b) judicious application of new drugs for children; and (c) careful record-keeping and recording of adverse reactions.

deviancy   Condition that departs from the norm (e.g., sexual deviancy is sexual behavior that is either illegal or against social mores in relation to the nature of the act or certain characteristics of the victim).

deviation, mean   See **mean deviation.**

deviation, median   See **median deviation.**

deviation, probable   See **median deviation.**

dexamethasone   (Decadron) (DEX) Synthetic glucocorticoid developed by chemical modification of naturally-occurring steroids, the principal aim of which was to potentiate therapeutic effect and adjust mineral corticoid and glucocorticoid properties of the steroid. It was designed to be a very potent "long-acting" corticosteroid; duration of action is, in part, due to its slow metabolism. DEX acts similarly to cortisol in normally suppressing adrenocorticotropic hormone and cortisol secretion in normal subjects for 24–36 hours by means of a "slow feedback" mechanism. This action forms the basis of the "normal suppressor" pattern on the DEX suppression test (Ritchie JA, Owens MJ, Mayer H, et al. Preliminary studies of 6-beta-hydroxydexamethasone and its importance in the DST. *Biol Psychiatry* 1992; 32:825–833).

dexamethasone suppression test   (DST) Widely studied biological marker of hypothalamic/pituitary/adrenal (HPA) disinhibition that has been suggested as a test for depression and as a predictor of outcome. It seemed to herald a new era in psychiatric diagnosis when it was reported in 1976 that 48% of primary depressive but only 2% of other psychiatric patients showed early escape from dexamethasone suppression of the HPA axis. Conflicting reports have since obscured the significance of the test; some confirm its clinical utility, whereas others argue that it may be regarded as a very sensitive indicator of stress rather than a diagnostic tool for everyday practice. It involves serum cortisol sampling after a dose of dexamethasone (DEX) to see if cortisol levels have been suppressed. DEX, a potent glucocorticoid that suppresses endogenous adrenocorticotropic hormone (ACTH) and cortisol production for up to 24 hours in normal subjects, is administered as follows: Day 1: 1 mg given orally at 11 pm. Day 2: blood is

drawn at 8 am, 3 or 4 pm, and 10 or 11 pm for serum cortisol determinations. Normally, plasma cortisol is suppressed below 5 mg/dl, but in many depressed patients levels are much higher than 5 mg/dl. Results are considered abnormal if elevated cortisol level is not suppressed by DEX (1 mg) given 16–24 hours before withdrawal of the blood sample for cortisol estimation. The DST is considered a useful indicator of HPA axis abnormalities associated with depressive illness. Abnormal DST results after apparent clinical recovery may be associated with a high likelihood of relapse. If cortisol hypersecretion and the DST are independently measured, however, they do not invariably identify identical patients; some depressed patients with cortisol hypersecretion are not DST nonsuppressors, and not all DST nonsuppressors show cortisol hypersecretion. Serum cortisol concentrations following the DST vary with the subtype of mood disorder and with higher postdexamethasone cortisol levels in patients with psychotic depression compared to patients with nonpsychotic major depression. Thus, cortisol nonsuppression following DEX challenge may be a marker for severity of affective illness, or may define a biologically distinct group of mood disorder patients (Carroll BJ, Feinberg M, Greden JF, et al. A specific laboratory test for the diagnosis of melancholia: standardization, validation, and clinical utility. *Arch Gen Psychiatry* 1981;38:15–22). Whereas nonsuppression is seen in one of five cases of schizophrenia, it is found in two of three patients with severe, endogenous, unipolar depression. However, depressive patients who were nonsuppressors were 5 times more likely than suppressors to be free of psychotic features and to exhibit insight when interviewed 8 years after initial assessment (Breathnach C. Endocrinology and the psychiatrist. *Ir J Psychol Med* 1993;10:110–113). The DST ultimately may prove more useful as a measure of clinical outcome or the need for continued treatment. Its administration does not have a statistically significant effect on depressive symptoms and thus does not interfere with study results and interpretation (Lafer B, Fava M, Hammerness P, Rosenbaum JF. The influence of DST and TRH test administration on depression assessments: a controlled study. *Biol Psychiatry* 1993;34:650–653).

dexamethasone suppression test (DST)/children/ adolescents   A few studies of relatively small samples of patients have shown that a clinical diagnosis of endogenous depression in prepubertal children is associated with positive DST results. Others have not found a clear relationship between the diagnosis of depression and positive DST results and are doubtful about the specificity of the test in children. In children, dexamethasone (DEX) is given, as near as possible to 10 pm, according to weight (1 mg in those weighing 49 kg or more, 0.5 mg in those weighing less than 49 kg). Blood is taken for plasma cortisol at 3 pm the next afternoon. DEX is given at 10 pm to avoid sleep interruption that administration at 11 pm may necessitate; stress may cause increased cortisol escape following DEX administration. Validity studies of the DST as a diagnostic test in children suggest that it is not of great value in identifying depression in children attending an outpatient clinic; they show a high rate of nonsuppression of plasma cortisol irrespective of the diagnosis of depression, however this is classified (Tyrer SP, Barrett ML, Berney TP, et al. The dexamethasone suppression test in children: lack of an association with diagnosis. Br J Psychiatry 1991;159[suppl 11]:41–48). Other reviews indicate that DST sensitivity appears to be higher among children than among adolescents (58% vs. 44%), higher in subjects from inpatient settings than subjects in outpatient settings (61% vs. 29%), and more specific in adolescent samples (84% vs. 74%). Computation of specificity rates for different diagnostic psychiatric control groups has shown that within samples of child inpatients, approximately 40% of children with dysthymia, anxiety disorders, or schizophrenia spectrum disorders were DST nonsuppressors. Within adolescent inpatient samples, approximately 16% of all psychiatric control subjects, regardless of diagnosis, were DST nonsuppressors. These data raise important questions regarding the appropriateness of the current standard DEX dose used with adolescents, and the need to consider the "quantity of stress" associated with DST administration (Dahl RE, Kaufman J, Ryan ND, et al. The dexamethasone suppression test in children and adolescents: a review and a controlled study. Biol Psychiatry 1992;32:109–126).

dexamethasone suppression test (DST)/elderly Plasma cortisol levels do not increase significantly with normal aging (Weiner MF, Davis BM, Mohr RC, et al. Influence of age and relative weight on cortisol suppression in normal subjects. Am J Psychiatry 1987;144:646–649). DST nonsuppression may occur normally with advanced age, because the elderly often fail to obtain adequate plasma dexamethasone (DEX) levels (Weiner MF. Age and cortisol suppression by dexamethasone in normal subjects. J Psychiatr Res 1989;23:163–168). A valid DST in elders requires simultaneous determination of plasma DEX concentration.

dexamethasone suppression test (DST), false-negative/drugs May be due to high dose benzodiazepine treatment, high-dose cyproheptadine treatment, indomethacin, or long-term synthetic steroid therapy.

dexamethasone suppression test (DST), false-positive/drugs Drugs that induce hepatic microsomal enzymes increase the rate of dexamethasone metabolism, potentially resulting in a false-positive DST. These include certain anticonvulsants (phenytoin, carbamazepine), sedative hypnotics (barbiturates, meprobamate, glutethimide, methyprylon), alcohol in large quantities, and possibly narcotics and reserpine.

dexamethasone suppression test (DST), false-positive/medical causes Many conditions, especially severe, acute illnesses (medical and psychiatric), may lead to hypothalamic-pituitary-adrenocortical hyperactivity and thus positive DST results. These conditions include acute psychoses, advanced age, hypertension, cardiac or renal failure, fever, nausea, dehydration, pregnancy, severe weight loss, malnutrition, and eating disorders (anorexia and bulimia nervosa).

dexamphetamine See **dextroamphetamine.**

Dexamyl See **amobarbital; amphetamine.**

Dexedrina See **dextroamphetamine.**

Dexedrine See **dextroamphetamine.**

Dexedrine Spansule See **dextroamphetamine sulfate.**

dexfenfluramine (Adifax; D-Fenfluramine; Dipondal; Isomeride; Obedial) (D-FEN) Dextroisomer of fenfluramine that is not chemically related to the amphetamine-like anorexiants. It is a potent anorectic drug that inhibits reuptake and increases release of serotonin (5-HT). It is not a stimulant and is said to have no significant abuse potential. It has been used to study 5-HT function in depression and obsessive-compulsive disorder (Dinan TG, O'Keane V. d-Fenfluramine/prolactin responses in depressed subjects before and after treatment. Clin Neuropharmacol 1990;13[suppl 1]:412; Lucey JV, O'Keane V, Butcher G, et al. Cortisol and prolactin responses to D-fenfluramine in nondepressed patients with obsessive-compulsive disorder: a comparison with depressed and healthy controls. Br J Psychiatry 1992;161:517–521). It has been suggested as adjunctive therapy for obesity unresponsive to nonpharmacological treatments. Common adverse effects are drowsiness, depressed mood, asthenia, dizziness, dry mouth, polyuria, and diarrhea. A study showing that D-FEN can cause brain damage in monkeys raises concern about its use in humans. Half-life is 7–8 hours; since patients take one pill every 21 hours or less for 12 weeks to 1 year, the drug could accumulate and reach toxic levels over time. D-FEN is currently approved for marketing in 31 countries outside the United States. Application for marketing approval has been filed with the U.S. Food and Drug Administration (FDA) by Liz Laboratoiries Servier. See **fenfluramine.**

dexoxadrol   Compound structurally related to phencyclidine (PCP).

dextroamphetamine   (D-Amphetamine; Desoxyn; Dexadrina; Dexedrine; Ferndex; Oxydess II; Spancap No. 1) (D-AMPH) Sympathomimetic amine with central nervous system stimulant activity thought to be due to its ability to release and block reuptake of dopamine and norepinephrine from central noradrenergic and dopaminergic neurons. At high doses it also increases dopamine release in the mesolimbic portion of the brain. It is useful in narcolepsy and for the treatment of childhood behavioral disorders such as attention-deficit hyperactivity disorder (ADHD). ADHD-affected boys improve in reading and math, particularly the latter, during D-AMPH treatment. Although not Food and Drug Administration (FDA)-approved for it, D-AMPH may also be useful in the treatment of negative schizophrenic symptoms (Angrist B, Peselow E, Rubinstein M, et al. Partial improvement in negative schizophrenic symptoms after amphetamine. *Psychopharmacology* 1982;78:128–130). Side effects include sleeplessness, restlessness, irritability, dizziness, dry mouth, loss of appetite, sweating, and stimulation of the heart. Dependence is a hazard. Pregnancy risk category C; Schedule II .

dextroamphetamine + fluoxetine   Adding dextroamphetamine to fluoxetine (FLX) in patients with refractory depression characterized by anergy, anhedonia, weight gain, and hyperphagia may augment FLX antidepressant effects (Linet LS. Treatment of refractory depression with a combination of fluoxetine and d-amphetamine. *Am J Psychiatry* 1989;146:803–804).

dextroamphetamine + monoamine oxidase inhibitor (MAOI)   Co-administration is generally considered contraindicated because of the risk of hypertensive crisis or hyperthermia. However, some investigators have suggested that it could be a safe and effective intervention for treatment-resistant depression (Sovner R. Amphetamine and tranylcypromine in treatment-resistant depression. *Biol Psychiatry* 1990;28:1011–1013). Dextroamphetamine (D-AMPH) (5–40 mg/day) has been given to patients partially responsive to an MAOI without significantly serious adverse interactions and with robust therapeutic effects (Fawcett J, Kravitz HM, Zajecka JM, et al. CNS stimulant potentiation of monoamine oxidase inhibitors in treat-

ment-refractory depression. *J Clin Psychopharmacol* 1991;11:127–132). However, since norepinephrine accumulates during MAOI therapy, addition of D-AMPH can liberate large amounts of intraneuronal norepinephrine, resulting in elevations in blood pressure, hyperpyrexia, and headache. Hypertensive emergency with intracerebral hemorrhage may ensue if hypertension is not quickly controlled with an alpha-adrenergic blocking agent such as phentolamine. In recent years, nifedipine has been shown to be an effective treatment for MAOI-induced hypertensive crisis (Stockley I. Chewing nifedipine to treat MAOI-cheese reaction. *Pharm J* 1991;247:784). See **nifedipine.**

dextroamphetamine + morphine   Dextroamphetamine antagonizes morphine-associated respiratory depression and sedation and may potentiate morphine analgesia (Bourke DL, Allan PD, Rosenberg M, et al. Dextroamphetamine with morphine: respiratory effects. *J Clin Pharmacol* 1983;23:65–70).

dextroamphetamine sulfate   (Dexedrine Spansule) Long-acting form of dextroamphetamine used for the treatment of attention deficit-hyperactivity disorder in children.

dextroamphetamine + tranylcypromine   Transient response to dextroamphetamine (D-AMPH) in treatment-resistant depression may predict response to D-AMPH plus tranylcypromine. Even though some patients have been safely treated, potentially fatal adverse reactions have occurred with the combination of monoamine oxidase inhibitors and psychostimulant therapy. It should be reserved for truly drug-resistant depressive disorders. See **dextroamphetamine + monoamine oxidase inhibitor.**

dextroamphetamine + warfarin   Co-administration decreases metabolism of dextroamphetamine and increases its plasma levels.

dextromethorphan   (Benylin) (DXM) Antitussive ingredient in at least 60 over-the-counter preparations. It is the dextrorotary isomer of the morphine congener, methylmorphinan. It can be used instead of debrisoquine in pharmacogenetic studies. Although it is associated with some abuse, the abuse is not due to opioid actions; DXM is demethylated in the body to dextrorphan, which can act at the phencyclidine (PCP) and sigma receptors. It has been reported to interact with monoamine oxidase inhibitors in a few cases, but sympathomimetic amines were also ingested.

dextromethorphan abuse/mania   Mania has occurred with dextromethorphan (DXM) abuse. Mania may improve with small doses of a neuroleptic (e.g., haloperidol) (Mendez MF. Mania self-induced with cough syrup. *J Clin Psychiatry* 1992;53:173–174; Walker J, Yatham

LN. Benylin [dextromethorphan] abuse and mania. *Br Med J* 1993;306:896).

dextromethorphan + fluoxetine See **fluoxetine + dextromethorphan.**

dextromethorphan + isocarboxazid See **isocarboxazid + dextromethorphan.**

dextromethorphan + moclobemide See **moclobemide + dextromethorphan.**

dextromethorphan + monoamine oxidase inhibitor (MAOI) See **monoamine oxidase inhibitor + dextromethorphan.**

dextromethorphan + phenelzine See **phenelzine + dextromethorphan.**

dextropropoxyphene (Darvocet; Darvon) (propoxyphene) Synthetic opioid-like narcotic that is chemically similar to methadone. It is chemically distinct from morphine, but seems to act via similar mechanisms and is cross-tolerant with morphine. Clinical data suggest that it is no more effective than aspirin. It is biotransformed to a potentially toxic metabolite (norpropoxyphene); both parent and metabolite can accumulate after repetitive dosing or overdose, in some cases producing convulsions or a toxic psychosis. Abuse, dependence, and withdrawal have been associated with its use. Schedule IV; pregnancy risk category C.

dextropropoxyphene + alprazolam See **alprazolam + dextropropoxyphene.**

dextropropoxyphene + carbamazepine See **carbamazepine + dextropropoxyphene.**

dextropropoxyphene + clomipramine See **clomipramine + dextropropoxyphene.**

dextropropoxyphene + moclobemide See **moclobemide + dextropropoxyphene.**

dextropropoxyphene + orphenadrine See **orphenadrine + dextropropoxyphene.**

dextropropoxyphene + phenelzine See **phenelzine + dextropropoxyphene.**

dextrorphan (DXT) N-methyl-D-aspartate (NMDA) antagonist.

"dexy" Street name for dextroamphetamine (Dexedrine).

D-fenfluramine See **dexfenfluramine.**

diacetylmorphine See **heroin.**

diacylglycerol (DAG) Second messenger generated by the ligand- dependent breakdown of the phosphoinositide (PIP_2). Another second messenger, inositol-1,4,5-triphosphate (IP_3), is also formed in the process.

diagnosis 1. Process of identifying specific mental or physical disorders. 2. Comprehensive evaluation not limited to identification of specific disorders.

diagnosis of organicity Diagnosis given to a psychiatric patient if symptoms are due to demonstrable structural damage of the brain instead of being functional or purely psychological.

diagnostic criteria Clearly articulated, exclusionary criteria for arriving at a diagnosis (e.g., Research Diagnostic Criteria [RDC] and DSM-IV criteria.) Development of these systems has greatly advanced psychiatric research by assuring greater homogeneity in study samples. Improving criteria to assure even greater homogeneity is an ongoing process; work is underway in developing DSM-IV criteria).

diagnostic molecular biology See **molecular diagnostics.**

Diahist See **diphenhydramine.**

dialectical behavior therapy See **behavior therapy, dialectical.**

dialysis delirium See **encephalopathy, progressive dialysis.**

dialysis dementia See **encephalopathy, progressive dialysis.**

dialysis encephalopathy See **encephalopathy, progressive dialysis.**

dialysis encephalopathy syndrome See **encephalopathy, progressive dialysis.**

diamorphine See **codeine.**

Diamox See **acetazolamide.**

Dianabol Anabolic steroid no longer available in the United States or Canada. See **methandrostenolone.**

diaschisis Phenomenon indicating that dysfunction of a given brain area can have repercussions for other brain areas. It appears to result from disrupted interaction among brain areas secondary to disruption in one of the areas of the communication pathway.

diathesis Constitutional or inborn predisposition to a disease or metabolic or structural anomaly.

diazepam (Apo-Diazepam; Assival; Disopam; E-Pam; Gewacalm; Horizon; Meval; Novodipam; Umbrium; Valium; Valrelease; Vivol) (DZ) GABA-mimetic benzodiazepine (BZD). Elimination half-life (including metabolites) in young adults is 48–96 hours. In the elderly, half-life of the parent compound may double to 50–60 hours. Diazepam is metabolized in the liver, producing N-desmethyldiazepam and N-methyloxazepam. The former, like DZ, has significant anticonvulsant, sedative, and anxiolytic properties. Use as a tranquilizer should be restricted to those with short-lived anxiety. As an anticonvulsant, major use is intravenous or rectal administration for status epilepticus. It is used intravenously for treatment of acute neuroleptic-induced dystonia and orally for neuroleptic-induced akathisia. It should not be administered intramuscularly because of poor absorption. DZ is highly protein-bound to albumen. Hypoalbuminemia may be associated with toxic symptoms resulting from relatively small doses. Side effects are the same as for other BZDs. DZ may induce dependency and may be responsible for withdrawal symptoms if discontinued abruptly. Pregnancy risk category D; Schedule IV.

diazepam + alcohol Additive or synergistic central nervous system depressant effects may occur when diazepam (DZ) is combined with acute ingestion of alcohol. Unpredictable DZ tolerance may occur with chronic alcohol use (Ciraulo DA, Shader RA, Greenblatt DJ, Creelman W [eds]. *Drug Interactions in Psychiatry.* Baltimore: Williams & Wilkins, 1989).

diazepam-binding inhibitor (DBI) Neuropeptide found in human brain and cerebrospinal fluid (CSF) that negatively modulates GABA-ergic neurotransmission. It binds to benzodiazepine receptors but inhibits, rather than potentiates, GABA effects. Positive correlation between CSF DBI and corticotropin-releasing factor (CRF) has been reported in normal control subjects, depressed patients, and pathological gamblers. DBI may be a potential endogenous anxiogenic ligand. Measurements of DBI-like immunoreactivity indicate that it may play a role in the pathophysiology of schizophrenia.

diazepam + cimetidine Co-administration increases steady-state concentrations of diazepam (DZ) and desmethyldiazepam, but apparently causes minimal, if any, alterations in therapeutic or potentially toxic drug effects (Greenblatt DJ, Abernathy DR, Morse DS, et al. Clinical importance of interaction of diazepam and cimetidine. *N Engl J Med* 1984;310: 1639–1643). Cimetidine can double DZ elimination half-life, presumably via inhibition of hepatic metabolism.

diazepam + clomipramine Diazepam does not appear to influence plasma levels or clinical efficacy of clomipramine (CMI) (Luscombe DK, Jones RB. Effects of concomitantly administered drugs on plasma levels of clomipramine and desmethylclomipramine in depressive patients receiving clomipramine therapy. *Postgrad Med J* 1977;53[suppl 4]:77–78). Co-administration (CMI 50–225 mg/day + diazepam 10–45 mg/day) has been used with benefit and good tolerance in phobic and obsessive-compulsive disorder (Cassano GB, Castrogiovanni P, Mauri M, et al. A multicenter controlled trial in phobic-obsessive psychoneurosis. The effect of chlorimipramine and of its combinations with haloperidol and diazepam. *Progr Neuro-Psychopharmacol* 1981;5: 129–138).

diazepam + clonidine + naltrexone Co-administration has been shown to significantly reduce average opioid withdrawal time from 3.3 to 2.3 days, despite lower clonidine dosage

and significantly lower diazepam dosage on the second day.

diazepam + digoxin Diazepam may decrease digoxin clearance; it may be prudent to monitor patients for symptoms of digoxin toxicity.

diazepam + fluoxetine Co-administration increases diazepam (DZ) blood levels and may result in toxicity due to fluoxetine's inhibiting metabolism and slowing clearance of DZ (Lemberger L, Rowe H, Bosomworth JC, Tenbarge JB, Bergstrom RF. The effect of fluoxetine on the pharmacokinetics and psychomotor responses of diazepam. *Clin Pharmacol Ther* 1988;43:412–419). Lowering of concentrations of desmethyldiazepam, which itself is active, may explain why no psychomotor impairment was noted with the drug combination (Ciraulo DA, Shader RI. Fluoxetine drug-drug interactions: II. *J Clin Psychopharmacol* 1990;10:213–217).

diazepam + haloperidol Co-administration may lower haloperidol serum levels and impair its therapeutic efficacy.

diazepam + levodopa Diazepam may inhibit the therapeutic effect of levodopa.

diazepam + methadone Co-use by some methadone-maintenanced patients occurred frequently in the late 1970s and early 1980s. Diazepam (DZ) was generally taken within an hour of the methadone dose; its desired effect was to "boost" methadone (Budd RD, Walkin E, Jain NC, et al. Frequency of use of diazepam in individuals on probation and in methadone maintenance programs. *Am J Drug Alcohol Abuse* 1979;6:511–514). In two methadone clinics, 65–70% of patients had urine samples positive for benzodiazepines in a 1-month period; the majority used DZ in a single daily dose, often in excess of 100 mg and up to 300 mg (Stitzer ML, Griffiths RR, McLellan AT, et al. Diazepam use among methadone maintenance patients: patterns and dosages. *Drug Alcohol Dependence* 1981;8:189–199). By the late 1980s, alprazolam had become more popular than DZ among methadone patients (Weddington WW, Carney AC. Alprazolam abuse during methadone maintenance therapy. *JAMA* 1987;257:3363). Although DZ has been reported not to alter methadone metabolism, in one case it inhibited hepatic metabolism of methadone, resulting in elevated plasma methadone concentrations (Pond SM, Benowitz NL, Jacob P, Rigod J. Lack of effect of diazepam on methadone metabolism in methadone-maintained addicts. *Clin Pharmacol Ther* 1982;31:139–143; Preston KL, Griffiths RR, Stitzer ML, et al. Diazepam and methadone interactions in methadone maintenance. *Clin Pharmacol Ther* 1984;36:534–541; Stimmel B. Prescribing psychotropic agents in opiate dependency: the need for caution. *Advances in Alcoholism and Substance Abuse* 1986;5:121–133). See **alprazolam + methadone.**

diazepam + neuroleptic   Co-administration of high doses of diazepam to patients with neuroleptic-resistant chronic schizophrenia may augment therapeutic response (Nestoros JN, Nair NPV, Pulman JR, et al. High doses of diazepam improve neuroleptic-resistant chronic schizophrenia patients. *Psychopharmacology* 1983;18:42–47).

diazepam + olanzapine   To date no adverse reactions have been reported.

diazepam + oral contraceptive   Co-administration may increase psychomotor and cognitive impairment (Ellinwood EH, Easter ME, Linoilla M, et al. Effects of oral contraceptives on diazepam-induced psychomotor impairment. *Clin Pharmacol Ther* 1984;35:360–366).

diazepam + pancuronium   Co-administration may (rarely) result in intensified and prolonged respiratory depression.

diazepam + paroxetine   No interactions have been demonstrated. Paroxetine concentrations were not increased by multiple-dose co-administration of diazepam (Bannister SJ, Houser VP, Hulse JD, et al. Evaluation of the potential for interactions of paroxetine with diazepam, cimetidine, warfarin and digoxin. *Acta Psychiatr Scand* 1989;80[suppl 350]:102–106).

diazepam/pregnancy   There are a few reports of cleft palate associated with diazepam (DZ) use during pregnancy. One report concluded that the defect may be due to chance (Rosenberg L, Mitchell AA, Parsells JL. Lack of relation of oral cleft to diazepam use during pregnancy. *N Engl J Med* 1983;309:1282–1285). Möbius syndrome was reported in a female infant whose mother took DZ (20 mg/day) from week 25 until delivery and oxazepam (20 mg/day) from the 7th month of gestation. The infant's serum DZ concentration on day 13 was greatly elevated. It has been suggested that because of the teratogenic potential of benzodiazepines (BZDs), in utero exposure to BZDs should be excluded in each case of Möbius syndrome, and that electromyography of the facial muscles be performed in infants whose mothers took BZDs during pregnancy (Courtens W, Vamos E, Hainaut M, Vergauwen P. Moebius syndrome in an infant exposed in utero to benzodiazepines. *J Pediatr* 1992;121:833–834).

diazepam + remoxipride   Diazepam (DZ) has no effect on remoxipride pharmacokinetics, but co-administration may augment DZ's decremental effects on cognitive and neuromotor functions (Yisak W, von Bahr C, Farde L, et al. Drug interaction studies with remoxipride.

Acta Psychiatr Scand 1990;82[suppl 358]:58–62; Matilla MJ, Mattila ME, Korno K, et al. Objective and subjective effects of remoxipride, alone and in combination with ethanol or diazepam, on performance in healthy subjects. *J Psychopharmacol* 1988;2:138–149; Mattila KN, Mattila ME. Effects of remoxipride on psychomotor performance, alone and in combination with ethanol and diazepam. *Acta Psychiatr Scand* 1990;82[suppl 358]:54–55).

diazepam + rifampin   Rifampin can hasten clearance of diazepam (DZ) and its metabolites, resulting in altered clinical or enhanced adverse effects. Dosage adjustment may be necessary during co-administration, and DZ dosage may have to be adjusted after rifampin discontinuation.

diazepam + sertraline   Sertraline has no clinically relevant effects on the pharmacokinetics of diazepam in healthy volunteers (Gaardner MH, Ronfeld RA, Wilner KD, et al. The effects of sertraline on the pharmacokinetics of diazepam in healthy volunteers. *Biol Psychiatry* 1991;29:354S).

diazepam + succinylcholine   Co-administration rarely may result in intensified and prolonged respiratory depression. In most patients, diazepam has no effect on the actions of succinylcholine.

diazepam + tacrine   Tacrine has no major impact on diazepam pharmacokinetics (Tacrine Package Insert, May 1993).

diazepam + valproate   Co-administration, even using a lower-than-normal dose of valproate, may produce a 1.4-fold higher serum concentration of free valproate. Valproic acid also displaces diazepam (DZ) from binding sites, increasing DZ plasma levels. Since valproate has a low therapeutic index, a dose lower than the standard 1500 mg/day should be used to avoid toxicity (Monfort S-Claude. Diazepam increases the serum level of free valproate. Presented at the 146th Annual Meeting of the American Psychiatric Association, San Francisco, May 27, 1993).

diazoxide   (Hyperstat) Nondiuretic benzothiadiazine that may be used to treat hypertensive crises associated with acute phencyclidine (PCP) intoxication.

dibenzepin   (Noveril; Victoril) Tertiary amine, dibenzodiazepine derivative antidepressant. Clinical effects of 480 mg/day appear to be similar to those of amitriptyline and imipramine, 150 mg/day. Not available in the United States.

dibenzothiazepine   (ICI-204,636) Experimental neuroleptic with apparently low propensity to cause extrapyramidal reactions.

dibenzoxazepine One of a class of antipsychotic drugs of which the prototype is loxapine.

dichotomous variable See **variable, dichotomous.**

diclofenac (Voltaren) Potent, well tolerated nonsteroidal anti-inflammatory drug (NSAID) introduced in the mid-1970s. It is a phenylacetic acid derivative. It has been reported to cause hepatotoxicity, a rare side effect that may occur in any patient receiving NSAIDs. If co-administered with lithium, diclofenac may decrease lithium excretion, thereby producing lithium intoxication. See **lithium + diclofenac.** Pregnancy risk category B.

diclofenac + lithium See **lithium + diclofenac.**

diclofensine Experimental antidepressant not available in the United States or Canada.

didactic Characteristic of therapeutic techniques that use teaching or lecture methods.

Didrex See **benzphetamine.**

diencephalon Anterior region of the brain that includes the thalamus, hypothalamus, and pituitary gland.

dietary fiber Carbohydrates and lignin in plant foods that are not digested by the enzymes of mammalian small intestines. It may be soluble or insoluble; each type has its own characteristics. Physiological responses associated with dietary fiber include increased fecal bulk, lowered levels of plasma cholesterol, reduced glycemic response to carbohydrate-containing meals, and decreased nutrient availability. Physical properties of fiber sources (e.g., water-holding capacity, viscosity, binding or absorption properties, fermentability) may influence physiological responses by affecting digestion and absorption. Increasing bulk, volume, and viscosity of small intestine contents may significantly slow or reduce digestion and absorption of nutrients and drugs. See **tricyclic antidepressant/high-fiber diet.**

diethazine (Deparcol) Predecessor of chlorpromazine that became available in France in 1946. It is a phenothiazine derivative with antihistaminic properties, including sedative side effects. It was used as a component of "lytic cocktails" in the early 1950s, and as an antiparkinson drug in neuroleptic-treated patients. See **"lytic cocktail."**

diethylpropion (Nobesine-75; Nu-Dispoz; Regibon; Ro-Diet; Tenuate; Tepanil) Sympathomimetic amine with some pharmacological activity similar to that of amphetamine. It is used as an anorexic for management of exogenous obesity as a short-term adjunct (a few weeks) in a regimen of weight reduction based on caloric restriction. It has abuse potential. Schedule IV, Pregnancy risk category C.

differential misclassification See **misclassification, differential.**

diffusion-weighted imaging (DWI) New magnetic resonance imaging (MRI) technique, technology for which is derived by measuring translational movement (diffusion) of water molecules over a short interval. Preliminary human application has documented that DWI can accurately localize acute brain lesions in stroke patients (Lebihan D. Molecular diffusion nuclear magnetic resonance imaging. *Magn Reson Q* 1991;7:1–30; Fisher M, Bogousslavsky J. Evolving toward effective therapy for acute ischemic stroke. *JAMA* 1993;270:360–364).

diflunisal (Dolobid) Peripherally acting, nonnarcotic, nonsteroidal drug with analgesic, anti-inflammatory, and antipyretic properties. Habituation, tolerance and addiction have been associated with its use. Pregnancy risk category C.

digitalis (Lanoxin) Powdered, dried leaf of the plant *digitalis purpurea* used in the treatment of some cardiac disorders (e.g., congestive heart failure).

digitalis + fluoxetine See **fluoxetine + digitalis.**

digitalis + lithium See **lithium + digitalis.**

digitalization See **rapid tranquilization.**

digital spectral analysis Improved method of recording and monitoring electroencephalographic background activity.

digit repetition test Measure of attention level in which the subject repeats previously presented digits after a 5-minute interval. The average subject can remember 5–7 digits.

digit vigilance Measure of sustained vigilance.

digoxin Glycoside derived from the leaves of *Digitalis lanata* used in the treatment of heart failure, atrial fibrillation, and atrial flutter.

digoxin + buspirone See **buspirone + digoxin.**

digoxin + carbamazepine See **carbamazepine + digoxin.**

digoxin + clomipramine See **clomipramine + digoxin.**

digoxin + diazepam See **diazepam + digoxin.**

digoxin + fluvoxamine See **fluvoxamine + digoxin.**

digoxin + lithium See **lithium + digoxin.**

digoxin + moclobemide See **moclobemide + digoxin.**

digoxin + paroxetine See **paroxetine + digoxin.**

digoxin + sertraline See **sertraline + digoxin.**

digoxin + tacrine See **tacrine + digoxin.**

dihydrexidine First high-potency, full-efficacy D_1 agonist that also has significant D_2 potency comparable to that of quinpirole. In monkeys it reduces 1-methyl-4-phenyl-1,2,3,6-tetrahydropyridine (MPTP)-induced parkinsonism.

dihydroergotamine   (DHE) Ergot alkaloid that may be effective in the treatment of acute migraine. It strongly binds to serotonin (5-HT)$_{1A}$ and 5-HT$_{1D}$ receptors. It also binds to the 5-HT$_{1C}$, 5-HT$_2$, alpha$_1$ and alpha$_2$ noradrenergic, and DA receptors. Pregnancy risk category X.

dihydroergotoxine   (Encephabol; Hydergine) Psychotropic agent claimed to produce changes in neuronal lipopigment. It is the most extensively studied of all drugs used in attempts to alleviate chronic cognitive impairment in the elderly. It has been claimed that it can minimize the harmful effects of cerebral anoxia. It is of little use in Alzheimer's disease (Thompson TL, Filley CM, Mitchell WD, et al. Lack of efficiency of Hydergine in patients with Alzheimer's disease. *N Engl J Med* 1990; 323:445–448). Also called "co-dergocrine."

dihydroindolone   Category of neuroleptics, the only representative of which is molindone. See **molindone**.

dihydropyridine   (DHP) Calcium channel antagonist that can reduce or prevent withdrawal symptoms and seizures in alcohol-dependent rats.

3,4-dihydroxyphenylacetic acid   (DOPAC) Dopamine metabolite in humans measured in blood, urine, and brain.

dihydroxyphenylalanine   See **levodopa**.

dihydroxyphenylamine   See **dopamine**.

dihydroxyphenylglycol   (DHPG) Deaminated compound that is one of the principal metabolites of norepinephrine (NE). Basal and stimulated levels of plasma NE and DHPG are believed to reflect intraneuronal disposition of NE and may be the most sensitive indices of sympathetic nervous activity.

5,7-dihydroxytryptamine   Neurotoxic drug that causes long-lasting, selective depletion of brain serotonin. It is used in preclinical research.

Dilantin   See **phenytoin**.

Dilaudid   See **hydromorphone**.

diltiazem   (Cardizem) Relatively short-acting calcium channel blocker and calcium antagonist used primarily in the treatment of cardiovascular disease. Doses up to 240 mg/day have effectively alleviated severe manic symptoms in a small number of patients. Such use is regarded as experimental and should be reserved for patients unresponsive to lithium or carbamazepine. Diltiazem is well tolerated; constipation and headache are its most common side effects. It is safe in patients without serious cardiac conduction defects.

diltiazem + carbamazepine   See **carbamazepine + diltiazem**.

diltiazem + lithium   See **lithium + diltiazem**.

dimer   Protein composed of two identical polypeptides (chain of amino acids).

dimethoxymethylamphetamine   (DOM) Synthetic, methoxylated amphetamine with structural resemblance to both amphetamine and mescaline. It is a designer drug more potent than mescaline that can provoke a lysergic acid diethylamide (LSD)-like reaction. Doses under 3 mg produce effects similar to those of mescaline. Higher doses cause hallucinations and unpleasant side effects (Snyder S, Failace L, Hollister L. 2,5-dimethoxy-4-methyl-amphetamine (STP): a new hallucinogenic drug. *Science* 1967;158:669–670). Street names include: peace, purple wedge, red barrel, serenity, STP ("serenity, tranquility, and peace"), sweet tart, tranquility, white wedge, and yellow wedge.

dimethracin   Tricyclic antidepressant studied extensively in Europe in the 1960s. Although found comparable in effectiveness to imipramine and amitriptyline, it is now considered obsolete.

2,5-dimethylamphetamine   See **methyl-2,5-dimethoxyamphetamine**.

dimethyltryptamine   (DMT) Hallucinogenic, psychotomimetic drug found in cohoba snuff from the seeds of *Pipradenia peregrina* and made synthetically for street sale. It has rapid onset of a lysergic acid diethylamide (LSD)-like effect and a short duration of action (1–2 hours). It may markedly elevate blood pressure.

Dinaplex   See **flunarizine**.

diphasic dyskinesia   See **dyskinesia, diphasic**.

Diphen   See **diphenhydramine**.

Diphenadril   See **diphenhydramine**.

diphenhydramine   (Beldin; Benadryl; Diahist; Diphen; Diphenadril; Fenylhist; Fynex; Hydramine; Hydril) Histamine H$_1$ antagonist with anticholinergic and nonspecific sedative effects often used as an anxiolytic, as a hypnotic, and for acute extrapyramidal reactions. Dose-dependent increase in hypnotic effect is significantly greater in patients who have not been treated previously; thus, appropriate dosage depends on previous medical treatment of insomnia (Kudo Y, Kurihara M. Clinical evaluation of diphenhydramine hydrochloride for the treatment of insomnia in psychiatric patients: double blind study. *J Clin Pharmacol* 1990;30:1041–1048). Diphenhydramine (50–150 mg/day) also has antiparkinson effects. It is useful for treating early tremor and rigidity, but is not as potent as levodopa in treating akinesia and bradykinesia and their associated slowness, stooping, and falls. It helps to control hypersalivation and drooling but may cause dry mouth with associated adverse effects. This and other anticholinergic side effects limit diphenhydramine's usefulness in treating moderate and advanced stages of parkinsonism. Pregnancy risk category B.

diphenhydramine + alcohol Combined use may result in additive central nervous system depressant effects.

diphenhydramine + anticholinergic Co-administration may cause severe anticholinergic symptoms or intoxication.

diphenhydramine/breast milk Diphenhydramine should not be used during breast feeding.

diphenhydramine + central nervous system depressant Co-administration may produce moderate to severe sedation or induce drowsiness and various degrees of sleep.

diphenhydramine + monoamine oxidase inhibitor (MAOI) MAOIs prolong diphenhydramine's central depressant and anticholinergic effects.

diphenhydramine/pregnancy Diphenhydramine should not be ingested during pregnancy, especially in the third trimester.

diphenoxylate Chemical congener of meperidine used in the management of diarrhea. In very high doses it effectively alleviates symptoms accompanying methadone detoxification and narcotic withdrawal. It has low abuse potential. It is available as a combination product containing low doses of atropine (Lomotil). Schedule V.

diphenylbutylpiperidine Class of antipsychotic drugs, one member of which is pimozide. Diphenylbutylpiperidines are structurally related to the butyrophenones and have similar properties. They have greater pharmacological specificity, acting largely if not exclusively on dopamine receptors with little effect on alpha$_1$ or histamine H$_1$ receptors. They are less sedative than butyrophenones and are less likely to cause drowsiness or hypotension. They are highly liquid-soluble and extensively distributed to tissues. Slow release from deep tissue compartments delays elimination, which occurs via hepatic metabolism and excretion of metabolites. Elimination half-life usually ranges from 50–200 hours. See **pimozide.**

diphenylhydantoin See **phenytoin.**

Dipiperon See **pipamperone.**

diploid cell Cell carrying a double set of chromosomes.

diploidy Having two complete sets of chromosomes, double the number found in the gametes (i.e., the full number resulting from the duplicating equation division, prior to their reduction to the halved or haploid number through the reduction division). The human diploid number is 46.

Dipondal See **dexfenfluramine.**

Diprivan See **propofol.**

dipropyltryptamine (DPT) Synthetic hallucinogen with rapid onset of a lysergic acid diethylamide (LSD)-like effect and a short duration of action (1–2 hours). It is used for a "businessman's trip" because of these properties. It may cause marked elevation of blood pressure. See **"businessman's trip"; "DPT."**

direct agonist See **agonist, direct.**

"dirt" Street name for heroin.

disability Restriction or lack (resulting from an impairment) of ability to perform an activity in the manner or within the range considered normal (International Classification of Impairments, Disabilities, and Handicaps [ICIDH], WHO, 1980). It may hinder mobility, occupation, communication, or ability to care for self. It can be continuous or intermittent and may be present from birth or acquired later.

disability, physical See **physical disability.**

disassortative mating See **negative assortative mating.**

discontinuation-emergent signs and symptoms (DESS) Any event during the post-treatment period that is new or worsened compared to the treatment period.

discordance Dissimilarity in a twin pair with respect to the presence or absence of a disease or trait. The discordance percentage in monozygotic twins in a systematic study provides a measure of the contribution of nongenetic factors operating within or outside the organism. It is also used in matched-pair case-control studies to describe a pair whose members had different exposures to the risk factor under study. Only the discordant pairs are informative about the association between exposure and the disease.

discrete scale Measurement of a numerical characteristic that has integer values.

discriminant analysis Multivariate analysis with continuous dependent variables (called "groups"). Given a set of variable values, it is used to study how a subject should be classified into one of several groups. It is sometimes used instead of regression analysis. Also called "discriminant function analysis."

discriminant function analysis See **discriminant analysis.**

discriminative validity Ability of an instrument to differentiate between two groups that in principle are expected to test differently.

disease concept of chemical dependency Recognition that chemical dependency is a chronic, progressive, potentially fatal biogenic and psychosocial disease characterized by tolerance, physical dependence, diverse personality changes, and adverse social consequences.

disease-related depression See **depression, disease-related.**

disease, subclinical   See **subclinical disease.**

disequilibrium   Sensation of dizziness most often caused by neurological disorders including: multiple sensory deficits, C-P angle or posterior fossa tumors, and cerebellar degeneration.

disinhibition   Complex behaviors that the subject knows are dangerous or inappropriate but feels incapable of resisting. It includes release of socially inappropriate behaviors by alcohol and benzodiazepines. Hostility and rage are the more dangerous manifestations of alcohol- or drug-induced disinhibition. See **behavioral dyscontrol.**

disinhibitor   Internal or external stimulus that may release certain types of physical, psychological, or behavioral processes.

Disipal   See **orphenadrine.**

Disopam   See **diazepam.**

disopyramide   (Norpace) Type A antiarrhythmic drug. If co-administered with cyclic antidepressants that retard conduction, toxic cardiac effects may occur. Because antipsychotic agents have quinidine-like actions, arrhythmias caused by overdoses should not be treated with disopyramide.

disorientation   Lack of awareness of one's relationship to the milieu, including persons, place, and time. It may be due to confusion or drug or alcohol withdrawal. It can range in severity from mild to severe. In severe disorientation the patient has no knowledge of his or her whereabouts, confuses the date by more than 1 year, and can name only one or two individuals in his or her current life.

disorganization   State of behavioral chaos often seen as a consequence of severe, particularly psychotic, disorders.

disorganized thinking   Inability to engage in goal-directed thinking; it often gives rise to thought disorder. See **circumstantiality; loosening of association; thought disorder.**

displacement   Mechanism in which the person generalizes or redirects a feeling about or response to an object onto another, usually less threatening, object (DSM-IV).

dispositional tolerance   Body's development of the capacity to degrade or metabolize a drug at a faster rate in the liver or elsewhere and/or to excrete it more efficiently into the urine. It results in reduced concentration of drug at its sites of action; thus, less drug is available to exert its critical effects. It is unlikely that dispositional tolerance accounts for much of the tolerance to drugs seen at the behavioral level.

disseminated intravascular coagulation   Dangerous phenomenon that can be associated with severe neuroleptic malignant syndrome. It can be initiated by sepsis, shock, trauma, rhabdomyolysis, and exertional heatstroke. In general, disorders involving hypotension, acidosis, and hypoxia pose a high risk (Addonizio G, Susman VL. *Neuroleptic Malignant Syndrome. A Clinical Approach.* St. Louis: Mosby Year Book, 1991).

dissimulation   Concealment or minimization of existing symptoms by a malingerer.

dissociation   Mechanism in which the person sustains a temporary alteration in the integrative functions of consciousness or identity (DSM-IV). Specific internal mental factors (e.g., memories, ideas, feelings, perceptions) are lost to conscious awareness and cannot be recalled voluntarily. Dissociation may be considered a psychological defense because it provides a way of banishing from consciousness unpleasant, painful, anxiety-provoking thoughts. See **dissociative disorder.**

dissociation constant   (K_d) Quantitative expression of the separation of a ligand from a receptor. In ligand-binding studies, it may be expressed as the reciprocal of the affinity constant.

dissociative amnesia   See **amnesia, psychogenic.**

dissociative anesthetic   Drug (e.g., ketamine, phencyclidine) that can alter thalamocortical interactions and noncompetitively block the effects of the excitatory amino acid neurotransmitters glutamate and aspartate at the N-methyl-D-aspartate (NMDA) subclass of their receptors. The drugs produce distortions in body image, analgesia, depersonalization, slowing or loss of time perception, amnesia, and other alterations in sensory perceptions.

dissociative disorder   (DD) One of five DSM-IV disorders: dissociative amnesia, dissociative fugue, dissociative identity disorder, depersonalization disorder, and dissociative disorder not otherwise specified. Dissociative amnesia is considered the most common, and dissociative identity disorder the most severe and chronic. Formerly called "hysterical neuroses of the dissociative type." Also called "conversion disorder."

dissociative fugue   See **psychogenic fugue.**

distractibility   Able to have one's attention drawn too frequently and/or easily to unimportant or irrelevant external stimuli.

distribution   Dissemination of drugs to body compartments. Distribution rate is a function of (a) regional blood flow to various tissues and organs; (b) the drug's lipid solubility; (c) degree of drug binding to plasma proteins; and (d) active transport of a drug across cell membranes. The ratio of lean body mass to adipose tissue mass can also affect a drug's distribution.

distribution phase   Period in a complex (multi-compartmental) pharmacokinetic model during which the drug concentration-time curve reflects the distribution of drug from one body compartment to another.

disulfiram   (Antabuse) Long-acting drug used in the treatment of alcoholism for over 35 years. It blocks normal metabolism of alcohol, including interfering with acetaldehyde breakdown, and causes very unpleasant reactions that can discourage further alcohol use. It is rapidly absorbed following oral administration. It also can be subcutaneously implanted into the abdominal wall, although there is no evidence this significantly extends pharmacological effects. The more alcohol consumed and the higher the dose of disulfiram, the more severe the adverse reaction. Disulfiram is a safe drug, particularly in comparison with the serious mortality of unchecked alcohol misuse (Heather N. Disulfiram treatment for alcoholism: deserves re-examination. *Br Med J* 1989;299:471–472). Although alcohol-sensitizing drugs can be a powerful clinical aid in initiating abstinence in alcoholic patients, reported long-term outcome results are disappointing (Institute of Medicine. *Prevention and Treatment of Alcohol Problems: Research Opportunities.* Washington, DC: Naval Academy Press, 1989). Compliance is a problem in clinical use; the major limiting factor is that disulfiram must be taken daily for the reaction to take place when alcohol is drunk. Because it also produces severe reactions if alcohol is absorbed, the patient must avoid any products containing alcohol (e.g., aftershave lotions, cough syrups). Disulfiram can raise dopamine and lower norepinephrine levels. Hence, although rare at normal doses, psychosis may occur (Rossiter SK. Psychosis with disulfiram prescribed under probation order. *Br Med J* 1992;305:763). Schizophrenic patients who abuse alcohol should be followed closely, particularly in the early stages of disulfiram therapy. See **disulfiram + alcohol.**

disulfiram + alcohol   After ingestion of a small amount (about 50 mg) of disulfiram, within 10 minutes of drinking alcohol flushing and a sensation of facial warmth occurs; by 20–30 minutes vasodilation of peripheral blood vessels is manifested by a red appearance; between 30 and 90 minutes the patient may have a throbbing headache, chest tightness, difficulty breathing, weakness, vertigo, nausea and vomiting, pallor, hypotension, tachycardia, and vomiting. Other interactions include blurred vision, sweating, thirst, and confusion. More severe reactions include hypotension, cardiovascular collapse, and, sometimes, convulsions.

disulfiram + alprazolam   No serious interactions have been reported (Diquet B, Gujadhur L, Lamiable D, et al. Lack of interaction between disulfiram and alprazolam in alcoholic patients. *Eur J Clin Pharmacol* 1990;38: 157–160).

disulfiram + benzodiazepine   Co-administration increases sedation and decreases benzodiazepine (BZD) clearance; BZD dosage adjustment may be necessary to avert toxicity. Disulfiram may also increase the half-lives of oxidatively metabolized BZDs. See **benzodiazepine grouping.**

disulfiram + carbamazepine   Carbamazepine does not appear to interact with disulfiram (Krag B, Dam M, Helle A, Christensen JM. Influence of disulfiram on the serum concentrations of carbamazepine in patients with epilepsy. *Acta Neurol Scand* 1981;63:395).

disulfiram + maprotiline   Co-administration may cause tachycardia and delirium.

disulfiram + marijuana   There is a single case report of a hypomanic-like reaction characterized by euphoria, hyperactivity, insomnia, and irritability (Lacoursiere RB. Swatek R. Adverse interaction between disulfiram and marijuana: a case report. *Am J Psychiatry* 1983;140:242–244).

disulfiram + methadone   Disulfiram inhibits clearance of methadone, possibly resulting in methadone toxicity.

disulfiram + neuroleptic   Co-administration decreases clearance of neuroleptics and requires decreased neuroleptic dosage to prevent toxicity.

disulfiram + oxazepam   Co-administration minimally alters oxazepam disposition. Oxazepam may be the drug of choice if benzodiazepine therapy is used for patients taking disulfiram (MacLeod SM, Sellers EM, Giles HG, et al. Interaction of disulfiram with benzodiazepines. *Clin Pharmacol Ther* 1978;24:583–589).

disulfiram + perphenazine   Co-administration may reduce perphenazine plasma levels (Hansen L, Larsen N. Metabolic interaction between perphenazine and disulfiram. *Lancet* 1982;2:1472).

disulfiram + phenytoin   Co-administration decreases phenytoin (PHT) clearance and markedly increases its serum levels. PHT toxicity has occurred when disulfiram was added to an anticonvulsant regimen (Kiorboe E. Phenytoin intoxication during treatment with Antabuse. *Epilepsia* 1966;7:246; Svendsen TL, Kristensen MB, Hansen JM, Skovsted L. The influence of disulfiram on the half-life and metabolic clearance rate of diphenylhydantoin and tolbutamide in man. *Eur J Clin Pharmacol* 1976;9:439).

disulfiram + tricyclic antidepressant (TCA)　Co-administration decreases TCA clearance, necessitating reduced TCA dosage to prevent toxicity.

diuretic + lithium　See **lithium + diuretic.**

diurnal　Occurring during the daytime. Whereas circadian events occur during the whole 24 hours of day and night, diurnal events occur in the day only.

divalproex　(Depakote; Epival) Divalproic acid, in the form of sodium valproate. See **valproate.**

divalproex + carbamazepine　Co-administration may result in sustained prophylaxis for bipolar disorder in patients who have had an inadequate response to either anticonvulsant alone (Ketter TA, Pazzaglia PJ, Post RM. Synergy of carbamazepine and valproic acid in affective illness: case report and review of literature. *J Clin Psychopharmacol* 1992;12:276–281; Keck PE Jr, McElroy SL, Vuckovic A, Freidman LM. Combined valproate and carbamazepine treatment of bipolar disorder. *J Neuropsychiatry Clin Neurosci* 1992;4:319–322; Schaff MR, Fawcett J, Zajecka JM. Divalproex sodium in the treatment of refractory depressive disorders. *J Clin Psychiatry* 1993;54:380–384).

divalproex + clozapine　Priapism has been reported with co-administration for about 5 weeks. Attempts to renew treatment resulted in recurrence of priapism (Seftel AD, Saenzde Tejada I, Szetela B, et al. Clozapine-associated priapism: a case report. *J Urol* 1992;147:146–148). Whether priapism was due to the combination is uncertain since priapism has been reported with clozapine monotherapy (Ziegler J, Behar D. Clozapine-induced priapism. *Am J Psychiatry* 1992;149:272–273).

Dixaret　See **clonidine.**

Dixeran　See **melitracen.**

dixyrazine　(Esucos) Piperazine phenothiazine not marketed in the United States or Canada.

dizocilpine　(MK-801) Phencyclidine (PCP) receptor ligand (PRL) marketed as a dissociative anesthetic. It is more potent than selective in binding to the PCP receptor than PCP itself. Like all PRLs, it is a potent N-methyl-D-aspartate (NMDA) receptor antagonist with neuroprotective effects in animal models of stroke. It is the most potent of a group of drugs that block the ion channel of the NMDA receptor. NMDA receptors are stimulated by certain amino acids that can be toxic when released in large amounts, as in the case of strokes. In rats, MK-801 prevents tolerance for or dependence on morphine, suggesting that it may also prevent morphine addiction in patients given the narcotic for pain. It causes a high incidence of emergence reaction in adult patients following ketamine anesthesia (Mar-

shall BE, Longnecker DE. General anesthetics. *In* Gilman AG, Rall TW, Nies AS, Taylor P [eds]. *Goodman and Gilman's The Pharmacological Basis of Therapeutics*, 8th ed. New York: Pergamon Press, 1990, p 307).

dizygotic　Twins who developed from two ova and have different genetic characteristics (i.e., nonidentical twins).

"DL"　Street name for oxymorphone.

D-loop synthesis　Mode of DNA replication in mitochondria in which staggered copying of the parenteral strands produces a displacement (D) loop.

2,5-DMA　See **dimethoxymethylamphetamine.**

D-m-I syndrome　In bipolar patients, episodes of depression with only hypomania or cyclothymia. Patients are more responsive to lithium than those with D-M-I syndrome.

D-M-I syndrome　In bipolar patients, occurrence of depression before mania. Patients are less likely to respond to lithium than those with D-m-I syndrome.

"DMT"　Street name for dimethyltryptamine.

DNA　See **deoxyribonucleic acid.**

DNA, junk　See **junk DNA.**

DNA marker　See **restriction fragment length polymorphism.**

DNA probe　Small fragment of single-strand DNA treated so it will be detectable.

DNA recombination　See **gene cloning.**

DNA replication　Capacity of DNA to produce an exact copy of itself. It constitutes the basis of hereditary transmission.

DNA sequence　Linear order of base pairs along a DNA molecule.

DNA transcription　Molecular process whereby the genetic code in a DNA molecule is used as a template to make a corresponding molecule of RNA.

DOB　See **4-bromo-2,5-dimethoxyamphetamine.**

DOD　(4-bromo-2,5-dimethoxyphenylisopropylamine) Hallucinogenic amphetamine derivative.

Do-Do　Over-the-counter preparation containing ephedrine (222 mg), caffeine (30 mg) and theophylline (50 mg) widely used in England for relief of "bronchial coughs, wheezing, and breathlessness." It has an amphetamine-like action. Abuse and withdrawal symptoms similar to those following cessation of amphetamines have been reported (Loosmore S, Armstrong D. Do-Do abuse. *Br J Psychiatry* 1990;157:278–281).

Dogmatyl　See **sulpiride.**

"doll"　Street name for barbiturates.

"dolly"　Street name for methadone.

Dolmatil　See **sulpiride.**

Dolobid　See **diflunisal.**

Dolophine   See **methadone.**

domain   Discrete portion of a protein with its own function. The combination of domains in a single protein determines its unique overall function.

domain, regulatory   See **regulatory domain.**

domain, transcribed   See **transcribed domain.**

domestic abuse   Behavior pattern in which a person repeatedly inflicts physical injury, pain, fear, or mental anguish on another family member. Trauma may be physical, psychological, sexual, or economic. Neglect occurs when a caregiver fails to provide basic necessities for a family member. Victims of abuse and neglect often come to the emergency department for treatment.

dominance   Expression of the phenotype of one gene of an allelic pair while the phenotype of the other, recessive allele does not appear in the characteristics of the organism.

dominant gene   See **gene, dominant.**

dominant inheritance   See **inheritance, dominant.**

dominant trait   See **trait, dominant.**

Domnamid   See **estazolam.**

domoic acid   (DOA) Environmental excitotoxant implicated in a 1987 food poisoning incident in Canada that killed some persons and left others demented. Excitotoxant activity is exerted exclusively at kainic acid receptors.

domperidone   (Motilium) Butyrophenone dopamine antagonist that does not cross the blood-brain barrier. It is used for gastrointestinal motility problems.

"done"   Street name for methadone.

"doobie"   Street name for a marijuana cigarette.

dopa   See **levodopa.**

DOPAC   See **3,4-dihydroxyphenylacetic acid.**

dopamine   (DA) Neurotransmitter in three major areas of the brain: the nigrostriatal system, which extends from the substantia nigra to the corpus striatum and basal ganglia; the mesocorticol system, which projects from the mesencephalon to the limbic system and cortex; and the tuberoinfundibular system, which projects from the hypothalamus to the median eminence. Although DA seems to be predominantly a type B substrate, it is converted to noradrenaline, a type A substrate for monoamine oxidase. Degeneration of DA neurons in the nigrostriatal pathway accounts for many of the symptoms of Parkinson's disease. Neuroleptic blockade of DA receptors in the corpus striatum produces extrapyramidal symptoms, and of those in the tuberoinfundibular system an elevation of serum prolactin. DA receptor blockade is believed to be related to antipsychotic effects. DA has been implicated in the reinforcing effects of psycho-stimulant drugs of abuse such as cocaine and amphetamine. Dietary precursors of DA are phenylalanine and l-tyrosine. See **dopamine HCl.**

dopamine autoreceptor   Type of dopamine receptor that can exist on most portions of dopamine cells, including the soma, dendrites, and nerve terminals. Stimulation in the somatodendritic region slows the firing rate of dopamine neurons; stimulation on nerve terminals inhibits dopamine synthesis and release. Somatodendritic and nerve terminal autoreceptors work in concert to exert feedback on dopaminergic transmission.

dopamine-beta-hydroxylase   (DBH) Enzyme in noradrenergic neurons that converts dopamine to noradrenaline (European nomenclature) or norepinephrine (American system).

dopamine blockade   Effect produced by most typical neuroleptics, to a lesser extent by some atypical neuroleptics, and by some non-neuroleptic antagonists (e.g., the anti-emetic metoclopramide). It results in early-onset acute extrapyramidal reactions (EPS) and possibly late-onset EPS (e.g., tardive dyskinesia).

dopamine HCl   (Intropin; Revimine) Hydrochloride salt of the naturally occurring catecholamine neurotransmitter dopamine. It does not cross the blood-brain barrier. It is an inotropic vasopressor agent that can be used to treat hypotension secondary to inadequate cardiac output.

dopamine hypothesis of depression   In the early 1970s, Danish researchers began to formulate this hypothesis based on the following clinical observations: (a) dopamine-blocking neuroleptics may cause depression in some patients; (b) these same drugs also may relieve depression in some depressed patients; (c) they can aggravate depression in patients with this affective disorder; (d) they can be quite helpful in relieving schizoaffective, agitated, and anxious depressions; (e) either alone or in combination with antidepressants, these neuroleptics can alleviate psychotic depression; and (f) depression occurs frequently in patients with dopamine-related neurological deseases (e.g., Parkinson's disease and Huntington's chorea). This evidence prompted these clinician/researchers to advance the hypothesis that brain dopamine plays an important role in the pharmacology and, probably, in the pathogenesis of depression (Randrup A, Munkvad I, Fog R, et al. Mania, depression, and brain dopamine. *In* Essman WB, Valzelli L [eds], *Current Developments in Psychopharmacology.* New York: Spectrum Publications, 1975, pp 207–229).

dopamine hypothesis of schizophrenia   Postulation of a functionally hyperactive central dopaminergic system in schizophrenia supported by some pharmacological and biochemical evidence. Amphetamine abuse or intoxication enhances dopamine (DA) transmission that may lead to psychosis characterized by delusions and hallucinations. It shares many features with agitated schizophrenia and is consistently reversed by DA blockade. Neuroleptic treatment of schizophrenia is associated with reduction in delusions and hallucinations, an effect correlated with DA-blocking properties of these drugs. An important limitation of the DA hypothesis is that amphetamine does not induce negative schizophrenic symptoms and generally spares cognitive functions. Furthermore, many schizophrenics are refractory to DA antagonists, and typical neuroleptics primarily alleviate positive symptoms and have less impact on negative symptoms. The hypothesis has been challenged on several accounts: (a) DA blockade cannot be directly equated with antipsychotic drugs; (b) DA agonists (e.g., amphetamines) exacerbate symptoms of actively psychotic schizophrenic patients and can produce transient exacerbation in remitted patients; (c) several predictions that should follow from excessive DA activity (e.g., low prolactin concentrations and incompatibility of Parkinson's disease with schizophrenic symptoms) are not borne out; (d) DA level in schizophrenia as measured by DA turnover from cerebrospinal fluid homovanillic acid is not consistently elevated except among those with motor hyperactivity; (e) postmortem studies of the brain of schizophrenic patients, taking into account their experience with neuroleptics, do not show clear-cut DA excess; (f) postmortem studies that do indicate increased number of D$_2$ type DA receptors are contaminated by recent use of antipsychotic drugs, which also increases D$_2$ receptor number; and (g) DA excess is not evident in patients who terminated drug treatment at least 1 month prior to death (Lader M. *Introduction to Psychopharmacology.* Kalamazoo, MI: Scope Publications, 1983). Positron emission tomography studies, which enable direct testing of D$_2$ receptor functioning, indicate no apparent abnormalities in the DA system or of the D$_2$ receptor in particular in schizophrenia. This has led a principle advocate of the DA hypothesis, Arvid Carlsson, to conclude that it is no longer tenable (Carlsson A. Early psychopharmacology and the rise of modern brain research. *J Psychopharmacol* 1990;4:120–126).

dopamine precursor   See **memantine.**

dopamine radioreceptor assay   Assay similar to a radioimmunoassay except that instead of using an antibody to recognize the radioactive tracer and the drug (antigen), it uses dopamine receptors. Like a radioimmunoassay, the dopamine (DA) radioreceptor assay is very sensitive; unlike a radioimmunoassay, it is not specific. The radioreceptor assay for neuroleptics detects DA receptor blocking activity but alone cannot identify the compound(s) causing the activity. Results from the DA radioreceptor assay for neuroleptics are expressed as chlorpromazine equivalents in nanograms per milliliter, which indicate the concentration of chlorpromazine that would produce the same degree of binding inhibition observed with serum samples.

dopamine receptor   Any of the multiple dopamine (DA) receptors (D$_1$–D$_5$) in the brain, each of which has a specific ligand. Drugs may have a selective or specific action on just one of the dopamine receptors. All neuroleptics that have antipsychotic action are DA antagonists that block DA actions. Studies of receptor occupancy indicate that all typical neuroleptics show substantially greater occupancy of D$_2$ than of D$_1$ receptors. Many patients with extrapyramidal side effects induced by typical neuroleptics show more than 80% occupancy of D$_2$ receptors. By contrast, the atypical neuroleptic clozapine has higher affinity for D$_1$ receptors than other marketed antipsychotics, and lower affinity for D$_2$ than other drugs. Current theories of schizophrenia etiology focus on D$_2$ receptors.

dopamine receptor, D$_1$ First dopamine receptor discovered. D$_1$ receptors are localized mainly on striatal neurons. Activation stimulates adenylate cyclase activity, blockade prevents stimulation of adenylate cyclase by D$_1$ agonists, and chronic administration of an antagonist increases receptor density. Its principle known agonist is the experimental drug SKF 38393. It remains to be seen whether pure D$_1$ antagonists (e.g., SCH 39166) are antipsychotic. The atypical antipsychotic clozapine upregulates D$_1$ receptors and is associated with much lower incidence of extrapyramidal reactions and tardive dyskinesia. The D$_1$ dopamine receptor was the first of the dopamine receptor subtypes for which a biochemical effector system was described. Positron emission tomography (PET) studies of patients treated with clozapine and flupenthixol show that D$_1$ occupancy by flupenthixol is 36–44%, whereas with clozapine it is 38–52%. D$_1$ occupancy induced by clozapine and flupenthixol may contribute to their antipsychotic effects. The D$_1$ group contains two receptors: D$_1$ and D$_5$.

dopamine receptor, D$_2$ Dopamine (DA) receptor that inhibits adenylate cyclase and occurs most prominently in the striatal and limbic structures in man. Stimulation inhibits forskolin-stimulated adenylate cyclase by D$_2$ agonists, and chronic administration of antagonist increases D$_2$ receptor density. Typical neuroleptics may exert their antipsychotic effect by blocking D$_2$ receptors. Such blockade is also associated with a high incidence of extrapyramidal reactions (EPS) and tardive dyskinesia. Haloperidol and sulpiride are D$_2$ antagonists. In patients treated with conventional dosages of typical neuroleptics, D$_2$ occupancy is 70–89%. Patients with acute EPS have higher D$_2$ occupancy than those without side effects, indicating that neuroleptic-induced EPS are related to the degree of central D$_2$ occupancy in the basal ganglia. By contrast, in positron emission tomography (PET) studies in patients treated with clozapine, D$_2$ occupancy is 38–63%. Hallucinations and positive symptoms are blocked when about 70% of D$_2$ receptors are occupied by neuroleptic drugs. An important pharmacological agonist is quinpirole; sulpiride is an antagonist. Other drugs with agonist effects include psychostimulants and L-dopa. D$_2$ receptors have been implicated in the pathogenesis of several neuropsychiatric disorders, especially schizophrenia. The recent cloning of the dopamine D$_2$ receptor gene allows more precise analysis of antipsychotic-induced up-regulation. D$_2$ receptor binding correlates with clinical antipsychotic potency. There are two D$_2$ subreceptors, D$_{2a}$ and D$_{2b}$ (Davis K, Khan R, Ko G, Davidson M. Dopamine in schizophrenia: a review and reconceptualization. *Am J Psychiatry* 1991;148:1474–1486).

dopamine receptor, D$_3$ Dopamine receptor anatomically limited to limbic areas, but resembling neither D$_1$ nor D$_2$. D$_3$ receptors have been implicated as a target for neuroleptic drugs based on affinity of atypical neuroleptics for the receptor and on its localization to limbic brain structures implicated in the etiology of schizophrenia (McAllister G, Knowles MR, Ward-Booth S, et al. The quest for a functionally coupled D3 dopamine receptor. *Neuropsychopharmacology* 1993;9:85S).

dopamine receptor, D$_4$ Recently cloned dopamine receptor that has a higher affinity for the atypical antipsychotic clozapine. D$_4$ receptors are high in limbic and cortex regions, but low in the normal human striatum, consistent with the clinical profile of clozapine. Thus, D$_4$ appears to be a promising target for future antipsychotic drugs. In schizophrenia, D$_4$ receptors are elevated by 500%, whereas the density of D$_2$ receptors is elevated only about 15% (Seeman P. Schizophrenia, antipsychotic drugs, and D$_4$. *Neuropsychopharmacology* 1993;9:13S).

dopamine receptor, D$_5$ Recently cloned dopamine receptor that has a higher affinity for the atypical antipsychotic clozapine. D$_5$ receptors resemble D$_1$ receptors, but have a higher affinity for dopamine.

dopamine receptor gene   One of two genes cloned in 1990. D$_1$ receptor gene is mapped to chromosome 5q31–34. D$_2$ receptor gene (DRD2) is mapped to chromosome 11 q22–q23 and placed in the genetic linkage map. It has been extensively studied genetically because of the pharmacological importance of D$_2$ receptors. Linkage studies have excluded mutation in DRD2 as a cause of schizophrenia and Tourette's syndrome in several families. A large number of linkage studies have been done; over 50% find some increase in A1 allele in alcoholism, but only a few have been published so far. Other studies have shown that the A1 allele of the DRD2 gene is associated with a number of behavior disorders in which it may act as a modifying gene rather than as the primary etiological agent.

dopamine supersensitivity hypothesis of tardive dyskinesia (TD)   Postulation by Klawans (1970) that chronic neuroleptic treatment produces supersensitivity of striatal dopamine (DA) receptors similar to denervation-induced supersensitivity seen in peripheral muscles. Supersensitivity has become a predominant theoretical construct guiding TD therapy. This construct is supported by numerous basic and clinical studies. However, it appears that supersensitive DA receptors only modulate TD to some degree and that additional factors independent of the DA receptor are probably involved as well.

dopamine synthesis   Like most neurotransmitters (NTs), dopamine (DA) is derived from an amino acid. The amino acid tyrosine is taken up by dopaminergic neurons, converted by the enzyme tryrosine hydroxylase to 3,4-dihydroxyphenylalanine (dopa), decarboxylated by the enzyme aromatic L-amino acid decarboxylase to DA, and stored in vesicles. Released DA interacts with dopaminergic receptors and is then re-uptaken into the prejunctional neurons. DA levels are held constant by changes in tyrosine hydroxylate activity and the enzyme monamine oxidase, which is localized in nerve terminals and metabolizes dopamine.

dopamine transporter   Newly cloned gene belonging to a family of transporters that move neurotransmitters back into the nerve terminals from which they were released. It is being called the "cocaine gene." See **cocaine gene.**

dopaminergic   Dopamine agonist (e.g., bromocriptine, piribedil, apomorphine, D-amphetamine). These drugs have been used to induce hypomania and mood elevation.

dopaminergic system   Five different dopamine (DA) receptors that can be divided into two subfamilies on the basis of their pharmacological properties. The D_2 subfamily contains the D_2, D_3, and D_4 receptors that bind with high affinity to typical neuroleptics. They differ, however, in their ability to recognize particular neuroleptics; D_3 and D_4 receptors have higher affinity for particular atypical neuroleptics and are found in brain tissues significantly different from the ones in which the D_2 receptor is found (Civelli O. Molecular characterization of the D_2, D_3, D_4 dopamine receptor family. *Neuropsychopharmacology* 1993;9: 35S).

Dopar   See **levodopa.**

"dope"   **1.** Street name for opioids, including heroin, morphine, and dilaudid. **2.** Street name for cannabis products in the United Kingdom.

Dopergin   See **lisuride.**

Dopergine   See **lisuride.**

Dopicar   See **levodopa/carbidopa.**

Dopram   See **doxapram.**

Doral   See **quazepam.**

Doriden   See **glutethimide.**

Doriglute   See **glutethimide.**

Dormalin   See **quazepam.**

Dormex   See **brotizolam.**

Dormicum   See **midazolam.**

Dormonoct   See **loprazolam.**

dosage   See **therapeutic dosage.**

dose comparison trial   Clinical drug trial, frequently done in phase II of drug development, designed to compare different drug doses with placebo.

dose dependence, therapeutic   See **therapeutic dose dependence.**

dose-escalation design   Study design in which drug doses are slowly increased in a predetermined manner. A typical design includes placebo administration to all subjects. After a predetermined period, the lowest active dose is given and the response is monitored. If response does not meet predefined criteria of a clinical endpoint and no unacceptable toxicity occurs, the dose is increased to the next highest active dose. If response is seen at any dose, it is maintained for the study duration, and response measurement continues. Study data consist of all responses from all subjects. The design allows gathering significantly more data than other designs at several dose levels and does not suffer from the ethical concerns of the crossover design. One problem is that period effects can be confounded with dose effects and with period-by-dose interactions (e.g., dependence of response on time).

dose-finding study   Phase II study in which subjects are given gradually escalating doses to assess minimal level for efficacy and level of tolerability.

dose-response curve   Chart in which drug dose or concentration is plotted on the horizontal (x) axis and a measurable drug response is plotted on the vertical (y) axis. It shows the percentage of subjects who respond or remit on drug therapy. In animal studies, it indicates the percent response to a specified (log) dose or less. The curve may represent an increasing percentage of animals responding to a drug or an increasing magnitude of response within an individual animal or tissue.

dose-response relationship   Important, commonly used concept in clinical pharmacology and epidemiology in which increase or decrease in intensity of an exposure results in increased or decreased response to a drug under study or risk of the disease.

dose-response study   Randomized, double-blind, placebo-controlled study with a minimum of three dosage levels of the study drug in order to fit various models.

dose titration within fixed ranges   Study design in which an experimental drug is randomized to one of three treatment groups: two dosage ranges each compared to placebo (e.g., a low-dose group treated with 50–300 mg/day, a high-dose group treated with 100–600 mg/day, compared to a placebo group treated with one to six capsules per day given for x weeks. Investigators continue dose titration to a maximum of six capsules within the first 2 weeks in the absence of side effects.

Dotazone   See **trazodone.**

dot-blot hybridization   Variation of Southern blotting in which total DNA is spotted directly on a solid support without prior gel fractionation.

dothiepin   (Idom; Prothiaden; Protiaden; Protiadene). Thio analog of amitriptyline marketed since 1964 in England and Europe, where it is used for depression and mixed anxiety depression. It inhibits noradrenergic and serotonergic uptake and is structurally similar to amitriptyline and doxepin. In overall therapeutic efficacy it is similar to amitriptyline, other heterocyclic antidepressants, fluoxetine, and trazodone. In anxiety associated with depression, efficacy is equivalent to amitriptyline and alprazolam. Most commonly reported side effects are dry mouth, drowsiness, gastrointestinal disorders, and dizziness. Dothiepin has fewer anticholinergic side effects than most tricyclics and has not been associated with cardiotoxicity at therapeutic doses (75–225 mg/day).

dothiepin/breast milk In women aged 28–40 taking orally administered dothiepin (25–225 mg/day), low levels of dothiepin and its metabolites were found in breast milk; no adverse effects were noted in their infants. Dothiepin is unlikely to be a significant hazard to breast-fed infants (Ilett KF, Lebedevs TH, Wojnar-Horton R, et al. Excretion of dothiepin and its primary metabolites in breast milk. *Br J Clin Pharmacol* 1992;33:635–639).

dothiepin + fluoxetine Changing from fluoxetine to dothiepin may cause agitation, tremulousness, sedation, and grand mal seizures (Lyndon RW. Fluoxetine-dothiepin interaction: seizures. *Pharmabulletin* 1993;17:9).

dothiepin + lithium Addition of lithium in depressed patients resistant to dothiepin therapy frequently produces a favorable clinical response.

"dot" Street name for lysergic acid diethylamide (LSD).

dot plot Graphic method for displaying frequency distributions of numerical observations for one or more groups.

double-blind trial Study in which one or more drugs and/or placebo are compared or active drugs are compared with each other in such a way that neither subjects nor those directly involved in administering and evaluating the treatment know which preparation is given to each subject. A third party holds the code identifying each medication packet; the code is not broken until all clinical data have been collected. Design criteria include the following: (a) compared drugs should be as physically identical and indistinguishable as possible; (b) the code should be accessible in case of emergency; and (c) strict precautions should be taken to avoid information leaks. Also called "double mask."

"double cross" Street name for amphetamines.

double crossover Type of experimental design in which treatments are switched back and forth between groups of subjects (e.g., ABA design).

double depression See **depression, double.**

double dummy design Clinical drug trial in which placebos are matched in appearance to two different active drugs. Blindness can be preserved if those taking one drug take matching dummies of the other drugs being studied; whatever active treatment is administered, drugs taken together look the same.

double helix Twisted ladder structure of DNA with complementary strands around each other and connected by bonds between base pairs.

double heterozygousness See **heterozygousness, double.**

double mask See **double-blind trial.**

"double trouble" **1.** Street name for the combination of amobarbital and secobarbital (Tuinal). **2.** Self-help group designed for patients with a dual diagnosis (e.g., alcoholism and substance abuse).

"down" Street name for central nervous system depressants.

"downer" Street name for barbiturates.

down-regulation Reduction of response following exposure of a receptor to a given concentration of an agonist. Chronic administration of a receptor agonist usually results in receptor down-regulation, as does chronic overexposure of receptors to the endogenous transmitter (e.g., after uptake inhibition). Down-regulation can involve decreases in density of receptors and/or change in the signal transducing system distal to the receptor. See **subsensitivity; up-regulation.**

Down syndrome Mental retardation arising from the meiotic nondisjunction of chromosome 21 (trisomy 21). Studies of 200 families, using multiple DNA polymorphisms, indicate maternal origin of the extra chromosome 21 in 95% of cases. Down syndrome can be detected in utero by determining the karyotype of fetal cells, but limited resources available for the test and morbidity associated with sampling fetal tissue restrict it to women thought to be at highest risk (over age 35 or genetic history). Formerly called "mongolism." See **trisomy 21.**

doxacurium + carbamazepine See **carbamazepine + doxacurium.**

doxapram (Dopram) Respiratory stimulant that apparently acts on the peripheral carotid oxygen receptors and on the respiratory center of the medulla oblongata. It may be a potentially useful probe for investigating the pathophysiology of panic disorder.

doxepin (Adapin; Curetin; Deptran; Gilex; Sinequan; Triadapin) Tricyclic antidepressant composed of a mixture of geometric isomers, *cis*-doxepin, and *trans*-doxepin, which are metabolized into *cis*-N-desmethyldoxepin and *trans*-N-desmethyldoxepin. Its active metabolite is N-desmethyldoxepin. Its general pharmacokinetic properties are similar to those of other tricyclic antidepressants; orthostatic potential is midway between that of imipramine and nortriptyline (Rouse SP, Dalack GW, Glassman A, et al. Is doxepin a safer tricyclic for the heart? *J Clin Psychiatry* 1991; 52:338–341). Pregnancy risk category C.

doxepin/breast milk Doxepin is excreted in breast milk. High daily doses (250 mg+) should not be taken during breastfeeding.

doxepin + carbamazepine Carbamazepine (CBZ) decreases doxepin serum concentration (Leinonen E, Lillsunde P, Laukkanen V,

Ylitalo P. Effects of carbamazepine on serum antidepressant concentration in psychiatric patients. *J Clin Psychopharmacol* 1991;11:313–318). If doxepin levels are monitored, the combination can be used for pain caused by cancer or other disorders. Doxepin (50 mg) plus CBZ (800 mg) produces serum concentrations in the therapeutic range (Storey P, Trimble M. Rectal doxepin and carbamazepine therapy in patients with cancer. *N Engl J Med* 1992;327:1318–1319).

doxepin + cimetidine   Cimetidine may double doxepin serum concentrations (Sutherland DL, Remillard AJ, Haight KR. The influence of cimetidine versus ranitidine on doxepin pharmacokinetics. *Eur J Clin Pharmacol* 1987; 32:159–164).

doxepin + fluoxetine   Low-dose (25–50 mg) doxepin can be combined with fluoxetine for night-time nervousness attributed to fluoxetine.

doxepin + lithium   Co-administration may augment the antiobsessional effect of chronic treatment with doxepin in patients with obsessive-compulsive disorder. Lithium also augments doxepin's antidepressant effects.

doxepin + monoamine oxidase inhibitor (MAOI)   Co-administration can be safe and effective for treatment-resistant depression (White K, Simpson G. Combined monoamine oxidase inhibitor-tricyclic antidepressant treatment: a reevaluation. *J Clin Psychopharmacol* 1981;1: 264–281).

doxepin + pergolide   Co-administration has been used in patients refractory to doxepin alone. Response is usually rapid, within a week, and without incremental improvement over the next month. Some patients tolerate the combination well; others develop nausea and vomiting that may or may not respond to lowering pergolide dose (Bouckoms A, Mangini L. Pergolide: an antidepressant adjuvant for mood disorders. *Psychopharmacol Bull* 1993;29:207–211).

doxepin + ranitidine   Ranitidine had no effect on doxepin serum concentration (Sutherland DL, Remillard AJ, Haight KR. The influence of cimetidine versus ranitidine on doxepin pharmacokinetics. *Eur J Clin Pharmacol* 1987; 32:159–164).

doxepin + sertraline   Low-dose doxepin (25–50 mg) has been added at bedtime for sertraline-treated patients with persistent pretreatment insomnia. The regimen has been safe and effective (Kline NA, Dow BM, Brown SA, Matloff JL. Sertraline efficacy in depressed combat veterans with posttraumatic stress disorder. Presented at the 146th Annual Meeting of the American Psychiatric Association, San Francisco, May 1993).

doxepin-N-oxide   Metabolite of doxepin in both humans and animals.

doxycycline + carbamazepine   See **carbamazepine + doxycycline.**

doxylamine   Sedative antihistamine often prescribed as a hypnotic.

DPAX   Computer program for case identification and diagnosis that refers to (a) essential features of a psychiatric syndrome; (b) pattern and frequency of associated symptoms; and (c) criteria for duration and level of functional impairment. DPAX also divides noncase patients into categories reflecting the degree to which they fail to meet case criteria (borderline, conceivable, or well) (Murphy JM, Neff RK, Sobol AM, et al. Computer diagnosis of depression and anxiety: the Stirling County Study. *Psychol Med* 1985;15:99–112).

"DPT"   Street name for dimethyltryptamine. See **also dipropyltryptamine.**

"draw"   Street name for cannabis products in the UK.

D_1 receptor   See **dopamine receptor, D_1.**

D_2 receptor   See **dopamine receptor, D_2.**

D_3 receptor   See **dopamine receptor, D_3.**

D_4 receptor   See **dopamine, receptor D_4.**

D_5 receptor   See **dopamine receptor, D_5.**

D_2 receptor agonist/antagonist   Chemical compound with relatively strong affinity for D_2 receptors.

D_2 receptor gene   See **dopamine D_2 receptor gene.**

drinking, acceptable   Level of alcohol consumption that does not lead to negative medical, psychiatric, or interpersonal consequences, and that conforms to the amounts of alcohol, types of alcohol, and settings acceptable to society at large, religious, or ethnic subgroups of society, and an individual's primary group. The Royal College of Physicians (1987) suggested the following guidelines for safe levels of alcohol consumption: "14 units of alcohol for women and 21 for men, per week. (A unit is 8 g pure alcohol, approximately equivalent to one glass of wine, half a pint of ordinary beer, one measure [1/6 gill] of spirits or one glass of sherry.)" It also suggested that drinking 14–35 units per week is hazardous, particularly for women, and that 35 or more units is definitely dangerous for anyone.

drinking/drugs   See **alcohol + other drugs.**

drinking, moderate   Drinking of alcohol that generally does not cause problems for either the drinker or society. Most experts consider moderate drinking to mean up to two drinks a day for men and one drink a day for women. Adverse consequences, however, still may occur, including stroke, motor vehicle accidents, interactions with medications, cancer, and birth defects (Anon. Moderate drinking. *Alcohol Alert* 1992;No. 16:1–4).

Drolban   See **dromostanolone propionate.**

Droleptan   See **droperidol.**

dromomania   **1.** Abnormal impulse to travel. **2.** Desire to escape from an unpleasant sexual situation.

dromostanolone propionate   (Drolban) Commonly abused anabolic steroid.

dronabinol   (Marinol) Stereochemical variant of delta-9-tetrahydrocannabinol, the active principle of cannabis, that is effective in the management of nausea and vomiting induced by cancer chemotherapy. Despite its high abuse potential, there are no reports of actual abuse of dronabinol. See **tetrahydrocannabinol.**

droperidol   (Droleptan; Inapsine) Butyrophenone neuroleptic administered intramuscularly or intravenously as a preanesthetic to calm preoperative patients or in emergency rooms or intensive care units to control agitated behavior in both psychotic and nonpsychotic patients. It differs structurally from haloperidol, the prototype butyrophenone, by having a benzimidazolinone group substituted at the para position of the piperidine ring. Half-life is short (2–4 hours) and onset of action is rapid (5–10 minutes). It produces marked tranquilization and sedation, is a potent antiemetic, and potentiates other central nervous system depressants (e.g., fentanyl). It can be used in the treatment of anxiety, agitation, and psychomotor excitement in both psychotic and nonpsychotic individuals. It may be superior to haloperidol for rapid treatment of acute psychosis, agitation, and disturbed behavior because of its potent calming effect and low incidence of cardiovascular or extrapyramidal side effects (Resnick M, Burton BT. Droperidol vs haloperidol in the initial management of acutely agitated patients. *J Clin Psychiatry* 1984;45:298–299). It also has been used to calm patients with recent myocardial infarction (Pall H. Neuroleptanalgesic beim frischen herzinfarck. *Wien Klin Wochenschr* 1986;85:804–806); Santos AB, Arana GW. Pharmacological approaches to the agitated ICU patients. *Clinical Advances in the Treatment of Psychiatric Disorders* 1993;7:1–3, 12). To control agitation, it is given in intravenous doses of 5–10 mg every 30–60 minutes. Extremely agitated patients may require repeated administration of 5–10 mg. Single intramuscular doses range from 1.5 to 10 mg, and single intravenous doses range from 10 to 100 mg twice daily. Droperidol's effects begin to wane within 2–4 hours, although some effects may persist as long as 10–12 hours. It is reasonably free from serious toxicity or adverse side effects. Intravenous doses, which should be given slowly and not as a bolus, may cause some mild transient hypotension and reflex tachycardia with some respiratory depression. It may cause acute extrapyramidal reactions, most frequently acute dystonic reactions and akathisia. See **neuroleptanalgesia.**

dropout   Study participant who becomes inaccessible or ineligible for follow-up because of inability or unwillingness to continue in the study. Dropouts can lead to biases in study results.

drowsiness   State of quiet wakefulness that typically occurs prior to sleep onset. If the eyes are closed, diffuse and slowed alpha activity is usually present in the electroencephalogram, followed by early features of stage 1 sleep.

drug   **1.** Chemical used for recreational purposes. Nonmedical use adversely affects the user's health. It is characterized by erratic intake of high doses, illegality (except adult alcohol use), and control only by the user. **2.** Chemical used with the intent of improving the user's health. Pattern of use is reasonable and steady, and control is shared with a physician. Drugs can be classified pharmacologically according to their main effects (e.g., hypnotic) or clinically according to syndromes or disorders best treated by them (e.g., antidepressant). Clinical effects may be divided into acute (e.g., improving behavior) and chronic (e.g., preventing deterioration of behavior). Also called "medication"; "medicine."

drug absorption   Drug movement from administration site toward the systemic circulation.

drug absorption rate   (T_{max}) Time between drug ingestion and occurrence of maximum plasma concentration (C_{max}). When T_{max} is short, absorption is relatively rapid and onset of drug action should also be rapid. When T_{max} is long, absorption is relatively slow and onset of action may be delayed. T_{max} can be influenced by many factors (e.g., drug solubility and circumstances of administration, as illustrated by differences between fasting and postprandial administration). See **maximum plasma concentration.**

drug abuse   **1.** Use of a mind-altering substance in a way that differs from generally approved medical or social practices. **2.** Psychoactive substance abuse (DSM-IV) characterized by drug-seeking behavior associated with problems with paroxysmal breaks in use and typically certain relapses; patterns of use do not meet criteria for any form of drug dependence. **3.** In government publications, any use (problematic or not) of a drug wholly illegal to use, including use of alcohol by those underage for legal use. Any use of drugs that causes physical, psychological, economic, legal, or social harm to the individual user or to others affected by the drug user's behavior is designated drug abuse.

Drug Abuse Warning Network   (DAWN) Surveillance system sponsored by the National Institute on Drug Abuse (NIDA) that records drug-related visits to emergency rooms in the United States. It was established to provide timely information about trends in drug-related mortality in communities with high levels of drug abuse. To address vital statistics problems of inconsistently reported data, it uses coding procedures and provides on-site training to personnel responsible for reporting data.

drug allergy   Adverse reaction evoked by drugs that activate the immune system in undesirable ways. Manifestations may include skin eruptions, edema, anaphylactoid reactions, fever, and eosinophilia. Four major types of hypersensitivity can be associated with an allergic drug reaction: type I: IgE mediated allergic reactions including anaphylaxis, urticaria, and angioedema; type II: autoimmune syndromes such as thrombocytopenia, purpura, and agranulocytosis; type III: serum sickness and vasculitic reactions; and type IV: cell-mediated allergy such as contact dermatitis from topically applied drugs.

drug assay   Measurement of the total amount of a drug, both protein-bound and free, in a body fluid or tissue. An assay that reveals only the total level of the parent drug and does not detect pharmacologically active metabolites can be misleading.

drug automatism   Condition reputedly the cause of accidentally self-administered overdose of a central nervous system depressant (e.g., barbiturate, benzodiazepine, sedative tricyclic antidepressant) taken as an hypnotic. The person fails to go to sleep after the first or second dose, may become confused or amnestic, and unwittingly ingests an overdose. After recovery, there is no recollection of taking more than the usually prescribed one or two doses. Scientifically proving the occurrence of automatism in any specific case has been emphasized in legal suits. In 1961, Janssen, after investigating 488 apparent suicide attempts, said that it could be shown that approximately one-fourth of the cases were classifiable as drug automatisms; they showed a noticeably higher proportion of cerebral lesions than did patients with suicidal intent and thus were probably more disposed to confusional states during mild intoxication.

drug biotransformation   Drug metabolism, usually resulting in metabolites that are more polar, less lipid-soluble, distribute less exten-

sively in tissues, and undergo faster elimination than the parent. However, many metabolites have pharmacodynamic activity that may contribute to the overall pharmacodynamic response of the parent or at times have a totally different effect (therapeutic or toxic) of their own until they are excreted or further metabolized. Biotransformation facilitates both drug elimination and inactivation.

drug co-use   Use of two or more drugs by the same individual, without specificity as to the temporal relationship.

drug craving   Irresistible urge that compels drug-seeking behavior. It is a subjective phenomenon that often accounts for relapse among treated drug abusers.

drug dependence   Condition that may be either psychological or physical. With psychological dependence, a drug produces a feeling of satisfaction and psychic drive that requires periodic or continuous administration of the drug to produce pleasure or avoid discomfort (Eddy NB, Halbach H, Isbell H, Seevers MH. Drug dependence, its significance and characteristics. *Bull WHO* 1965;32:721–723). It refers only to subjective need for the drug independent of tolerance or withdrawal symptoms and is reflected by fear of being without the medication. Physical dependence is an adaptive state characterized by intense physical disturbances (withdrawal or abstinence syndrome characteristic of the particular drug) when repeated drug administration is suspended (Eddy NB, Halbach H, Isbell H, Seevers MH. Drug dependence, its significance and characteristics. *Bull WHO* 1965;32:721–723). It is a state of cellular adaptation to the presence of a drug induced by repeated, continuous exposure to it. Also called "physiological dependence."

drug discrimination   Procedure in which animals are trained to emit one response when administered one drug and a different response when no drug or other drugs are administered.

drug disposition   Rates and extent of drug absorption, distribution, biotransformation, and elimination.

drug distribution   Transfer of drug from blood to extravascular fluids and various tissues. It is frequently rapid and usually reversible. The simplest pattern is the one-compartment model. Rate at which a drug enters and leaves a compartment is largely a function of its physiochemical properties, notably lipophilicity and dissociation constant. Distribution (alpha phase) can be distinguished from elimination (beta phase) on the serum concentration-time curve following intravenous administration. Distribution speed depends on (a) blood flow; (b) ease with which it traverses membrane; and (c) magnitude of concentration gradients. Distribution of lipophilic drugs occurs quickly from blood to brain (a well perfused lipid-rich organ) and more slowly from blood to less well perfused peripheral fatty tissue. Redistribution of a drug from the brain to peripheral fatty tissue terminates its action on the brain. Another important factor in drug distribution is protein binding. See **one-compartment model.**

drug-drug interaction Alteration of the effects of one drug (the target) by prior or concurrent administration of another drug (the protagonist). Most interactions are pharmacodynamic; the remainder are pharmacokinetic. As a rule, effects of one of the drugs are increased or decreased. Some desired drug-drug interactions are achieved with combination therapy in which two or more drugs are used to increase therapeutic effects or reduce toxicity. However, there may be inordinately high or low levels of the target drug and/or its metabolites, with consequent reduced efficacy and/or increased toxicity. Unwanted drug-drug interactions may be either an increase or a decrease in a known effect of either or both drugs, or a new effect not seen with either drug alone. See **pharmacodynamics; pharmacokinetics.**

drug efficacy See **efficacy.**

drug efficiency Capability of a drug to produce a desired effect at an acceptable cost.

drug elimination Major pharmacokinetic process in which a drug is eliminated from the body through clearance by renal, hepatic, and/or other processes. Appearance of a drug in the circulation and its presence at the site of action will be modified by the speed of drug elimination. Drugs may be eliminated through renal excretion in an unchanged form, or by biotransformation to metabolites that are eliminated in the urine. In nontoxic doses, elimination of most drugs is characterized by an apparent first-order process (i.e., elimination rate is proportional to how much drug is in the body). In some instances, elimination kinetics are nonlinear; in others, there is a linear relationship between dose and plasma concentration.

drug elimination half-life (t_p) Units of time that indicate rate of drug disappearance from plasma and brain *after* distribution has been attained and *after* the disappearance curve has entered its terminal phase. Elimination half-life is not equivalent to clearance or the time required for the plasma concentration to fall to 50% of its maximum value. It depends on both drug distribution and clearance, based

on the following relationship: elimination half-life = 0.693 × volume of distribution.

drug excretion Elimination from the body of a drug or metabolite without any further change in its chemical form.

drug fever Disorder characterized by fever coinciding with administration of a drug and disappearing after discontinuation of the drug when no other cause for the fever is evident after a careful physical examination and laboratory investigation. It has been reported with a variety of pharmacological agents, including several psychotropics. Causes have been divided into five subtypes: administration-related, pharmacological action, hypersensitivity, direct alteration of thermoregulation, and idiosyncratic susceptibility from a hereditary biochemical defect.

drug-food interaction Alteration of drug effect(s) by food. Food may delay or reduce absorption of many drugs. It may slow gastric emptying and it may affect absorption by binding with drugs, by decreasing their access to absorption sites, by altering their dissolution rates, or by altering the pH of the gastrointestinal contents.

drug-free Ongoing dissociation from use of any psychoactive substance.

drug habituation (*Obsolete*) Pattern of repetitious drug use considered distinct from dependence or addiction. According to a World Health Organization (WHO) expert committee (1964), it would include (a) desire (but not compulsion) to continue taking the drug for the sense of improved well-being it engenders; (b) little or no tendency to increase the dose; (c) some degree of psychic dependence on the effect of the drug, but absence of physical dependence and an abstinence syndrome; and (d) detrimental effects, if any, primarily on the individual. See **drug abuse; drug dependence.**

drug holiday Discontinuation of a therapeutic drug for a limited period to control dosage and side effects and/or evaluate baseline behavior. It is feasible for judiciously selected patients; the most suitable candidates are clinically stable on maintenance medication that has required no dosage variation for 3–6 months. Use of drug holidays is controversial; most experts now consider the best strategy to be continuous use of the lowest effective dose.

drug holiday/neuroleptic For many patients on maintenance neuroleptic therapy, drug holidays of 1–3 consecutive days a week may be used without ill effects. They are advocated to reduce total drug amount consumed and possibly lessen risk of serious side effects (e.g., tardive dyskinesia) associated with long-term neuroleptic therapy. Recent studies, however, have shown increased relapses or mini-relapses with intermittent treatment and no clear benefit in terms of side effects.

drug-induced cycling   Episodes of hypomania/mania and depression induced by antidepressant treatment of manic-depressive illness.

drug-induced depression   See **depression, drug-induced.**

drug-induced hypotension   See **hypotension, drug-induced.**

drug-induced hypothermia   See **hypothermia, drug-induced.**

drug-induced parkinsonism   See **parkinsonism, drug-induced.**

drug interaction   See **drug-drug interaction; drug-food interaction.**

drug interaction, additive   Combined effect is the sum of each drug.

drug interaction, adverse   See **adverse drug interaction.**

drug interaction, beneficial   Interaction in which one drug increases another's efficacy or decreases its toxicity.

drug interaction, idiosyncratic   Alteration of one drug's effect(s) by another drug; mechanism unknown.

drug interaction, pharmacokinetic   One drug altering what the patient's physiology does to another drug.

drug interaction, pharmacodynamic   One drug altering what another drug does to a patient's physiology. There are three types: receptor-mediated (e.g., use of flumazenil to stabilize the benzodiazepine (BZD) receptor and reverse BZD coma); physiologically linked (e.g., potentiation of the depressant effects of sedative/hypnotics and opiates by ethanol); and transport-related (e.g., inhibition of the monoamine uptake pump by cyclic antidepressants and neuroleptics, thus antagonizing the antihypertensive effects of guanethidine and bethanidine). Pharmacodynamic interactions between drugs with similar pharmacological effects are additive (e.g., use of the anticholinergic neuroleptic chlorpromazine plus the anticholinergic antiparkinson drug benztropine may produce excessive anticholinergic effects). Pharmacodynamic interactions between drugs with opposing pharmacological effects may counteract therapeutic effects of one or both drugs (e.g., a thiazide diuretic may elevate blood glucose levels and counteract the hypoglycemic effects of insulin).

drug interaction, potential   Interaction that has occurred in a previous patient or might be expected because it has been evoked by similar drugs.

drug interaction, synergistic   Combined effect greater than the sum of each drug effect.

drug intolerance   Nonimmunological reaction to a drug (e.g., overdose, side effect, secondary effect, drug interaction, idiosyncratic reaction, or teratogenetic reaction) (Anderson JA. Allergic reactions to drugs and biological agents. *JAMA* 1992;268:2845–2857). Overdose, side effects, secondary effects, and drug interactions are usually predictable adverse reactions in normal patients (DeSwarte R. Drug allergy. *In* Patterson R [ed], *Allergic Diseases, Diagnoses and Management.* Philadelphia: JB Lippincott, 1985, pp 505–661). Drug intolerance may account for over 90% of all adverse reactions to drugs.

drug intoxication   Disruptive changes in physiological and psychological functioning and mood states or cognitive processes as a consequence of excessive consumption of a drug.

drug level   Measured drug concentration in blood, serum, or plasma.

drug metabolism   Chemical changes undergone by drugs in the body. They can be divided into phase I (nonsynthetic) and phase II (synthetic). Phase I consists of biotransformation (oxidation or reduction) such as N-dealkylation, hydroxylation of carbon atoms, deamination, or hydrolysis of esters or ethers. Phase I oxidative reactions are catalyzed by the P450 hepatic enzyme system and result in active or toxic metabolites. Phase I oxidative metabolic pathways are more prone to inhibition. Phase II metabolism includes methylation reaction, acetylation, and conjugation. Phase II reactions result in biologically inactive metabolites that are water-soluble, facilitating renal excretion. Most drugs are first oxidized by phase I reactions. Metabolites formed in phase I then undergo phase II metabolism and are excreted in bile or by renal clearance.

drug misuse   Any drug use that varies from a socially or medically accepted use.

drug-naive   State of a patient or subject who has never been exposed to a particular drug or class of drugs.

drug/neonate   Pregnant women may take prescription and nonprescription drugs, some of which may have deleterious effects on the fetus, especially alcohol, tobacco, and some illicit drugs (e.g., cocaine). Not all drug-exposed neonates have demonstrable sequelae of their exposure. See **name of specific drug/neonate.**

drug of abuse   Any substance taken by any route of administration that alters mood (generally producing euphoria), level of perception, state of consciousness, or brain functioning in such a way that it can lead to drug abuse or dependence. Drugs of abuse range from prescribed medications to alcohol and solvents.

drug overdose death (DOD) Any case meeting the following criteria: (a) coroner's file documents use of opiates or illicit drugs; (b) cause of death is listed as unknown, the result of addiction to drugs, or the result of drug ingestion or overdose; (c) manner of death was other than suicide or homicide; and (d) there was no trauma to internal organs. A clinical picture consistent with drug overdose, but with low levels of traditional drugs of abuse, should prompt a search for designer drugs in the patient's history. In searching for the cause of DOD outbreaks, designer drugs cannot be ruled out solely because traditional drugs of abuse are detectable in body fluids.

drug overuse World Health Organization (WHO) classification for excessive medical or lay use of a drug, in terms of length of therapy or severity of the disorder treated, but always within the framework of use for diseases in which there is medically accepted evidence of therapeutic effect.

drug-refractory Partially or completely unresponsive to a drug known to be effective in the condition for which it is being prescribed. Apparent refractoriness to treatment with a single drug may be due to contributing factors: (a) poor treatment compliance; (b) wrong diagnosis (e.g., mistaking dysphoria for depression); (c) wrong drug; (d) inadequate dosage; (e) inadequate duration of treatment (i.e., less than 2–3 months); (f) psychosocial stressors requiring psychotherapy; and (g) illness for which the drug is prescribed is secondary to an undiagnosed medical disorder.

drug safety data In the United States, the two major sources are clinical trials supporting the New Drug Application (NDA) and Food and Drug Administration (FDA)-mandated reporting systems. Both are useful, but have serious limitations.

Drugs Anonymous (DA) Self-help group concentrating on problems generated by drug abuse.

drug-seeking behavior 1. Making frequent requests for dosage increases and being noncompliant ("doctor shopping"). 2. Fear of or being in acute withdrawal. 3. Buying illicit drugs. 4. Visiting physicians or the emergency service as an economical and legal source of prescription drugs for personal use or to sell on the street.

drug selection Choosing a treatment drug by using objective criteria.

drug therapy Use of chemical substances in the treatment of illness (e.g., chemotherapy, pharmacotherapy).

drug tolerance See **tolerance.**

drug use, simultaneous Use of two or more drugs at the same time.

drug utilization Marketing, distribution, prescription, and use of drugs with special emphasis on resulting medical, social, and economic consequences (World Health Organization [WHO]).

Drug Utilization Review (DUR) Procedure to determine the status of drug therapy and its conformity to accepted standards for appropriate pharmacotherapy. It is designed to improve drug use by intervening when inappropriate drug use is detected.

drug utilization study 1. Quantitative study to determine the present state, developmental trends, and time course of drug use at various levels of the health care system, whether national, regional, local, or institutional. 2. Qualitative study to assess the appropriateness of drug utilization, usually by linking prescription data to reasons for drug prescribing. Unlike quantitative studies, qualitative studies include the concept of appropriateness.

drug withdrawal 1. Purposeful termination of a medication regimen by a physician for either therapeutic or research purposes. 2. Reaction(s) experienced by the patient when a drug is stopped.

DSM-I The first Diagnostic and Statistical Manual published by the American Psychiatric Association (1952).

DSM-II The second Diagnostic and Statistical Manual published by the American Psychiatric Association (1968). The attempt to integrate it with the International Classification of Diseases (ICD-8) was a beginning step toward international nomenclature.

DSM-III The third Diagnostic and Statistical Manual published by the American Psychiatric Association (1980). It introduced multiaxial diagnosis.

DSM-III-R The fourth Diagnostic and Statistical Manual published by the American Psychiatric Association (1987). It incorporated much of the classification and principles found in DSM-III, retained the 10 syndromes of DSM-III, and added organic anxiety syndrome. The general approach to diagnosis multiaxial: Axes I and II (mental disorders), Axis III (physical disorders substantially related to Axes I or II), Axis IV (significant psychosocial stressors), and Axis V (highest level of adaptational functioning in the previous year). It is used by most psychiatrists and many other mental health professionals and lawyers. Many insurance forms now require a DSM-III-R diagnosis.

D-tubocurarine (Tubarine) Muscle relaxant that causes postsynaptic blockade at neuromuscular junctions. It is sometimes used just prior to electroconvulsive therapy to prevent muscle fasciculations and secondary myalgias that may result from use of succinylcholine to reduce muscular contractions.

dual diagnosis Substance abuse plus a psychiatric disorder. Patients tend to be younger, are more often male, and have poorer medication compliance histories. Any DSM-IV disorder may be included. Other Axis I disorders commonly found include affective disorders, anxiety disorders, and schizophrenic disorders. Relative frequency varies with individual drugs of abuse, including alcohol and nicotine. Prognosis in treatment is not good unless specific treatment for the co-existing psychiatric disorder is given. Multiple dependence adds to problems of disruptive, disinhibited, and noncompliant behaviors in the chronically mentally ill.

dually diagnosed alcoholism See **alcoholism, dually diagnosed.**

Duarte protein Mutant protein, Pc 1 Duarte (Pc for perchloric acid extract), that has been identified in brain specimens taken at autopsy from individuals with affective disorder and/or alcoholism. It is most common in caudate, putamen, thalamus, pons, and brain stem. No increased frequency was found in samples from schizophrenics. It is the first report claiming to document an abnormal brain protein in persons with a psychiatric disorder and invites speculation that affective disorder is associated with increased susceptibility to viral central nervous system infection.

Duchenne muscular dystrophy (DMD) Progressive muscular dystrophy due to a sex-linked recessive gene. It typically presents in boys aged 3–7 years as proximal muscle weakness causing waddling gait, toe-walking, lordosis, frequent falls, and difficulty in standing up and climbing stairs. It is very rare in females. It leads to progressive muscle degeneration and wasting; 90% of patients die before age 20 (Emery AEH. *Duchenne Muscular Dystrophy.* Oxford: Oxford University Press, 1987).

Dumirox See **fluvoxamine.**

dummy coding In regression analysis, assignation of a code (*0* or *1*) to a nominal predictor variable.

"dummy mist" Street name for phencyclidine (PCP).

Dumyrox See **fluvoxamine.**

Dunnett's procedure Method for comparing multiple treatment groups with a single control group following a significant F test in analysis of variance.

Dunnett's "T" distribution Distribution of the comparison of at least two treatment groups with only one control (reference) group.

Dunn multiple-comparison procedure See **Bonferroni t procedure.**

DuP 996 Cognitive enhancer identified after enhancing the stimulus-induced release of acetylcholine. It is in phase II clinical studies for Alzheimer's disease and age-associated memory impairment.

duplication In genetics, an extra copy of one or more genes in the DNA.

Durabolin See **nandrolone phenpropionate.**

Duragesic See **fentanyl transdermal system.**

Duralith See **lithium.**

Duramorph See **morphine.**

Durapam See **flurazepam.**

Duratest See **testosterone cypionate.**

Durathate See **testosterone enanthate.**

duration-response relationship Longer exposure increasing risk of the disease (e.g., tardive dyskinesia).

Durolith See **lithium.**

Duromine See **phentermine.**

"dust" Street name for cocaine or phencyclidine (PCP).

Dyazide See **triamterene/hydrochlorothiazide.**

dydrogesterone Synthetic orally active progestogen (6-dehydro-retroprogesterone) that has been advocated for treatment of premenstrual syndrome.

Dymyrox See **fluvoxamine.**

dynamic disease Disease that occurs in an intact physiological control system operating in a range of control parameters that lead to abnormal dynamics (Mackey MC, Milton JG. Dynamical diseases. *Ann N Y Acad Sci* 1987; 504:16–32). Bipolar affective disorder is an example.

dynorphin (DYN) Endogenous opioid peptide derived from one of the three precursor protein families that make up the opioid peptide superfamily. The peptides appear to be part of the signaling system relating to pain perception, mood regulation, and learning. Dynorphin constitutes the endogenous ligand for kappa opiate receptors. It has been given intravenously (60 mg/kg) to heroin addicts during withdrawal periods and found to be transiently effective (Wen HL, Ho WKK. Suppression of withdrawal symptoms by dynorphin in heroin addicts. *Eur J Pharmacol* 1982; 82:183–186).

Dyrenium See **triamterene.**

dysarthria Disturbance of speech articulation due to emotional stress, brain injury, or impairment of the speech mechanism, including muscle weakness. It is manifested by slurred pronunciation.

dysarthria, hypophonic Defective speech due to lack of phonation and manifested by whispering. It is often a symptom of Parkinson's disease.

dysautonomia   Abnormal functioning of the autonomic nervous system as a result of a brain abnormality. It is often familial. The affected child is tense, irritable, subject to recurrent physical crises, and defective in organizing complex behavior and adapting to change. There may be a number of emotional disturbances.

dyscontrol, episodic   See **episodic dyscontrol.**

dyscrasia   Blood abnormality (e.g., leukopenia, agranulocytosis, aplastic anemia) that may be caused by certain psychoactive drugs (e.g., carbamazepine and chlorpromazine).

dysdiadochokinesia   Difficulty in performing rapid alternating movements. It is a sign of damage to, or abnormality of, the cerebellum.

dyskinesia   Impairment of voluntary movements, including certain types of abnormal involuntary movements or hyperkinesias, especially those induced by drugs. Dyskinesias may be choreiform (nonrepetitive, rapid, jerky, quasipurposive), athetoid (continuous, slow, sinuous, purposeless), or rhythmic movements in certain areas of the body that are reduced by voluntary movement of the affected part and increased by voluntary movement of an unaffected part. Dyskinesias are well known side effects of neuroleptics, but have been reported in association with a number of other drugs, although cause/effect has not been clearly established in most cases: L-dopa, amphetamine, apomorphine, methylphenidate, fenfluramine, amantadine, monoamine oxidase inhibitors, metoclopramide, tricyclic antidepressants, fluoxetine, antihistamines, anticonvulsants, lithium, and estrogens. Dyskinesias caused by most of these drugs are almost always reversible. Dyskinesia intensity depends highly on vigilance: the more alert the individual, the more pronounced the dyskinesia; the more drowsy the individual, the less pronounced the dyskinesia. Symptoms of tardive dyskinesia disappear during sleep. Movements *not* considered dyskinesias include continuous partial seizures, mannerisms, myoclonus, stereotypy, and tremors; also excluded are drug-induced tics, chronic dystonias, and akathisia because their pathology, phenomenology, outcome, and treatment are different from those of tardive dyskinesias. Although dyskinesias may arise spontaneously in the elderly in the absence of drugs or medical illnesses, they are infrequent and account for only a very few orofacial dyskinesias.

dyskinesia, diphasic   Type of dyskinesia that appears as levodopa begins to take effect and as the drug effects wane. It consists of choreoathetotic, dystonic, stereotyped, or ballistic movements. It can be extremely severe; ballistic movements may be accompanied by marked sweating, hypertension, tachycardia, and sudden death attributable to cardiac arrhythmias (Marsden CD, Parkes JD, Quinn N. Fluctuations of disability in Parkinson's disease: clinical aspects. *In* Marsden CD, Fahn S [eds], *Movement Disorders*. London: Butterworths, 1981, pp 96–122).

dyskinesia, intermittent   Putative subtype of tardive dyskinesia (TD) manifested by remissions and relapses of dyskinesia for periods of weeks to months that are not attributable to changes in medication. It is not known whether patients will ultimately develop TD. Patients with intermittent dyskinesias should not be included in therapeutic trials on TD as they may largely account for false-positive and false-negative results. See **dyskinesia, state-dependent.**

dyskinesia, orofacial   Abnormal, involuntary movements of facial muscles, typically involving continual, repetitive lip smacking, licking, grimacing, and chewing. It is most commonly seen as a consequence of long-term neuroleptic treatment (so-called tardive orofacial dyskinesia), but may also be spontaneous or a feature of long-standing Huntington's disease. It may respond to tetrabenazine.

dyskinesia, persistent   Abnormal involuntary movement disorder that is one of the most serious complications of protracted neuroleptic therapy. It does not respond to neuroleptic withdrawal or to most other available treatments. Data to date suggest that over long periods there is often no worsening of symptoms. Rapidly deteriorating course suggests possible progressive brain disease warranting complete neurological and medical evaluations.

dyskinesia, respiratory   Abnormal involuntary movement disorder induced by neuroleptic therapy, usually in patients with tardive dyskinesia (TD), although it may be a neuroleptic-induced, early-onset extrapyramidal reaction. It is characterized by irregularity in the rate, rhythm, and depth of breathing and may be accompanied by grunting, snorting, or puffing (Chiang E, Pitts WM, Rodriquez-Garcia M. Respiratory dyskinesia: review and reports. *J Clin Psychiatry* 1985;46:232–234; Chiu HFK, Lam LCW, Chan CHS, et al. Clinical and polygraphic characteristics of patients with respiratory dyskinesia. *Br J Psychiatry* 1993;162:828–830). In addition to the respiratory abnormality, there is restlessness and hyperkinesia, but no parkinsonism. Symptoms may appear in the first few days or weeks of oral or depot neuroleptic therapy and usually are promptly relieved by either neuroleptic dosage reduction and/or antiparkinson drug therapy, especially when the latter is administered parenterally. Respiratory dysfunction associated with TD primarily includes irregular respiration (usually dyspnea) and orofacial, limb, and truncal dyskinetic movements. Characteristically, respiratory symptoms do not appear until after the dose of the responsible neuroleptic has been decreased. In some cases, respiratory dysfunction precedes appearance of orofacial dyskinesia; in others, it evolves after other TD manifestations emerge. Acute dyspnea and chest pain not due to cardiac or pulmonary disorders can be symptoms of severe involuntary respiratory dyskinesias associated with TD. Potentially life-threatening ventilatory and gastrointestinal disturbances have occurred (rarely) in TD patients.

dyskinesia, reversible Dyskinetic symptoms that ameliorate following discontinuation of the responsible neuroleptic(s). Reversibility rate is highest during the first 3 months after stopping the neuroleptic. The longer the period of drug discontinuation, the greater the chance that dyskinetic symptoms will cease. Symptom relief within 3 months of neuroleptic discontinuation may be used as a test for reversibility of tardive dyskinesia.

dyskinesia, spontaneous Movements phenomenologically similar to neuroleptic-induced dyskinesia. It was known for over a century prior to the advent of neuroleptics; over 25% of patients with schizophrenia in the 19th century are estimated to have had involuntary movements that today would be described as tardive dyskinesia (TD). Spontaneous dyskinesias are clinically indistinguishable from TD; the only differential diagnostic clue is time of onset (before or after initiation of neuroleptic medication). Prevalence of spontaneous dyskinesia is estimated at 0–53% and increases with age. Prevalence estimates based on observations not adjusted for spontaneous dyskinesia are inflated. After age 40, prevalence is sufficiently high to warrant neurological examination of patients before neuroleptic treatment is started. Many patients with diagnoses of TD have abnormal movements attributable to causes other than neuroleptics (Khot V, Wyatt RJ. Not all that moves is tardive dyskinesia. *Am J Psychiatry* 1991;148:661–666). Oral dyskinesia and choreoathetoid movements of the extremities (senile chorea) occur spontaneously in a significant percentage of elderly persons; cellular loss in the caudate nucleus has been found in some postmortem studies.

dyskinesia, state-dependent Fluctuations in tardive dyskinesia (TD) severity, not attributable to changes in medication, that occur during or preceding an episode of an affective illness.

For example, TD symptoms may increase before or during a depressive episode and decrease during mania (Cutler NR, Post RM. State-related cyclical dyskinesias in manic-depressive illness. *J Clin Psychopharmacol* 1982;2: 350–354).

dyskinesia, tardive See **tardive dyskinesia.**

dyskinesia, truncal See **hyperkinesia, axial.**

dyskinesia, withdrawal Abnormal involuntary movements following abrupt discontinuation of high doses of a neuroleptic. They occur most often in young patients, especially children. Manifestations resemble tardive dyskinesia (TD), which often worsens after sudden neuroleptic discontinuation. Withdrawal-emergent dyskinesias are transient and usually subside or disappear within 1–3 weeks of stopping medication. They also may remit if neuroleptics are readministered. If symptoms persist for several weeks after neuroleptic withdrawal or reinstitution, the condition would be TD, not withdrawal dyskinesia (Engelhardt DM, Polizos P, Waizer J. CNS consequences of psychotropic drug withdrawal in autistic children: a follow-up report. *Psychopharmacol Bull* 1975;11:6–7; Winsberg BG, Hurwic MJ, Perel J. Neurochemistry of withdrawal emergent symptoms in children. *Psychopharmacol Bull* 1977;13:38–40). Also called "transient tardive dyskinesia-like reaction"; "withdrawal emergent syndrome."

dyskinetic dysphagia See **dysphagia, dyskinetic.**

dyslexia Difficulty in reading. The most common cause worldwide is never having been taught to read. Other cases arise from defective vision and disease of the nervous system, including mental handicap and brain damage. There is often a tendency to reverse letters and words in reading and writing. Dyslexia appears to be both familial and heritable, but mode of genetic transmission remains unclear. Dyslexia is more common in boys and tends to be associated with clumsiness and poor concentration.

dysmenorrhea Painful menstruation, one of the most frequently encountered gynecological disorders. In primary dysmenorrhea, there is no visible disease to account for the pain. In secondary dysmenorrhea, pain is secondary to an identifiable pelvic lesion. Primary dysmenorrhea is estimated to affect more than 50% of menstruating women, 10% of whom have pain severe enough to cause absenteeism for 1–3 days each month. Although it does not give rise to any documented mortality, dysmenorrhea is sufficiently disruptive that optimal pain relief is desirable. Effective medical management should be directed at correcting the biochemical abnormality underlying the condition (Dawood MY. Dysmenorrhea. *In* Max M, Portenoy R, Laska E [eds], *Advances in Pain*

Research and Therapy, vol 18:. New York: Raven Press, 1991).

dysmentia, tardive   See **tardive dysmentia.**

dysmetria   Cerebellar disturbance that causes impaired meaning of distance, spatial disorientation, and inability to reach accurately for a target. Patients may touch in front of, behind, or to either side of a target.

dysmorphophobia   See **body dysmorphic disorder.**

dysphagia   Difficulty swallowing. It is the most common complication of cervical dystonia and a common complication of tardive dyskinesia (TD), particularly bucco-oral-lingual dyskinesia. It also may develop many years after an attack of acute paralytic poliomyelitis in what is now called the postpolio syndrome. Any patient who complains of difficulty swallowing should be evaluated for dysphagia (Bazemore PH, Tonkonogy J, Ananth R. Dysphagia in psychiatric patients: clinical and videofluoroscopic study. *Dysphagia* 1991;6:2–5). Patients with dysphagia may be unable to swallow tablets or capsules and need to be treated with a liquid form of medication. See **fast eating syndrome; globus hystericus.**

dysphagia, bradykinetic   Hypokinesia affecting the oral-pharyngeal and esophageal phases of swallowing. It is a common cause of choking incidents in patients with drug-induced or idiopathic Parkinson's disease who often are being treated with neuroleptic drugs that have induced akinesia, rigidity, resting tremor, reduced lingual range of motion, delayed initiation of swallow reflex, and other bradykinetic symptoms. Choking incidents secondary to bradykinetic dysphagia are believed to be more severe than those due to other causes, except those due to paralytic dysphagia. They may be fatal unless resolved by prompt application of the Heimlich maneuver. Bradykinetic dysphagia can be treated most effectively with adjustment of the dosage (preferably reduction) of the causative neuroleptic (Bazemore PH, Tonkonogy J, Ananth R. Dysphagia in psychiatric patients: clinical and videofluoroscopic study. *Dysphagia* 1991;6:2–5).

dysphagia, dyskinetic   Manifestation of tardive dyskinesia (TD) in which involuntary, abnormal tongue movements and hyperkinetic movements of pharyngeal and esophageal musculature affect mastication, bolus formation, and esophageal transport of solids and liquids. It is the result of long-term treatment with neuroleptics and other dopamine-blocking drugs. The major problem is in the oral phase of swallowing and is due to interference with proper bolus propulsion, which accounts for the relatively low incidence of choking incidents (Bazemore PH, Tonkonogy J,

Ananth R. Dysphagia in psychiatric patients: clinical and videofluoroscopic study. *Dysphagia* 1991;6:2–5).

dysphagia, medical   Obstructing lesion in the pharynx or esophagus, or an inflammatory lesion in the esophagus. It is an infrequent cause of choking incidents.

dysphagia, paralytic   Lesion-induced hemiparesis causing asymmetry or weakness of the tongue, palate, or pharynx. It is often responsible for severe choking incidents, the majority of which require treatment with the Heimlich maneuver.

dysphasia   Difficulty with speech due to a lesion in the central nervous system. It may be *receptive,* in which the person, despite normal hearing, can make limited or no sense of the language heard; or *expressive,* in which the person understands but cannot easily put ideas into spoken words. Some people have a mixed dysphasic disability.

dysphonia   See **aphonia.**

dysphonia, spasmodic   See **dystonia, laryngeal.**

dysphoria   Acute transient changes in mood (e.g., feelings of sadness, sorrow, anguish, misery, mental malaise accompanied by verbal complaints of feeling depressed, sad, blue, gloomy, down in the dumps, and empty (Spitzer RL, Endicott J. *Schedule for Affective Disorders and Schizophrenia.* New York: New York State Psychiatric Institute, 1978). The relationship between severe, persistent dysphoric mood and the persistent dysphoric affect seen in major depression and other psychiatric diseases is unknown. Positron emission tomographic (PET) measurement of regional cerebral blood flow in psychiatrically healthy subjects suggests that the inferior and orbitofrontal cortices play an important role in normal emotional cognitive processes (Pardo JV, Pardo PJ, Raichle ME. Neural correlates of self-induced dysphoria. *Am J Psychiatry* 1993;150:713–719).

dysphoria, chronic   See **dysthymic disorder.**

dysphoria, hysteroid   See **hysteroid dysphoria.**

dyspnea   Difficulty breathing; shortness of breath.

dyspnea, paroxysmal nocturnal   (PND) Respiratory distress and shortness of breath due to pulmonary edema that appears suddenly and often causes awakening.

dyspraxia   Partial impairment of ability to perform coordinated skilled movement in the absence of a defect in the basic motor system.

dys-somnia   One of a group of primary sleep disorders in which there is a disturbance in the amount, quality, or timing of sleep. It includes various types of insomnia, hypersomnia, narcolepsy, and disturbances in the sleep/wake schedule.

dysthymia Mild form of affective disorder that frequently responds to treatment with antidepressant medication. It is a common condition, affecting approximately 3% of the adult population. It is more common in women under 65, unmarried persons, and young persons with low income. It is associated with increased use of general health and psychiatric services and psychotropic drugs. A subgroup of dysthymics may have an attenuated form of major depression. Dysthymia differs from major depression in that it is less stringent in terms of number of symptoms, but requires much longer duration. It is possible to meet criteria for both major depression and dysthymia.

dysthymia, pure Dysthymia in which no major depression is superimposed.

dysthymic disorder (DD) Chronic mild depression formally introduced into psychiatric nomenclature in 1980 with the publication of DSM-III. It is frequently unresponsive to antidepressant pharmacotherapy. Previously called chronic minor depression, neurotic depression, depressive neurosis, characterologic depression, depressive personality, chronic dysphoria, intermittent depression. All are characterized by chronic depression less severe than melancholia.

dysthymic subictal mood disorder Syndrome characterized by (a) chronic depressive baseline; (b) brief euphorias, often with beatific religious coloration; (c) brief severe depressive dips with impulsive suicide attempts (frequently wrist cutting); (d) unusual amount of irritability and hostile outbursts; (e) marked premenstrual exacerbation in women; (f) paradoxical reactions to standard mood-active drugs. Severe cases are often diagnosed as severe and/or rapid cycling bipolar affective disorder, schizoaffective disorder, or (rarely) delusional depression. Milder cases are often diagnosed as dysthymic disorder, atypical or hysteroid depression, or cyclothymia. In some patients the electroencephalogram (EEG) is normal. In others, there may be frank temporal lobe epilepsy or behavioral disorders with paroxysmal EEG (Himmelhoch JM. Major mood disorders related to epileptic changes. *In* Blumer D [ed], *Psychiatric Aspects of Epilepsy.* Washington, DC: American Psychiatric Press, 1984). Also called "subictal affective disorder."

dystonia Neurological condition characterized by slow, tonic, sustained muscle contractions, often of the tongue, jaw, eyes, and neck, and sometimes of the whole body, frequently causing twisting and repetitive movements, or abnormal postures. There are five main types: (a) *focal:* affecting one body area only; (b)

segmental: affecting two or more contiguous body areas; (c) *multifocal:* affecting two or more noncontiguous body areas; (d) *generalized:* affecting multiple, disparate body areas; and (e) *hemidystonia:* affecting ipsilateral limbs, with or without involvement of ipsilateral trunk or face. Clinical, pharmacological, and biochemical studies indicate noradrenergic predominance in dystonia; this neurochemical abnormality may be genetically determined. Dystonia can be caused by the catecholamine-depleting agent alpha-methylparatyrosine (AMPT) (McCann JD, Penetar DM, Belenky G. Acute dystonic reaction in normal humans caused by catecholamine depletion. *Clin Neuropharmacol* 1990;13:565–568). Acute dystonia occurs in 2–10% of patients receiving neuroleptic drugs, more often in young males. Most common manifestations are oculogyric crisis, cervical dystonia (torticollis), tongue contraction, trismus, and opisthotonus. Dystonic dysphagia is an infrequent manifestation of neuroleptic-induced dystonia. Laryngeal dystonia can compromise the airway and lead to severe respiratory distress. Treatment of an acute neuroleptic-induced dystonic reaction consists of prompt intravenous administration of an antiparkinson drug (e.g., biperiden or benztropine, 2 mg). If necessary, the same dose can be repeated after 5 minutes. Thereafter, patients should be given oral antiparkinson medication 3 times a day for 3 days. Botulinum toxin can be used to successfully treat cervical dystonia, oromandibular dystonia, and laryngeal dystonia. In patients with focal dystonia and in some with segmental dystonia unresponsive to pharmacological therapy, injections of botulinum toxin into the contracting muscles provide the most effective temporary relief. See **botulinum toxin.**

dystonia, action Dystonic movements and postures that are often related to selected actions. Many patients are able to use a variety of peculiar tricks to lessen the severity of the dystonia.

dystonia, acute Early-onset extrapyramidal reaction usually regarded as idiosyncratic, but which can also be dose-dependent. It is characterized by sustained abnormal posture or muscle spasm involving any part of body musculature. Severity may range from a feeling of muscular cramp or tightness to gross abnormal movements. Probability of occurrence increases with rising doses of the responsible neuroleptic or dopamine-blocking non-neuroleptic agent. Approximately 50% of acute dystonias occur within 48 hours, and about 90% within 5 days, of starting therapy by the oral route. It can start earlier with parenteral drug use. It is more likely to occur in children and young adults following parenteral or rectal administration. Treatment consists of prompt administration of an intravenously or intramuscularly administered antiparkinson drug (e.g., biperiden or benztropine, 2 mg). If necessary, the same dose can be repeated after 5 minutes. Thereafter, patients may need additional ongoing antiparkinson medication if the neuroleptic or other agent that caused the reaction is continued. Acute dystonic reactions can readily be reversed by parenteral administration of diazepam. Abusers of antiparkinson medication may feign an acute dystonic reaction to acquire a prescription for an antiparkinson drug.

dystonia, axial   Fixed rotational lateral tilt to the trunk. It can be induced as an extrapyramidal effect of neuroleptics. Unilateral axial dystonia has been called the "Pisa syndrome" because of characteristic truncal lean. See **"Pisa" syndrome.**

dystonia, cervical   Focal dystonia affecting the neck muscles that causes patterned, repetitive, clonic (spasmodic) head movements or tonic (sustained) abnormal postures of the head as a result of twisting (torticollis), tilting toward one shoulder (laterocollis), flexing (anterocollis), or extending (retrocollis). Although uncommon, idiopathic cervical dystonia is the most prevalent of the focal dystonias. Spontaneous remissions occur in up to 20% of patients, but are usually transient. It is frequently induced by neuroleptic therapy. Botulinum toxin is a safe and effective treatment. Also called "torticollis." See **botulinum toxin.**

dystonia, cranial   Movement disorder predominantly characterized by spasms involving head musculature. It is usually idiopathic and is thought to represent an adult-onset form of torsion dystonia. It tends to remain focal or segmental in distribution. A number of focal dystonias (e.g., blepharospasm, laryngeal dystonia, lingual dystonia, oromandibular dystonia) may occur in a cranial distribution.

dystonia, laryngeal   Action-induced dystonia, of which there are two distinct types: abductor and adductor. Abductor is due to intermittent separation of the vocal folds; patients have a voice that is breathy and whispery. Adductor is due to approximation of the vocal folds; patients have a voice that sounds choked, strained, or strangled, and an abrupt manner of initiating and terminating their speech, resulting in short breaks in phonation. Treatment of laryngeal dystonia was unrewarding until the advent of local injections of botulinum toxin. Also called "spasmodic dysphonia." See **botulinum toxin.**

dystonia, laryngopharyngeal   Neuroleptic-induced focal dystonia involving the laryngopharyngeal muscles. It can cause dysphonia and dysphasia. Speech is strained, hoarse, and staccato, and there may be a sense of tightness in the throat.

dystonia musculorum deformans   See **dystonia, torsion.**

dystonia, oromandibular   Dystonia involving masticatory, lower facial, and tongue muscles. It results in trismus, bruxism, involuntary tongue movement, and opening, closure, or deviation of the jaw. Anticholinergic drugs, baclofen, benzodiazepines, and tetrabenazine may be helpful, but pharmacotherapy is usually ineffective. Injections of botulinum toxin into the masseter, temporalis, and internal pterygoid muscles result in reduction in the oromandibular and lingual spasms and improved chewing and speech in approximately 70% of patients with jaw closure due to oromandibular dystonia. See **botulinum toxin.**

dystonia, paroxysmal hypnogenic   Sleep disorder characterized by nocturnal episodes of twisting or thrashing dystonic movements associated with screaming and panic. It may represent a form of frontal lobe complex partial epilepsy. Without a sleep electroencephalographic evaluation, it may be difficult at times to distinguish it from the panic and agitation of pavor nocturnus and rapid eye movement (REM) sleep behavior disorder. Imipramine and carbamazepine may be effective treatment. See **REM sleep behavior disorder.**

dystonia, tardive   See **tardive dystonia.**

dystonia, torsion   Sustained, irregular muscle spasms distorting the body into characteristic postures: (a) neck twisted to one side (torticollis), extended (retrocollis) or flexed (anterocollis); (b) trunk forced into excessive lordosis or scoliosis; (c) arm extended and hyperpronated, wrist flexed, and fingers extended; and (d) leg extended with the foot plantar flexed and inverted. Initially, spasms may occur only on certain actions, so that patients may walk on their toes or develop the characteristic arm posture on writing.

dystrophin   Protein identified by molecular genetic studies of patients affected with Duchenne muscular dystrophy. Named by Kurikel and his colleagues in December 1987.

E

early sexual abuse See **sexual abuse, early.**

"earth" Street name for phencyclidine (PCP).

eating disorder/laxative abuse Eating disorder patients frequently abuse over-the-counter laxatives such as cascara sagrada (Peri-Colace), senna (Senokot), bisacodyl (Dulcolax), and phenolphthalein (Correctol; Ex-Lax; Feen-A-Mint). Abuse is associated with loss of intestinal fluid and electrolytes causing dizziness, lightheadedness, electrocardiogram changes, dehydration, and weakness. Medical problems associated with abuse of stimulant laxatives are more serious than those caused by misuse of other types of laxatives (bulk, emollient, and osmotic).

eating disorder/neonate Limited research has produced conflicting data. Some investigators report that infants of mothers with eating disorders have increased perinatal mortality and incidence of anomalies, as well as lower birth weight and Apgar scores. Others found no impact on pregnancy outcome.

eating disorder/pregnancy The literature is divided on the impact of pregnancy on eating disorders. In many studies, eating behavior improved during pregnancy and remained improved in a minority of women. Others found that symptoms continued or worsened during pregnancy and concluded that women should be counseled to delay pregnancy until remission of the eating disorder is achieved. Almost all studies on the impact of eating disorders and pregnancy on maternal and fetal health are flawed. A prospective, controlled study with adequate sample size is needed.

ecgonine methyl ester Major, de-esterified, inactive metabolite of cocaine formed by the action of liver and plasma cholinesterases. It may account for 25–50% of a dose of ingested cocaine.

echoencephalography Neurodiagnostic procedure in which ultrasound is transmitted to the brain and its echo is recorded on an oscilloscope. A shift in echo may indicate a possible space-occupying mass.

echokinesia Imitation of the movements of others. It is sometimes seen in Gilles de la Tourette's syndrome.

echolalia Repetition (echoing) of the words or phrases of others. Typical echolalia tends to be repetitive and persistent. The echo is often uttered with a mocking, mumbling, or staccato intonation. Echolalia is observed in some pervasive developmental disorders, organic mental disorders, and schizophrenia. It should not be confused with habitual repetition of questions, apparently to clarify the question and formulate its answer.

echo planar magnetic resonance imaging (MRI) Neuroimaging technique that allows measurement of brain metabolism each 30 ms, a temporal resolution comparable to the electroencephalogram (EEG) with the advantage of the excellent three-dimensional spatial resolution of MRI. It may be able to provide both functional and morphological imaging data.

ecologic illness Chronic multisystem disorder in which individuals react adversely to foods, some chemicals, and environmental agents at levels generally tolerated by the majority. Also called environmental illness, twentieth century disease, and total allergy syndrome. See **multiple chemical sensitivity syndrome.**

ecologic study See **analysis of secular trends.**

ecological validity Extent to which results of controlled ecological studies can be generalized beyond the confines of the particular experimental context of a variety of geographic and environment contexts in the real world.

ecology Relationship between living things and their environment. It includes studies of the differential incidence of mental disorders in various populations and the distribution of crime and delinquency within a specified geographical area. The psychiatric ecologist, also called a "social psychiatrist," is interested in why one person becomes ill while a neighbor retains good health. See **social psychiatry.**

economic evaluation Comparative analysis of alternative courses of action in terms of costs and consequences (Anon. Glossary of methodologic terms. *JAMA* 1992;268:43–44).

"ecstasy" Street name for 3,4-methylenedioxymethamphetamine (MDMA).

ED$_{50}$ See **effective dose-50.**

Edecrin See **ethacrynic acid.**

educational neglect Parent-permitted long-term truancy, failure to enroll a child in school, and inattention to special educational needs (US Dept. of Health and Human Services. *Study Findings: Study of National Incidence and Prevalence of Child Abuse and Neglect: 1988.* Washington, DC: US Dept. of Health and Human Services, 1988).

effect size In meta-analysis, a measure of the magnitude of a particular treatment effect while controlling for the sample size in each study.

effect size index   Difference between mean rating scale scores for the treatment under study and the control group divided by the standard deviation of the control group at the end of a short-term trial (4–6 weeks). With respect to antidepressants, it is the difference at the end-point of the mean Hamilton Rating Scale for Depression score for the drug investigated and the control drug divided by the standard deviation of the control drug (Quality Assurance Project. A treatment outline for depressive disorders. *Aust N Z Psychiatry* 1983; 17:129–146; Kasper S, Fuger J. Moller HJ. Comparative efficacy of antidepressants. *Drugs* 1992;43[suppl]:11–23).

effective dose-50   (ED_{-50}) **1.** Drug dose that produces 50% of a maximal effect (preferred definition). **2.** Drug dose that produces an effect in 50% of test subjects.

effective sample size   Sample size after dropouts, deaths, and other specified exclusions from an original sample.

effectiveness   Extent to which a specific item does what it is intended to do in a specific situation.

effector   In molecular neuropharmacology, the element involved in the biological response of the receptor.

Effexor   See **venlafaxine.**

efficacy   Extent to which a treatment does what it is intended to do. To be sure that a treatment is associated with unequivocal efficacy, it is customary to use placebo-controlled studies. Efficacy is usually accepted when there are two positive placebo-controlled studies. It is ideally determined by rejecting the null hypothesis in randomized controlled trials. This is achieved by selecting key end-points, designing trials with adequate power to detect a difference between treatment groups, and conducting those trials with the objective of rejecting the hypothesis that no difference exists between the assigned treatment groups. Efficacy is the performance of the intervention or treatment under trial conditions; it is distinguished from effectiveness, which is the performance of the treatment under ordinary clinical circumstances.

ego   In psychoanalysis, the part of the psyche that mediates reality testing, environment and object relations, defenses, impulse control, and thought content. It mediates between the id and the superego.

ego-alien   See **ego-dystonic.**

ego-dystonic   Anything unacceptable to the ego. Its opposite is ego-syntonic.

ego-syntonic   Anything acceptable to the ego. Its opposite is ego-dystonic.

E-10-hydroxynortriptyline   See **hydroxynortriptyline.**

eicosanoid   Any of the physiologically active substances derived from arachidonic acid (prostaglandins, thromboxanes, and leukotrienes, also called "arachidonic acid metabolites"). Eicosanoids, particularly the prostaglandin series, play an important modular role in nervous tissue, but how and where they act is not precisely known. They are not stored in tissue, but are synthesized on demand, particularly in pathophysiological conditions. They act briefly (some with a half-life of seconds) and at extremely low concentrations (10^{-10} M). They can act as second messengers. Arachidonic acid and its metabolites also can leave the cell to act extracellularly as first messengers on neighboring cells.

eidetic   Relating to the ability to visualize objects previously seen or imagined. Eidetic images are clearer and richer in detail than usual memory images. Since they are recognized as a memory experience, they are not an hallucination.

Ekbom's syndrome   See **restless legs syndrome.**

elation   Affect characterized by euphoria and the feeling or expression of excitement or gaiety. Prolonged and intense elation is characteristic of mania.

Elatrol   See **amitriptyline.**

Elavil   See **amitriptyline.**

Eldepryl   See **selegiline.**

elder abuse   Psychological (verbal), financial, sexual, and or violent abuse causing distress to a person past retirement age. It may be active or by neglect; it may occur in the home, an institution or a hospital. Prevalence ranges from 5% to 65%, depending on criteria. In the United States, incidence of the battered elder syndrome is estimated to be 4%. If abuse is confirmed, priorities are (a) safety of the victim; (b) physical and psychological health of the victim; (c) physical and psychological health of the abuser; and (d) a plan to prevent recurrence. Protective measures include self-help support groups or supervised and specialist teams from health authorities to detect, intervene in, and prevent elder abuse (Pitt B. Abusing old people. *Br Med J* 1992;305:968–969).

ELECT   Lilly term dictionary based on the Food and Drug Administration (FDA) COSTART dictionary which contains over 1,100 terms that may be used to classify adverse drug events.

elective mutism   See **mutism, elective.**

electrical kindling   See **kindling.**

electroconvulsive therapy   (ECT) Use of an electrical stimulus instead of a pharmacological one (e.g., subcutaneous insulin, intravenous metrazol, or inhaled flurothyl) to elicit an epileptiform seizure in the brain; it is this seizure that is therapeutic. ECT is in no sense electrical treatment or electrotherapy. Before 1980, most ECT treatments were given with a sine wave stimulus from constant current apparatus. This has been refined to a pulsed square wave stimulus of constant current with attention to technical aspects, such as electrode placement and monitoring seizure duration. Safety has been enhanced by the use of barbiturates to induce amnesia, succinylcholine to paralyze muscles, and continuous ventilation with oxygen. Treatments are administered usually every other day, 3 times a week. Seizures are usually monitored on a two-lead single-channel electroencephalograph (EEG). Electrodes may be placed in one of three nondominant, unilateral, temporoparietal positions. Especially with unilateral treatments, inadequate seizures may be very common; thus the trend toward monitoring electrode placement, seizure duration, and concurrent medications. Seizure activity less than 25 seconds is considered a brief seizure. Since during an ECT series the seizure threshold is increased secondary to the anticonvulsant properties of ECT itself, either increased power settings (stimulus intensity dosing) or epileptogenic agents must be used to maintain therapeutic treatments. The first option may result in increased morbidity (cognitive deficits), the latter requires intravenous caffeine augmentation, which may pose cardiovascular complications. Lately, trazodone and bupropion have been used as the epileptogenic agent without complications. Patients taking benzodiazepines may not respond to unilateral ECT because of their effect on seizure duration. ECT activation of the sympathetic nervous system can result in marked increases in blood pressure and pulse during and immediately after the seizure. These hyperdynamic states are typically transient and well tolerated by most patients. Contemporary advances in equipment and anesthesia have made it possible to conclude that there are no longer any "absolute" contraindications for ECT (American Psychiatric Association Task Force on ECT. *The Practice Of ECT: Recommendations for Treatment, Training and Privileging.* Washington, DC: American Psychiatric Press, 1990).

electroconvulsive therapy (ECT) + alprazolam Therapeutic response to unilateral electroconvulsive therapy (ECT) is much diminished in patients receiving concurrent alprazolam. In addition, there can be difficulties in evoking seizures. Alprazolam offers little benefit and may predispose patients to adverse effects during ECT. There also should be concern about provoking further impairment of cog-

nitive and memory function (Jarvis MR, Goewert AJ, Zorumski CF. Novel antidepressants and maintenance electroconvulsive therapy. A review. *Ann Clin Psychiatry* 1992;4:275–284).

electroconvulsive therapy (ECT) + amoxapine Amoxapine's predilection to cause seizures raises concern that serious adverse effects could occur if it is taken during ECT (Jarvis MR, Goewert AJ, Zorunski CF. Novel antidepressants and maintenance electroconvulsive therapy. A review. *Ann Clin Psychiatry* 1992;4: 275–284).

electroconvulsive therapy (ECT) + anticonvulsant An anticonvulsant should probably be discontinued, if possible, before starting ECT because it can markedly increase the amount of current necessary to produce a seizure (Roberts MA, Attah JR. Carbamazepine + ECT. *Br J Psychiatry* 1988;153:418).

electroconvulsive therapy (ECT) + benzodiazepine It is often asserted that patients being treated with benzodiazepines (BZDs) should not be given ECT because the BZD's anticonvulsant properties might modify seizures and decrease the antidepressant efficacy of ECT. A BZD may shorten an ECT-induced seizure, but there are no substantive data indicating that BZD therapy diminishes ECT efficacy. On the other hand, BZD therapy may impede the full therapeutic effect of unilateral ECT and should be discontinued before unilateral ECT is administered (Pettinati HM, Stephens SM, Willis KM, Robin SE. Evidence for less improvement in depression in patients taking benzodiazepines during unilateral ECT. *Am J Psychiatry* 1990;147:1029–1035; Cohen SI, Lawton C. Do benzodiazepines interfere with the action of electroconvulsive therapy? *Br J Psychiatry* 1992;160:545–546).

electroconvulsive therapy (ECT)/bilateral ECT in which electrodes are placed in both temple areas. It induces both retrograde and anterograde amnesia, which are a function of the number and frequency of induced seizures. Amnesias completely subside in almost all patients within a month or two of treatment termination. Also called "bitemporal ECT." See **electroconvulsive therapy, unilateral.**

electroconvulsive therapy (ECT)/bitemporal See **electroconvulsive therapy/bilateral.**

electroconvulsive therapy (ECT)/brain structure It has been alleged that ECT causes brain damage. This was based on such findings as abnormal pneumoencephalograms in some ECT-treated patients (Friedberg J. Shock treatment, brain damage and memory loss. A neurological perspective. *Am J Psychiatry* 1977; 134:1010–1014). However, early studies of ECT effects on central nervous system (CNS) structure were done without the present knowledge of the association among CNS changes, age, and mental illness. Since the development of technologies such as computed tomography (CT) and magnetic resonance imaging (MRI), retrospective and prospective studies have shown that ECT does not cause permanent morphological changes in the brain. Many elderly patients who are referred for ECT have a variety of brain abnormalities, including cortical atrophy, white matter lesions, caudate lesions, and basal ganglion lesions. These have not been shown to worsen after ECT. All of these findings argue against the claim that ECT causes neuronal damage (Black JL. ECT: lessons learned about an old treatment with new technologies. *Psychiatr Ann* 1993;23:7–14).

electroconvulsive therapy (ECT) + bupropion Like tricyclic antidepressants, trazodone, and fluoxetine, bupropion (BUP) has been reported to prolong seizures associated with ECT. Thus, some clinicians have speculated that BUP might be used beneficially to assure adequate seizure length during ECT in patients with short seizures and high seizure thresholds, similar to the way in which caffeine sodium benzoate is now often used (Figiel GS, Jarvis MR. Electroconvulsive therapy in a depressed patient receiving bupropion. *J Clin Psychopharmacol* 1990;10:376). However, delirium was reported in a 75-year-old man given BUP (75 mg twice a day) after a course of ECT, suggesting that risks of concurrent use may outweigh any potential benefit (Libergon I, Deguardo JR, Silk KR. Bupropion and delirium. *Am J Psychiatry* 1990; 147:1689–1690).

electroconvulsive therapy (ECT) + buspirone No interactions have been reported.

electroconvulsive therapy (ECT) + caffeine Caffeine augmentation has been used successfully to lengthen seizures in ECT. A dose of 500–2000 mg of caffeine sodium benzoate is given intravenously prior to unilateral or bilateral ECT. It is well tolerated even in elderly patients with pre-existing cardiovascular disease (Coffey CE, Figel GS, Weiner RD, Saunders WB. Caffeine augmentation of ECT. *Am J Psychiatry* 1990;147:579–585). Orally administered caffeine also has been reported to decrease frequency of missed or inadequate seizures without increasing adverse effects, thus minimizing the need for higher stimulus dosing and a protracted course of ECT (Ancill RJ, Carlyle W. Oral caffeine augmentation of ECT. *Am J Psychiatry* 1992;149:137). Cardiovascular complications, however, have been reported (Jaffe R, Brubaker G, Dubin WR, Roemer R. Caffeine-associated cardiac dys-

rhythmia during ECT: report of three cases. *Convulsive Ther* 1990;6:308–313).

electroconvulsive therapy (ECT) + carbamazepine Carbamazepine (CBZ) may interact with pre-ECT anesthetic(s) and may prevent seizure induction. Many experts advise stopping CBZ during ECT therapy (Roberts MA, Attah JR. Carbamazepine and ECT. *Br J Psychiatry* 1988;153:418).

electroconvulsive therapy (ECT)/children and adolescents Very little is known about use of ECT in children and adolescents; the published literature consists almost entirely of case reports (Bertagnoli MW, Borchardt CM. A review of ECT for children and adolescents. *J Am Acad Child Adolesc Psychiatry* 1990;29:302–307). Use in those under age 16 is rare; this may in part reflect the fact that disorders thought to respond to ECT (e.g., psychotic depression) are relatively uncommon among children and adolescents. Among psychiatrists working with this age group, reluctance to use ECT does not appear to result from widespread disagreement with the concept of depressive disorder among the young or general reluctance to use physical treatments; rather, it seems to be related to concern about lack of knowledge about ECT side effects in this age group (Parmar R. Attitudes of child psychiatrists to electroconvulsive therapy. *Psychiatr Bull* 1993;17:12–13).

electroconvulsive therapy (ECT)/clinical indications Most frequent psychiatric reasons for ECT referral include: inadequate rate of improvement with pharmacotherapy; history of prior response to ECT; urgent need for rapid improvement from severe depression; and intolerance of antidepressant medication. ECT should be considered initial treatment for severely depressed, delusional, suicidal patients; patients with severe mania; and for patients with some acute psychotic illnesses and catatonic conditions. ECT is effective for depression in patients with concurrent neurological diseases, Parkinson's disease, acquired encephalopathies, primary degenerative dementias, cerebrovascular disease, and seizure disorders. Patients with degenerative brain diseases and diffuse encephalopathies may be prone to ECT-induced delirium. In patients with human immunodeficiency virus (HIV) infection, ECT has been used successfully in psychotic depression and prophylaxis of bipolar affective disorder. ECT has been beneficial in some patients with neuroleptic malignant syndrome (NMS), particularly if intervention is early. ECT also has been used as an alternative to reintroducing neuroleptic drugs to psychotic patients who have experienced NMS (Black JL. ECT: lessons learned about an old treatment with new technologies. *Psychiatr Ann* 1993;23:7–14).

electroconvulsive therapy (ECT) + clozapine
Clozapine (CLOZ) is associated with increased seizure risk as daily dosage increases (Haller E, Binder RL. Clozapine and seizures. *Am J Psychiatry* 1990;147:1069–1071). Spontaneous seizures following one ECT treatment was reported in a patient receiving CLOZ 800 mg/day, propranolol 60 mg/day, and diazepam 20 mg/day. CLOZ and propranolol were tapered over 14 days and stopped 4 days before ECT administration; diazepam was reduced to 5 mg/day 72 hours before ECT. It is unclear whether CLOZ contributed to seizures in this case. A 1-in-500 incidence of tardive seizure phenomenon following ECT has been reported (Fink M. CNS sequelae of electroseizure therapy: risks of therapy and their prophylaxis. *In* Shagass C, Friedhoff A [eds], *Psychopathology and Brain Dysfunction.* New York: Raven Press, 1977). Relatively rapid tapering of long-term diazepam treatment also may have been a factor. It is recommended that 7–10 days should elapse between clozapine discontinuation and ECT administration (Masiar SJ, Johns CA. ECT following clozapine. *Br J Psychiatry* 1991;158:135).

electroconvulsive therapy (ECT)/delirium   See **delirium/electroconvulsive therapy.**

electroconvulsive therapy (ECT) + fluoxetine
There are reports indicating no additional antidepressant benefit from concurrent use of fluoxetine (FLX) and ECT. Co-administration also has been reported both to prolong seizure duration and not to prolong it (Elizon A, Steinbok M, Levin Y. Fluoxetine prevents increase of seizure threshold and shortening of seizure duration in depressive patients treated by ECT. Presented at the 146th Annual Meeting of the American Psychiatric Association, San Francisco, May 1993). The possibility of complications from FLX-induced elevations of anesthetic agents and the theoretical possibility of provoking a serotonin syndrome with ECT-induced elevations of brain serotonin have prompted the recommendation that patients not take FLX during ECT (Jarvis MR, Goewert AJ, Zorineski CF. Novel antidepressants and maintenance electroconvulsive therapy. A review. *Ann Clin Psychiatry* 1992;4: 275–284).

electroconvulsive therapy (ECT) + labetalol   Labetalol, a beta-blocker, is commonly prescribed to modify the hypertensive/tachycardia response to an ECT-induced seizure. Since beta-blockers may increase the risk of bradycardia or asystole if a subconvulsive electrical stimulus is administered, pretreatment with an anticholinergic agent (e.g., glycopyrrolate

or atropine) is indicated (Kellner CH. Labetalol and ECT. *J Clin Psychiatry* 1991;52:386–387).

electroconvulsive therapy (ECT) + lithium
Lithium levels should be carefully determined and lowered to half therapeutic levels in patients referred for ECT (American Psychiatric Association Task Force on Electroconvulsive Therapy. *The Practice of Electroconvulsive Therapy: Recommendations for Treatment, Training, and Privileging.* Washington, DC: American Psychiatric Press, 1990). It is prudent to stop lithium 1 week prior to ECT, which seems to be sufficient to prevent complications. It also is prudent not to restart lithium until 4–7 days after ECT is completed (Small JG, Milstein V. Lithium interactions: lithium and electroconvulsive therapy. *J Clin Psychopharmacol* 1990;10:346–350). Available data suggest that the higher the serum lithium concentration when ECT is administered, the greater the risk of cerebral toxicity. Even therapeutic lithium levels may be associated with organic brain syndromes, particularly in patients who become severely depressed during maintenance lithium therapy and who are given ECT either along with lithium or within a day or two after it was discontinued. The American Psychiatric Association Task Force Report warns of the potential increased risk of delirium when ECT and lithium are given concurrently. Co-administration also has been reported to cause nonconvulsive status epilepticus 2 days after the fifth ECT treatment (Weiner RD, Whanger AD, Ervin CW, et al. Prolonged confusional state and EEG seizure activity following concurrent ECT and lithium use. *Am J Psychiatry* 1980;137:1452–1453).

electroconvulsive therapy (ECT), maintenance
(MECT) Continuing treatment with ECT is considered an effective alternative treatment for several psychiatric illnesses. Use, especially in chronic unipolar depression, has increased steadily since 1970 (Kramer BA. Maintenance ECT: a survey of practice [1986]. *Convulsive Ther* 1987;3:260–268). Several studies have demonstrated efficacy and diminished relapse rates of affective illness in selected patients. It can be particularly effective for patients either intolerant of or poorly responsive to psychotropic medications; patients unresponsive to medications prior to ECT are unlikely to respond to maintenance pharmacotherapy after completing a beneficial course of ECT (Sackeim HA, Prudic J, Devanand DP, et al. The impact of medication resistance and continuation pharmacotherapy on relapse following response to electroconvulsive therapy in major depression. *J Clin Psychopharmacol* 1990;

10:96–104). MECT may keep these patients' illnesses in remission (Jarvis MR, Goewert AJ, Zorumski CF. Novel antidepressants and maintenance electroconvulsive therapy. A review. *Ann Clin Psychiatry* 1992;4:275–284).

electroconvulsive therapy (ECT)/mania   ECT has been found to be as effective as lithium in the treatment of acute mania. It is an appropriate alternative for patients who require rapid control of severe manic symptoms or who are unresponsive to available antimanic agents. It also should be considered for those with mixed mania at high risk of suicide (Black DW, Winokur G, Nasrallah A. Treatment of mania: a naturalistic study of electroconvulsive therapy versus lithium in 438 patients. *J Clin Psychiatry* 1987;48:132–139). ECT has been used successfully in the treatment of mania in children (Carr V, Donington C, Schrader G. The use of ECT for mania in childhood bipolar disorder. *Br J Psychiatry* 1983;143:411–415). Whether ECT for mania requires bitemporal electrode placement is controversial; in one study unilateral ECT was as effective as bilateral ECT (Black DW, Winokur G, Nasrallah. Treatment of mania: a naturalistic study of electroconvulsive therapy versus lithium in 438 patients. *J Clin Psychiatry* 1987;48:132–139).

electroconvulsive therapy (ECT)/medication impact   Medications during the course of ECT may (a) increase or decrease seizure activity; (b) increase risk of post-ECT organic brain syndrome; and (c) modify cardiovascular response to ECT (Jowsey SG. The effect of medications on ECT. *Psychiatr Ann* 1993;23:33–37). All ongoing psychotropic and medical agents should be reviewed as part of the pre-ECT evaluation (American Psychiatric Association Task Force on Electroconvulsive Therapy. *The Practice of Electroconvulsive Therapy: Recommendations for Treatment, Training, and Privileging.* Washington, DC: American Psychiatric Press, 1990).

electroconvulsive therapy (ECT)/medications + seizure duration   To be efficacious, the seizure induced during ECT must be of sufficient duration (25 seconds). Many psychotropic, anesthetic, and anticonvulsant medications may affect ECT efficacy by altering seizure threshold or increasing or decreasing seizure activity. Drugs that increase seizure activity include theophylline, caffeine, lithium, tricyclic antidepressants, neuroleptics, trazodone, bupropion, and fluoxetine. Drugs that decrease seizure activity include benzodiazepines, anticonvulsants, barbiturates, lidocaine, and propofol (Jowsey SG. The effect of medications on ECT. *Psychiatr Ann* 1993;23:33–37).

electroconvulsive therapy (ECT) + monoamine oxidase inhibitor (MAOI)   ECT administration to patients receiving *chronic* MAOI therapy has been safe and effective. Little data are available to indicate whether co-administration enhances ECT's antidepressant effect. Concerns about adverse interactions between ECT anesthesia and an MAOI have prompted many to recommend that the MAOI be discontinued up to 2 weeks prior to ECT.

electroconvulsive therapy (ECT), multiple monitored   (MMECT) Administration in a single treatment session of several ECTs (two to eight seizures at 3-minute intervals) while monitoring the patient's electrocardiogram and electroencephalogram. The goal is to shorten the time needed for a course of treatment. MMECT appears to be as safe as conventional ECT, requires less exposure to anesthesia, allows a shorter hospital stay, and may produce less memory impairment. There may be increased risk of treatment-related reversible confusion.

electroconvulsive therapy (ECT) + neuroleptic   Co-administration may be effective in the treatment of psychotic symptoms in drug-resistant schizophrenia.

electroconvulsive therapy (ECT)/parkinsonism   ECT may relieve drug-induced parkinsonism, whether administered therapeutically or prophylactically (Goswani U, Dutta S, Kuruvilla K, et al. Electroconvulsive therapy in neuroleptic-induced parkinsonism. *Biol Psychiatry* 1989;26:234–238; Gangadhar BN, Choudhary JR, Channabasavanna SM. ECT and drug-induced parkinsonism. *Ind J Psychiatry* 1983;25:212–213).

electroconvulsive therapy (ECT)/Parkinson's disease   ECT is effective in reducing psychiatric and neurological symptoms, particularly depression and rigidity, of Parkinson's disease (PD) (Andersen K, Balldin J, Gottfries CG, et al. A double-blind evaluation of electroconvulsive therapy in Parkinson's disease with "on-off" phenomena. *Acta Neurol Scand* 1987;76:191–199). Patients with cognitive impairment prior to ECT should be given ECT cautiously and with close monitoring for signs of worsening cognitive status. Should the latter be detected, ECT should be terminated promptly. PD patients with cognitive decline experience more ECT morbidity in the form of post-ECT delirium (Rummans TA. Medical indications for electroconvulsive therapy. *Psychiatr Ann* 1993,23:27–32). Risk of delirium may be higher in patients continuing to receive dopaminergic drug treatment (usually Sinemet) for parkinson symptoms. Risk can be minimized if dopaminergic treatment is reduced before beginning ECT (Zervas IM, Fink M. ECT and delirium in Parkinson's disease. *Am J Psychiatry* 1992;149:1758).

electroconvulsive therapy (ECT) + paroxetine Some interactions may occur. At steady-state concentrations, paroxetine can inhibit and saturate the high affinity components of the hepatic P450 enzyme system, resulting in potentially higher plasma levels of compounds metabolized by these pathways and possible interference with the metabolism of anesthetics used during ECT. Because paroxetine is a selective inhibitor of serotonin uptake, there is a theoretical possibility of its provoking a serotonin syndrome with ECT-induced elevations of brain serotonin. Paroxetine should be discontinued prior to ECT (Jarvis MR, Goevert AJ, Zorumski CF. Novel antidepressants and maintenance electroconvulsive therapy. A review. *Ann Clin Psychiatry* 1992;4:275–284).

electroconvulsive therapy (ECT)/poststroke depression ECT is a very effective and generally well tolerated therapeutic option for post-stroke depression patients who (a) are intolerant of or nonresponsive to pharmacotherapy; (b) have severe cardiovascular disease precluding the use of pharmacotherapy; or (c) have life-threatening depressive symptoms (e.g., dehydration due to refusal to eat) (Currier MB, Murray GB, Welch CC. Electroconvulsive therapy for post-stroke depressed geriatric patients. *J Neuropsychiatry Clin Neurosci* 1992;4:140–144).

electroconvulsive therapy (ECT) seizure monitoring Electroencephalogram (EEG) monitoring to ensure that a seizure of sufficient duration has occurred (an arbitrary minimum of 25 seconds is now generally agreed upon). Seizure monitoring can also be done with a blood pressure cuff. For unilateral ECT, the ipsilateral limb is monitored to assure seizure generalization. The duration of muscular convulsion in the cuffed limb correlates with the simultaneously recorded EEG.

electroconvulsive therapy (ECT) + sertraline There is currently (1994) insufficient experience to indicate whether co-administration is safe. Because potential interactions could include provocation of a serotonin syndrome, sertraline should be avoided during ECT (Jarvis MR, Goewert AJ, Zorumski CF. Novel antidepressants and maintenance electroconvulsive therapy. A review. *Ann Clin Psychiatry* 1992;4:275–284).

electroconvulsive therapy (ECT)/tardive dyskinesia (TD) Whether ECT has a direct effect on TD is unclear. ECT has been reported to both improve and worsen TD (Gosek E, Weller RA. Single case study: improvement of tardive dyskinesia associated with electroconvulsive therapy. *J Nerv Ment Dis* 1988;176:120–122;

Uhrbrand L, Faurbye A. Reversible and irreversible dyskinesia after treatment with perphenazine, chlorpromazine, reserpine, and ECT. *Psychopharmacologia* 1960;1:408–418). It has been suggested that ECT is a risk factor for TD, although the majority of studies have not found a correlation (Gurrje O. The significance of subtyping tardive dyskinesia: a study of prevalence and associated factors. *Psychol Med* 1989;19:121–128). Some clinicians have used adjunctive ECT to reduce the need for neuroleptic therapy for some patients with severe TD (Gujavarty K, Greenberg LB, Fink M. Electroconvulsive therapy and neuroleptic medication in therapy-resistant positive-symptom psychosis. *Convulsive Ther* 1987;3:185–195).

electroconvulsive therapy (ECT) + theophylline Deciding whether to use ECT in patients with severe pulmonary conditions treated with theophylline is a fairly common clinical problem. Initiating a course of ECT in patients taking theophylline has been associated with status epilepticus and consequent brain damage or even death. Although theophylline is a risk factor for prolonged seizures in patients given ECT, ECT can be given safely if the patient cannot be safely tapered off theophylline, is intolerant of or resistant to antidepressant pharmacotherapy, and the pre-ECT theophylline level is not greater than 20.0 µg/ml. ECT can be administered provided intravenous anticonvulsants to terminate prolonged seizures are used earlier than usual (i.e., to stop the seizure after 90 seconds rather than after the customary 180 seconds) (Rasmussen KG, Zorumski CF. Electroconvulsive therapy in patients taking theophylline. *J Clin Psychiatry* 1993;54:427–431).

electroconvulsive therapy (ECT) + tranylcypromine Data are sparse, but no adverse side effects or any enhancement of ECT by tranylcypromine have been reported.

electroconvulsive therapy (ECT) + trazodone Co-administration has been reported to cause prolonged seizures to the point of status epilepticus that required intravenous diazepam intervention (Kaufman KR, Finstead B, Kaufman ER. Status epilepticus following electroconvulsive therapy. *Mt Sinai J Med* 1986;53:119–122). Thus, some clinicians feel that trazodone should be withheld in patients while they are receiving ECT. However, since during a series of ECTs the seizure threshold is increased secondary to the anticonvulsant properties of ECT itself, the therapist must use either increased power settings or epileptogenic agents in order to assure therapeutic treatments. The first option results in increased morbidity (cognitive defects), whereas the second has other complications when caffeine is used. In the latter case, trazodone can be used as the epileptogenic agent without complications (Kaufman KR, Finstead B, Kaufman ER. Electroencephalography and electroconvulsive therapy. *Electroencephalogr Clin Neurophysiol* 1985;61:S178).

electroconvulsive therapy (ECT) + tricyclic antidepressant (TCA) Although there is hope that a beneficial additive or synergistic effect could lead to faster, more complete recovery, co-administration could result in adverse interactions, mainly cardiovascular, between a TCA and ECT or anesthetic agents used during ECT. Most experts recommend that antidepressants be stopped prior to ECT (American Psychiatric Association Task Force on Electroconvulsive Therapy. *The Practice of Electroconvulsive Therapy: Recommendations for Treatment, Training, and Privileging.* Washington, DC: American Psychiatric Press, 1990).

electroconvulsive therapy (ECT)/unilateral ECT preferentially administered to the hemisphere nondominant for language. A variety of electrode placements have been used for unilateral ECT. Current consensus is that the lower electrode should be placed exactly as for bilateral ECT, while the upper electrode is placed on the same side of the head adjacent to the vertex of the skull. It has been recommended that unilateral ECT, with its relative paucity of cognitive side effects, be given an initial trial in every patient except agitated, delusional, or suicidal melancholic patients; acutely manic patients; catatonic patients; and high-risk medically ill patients. Switching to bilateral ECT is recommended if four to six unilateral treatments have not been beneficial. See **electroconvulsive therapy, bilateral.**

electroconvulsive therapy (ECT) + valproate Since valproate may prevent seizure induction, many experts advise stopping it during ECT therapy (Roberts MA, Attah JR. Carbamazepine and ECT. *Br J Psychiatry* 1988;153: 418).

electrocorticogram Recording directly from the cortex of the four different physiological brain rhythms: alpha, beta, theta, and delta.

electrodermal activity (EDA) Measure of sweat gland activity, a sympathetic nervous system measure with a cholinergic instead of adrenergic end-organ synapse. Also called "skin conductance activity"; "skin conductance level (SCL)", "skin conductance response (SC)."

electrodermal response (ED) See **galvanic skin response.**

electroencephalogram (EEG) Graphic (voltage and frequency vs. time) depiction of the brain's electrical potentials recorded by scalp electrodes. Since 1929, it has been used to diagnose a variety of brain diseases. Constituent rhythms are alpha (10–12 Hz), slower delta (4–6 Hz) and intermediate theta associated with drowsiness or sleep, slow beta with arousal or sleep spindles (stage II), and fast beta associated with mental activity. Characteristic changes in the type, frequency, and potential of brain waves occur in altered brain states. Different rhythms are characteristic of various stages of alertness, sleep, and age. Proportion of each rhythm is particularly sensitive to psychoactive medications. Techniques such as stroboscopic light, hyperventilation, sleep deprivation, and sleep induction are used to accentuate abnormal waves or bring out latent abnormalities. An EEG is often necessary to classify disorders. In about a third of seizure patients, a routine EEG may not be abnormal; in these patients hyperventilation, sleep deprivation, and photic stimulation may be necessary to evoke epileptic discharges.

electroencephalograph Apparatus used to make a graphic record of the electrical activity of the brain (electroencephalogram).

electroencephalographic brain mapping Use of multiple electrodes to provide a topographic map of various frequencies and voltages. It is a readily available, inexpensive, high time-resolution method for objective and quantitative evaluation of the neurophysiological basis of psychiatric disorders and their respective treatment. Also called "electroencephalographic topography."

electroencephalographic coherence Co-variation by frequency between two recording channels that may reflect underlying patterns of brain activity.

electroencephalographic topography See **electroencephalographic brain mapping.**

electrolytic lesion Destruction of a specific nerve pathway by passing a current between electrodes inserted into the brain region innervated by the nerve pathway.

electromyogram (EMG) Electrophysiological recording that measures the amount and nature of muscle activity at the site from which the recording is taken.

electromyography (EMG) Measurement of electrical signals emitted during muscle contractions. Electrode placement is important for accurate detection of electrical activity. Surface electrodes are useful for detecting EMG activity from large superficial muscles, but they cannot discriminate muscle activity from small or deep muscles. The relative ease of using surface electrodes in a clinical setting often outweighs loss of discriminatory ability. Needle or wire electrodes have greater muscle specificity than surface electrodes and are better suited for studying facial and hand muscle activity, but are more invasive. EMG is being used for the instrumental quantification of tardive dyskinesia.

electronarcosis Obsolete form of somatic treatment, introduced in 1944, for certain psychiatric illnesses that involves application of an electrical stimulus. Technically, it lies somewhere between electrosleep and electroconvulsive therapy (ECT). It is more dangerous and less effective than ECT.

electron transport chain Group of enzyme complexes that contain electron carriers (e.g., flavins, cytochromes, iron-sulfur centers). As electrons are transferred from donor to acceptor, energy is released and used to synthesize adenosine triphosphatase.

electronystagmograph (ENG) Electrical recording of the characteristic rapid conjugate movement of the eyes from leads placed over the extraocular muscles.

electro-oculogram (EOG) Electromyogram of the ocular muscles. The EOG is altered in diseases affecting the retinal pigment epithelial layer. It is one of a number of visual electrophysiological tests.

electro-oculography (EOG) Measurement of eye movement. Electrodes attached to the skin beside the outer corners of the eyes measure the standing potential that exists between the front and back of the eye and generated by the retinal pigment epithelial layer. This electrical potential increases when the retina is exposed to light. The electrical potential in the light-adapted eye, divided by the potential in adaptation to the dark, is called the EOG (or Arden) ratio and is an indirect measure of light-induced electrical changes. See **EOG ratio.**

electrophoresis Laboratory method in which a controlled electric current is used to separate molecules of proteins and nucleotides (DNA and RNA) through a gelatinous matrix (a gel) based on their size and/or charge. The gels can be used either analytically to characterize the size or chemical nature of proteins and nucleic acids (often in conjunction with autoradiography) or preparatively for Southern, northern, and western blots. The 1990s may be the decade of capillary electrophoresis of neuropeptides. By combining capillary electrophoretic separations with ultraviolet or fluorescence detection, enhancements in sensitivity have been impressive. Capillary zone electrophoresis, which makes possible the ability to separate and detect picogram and nanogram levels, can also be applied to large mixtures of peptides and proteins, thus providing an important analytical tool for the study of peptide biochemistry.

electrophysiological test Any of several tests used in the diagnosis and assessment of therapy of neuromuscular disorders. Neurophysiological evaluation of patients with a neuromuscular disorder consists of four parts: (a) testing motor conduction velocity; (b) testing sensory conduction velocity; (c) testing late responses by the Hoffman reflex (H reflex) and measuring response in the upper and lower extremities; and (d) electromyographic (EMG) assessment of the electrical characteristics of muscle.

electroplexy Obsolete British term for electroconvulsive therapy. See **electroconvulsive therapy.**

electroretinogram (ERG) Measurement of electric potentials generated by the photoreceptors of the eye. A signal generated by the retina in response to a flash of light is recorded (after topical anesthesia) by a contact lens or fork electrode on the surface of the eye. The electrical potential in the light-adapted eye, divided by the potential in adaptation to the dark, is known as the EOG (or Arden) ratio and is an indirect measure of light-induced electrical changes. The ERG is one of several visual electrophysiological tests (Berson EL. Electrical phenomena in the retina. *In* Hart D, Moser R [eds], *Adler's Physiology of the Eye*, 8th ed. St. Louis: CV Mosby, 1987).

electroshock therapy See **electroconvulsive therapy (preferred term).**

electroshock therapy, regressive (REST) Form of electroconvulsive therapy in which seizures are induced several times daily until the patient is out of contact and incontinent of urine. Recovery from the organic brain syndrome produced by this treatment is gradual. REST is seldom used today.

electrosleep Transcutaneous electrical stimulation with relatively low-intensity electrical pulses through the brain. Current is generally applied in an anteroposterior direction using electrodes bilaterally placed over the eyes and the mastoid or neck region. It has been studied as a nonpharmacological treatment for depression, anxiety disorders, and insomnia. It has also been proposed as an alternative treatment for hypnotic drug withdrawal in benzodiazepine-dependent patients. Based on double-blind studies, it is a questionable therapy. Also called "cerebral electrostimulation"; "cerebral electrotherapy (CET)"; "transcerebral electrotherapy."

electrostimulation Application of an electroshock of painful intensity as a technique of negative conditioning in aversion therapy.

elimination See **drug elimination.**

elimination half-life   See **drug elimination half-life.**

Elisal   See **sulthiame.**

Elston's method   Method of calculating likelihoods for various modes of genetic transmission.

Eltioxin   See **thyroxine**

eltoprazine   Selective serotonin $(5\text{-}HT)_{1AB}$ agonist that in animals induces dose-dependent inhibition of offensive aggression without causing sedation, motor impairment, sensory incapacity, or reduction in social interaction (Rasmussen DL, Olivier B, Raghoebar M, Mos J. Possible clinical application of serenics and some implications of their preclinical profile for their clinical use in psychiatric disorders. *Drug Metab Drug Interact* 1990;8:159–186). Results in the treatment of self-injurious behavior (SIB) have been conflicting. In doses up to 40 mg/day for 2 weeks it dramatically reduced SIB and increased cooperativeness, a feeling of well-being, alertness, and activity, supporting the hypothesis that serotonin is involved in the pathogenesis of self-injury. Effects seemed to diminish after 6 weeks (Verhoeven WMA, Tuinier S, Sijben NOA, et al. Eltoprazine in mentally retarded self-injuring patients. *Lancet* 1992;340:1037–1038). In a placebo-controlled multicenter trial, however, there was no change in SIB, and study patients did tolerate eltoprazine well with no medical, neurological, or psychiatric side effects or increased frequency or duration of epilepsy (Kohen D. Eltoprazine for aggression in mental handicap. *Lancet* 1993;341:628–629). It may be effective in patients who are aggressive, violent, and resistant to other antiaggressive therapies (Tiihonen J, Hakola P, Paanila J, Turtiainen M. Eltoprazine for aggression in schizophrenia and mental retardation. *Lancet* 1993;341:307). Sleep studies indicate a dose-dependent suppression of rapid eye movement (REM) sleep and ponto-geniculo-occipital activity, increases in S sleep, and no effect on waking. Eltoprazine shifts the balance between REM sleep and S sleep but does not change the balance of sleep and waking. It thus may be useful for investigating serotonergic-cholinergic interaction (Quattrochi JJ, Mamelak AN, Binder D, et al. Dose-related suppression of REM sleep and PGO waves by the serotonin-1 agonist eltoprazine. *Neuropsychopharmacology* 1993;8:7–13).

embryogenesis   Formation and development of the embryo.

Emdalen   See **lofepramine.**

emergence delirium   See **delirium, emergence.**

emergence phenomena   Reaction induced by the anesthetic ketamine manifested by disorientation, sensory and perceptual illusions, and vivid dreams following anesthesia. See **ketamine.**

emergency IND   See **Investigational New Drug, emergency.**

Emeside   See **ethosuximide.**

Emflex   See **acemetacin.**

emission computed tomography   (ECT) Form of tomography in which emitted decay products (e.g., positrons or gamma rays) of an ingested radioactive pharmaceutical are recorded in detectors outside the body. Computer data reconstruction yields a cross-sectional image of any portion of the body.

Emitrip   See **amitriptyline.**

emotional blunting   See **affect, flattened.**

emotional incontinence   Behavioral syndrome characterized by involuntary expression of feelings, such as weeping, grimacing, and/or laughter. It is frequently associated with neurological disease; it has been described in stroke, multiple sclerosis, head injury, central pontine myelinolysis, and anoxia. It has been successfully treated with fluoxetine. See **emotionalism.**

emotional lability   Pattern of abrupt mood shifts from normal to one or more dysphoric states, most commonly depression, irritability, anger, and anxiety (Spitzer RL, Endicott J. *Schedule for Affective Disorders and Schizophrenia.* New York: New York State Psychiatric Institute, 1978).

emotional neglect   Inadequate nurturance/affection, long-term or extreme spouse abuse, permitted alcohol/drug abuse or other maladaptive behavior, and refusal or delay in psychological care (US Dept. of Health and Human Services. *Study Findings: Study of National Incidence and Prevalence of Child Abuse and Neglect: 1988.* Washington, DC: US Dept. of Health and Human Services, 1988).

emotional withdrawal   Lack of interest in, involvement with, and affective commitment to life events. It may range from mild to extreme. When extreme, the patient is almost totally withdrawn, uncommunicative, and neglectful of personal needs.

emotionalism   After a stroke or some other type of brain injury, increased tearfulness with episodes of crying or laughing that are sudden or unheralded and not under normal social control. See **emotional incontinence.**

empathy   Capacity to understand what another person is experiencing from within the other's frame of reference (standing in the other's shoes). In empathy one feels as the other person does, but recognizes that other feelings are possible; there is no fusion or identification with the patient. Empathy is not *sympathy*, in which one person identifies with another while suspending critical intellect.

Emperal   See **metoclopramide.**

empirical   Based on experience (observation or experiment), rather than on reasoning alone. An empirical problem can be solved by collection and analysis of appropriate data using relevant statistical techniques.

employee assistance program   Comprehensive, worksite-based program to assist in early identification and resolution of productivity problems associated with impairment due to physical, mental, behavioral, or addictive problems. These include, but are not limited to, health, marital, family, financial, alcohol, drug, legal, emotional, stress-related, or other problems that may adversely affect employee job performance or well-being.

enabling behavior   Any action by another person or an institution that intentionally or unintentionally has the effect of facilitating the continuation of abuse or dependence.

enalapril   (Vasotec) Angiotensin-converting enzyme (ACE) inhibitor antihypertensive.

enalapril + lithium   See **lithium + enalapril.**

enantiomer   One of a pair of molecules that are mirror images of each other. Many psychoactive drugs have enantiomers (e.g., fluoxetine enantiomers are R(2)- and S(+)-fluoxetine). They differ in both their pharmacokinetic and pharmacodynamic properties.

Encephabol   See **dihydroergotoxine.**

encephalography, radioisotopic   Measurement of brain function based on uptake of radioisotopes by different cerebral structures. The procedure includes injection of an isotope, scanning of the brain by an isotope-sensitive probe, recording the intensity of reaction in graphic form, and comparing it with normal patterns. It is useful in detecting neoplasms, subdural hematomas, arteriovenous malformations, brain abscess, and cerebral infarcts.

encephalopathy   Any degenerative brain disease that is general and widespread rather than localized to one area. It may be due to alcohol, hypertension, lead, or conditions such as Wernicke's syndrome.

encephalopathy, hypertensive   Diffuse, increased intracranial pressure that may complicate the course of arterial hypertension. Symptoms include papilledema, raised cerebrospinal fluid pressure, headaches, vomiting, convulsions, and coma. Onset is usually subacute with focal signs (e.g., visual disturbances, aphasia, hemiplegia), but may be chronic and characterized by personality changes, poor judgement, and anxiety.

encephalopathy, progressive dialysis   (PDE) Encephalopathy due to aluminum accumulation that occurs in some patients being dialyzed for end-stage renal disease (ESRD). Exposure occurs via chronic ingestion of aluminum-containing dialysate and/or aluminum-containing antacids as a concomitant of ESRD therapy. Onset is usually subtle; initial symptoms occur after a mean of 37 months from first dialysis. It progresses rapidly from personality changes to global intellectual impairment, accompanied by seizures, gait problems, asterixis, dysarthria, apraxia, and myoclonus. There may be electroencephalograph (EEG) and/or computed tomography (CT) abnormalities. Severity is correlated with brain aluminum concentration (detected at autopsy). It is a leading cause of mortality among patients undergoing chronic hemodialysis (Rosati G, De Bastiani P, Gilli P, et al. Oral aluminum and neuropsychological functioning. *J Neurol* 1980;223:251–257). Clinical experience suggests that PDE is reversible when treated early (i.e., before a critical but yet to be determined point) with benzodiazepines (especially clonazepam and diazepam) and irreversible or progressive beyond that point. Also called "dialysis delirium"; "dialysis dementia"; "dialysis encephalopathy"; "dialysis encephalopathy syndrome."

encoding   **1.** Transformation of messages into signals that can be transmitted by a communications channel. **2.** Transformation of information by an individual into behavior that can function as a signal in a communications system.

encopresis   Involuntary functional fecal incontinence. Most children attain bowel control before age 5, but severely mentally handicapped children may take longer to learn it. Encopresis is associated with poor toilet training or emotional problems when it occurs in children. Another common cause is constipation with overflow soiling. Encopresis during the night is sometimes referred to as "nocturnal encopresis." See **enuresis.**

Endep   See **amitriptyline.**

endocrine system   Glandular system that secretes hormones into the blood to influence metabolism and other body processes (e.g., epinephrine affects small-vessel blood flow to tissues, air-passage regulation, and gastric secretion). It is susceptible to changes in emotion.

endogenous   Originating within the organism.

endogenous depression   See **depression, endogenous.**

endogenous opiate   See **opiate, endogenous.**

endonuclease   Enzyme that digests DNA molecules at specific nucleotide sequences. Originally used by bacteria to get rid of harmful viral DNA (which has sequences not present in the bacteria), restriction endonucleases have been taken over by molecular biologists to manipulate pieces of DNA for recombinant DNA engineering.

endorphin   Any of the endogenous opiate-like peptides secreted or activated by the brain. They are composed of amino-acid chains located in the spinal cord and limbic system. Endorphins have the same properties as morphine: pain relief, euphoria, sedation, and respiratory depression. Their discovery has led to considerable research relating mental illness, particularly schizophrenia, to possible disturbances of endorphinergic systems. Endorphins may modulate the rewarding effects of addictive drugs.

endozepine   One of a group of endogenous ligands for the benzodiazepine (BZD) binding site of the gamma-aminobutyric acid A receptor ($GABA_A$). They are nonpeptide, non-BZD substances that appear to have a quinoline core. Experimental observations indicate that they may play a part in normal central nervous system processes (e.g., memory, learning) and in pathological processes (e.g., panic disorders, hepatic encephalopathy). Endozepine-4 may contribute to or cause idiopathic recurring stupor (Rothstein JD, Guidotti A, Tinuper P, et al. Endogenous benzodiazepine receptor ligands in idiopathic recurring stupor. *Lancet* 1992;340:1002–1004).

end-point   See **outcome.**

end-point, surrogate   Proximal event that might equally well (or even better) reflect therapeutic benefit, used to rapidly evaluate new drugs for fatal and nonfatal diseases. Examples are blood pressure for cardiovascular mortality and intraocular pressure as a surrogate for long-term visual function. End-points are generally accepted as valid for assessing therapeutic efficacy and have served as the basis for the approval of drugs by regulatory agencies. Clinical investigators of acquired immunodeficiency syndrome (AIDS) are using surrogate end-points such as the effect of a drug on progression of disease rather than death as the primary end-point.

end-point modal dose   Daily drug dose taken on most days during the last week of treatment.

end-stage dementia   See **dementia, end stage.**

Engramon   See **zotepine.**

enhancer   In genetics, a term applied to a major type of regulatory sequence in the region of DNA responsible for regulating transcription of the corresponding gene. See **promoter; regulatory sequence.**

enkephalin   Originally described as an endogenous opioid peptide modulating pain perception, but more recently recognized as an immunomodulator that activates T cells in rodents and humans. Two well known en-

kephalins are methionine-enkephalin (Met-enkephalin) and leucine-enkephalin (Leu-enkephalin), which are cleavage products of proenkephalin. The distribution of enkephalin is uneven and closely resembles that of opiate receptors.

Enordin   See **amisulpride.**

Enovil   See **amitriptyline.**

entactogen   Possible new class of psychoactive drugs currently represented by 3,4-methylenedioxymethamphetamine (MDMA, "ecstasy," "Adam," "XTC") and 3,4-methylenedioxyethamphetamine (MDEA, "Eve"). Entactogens are reported to exert unique psychological effects in humans, discriminating them from chemically related substances such as amphetamine and the hallucinogens 3,4-methylenedioxyamphetamine (MDA) and 3,4,5-trimethoxyphenethylamine (mescaline). Data on the psychological effects of MDMA and MDEA are limited. Two double-blind placebo-controlled psychometric trials with normal control subjects found that these drugs produce a partially controllable state of enhanced insight, empathy, and peaceful feelings. All subjects displayed a general stimulation with increased psychomotor drive, logorrhea, and facilitation of communication. One volunteer developed a toxic psychosis, another had a dysphoric reaction, and a third had episodes of anxiety for some days after the experiment. The findings support the hypothesis that MDMA and MDEA represent a novel pharmacological class. Despite reports that entactogens are generally safe, and even despite the conceivable beneficial effects, available data suggest that their safety may depend on the setting in which they are used. There are no reports of individuals who take frequent or large amounts of MDMA or MDEA for extended periods because its "positive" effects seem to diminish and its "negative" effects seem to increase with time. There are some reports of panic reactions and bizarre and risky behavior during peak intoxication from the drug (Hermle L, Spitzer M, Borchardt D, et al. Psychological effects of MDE in normal subjects. Are entactogens a new class of psychoactive agents? *Neuropsychopharmacology* 1993;8:171–176; Nichols DE. Differences between the mechanism of action of MDMA, MBDB, and the classic hallucinogens. Identification of a new therapeutic class: entactogens. *J Psychoactive Drugs* 1986;18:305–313).

enterohepatic recirculation   Reabsorption and eventual entering into the systemic circulation of either active or inactive metabolites.

entrainment   Synchronization of a biological rhythm by a forcing stimulus such as an environmental time cue (zeitgeber). During entrainment the frequencies of the two cycles are the same or integral multiples of each other.

Entrix   See **prazepam.**

enuresis   Involuntary passage of urine, usually at night during sleep, in the absence of a urological or neurological disorder. It occurs commonly 30 minutes to 3 hours after sleep onset, is more common in males, and may persist into adulthood in 1% of patients. Most 2-year-olds are able to remain dry during the day;. by age 3, nearly 75% of children also remain dry during the night. Nocturnal enuresis affects 10% of 5-year-olds, 7% of 10-year-olds, and 1% of 15-year-olds. Frequency shows no signs of diminishing; most of these children wet the bed several nights a week. At least 90% of children with nocturnal enuresis are reliably dry during the day. Since such a large proportion of young children wet their beds, the term *enuresis* should not be used until a child is 4–5 years old. There are wide variations in reported prevalence rates. Nocturnal enuresis alone, particularly if primary, is both a disorder of maturation and a genetic trait. Patients are 3–4 times more likely to have a parent who had been enuretic than are control subjects. They are also more likely to have excessive diffuse slow background activity on the electroencephalogram. Minor neurological dysfunction is common, including mild hypotonia, problems with coordination or fine manipulation, and mild dyskinesias. Many also have learning problems, emotional difficulties, and problems with relationships. The most effective treatment is dry bed training. Some therapists use conditioning techniques (e.g., alarms) and pharmacotherapy (e.g., imipramine). Imipramine (25–100 mg) can reduce enuresis within 1 week, but long-term success is poor: only 15% of children remain dry after drug discontinuation. Most relapse after 3 months. Successful treatment of enuresis is more likely when the problem is maturational, and less likely when there is a psychiatric disorder in the child, severe family stress, absence of concern by child and parents, urological dysfunction, and developmental delay. Day wetting and maternal intolerance of enuresis are poor prognostic signs. See **desmopressin; encopresis.**

environmental illness   See **ecologic illness.**

enzyme   Protein that takes apart or puts together other molecules. Enzymes are responsible for the overall active metabolism of the cell, including biosynthetic and degradative processes that produce and use energy. Each enzyme is responsible for just one specific reaction. Absence of an enzyme may prevent important biochemical reactions and may also lead to build-up of abnormal substances that can act as "poisons." Enzymes are the products of gene expression. Each enzyme is specified (coded for) by a particular gene in the genome. When the body does not manufacture a needed enzyme, it is usually because of recessive inheritance (e.g., phenylketonuria, an inherited condition that leads to mental retardation, is due to reduced activity of the enzyme phenylalanine hydroxylase).

enzyme immunoassay   (EIA) Sensitive screening test for prescription drugs and drugs of abuse based on antibody-antigen reaction detection technology. Cross-between compounds can be problematic and lead to false-positive results. See **enzyme multiplied-immunoassay test.**

enzyme induction   Increase in liver enzyme activity due to chronic use of a drug (e.g., barbiturates, meprobamate, methyprylon, glutethimide). Enzyme induction has little effect on the peak intensity of drug action, but decreases the drug's duration of action. On cessation of the drug, enzyme activity declines over a period of 6–8 weeks.

enzyme-linked and fluorescent immunoassay (ELISA) Widely available, frequently used test in the screening of both symptomatic and asymptomatic cases of human immunodeficiency virus (HIV) infection. Its sensitivity is equal to that of other immunological procedures with a simple protocol and quick results (Green S. Use of a toxicology laboratory. *Crit Care Q* 1982;2:19–23).

enzyme multiplied-immunoassay test   (EMIT) Test using an enzyme-labeled tracer that can detect the presence of most drugs for up to 72 hours after last use. It is a faster, more automated technology than EIA. Experts advise against drawing definite conclusions about illicit drug use based on EMIT alone (Verebey K. Cocaine abuse: detection by laboratory methods: *In* Washton AM, Gold MS [eds], *Cocaine: A Clinician's Handbook.* New York: Guilford, 1987, pp 214–218).

EOG ratio   Electrical potential in the light-adapted eye divided by the potential in adaption to the dark. It is an indirect measure of light-induced electrical changes recorded by an electroretinogram. Also called "Arden ratio." See **electro-oculography.**

eosinophilia myalgia syndrome   (EMS) Toxic, potentially fatal disorder attributed to a contaminant in or of tryptophan, accidentally produced by one manufacturer. This newly recognized disorder occurred in epidemic proportions during 1989. More than 1,500 persons in the United States became ill; at least 27 died. Hallmarks are eosinophilia and myalgia, principally in the proximal limbs, that is often disabling. Other acute symptoms include malaise, fatigue, irritability, fever, dyspnea, edema, arthralgia, neuropathy, and rashes. In some respects the illness resembles the toxic oil syndrome that occurred in Spain in 1981, after use of denatured rapeseed oil. A prospective follow-up (16–30 months) on 32 EMS patients from the 1989 cohort found that since illness onset, three had died and 93% of survivors continued to have symptoms. Features most commonly associated with long-term disability are scleroderma (skin thickening), sensorimotor polyneuropathy, proximal myopathy, and severe episodic myalgia.

E-Pam See **diazepam.**

ephedrine Orally active sympathomimetic drug used mainly as a nasal decongestant and pressor agent. It causes mild amphetamine-like stimulation effect; increased blood pressure, heart rate and circulation; heart palpitations; nervousness; anxiety; and insomnia. Some clandestine laboratories use it as a precursor in the illicit production of amphetamine and methamphetamine. Others use it as a common ingredient in look-alike amphetamine that is sold as a street drug. Long term illicit use may cause a toxic psychosis.

ephedrine + moclobemide See **moclobemide + ephedrine.**

ephedrone Drug of abuse (street name, "jeff") synthesized from ephedrine. It apparently originated in the USSR, spreading from there to parts of Europe and elsewhere. Fatal overdoses have been reported, but little is known of its pathology or clinical pharmacology (Zhingel K, Dovensky W, Crossman A, Allen A. Ephedrone: 2-methylamino-1-phenylpropan-1-one [Jeff]. *J Forens Sci* 1991;36:915–920).

epidemiologic catchment area survey (ECA) Multisite, general population study of prevalence and rates of psychiatric disorders and associated health services utilization conducted in the United States in the early 1980s in collaboration with the staff of the National Institute of Mental Health (NIMH). Approximately 18,000 general population respondents 18 years of age and older, living in five U.S. communities, were personally interviewed at index (structured interviews for the recognition of mental disorders), contacted by telephone approximately 6 months later, and personally reinterviewed 1 year later. Each ECA site used the Diagnostic Interview Schedule (DIS), which generated DSM-III definitions of psychiatric disorders. Results show that about 15.4% of the general U.S. population had one or more DSM-III disorders 1 month before the interview. A substance abuse problem was noted in 11.5%. The ECA pro-

vides the most complete data about the prevalence of mental disorders in persons of all ages.

epidemiological psychiatry Investigation of the causes and control of rapidly spreading psychiatric disorders (e.g., adolescent suicide) suddenly erupting in a local community.

epidemiological study designs Case reports; case series; cross-sectional, ecological, case-control, cohort, and randomized clinical trials (experimental studies).

epidemiology Study of the etiology, natural course, frequency, distribution, and prognosis of disease and disability in defined populations. It includes (a) establishing dimensions of morbidity and mortality as a function of person, place, and time; (b) quantifying risk of developing a disorder as a function of post-agent and environmental factors; (c) identifying and defining syndromes; (d) describing the natural history in terms of onset, duration, recurrence, complications, disability, and mortality; (e) identifying factors that influence or predict clinical course; (f) identifying causes of disorders and relating disabilities; and (g) evaluating specific methods of prevention and control. In the last 15 years, the scope of epidemiology has broadened to include clinical epidemiology, decision analysis, health services research, clinical intervention, and outcomes research. Epidemiological research can contribute to clinical decision making by identifying patients at risk and helping the clinician determine when appropriate clinical interventions are warranted. The epidemiologist's "patients" are whole populations, in which illnesses are measured by averages, percentages, rates, and risks. In public health schools, epidemiology and statistics are usually taught in parallel.

epilepsy Paroxysmal, transitory disturbance of brain function that develops suddenly, ceases spontaneously and exhibits a conspicuous tendency to recurrence. Clinically it consists of sudden onset of loss of consciousness, with or without tonic spasm and clonic contractions of the musculature. Forms vary depending on site of origin, extent of the area involved, and nature of etiological factors. Epilepsy is a symptom, not a disease.

epilepsy, automatic See **seizure, complex partial** (preferred term).

epilepsy/electroencephalography The most helpful laboratory test in the diagnosis of epilepsy, because an abnormal tracing with epileptiform features supports the diagnosis of epileptic seizures and often gives clues to the location and type of disturbance. However, an abnormal electroencephalogram (EEG) is inadequate for the diagnosis of epileptic seizures, and a normal EEG does not rule out the diagnosis.

epilepsy, Jacksonian   Form of partial seizures that begins with clonic movements (in the thumb and index finger, the angle of the mouth, or the great toe) and increases in severity and spreads to involve large segments of the limb, and then other portions of the body, at which point consciousness is usually lost. This type of seizure almost always indicates organic disease of the precentral cortex. See **seizure, focal motor.**

epilepsy, juvenile myoclonic   (JME) Common, idiopathic generalized epileptic syndrome that accounts for between 5.4% and 10.2% of epilepsy cases. Patients may experience generalized tonic-clonic seizures, myoclonic jerks, and typical absences. It typically occurs in a teenager who has a generalized tonic-clonic seizure on rising early in the morning after a late-night party, possibly with alcohol. Neurological examination shows no abnormality, but there is a family history of seizures. Myoclonic jerks generally appear in the mid-teens, preceding generalized tonic-clonic seizures by a few months. Jerks occur mainly on awakening, are usually but not always bilateral, and are not associated with impairment of consciousness. They may be so severe that the patient drops objects or falls, but often are mild and interpreted as clumsiness or tremor. A series of jerks may herald a generalized tonic-clonic seizure. About one-third of patients experience typical absences that may antedate myoclonic jerks by several years. Seizure-precipitating factors include sleep deprivation, alcohol, stress, menstruation, and flashing lights. Over 80% of patients are well controlled by sodium valproate alone or in combination with clonazepam or phenobarbital, but relapse is the norm on discontinuation of antiepileptic medication even after many years seizure-free. Carbamazepine is not effective (Anon. Diagnosing juvenile myoclonic epilepsy. *Lancet* 1992;340:759–760; Grunewald RA, Panayiotopoulos CP. Juvenile myoclonic epilepsy. A review. *Arch Neurol* 1993; 50:594–598).

epilepsy, nocturnal   Movement disorder that can be distinguished from nocturnal myoclonus and restless legs syndrome by sleep electroencephalographic evaluation.

epilepsy, post-traumatic   Occurrence of tonic-clonic seizure following head injury. Onset may be immediate (seconds after an acute head injury); on the second day after the trauma, usually at the height of cerebral edema; or late (between 2 and 3 months after the injury).

epilepsy, psychomotor   See **seizure, complex partial** (preferred term).

epilepsy, temporal lobe   See **seizure, complex partial** (preferred term).

epilepsy, visceral   Form of focal epilepsy manifested by visceral sensations, usually referable to the gastrointestinal, cardiorespiratory, or genitourinary systems.

epileptic absence   See **absence, epileptic.**

epileptic equivalent   Behaviors occurring in people with epilepsy that are inappropriate, unpredictable, and without apparent environmental cause. Complex partial seizures might account for the behaviors in some individuals, as there is an association between such seizures and behavior disorders. A small number of people with epilepsy tend to be more irritable before, or sometimes after, seizures.

epileptic neuron   Major features are autonomous, sustained abnormal firing and increased electrical activity. Instability of the membrane, producing paroxysmal depolarization shifts, has been ascribed to the epileptic neurons. An epileptogenic focus contains both strongly and weakly epileptic cells (groups 1 and 2 epileptic neurons). Group 1 generates the epileptic activity, whereas group 2 gradually follows the lead and produces synchronous epileptic firing.

epileptic psychosis   Episodic or chronic alteration of reality contact frequently associated with clearly visible or subtle seizure manifestations and deficits in higher cerebral functions. Psychosis may be manifested by delusions, illusions, hallucinations, mood disturbances, and irrational behavior, often of an aggressive type. There is a temporal relationship between seizures and psychosis, with a prolonged (e.g., 14 years) interval between onset of the seizure disorder and that of psychosis. The term *epileptic psychosis* is preferred to *schizophrenia-like* and *schizophrenia* to describe psychotic symptoms in patients with epilepsy.

epileptic seizure   See **seizure, epileptic.**

epileptiform   Resembling epilepsy.

epileptiform seizure   See **seizure, epileptiform.**

epileptoid   Resembling epilepsy.

Epilim   See **valproate.**

epinephrine   (EPI) Member of the catecholamine family that is a hormone and a beta-adrenergic agonist neurotransmitter. It is a powerful stimulator of the sympathetic nervous system, producing many of the physiological changes associated with states of fear or anxiety. It is contraindicated for phenothiazine-induced hypotension. Also called "adrenaline."

epinephrine + amoxapine   See **amoxapine + epinephrine.**

episode Period (onset to resolution) during which an illness exists.

episodic dyscontrol Episodic, violent outbursts with loss of control over aggressive behavior, on minimal provocation. It is often related to alcohol ingestion in those with a history of childhood hyperkinesis and truancy. It is best understood as epilepsy-like dysfunction of limbic structures in the temporal lobe that responds well to diphenylhydantoin, carbamazepine, and other anticonvulsants (Lewin J, Sumners D. Successful treatment of episodic dyscontrol with carbamazepine. *Br Med J* 1992; 161:261–262).

episodic memory See **memory, episodic.**

epistasis Interaction between the products of two genes at different loci, in which one gene prevents the phenotypic expression of the other.

Epital See **carbamazepine.**

Epitol See **carbamazepine.**

epitope Portion of a protein molecule that elicits an antibody response. Any protein contains many epitopes. Monoclonal antibodies can be produced that will recognize only a specific epitope of a protein. Thus, alterations of an epitope (for example, by phosphorylation) can be manifested in altered antigenicity to a monoclonal antibody. The ALZ 50 monoclonal antibody recognizes a phosphorylation event on a specific epitope of the tau protein.

Epival See **valproate.**

epoch Measure of duration of the sleep recording. It is typically 20 or 30 seconds, depending on the paper speed of the polysomnograph, and corresponds to one page of the polysomnogram.

epoetin Genetically engineered human recombinant erythropoietin (protein that enhances red blood cell formation) that is chemically identical to endogenous erythropoietin. It can be abused for its ergogenic potential. Endurance athletes who abuse it may be at greater risk for toxic effects through fluid loss during competition; hematocrits may increase by 0.1 or more during a marathon race. Toxic reaction potential is greater than with blood doping, since continued, inappropriate use of epoetin will lead to higher pre-event hematocrits than is possible with blood doping. In addition, blood doping requires assistance of trained medical personnel for withdrawal, storage, and reconstitution of red blood cells; "black market" epoetin can be self-administered without medical supervision, further increasing risk. Council on Scientific Affairs of the American Medical Association opposes use of epoetin to enhance athletic performance and urges physicians not to prescribe it for this purpose and not to assist endurance

athletes to obtain and self-administer it to enhance performance (Flaherty KK, Gremin AM, Vlasses PH. Epoetin: human recombinant erythropoietin. *Clin Pharm* 1989;8:769–782; Adamson JW, Vaponek D. Recombinant erythropoietin to improve athletic performance. *N Engl J Med* 1991;324:698–699; Scott WC. The abuse of erythropoietin to enhance athletic performance. *JAMA* 1990;264:1660). See **blood doping; ergogenic drug.**

epsilon Specific opioid receptor for beta-endorphin.

Epstein-Barr virus Naturally occurring virus used to immortalize lymphocytes taken from individuals so that their DNA can be permanently saved by deep freezing the cells. In this way, a cell bank representing the genomes of all members of many families can be produced. The DNA samples are used for molecular genetic analysis (e.g., restriction fragment length polymorphism determinations).

Equanil See **meprobamate.**

equilibrium State of being evenly balanced.

Equilium See **tiapride.**

Equipoise See **boldenone undencyclate.**

ergogenic drug Performance-enhancing agent used by athletes to gain an athletic advantage in strength or endurance. Strength enhancers include anabolic/androgenic steroids; endurance enhancers include amphetamines and epoetin. These drugs are banned by the National Collegiate Athletic Association and International Olympic Committee.

ergoline Any of a recently developed group of dopamine agonists including bromocriptine, lisuride, and pergolide. They are ergot derivatives and appear to be partial agonists at presynaptic dopamine D_2 receptors.

ergoloid mesylate See **dihydroergotoxine.**

ergot Product of a fungus that grows on grains; it consists of ergot alkaloids and amines such as histamine and tyramine.

ergot alkaloid One of a group of compounds that were the first adrenergic blocking agents discovered. They act as partial agonists or antagonists at alpha-adrenergic and dopaminergic receptors. They possess antiparkinson activity because they directly activate dopamine receptors in the basal ganglia. Bromocriptine and pergolide are examples.

erotomania See **compulsive sexual behavior.**

error, alpha False-positive result. The error is made when the null hypothesis is true, because the result of the test of significance is rejected or declared false. It consists of concluding that there is a difference when in fact one does not exist. Also called "type I error."

error, beta False-negative result. The error is made when the null hypothesis is false, but because of the results of the test of significance, it is not rejected or declared false. It consists of concluding that there is no difference, when in fact one does exist. It frequently occurs as a result of insufficient N's and/or relatively insensitive measures of change. Also called "type II error."

error, inborn · See **inborn error.**

error mean square Over-group summation of square of variation between group means and the observed values within those groups, divided by the associated degree of freedom. Usually it is the denominator of the F test in analysis of variance (ANOVA).

error, probable See **median deviation.**

error, random In statistics, noise that accompanies observations carrying the desired information.

error, systematic Error that often has a recognizable source (e.g., faulty measuring instrument or pattern) and is consistently wrong in a particular direction.

error, type I See **error, alpha.**

error, type II See **error, beta.**

erythrocyte choline Potential indirect measure of cholinergic function in the central nervous system. It is elevated modestly in patients with affective illnesses, psychoses, dementia, and other neuropsychiatric disorders when compared to controls. Investigators have documented a dramatic rise in erythrocyte choline concentration during lithium therapy, which probably does not parallel a similar rise in the brain. There is a need for much more study to answer this question. Lithium is the only drug known to produce such an effect. It is possible that pretreatment or post-treatment erythrocyte choline concentrations may predict response to lithium, even though plasma levels are relatively low. This is especially true in geriatric patients.

erythromycin + benzodiazepine See **benzodiazepine + erythromycin.**

erythromycin + carbamazepine See **carbamazepine + erythromycin.**

erythromycin + midazolam See **midazolam + erythromycin.**

Eserine See **physostigmine.**

Esilgan See **estazolam.**

Eskalith See **lithium.**

Eskalith CR See **lithium.**

Eskapar See **tranylcypromine.**

Eskazine See **trifluoperazine.**

esmolol (Brevibloc) Beta$_1$ selective (cardioselective) adrenergic receptor blocking agent with a very short duration of action (elimination half-life is approximately 9 minutes). It is commonly used to control the hyperdynamic response to electroconvulsive therapy (ECT). It significantly reduces heart rate, systolic and diastolic pressure, and length of ECT-induced seizure. Since esmolol and other beta-blockers may increase risk of bradycardia or asystole if a subconvulsive electrical stimulus is administered, it is generally agreed that pretreatment with an anticholinergic agent (usually glycopyrrolate or atropine) is indicated when beta-blockers are administered with ECT (Kellner CH, Nixon DW, Bernstein HJ. ECT-drug interactions: a review. *Psychopharmacol Bull* 1991;27: 595–609).

"essence" Street name for analog of methamphetamine.

essential tremor See **tremor, essential.**

estazolam (Cannoc; Domnamid; Esilgan; Eurodin; Julodin; Kainever; Nuctalon; Prosom; Somnatrol; Tasedan) Triazolo-benzodiazepine hypnotic with intermediate half-life (10–24 hours). Clearance can be accelerated in smokers compared with nonsmokers; decrease in half-life is presumably due to liver P450 enzyme reduction by smoking. It is an effective and safe hypnotic in insomniacs with concomitant psychiatric illness, including major depression. In the insomniacs with major depression, it may not only relieve depression-related insomnia, but contribute to improvement of depressive symptoms. Initial dose for adults and healthy elderly patients is 1–2 mg at bedtime. An initial dose of 0.5 mg is recommended for small or debilitated older patients. Like other benzodiazepines, its effects may be potentiated by anticonvulsants, antihistamines, alcohol, barbiturates, monoamine oxidase inhibitors, narcotics, neuroleptics, or other drugs that produce central nervous system depression. Most common adverse effects are somnolence, hypokinesia, dizziness, and abnormal coordination. Dosage increase should be done slowly in the elderly (Vogel GW, Morris D. Effects of estazolam on sleep, performance, and memory: long-term sleep laboratory study of elderly insomniacs. *J Clin Pharmacol* 1992;32:647–651). Schedule IV; pregnancy risk category X.

estimation In epidemiology, process of using information from a sample to draw conclusions about the parameter values in a population.

Estrace See **estradiol.**

estradiol (Estrace) Potent, naturally occurring estrogen in mammals. It is used therapeutically as estrogen replacement therapy. See **catecholestrogen.**

estrogen antagonist See **antiestrogen.**

estrone Metabolite of estradiol that is less potent than the parent.

"estupefaciente" Chemical families of drugs (e.g., morphine, cocaine, lysergic acid diethylamide [LSD]) with pharmacological effects on the central nervous system without links other than the potential for drug dependence. The term is used in Europe and widely in Spain by the general population, police, lawyers, politicians, toxicologists, and medical practitioners. It should be abandoned, since it serves no useful purpose (Alloza J-L. Opiophobia and cancer pain. *Lancet* 1993;341:1473–1474).

Esucos   See **dixyrazine.**

ethacrynic acid   (Edecrin) Potassium-retaining diuretic that over time may moderately increase lithium blood level. See **lithium + ethacrynic acid.**

ethanol   (ethyl alcohol) See **alcohol.**

ethchlorvynol   (Avenol; Normoson; Placidyl) Tertiary carbinol, nonbarbiturate, nonbenzodiazepine hypnotic, possibly the only one that does not stimulate hepatic microsomal oxidizing systems. It is as effective (750 mg) as a short-acting barbiturate (100 mg). Abuse and dependence have occurred. Schedule IV; pregnancy risk category C.

ethchlorvynol + maprotiline   Co-administration may cause tachycardia and delirium.

ethinamate   (Valmed; Valmid) Short-acting, nonbenzodiazepine hypnotic that is rapidly absorbed after oral administration. It is best used for limited periods. Abuse and dependence have occurred. Schedule IV; pregnancy risk category C.

Ethmozine   See **moricizine.**

ethnomedicine   Study of how illness problems are realized and dealt with in different societies with emphasis on social and cultural factors (Hughes CC. Medical care, section I: ethnomedicine. *In* Sills DL [ed], *International Encyclopedia of the Social Sciences*, vol 10. New York: Macmillan, 1968).

ethology   Study of the characteristic behavior patterns of animals.

ethopharmacology   Study of drugs in humans.

ethopropazine   (Parsidol) Antihistaminic/anticholinergic drug used for the treatment of parkinsonism and acute early-onset extrapyramidal reactions induced by neuroleptics. Daily doses are 50–200 mg.

ethopropazine + fluoxetine   No adverse interaction in depressed Parkinson8s disease patients has been reported.

ethosuximide   (Emeside; Zarontin) Anticonvulsant used in the treatment of absence (petit mal) epilepsy. Initial dose is low; it is gradually adjusted according to number of seizures and presence of any side effects. Usual adult dose is 750–2250 mg/day; optimum daily dose is around 20 mg/kg. It can be given 2 or 3 times daily. Therapeutic serum concentration range is 40–100 µg/ml. Mild, usually transient side effects may occur initially. These include apathy, drowsiness, headache, unsteadiness, loss of appetite, nausea, and vomiting. Skin rashes rarely develop. Changes in blood cells, also reported very rarely, include anemia and lowered resistance to infection. Ethosuximide should not be combined with other agents known to cause blood dyscrasias (e.g., carbamazepine). Blood tests are recommended to minimize risk of adverse hematologic effects. Pregnancy risk category D. See **absence, epileptic.**

ethosuximide + carbamazepine   See **carbamazepine + ethosuximide.**

ethotoin   Hydantoin derivative anticonvulsant. See **hydantoin.**

ethrohydrobupropion   Pharmacologically active metabolite of bupropion.

ethyl alcohol   See **alcohol.**

ethyl chloride   (Ethyl Gaz; Ethyl Four Star) Drug used in spray form by physical therapists, sports trainers, etc., for treating musculotendinous pathology. It is a widely available volatile liquid that may be abused. It can produce anesthesia, coma, and death when inhaled.

Ethyl Gaz   See **ethyl chloride.**

Ethyl Four Star   See **ethyl chloride.**

ethylene glycol   Abused "household" intoxicant that has proven to be lethal in almost a third of poisoning cases. In Poland between 1980 and 1990, of 332 ethylene glycol poisoning patients brought to the Warsaw Poison Control Center, 98 died (Poland RV. Curbing ethylene glycol abuse. *Lancet* 1993;341:169).

ethylestrenol   (Maxibolan) 17-alpha-ethyl testosterone derivative anabolic steroid.

etiology   Scientific study of the causes of diseases.

etiracetam   (Soften) Drug with nootropic properties. See **nootropic drug.**

etizolam   (Depas; Pasaden) New benzodiazepine anxiolytic with a therapeutic effect comparable to that of alprazolam.

etomidate   (Amidate) Nonbarbiturate, ultrashort acting anesthetic that enhances seizure activity in humans. It is only given intravenously. Onset of action is rapid, beginning in 60 seconds, and duration of action is usually 3–5 minutes. It is compatible with commonly used preanesthetic agents. Studies to date indicate that it is safe, with few complications, for unilateral and bilateral electroconvulsive therapy (ECT). Etomidate allows for longer seizures during ECT. It is equivalent to methohexital and thiopental (Greenberg L, Boccio R, Fink M. A comparison of etomidate and methohexital anesthesia for electroconvulsive therapy. *Ann Clin Psychiatry* 1989;1:39–42; Chirstensen P, Kragh-Sorenson P, Sonerson C, et al. EEG-monitored ECT. A comparison of the seizure duration under anaesthesia with hydnomidat-etomidate and thiopentone. *Con-*

vuls Ther 1986;2:145–150; Kovac AL, Pardo M. A comparison between etomidate and methohexital for anesthesia in ECT. *Convuls Ther* 1993;8:118–125; Trzepacz PT, Weniger FC, Greenhouse J. Etomidate anesthesia increases seizure duration during ECT. *Gen Hosp Psychiatry* 1993;15:115–120). It is an acceptable alternative to methohexital, especially when barbiturates may be contraindicated; however, it is infrequently used by anesthesiologists because of reports of cortical adrenal collapse, arrhythmias, and death. Pregnancy risk category C.

etoperidone   M-halophenylpiperazine that affects serotonergic function and may have psychotropic functions. Compared with other commonly used antidepressants, efficacy is similar and tolerability is better.

etorphine   (M99) Potent opioid produced from thebaine that is used mainly in the immobilization of large animals.

Etrafon   See **amitriptyline + perphenazine.**

Etrafon-A   perphenazine 4 mg + amitriptyline 10 mg.

Etrafon-D   perphenazine 2 mg + amitriptyline 25 mg.

Etrafon-F   perphenazine 4 mg + amitriptyline 25 mg.

Etrafon-M   perphenazine 2 mg + amitriptyline 10 mg.

Etrafon-2-10   perphenazine 2 mg + amitriptyline 10 mg.

euchromatin   Substance that shows the staining behavior characteristic of the majority of chromosomal material.

eugenics   Attempt to improve a species by controlling hereditary factors in mating.

eugenics, negative   Policies and programs intended to reduce the occurrence of genetically determined disease.

eugenics, positive   Systematic, planned genetic changes to improve individuals or their offspring.

Euhypnos   See **temazepam.**

eukaryote   Nuclear material surrounded by a membrane.

Eunal   See **lisuride.**

Eunerpan   See **melperone.**

euphoria   Morbid or abnormal sense of well-being.

euphoriant   Agent capable of producing a sense of euphoria or well-being.

Eurodin   See **estazolam.**

Euthroid   See **thyroxine.**

euthymia   Normal range of mood that is intermediate between an elevated mood (more cheerful than normal, associated with feelings of confidence and well-being that are not excessive or pathological) and depression.

Eutonyl   See **pargyline.**

Evamyl   See **lormetazepam.**

"Eve"   See **3,4-methylenedioxyethamphetamine (MDEA).**

event   Single outcome (or set of outcomes) from an experiment.

event-related potential   (ERP) Computer-averaged brain waves measuring electrophysiological brain reactions to stimuli. It is a powerful tool to investigate information and linguistic processing. ERPs provide information about the nature and timing of neuronal events independent of behavioral data such as reaction time. They also provide information about the topographic distribution of neuronal events, which is particularly important because language functions are believed to be largely lateralized.

Everone   See **testosterone enanthate.**

E-Vista   See **hydroxyzine.**

evoked potential   (EP) Electrophysiological measurement in which a sensory (flash of light, tone) or cognitive signal stimulates a response that is detected from the scalp or cerebral cortex and presumably represents brain responsiveness to a stimulus. The EP is reproduced as an averaged tracing with latency (stimulus onset to response) and amplitude (height of response) within a series of generated waveforms. The reaction of the nervous system or the evoked potential to the stimulation may then be assessed. EPs appear as stable sequences of electroencephalograph peaks after appropriate stimuli and abnormalities reflect subclinical impairment of central sensory pathways. Also called "evoked response."

evoked response   See **evoked potential.**

evolution   1. Development process in which an organ or organism becomes more complex by the differentiation of its parts. 2. Theory that all forms of life developed from earlier forms by hereditary transmission of slight or large variation in successive generations.

exact test   Statistical test based on the actual null probability distribution of study data rather than normal approximation. The most common exact test is Fisher's.

excess risk   Statistic, calculated from epidemiologic studies, that is the arithmetic difference between incidence rates. Also called "risk difference."

excessive sleepiness   See **sleepiness, excessive.**

excitatory amino acid   (EAA) See **glutamate.**

excitement   Hyperactivity as reflected in accelerated motor behavior, heightened responsivity to stimuli, hypervigilance, or excessive mood lability. It may range from mild to extreme; the latter seriously interferes with eating and sleeping, and makes interpersonal interactions virtually impossible. Acceleration of speech and motor activity may result in incoherence and exhaustion. These states typically are associated with drug intoxication, mania, and catatonia.

excitotoxin   Substance that induces toxic excitement.

executive deficit   See **executive function.**

executive function   Ability, mediated primarily by the prefrontal cortex, to initiate an appropriate set of responses to the environment, maintain these responses and shift to a new set of responses when necessary (e.g., planning, sequencing, concept formation, cognitive set shifting, and cognitive set maintenance). Without executive functions, behaviors important for independent living (cooking, dressing, self-care) may break down. Executive deficits undermine the independence of many elderly patients and lead to common behavior problems. Schizophrenic patients are particularly deficient on measures of executive functioning; deficits may be in formation of concepts, not their application (Goldman RS, Axelrod BN, Tompkins LM. Effect of instructional cues on schizophrenic patients' performance on the Wisconsin Card Sorting Test. *Am J Psychiatry* 1992;149:1718–1722). Bipolar disorder patients also have deficits in executive functions, indicating that frontal lobe pathology is not specific to schizophrenia, although the specific nature of the pathology may be.

executive function assessment   Tests include (a) Executive Interview; (b) Mini-Mental State Test; (c) Wisconsin Card Sorting Test; (d) Trail Making Test parts A and B; and (e) verbal fluency test.

exhibitionism   Sexual deviation in which sexual stimulation or gratification is gained from exposing genitals to a person of the opposite sex in a public place. The exposure may be accompanied by masturbation.

existential   Relating to the philosophy that a person ultimately must accept responsibility for his or her own actions. The responsibility may be the source of great anxiety (Bloch S, Crouch E. *Therapeutic Factors in Group Psychotherapy.* Oxford: Oxford University Press, 1985).

exogenous depression   See **depression, exogenous.**

exogenous metabolic brain disease   See **delirium.**

exon   Part of a gene that encodes information present in messenger ribonucleic acid (mRNA). RNA is generated in the process called transcription, in which information present in a gene is converted to an RNA molecule that is colinear with DNA of the gene. The RNA molecule, referred to as the primary transcript, undergoes a series of reactions (capping, polyadenylation, splicing) that ultimately results in formation of the mRNA. RNA splicing is the process whereby certain sequences (called introns) are removed from the primary transcript. Generally, exons code for functional domains of the final protein product. For example, the portion of many neurotransmitter receptors that span the membranes (transmembrane domain) is coded for within one discrete exon. Often, one gene can produce more than one protein by altering the exons present in the mRNA. These "splice variants" lead to proteins with different properties. Examples include the various forms (isotypes) of the amyloid precursor protein gene and the long and short forms of the D_2 dopamine receptor. See **intron.**

expected frequency   In contingency tables, frequency observed if the null hypothesis is true.

experiment   Test or trial with a planned process of data collection concerning a hypothesis.

experimental design   Logical framework of an experiment that maximizes the probability of obtaining or detecting real effects and minimizes the likelihood of ambiguities regarding the significance of the experimentally observed differences.

experimental illicit drug use   World Health Organization (WHO) classification of drug use defined as short-term, nonpatterned trials of a drug, primarily motivated by curiosity and a desire to experience anticipated effects. It generally begins among close friends. After the first few uses, the person may lose interest or begin the next phase in chemical use—recreational use. See **recreational illicit drug use.**

experimental therapeutic study   See **study, experimental therapeutic.**

experimenter bias   See **bias, experimenter.**

explicit memory   See **memory, explicit.**

exposure in imagination   Form of exposure therapy for agoraphobia in which the patient must imagine returning to avoided situations. It is not as effective as exposure in practice. Also called "in vitro exposure."

exposure in practice   Form of exposure therapy for agoraphobia in which the patient returns to actual avoided situations. It is more effective than exposure in imagination. Also called "in vivo exposure."

exposure therapy   Treatment for agoraphobia in which patients are repeatedly exposed to any anxiety-provoking situations that have persistently been avoided. Methods include desensitization, exposure in imagination, exposure in practice, and flooding.

expressed emotion (EE) Concept introduced by Brown and colleagues (1958) to explain why some schizophrenic patients relapse despite adequate drug therapy. These authors observed that the relapse rate in patients who lived with critical, overly involved, or hostile families was more than double that in patients whose families did not show these characteristics (Brown GW, Carstairs GM, Topping G. Post-hospital adjustment of chronic mental patients. *Lancet* 1958;2:685–689). The effect of EE on schizophrenics was more pronounced if patients spent more than 35 hours a week in close contact with their family (Brown GW, Monk EM, Carstairs GM, Wing JK. Influence of family life on the course of schizophrenic illness. *Br J Prev Soc Med* 1962;16:55–68). Evidence for a relationship between EE and relapse has remained strong. In a review of 26 studies involving more than 1300 patients in several countries, median relapse rate for patients from high-EE families was 48% at 6–9 months after discharge from the hospital, versus 21% for patients from low-EE families. In some cases, the difference persisted for 2 years (Kavanaugh DJ. Recent developments in expressed emotion and schizophrenia. *Br J Psychiatry* 1992;160:601–620). A relationship between EE and relapse does not necessarily mean that high EE is causal; families could become critical in response to a patient who is very ill and more likely to relapse. If this were so, a correlation could be expected between EE and symptom severity, yet such a correlation is not typical. Even when compliance is assured with long-acting depot antipsychotic drugs, relapse rates in patients from high-EE families greatly exceed those in patients from low-EE families. Thus, it is hard to avoid the conclusion that emotional climate can alter the course of a schizophrenic illness (Anon. Expressed emotion in schizophrenia. *Lancet* 1992;340:1007–1008). To improve relapse rates, various types of psychosocial family interventions are now used. In most cases, they not only diminish EE levels, but lower relapse rates to levels seen in low-EE families (Lam DH. Psychosocial family intervention in schizophrenia: a review of empirical studies. *Psychol Med* 1991;21:423–441).

expression 1. Way in which information contained in a gene is converted into a trait manifested by the cell. 2. Process in which the DNA nucleotide sequence of a gene is converted by transcription and translation into the protein, which serves a unique function in the cell.

expression vector Specific class of recombinant constructs engineered so that the specific cDNA cloned into the plasmid will be expressed in either bacterial or eukaryotic cell types. Bacterial expression vectors contain the requisite control elements to enable expression of a cDNA in strains of *Escherichia coli* for purposes of generating large amounts of a recombinant protein. Eukaryotic expression vectors contain the regulatory elements necessary to allow expression of a cloned cDNA in an appropriate eukaryotic cell. The eukaryotic expression vectors generally contain a promoter/enhancer system (such as that from cytomegalovirus) that drives the expression of the inserted cDNA.

expressivity Extent to which a gene is expressed. It is a characteristic of autosomal traits because the same gene may result in clinical manifestations of varying degrees of severity in different individuals. A trait with variable expressivity may range in expression from mild to severe.

extensive metabolizer See **acetylator, rapid.**

external validity How well a test measures what it is supposed to measure and identifies what it is supposed to identify.

exteroception Perception of a cognitive input.

exteroceptive system External surface field of distribution of receptor sense organs.

extinction Behavior modification technique that attempts to reduce the frequency of an undesirable behavior by stopping any reinforcements that have been maintaining the behavior. Depending on the circumstances, it may take some time for extinction to be effective; there is often an initial increase in the behavior followed by gradual decline. Extinction has been widely used with "nuisance" behaviors (e.g., excessive attention-seeking, tantrums, spitting, property destruction).

extraction ratio Ratio of drug clearance to liver blood flow.

extrapyramidal dyskinesia Movement disorder caused by dysfunction of the extrapyramidal motor system. It is manifested by a variety of involuntary movements and postures; muscular rigidity, tremor, and gait disturbance; parkinsonism; chorea; athetosis; and hemiballismus. It may occur as a side effect of neuroleptic and other drugs affecting the dopaminergic system; reactions include akinesia, acute dystonic reactions, akathisia, parkinsonism, and various forms of tardive dyskinesia.

extrapyramidal side effects (EPS) Tremor of the hands, tongue, and facial muscles; paucity of movements; shuffling gait; and acute dystonia that may manifest as muscle spasms and cramps sometimes associated with pain and akathisia. Oculogyric crises may occur in which there is involuntary rolling upward of the eyes for minutes or hours. Occurrence depends, among other things, on the pharmacological structure and dosage of administered neuroleptics and on concomitant use of anticholinergic agents. Age, sex, and individual predisposition also are important factors. See **extrapyramidal dyskinesia.**

extrapyramidal system Polysynaptic neural pathways involving the basal ganglia and related subcortical nuclei that influence motor behavior. The system is mainly responsible for static, postural activities; the pyramidal system is principally involved in voluntary movements.

extreme problematic behavior Term used by Dutch investigators to describe patients who, when no measures are taken, seriously damage themselves or others mentally or physically with the possibility of lasting consequences (intense aggression, serious self-mutilation, or strong suicidal tendency), for whom measures taken to prevent the behavior can have considerable negative consequences (isolation, tying up, being given large dosages of psychopharmaceutical drugs) and for whom an effective treatment is not available.

extrinsic sleep disorder See **sleep disorder, extrinsic.**

eye blink rate Dopamine-mediated clinical sign. Spontaneous eye blink rates are decreased in Parkinson's disease (in which there is decreased central dopamine activity), but increased in Gilles de la Tourette's syndrome and some schizophrenias (in which increased dopamine activity has been implicated). The dopamine agonist amorphine increases blink rates in monkeys and humans. Men blink more frequently than women, whose circulating estrogens are dopamine antagonists. Reduced blink rate has been correlated with reduction of positive symptoms of schizophrenia, especially thought disturbance, in haloperidol-treated chronic schizophrenics. The correlation was particularly clear in patients with normal cerebral ventricles (Karson CN, Bieglow LB, Kleinman JE, et al. Haloperidol-induced changes in blink rate correlate with changes in BPRS score. *Br J Psychiatry* 1982; 140:503–507).

eye tracking, impaired Inability to follow a moving target smoothly with both eyes. It is a fairly common biological correlate of schizophrenia, but may occur in other psychoses, including bipolar disorder, and is found in 7% of control subjects. Impairment persists in schizophrenia during remission and is increased in prevalence among relatives of schizophrenic patients. Eye tracking impairment is a state-independent correlate of schizophrenia that may reflect a genetic diathesis to schizophrenic-related disorders. It also may be a nonspecific, "soft sign" of brain damage that may be caused by many factors (Holzman PS, Kringlen E, Matthysse S, et al. A single dominant gene can account for eye tracking dysfunctions in schizophrenia in offspring of discordant twins. *Arch Gen Psychiatry* 1988;45:641–647).

F

face recognition   Test of cognitive processes that assesses ability to recognize faces.

face validity   Whether a test instrument looks as if it will measure what the researcher wishes it to measure. Lack of face validity could make the items appear irrelevant to the patient. Reliance on the apparent validity of a test has been derided as being the equivalent of "faith validity." See **construct validity; content validity.**

factitious disorder   Feigning physical or psychological symptoms because of a need to assume the sick role.

factor   Characteristic that is the focus of inquiry in a study; used in analysis of variance.

factor analysis   Multivariate statistical technique based on observed patterns of correlations between variables. It is sensitive to sample variations in each correlation occurring by chance. It aims at generating hypothetical variates that are weighted sums of observed variates. The former, fewer in number than the latter, are usually expected to describe, summarize, or explain the latter.

factorial design   In analysis of variance, a design in which each subject (or object) receives one level of each factor.

factorial-design trial   Several doses of the test drug, or placebo, combined with several doses of a second drug in a multicelled array. It provides a more complete evaluation of the various doses of the combination and permits unbiased selection of the most effective combination of any two drugs.

factorial design, two-by-two   Design with two factors, each with two levels, measured against each other to ascertain their similarities and differences.

factorial validity   Demonstration that a test or scale is composed of the same factors that it purports to measure.

failed discharge   Readmission to a hospital within a relatively short period of discharge. It is often associated with noncompliance, multiple previous admissions, and personality abnormality, but not other demographic or diagnostic factors.

falls   Every year, thousands of hospitalized psychiatric patients are victims of falls that may or may not result in injury. Factors associated with increased risk include age and medication side effects. Risk of falling increases at ages 60–65; one-third of falls occur in patients over age 70. Falls are a major health problem in old age because of their frequency and physical (e.g., hip fractures), psychological, and social consequences. Medications associated with increased risk include diuretics, sedatives, antihypertensives, and psychotropics (e.g., tricyclic antidepressants and certain phenothiazines) that may produce orthostatic hypotension, especially in the elderly. Demented patients treated with these drugs have a higher rate of falls than comparable, unmedicated patients. Benzodiazepines, especially those with long half-lives, may contribute to falls (Ray WA, Griffin MR, Schaffner W, et al. Psychotropic drug use and the risk of hip fracture. *N Engl J Med* 1987;316:363–369; Sorock GS, Shimkin EE. Benzodiazepine sedatives and the risk of falling in a community-dwelling elderly cohort. *Arch Intern Med* 1988; 148:2441–2444). Drugs and mental disorders may decrease awareness of environmental hazards such as unstable furniture, wet or glossy floors, and poorly soled or ill-fitting shoes (Poster EC, Pelletier LR, Lay K. A retrospective cohort study of falls in a psychiatric inpatient setting. *Hosp Community Psychiatry* 1991; 42:714–720).

false negative   1. Diagnosing an affected individual as unaffected. 2. In genetics, lack of expression of a gene (i.e., incomplete penetrance). 3. In research, concluding that a treatment has no effect when it actually is effective (beta or type II error).

false positive   1. Diagnosing an unaffected individual as affected. 2. In research, concluding that a treatment is effective, when it actually is not (alpha or type I error).

falsifiable hypothesis   See **hypothesis, falsifiable.**

familial   Affecting several members of the same family. The term is commonly but incorrectly used to mean "genetic." See **familial aggregation.**

familial aggregation   Appearance of a syndrome or disorder in several members of the same family. It includes expression of learned family behavior and social and moral values. It appears to be valid for alcoholism, manic-depressive disorders, schizophrenia, and other illnesses.

familial alcoholism   See **alcoholism, familial.**

familial pure depressive disorder   (FPDD) Subtype of primary unipolar depression that occurs in a person with a family history of primary depression but no family history of alcoholism, antisocial personality, or mania. It is the prototype for comparison because it shows both a clinical picture and a family history of primary unipolar depression. FPDD patients are far more likely than depression spectrum disorder patients to have positive results with a dexamethasone suppression test and a higher rate of good response to tricyclic antidepressants (Winokur G, Coryell W. Familial subtypes of unipolar depression: a prospective study of familial pure depressive disease compared to depression spectrum disease. *Biol Psychiatry* 1992;32:1012–1018).

family history method   Obtaining information about the history of psychiatric illness in relatives. It is widely used in psychiatric research. It should be distinguished from direct evaluation of individual relatives (family study method).

family intervention   Specific form of intervention involving family members of alcohol and drug addicts designed to benefit the target patient as well as the family.

family re-enactment   In group therapy, corrective recapitulation of the primary experience within the group (Bloch S, Crouch E. *Therapeutic Factors in Group Psychotherapy*. Oxford: Oxford University Press, 1985).

family risk study   Study to determine the rate of a disorder or trait among the relatives of identified index cases who are affected with the condition.

family study method   Obtaining information on the psychopathological status of the relatives of psychiatric patients by direct evaluation of individual relatives.

family tree   See **genogram.**

famotidine   (Pepcid) Histamine H_2-receptor antagonist used for the treatment of peptic ulcer. At doses used to treat ulcer disease (40 mg/day), it penetrates the blood-brain barrier. It has been reported to improve deficit symptoms in chronic schizophrenias.

Farlotal   See **medroxyprogesterone.**

Farr's law of epidemics   Principle promulgated by William Farr (1840) that epidemics tend to rise and fall in a roughly symmetrical pattern that can be approximated by a normal bell-shaped curve. Its most recent application has been to study the U.S. acquired immunodeficiency syndrome (AIDS) epidemic.

fasciculations   Twitching, undulating muscle movements that are not widespread, coordinated, or sustained enough to cause limb movement. They may follow prolonged muscle activity or be exacerbated by anxiety or caffeine. They may be benign or an early sign of anterior horn cell disease.

fast eating syndrome   Rapid meal consumption, characterized by taking large bites of food and pocketing them in the cheeks. Because mastication is incomplete, large boluses are forced into the pharynx. It is a very common cause of dysphagia and choking incidents among psy-

chiatric inpatients, especially the mentally retarded.

Fastin   See **phentermine.**

fatal toxicity index   (FTI) Number of deaths due to poisoning per million National Health Service prescriptions of a given antidepressant drug in the United Kingdom from 1975 to 1984. Older antidepressants (those introduced before 1970) had a significantly higher FTI (desipramine, 80.2; amitriptyline, 46.5; imipramine, 28.4; nortriptyline, 39.2) than newer antidepressants (those introduced after 1974) (trazodone, 13.6; mianserin, 5.6; nomifensine, 2.5). The change in index scores could be due to differences in the efficacies of the antidepressants in suicidal patients or to differences in toxicity when the antidepressant is taken in overdose as a method of suicide. Whatever the reason, newer antidepressants appear to be associated with a lower incidence of fatalities (Cassidy S, Henry J. Fatal toxicity of antidepressant drugs in overdose. *Br Med J* 1987;295:1021–1024).

fatigue   Abnormal tiring during prolonged mental or physical activity. It is a symptom of many illnesses that makes it difficult for the patient to sustain the same level of activity as normal. Moderate to severe fatigue can be incapacitating.

"fatty"   Street name for a larger than normal marijuana cigarette made of impotent marijuana.

Faverin   See **fluvoxamine.**

Favoxil   See **fluvoxamine.**

F distribution   Ratio of two independent random variables divided by the associated degree of freedom. Each variable has a chi-squared distribution with n and m degrees of freedom. It is the distribution used with the F test in analysis of variance.

febarbamate   (Tymium) Meprobamate derivative anxiolytic that has been used successfully in the treatment of agitated and aggressive states in demented patients, reportedly without causing adverse cognitive effects.

febrile convulsion   See **convulsion, febrile.**

fecal incontinence   Inability to control defecation. It may be functional or organic. Most common causes are constipation and laxative use, neurological disorders, and colorectal disorders. It is less common than urinary incontinence. When it coexists with urinary incontinence in the elderly, there may be common pathophysiological mechanisms. Fecal incontinence from neurological disorders is sometimes amenable to biofeedback therapy. See **encopresis.**

feeblemindedness   See **mental retardation.**

feedback   Giving information to patients about the nature and effects of their behavior. It can be done by such means as direct communication, videotaped replays, and role-playing.

feedback inhibition Capacity of neurons to turn themselves off once activated.

feeling of passivity First-rank symptom of schizophrenia in which emotions, specific bodily movements, or specific sensations are experienced as being caused by an external agency or being under some external control.

feeling of unreality See **depersonalization.**

feigned seizure See **seizure, feigned.**

felbamate (Felbamyl; Felbatol) (FBM) Dicarbamate, related to meprobamate, marketed as an anticonvulsant. It has been reported effective in partial seizures, Lennox-Gestaut syndrome, and atypical absence seizures (Leppik IE, Dreifuss FE, Pledger GW, et al. Felbamate for partial seizures: results of a controlled clinical trial. *Neurology* 1991;41:785–789; The Felbamate Study Group in Lennox-Gestaut Syndrome: efficacy of felbamate in childhood epileptic encephalopathy [Lennox-Gestaut syndrome]. *N Engl J Med* 1993;328:29–33; Thompson G, Kuzniecky R, Faught E. Long-term felbamate add-on therapy in intractable atypical absence seizures. *Neurology* 1993;43[suppl]: A308). In newly diagnosed patients or those who have not taken antiepileptic medications for an extended period, FBM should be started at 1,200 mg/day in divided doses and increased in increments of 600 mg/day every 2 weeks until clinical response is obtained (Sachdeo RC, Sachdeo SK. Tolerability of felbamate [Felbatol, FBM] in newly diagnosed epileptics. *Neurology* 1993;43[suppl]:A308; Sachdeo RC, Kramer LD, Rosenberg A, Sachdeo S. Felbamate monotherapy: controlled trial in patients with partial-onset seizures. *Ann Neurol* 1992;32: 386–392; Sachdeo RC. Felbamate. *Lancet* 1993; 342:300). Seizure control may decrease in some patients at 3,600 mg/day. Co-administration with phenytoin or carbamazepine may reduce seizure frequency.

felbamate + carbamazepine Co-administration increases carbamazepine (CBZ) clearance and decreases CBZ plasma concentration by 28%. If the CBZ pharmacodynamic effect is linear, 20% reduction of CBZ level would be associated with a 20% increase in seizure frequency. Patients treated with the combination may need increased CBZ dosage (Fuerst RH, Graves NM, Leppik IE, et al. A preliminary report on alteration of carbamazepine and phenytoin metabolism by felbamate. *Drug Intell Clin Pharm* 1986;20:465–466; Fuerst RH, Graves NM, Leppik IE, et al. Felbamate increases phenytoin but decreases carbamazepine concentrations. *Epilepsia* 1988;29:488–491). Interaction between felbamate and CBZ may not be as important as that between

felbamate and other anticonvulsants because concentration of CBZ's active epoxide metabolite rises in parallel with the fall in the concentration of the parent drug (Albani F, Theodore WH, Washington P, et al. Effect of felbamate on plasma levels of carbamazepine and its metabolite. *Epilepsia* 1991;32:130–132). CBZ induces felbamate metabolism, resulting in lower-than-expected steady-state concentrations (Wagner ML, Leppik IE, Graves NM, et al. Felbamate serum concentrations: effect of valproate, carbamazepine, phenytoin and phenobarbital. *Epilepsia* 1990;31:642).

felbamate + phenytoin Co-administration increases phenytoin (PHT) plasma concentrations; PHT dosage may have to be reduced 10–30% to maintain stable PHT levels. Felbamate (FBM) is a competitive inhibitor of PHT metabolism since PHT concentrations increase primarily at higher (> 20 mg/kg) FBM doses (Graves RM, Holmes GB, Fuerst GP, Leppik IE. Effect of felbamate on phenytoin and carbamazepine serum concentrations. *Epilepsia* 1989;30:225–229; Leppik IE, Dreifuss FE, Pledger GW, et al. Felbamate for partial seizures: results of a controlled clinical trial. *Neurology* 1991;41:785–789). PHT induces FBM metabolism to give lower-than-expected steady-state concentrations (Wagner ML, Leppik IE, Graves NM, et al. Felbamate serum concentrations: effect of valproate, carbamazepine, phenytoin and phenobarbital. *Epilepsia* 1990;31:642).

felbamate + valproate Felbamate (FBM) increases valproate plasma concentration by about one-third (Wagner ML, Graves NM, Leppik IE, et al. The effect of felbamate on valproate disposition. *Epilepsia* 1991;32[suppl 3]:15). Valproate does not seem to influence FBM clearance (Ward DL, Wagner ML, Perlach JL, et al. Felbamate steady-state pharmacokinetics during co-administration of valproate. *Epilepsia* 1991;32[suppl 3]:8).

Felbamyl See **felbamate.**

Felbatol See **felbamate.**

Feldene See **piroxicam.**

felodipine + carbamazepine See **carbamazepine + felodipine.**

felodipine + oxcarbazepine See **oxcarbazepine + felodipine.**

femoxetine (Malexil) Selective serotonin uptake inhibitor being tested as an antidepressant, primarily in Europe. To date it has not proven effective in treating depression.

femoxetine + alcohol Therapeutic doses do not interact with alcohol (Stromberg C, Mattila MJ. Acute and subacute effects on psychomotor performance of femoxetine alone and with alcohol. *Eur J Clin Pharmacol* 1985;28:641–647).

fenfluramine (Ponderal; Ponderax; Pondimin) (FEN) Halogenated phenylethylamine derivative marketed as an anorectic. It is an indirect serotonin (5-HT) agonist and may have dopaminergic effects. It increases central 5-HT release and inhibits its reuptake. The racemic mixture FEN stimulates all five 5-HT receptor subtypes through release of 5-HT from the presynaptic neuron. Because its active metabolite, norfenfluramine, has direct effects on postsynaptic sites, the combined effects of parent and metabolite make FEN a good probe to assess overall central 5-HT function. In healthy subjects, FEN induces a dose-dependent increase in plasma prolactin levels. It appears to be effective in treating bulimia nervosa. Dosage for appetite suppression is 20 mg 3 times a day before meals. Its major behavioral effect is to reduce meal size and prolong duration of satiety after a meal (Chua A, Keating J, Hamilton D, et al. Central serotonin receptors and delayed gastric emptying in non-ulcer dyspepsia. *Br Med J* 1992; 305:280–282). FEN has not been found to be an effective augmenter in tricyclic refractory depression, but it has been reported to augment 5-HT uptake inhibition effects in obsessive-compulsive disorder. It has been used as an antiaggressive agent in the treatment of autism. Schedule IV; pregnancy risk category C. See **fenfluramine challenge test.**

fenfluramine challenge test Endocrine procedure used to study putative differences in central neurotransmitter function in depressive subtypes by measuring serum cortisol and prolactin responses to fenfluramine (FEN) challenge. Blunted prolactin response to FEN has been observed in adult patients with major depressive disorder and personality disorder patients with a history of suicide attempts. In normal and suicidal adolescents, FEN challenge induces a prolactin response significantly different from the response seen with placebo. Subjects fasting from midnight undergo intravenous cannula insertion. After 15 minutes, serial blood samples are taken for prolactin and cortisol estimation. FEN (60 mg) is administered orally at zero time, and blood samples are taken at 215, 0, +60, +120, +180, +240, and +300 mins (McBride PA, Anderson GM, Hertzig ME, et al. Serotonergic responsivity in male young adults with autistic disorder: results of a pilot study. *Arch Gen Psychiatry* 1989;46:213–221; Dinan TG, O'Keane V. D-fenfluramine/prolactin responses in depressed subjects before and after treatment. *Clin Neuropharmacol* 1990;13[suppl 1]:412).

fenfluramine + clomipramine Fenfluramine has been reported to potentiate effects of clomipramine (CMI) in a few obsessive-compulsive disorder patients partially responsive to CMI. In one patient, the combination was discontinued because of marked postural hypotension (Judd FK, Chua P, Lynch C, Norman T. Fenfluramine augmentation of clomipramine treatment of obsessive compulsive disorder. *Aust N Z J Psychiatry* 1991;25:412–414; Hollander E, DeCaria CM, Schneier FR, et al. Fenfluramine augmentation of serotonin reuptake blockade antiobsessional treatment. *J Clin Psychiatry* 1990;51:119–123).

fenfluramine + desipramine Co-administration increases desipramine levels, but does not produce additional amelioration of depressive symptoms (Price LH, Charney DS, Delgado PL, Heninger GR. Fenfluramine augmentation in tricyclic-refractory depression. *J Clin Psychopharmacol* 1990;10:312–317).

fenfluramine + fluoxetine Co-administration may augment the antiobsessional effects of fluoxetine (FLX). In obsessive compulsive disorder patients only partially responsive to FLX, fenfluramine (20–60 mg/day) further decreased obsessions and compulsions and was well tolerated (Hollander E, DeCaria CM, Schneier FR, et al. Fenfluramine augmentation of serotonin reuptake blockade antiobsessional treatment. *J Clin Psychiatry* 1990;51:119–123).

fenfluramine + fluvoxamine Fenfluramine (FEN) augmented antiobsessional response in six of seven patients being treated with a serotonin uptake inhibitor. FEN augmentation was well tolerated (Hollander E, DeCaria CM, Schneier FR, et al. Fenfluramine augmentation of serotonin reuptake blockade antiobsessional treatment. *J Clin Psychiatry* 1990;51: 119–123). Use is limited, however, by evidence from preclinical data strongly suggesting that neurotoxicity may occur when fenfluramine is co-prescribed with fluvoxamine.

fenfluramine + neuroleptic Co-administration has no effect on the steady-state plasma concentrations of fenfluramine, neuroleptics, and metabolites (Hubbard JW, Marshall BD, Srinivas NR, et al. Pharmacokinetics of fenfluramine and neuroleptics in the treatment of refractory schizophrenia. *Drug Invest* 1992;4: 99–111).

fenfluramine + phentermine Co-administration in 150 obese patients produced significant weight loss, minimal side effects, and a dropout rate of less than 20%. In 11 of 12 consecutive alcoholics, fenfluramine (80 mg) + phentermine (30 mg) produced marked or total decrease in alcohol craving and consumption, usually in less than 24 hours (Hitzig P. Combined dopamine and serotonin agonists: a synergistic approach to alcoholism and other addictive behaviors. *Maryland Med J* 1993;42: 153–157).

fenfluramine + serotonin uptake inhibitor Addition of fenfluramine (FEN) to serotonin uptake inhibitor (SUI) therapy of obsessive compulsive disorder may enhance therapeutic response (Hollander E, DeCaria CM, Schneier FR, et al. Fenfluramine augmentation of serotonin reuptake blockade antiobsessional therapy. *J Clin Psychiatry* 1990;51:119–123). Although FEN is neurotoxic in laboratory animals, an SUI may neutralize neurotoxic damage by blocking FEN entry into serotonin nerve terminals (Clineschmidt BV, Jacekei AG, Totaro JA, et al. Fenfluramine and brain serotonin. *Ann N Y Acad Sci* 1978;305:222–241).

fengabine (SL-79229) Drug undergoing testing as an antidepressant, primarily in Europe. It enhances gamma-aminobutyric acid (GABA)-B function, increases norepinephrine turnover, and causes desensitization of beta-adrenergic receptor-linked adenylate cyclase. It does not modify beta, alpha, or $alpha_2$ receptors and does not inhibit monoamine oxidase. It has been found to be as effective as clomipramine, amitriptyline, and imipramine, but is better tolerated, particularly with regard to anticholinergic side effects. Daily dose ranges from 600 to 2,400 mg (Lloyd KG, Zivkovic B, Scatton B, et al. The GABAergic hypothesis of depression. *Prog Neuropsychopharmacol Biol Psychiatry* 1989;13:341–351).

fenobam Imidazole derivative that in animals has antianxiety activity without relaxant or sedative/hypnotic activity, and minimal interaction with alcohol. In clinical trials, it is an effective antianxiety agent compared to placebo and as effective as diazepam with minimal side effects and little sedation.

fentanyl (Innovar; Sublimaze) Synthetic opioid used mainly as an anesthetic. It is a mu-agonist closely related in structure to meperidine. Analgesic potency is 1,000 times that of meperidine and 80–100 times that of morphine. It has a rapid onset of sedation and analgesia, and a relatively short duration of action (approximately 30–40 minutes) because of rapid redistribution. Its actions are quickly reversed by opioid antagonists. High doses produce marked muscular rigidity that is naloxone-reversible and may be due to dopaminergic action in the corpus striatum. Fentanyl transdermal is indicated in the management of chronic pain. It is not currently used for acute analgesia. It accumulates when given in large or repeated doses and can produce drug dependence similar to that produced by morphine. More than 100 deaths from fentanyl or one of its illicit homologs have been reported

(Henderson G. Fentanyl-related deaths: demographics, circumstances and toxicology of 112 cases. *J Forens Science* 1991;36:422–433). Schedule II.

fentanyl analog At least 12 different analogs are known to have been sold on the illicit drug market (World Health Organization. *Fentanyl Analogs. Information Manual on Designer Drugs.* Geneva: World Health Organization, 1990).

fentanyl + heroin In 1991, a mixture of heroin and fentanyl was sold on the illicit market in New York, resulting in the hospitalization of 200 drug abusers and at least 22 deaths.

fentanyl transdermal system (Duragesic) Transdermal patch for chronic pain that releases fentanyl at a slow, controlled rate. Once treatment is established, it provides sustained, consistent fentanyl plasma levels for 72 hours.

Fenylhist See **diphenhydramine**

Ferndex See **dextroamphetamine.**

festination Involuntary tendency to accelerate gait; it is a typical symptom of Parkinson's disease.

fetal alcohol effects (FAE) Presence of two of the following criteria in a child with a history of maternal alcohol abuse: (a) prenatal or postnatal growth retardation (height and weight below the 10th percentile for age or gestational age); (b) any neurological abnormality, developmental delay, or intellectual impairment; and (c) at least two characteristic craniofacial abnormalities (microcephaly, microphthalmia or short palpebral fissures, poorly developed philtrum, thin upper lip, and flattening of the maxillary area). FAE, a less serious diagnosis than fetal alcohol syndrome (FAS), is estimated to occur in 3–5 per 1,000 live births (Sokol RJ, Clarren SK. Guidelines for use of terminology describing the impact of prenatal alcohol on the offspring. *Alcoholism* 1989;13:597–598; Spohr H-L, Willms J, Steinhausen HC. Prenatal alcohol exposure and long-term developmental consequences. *Lancet* 1993;341:907–910). See **fetal alcohol syndrome.**

fetal alcohol syndrome (FAS) Specific, recognizable pattern of malformation in children born to alcoholic mothers. It is diagnosed when there is a positive history of maternal alcohol abuse during pregnancy and (a) prenatal or postnatal growth retardation (height and weight below the 10th percentile for age or gestational age); (b) any neurological abnormality, developmental delay, or intellectual impairment (seizures, attention and/or intellectual deficits, hyperactivity, learning disabilities); and (c) a pattern of specific craniofacial anomalies (microcephaly, short palpebral fissures, midface hypoplasia, smooth and/or long philtrum, and thin upper lip). Not only are the facial features associated with FAS difficult to recognize, but central nervous system dysfunction, including mental retardation, may not be identified until several years after birth (Anon. Fetal alcohol syndrome. *Alcohol Alert* 1991, No.13, pp 1–4). Facial deformities may fade, but adolescents and adults with FAS continue to manifest a recognizable pattern of low IQ (particularly in mathematics), attentional deficits, and problems with abstraction that frequently contribute to significant conduct disorder (Cermak T. *Evaluating & Treating Adult Children of Alcoholics,* vols I and II. Minneapolis: Johnson Institute Publications, 1990 and 1991). It is estimated that in the United States, nearly 1 in every 750 babies is born with FAS; mental handicap occurs in 85% of FAS-affected babies. FAS is now recognized as the leading known cause of mental retardation in the United States, surpassing Down syndrome and spina bifida. FAS is the second most common entity associated with agenesis of the corpus callosum, a rare abnormality present in 2.3% of developmentally disabled individuals, an incidence 10–20 times greater than in the general population. FAS represents the severe end of the continuum of disabilities caused by maternal alcohol use during pregnancy. It occurs in children whose mothers consume more than 80 g of alcohol (approximately six to eight alcoholic beverages) per day during pregnancy. Not all those affected by alcohol in utero have FAS; however, subtle signs can be found in the children of "social drinkers" and there is some evidence that even the occasional "binge" can be harmful. In children with an intelligence quotient in the normal range, there still may be deficits in cognitive skills and language development. See **fetal alcohol effects.**

fetal alcohol syndrome (FAS)/long-term effects
In 60 FAS children (ages 6–137 months at first assessment) followed over a 10-year period, craniofacial anomalies diminished with time. Microcephaly, short stature, and underweight status (in boys) persisted; in female adolescents, body weight normalized. Persistent mental retardation was the major sequela in many cases; environmental and educational factors did not have strong compensatory effects on the intellectual development of affected children (Spohr HL, Willms J, Steinhausen HC. Prenatal alcohol exposure and long-term developmental consequences. *Lancet* 1993;341:907–910).

fetal hydantoin syndrome Occurrence of congenital malformations (cleft lip, cleft palate, congenital heart defect) in infants whose mothers were treated with hydantoin during pregnancy. Not all exposed infants are at risk; approximately 5–10% will have the clinical phenotype of the full-blown fetal hydantoin syndrome (Buehler BA, Delimont D, van Waes M, Finnell RH. Prenatal prediction of risk of the fetal hydantoin syndrome. *N Engl J Med* 1990;322:1567–1572). The teratogenicity of phenytoin and probably of other anticonvulsants (e.g., carbamazepine, phenobarbital) is mediated not by the parent compound but by toxic intermediary metabolites (e.g., epoxides) produced as a result of the biotransformation of the parent.

fetal narcotic withdrawal Narcotic use during pregnancy may result in fetal addiction and a withdrawal syndrome in the first few days of life in about 80%. Symptoms include hyperactivity, irritability, tremors, regurgitation, poor feeding, diarrhea, and (occasionally) convulsions. Seizures are more common in newborns addicted to methadone than to other narcotics.

fetal solvent syndrome There is little direct information regarding effects due to solvent exposure during pregnancy. Concomitant influence of maternal undernutrition, abuse of other substances, and genetic predisposition remain to be clarified (Sharp CW, Rosenberg NL. Volatile substance. *In* Lowinson JH, Ruiz P, Millman RB, Langrod JG [eds], *Substance Abuse. A Comprehensive Textbook,* 2nd ed. Baltimore: Williams & Wilkins, 1992, pp 303–327).

fetishism Use of inanimate objects for sexual arousal. It has a multifactorial cause, with psychodynamic, behavioral, and cultural components. Biological abnormalities are rare, but fetishism has been reported in association with temporal lobe damage and temporal lobe epilepsy.

fetotoxin Substance poisonous to the unborn child.

Fevarin See **fluvoxamine.**

FG 7142 Partial inverse benzodiazepine agonist that produces a state of severe anxiety in humans. With acute dosage it is proconvulsant; chronic dosing leads to full seizures. Even a single dose can lead to long-term behavioral and receptor changes.

[^{18}F]haloperidol A positron emission tomography (PET) ligand that labels for haloperidol brain receptors.

fibromyalgia Chronic, poorly understood syndrome of widespread musculoskeletal aching, pain, and stiffness that invariably causes sleep disturbance. Pain and insomnia can be treated with amitriptyline (10–25 mg at bedtime) and/or temazepam (15–30 mg at bedtime). Intermittent use of sedative benzodiazepines also can produce good clinical response.

field survey   Collection of data in the field (usually the generalized population).

filgrastim   See **granulocyte-macrophage colony–stimulating factor.**

FilmFAX System   Use of telephone lines to transmit high-quality radiographic, computed tomography (CT), and magnetic resonance imaging (MRI) scans. Images can be zoomed, panned, and enlarged, allowing radiologists to make diagnoses directly from the FilmFAXed images.

"fine stuff"   Street name for marijuana.

Finiject 30   See **bolasterone.**

fipexide   See **nootropic drug.**

"firing"   Street term for intravenous injection or mainlining of cocaine.

first-night effect   In sleep laboratory studies, the effect of the environment and polysomnographic recording apparatus on the quality of the subject's sleep the first night of recording. Sleep is usually of reduced quality compared to what would be expected in the subject's usual sleeping environment. Subjects usually adjust to the laboratory by the second night of recording.

first order kinetics   See **kinetics, linear.**

first-pass effect   Amount of drug removed from the systemic circulation by metabolism in the liver. An appreciable portion of an oral dose never reaches the general circulation, even if there has been virtually complete absorption from the intestines. Drugs with a high hepatic extraction ratio are sensitive to hepatic blood flow rather than hepatic enzyme activity. First-pass effect can be affected by diseases, especially those affecting liver function (e.g., cirrhosis, hepatitis, congestive heart failure). Decreased bioavailability is a significant factor in determining the plasma levels of a considerable number of drugs. First-pass effect is bypassed by intramuscular or intravenous drug administration. In contrast to most orally administered neuroleptics, haloperidol and pimozide undergo relatively little first-pass metabolism. Also called "hepatic extraction."

first-rank symptom   Any of a group of symptoms selected and used by Kurt Schneider and his followers as a basis for making a diagnosis of schizophrenia. They include hallucinations, changes in thought process, delusional perceptions, and somatic passivity.

Fisher's exact probability test   Test for association in a two-by-two table based on the exact hypergeometric distribution of the frequencies within the table.

Fisher's z transformation   Transformation applied to the correlation coefficient so that it is normally distributed.

fit, uncinate   See **seizure, uncinate.**

fitness (Darwinian)   Species characteristics that influence likelihood of survival.

"fix"   Street term for intravenous injection of heroin.

fixated pedophile   See **pedophile, fixated.**

fixed combination drug   Fixed amounts of two different drug classes (e.g., Triavil = perphenazine [Trilafon] plus amitriptyline [Elavil]) for the treatment of specific disorders (e.g., psychotic depression or mixed anxiety/depression). General policy of the U.S. Food and Drug Administration (FDA) is: two or more drugs may be combined in a single dosage form when each contributes to claimed effects, and dosage of each (amount, frequency, duration) is such that the combination is safe and effective for a significant patient population requiring such concurrent therapies. In addition, the FDA requires that a combination drug be demonstrated superior to each of its separate components. This has given rise to a three-arm design in which patients are randomly assigned to the combination and to each of its two components. Separate tests of significance are then accomplished to evaluate superiority of the combination over the components. To satisfy FDA requirements, the smaller of the two treatment effects must be deemed statistically significant (implying that the larger of the two also is significant).

fixed dose design   Drug trial in which efficacy and safety of predetermined doses are compared to each other and placebo. Objective is usually to determine therapeutic efficacy and safety of a dose not yet established.

fixed pupil   Ocular pupil nonreactive to light, accommodation, or convergence.

"fixing"   Street term for intravenous injection ("mainlining") of a drug.

"flake"   Street name for cocaine.

"flakes"   Street name for phencyclidine (PCP).

flame emission spectrophotometry   See **flame photometry.**

flame photometry   Analytic method for drug concentration measurement in which a solution containing the drug (e.g., lithium) is sprayed into a flame. An electron absorbs energy and is displaced to a position of higher energy, further away from the nucleus. Also called "flame emission spectophometry."

flapping tremor   See **asterixis.**

flashback   Spontaneous occurrence of previously experienced drug effects (e.g., hallucinations, delusions, depersonalization) or distressing emotions originally associated with trauma. Flashbacks are generally associated with LSD-like drugs and occasionally with marijuana. Drug-associated flashbacks are usually brief (seconds to hours). They may occur during a drug-free period (often several months after the last drug ingestion), but also can be precipitated by stress, use of other drugs (e.g., marijuana), or environmental stimuli reminiscent of the original hallucinogenic experience. They may be accompanied by panic attacks. Flashbacks are reported by patients with post-traumatic stress disorder who are not drug abusers; treatment with the opiate antagonist naltrexone may be effective (Bills LJ, Kreisler K. Treatment of flashbacks with naltrexone. *Am J Psychiatry* 1993;150: 1430).

"flasher"   Exhibitionist who exposes the genitals by quickly opening clothing (e.g., bathrobe, raincoat).

"flash house"   Street term for a place where substance abusers inject drugs. Also called "galleria" or "shooting gallery."

flattened affect   See **affect, flattened.**

flesinoxan   Highly potent, selective serotonin (5-HT)$_{1A}$ agonist with affinity for any other receptor that is at least 80 times weaker. Animal testing indicates potentially strong anxiolytic and antidepressant properties. In healthy male volunteers, tolerance for flesinoxan (1 mg) was excellent; it was associated with a pleasant feeling of relaxation and slight drowsiness without gastrointestinal side effects (Moreno AG, Ansseau M, Pitchot W, et al. Effect of pindolol on the neuroendocrine and temperature responses to flesinoxan. *Neuropsychopharmacology* 1993;9:98S).

Flexeril   See **cyclobenzaprine.**

Flexoject   See **orphenadrine.**

Flexon   See **orphenadrine.**

flexibilitas cerea   See **catalepsy.**

flexibility, waxy   See **catalepsy.**

flicker fusion threshold   Widely used measure of central nervous system drug effects that assesses a narrow bandwidth of temporal information processing in the visual system (the threshold for flicker detection at high frequencies [> 30 Hz]).

flight of ideas   Rapid, continuous flow of thought or speech that is a frequent symptom of mania. The person jumps from one topic to another, each topic being only superficially related to the previous one.

"flipping"   Lay term for frequent bingeing and purging among professional jockeys.

flooding   Therapy for agoraphobia in which exposure to avoided situations is carried out repeatedly to reduce anxiety. Also called "implosion." See **implosive therapy.**

floppy infant syndrome   Syndrome characterized by lethargy, flaccid muscles, and poor suckling in newborns, especially premature infants, exposed to a central nervous system depressant (e.g., diazepam) during the last trimester of pregnancy. It appears to be asso-

ciated with the newborn's not fully developed hepatic and renal capacity to process parent drug and active metabolites. Diazepam, for example, persists in neonatal plasma several days, causing prolonged lethargy. Recovery usually occurs with supportive measures and the passage of time. If the condition is critical and definitely due to a benzodiazepine, low-dose flumazenil therapy may rapidly reverse it.

Florinef   See **fludrocortisone.**

"flower power"   Street name for morning glory seeds.

Floxyfral   See **fluvoxamine.**

Floxytal   See **fluvoxamine.**

Fluanxol   See **flupenthixol; flupenthixol decanoate.**

fluconazole + nortriptyline   See **nortriptyline + fluconazole.**

Fluctin   See **fluoxetine.**

Fluctine   See **fluoxetine.**

Fludecate   See **fluphenazine decanoate.**

fludrocortisone   (Florinef) Corticosteroid that may be used to treat symptomatic orthostatic hypotension induced by psychotropic drugs such as tricyclic antidepressants and neuroleptics. Usual dose is 0.2–0.3 mg/day for 2 weeks. Its use requires close monitoring for supine hypertension, congestive heart failure, and hypokalemia. Its antihypertensive and salt-retaining effect may be potentiated by indomethacin. See **hypotension, postural.**

Flugeral   See **flunarizine.**

flumazenil   (Anexate; Lanexate; Mazicon) (FLU) 1,4-Imidazobenzodiazepine that competitively blocks benzodiazepine (BZD) activation of inhibitory GABAergic synaptic transmission, thereby preventing or abolishing all known pharmacological effects of BZDs and non-BZD agonists of BZD receptors. FLU is a very valuable tool in the diagnosis and treatment of intoxications involving BZDs. Because of first-pass metabolism, FLU is most effective when given intravenously. After an initial bolus of 0.2 mg (minimum effective dose), it is usually titrated in increments of 0.1 mg/minute until the patient is awake and cooperative; when an appropriate state of alertness is reached, FLU is immediately discontinued. In monointoxications with high BZD doses, FLU (1–2 mg) usually reverses the effect of the agonist completely. If there is no response within 2–3 minutes of the end injection, factors and circumstances other than BZDs may be involved. When different sedative drugs contribute to the comatose state, much higher FLU doses (over 10 mg) may be needed. Because of FLU's short half-life, which is exceeded by that of all BZD agonists, reinjections after 45–60 minutes are often needed to maintain alertness (Kulka PJ, Lauven PM.

Benzodiazepine antagonists. An update of their role in the emergency care of overdose patients. *Drug Safety* 1992;7:381–386). Even when reversal of unconsciousness is incomplete, it often improves to the point at which an ingestion history can be obtained and invasive procedures can be avoided (Hojer J, Baehrendtz S, Matell G, Gustafsson LL. Diagnostic utility of flumazenil in coma with suspected poisoning: a double-blind, randomised controlled study. *Br Med J* 1990;301:1308–1311). Preclinical studies suggest that FLU can reverse BZD dependence. It can be useful in the management of anesthesia by shortening the postoperative period and reducing sedation-related adverse effects; it significantly improves postoperative recall after midazolam anesthesia. In patients with various seizure disorders, FLU's effects on clinical seizures are similar to those of diazepam in magnitude and duration. It also has been shown to improve neurological symptoms in patients with hepatic encephalopathy, probably by inhibiting the binding of endogenous ligands, without specific side effects. Adverse effects and complications of FLU are usually mild, consisting mainly of nausea and vomiting (Galletly DC, Ure R, Turley A. Flumazenil: a twelve month survey of use in a New Zealand public hospital. *Anaesth Intensive Care* 1990;18:229–233). Agitation, discomfort, anxiety, flushing, and coldness have been reported in patients receiving FLU for BZD overdoses, usually when the FLU dose exceeds 5 mg (Amrein R, Leishman B, Bentzinger C, Roncari G. Flumazenil in benzodiazepine antagonism: actions and clinical use in intoxications and anesthesiology. *Med Toxicol* 1987;2:411–429). More serious adverse effects include precipitation of a BZD withdrawal syndrome that may include absence status and other seizures (Thomas P, Lebrun C, Chatel M. De novo absence status epilepticus as a benzodiazepine withdrawal syndrome. *Epilepsia* 1993;34:355–358; Analgesic and anesthetic drugs. *In Drug Evaluations Subscription*, vol 1. Chicago: American Medical Association, 1992, pp 21–22). Cardiac arrest attributed to FLU (0.4 mg) given to reverse diazepam sedation in a 60-year-old man has been reported (Katz Y, Boulos M, Singer P, Rosenberg B. Cardiac arrest associated with flumazenil. *Br Med J* 1992;304:1415). A severe acute psychotic disorder associated with FLU was reported in a patient with hepatic encephalopathy. Intravenously administered FLU produced dizziness and lightheadedness in normal subjects, but provoked panic in 8 of 10 patients with untreated panic disorder; several reported that FLU-related panic differed from clinical attacks by absence of respiratory symptoms (Klein DF. False suffoca-

tion alarms, spontaneous panics, and related conditions. *Arch Gen Psychiatry* 1993;50:306–317).

flumazenil/alcohol intoxication   Data on flumazenil (FLU) reversal of alcohol effects are contradictory. In some studies, it has been effective in cases of alcohol or benzodiazepine and alcohol poisoning (Hojer J, Baehrendtz S. The effect of flumazenil [Ro 15-1788] in the management of self-induced benzodiazepine poisoning: a double-blind controlled study. *Acta Med Scand* 1988;224:357–365). In others, it did not reverse alcohol-induced sedation and prolongation of choice reaction time (Kulka PJ, Lauven PM. Benzodiazepine antagonists. An update of their role in the emergency care of overdose patients. *Drug Safety* 1992;7:381–386).

flumazenil/benzodiazepine withdrawal   Intravenous flumazenil (FLU) has been used to treat protracted benzodiazepine (BZD) withdrawal symptoms. Despite FLU's short half-life (1 hour), benefits last a few hours to several days. Improvement was observed in some long-standing BZD withdrawal symptoms, including clouded thinking, tiredness, muscular symptoms, and perceptual symptoms (e.g., "pins and needles" feeling, pain, subjective sensations of body distortion). Mood disorder, when present, also improved. Side effects typically were mild or absent (Lader M, Morton S. Benzodiazepine withdrawal syndrome. *Br J Psychiatry* 1991;158:435–436).

flumazenil/cannabis   Flumazenil has been used to reverse coma in children (ages 18 months and 4.5 years) who had ingested cannabis. Both regained consciousness within 1 minute of flumazenil (0.2 mg) injection (Rubio F, Quintero S, Hernandez A, et al. Flumazenil for coma reversal in children after cannabis. *Lancet* 1993;341:1028–1029).

flumazenil/seizures   Seizures have been reported in patients prone to convulsions, including benzodiazepine (BZD)-dependent patients, epileptic patients treated with BZDs, patients with central nervous system trauma, and patients intoxicated with tricyclic antidepressants or isoniazid (Gaudreault P, Guay J, Thivierge RL, Verdy I. Benzodiazepine poisoning. Clinical and pharmacological considerations and treatment. *Drug Safety* 1991;6:247–265).

flumazenil/zopiclone overdose   Flumazenil has been effective in reversing zopiclone overdose effects.

Flunanthate   See **fluphenazine enanthate.**
Flunar   See **flunarizine.**
Flunarizina   See **flunarizine.**
flunarizine   (Bercetina; Dinaplex; Flugeral; Flunar; Flunarizina; Flunarl; Gradient; Sibelium;

Vasculoflex; Vertex). Class IV calcium antagonist with antihistaminic, antiserotonergic, and antidopaminergic activity. Terminal elimination half-life averages 18 days. It does not alter carbamazepine or phenytoin steady-state concentrations. It has been reported to be an effective maintenance treatment for bipolar patients and may be useful in patients unable to tolerate lithium side effects (Lindelius R, Nilsson CG. Flunarizine as maintenance treatment of a patient with bipolar disorder. *Am J Psychiatry* 1992;149:139). It is an effective prophylactic treatment for common or classic migraine in children and adults (Germain H, Neron A. Flunarizine in headache. *Headache Q Curr Treat Res* 1990;1:320–323). Anticonvulsant efficacy is still being evaluated. Flunarizine is sedating and can produce extrapyramidal reactions.

Flunarl See **flunarizine**.

flunitrazepam (Hypnodorm; Rohypnol) Potent 1,4 intermediate-acting benzodiazepine hypnotic. Not available in the United States.

flunoxaprofen (Priaxim) New, nonsteroidal anti-inflammatory drug. It should be prescribed with caution in the elderly, particularly those with decreased renal function, because of the risk of significant prolongation of its elimination half-life.

fluorescence polarization immunoassay (FPI) Single immunoassay test for drug detection that is relatively inexpensive.

fluorescent banding Use of chemical staining to identify chromosomes.

fluorescent in situ hybridization (FISH) Use of fluorescin-labeled DNA probes to hone in on five regions of the five chromosomes (21, 18, 13, X, and Y) that account for 95% of chromosomal defects. It may be as reliable as conventional cytogenetic analysis (*Science* 1991;254:378–379).

fluorescent polarization (FPIA) Immunoassay using a fluorescent-labeled tracer to measure drug concentration.

fluorescent polarization, particle concentration (PCFIA) Immunoassay method for measuring drug levels.

fluorescent treponemal antibody absorption test for syphilis (FTA-ABS) Extremely sensitive, highly specific test for syphilis with a less than 1% incidence of false-positive reactions.

fluorination Addition of a fluorine atom to a basic molecular structure.

4-fluorotranyl-cypromin (FTCP) Monoamine oxidase inhibitor (MAOI) synthesized with the hope that it might have improved pharmacokinetic and side effect profiles compared to the parent antidepressant tranylcypromine. Animal testing indicates that it may be a useful MAOI antidepressant with limited interac-

tions (McKenna S, Lynn R, Baker GB, et al. *Neuropsychopharmacology* 1993;9:159–160).

fluoxetine (Fluctin; Fluctine; Fontex; Ladose; Lovan; Prozac; Saurat) (FLX) Bicyclic, serotonin (5-HT) uptake inhibitor antidepressant chemically distinct from tricyclic, tetracyclic, and other antidepressants. It does not significantly affect noradrenergic, cholinergic, alpha-adrenergic, or histaminergic pathways. It seems to work by desensitizing both inhibitory somatodendritic and terminal 5-HT autoreceptors, thus increasing central nervous system 5-HT synaptic transmission. It has been reported to reduce dopamine synthesis in a variety of brain areas, including the striatum, and thus may have significant antidopaminergic effects. Half-life is long (2–3 days). Because its active metabolite norfluoxetine has a half-life of 7–9 days, FLX can be considered a prodrug for norfluoxetine. The active metabolite, however, may be a kinetic disadvantage; its long half-life increases risk of drug interactions, even after FLX is discontinued. Steady state of each is achieved only at 4–6 weeks. Therapeutic blood levels have not been established, but reasonable maximum daily dose, if tolerated, is 80 mg. FLX is effective in the treatment of typical and atypical depressions, including depressed patients on hemodialysis. It also has been reported effective in premenstrual syndrome (PMS), fibromyalgia, hypochondriasis, paraphilias, trichotillomania, depersonalization disorder, and borderline personality disorder (Perilstein RD, Lipper S, Friedman LJ. Three cases of paraphilias responsive to fluoxetine treatment. *J Clin Psychiatry* 1991;52:169–170; Stanley MA, Bowers TC, Swann AC, Taylor DJ. Treatment of trichotillomania with fluoxetine. *J Clin Psychiatry* 1991; 52:282; Fichtner CG, Horevitz RP, Braun BG. Fluoxetine in depersonalization disorder. *Am J Psychiatry* 1992;149:1750–1751; Markovitz PJ, Schulz SC. Drug treatment of personality disorders. *Br J Psychiatry* 1993;162:122). It may decrease anger and hostility in certain unipolar patients and impulsive, labile, acting-out behavior and self-injurious behavior in mentally retarded persons. Preliminary research data also suggest that FLX may be useful in the treatment of cocaine (COC) abuse because it reduces COC8s reinforcing effects. FLX has been linked with akathisia, parkinsonism, marked generalized rigidity, and truncal dyskinesia (Bouchard RH, Pourcher E, Vincent P. Fluoxetine and extrapyramidal side effects. *Am J Psychiatry* 1990;146:1352–1353; Lipinski JF, Mallya G, Zimmerman P, Pope HG. Fluoxetine-induced akathisia: clinical and theoretical implications. *J Clin Psychiatry* 1989; 50:339–342). Clinicians should be aware of the possible increased risk of extrapyramidal side effects when FLX is prescribed in conjunction with dopamine-blocking agents. In some patients, FLX reportedly has induced an akathisia-like reaction manifested by agitation, restless motor movement, dysphoria, pacing, an internal sense of desperation, and suicidal ideation. High doses may cause a syndrome resembling a frontal lobe syndrome manifested by apathy, indifference, inattention, and perseveration. There have been a number of anecdotal reports about FLX-induced anorgasmia and paranoid reactions. It also should be considered a possible cause of the syndrome of inappropriate secretion of antidiuretic hormone. FLX may interact with many other drugs and may be lethal in combination with a monoamine oxidase inhibitor. Pregnancy risk category B.

fluoxetine + acetaminophen   No serious adverse interactions have been reported.

fluoxetine/akathisia   Fluoxetine's capacity to evoke akathisia is well recognized. Neurological and psychological manifestations are as subjectively distressing as neuroleptic-induced akathisia. Treatment with propranolol may be effective. See **fluoxetine + propranolol.**

fluoxetine + alcohol   Available evidence indicates that fluoxetine (FLX) in therapeutic doses does not interact with alcohol (Allen D, Lader M, Curran HV. A comparative study of the interactions of alcohol with amitriptyline, fluoxetine and placebo in normal subjects. *Prog Neuropsychopharmacol Biol Psychiatry* 1988; 12:63–80; Schaffler K. Study on performance and alcohol interaction with the antidepressant fluoxetine. *Int Clin Psychopharmacol* 1989; 4[suppl I]:15–20). FLX can alter alcohol intake, indicating a potential role in treating alcoholics (Naranjo CA, Kadlec KE, Sanhueza P, et al. Fluoxetine differentially alters alcohol intake and other consummatory behaviors in problem drinkers. *Clin Pharmacol Ther* 1990; 47:490–498). There is no evidence that FLX inhibits the metabolism of alcohol (Leonard BE. The comparative pharmacology of new antidepressants. *J Clin Psychiatry* 1993;54[suppl 3]:3–15).

fluoxetine + alprazolam   Co-administration may increase psychomotor impairment, but usually it is insufficient to warrant modifying the dose of either agent if the combination is clinically effective. Clinical studies show decreased alprazolam (ALP) clearance. In vitro studies suggest that the oxidative metabolite norfluoxetine is responsible for inhibition of ALP metabolism, thus explaining the lag in recovery of ALP clearance after fluoxetine levels have fallen to almost zero with norfluoxetine levels remaining high. In one double-

blind parallel study, co-administration increased ALP plasma levels about 30%. No significant changes were observed in mood status (Anon. *A Pharmacokinetic/Pharmacodynamic Evaluation of the Combined Administration of Alprazolam and Fluoxetine.* Kalamazoo, MI: The Upjohn Company, 1990).

fluoxetine + amantadine   Fluoxetine may elevate amantadine plasma levels, which may produce delirium (Baker RW. Fluoxetine and schizophrenia in a patient with obsessional thinking. *J Neuropsychiatry Clin Neurosci* 1992; 4:232–233).

fluoxetine + amitriptyline   Fluoxetine inhibits hepatic metabolism of amitriptyline (AMI), producing elevated AMI plasma levels and side effects consistent with AMI toxicity.

fluoxetine + amphetamine   Fluoxetine (FLX) (60 mg/day) plus amphetamine (45 mg 3 times a day) (well in excess of conventional doses) potentiated FLX's antidepressant effects in a patient refractory to FLX alone and combined imipramine/amphetamine. Relapse occurred on four occasions when d-amphetamine was not used (Linet LS. Treatment of refractory depression with a combination of fluoxetine and d-amphetamine. *Am J Psychiatry* 1989; 146:803–804).

fluoxetine/appetite suppression   Fluoxetine is an effective appetite suppressant for the treatment of obesity. Dosage range is 40–60 mg/day, higher than the usual antidepressant dose.

fluoxetine + atenolol   Co-administration apparently produces no adverse interactions (Walley T, Pirmohamed M, Proudlove C, Maxwell D. Interaction of metoprolol and fluoxetine. *Lancet* 1993;341:967–968).

fluoxetine/attention deficit hyperactivity disorder   In a preliminary open-label trial with 19 children and adolescents (ages 7–15, mean age 11) diagnosed with attention deficit hyperactivity disorder, 58% showed moderate improvements in clinician, teacher, and parental behavioral ratings with fluoxetine (FLX) (20–60 mg/day). Clinical response was rapid, usually within 1 week, in contrast to the longer time necessary (3–4 weeks) for FLX's antidepressant effects to appear (Barrickman L, Noyes R, Kuperman S, et al. Treatment of ADHD with fluoxetine: a preliminary trial. *J Am Acad Child Adolesc Psychiatry* 1991;30:762–767). See **fluoxetine/children, adolescents/side effects; fluoxetine + methylphenidate.**

fluoxetine + benzodiazepine   Fluoxetine (FLX) inhibits hepatic microsomal enzymes and may reduce hepatic clearance and increase plasma concentrations of benzodiazepines metabolized by oxidation (e.g., alprazolam, chlordiazepoxide, clorazepate, diazepam, estazolam, flurazepam, halazepam, prazepam, quazepam, temazepam, and triazolam). FLX does not affect glucuronidated BZDs (e.g., lorazepam, oxazepam, and clonazepam).

fluoxetine + benztropine   Fluoxetine may elevate benztropine plasma levels, possibly causing delirium (Baker RW. Fluoxetine and schizophrenia in a patient with obsessional thinking. *J Neuropsychiatry Clin Neurosci* 1992; 2:232–233).

fluoxetine + beta-blocker   Fluoxetine may inhibit oxidative metabolism of metoprolol and other lipophilic beta-blockers that undergo extensive hepatic metabolism, resulting in higher plasma concentrations of the beta-blocker and adverse cardiovascular effects (Walley T, Pirmohamed M, Proudlove C, Maxwell D. Interaction of metoprolol and fluoxetine. *Lancet* 1993;341:967–968). Patients who require beta-blockade while on fluoxetine should be prescribed water-soluble drugs (e.g., atenolol, sotalol).

fluoxetine/breast milk   Secretion of fluoxetine (FLX) in breast milk is minimal (Isenberg KE. Excretion of fluoxetine in human breast milk. *J Clin Psychiatry* 1990;51;169). Breast milk concentrations of FLX and norfluoxetine were measured after 53 days of maternal FLX therapy (20 mg/day). Total drug ingested (FLX and norfluoxetine) by the infant was calculated to be no more than 15–20 μg/kg/day. There were no adverse behavioral or developmental outcomes (Burch KJ, Wells BG. Fluoxetine/norfluoxetine concentrations in human milk. *Pediatrics* 1992;89:676–677). There is a report of a 6-week-old, breast-fed infant referred for colic whose mother was taking FLX. When the infant was switched to a commercial formula, crying decreased dramatically. Analysis of breast milk showed concentrations of 69 ng/ml for FLX, 90 ng/ml for norfluoxetine. After the infant was switched back to breast milk, infant blood serum/plasma level concentrations were 340 ng/ml for FLX and 208 ng/ml for norfluoxetine (Lester BM, Cucca J, Andreozzi L, et al. Possible association between fluoxetine hydrochloride and colic in an infant. *J Am Acad Child Adolesc Psychiatry* 1993;32:1253–1255).

fluoxetine + bromocriptine   No adverse interactions in depressed Parkinson8s disease patients have been reported (Lauterbach EC. Dopaminergic hallucinosis with fluoxetine in Parkinson's disease. *Am J Psychiatry* 1993;150:1750).

fluoxetine/bulimia nervosa   In an 8-week, placebo-controlled trial in 387 bulimic outpatients, FLX (60 mg/day) reduced binge eating, vomiting, depression, carbohydrate craving, and pathological eating attitudes and behaviors. There was a low occurrence of adverse effects and small but statistically significant weight loss compared with weight gains reported with other antidepressant agents (Fluoxetine Bulimia Nervosa Collaborative Study Group. Fluoxetine in the treatment of bulimia nervosa. A multicenter placebo-controlled, double-blind trial. *Arch Gen Psychiatry* 1992;49:139–147).

fluoxetine + bupropion   Fluoxetine (FLX) can augment therapeutic response to bupropion (BUP) and vice versa. Co-administration is usually well tolerated and may sometimes be effective in patients refractory to FLX. In a controlled trial, BUP treatment was associated with moderate to marked improvement in 10 of 22 patients who had not responded to a previous trial of FLX. FLX inhibits BUP metabolism, leading to a threefold and eightfold increase in plasma levels of the metabolites hydroxybupropion and threohydroxybupropion, respectively. There can be a pharmacokinetic interaction between these compounds, interfering with BUP clearance and resulting in a severe extrapyramidal syndrome with ataxia, impaired psychomotor coordination, and catatonic symptoms (Preskorn SH. Selected topics on the pharmacokinetics and drug interactions of serotonin-selective reuptake inhibitors. *Curr Psychopharmacol* 1992; 11:5–12). Addition of BUP to FLX-resistant obsessive-compulsive disorder patients may reduce symptoms in some patients and worsen them in others (Goodman WK, McDougle CJ, Price LH. Pharmacotherapy of obsessive compulsive disorder. *J Clin Psychiatry* 1992;53 [suppl]:29–37). The combination causes the same type of side effects seen with either drug alone. No seizures have been reported with combined therapy (Boyer WF, Feighner JP. The combined use of fluoxetine and bupropion. Presented at the 146th Annual Meeting of the American Psychiatric Association, San Francisco, May 1993).

fluoxetine + buspirone   Buspirone may augment response in obsessive-compulsive child and adult patients refractory or only partially responsive to fluoxetine (FLX) (Alessi N, Bos T. Buspirone augmentation of fluoxetine in a depressed child with obsessive-compulsive disorder. *Am J Psychiatry* 1991;148:1605–1606; Jenike MA, Baer L, Buttolph L. Buspirone augmentation of fluoxetine in patients with obsessive-compulsive disorder. *J Clin Psychiatry* 1991;1:13–14). In a double-blind, crossover study, 13 FLX-treated (80 mg/day for a minimum of 10 weeks) obsessive-compulsive disorder patients were given adjuvant buspirone and placebo for 4 weeks each. Buspirone dosage was gradually increased over 2 weeks;

all patients reached a stable dose of 60 mg/day for the final 2 weeks of active treatment. There were no significant differences between buspirone and placebo in obsessive-compulsive, depressive, or anxiety symptoms (Grady TA, Pigott TA, L'Heureux F, et al. Double-blind study of adjuvant buspirone for fluoxetine-treated patients with obsessive-compulsive disorder. *Am J Psychiatry* 1993;150:819–821). Co-administration appears to have more potent antidepressant activity than either drug alone in patients with severe depression (Jacobsen FM. A possible augmentation of antidepressant response by buspirone. *J Clin Psychiatry* 1991;52:217–220; Bakish D. Fluoxetine potentiation by buspirone: three case histories. *Can J Psychiatry* 1991:36:749–750; Joffe RT, Schuller DR. An open study of buspirone augmentation of serotonin reuptake inhibitors in refractory depression. *J Clin Psychiatry* 1993;54:269–271). However, sequential use of buspirone followed by FLX may interfere with FLX8s antidepressant effect (Markovitz PJ, Stagno SJ, Calabrese JR. Buspirone augmentation of fluoxetine in obsessive-compulsive disorder. *Am J Psychiatry* 1990;147:798–800; Bakish D. Fluoxetine potentiation by buspirone: three case histories. *Can J Psychiatry* 1991;36: 749–750). Sequential administration also may cause a serotonin syndrome, seizures, and antagonism of buspirone's anxiolytic effects (Sternbach H. Danger of MAOI therapy after fluoxetine withdrawal. *Lancet* 1988;2:850; Bodkin JA, Teicher MH. Fluoxetine may antagonize the anxiolytic action of buspirone. *J Clin Psychopharmacol* 1989;9:150). Seizure has been reported with the combination in the absence of the serotonin syndrome (Grady TA, Pigott TA, L'Heureux F, et al. Seizure associated with fluoxetine and adjuvant buspirone therapy. *J Clin Psychopharmacol* 1992;12:70–71). Simultaneous administration or low doses of buspirone (30 mg/day) after FLX discontinuation (20 mg/day) may cause euphoria, pressured speech, disinhibition, and motor hyperactivity (Lebert F, Pasquier F, Goudemand M, et al. Euphoria with buspirone after fluoxetine treatment. *Am J Psychiatry* 1993;150: 167). A paradoxical reaction to buspirone augmentation of FLX was reported (Tanquary J, Masand P. Paradoxical reaction to buspirone augmentation of fluoxetine. *J Clin Psychopharmacol* 1990;10:377).

fluoxetine + carbamazepine   There are mixed data on fluoxetine's (FLX) effect on carbamazepine (CBZ) plasma levels. Co-administration should be cautious, with frequent monitoring of CBZ levels. FLX inhibits CBZ metabolism, possibly resulting in clinically important interaction effects. There have been a few reports that addition of FLX to CBZ resulted in increased plasma levels of CBZ (27%) and its active metabolite, 10,11 epoxide (31%), increasing the risk of neurotoxicity and/or cardiotoxicity (Grimsley SR, Jann MW, Carter G, et al. Increased carbamazepine plasma concentrations after fluoxetine co-administration. *Clin Pharmacol Ther* 1991;50: 10–15; Pearson HT. Interaction of fluoxetine with carbamazepine. *J Clin Psychiatry* 1990;51: 126). Interactions may be due to FLX inhibition of CYP3A, which metabolizes CBZ (Pirmohamed M, Kitteringham N, Breckenridge A, Park BK. The effect of enzyme induction on the cytochrome P450-mediated bioactivation of carbamazepine by mouse liver microsomes. *Biochem Pharmacol* 1992;44:2307–2314). Addition of FLX to CBZ may cause parkinsonism. Clinical observations and neuroscientific and pharmacological data suggest that any drug that potentiates 5-HT effects, presumably by inhibiting dopaminergic nigrostriatal projections, may precipitate parkinsonism, especially when combined with neuroleptics or other 5-HT–enhancing drugs or when used in patients with subclinical or mild parkinsonism (Gernaat HBPE, van de Woude J, Touw DJ. Fluoxetine and parkinsonism in patients taking carbamazepine. *Am J Psychiatry* 1991;148; 1604-1605; Touw DJ, Gernaat HBPE, van der Woude J. Parkinsonisme na toevoeging van fluoxetine aan de behandeling met neuroleptica of carbamazepine. *Ned Tijdschr Geneeskd* 1992;136:332–333). A toxic serotonin syndrome was reported in an affective disorder patient treated with CBZ (200 mg/day) who had FLX (20 mg/day) added for 14 days. She also had leukopenia and thrombocytopenia. Following FLX discontinuation, all symptoms of toxicity subsided after 72 hours (Dursun SM, Mathew VM, Reveley MA. Toxic serotonin syndrome after fluoxetine plus carbamazepine. *Lancet* 1993;342:442–443). CBZ plasma concentrations should be monitored closely for up to 3–5 weeks in any patient who has FLX added to the drug regimen. No apparent interaction occurred when FLX was added to a stable CBZ regimen in patients with epilepsy. There were no significant changes in steady-state CBZ or its metabolites during seizures; nor were there any changes in seizure frequency, possibly because FLX and CBZ are metabolized by different hepatic isoenzymes (Spina E, Avenoso A, Pollicino AM, et al. Carbamazepine co-administration with fluoxetine or fluvoxamine. *Ther Drug Monit* 1993;15:247–250).

fluoxetine/cardiovascular effects   Fluoxetine can slow the heart rate, and in a few patients it has been associated with clinically significant bradycardia (Ellison JM, Milofsky JE, Ely E. Bradycardia and syncope induced by fluoxetine in two patients. *J Clin Psychiatry* 1990;51: 385–386; Feder R. Bradycardia and syncope induced by fluoxetine. *J Clin Psychiatry* 1991; 52:139).

fluoxetine/children, adolescents/side effects Early studies reported significant problems with side effects such as agitation and gastric distress (King RA, Riddle MA, Chappell PB, et al. Emergence of self-destructive phenomena in children and adolescents during fluoxetine treatment. *J Am Acad Child Adolesc Psychiatry* 1991;30:179–186). Most early studies used a fixed starting dose (20 mg/day) without gradual titration, however, and adverse effects may have been dose-related (Boulos C, Kutcher S, Gardner D, Young E. An open naturalistic trial of fluoxetine in adolescents and young adults with treatment-resistant major depression. *J Child Adolesc Psychopharmacol* 1992;2:103–111). It now appears that 20 mg/ day initially is excessive. Even in those who eventually may benefit from 20 mg/day or more, side effects are likely to be minimized if low starting doses are used and slowly titrated. Behavioral side effects reported include motor restlessness; subjective dysphoric excitation (inner restlessness, agitation, excessive energy); insomnia and/or vivid dreams; uncharacteristic social disinhibition (garrulousness, silliness, subtle impulsivity); and aggressive, irritable affects with self-destructive ideation/gestures (Ambrosini PJ, Bianchi MD, Rabinovich H, Elia J. Antidepressant treatments in children and adolescents: II. Anxiety, physical, and behavioral disorders. *J Am Acad Child Adolesc Psychiatry* 1993;32:483–493; Jafri AB, Greenberg WM. Fluoxetine side effects. *J Am Acad Child Adolesc Psychiatry* 1991;30:852; King RA, Riddle MA, Chappell PB, et al. Emergence of self-destructive phenomena in children and adolescents during fluoxetine treatment. *J Am Acad Child Adolesc Psychiatry* 1991;30:179–186; Koizumi H. Fluoxetine and suicidal ideation. *J Am Acad Child Adolesc Psychiatry* 1991;30:695; Matthews MB, Quinn D, Marcoux GS, Falkenberg K. Fluoxetine and neuroleptic synergistic effects. *J Am Acad Child Adolesc Psychiatry* 1991;30:154–155; Riddle MA, King RA, Hardin MT, et al. Behavioral side effects of fluoxetine in children and adolescents. *J Child Adolesc Psychopharmacol* 1990/ 1991;1:193–198). Neuropsychiatric disturbances include possible delusional ideation and hypomanic/manic symptoms with fluoxetine alone or in combination with lithium (Achamallah NS, Decker DH. Mania induced by fluoxetine in an adolescent patient. *Am J Psychiatry* 1991;148:1404; Hersh CB, Sokol MS,

Pfeffer CR. Transient psychosis with fluoxetine. *J Am Acad Child Adolesc Psychiatry* 1991;30: 851; Jerome L. Hypomania with fluoxetine. *J Am Acad Child Adolesc Psychiatry* 1991;30:850– 851; Venkarataman S, Naylor MW, King CA. Mania associated with fluoxetine treatment in adolescents. *J Am Acad Child Adolesc Psychiatry* 1992;31:276–281).

fluoxetine + chloral hydrate Co-administration causes moderate, prolonged drowsiness, possibly due to fluoxetine interference with the metabolic degradation of chloral hydrate or to fluoxetine displacement of chloral hydrate from its binding sites (Devarajan S. Interactions of fluoxetine and chloral hydrate. *Can J Psychiatry* 1992;37:590–591).

fluoxetine + chlorpromazine Even small doses of fluoxetine (< 10 mg) added to chlorpromazine may produce dry mouth and pronounced orthostatic hypotension.

fluoxetine + clomipramine Fluoxetine (FLX) inhibits the metabolic pathways involved in tricyclic antidepressant biotransformation (Bertschy G, Vandel S, Francois T, et al. Metabolic interaction between tricyclic antidepressant and fluvoxamine and fluoxetine, a pharmacogenic approach. *Clin Neuropharmacol* 1992;15[suppl 1/A]:78A–79A). Co-administration was effective in adult patients with severe obsessive-compulsive disorder (OCD) refractory to FLX or clomipramine (CMI) alone. In other cases, adjunctive FLX produced benefits with no additional side effects (Brownc M, Horn E, Jones TT. The benefits of clomipramine-fluoxetine combination in obsessive compulsive disorder. *Can J Psychiatry* 1993;38: 242–243). Similar benefits have been reported in adolescents with OCD (Simeon JG, Thatte S, Wiggins D. Treatment of adolescent obsessive-compulsive disorder with a clomipramine-fluoxetine combination. *Psychopharmacol Bull* 1990;26:285–290). Combined use of these two serotonergic agents did not produce the serotonin syndrome. FLX may potentiate CMI's capacity to induce convulsions either by increasing its serum concentration or by some additive effect. Drugs with known seizure potential should be administered very cautiously in conjunction with high-dose FLX.

fluoxetine + clonazepam No serious adverse interactions have been reported. Adjuvant clonazepam (CNP) may be associated with additional antianxiety and possible antiobsessive effects when combined with fluoxetine (FLX) in the treatment of obsessive-compulsive disorder (OCD). CNP (0.5 mg 2 or 3 times a day) added to FLX in seven OCD patients resistant to behavior therapy produced improvement of more than 20% in only one patient (Jenicke MA. Augmentation strategies for treatment-resistant obsessive compulsive disorder. *Harvard Rev Psychiatry* 1993;1:17–26).

fluoxetine + clonidine   Co-administration is ineffective in the treatment of obsessive compulsive disorder. Side effects, mainly excessive sedation and unsteadiness, necessitated clonidine discontinuation before the end of a 1-month trial in over 50% of patients (Jenike MA. Augmentation strategies for treatment-resistant obsessive-compulsive disorder. *Harvard Rev Psychiatry* 1993;1:17–26).

fluoxetine + clozapine   Co-administration may be useful in the treatment of schizophrenia (Cassady SL, Thaker GK. Addition of fluoxetine to clozapine. *Am J Psychiatry* 1992;149:1274). Obsessive-compulsive symptoms have developed during clozapine (CLOZ) treatment of chronic schizophrenia (Patil VJ. Development of transient obsessive-compulsive symptoms during treatment with clozapine. *Am J Psychiatry* 1992;149:272). In some patients, symptoms did not resolve spontaneously, but responded to fluoxetine (FLX) (20–40 mg/day) with no compromise of CLOZ effectiveness (Patel B, Tandon R. Development of obsessive-compulsive symptoms during clozapine treatment. *Am J Psychiatry* 1993;150:836). FLX may potentiate CLOZ's capacity to induce convulsions either by increasing its serum concentration or by some additive effect. Drugs with known seizure potential should be administered very cautiously in conjunction with high-dose FLX. Co-administration also may result in CLOZ toxicity associated with elevated plasma levels.

fluoxetine/cocaine dependence   In an open prospective study, 16 cocaine (COC)-dependent methadone maintenance patients were treated with fluoxetine (FLX) at a mean dose of 45 mg/day for 9 weeks. Eleven (69%) had the human immunodeficiency virus (HIV). COC use was significantly reduced by the end of treatment, although most subjects did not achieve abstinence. FLX was well tolerated in combination with methadone and did not appear to alter methadone plasma concentrations. Few adverse effects were noted and none required FLX discontinuation. Study data also indicate that quantitative determination of exact COC and benzoylecgonine concentrations in biofluids may be a more accurate method of measuring COC use outcome than qualitative urinalysis (Batki SL, Manfredi LB, Jacob P, Jones RT. Fluoxetine for cocaine dependence in methadone maintenance: quantitative plasma and urine cocaine/benzoylecgonine concentrations. *J Clin Psychopharmacol* 1993;13:243–250).

fluoxetine + cyclobenzaprine   Fluoxetine inhibits hepatic metabolism of cyclobenzaprine, producing elevated cyclobenzaprine plasma levels and side effects consistent with cyclobenzaprine toxicity.

fluoxetine + cyproheptadine   Cyproheptadine may reverse fluoxetine (FLX)-induced anorgasmia, but may also reverse FLX's antidepressant activity (Feder R. Reversal of antidepressant activity of fluoxetine by cyproheptadine in three patients. *J Clin Psychiatry* 1991;52:163–164; Goldbloom DS, Kennedy SH. Adverse interaction of fluoxetine and cyproheptadine in two patients with bulimia nervosa. *J Clin Psychiatry* 1991;52:261–262).

fluoxetine + deprenyl   See **fluoxetine + selegiline.**

fluoxetine + desipramine   Combined use downregulates beta-adrenergic receptors more rapidly than either drug alone and may be rapidly effective in the treatment of major depression, supporting the recent hypothesis of noradrenergic-serotonergic synergism (Eisen A. Fluoxetine and desipramine: a strategy for augmenting antidepressant response. *Pharmacopsychiatry* 1989;22:272–273; Nelson JC, Mazure CM, Bowers MB, Jatlow PI. Augmentation of desipramine with fluoxetine. Presented at the 146th Annual Meeting of the American Psychiatric Association, San Francisco, May 1993; Nelson JC, Mazure CM, Bowers MB, Jatlow PI. A preliminary open study of the combination of fluoxetine and desipramine for rapid treatment of major depression. *Arch Gen Psychiatry* 1991;48:303–307; Baron BM, Ogden AM, Siegel BW, et al. Rapid down regulation of beta-adrenoceptors by co-administration of desipramine and fluoxetine. *Eur J Pharmacol* 1988;154:125–134; Vaughan DA. Interaction of fluoxetine with tricyclic antidepressants. *Am J Psychiatry* 1988;145:1478; Blier P, De Montigny CA. Basis for augmentation strategies in depression. Presented at the 146th Annual Meeting of the American Psychiatric Association, San Francisco, May 1993). The combination should be given for 4 weeks for optimal results. One week after treatment begins, there is a rise in desipramine (DMI) plasma level, as well as a mean change in Hamilton Depression Rating Scale (HAM-D) scores (42%). After 2 weeks, mean change in the HAM-D is about 60%. DMI and hydroxydesipramine plasma levels increase, but the higher the level, the less favorable the result. In one study, addition of FLX resulted in mean DMI levels 2.5 times higher than expected (Suckow RF, Roose SP, Cooper TB. Effect of fluoxetine on plasma desipramine and 2-hydroxydesipramine. *Biol Psychiatry* 1992;31:200–204). In another, FLX caused an average 350% increase in plasma DMI by the third week in normal volunteers receiving FLX (20 mg/day) or DMI (50 mg/day). The effect persisted for more than 21 days after discontinuation and was attributed to the longer half-life of FLX (and norfluoxetine, its major metabolite) (Preskorn SH. Unpublished data). Co-prescribing FLX and DMI or switching immediately from FLX to DMI may cause potentially toxic DMI plasma levels (van Ameringen M, Mancini C. Adverse effects of switching from fluoxetine to desipramine. *Can J Psychiatry* 1992;37:278). In some patients, a trial of FLX with low-dose DMI caused excessive anticholinergic effects (Murray MJ, Hooberman D. Fluoxetine and prolonged erection. *Am J Psychiatry* 1993;150:167–168). If FLX is given with DMI, 40% of the DMI dose, calculated using 24-hour levels, should be sufficient to attain the desired target level. The combination has not caused any serious side effects; type and frequency of side effects are similar to those reported with DMI alone.

fluoxetine + desipramine + lithium Lithium augmentation may be beneficial in patients being treated with desipramine and fluoxetine for refractory depression (Fontaine R, Ontiveros A, Elie R, et al. Lithium carbonate augmentation of desipramine and fluoxetine in refractory depression. *Biol Psychiatry* 1991; 29:946–948).

fluoxetine + dextroamphetamine Adding dextroamphetamine to fluoxetine (FLX) in patients with refractory depression characterized by anergy, anhedonia, weight gain, and hyperphagia may augment FLX antidepressant effects (Linet LS. Treatment of refractory depression with a combination of fluoxetine and d-amphetamine. *Am J Psychiatry* 1989;146: 803–804).

fluoxetine + dextromethorphan Visual hallucinations were reported in a patient taking fluoxetine (20 mg/day) for 17 days who used 4 teaspoons of cough syrup containing dextromethorphan in a 24-hour period. Hallucinations occurred 2 hours after the last dose of the cough syrup, lasted 6–8 hours, and were very similar to an experience with lysergic acid diethylamide (LSD) 12 years earlier (Achamallah NS. Visual hallucinations after combining fluoxetine and dextromethorphan. *Am J Psychiatry* 1992;149:1406).

fluoxetine + diazepam Co-administration increases diazepam (DZ) blood levels and may result in toxicity due to fluoxetine's inhibiting metabolism and slowing clearance of DZ (Lemberger L, Rowe H, Bosomworth JC, Tenbarge JB, Bergstrom RF. The effect of fluoxetine on the pharmacokinetics and psychomotor responses of diazepam. *Clin Pharmacol Ther* 1988;43:412–419). Lowering of concentrations

of desmethyldiazepam, which itself is active, may explain why no psychomotor impairment was noted with the drug combination (Ciraulo DA, Shader RI. Fluoxetine drug-drug interactions: II. *J Clin Psychopharmacol* 1990;10:213–217).

fluoxetine + digitalis Co-administration may alter digitalis serum concentration.

fluoxetine + dothiepin Changing from fluoxetine to dothiepin may cause agitation, tremulousness, sedation, and grand mal seizures (Lyndon RW. Fluoxetine-dothicpin interaction: seizures. *Pharmabulletin* 1993;17:9).

fluoxetine + doxepin Low-dose (25–50 mg/day) doxepin can be combined with fluoxetine for night-time nervousness attributed to fluoxetine.

fluoxetine + electroconvulsive therapy (ECT) There are reports indicating no additional antidepressant benefit from concurrent use of fluoxetine (FLX) and ECT. Co-administration also has been reported both to prolong seizure duration and not to prolong it (Elizon A, Steinbok M, Levin Y. Fluoxetine prevents increase of seizure threshold and shortening of seizure duration in depressive patients treated by ECT. Presented at the 146th Annual Meeting of the American Psychiatric Association, San Francisco, May 1993). The possibility of complications from FLX-induced elevations of anesthetic agents and the theoretical possibility of provoking a serotonin syndrome with ECT-induced elevations of brain serotonin have prompted the recommendation that patients not take FLX during ECT (Jarvis MR, Goewert AJ, Zorineski CF. Novel antidepressants and maintenance electroconvulsive therapy. A review. *Ann Clin Psychiatry* 1992;4: 275–284).

fluoxetine + ethopropazine No adverse interaction in depressed Parkinson8s disease patients has been reported.

fluoxetine + fenfluramine Co-administration may augment the anti-obsessional effects of fluoxetine (FLX). In obsessive-compulsive disorder patients only partially responsive to FLX, fenfluramine (20–60 mg/day) further decreased obsessions and compulsions and was well tolerated (Hollander E, DeCaria CM, Schneier FR, et al. Fenfluramine augmentation of serotonin reuptake blockade antiobsessional treatment. *J Clin Psychiatry* 1990;51:119–123).

fluoxetine + fluphenazine Co-administration of fluoxetine (40 mg/day) and fluphenazine (2.5 mg) caused acute laryngeal dystonia manifested by painful jaw tightness and a feeling that the throat was "closing up." Symptoms responded promptly to intravenous diphenhydramine (Ketai R. Interaction between fluoxetine and neuroleptics. *Am J Psychiatry* 1993,150:836–837).

fluoxetine + haloperidol Fluoxetine (FLX) inhibits haloperidol (HAL) metabolism and raises its blood level. Addition of FLX (20 mg/day) for 7–10 days to stable HAL doses increased mean HAL concentration by 20%, but extrapyramidal symptoms (EPS) did not increase appreciably (Levinson ML, Lipsy RJ, Fuller DK. Adverse effects and drug interactions associated with fluoxetine therapy. *Drug Intell Clin Pharm* 1991;25:657–661). Examination of FLX effects on ongoing HAL treatment in eight subjects disclosed substantial increase in blood levels in three who had low initial HAL levels and appeared to be rapid metabolizers of the drug. Slow HAL metabolizers were unaffected (Goff DC, Midha KK, Brotman AW, et al. Elevation of plasma concentrations of haloperidol after the addition of fluoxetine. *Am J Psychiatry* 1991;148:790–792). It is not clear whether these interactions have a pharmacokinetic or a pharmacodynamic basis, or both. Increased HAL levels may lead to toxicity, sometimes manifested by EPS such as akathisia and parkinsonism (Tate JL. Extrapyramidal symptoms in a patient taking haloperidol and fluoxetine. *Am J Psychiatry* 1989;146:399–400). Tardive dyskinesia also has been reported (Stein M. Tardive dyskinesia in a patient taking haloperidol and fluoxetine. *Am J Psychiatry* 1991;148:683).

fluoxetine + imipramine Elevated imipramine serum levels were reported in a patient 3 days after fluoxetine discontinuation (Hahn SM, Griffin JH. Comment: Fluoxetine adverse effects and drug interactions. *Ann Pharmacother* 1991;25:1273–1274).

fluoxetine + levodopa Fluoxetine may be responsible for hallucinations in patients being treated with levodopa (Lauterbach EC. Dopaminergic hallucinosis with fluoxetine in Parkinson's disease. *Am J Psychiatry* 1993;150:1750).

fluoxetine + levodopa/carbidopa See **fluoxetine + levodopa.**

fluoxetine + lithium Co-administration may augment antidepressant effects of fluoxetine (FLX) and may benefit some patients unresponsive to other antidepressants. There were no adverse interactions, possibly because patients were started on FLX and lithium (900–1200 mg/day) was added later (Pope HG, McElroy SL, Nixon RA. Possible synergism between fluoxetine and lithium in refractory depression. *Am J Psychiatry* 1988; 145:1292–1294). Addition of lithium to ongoing FLX treatment has been reported to improve obsessive compulsive disorder symptoms (Ruegg RG, Evans DL, Comes WS, et al. Lithium and fluoxetine

treatment of obsessive compulsive disorder. *In* New Research Programs and Abstracts of the 143rd Annual Meeting of the American Psychiatric Association, New York, May 14 1990; Abstract NR 92). Although there is evidence that FLX is unlikely to produce clinically significant changes in lithium blood concentrations (Hopwood SE, Bogle S, Wildgust HJ. The combination of fluoxetine and lithium in clinical practice. *Int Clin Psychopharmacol* 1993;8:325–327), addition of FLX may elevate serum lithium level and result in neurotoxicity (Salama AA, Shafey M. A case of severe lithium toxicity induced by combined fluoxetine and lithium carbonate. *Am J Psychiatry* 1989;146:278; Wright P, Seth R. Lithium toxicity, hypomania and leucocytosis with fluoxetine. *Ir J Psychol Med* 1992;9:59–60). Mania, seizures, and hyperpyrexia have been reported (Committee on the Safety of Medicines. Fluvoxamine and fluoxetine—interaction with monoamine oxidase inhibitors, lithium and tryptophan. *Curr Prob* 1989;26:61; Hadley A, Cason MP. Mania resulting from lithium-fluoxetine combination. *Am J Psychiatry* 1989;146:1637–1638). Toxicity has also been observed when lithium was added to FLX, although lithium serum level was well within the therapeutic range. Other adverse reactions reported with combined use include absence seizures and a toxic encephalopathy-like state (Saeristan JA, Iglesias G, Aurellano F, et al. Absence seizures induced by lithium: possible interaction with fluoxetine. *Am J Psychiatry* 1991;148:146–147; Noveske FG, Hahn KR, Flynn RJ. Possible toxicity of combined fluoxetine and lithium. *Am J Psychiatry* 1989; 146:1515). An acute confusional state was reported in a 60-year-old woman taking amitriptyline (AMI) (100 mg/day) and lithium (600 mg/day). AMI was discontinued and FLX (20 mg/day) was started, at which time serum lithium was 0.6 mmol/L. She developed clouding of consciousness, perplexity, disorientation to time and place, reduced attention and concentration, impaired short-term memory, and visual hallucinations. Physical examination was normal and serum lithium was 0.5 mmol/L. FLX and lithium were stopped; within 3 days the confusional state improved and depression gradually returned. Lithium (600 mg/day) was reintroduced with no adverse cognitive effects (Shah AK, McClosky O. Case report: acute confusional state secondary to a combination of fluoxetine and lithium. *Int J Geriatr Psychiatry* 1992;7:68–69).

fluoxetine + lithium/serotonin syndrome Symptoms of a serotonin syndrome (restlessness, increased myoclonus, hyperreflexia, shivering, tremor, diarrhea, and incoordination) appeared in a 36-year-old woman after lithium

(900 mg/day) was added to fluoxetine (40 mg/day). This is the first report of a serotonin syndrome attributed to this combination (Muly E, McDonald W, Steffens D, Book S. Serotonin syndrome produced by a combination of fluoxetine and lithium. *Am J Psychiatry* 1993;150:1565).

fluoxetine + tryptophan   Fluoxetine increases tryptophan blood level and may result in toxicity. A serotonin-like syndrome manifested by agitation, restlessness, insomnia, nausea, and abdominal cramps was reported with the combination (Steiner W, Fontaine R. Toxic reaction following the combined administration of fluoxetine and L-tryptophan: five case reports. *Biol Psychiatry* 1986;21:1067–1071). See **serotonin syndrome.**

fluoxetine + lysergic acid diethylamide (LSD) Fluoxetine (20 mg/day) may markedly decrease sensitivity to LSD; doses that had been able to elicit a full hallucinogenic effect become approximately one-half to one-third as effective in producing the desired hallucinogenic results (Strassman RJ. Human hallucinogen interactions with drugs affecting serotonergic neurotransmission. *Neuropsychopharmacology* 1992;7:241–243). Grand mal convulsions were reported in a patient taking FLX (20 mg/day) for 1 year, who then took two doses of "blotter" LSD. The patient had taken about 30 single doses of LSD during the preceding year's treatment with FLX (Picker W, Lerman A, Hajal F. Potential interaction of LSD and fluoxetine. *Am J Psychiatry* 1992;149:843–844).

fluoxetine/mania   Since 1972, there have been a number of reports of fluoxetine-induced mania. A study of time to onset found an average of 59 days; individual patients relapsed on days 154, 149, 77, 73, 56, 51, 42, 42, 40, 28, 28, 14, and 10 (Terao T. Comparison of manic switch onset during fluoxetine and trazodone treatment. *Biol Psychiatry* 1993;33:477–478).

fluoxetine + marijuana   Combined use has been reported to cause mania, which may be due to marijuana potentiating the action of fluoxetine at central serotonergic neurons (Stoll AL, Cole JO, Lukas SE. A case of mania as a result of fluoxetine-marijuana interaction. *J Clin Psychiatry* 1991;52:280–281).

fluoxetine + methadone   Co-administration is associated with increased plasma methadone concentrations. Prescription of fluoxetine (FLX) for patients in a methadone-maintenance treatment program has had positive results in reducing cocaine (COC) use (Pollack MH, Rosenbaum JF. Fluoxetine treatment of cocaine abuse in heroin addicts. *J Clin Psychiatry* 1991;52:31–33). In an open prospective study, 16 COC-dependent methadone

maintenance patients took FLX (mean dose, 45 mg/day) for 9 weeks. It was well tolerated and did not appear to alter methadone plasma concentrations. Few adverse effects were noted; none required FLX discontinuation (Batki SL, Manfredi LB, Jacob P, Jones RT. Fluoxetine for cocaine dependence in methadone maintenance: quantitative plasma and urine cocaine/benzoylecgonine concentrations. *J Clin Psychopharmacol* 1993;13:243–250).

fluoxetine + methamphetamine   An 11-year-old child with obsessive-compulsive disorder, major depression, and attention deficit hyperactivity disorder was successfully treated with fluoxetine (mean 30 mg/day) and methamphetamine (sustained release 10 mg/day). Methamphetamine was selected to avoid stimulations with commercial formulations containing food dyes because this child was sensitive to tartrazine. There did not appear to be any significant adverse effects (Bussing R, Levin GM. Methamphetamine and fluoxetine treatment of a child with attention-deficit hyperactivity disorder and obsessive-compulsive disorder. *J Child Adolesc Psychopharmacol* 1993; 3:53–58).

fluoxetine + methylphenidate   Addition of methylphenidate (10–40 mg/day) to fluoxetine (FLX) (20–80 mg/day) produced definite and sustained (6 months) antidepressant response in patients refractory to FLX alone (Zajecka JM, Fawcett J. Antidepressant combination and potentiation. *Psychiatr Med* 1991;9:55–75). Some attention deficit disorder patients unresponsive to methylphenidate may benefit from FLX augmentation (Gammon GD, Brown TE. Fluoxetine and methylphenidate in combination for treatment of attention deficit disorder and co-morbid depressive disorder. *J Child Adolesc Psychopharmacol* 1993;3:1–10).

fluoxetine + metoclopramide   Co-administration may increase risk of extrapyramidal side effects. This may be caused indirectly by increased plasma level of either drug or more directly by an interactive effect on the extrapyramidal system.

fluoxetine + metoprolol   Profound lethargy and bradycardia (36 beats/minute) occurred in a 54-year-old man 2 days after fluoxetine (FLX) (20 mg/day) was started. He had taken metoprolol (100 mg/day) for 1 month when FLX was added. FLX was discontinued; over the next 5 days heart rate returned to its previous rate. Metoprolol was withdrawn and replaced with sotalol (160 mg/day). FLX was reintroduced a week later with no recurrence of bradycardia. FLX may have inhibited the oxidative metabolism of metoprolol, leading to higher metoprolol concentrations and symptomatic bradycardia (Walley T, Pirmohamed M, Proudlove C, Maxwell D. Interaction of metoprolol and fluoxetine. *Lancet* 1993;341: 967–968).

fluoxetine + moclobemide Adverse events during co-administration are similar to those seen when each drug is given separately (Dingemanse J. An update of recent moclobemide interaction data. *Int Clin Psychopharmacol* 1993; 7:167–180).

fluoxetine + monoamine oxidase inhibitor (MAOI) Co-administration reportedly helped two treatment-resistant patients (Peterson G. Strategies for fluoxetine-MAOI combination therapy. *J Clin Psychiatry* 1991;52:87). Co-administration, either together or in close succession, generally should be avoided because of the very high incidence of adverse effects, especially the serotonin syndrome. Because of the long duration of action of norfluoxetine, it has been recommended that an MAOI not be taken for at least 4–5 weeks after fluoxetine (FLX) has been discontinued (Feighner JP, Boyer WF, Tyler DL, Neborsky RJ. Adverse consequences of fluoxetine-MAOI combination therapy. *J Clin Psychiatry* 1990;51:222–225). A longer period between these drugs, however, may be necessary. A serotonin syndrome developed after tranylcypromine was started in a patient who had discontinued FLX for over 5 weeks. Thus, if FLX is discontinued 5 weeks before an MAOI is started, a FLX and norfluoxetine level should be determined, or the MAOI should be started with caution (Doplan JK, Gorman JM. Detectable levels of fluoxetine metabolites after discontinuation: an unexpected serotonin syndrome. *Am J Psychiatry* 1993;150:837). See **serotonin syndrome.**

fluoxetine + moricizine No interactions have been reported.

fluoxetine + morphine Fluoxetine increases morphine blood level and may result in toxicity.

fluoxetine + naltrexone In open trials, fluoxetine (FLX) has been effective as an "anticraving" drug in heroin patients on naltrexone (Maremmani I, Castrogiovanni P, Daini L, Zolesi O. Use of fluoxetine in heroin addiction. *Br J Psychiatry* 1992;160:570–571). Co-administration also was used to treat a 9-year-old boy with Prader-Willi syndrome manifested by compulsive eating, severe skin picking, mild mental retardation, and behavioral problems who had been refractory to various pharmacotherapies, including FLX (60 mg/day) for a year. Naltrexone (12.5–50 mg) was added to FLX, and the patient was placed on a strict behavioral program, a 900-kcal American Diabetic Association (ADA) diet, wound care, and treatment with bactroban. At 9-month follow-up, there was continued improvement in behavior and social interactions, decreased self-mutilation, continued weight control, and continued academic progress in school (Benjamin E, Buot-Smith T. Naltrexone and fluoxetine in Prader-Willi syndrome. *J Am Acad Child Adolesc Psychiatry* 1993; 32:870–873).

fluoxetine + neuroleptic In neuroleptic-resistant schizophrenia, addition of fluoxetine (FLX) (20 mg/day) to ongoing neuroleptic therapy may improve both positive and negative schizophrenic symptoms and depressive symptoms (Goff DC, Brotman AW, Waites M, et al. Trial of fluoxetine added to neuroleptics for treatment-resistant schizophrenic patients. *Am J Psychiatry* 1990;147:492–494). Co-administration may exacerbate any neuroleptic-induced extrapyramidal effects (EPS) and may potentiate FLX's ability to cause extrapyramidal disorders such as akathisia (Chouinard G. Fluoxetine and preoccupation with suicide. *Am J Psychiatry* 1991;148:1258–1259). Some evidence suggests that FLX precipitation of EPS may be more likely during the early stages of neuroleptic treatment when serotonergic modulation of dopamine activity may be greatest and when dopamine levels are elevated above resting conditions (Goff DC, Baldessarini RJ. Drug interactions with antipsychotic agents. *J Clin Psychopharmacol* 1993;13:57–65).

fluoxetine + nortriptyline Co-administration may be effective in patients resistant to a standard antidepressant and a full course of electroconvulsive therapy (Seth R, Jennings AL, Bindman J, et al. Combination treatment with noradrenaline and serotonin uptake inhibitors in resistant depression. *Br J Psychiatry* 1991;161:562–569). Fluoxetine (FLX) can markedly elevate nortriptyline plasma level at steady state (2–11 times), apparently through inhibition of the P450 enzyme system. The interaction may result in hypotension, adverse cardiovascular effects (prolongation of PR, QRS, and QT intervals), a grand mal seizure, and anticholinergic delirium. Thus, nortriptyline plasma levels should be monitored during co-administration (Vaughan DA. Interaction of fluoxetine with tricyclic antidepressants. *Am J Psychiatry* 1988;145:1478; Kahn DG. Increased plasma nortriptyline concentration in a patient cotreated with fluoxetine. *J Clin Psychiatry* 1990;51:36).

fluoxetine/obsessive-compulsive disorder Fluoxetine (FLX) (40 mg+/day) has been shown to be effective in obsessive-compulsive disorder (Turner SM, Jacob RG, Beidel DC, et al. Fluoxetine treatment of obsessive-compulsive disorder. *J Clin Psychopharmacol* 1985;5:207–

212; Pigott TA, Pato MT, Bernstein SE, et al. Controlled comparisons of clomipramine and fluoxetine in the treatment of obsessive-compulsive disorder. *Arch Gen Psychiatry* 1990;47: 926–932). Obsessions may transiently increase at the beginning of treatment (Papp LA, Gorman JM. Suicidal preoccupation during fluoxetine treatment. *Am J Psychiatry* 1990;147: 1380).

fluoxetine + other drugs   Fluoxetine (FLX) appears to interact pharmacokinetically with other drugs, either by inhibiting their oxidative metabolism or by displacing them from protein-binding sites. Pharmacodynamic interactions between FLX and other psychotropic drugs cannot be excluded, since they may have similar actions on neurotransmitter receptor systems (Ciraulo DA, Shader RI. Fluoxetine drug-drug interactions: I. Antidepressants and antipsychotics. *J Clin Psychopharmacol* 1990;10:48–50; Ciraulo DA, Shader RI. Fluoxetine drug-drug interactions. II. *J Clin Psychopharmacol* 1990;10:213–217).

fluoxetine overdose   Serotonin reuptake inhibitors are associated with very low fatal toxicity (number of deaths: 0–6 per 1 million prescriptions) in comparison with tricyclic antidepressants (25–52) and monoamine oxidase inhibitors (21–61), and thus appear to be relatively safe in overdose (Leonard BE. Pharmacological differences of serotonin reuptake inhibitors and possible relevance. *Drugs* 1992;43 [suppl 2]:3–10). On an estimated database of 5 million patients worldwide, reports of death attributed to overdosage of fluoxetine (FLX) alone have been extremely rare (Harrison D. Safety of 5-HT reuptake inhibitors. *Br J Psychiatry* 1992;160:866).

fluoxetine + oxycodone   No serious adverse interactions have been reported.

fluoxetine/Parkinson's disease   Fluoxetine (FLX) up to 40 mg/day may be used for depression without adverse consequences in most outpatients with Parkinson's disease (PD) being treated with levodopa/carbidopa, amantadine, bromocriptine, deprenyl, pergolide, and ethopropazine (Brod TM, Fluoxetine and extrapyramidal side effects. *Am J Psychiatry* 1989;146:1352–1353; Bouchard RH, Pourcher E, Vincent P. Fluoxetine and extrapyramidal side effects. *Am J Psychiatry* 1989; 146:1352–1353; Tate JL. Extrapyramidal symptoms in a patient taking haloperidol and fluoxetine. *Am J Psychiatry* 1989;146:399–400; Caley CF, Friedman JH. Does fluoxetine exacerbate Parkinson's disease? *J Clin Psychiatry* 1992;53:278–282; Steur ENHJ. Increase of Parkinson disability after fluoxetine medication. *Neurology* 1993;43:211–213). FLX treatment requires caution, however, because it may be

associated with induction or exacerbation of parkinsonism. There is a case report of a PD patient suffering acute worsening of symptoms when treated with FLX alone for major depression. Exacerbation coincided with improvement in depression after 3 weeks' treatment with FLX and returned to baseline 1 month after FLX discontinuation (Chouinard G, Sultan S. A case of Parkinson's disease exacerbated by fluoxetine. *Hum Psychopharmacol* 1992;7:63–66).

fluoxetine + paroxetine   Co-administration may require doses lower than usually prescribed for either drug alone.

fluoxetine + pemoline   Co-administration has been used successfully to treat depressed patients partially responsive or unresponsive to fluoxetine (FLX) alone. Potential side effects include agitation, anxiety, insomnia, anorexia, and weight loss (Metz A, Shader R. Combination of fluoxetine with pemoline in the treatment of major depressive disorder. *Int Clin Psychopharmacol* 1991;6:93–96). FLX (80 mg/ day) was reported to potentiate therapeutic response to pemoline (75 mg/day) without causing adverse effects (Zajecka JM, Fawcett J. Antidepressant combination and potentiation. *Psychiatr Med* 1991;9:55–75).

fluoxetine + pentazocine   Co-administration may cause excitatory toxicity resembling the serotonin syndrome (Hansen TE, Dieter K, Keepers GA. Interaction of fluoxetine and pentazocine. *Am J Psychiatry* 1990;147:949–950).

fluoxetine + pergolide   Co-administration has been used to treat patients refractory to fluoxetine (FLX) alone. Response is usually rapid (within a week), but without incremental improvement over the next month. Some patients tolerate the combination well; others develop nausea and vomiting that may or may not respond to lowered pergolide dose (Bouckoms A, Mangini L. Pergolide: an antidepressant adjuvant for mood disorders. *Psychopharmacol Bull* 1993;29:207–211). No adverse interaction in depressed parkinson patients has been reported.

fluoxetine + perphenazine   Co-administration has been found effective in depression with psychotic features (Rothschild AJ, Samson JA, Bessette MP, Carter-Campbell J. Efficacy of the combination of fluoxetine and perphenazine in the treatment of psychotic depression. *J Clin Psychiatry* 1993;54:338–342). An increase in extrapyramidal symptoms has been reported (Lock JD, Gwirtsman HE, Targ EF. Possible adverse drug interactions between fluoxetine and other psychotropics. *J Clin Psychopharmacol* 1990;10:383–384). It is not clear whether the interactions have a pharmacokinetic or pharmacodynamic basis, or both.

fluoxetine + phenelzine   Co-administration may cause symptoms of the serotonin syndrome and should always be avoided. See **fluoxetine + monoamine oxidase inhibitor; serotonin syndrome.**

fluoxetine + phenytoin   Signs and symptoms of phenytoin intoxication occurred in 2 patients 5 and 10 days, respectively, after fluoxetine (20 mg/day) was started. Symptoms included gait ataxia, vertigo, diplopia, altered consciousness, vomiting, difficulty getting up, and increased serum phenytoin concentrations (Jalil P. Toxic reaction following the combined administration of fluoxetine and phenytoin: two case reports. *J Neurol Neurosurg Psychiatry* 1992;55:412–413).

fluoxetine + phototherapy   Combined treatment may be helpful in otherwise refractory bulimia nervosa patients (Schwitzer J, Neudorfer C, Fleishhacker WW. Seasonal bulimia treated with fluoxetine and phototherapy. *Am J Psychiatry* 1993;150:1752).

fluoxetine + pimozide   Pimozide (1–4 mg/day) may augment therapeutic response in patients with trichotillomania refractory or partially responsive to fluoxetine (FLX) (Stein DJ, Hollander E. Low-dose pimozide augmentation of serotonin reuptake blockers in the treatment of trichotillomania. *J Clin Psychiatry* 1992;53:123–126). Pimozide (5 mg/day) plus FLX (20 mg/day) led to a potentially life-threatening bradycardia in a 77-year-old man (Ahmed I, Dagincourt PG, Miller LG, Shader RI. Possible interaction between fluoxetine and pimozide causing sinus bradycardia. *Can J Psychiatry* 1993;38:62–63). Co-administration may worsen extrapyramidal symptoms (Bouchard RH, Pourcher E, Vincent P. Fluoxetine and extrapyramidal side effects. *Am J Psychiatry* 1989;146:1352–1353). A patient receiving pimozide (6 mg) experienced marked mental status changes 4 days after FLX dosage was increased to 40 mg/day. Sensorium cleared completely within a week after pimozide was discontinued (Hansen-Grant S, Silk KR, Guthrie S. Fluoxetine-pimozide interaction. *Am J Psychiatry* 1993;150:1751–1752).

fluoxetine/plasma level/clinical response   There are conflicting data on the relationship between clinical response and plasma concentrations of fluoxetine (FLX) and norfluoxetine. Some investigators have found no significant relationship (Kelly MW, Perry PJ, Holstad SG, Garvey MJ. Serum fluoxetine and norfluoxetine concentrations and antidepressant response. *Ther Drug Monit* 1989;11:165–170; Beasley CM, Bosomworth IC, Wernicke JF. Fluoxetine relationships among dose, re-

sponse, adverse events and plasma concentrations in the treatment of depression. *Psychopharmacol Bull* 1990;26:18–24), whereas others have reported an association between increased norfluoxetine concentration and poor clinical response (Montgomery SA, Baldwin D, Shah A, et al. Plasma-level response relationships with fluoxetine and zimelidine. *Clin Neuropharmacol* 1990;13:S71–S75; Tyrer SP, Marshall EF, Griffiths HW. The relationship between response to fluoxetine, plasma drug levels, imipramine binding to platelet membranes and whole-blood 5-HT. *Progr Neuropsychopharmacology Biol Psychiatry* 1990;14:797–805). A study of plasma concentration, clinical outcome, and side effects revealed no significant differences for plasma FLX or norfluoxetine concentrations between responders and nonresponders. FLX and norfluoxetine plasma concentrations were not significantly different between patients with and without side effects (Norman TR, Gupta RK, Burrows GD, et al. Relationship between antidepressant response and plasma concentrations of fluoxetine and norfluoxetine. *Int Clin Psychopharmacol* 1993;8:25–29).

fluoxetine/post-traumatic stress disorder   There are reports suggesting that fluoxetine may benefit patients with post-traumatic stress disorder (Davidson J, Roth S, Newman E. Fluoxetine in post-traumatic stress disorder. *J Traumatic Stress* 1991;4:419–425; March JS. Fluoxetine and fluvoxamine in PTSD. *Am J Psychiatry* 1992;149:413).

fluoxetine + prednisone   Fluoxetine may alleviate corticosteroid-induced depression without interrupting prednisone therapy (Wyszynski AA, Wyszynski B. Treatment of depression with fluoxetine in corticosteroid-dependent central nervous system Sjogren's syndrome. *Psychosomatics* 1993;34:173–177).

fluoxetine/pregnancy   Available data on fluoxetine (FLX) use early in pregnancy indicate that it does not pose a high risk to the fetus. Postmarketing data (December 1991) covering 219 outcomes of 610 prospective reports show 128 births considered to be within normal limits (no malformations and any problems seen were minor). There were 10 premature births and 29 spontaneous abortions; the latter is slightly higher than the rate usually reported for the general population in the United States (about 15%). One woman had three pregnancies; two ended in spontaneous abortions and 1 produced a normal child. Another had two pregnancies; one ended in spontaneous abortion and the other was a normal child. In six pregnancies there were major malformations, but no pattern (e.g., one atrial septal defect, one bilateral hydroceles, one pyloric stenosis). Six major malformations among 219 pregnancy outcomes is not an excessive rate. In a study of 128 women exposed to FLX (10–80 mg/day) during the first trimester, there was no increased risk of major birth malformations and there were no statistical differences in pregnancy outcome, maternal weight gain, gestational age at delivery, or birth weight (Pastuszak A, Schick-Boschetto B, Zuber C, et al. Pregnancy outcome following first trimester exposure to fluoxetine [Prozac]. *JAMA* 1993;269:2246–2248). These data indicate that FLX should not be automatically discontinued during pregnancy. The data should be shared with the patient, with a review of the risk of remaining untreated, so that the patient can make a reasonably informed decision about continuing FLX therapy (Shader RI. Does continuous use of fluoxetine during the first trimester of pregnancy present a high risk for malformation or abnormal development to the exposed fetus? *J Clin Psychopharmacol* 1992;12:441).

fluoxetine + propranolol Propranolol (60–90 mg/day) produces prompt (within 36–48 hours) relief of fluoxetine (FLX)-induced akathisia (Fleischhacker WW. Propranolol for fluoxetine-induced akathisia. *Biol Psychiatry* 1991;30:531–532; Lipinski VF, Mallya G, Zimmerman P, Pope HG. Fluoxetine-induced akathisia: clinical and theoretical implications. *J Clin Psychiatry* 1989;50:339–342). There is a case report of complete heart block 2 weeks following FLX initiation in a man who had been taking propranolol for several years (Drake WM, Gordon GD. Heart block in a patient on propranolol and fluoxetine. *Lancet* 1994;343:425–426).

fluoxetine/red cell-plasma concentration Red cell and plasma levels of fluoxetine (FLX) and norfluoxetine after their addition to human blood (500 ng/ml each) were compared with levels in six patients treated with FLX (20–80 mg/day). Mean red cell and plasma FLX levels were 493 and 454 ng/ml, respectively; for norfluoxetine they were 533 and 446 ng/ml, respectively. In four patients, FLX and norfluoxetine levels in red cells and plasma were comparable; in the other two patients, levels of both were about twofold higher. Variations in FLX and norfluoxetine distribution in blood compartments were relatively small, indicating that their partitioning blood compartments are quite homogeneous (Amital Y, Kennedy E, DeSandre P, et al. Red cell and plasma concentrations of fluoxetine and norfluoxetine. *Vet Hum Toxicol* 1993;35:134–136).

fluoxetine/seizures Even in large fluoxetine (FLX) overdoses, spontaneous seizures are rare (Jarvis MR, Goewert AJ, Zoremski CF. Novel antidepressants and maintenance electroconvulsive therapy. A review. *Ann Clin Psychiatry* 1992;4:275–284). A possible spontaneous seizure was reported after a 12-day course of 30 mg/day (Lemberger L, Rowe H, Carmichael R, et al. Fluoxetine, a selective serotonin uptake inhibitor. *Clin Pharmacol Ther* 1978;23:421–429). No seizure abnormality was detected on electroencephalography despite unchanged FLX blood levels.

fluoxetine + selegiline Co-administration of fluoxetine (FLX) and selegiline (10 mg/day) may be safe for treatment of Parkinson's disease patients, many of whom have tolerated the combination well (Caley CF, Friedman JH. Does fluoxetine exacerbate Parkinson's disease? *J Clin Psychiatry* 1992;53:278–282). It has been reported to cause mania and episodes of diaphoresis and hypertension. A reaction manifested by shivering and sweating; coldness, clamminess, and vasoconstriction of the hands; blue and mottled fingers; and persistently elevated blood pressure (200/120 mm Hg) was reported with selegiline (5 mg/day) plus FLX (20 mg/day). Symptoms abated a few days after both were discontinued (Suchowersky O, de Vries JD. Interaction of fluoxetine and selegiline. *Can J Psychiatry* 1990; 35:571–572). A Parkinson8s disease patient treated with selegiline (10 mg/day) and FLX (20 mg/day) developed headaches, flushes, and palpitations twice a day for 4 weeks, followed by a probable generalized tonic-clonic seizure associated with hypertension (250/130 mm Hg) (Montaastruc JL, Chamontin B, Senard JM, et al. Pseudophaeochromocytoma in parkinson patient treated with fluoxetine plus selegiline. *Lancet* 1993;341: 555). A 66-year-old woman with Parkinson's disease taking selegiline (10 mg/day) experienced ataxia after receiving FLX (20 mg/day) for 1 month. Selegiline was discontinued. Six weeks later, the patient reported no depressive symptoms, and ataxia had lessened significantly. FLX was decreased to 10 mg/day and discontinued 4 weeks later. Within 1 month, the ataxia was completely resolved. This case suggests that ataxia may be the result of an interaction between fluoxetine and selegiline (Jermain DM, Hughes PL, Follender AB. Potential fluoxetine-selegiline interaction. *Ann Pharmacother* 1992;26:1300). Despite selectivity and reversibility, selegiline and similar "new" reversible monoamine oxidase inhibitors (MAOIs) are not immune to the usual interactions of "old" MAOIs.

fluoxetine + sertraline Co-administration may increase sertraline plasma level.

fluoxetine/sexual dysfunction Fluoxetine (FLX) at therapeutic doses may cause changes in sexual desire and orgasmic and erectile difficulties within the first 2 months of treatment. FLX-induced sexual dysfunction persists as long as FLX therapy is continued, tends to diminish upon dose reduction, and usually remits within 3–4 weeks after FLX discontinuation. Addition of yohimbine may produce partial or complete relief. See **fluoxetine + yohimbine.**

fluoxetine + sotalol Co-administration apparently produces no adverse interactions (Walley T, Pirmohamed M, Proudlove C, Maxwell D. Interaction of metoprolol and fluoxetine. *Lancet* 1993;341:967–968).

fluoxetine/suicidal ideation Fluoxetine (FLX) has been reported to provoke long-lasting suicidal ideation and behavior in some depressed patients, possibly due to impaired ability to reverse initially decreased serotonergic transmission (Teicher MH, Glod C, Cole JO. Emergence of intense suicidal preoccupation during fluoxetine treatment. *Am J Psychiatry* 1990;147:207–210). This sparked a number of reports of similar occurrences; it also sparked controversy regarding the validity of the findings. To determine if treatment with antidepressants in general and FLX in particular is associated with emergence or worsening of suicidality, a meta-analysis was performed on data from 17 double-blind trials in patients treated with FLX, tricyclic antidepressants (TCAs), or placebo; it was concluded that FLX is not associated with increased risk of suicidality among depressed patients treated for 6 weeks (Beasley CM Jr, Dornseif BE, Bosomworth JC, et al. Fluoxetine and suicidality: a meta-analysis of controlled trials of treatment of depression. *Br Med J* 1991;303:685–692). An analysis of clinical trials with several serotonin uptake inhibitors (SUIs) disclosed no increased incidence of suicide attempts or completions in comparison to random assignment to placebo or a TCA (Mann JJ, Kapur S. The emergence of suicidal ideation and behavior during antidepressant pharmacotherapy. *Arch Gen Psychiatry* 1991;48:1027–1033; Fava M, Rosenbaum J. Suicidality and fluoxetine: is there a relationship? *J Clin Psychiatry* 1991;52:108–111). There may be a subgroup of patients more susceptible to certain adverse effects of SUIs (e.g., agitation, akathisia), perhaps predisposing them to a paradoxical increase in suicidal ideation or behavior (Rothschild AJ, Locke CA. Reexposure to fluoxetine after serious suicide attempts by three patients: the role of akathisia. *J Clin Psychiatry* 1991;52:491–493). If there is an association between suicidality and akathisia in FLX-treated patients, a number of factors may

be involved, including previous history of suicidal ideation and rapid dosage increase. High FLX doses are associated with an increased likelihood of side effects, one of which may be akathisia in some patients (Ayd FJ Jr. Fluoxetine, akathisia, and suicidal ideation. *Int Drug Ther Newsl* 1992;27:5–6). Depressive illness is a major risk factor for suicide, suicidal behavior, and suicidal ideation. Given the difficulty in determining if a symptom of a disorder may also be a side effect of treatment for that disorder, the best advice for any use of an antidepressant is vigilance on the part of the physician and careful patient/family education.

fluoxetine + sulpiride Co-administration can evoke acute extrapyramidal reactions (Dinan TG, O'Keane V. Acute extrapyramidal reactions following lithium and sulpiride co-administration. *Hum Psychopharmacol Clin Exp* 1991;6:67–69).

fluoxetine + sumatriptan Co-administration may increase sumatriptan effects (Anon. Sumatriptan: a new approach to migraine. *Drug Ther Bull* 1992;30:85–87).

fluoxetine test After one night of fasting, FLX (80 mg) is administered orally. Serum cortisol samples are taken every 30 minutes, starting 90 minutes after drug administration, for a total of 270 minutes. Depressed subjects have a statistically significant difference in cortisol plasma levels compared to normal control subjects. Results suggest a serotonergic dysfunction that may be used as a marker for depression.

fluoxetine + tolbutamide No adverse interactions have been reported (Lemberger L, Rowe H, Bosomworth JC, et al. The effect of fluoxetine on the pharmacokinetics and psychomotor responses of diazepam. *Clin Pharmacol Ther* 1988;43:412–419).

fluoxetine + tranylcypromine Death was reported following initiation of tranylcypromine shortly after fluoxetine (FLX) treatment was discontinued (Prozac. *In Physicians' Desk Reference.* Oradell, NJ: Medical Economics; 1990, pp 905–908). A serotonin-like syndrome manifested by fevers, chills, flushes, disorientation, diplopia, memory loss, confusion, incoordination, abdominal cramping and diarrhea, paresthesias, insomnia, and a hypomanic mood occurred in a patient who was started on tranylcypromine (20 mg/day) 6 weeks after discontinuing FLX. Symptoms remitted 48 hours after tranylcypromine was discontinued 3 weeks later. The reaction is attributed to interaction between tranylcypromine and residual norfluoxetine (Coplan JD, Gorman JM. Detectable levels of fluoxetine metabolites after discontinuation: an unexpected serotonin syndrome. *Am J Psychiatry* 1993;150:837; Sternbach H. Danger of MAOI therapy after fluoxetine withdrawal [letter]. *Lancet* 1988;2: 850–851).

fluoxetine + trazodone   Trazodone may augment fluoxetine's (FLX) antidepressant effect, counteract its stimulant effect, and overcome its delayed sleep onset effect (Jacobsen FM. Low-dose trazodone as a hypnotic in patients treated with MAOIs and other psychotropics: a pilot study. *J Clin Psychiatry* 1990;51: 298–302; Nierenberg AA, Cole JO, Glass L. Possible trazodone potentiation of fluoxetine. A case series. *J Clin Psychiatry* 1992;53:83–85). In some patients the combination may cause intolerable headaches, dizziness, or daytime sedation and fatigue possibly due to FLX's reducing trazodone clearance (Aranow RB, Hudson JI, Pope HG Jr, et al. Elevated antidepressant plasma levels after addition of fluoxetine. *Am J Psychiatry* 1989;46:911–913; Metz A, Shader RI. Adverse interactions encountered when using trazodone to treat insomnia associated with fluoxetine. *Int Clin Psychopharmacol* 1990;5:191–194). In 4 of 13 obsessive-compulsive disorder patients, rating scale scores dropped by more than 20% when trazodone was added to ongoing FLX, but trazodone caused excessive daytime sedation (Jenike MA. Approaches to the patient with treatment-refractory obsessive-compulsive disorder. *J Clin Psychiatry* 1990;51[suppl 2]:15–21; Jenike MA. Management of patients with treatment-resistant obsessive-compulsive disorder. *In* Pato MT, Zohar J [eds], *Obsessive-Compulsive Disorders*. Washington, DC: APA Press, 1991, pp 135–156).

fluoxetine + triazolam   No pharmacokinetic interactions occur (Wright CE, Lasher-Sisson TA, Steenwyck RC, Swanson CN. Pharmacokinetic evaluation of the combined administration of triazolam and fluoxetine. *Pharmacotherapy* 1992;12:103–106).

fluoxetine + tricyclic antidepressant (TCA)   Co-administration may benefit patients unresponsive to either drug alone (Weillburg JG, Rosenbaum JF, Biedermann J, et al. Fluoxetine added to non-MAOI antidepressants converts non-responders to responders: a preliminary report. *J Clin Psychiatry* 1989;50:477–479). Fluoxetine (FLX) inhibits hepatic metabolism of TCAs and may cause a twofold increase in TCA plasma level. If a TCA overdose is taken by a FLX-treated patient, side effects are consistent with TCA toxicity (Bergstrom RF, Peyton AL, Lemberger L. Quantification and mechanism of fluoxetine and tricyclic antidepressant interaction. *Clin Pharm Ther* 1992;51: 239–248). FLX also can prolong TCA elimination so that TCA levels may remain elevated

for a prolonged period following overdose. Recent treatment with FLX may significantly influence metabolism of subsequently prescribed TCAs, requiring dosage adjustments over time to establish and maintain TCA therapeutic levels and clinical response. It has been suggested that TCA dosage should be reduced by 75% when FLX is added, and that about 3 months must be allowed for a new steady-state TCA blood concentration to be reached. Co-administration without monitoring TCA plasma levels may be associated with more side effects and/or poor response. TCA levels may fall as FLX's inhibition of TCA metabolism dissipates; thus, TCA dosage may need to be increased to maintain therapeutic plasma levels and achieve clinical response. Failure to increase TCA dosage may lead to some patients being falsely labeled as TCA nonresponders (Westermeyer J. Fluoxetine-induced tricyclic toxicity: extent and duration. *J Clin Pharmacol* 1991;31:388–392; Suckow RF, Roose SP, Cooper TB. Effect of fluoxetine on plasma desipramine and 2-hydroxydesipramine. *Biol Psychiatry* 1992;31:200–204).

fluoxetine + tri-iodothyronine (T$_3$)   T$_3$ has been reported to augment fluoxetine's antidepressant effect (Crowe D, Collins JP, Rosse RB. Thyroid hormone supplementation of fluoxetine treatment. *J Clin Psychopharmacol* 1990; 10:150–151; Jaffe R. Triiodothyronine potentiation of fluoxetine in depressed patients. *Can J Psychiatry* 1992;37:48–50).

fluoxetine + tri-iodothyronine (T$_3$) + lithium   Lithium may act synergistically (perhaps via separate mechanisms) with fluoxetine and T$_3$ to enhance mood (Geracioti TD, Loosen PT, Gold PW, Kling MA. Cortisol, thyroid hormone, and mood in atypical depression: a longitudinal case study. *Biol Psychiatry* 1992;31: 515–519).

fluoxetine + tryptophan   Co-administration may produce an adverse reaction manifested by agitation, restlessness, and gastrointestinal distress (Steiner W, Fontaine R. Toxic reaction following the combined administration of fluoxetine and L-tryptophan: five case reports. *Biol Psychiatry* 1986;21:1067–1071).

fluoxetine + valproate   Sodium valproate may augment fluoxetine (FLX) in the treatment of refractory depression (Corrigan FM. Sodium valproate augmentation of fluoxetine or fluvoxamine effects. *Biol Psychiatry* 1992;31:1178–1179). FLX-mediated inhibition of hepatic valproic acid metabolism may increase valproate plasma level as much as 50%, exposing the patient to increased risk of drug-related side effects (Sovner R, Davis JM. A potential drug interaction between fluoxetine and valproic acid. *J Clin Psychopharmacol* 1991;11: 389).

fluoxetine + warfarin   Co-administration may alter warfarin serum concentration, resulting in increased bleeding time, a coagulation disorder, or increased coagulation time manifested by severe bruising and other complications (Claire RJ, Servis ME, Cram DL: Potential interaction between warfarin sodium and fluoxetine. *Am J Psychiatry* 1991;148:1604; Woolfrey S, Gammack NS, Dewar MS, Brown PJE. Fluoxetine-warfarin interaction. *Br Med J* 1993;307:241).

fluoxetine/withdrawal   Withdrawal from fluoxetine may be manifested by symptoms such as dizziness, sweating, nausea, insomnia, tremor, and confusion. Symptoms are mild and transient, and similar to withdrawal symptoms noted with other serotonin uptake inhibitors (Anon. *Current Problems in Pharmacovigilance* 1993;19:1).

fluoxetine + yohimbine   Yohimbine (5.4 mg 3 times a day) may produce partial or complete relief of fluoxetine (FLX)-induced sexual dysfunction in up to 90% of those treated. Favorable response occurs within the first treatment week and persists as long as yohimbine is continued. It is usually well tolerated; most common side effects are nausea, anxiety, insomnia, and urinary frequency (Jacobsen FM. Fluoxetine-induced sexual dysfunction and an open trial of yohimbine. *J Clin Psychiatry* 1992; 53;119-122). Combined use has been reported to negate FLX's antidepressant effect. See **fluoxetine/sexual dysfunction.**

fluoxymesterone   (Android F; Halotestin; Ora Testryl) 17-Alpha-methyl testosterone derivative anabolic steroid.

Fluoxytal   See **fluvoxamine.**

flupenthixol   (Depixol; Fluanxol; Fluxanol) (FPX) Thioxanthene antipsychotic that is a mixed dopamine D_1/D_2 antagonist. Pharmacological effects closely resemble those of phenothiazines and butyrophenones. In addition to effectiveness in schizophrenia, FPX may be useful for treatment of a variety of mood disorders. The injectable form may reduce craving for crack cocaine. Side effect profile is similar in many respects to that of other neuroleptics.

flupenthixol decanoate   (Depixol Injection; Fluanxol) Depot form of flupenthixol in a concentration of 20 mg/ml used in Europe for the same clinical indications as other depot neuroleptics. Therapeutic efficacy and side effects are comparable to those of most depot neuroleptics. Clinical studies suggest that flupenthixol decanoate may be advantageous in schizophrenia with marked negative symp-

toms. It also has been reported to reduce craving for crack cocaine and alleviate depression (Gawin FH, Allen D, Humblestone B. Outpatient treatment of "crack" cocaine smoking with flupenthixol decanoate: a preliminary report. *Arch Gen Psychiatry* 1989;46: 322–325). Not available in the United States.

flupenthixol + lithium   Neurotoxicity has been reported (West A. Adverse effects of lithium treatment. *Br Med J* 1977;2[6087]:642).

flupenthixol + melitracen   (Deanxit) Combination product not available in the United States.

fluperlapine   See **neuroleptic, atypical, type A.**

fluphenazine   (Moditen; Permitil; Prolixin; Sediten; Selectin) (FLU) Piperazine phenothiazine neuroleptic, the most potent phenothiazine available on a milligram per milligram basis. Metabolites include fluphenazine sulfoxide (FS), 7-hydroxyfluphenazine (7OHFLU), and fluphenazine N-oxide (FNO). Side effects include extrapyramidal reactions, tardive dyskinesia, drowsiness, and lethargy. It can be given orally, intramuscularly, intravenously, or in a long-acting depot injectable formulation. There are differences in the amount of active medication in depot neuroleptic formulations. In patients receiving FLU orally, 7OHFLU plasma levels are significantly higher than those of the parent compound. With FLU decanoate, levels of this metabolite are significantly lower than FLU levels. Pregnancy risk category C.

fluphenazine + benztropine   Co-administration in a woman with tardive dyskinesia resulted in dysphagia. Attempts to decrease neuroleptic dosage worsened the dysphagia and produced acute dyspnea. When the fluphenazine dose was increased, symptoms quickly resolved (Weiden P, Harrigan M. A clinical guide for diagnosing and managing patients with drug-induced dysphagia. *Hosp Community Psychiatry* 1986;37:396–398).

fluphenazine + carbamazepine   Carbamazepine's (CBZ) microsomal enzyme-inducing action decreases fluphenazine steady-state plasma concentration by approximately 50% and increases its hepatic clearance; clinical results range from improvement to deterioration (Jann MW, Fidone GS, Hernandez JM, Amrung JE, Davis CM. Clinical implications of increased antipsychotic plasma concentrations upon anticonvulsant cessation. *Psychiatry Res* 1989;28:153–159).

fluphenazine + fluoxetine   Co-administration of fluoxetine (FLX) (40 mg/day) and fluphenazine (2.5 mg) caused acute laryngeal dystonia manifested by painful jaw tightness and a feeling that the throat was "closing up." Symptoms responded promptly to intravenous diphenhydramine (Ketai R. Interaction between fluoxetine and neuroleptics. *Am J Psychiatry* 1993,150:836–837).

fluphenazine + idazoxan　In a placebo-controlled, double-blind trial, idazoxan added to chronic fluphenazine in 12 patients with schizophrenia significantly decreased global psychosis (p < 0.03); Brief Psychiatric Rating Scale (BPRS) total symptoms (p < 0.04); and specific BPRS positive symptoms such as suspiciousness/paranoia (p < 0.003), unusual thought content (p > 0.04), and negative symptoms (p < 0.06). Improvement did not appear to be related to idazoxan-induced changes in fluphenazine plasma levels or effects on extrapyramidal symptoms (Litman RE, Hong WW, Weissman EM, et al. Idazoxan, an alpha2 antagonist, augments fluphenazine in schizophrenic patients: a pilot study. *J Clin Psychopharmacol* 1993;13:264–267).

fluphenazine + lithium　Co-administration may be associated with neurotoxicity, including extrapyramidal symptoms (Alevegor B. Toxic reactions to lithium and neuroleptics. *Br J Psychiatry* 1979;135:482; Sachdev PS. Lithium potentiation of neuroleptic-related extrapyramidal side effects. *Am J Psychiatry* 1986;143:942).

fluphenazine + nalmefene　Co-administration successfully augmented effects of fluphenazine (mean dose, 28 mg/day) (Rapaport MH, Wolkowitz O, Kelsoe JR, et al. Beneficial effects of nalmefene augmentation in neuroleptic-stabilized schizophrenic patients. *Neuropsychopharmacology* 1993;9:111–115).

fluphenazine + nicotine　Smoking significantly increases fluphenazine (oral and decanoate) clearance, decreases plasma level, and shortens half-life (Ereshefsky L, Jann MW, Saklad FR, et al. Effect of smoking on fluphenazine clearance in psychiatric inpatients. *Biol Psychiatry* 1985;20:329–332).

fluphenazine + propranolol　Delirium was reported during treatment with fluphenazine decanoate, benztropine, and propranolol (Lima BR, Vanneman D. Propranolol, benztropine, fluphenazine decanoate and delirium. *Am J Psychiatry* 1983;140:659–660).

fluphenazine decanoate　(Fludecate; Modecate; Prolixin Decanoate) (FD) Depot formulation used primarily for maintenance neuroleptic therapy and occasionally for acute psychotic episodes. Duration of action is 3–4 weeks. Whereas haloperidol decanoate (HAL-D) is labeled as to the content of active constituent, FD is labeled as to content of the salt form (1 ml of FD contains 25 mg of decanoate salt and 21.5 mg of fluphenazine). Patients unresponsive to one depot preparation are often switched to another. Since HAL-D and FD are not exactly equipotent, the difference in label-

ing and content of active constituent should be taken into account when switching. Pregnancy risk category C.

fluphenazine decanoate + clomipramine　Addition of clomipramine (CMI) (300 mg/day) to ongoing treatment with fluphenazine decanoate (25 mg) every 2 weeks produced marked improvement in both schizophrenic and obsessive-compulsive symptoms in a patient with a 7-year history of undifferentiated schizophrenia (Zohar J, Kaplan Z, Benjamin J. Clomipramine treatment of obsessive-compulsive symptomatology in schizophrenic patients. *J Clin Psychiatry* 1993;54:385–388).

fluphenazine decanoate + nicotine　See **fluphenazine + nicotine.**

fluphenazine enanthate　(Flunanthate; Moditen Enanthate; Prolixin Enanthate) Depot formulation used primarily for maintenance neuroleptic therapy and occasionally for acute psychotic episodes. Duration of action is 2 weeks. Pregnancy risk category C.

fluphenazine N-oxide　(FLUNO) Fluphenazine metabolite; plasma level is significantly lower than fluphenazine's in patients treated with fluphenazine decanoate.

fluphenazine sulfoxide　(FS) Inactive fluphenazine metabolite.

Flupidol　See **penfluridol.**

flurazepam　(Apo-Flurazepam; Benozil; Dalmane; Durapam; Novoflupam; Som-Pam) (FZP) First benzodiazepine hypnotic marketed in the United States. Sleep is significantly improved on the first night; peak improvement occurs on the 2nd and 3rd consecutive nights because of carryover effects of the long half-life (37–289 hours) of the active metabolite, N-desalkylflurazepam. FZP is effective for both inducing and maintaining sleep for up to a month of consecutive nightly administration. Side effects include drowsiness, sedation, unsteadiness, and confusion. Mild rebound insomnia may occur 4–14 nights after drug discontinuation. Dependence and withdrawal reactions may occur if FZP is taken for prolonged periods. Schedule IV; pregnancy risk category D.

flurazepam + cimetidine　Co-administration inhibits flurazepam (FZP) hydroxylation, producing FZP accumulation and potential toxicity (Greenblatt DJ, Marmatz JS, Engelhardt N, et al. Pharmacokinetic determinants of dynamic differences among three benzodiazepine hypnotics. *Arch Gen Psychiatry* 1989;46:326–332).

flurazepamaldehyde　Flurazepam metabolite.

flurbiprofen　(Ansaid) Potent nonsteroidal anti-inflammatory analgesic used in chronic pain syndromes.

flush reaction Inflammatory skin redness in patients taking certain drugs and consuming alcohol at the same time. Symptoms appear very soon after alcohol ingestion and may be accompanied by dyspnea and headache. They can be blocked by naloxone and aspirin. Alcohol may enhance the release of prostaglandins centrally, either directly or through the release of encephalins, which would initiate the flush reaction and also explain the blocking action of aspirin. Flush reactions are distinct from disulfiram reactions (Strakosch CR, Jeffreys DB, Keen H. Blockade of chlorpropamide alcohol flush by aspirin. *Lancet* 1980;1:394–396; Williams L, Davis JA, Lowenthal DT. The influence of food on the absorption and metabolism of drugs. *Med Clin North Am* 1993;77:815–829).

fluspirilene (Imap) Long-acting depot neuroleptic used in low doses for anxiety and other psychosomatic disorders. Available in some European countries; not available in the United States.

Flutan See **flutoprazepam.**

flutazolam Benzodiazepine currently available in Japan.

flutoprazepam (Flutan; Restas) Benzodiazepine effective in the treatment of generalized anxiety disorders. In healthy subjects, driving skills are markedly impaired 2 hours after taking 4 mg, but only slightly impaired 2 hours after taking 2 mg (these findings are valid only for the period from 2 to 3 hours after drug ingestion). Kinetic and metabolic behavior of flutoprazepam may differ between Japanese and non-Japanese subjects.

fluvoxamine (Avoxin; Dumirox; Dumyrox; Dymyrox; Faverin; Favoxil; Fevarin; Floxyfral; Floxytal; Fluoxytal; Luvox; Maveral) (FVX) Potent presynaptic serotonin (5-HT) uptake inhibitor with high 5-HT2 receptor affinity and little norepinephrine uptake inhibition at normal doses. It is effective in the treatment of depression as well as mixed anxiety and depression (Laws D, Ashford JJ, Anstee JA. A multicentre double-blind comparative trial of fluvoxamine versus lorazepam in mixed anxiety and depression treated in general practice. *Acta Psychiatr Scand* 1990;81:185–189). FVX is nonepileptogenic and therefore an antidepressant of choice for patients with epilepsy. Pharmacokinetic parameters in the elderly do not differ significantly from younger patients. It therefore appears to be appropriate for elderly patients. Therapeutic blood levels have not been established, but a reasonable maximum daily dose, if tolerated, is 300 mg. FVX has antiobsessional and antipanic effects (Goodman WK, Price LH Rasmussen SA, et al. Efficacy of FVX in obsessive-compulsive disor-

der: a double-blind comparison with placebo. *Arch Gen Psychiatry* 1989;46:36–44; Price LH, Goodman WK, Charney DS, et al. Treatment of severe obsessive-compulsive disorder with fluvoxamine. *Am J Psychiatry* 1987;144:1059–1061; Black DW, Wesner R, Bowers W, Gabel J. A comparison of fluvoxamine, cognitive therapy, and placebo in the treatment of panic disorder. *Arch Gen Psychiatry* 1993;50:44–50). Preliminary findings indicate FVX may be valuable in the treatment of alcohol amnestic disorder (Korsakoff's syndrome). It improves episodic memory in this disorder, but not in dementia associated with alcoholism or compensated alcoholic liver disease. Memory improvement is significantly correlated ($p < 0.05$) with reductions in cerebrospinal fluid 5-hydroxyindoleacetic acid, suggesting that facilitation of serotonergic neurotransmission may ameliorate episodic memory failure and alcohol amnestic disorder. Addition of FVX to ongoing antipsychotic and anticholinergic therapy for chronic schizophrenia may improve negative symptoms. Dosage should be no higher than 100 mg/day to reduce risk of evoking a late-onset confusional state (Silver H, Nassar A. Fluvoxamine improves negative symptoms in treated chronic schizophrenia: an add-on double-blind, placebo-controlled study. *Biol Psychiatry* 1992;31:698–704). FVX produces very few anticholinergic side effects and apparently has no significant effect on the cardiovascular system (Laird LK, Lydiard RB, Morton WA, et al. Cardiovascular effects of imipramine, fluvoxamine, and placebo in depressed outpatients. *J Clin Psychiatry* 1993;54:224–228). In normal volunteers, 50 mg twice a day decreased mood ratings of calmness and increased feelings of anxiety, sweating, trembling, nausea, loss of appetite, restlessness, muscular tension, and irritability; effects tended to be maximal by day 4 and then to wane. High doses may cause symptoms resembling a frontal lobe syndrome (apathy, indifference, inattention, and perseveration).

fluvoxamine + alcohol In a set of psychometric tests, fluvoxamine (FVX) (75 mg/day) taken with sufficient alcohol to produce a blood alcohol level of 50 mg/100 ml caused no more impairment than alcohol and placebo. FVX (150 mg/day) + alcohol caused more impairment of vigilance, orientation capacity, and continuous attention span than did alcohol alone. FVX (50 or 100 mg) alone and in combination with alcohol produced no serious psychomotor or cognitive impairment or alterations in autonomic nervous system functioning (Linnoila M, Stapleton JM, George DT, et al. Effects of fluvoxamine, alone and in combination with ethanol, on psychomotor and cognitive performance and on autonomic nervous system reactivity in healthy volunteers. *J Clin Psychopharmacol* 1993;13:175–180). In healthy male volunteers (ages 20–32 years), FVX did not affect the pharmacokinetics of alcohol. It did not potentiate alcohol-induced impairment of cognitive function and in some instances appeared to reverse the effects or reduce their duration (Van Harten J, Stevens LA, Raghoeber M, et al. Fluvoxamine does not interact with alcohol or potentiate alcohol-related impairment of cognitive function. *Clin Pharmacol Ther* 1992;52:427–435). Despite FVX's negligible effects on alcohol kinetics, patients should be urged to use caution if both are ingested.

fluvoxamine + amitriptyline   Co-administration markedly enhances amitriptyline (AMI) plasma level due to inhibition of demethylation by fluvoxamine (FLV). AMI produces a higher plasma level of FLV than occurs with FLV monotherapy. Increased plasma levels of each drug may potentiate antidepressant effects in some patients, but also may cause adverse reactions; serum level monitoring is indicated (Bertschy G, Vandel S, Vandel B, et al. Fluvoxamine-tricyclic antidepressant interaction: an accidental finding. *Eur J Clin Pharmacology* 1991;40:119–121). Inhibitory effects of FLV on AMI metabolism disappear within 1–2 weeks of FLV discontinuation (Haertter S, Wetzel H, Hammes E, Hiemke C. Inhibition of antidepressant demethylation and hydroxylation of fluvoxamine in depressed patients. *Psychopharmacology* 1993;110:302–308).

fluvoxamine + anticoagulant   Bleeding disorder was reported in a patient taking the anticoagulant nicoumalone, fluvoxamine (FVX) (100 mg/day) for 17 days, and ibuprofen (600 mg/day) on days 14 to 17. Symptoms included multiple bruises, hematoma in limbs, marked anemia, and hypotension. FVX and nicoumalone were stopped on day 22, and the patient made a full recovery. Since ibuprofen may interact with anticoagulants, the exact role of FVX cannot be established, but co-administration with coumarin derivatives should be carefully monitored (Rahman MK, Akhtar MJ, Savla NC, et al. A double-blind, randomised comparison of fluvoxamine with dothiepin in the treatment of depression in elderly patients. *Br J Clin Pract* 1991;45:255–258).

fluvoxamine + atenolol   Fluvoxamine apparently has no significant effect on serum levels, volume of distribution, elimination half-life, or total body clearance of atenolol (Benfield P, Ward A. Fluvoxamine: a review of its pharmacokinetic properties and therapeutic efficacy in depressive illness. *Drugs* 1986;32:313–334).

fluvoxamine + benzodiazepine   In open and controlled studies, fluvoxamine has been combined with benzodiazepines and lithium with no report of interactions (Stimmel GL, Skowron DM, Chameides WA. Focus on fluvoxamine: a serotonin reuptake inhibitor for major depression and obsessive-compulsive disorder. *Hosp Formul* 1991;26:635–643).

fluvoxamine/breast milk   Fluvoxamine (FVX) is excreted in breast milk in a concentration much lower than its plasma concentration (Wright S, Dawling S, Ashford JJ. Excretion of fluvoxamine in breast milk. *Br J Clin Pharmacol* 1991;31:209; Isenberg KC. Excretion of fluoxetine in human breast milk. *J Clin Psychiatry* 1990;51:169). Although clinical evidence to date indicates little or no risk to the infant, women being treated with FVX should avoid breastfeeding unless there are compelling reasons for FVX therapy during nursing.

fluvoxamine + bromazepam   Bromazepam plasma concentrations increased by 2.4 times after multiple doses of fluvoxamine (Van Harten J, Holland RL, Wesnes K, et al. Kinetic and dynamic interaction study between fluvoxamine and benzodiazepines. Poster presented at the Second Jerusalem Conference on Pharmaceutical Sciences and Clinical Pharmacology, Jerusalem, May 24–29, 1992).

fluvoxamine + buspirone   Addition of buspirone in fluvoxamine treatment-resistant depression may produce augmentation effects. The combination appears to be safe (Joffe RT, Schuller DR. An open study of buspirone augmentation of serotonin reuptake inhibitors in refractory depression. *J Clin Psychiatry* 1993;54:269–271).

fluvoxamine + carbamazepine   Co-administration may result in increased carbamazepine (CBZ) plasma concentration with resultant toxicity (Fritze J, Unsorg B, Lanczik M. Interaction between carbamazepine and fluvoxamine. *Acta Psychiatr Scand* 1991;84:583–584). Fluvoxamine (FLX) (250 mg/day) plus CBZ (60 mg/day) significantly reduced obsessive-compulsive symptoms without adverse effects in a 26-year-old woman with a history of tonic-clonic seizures induced by combined levomepromazine-FLX treatment (Grinspoon A, Berg Y, Mozes T, et al. Seizures induced by combined levomepromazine-fluvoxamine treatment. *Int Clin Psychopharmacol* 1993;8:61–62). No apparent interaction occurred when FLX was added to a stable CBZ regimen in patients with epilepsy. There were no significant changes in steady-state CBZ or its metabolites, nor were there any changes in seizure frequency, possibly because of the drugs' metabolism by different hepatic isoenzymes (Spina E, Avenoso A, Pollicino AM, et al. Carbamazepine co-administration with fluoxetine or fluvoxamine. *Ther Drug Monit* 1993;15:247–250).

fluvoxamine + chloral hydrate Chloral hydrate (500–1500 mg) has been prescribed for insomnia in fluvoxamine-treated patients without adverse effects (Mallya GK, White K, Waternaux C, et al. Short- and long-term treatment of obsessive-compulsive disorders with fluvoxamine. *Ann Clin Psychiatry* 1992;4:77–80).

fluvoxamine + clomipramine Fluvoxamine (FVX) inhibits clomipramine (CMI) demethylation, markedly enhancing plasma levels of CMI and its metabolite desmethylclomipramine. The increase may lead to a potentiation of the antidepressant effect in some patients, but also may cause adverse reactions. CMI also increases FVX plasma level. During co-administration, serum level monitoring of both drugs is indicated (Bertschy G, Vandel S, Vandel B, et al. Fluvoxamine-tricyclic antidepressant interaction: an accidental finding. *Eur J Clin Pharmacol* 1991;40:119–120). Comedication appears to be well tolerated without signs of cardiotoxic or central nervous system side effects. FVX inhibitory effects on CMI metabolism disappeared within at least 1–2 weeks of FVX discontinuation (Haertter S, Wetzel H, Hammes E, Hiemke C. Inhibition of antidepressant demethylation and hydroxylation by fluvoxamine in depressed patients. *Psychopharmacology* 1993;110:302–308). Following cingulotomy, one patient had seizures on one occasion while taking both CMI and FVX (Jenike MA, Baer L, Ballantine HT, et al. Cingulotomy for refractory obsessive-compulsive disorder. A long-term follow-up of 33 patients. *Arch Gen Psychiatry* 1991;48:548–555).

fluvoxamine + desipramine Addition of fluvoxamine (FVX) (100 mg/day) to desipramine (DMI) (100–150 mg/day) dramatically increased DMI plasma concentration and was associated with adverse effects including confusion, tremor, dizziness, and seizures. The interaction is attributed to FVX's inhibition of DMI hydroxylation (Spina E, Campo GM, Avenosa A, et al. Interaction between fluvoxamine and imipramine/desipramine in four patients. *Ther Drug Monit* 1992;14:194–196).

fluvoxamine + desmethylclomipramine Fluvoxamine increases desmethylclomipramine plasma concentration. This may potentiate antidepressant effects in some patients, but also may cause adverse reactions (Bertschy G, Vandel S, Vandel B, et al. Fluvoxamine-tricyclic antidepressant interaction. *Eur J Clin Pharmacol* 1991; 40:119–120).

fluvoxamine + digoxin Fluvoxamine has no effect on serum levels, volume of distribution, elimination half-life, or total body clearance of digoxin (Ochs HR, Greenblatt DJ, Verburg-Ochs B, Labedski L. Chronic treatment with fluvoxamine, clovoxamine and placebo: interaction with digoxin and effects on sleep and alertness. *J Clin Pharmacol* 1989;29:91–95).

fluvoxamine/dystonic reaction An acute dystonic reaction, manifested by a gradual tightening and stiffening of her jaw muscles that interfered with speaking and eating, occurred in a 36-year-old woman after 4 weeks of treatment with fluvoxamine (FVX) (average dose, 200 mg/day). Symptoms resolved with dosage reduction to 100 mg/day and recurred when FVX was increased again to 200 mg/day. Dose reduction and diphenhydramine (50 mg/day) promptly relieved the symptoms. FVX at 150 mg/day did not cause a dystonic reaction (George MS, Trimble MR. Dystonic reaction associated with fluvoxamine. *J Clin Psychopharmacol* 1993;13:220–221).

fluvoxamine/extrapyramidal reactions Serotonin uptake inhibitors may evoke various types of extrapyramidal reactions and/or aggravate idiopathic or drug-induced extrapyramidal disorders. An extrapyramidal syndrome was reported with fluvoxamine in a 77-year-old woman who had a prior history of tardive dyskinesia (Wils V. Extrapyramidal symptoms in a patient treated with fluvoxamine. *J Neurol Neurosurg Psychiatry* 1992;55:330–331). See **fluvoxamine/dystonic reaction.**

fluvoxamine + fenfluramine Fenfluramine (FEN) augmented antiobsessional response in six of seven patients being treated with a serotonin uptake inhibitor. FEN augmentation was well tolerated (Hollander E, DeCaria CM, Schneier FR, et al. Fenfluramine augmentation of serotonin reuptake blockade antiobsessional treatment. *J Clin Psychiatry* 1990;51: 119–123). Use is limited, however, by evidence from preclinical data, strongly suggesting that neurotoxicity may occur when FEN is co-prescribed with fluvoxamine.

fluvoxamine + haloperidol Up to 50% of obsessive compulsive disorder (OCD) patients remain clinically unchanged after an adequate trial with serotonin uptake inhibitors. Because brain dopamine systems may also contribute to obsessive compulsive phenomena, haloperidol may potentiate response to fluvoxamine (FVX) in OCD patients resistant or partially responsive to FVX without causing any adverse interactions (Dominguez RA. Serotonergic antidepressants and their efficacy in obsessive compulsive disorder. *J Clin Psychiatry* 1992; 53[suppl 10]:56–59; McDougle CJ, Goodman WK, Price LH et al. Neuroleptic addition in fluvoxamine-refractory obsessive-compulsive disorder. *Am J Psychiatry* 1990;147:652–654).

fluvoxamine + imipramine Co-administration markedly enhances imipramine (IMI) plasma level because of inhibition of demethylation by fluvoxamine (FVX), possibly resulting in toxicity manifested by severe anticholinergic effects, tremor, and confusion. IMI also increases FVX plasma level. Serum level monitoring is indicated during co-administration (Spina E., Campo GM, Avenoso A, et al. Interaction between fluvoxamine and imipramine/desipramine in four patients. *Ther Drug Monit* 1992;42:194–196).

fluvoxamine + levomepromazine In a 26-year-old woman with schizotypal personality disorder and obsessive-compulsive disorder, addition of fluvoxamine (50 mg/day) to maintenance treatment (1.5 years) with levomepromazine (800 mg/day) led to development of tonic-clonic seizures (Grinspoon A, Berg Y, Mozes T, et al. Seizures induced by combined levomepromazine-fluvoxamine treatment. *Int Clin Psychopharmacol* 1993;8:61–62).

fluvoxamine + lithium Co-administration may be helpful in treatment-resistant depression and obsessive-compulsive disorder (OCD) partially responsive or refractory to fluvoxamine (FVX). Co-administration may rarely cause convulsions or hyperpyrexia (Committee on the Safety of Medicines. Fluvoxamine and fluoxetine—interaction with monoamine oxidase inhibitors, lithium and tryptophan. *Curr Prob* 1989;26:61; Goodman WK, Price LH, Rasmussen SA, et al. Efficacy of fluvoxamine in obsessive-compulsive disorder. *Arch Gen Psychiatry* 1989;46:36–44). Since lithium enhances FVX's serotonergic effects, the combination should be used with caution. In some bipolar patients, it has resulted in a manic episode (McDougle CJ, Price LH, Goodman WK, et al. A controlled trial of lithium augmentation in fluvoxamine-refractory obsessive-compulsive disorder: lack of efficacy. *J Clin Psychopharmacol* 1991;11:175–184; Hendricks B, Floris M. A controlled study of the combination of fluvoxamine and lithium. *Curr Therapeut Res* 1991;49:106–110).

fluvoxamine + lorazepam Lorazepam (1–2 mg) may relieve insomnia in fluvoxamine-treated patients without adverse effects (Mallya GK, White K, Waternaux C, et al. Short- and long-term treatment of obsessive-compulsive disorders with fluvoxamine. *Ann Clin Psychiatry* 1992;4:77–80).

fluvoxamine + maprotiline Co-administration has been effective in depression refractory to either drug alone.

fluvoxamine + moclobemide In 25 healthy volunteers, fluvoxamine (FVX) (100 mg) plus moclobemide caused adverse effects similar to those of FVX monotherapy. High FVX doses were not tested because they are poorly tolerated by healthy volunteers. There was no indication of the serotonin syndrome during combined treatment (Dingemanse J. An update of recent moclobemide interaction data. *Int Clin Psychopharmacol* 1993;7:167–180). See **moclobemide + serotonin uptake inhibitor.**

fluvoxamine + monoamine oxidase inhibitor (MAOI) Because the serotonin syndrome has occurred with fluoxetine plus an MAOI, a similar reaction could occur with fluvoxamine. Co-administration is not recommended.

fluvoxamine + neuroleptic Co-administration has been used with some success in obsessive compulsive disorder refractory to fluvoxamine alone.

fluvoxamine + nortriptyline Fluvoxamine increases nortriptyline plasma concentration. This may potentiate antidepressant effects, but also may cause adverse reactions (Bertschy G, Vandel S, Vandel B, et al. Fluvoxamine-tricyclic antidepressant interaction. *Eur J Clin Pharmacol* 1991;40:119–120).

fluvoxamine/overdose In three cases involving overdoses of 600–1,500 mg, there were no serious medical sequelae after gastric lavage or vomiting. An overdose of fluvoxamine (FVX) (2,500 mg,) brompheniramine (100 mg), LA tablets, and six flurazepam capsules resulted in elevated temperature and pulse with hypomanic symptoms. After gastric lavage, a sedative was given for restlessness and disturbed behavior (Benfield P, Ward A. Fluvoxamine: a review of its pharmacodynamic and pharmacokinetic properties, and therapeutic efficacy in depressive illness. *Drugs* 1986;32:313–334). An elderly patient who ingested FVX (3 g) and temazepam (250 mg) was unconscious for 5 days, but recovered fully (Banerjee AK. Recovery from prolonged cerebral depression after fluvoxamine overdose. *Br Med J* 1988;296:1774). No deaths have been reported with FVX overdose alone, even after ingestion of 30 times the recommended daily dose (Freeman CP. Fluvoxamine: clinical trials and clinical use. *J Psychiatr Neurosci* 1991;16: 19–25). Ten overdoses involving FVX plus other drugs have been fatal. In an analysis of 298 cases of deliberate acute overdose with FVX, 77% involved co-ingestion of other drugs (mainly benzodiazepines, neuroleptics, other antidepressants, and alcohol). The acute toxicity that could be attributed to FLX alone was rarely severe. Symptoms observed (drowsiness, tremor, nausea, vomiting, abdominal pain, bradycardia, and/or anticholinergic effects) were always benign when the FVX dose was below 1,000 mg. Seizures occurred in a few cases after high doses (generally > 1,500 mg). Cardiotoxicity was not a serious problem; sinus bradycardia was noted with doses less than 1,000 mg, but was always moderate and required no treatment. Conduction abnormalities were rare (Garnier R, Azoyan P, Chataigner D, et al. Acute fluvoxamine poisoning. *J Int Med Res* 1993;21:197–208).

fluvoxamine/panic disorder   Fluvoxamine is as effective as clomipramine and more effective than maprotiline in the treatment of panic disorder (Den Boer JA, Westenberg GM, Kanerbeek WDJ, et al. Effect of serotonin uptake inhibitors in anxiety disorders: a double-blind comparison of clomipramine and fluvoxamine. *Int Clin Psychopharm* 1987;2:21–32; De Boer JA, Westenberg GM. Effect of serotonin and noradrenaline uptake inhibitor in panic disorders: a double-blind comparative study with fluvoxamine and maprotiline. *Int Clin Psychopharm* 1988;3:59–74).

fluvoxamine + pimozide   Co-administration may be effective in the treatment of obsessive-compulsive symptoms with concurrent Tourette's syndrome (McDougle CJ, Goodman WK, Price LH, et al. Neuroleptic addition in fluvoxamine-refractory obsessive compulsive disorder: an open case series. *Am J Psychiatry* 1990;147:552–554; Delgado PL, Goodman WK, Price LH, et al. Fluvoxamine/pimozide treatment of concurrent Tourette's and obsessive-compulsive disorder. *Br J Psychiatry* 1990;157:762–765).

fluvoxamine/post-traumatic stress disorder   Fluvoxamine has improved post-traumatic stress disorder symptoms in some patients with or without depression (March JS. Fluoxetine and fluvoxamine in PTSD. *Am J Psychiatry* 1992; 149:413).

fluvoxamine/pregnancy   There is a single report of fluvoxamine use (100 mg/day) throughout an entire pregnancy. The pregnancy was uneventful and the child was healthy (Szabadi E. Fluvoxamine withdrawal syndrome. *Br J Psychiatry* 1992;160:283–284).

fluvoxamine + propranolol   Co-administration increases bioavailability of oral propranolol, resulting in substantially higher propranolol serum levels (up to 5 times higher). Fluvoxamine (FVX) slightly potentiated propranolol-induced reductions in heart rate (by 3 beats/minute) and exercise diastolic blood pressure, but did not interfere with its blood-pressure-lowering effect. Propranolol dosage may have to be lowered if it is co-administered with FVX (Benfield P, Ward A. Fluvoxamine: a review of its pharmacokinetic properties, and therapeutic efficacy in depressive illness. *Drugs* 1986;32:313–334).

fluvoxamine/seizures   Myoclonus and focal and generalized seizures have been reported with a wide range of antidepressants. The proconvulsive activity of serotonin uptake inhibitors (SUIs) is reputed to be less than that of tricyclic and other cyclic antidepressants and monoamine oxidase inhibitors. However, seizures have been reported with therapeutic doses of SUIs in patients with no predisposing factors receiving no other medication. There are approximately 20 reports of seizures related to therapeutic doses of fluvoxamine; whether it has more or less epileptogenic potential than other SUIs has yet to be determined. It should be used with caution in epileptics and the seizure-prone, even though it has been used successfully and safely in depressed epileptic patients.

fluvoxamine + theophylline   Fluvoxamine (FVX) may increase theophylline plasma concentration (Wagner W, Plekkenpol B, Grag TE, et al. Review of fluvoxamine safety database. *Drugs* 1992;42[suppl 2]:48–54; Diot P, Jonville AP, Gerard F, et al. Possible interaction entre theophylline et fluvoxamine. *Therapie* 1991;46:169–171). Co-administration may produce toxic symptoms (headache, fatigue, vomiting) secondary to increased serum theophylline concentrations (Sperber AD. Toxic interaction between fluvoxamine and sustained release theophylline in an eleven year old boy. *Drug Safety* 1991;6:460–462; Thomson AH, McGovern EM, Bennie P, et al. Interaction between fluvoxamine and theophylline. *Pharmaceut J* 1992;249:127).

fluvoxamine + tricyclic antidepressant (TCA)   Fluvoxamine can increase previously stable TCA plasma levels (Bertschy G, Vandel S, Vandel B, et al. Fluvoxamine-tricyclic antidepressant interaction. *Eur J Clin Pharmacol* 1991; 40:119–120).

fluvoxamine + valproate   Sodium valproate may augment fluvoxamine effects in the treatment of refractory depression (Corrigan FM: Sodium valproate augmentation of fluoxetine or fluvoxamine effects. *Biol Psychiatry* 1992;31: 1178–1179).

fluvoxamine + warfarin   Fluvoxamine inhibits warfarin metabolism, increasing warfarin serum levels (about 65%) and lengthening prothrombin time (Benfield P, Ward A. Fluvoxamine: a review of its pharmacokinetic properties and therapeutic efficacy in depressive illness. *Drugs* 1986;32:313–334). Warfarin dosage may have to be adjusted (*British National Formulary Number 24*. London: British Medical Association and the Royal Pharmaceutical Society of Great Britain, 1992; 5-Hydroxytryptamine reuptake inhibitors. *MeReC Bull* 1991;2:29–32).

fluvoxamine/withdrawal syndrome   Fluvoxamine (FVX) discontinuation may be associated with symptoms such as dizziness, sweating, nausea, insomnia, tremor, and confusion. Symptoms are mild and transient and similar to those with other serotonin uptake inhibitors (Anon. *Current Problems in Pharmacovigilance* 1993;19:1). In one report, 12 of 14 subjects (86%) developed new symptoms within 24 hours after FVX (up to 300 mg/day) was abruptly discontinued. Symptoms peaked on the 5th day following discontinuation, then tapered off. The most frequent symptoms were dizziness/incoordination, headaches, nausea, and irritability. Panic recurred in one subject, and another developed anxiety and depression (Black DW, Wesner R, Gabel J. The abrupt discontinuation of fluvoxamine in patients with panic disorder. *J Clin Psychiatry* 1993;54:146–149; Mallya G, White K, Gunderson C. Is there a serotonergic withdrawal syndrome? *Biol Psychiatry* 1993;33:849–855). There is another report of a woman with severe obsessive-compulsive disorder who had a good response to FVX (100 mg/day). After a year, she reported being unable to stop FVX because of overwhelming feelings of aggression whenever she tried to do so. When FVX was later increased to 150 mg/day, she reported new symptoms after discontinuation. On the first day she felt elated and had general features of hypomania (overactivity, racing thoughts, lack of fatigue). On the second day, aggressive feelings and thoughts appeared, which she described as unbearably distressing (Szabadi E. Fluvoxamine withdrawal syndrome. *Br J Psychiatry* 1992;160:283–284).

Fluxanol   See **flupenthixol.**

"fly"   Street name for muscarine.

"fly catcher's tongue"   Infrequent lingual dyskinesia seen in patients with tardive dyskinesia in which the tongue is rapidly projected and retracted at irregular intervals.

focal motor seizure   See **seizure, focal motor.**

focal onset grand mal seizure   See **seizure, secondary generalized.**

folate   Ester of folic acid that may play a role in the genesis of psychiatric problems associated with epilepsy. Many reports link folate deficiency to chronic anticonvulsant intake and psychiatric symptoms, especially depression. Lower folate levels are more common in patients with epilepsy than in the general population; levels lower than 3 ng/ml are associated with a significant degree of depression on psychological tests. Folate and vitamin B12 levels are not significantly correlated. Folate supplements (1 5 mg/day) can be safe if anticonvulsant levels are kept stable.

folie a deux   Term coined by LaSegue and Falret (1873) for a rare paranoid delusional system that develops in one person as a result of a close relationship with another who has an established delusional system (Enoch MD, Trethowan WH. *Uncommon Psychiatric Syn-*

dromes. Bristol, England: Wright, 1979). Extended conditions involving three, four, or five persons, or even a whole family, have been reported. Over 90% of cases are blood relatives. Most frequently, two sisters are affected. A mother and child combination is found more often than one of father and child. Entire families are affected only very rarely (LaSegue C, Falret J. La folie a deux. *Annales Medico-Psycholoques* 1877;18:321–355; translated: Michaud R. *Am J Psychiatry* 1964;121 [suppl 4]:1–23). Also called "induced psychosis."

follicle-stimulating hormone   (FSH) Gonadotropic hormone that increases estradiol secretion. See **estradiol.**

follow-back study   Study using data from medical and academic records established before the clinical onset of the patient's illness. Chief weakness is the need to rely on indirect sources of information that may be incomplete and nonspecific.

follow-through   Research technique in which subjects are examined in childhood and periodically reevaluated until they reach the point at which outcome of interest is measured.

follow-up   Continued observation of patients or study populations to note changes in health status or health-related variables.

follow-up history   See **catamnesis.**

follow-up study   Investigation that relies on archival data on subjects presumed to be at high risk for adult psychiatric disorders. The first step is often obtaining childhood medical records from psychiatric treatment centers. Subjects are then located to determine adult outcome. Problems include failure to locate subjects (some of whom may represent a more deviant subgroup) and the nonrepresentativeness of the sample.

Foltran   See **zopiclone.**

Fontex   See **fluoxetine.**

Food and Drug Administration   (FDA) U.S. government agency responsible for setting and enforcing guidelines for food, food additive, and drug safety evaluation; licensing; and marketing.

"football"   Street name for central nervous system stimulant drugs.

forced diuresis   Technique to enhance removal of psychotropic drugs that are excreted unchanged in the urine (phenobarbital, butabarbital, meprobamate, tranylcypromine, amphetamines, lithium). After an indwelling Foley catheter is inserted, furosemide (20–40 mg) is given intravenously along with an intravenous solution of dextrose (5%), saline (0.23–0.45%), and potassium (10–20 mEq/

L). Urine output is measured hourly, and electrolytes are measured at least every 12 hours.

forced feeding   Feeding against a person's will. It is done in the treatment of anorexia nervosa, in patients trying to commit suicide through starvation, and in prisoners on hunger strike. It was frequently used to feed psychotic patients in the days before modern somatic and pharmacological treatments.

forced treatment   Imposition of therapy against a person's will.

forensic   Pertaining to or connected with the criminal justice system.

forensic psychiatry   Subspecialty concerned with diagnosis and treatment and preparing reports for courts regarding defense on mentally abnormal offenders. Forensic psychiatrists spend considerable time with attorneys, the courts, and probation officers.

formal thought disorder   Disturbance in the form of thought as distinguished from the content of thought. Because the boundaries of the concept are unclear and there is no consensus as to which disturbances in speech or thought are included, "formal thought disorder" is not used as a specific descriptive term in DSM-IV.

forme fruste   Partial expression of a disorder, disease, or genetic trait.

formication   Tactile hallucination involving the sensation of small insects creeping in or under the skin. It occurs in psychogenic mental states, but is most common in organic psychiatric syndromes associated with use/abuse of such substances as narcotics, alcohol, and cocaine. It may occur in alcohol withdrawal delirium and the withdrawal phase of cocaine intoxication.

Fortral   See **pentazocine.**

forward genetics   See **genetics, forward.**

fos   Protein product of the proto-oncogene c-fos. Its localization can serve as an index of the metabolic activation of individual neurons. Immunohistochemical studies of c-fos protein expression are useful in assessing the activation of central monoaminergic neurons. See **c-fos; oncogene.**

fos protein   Product of c-fos. A single dose of cocaine may cause up to an eightfold increase in fos proteins that may affect regulation of a number of target genes within striatal neurons.

founder effect   Deviation of gene frequencies from the norm in an isolated population due to presence or absence of certain genes in the founding ancestors of the population.

"fours and doors"   Street term for a combination of four acetaminophen-with-codeine tablets and two glutethimide tablets, which are crushed, mixed with water, and injected.

fragile chromosome site   Nonstaining gap that involves both chromatids and is always at exactly the same band region on a specific chromosome from an individual or kindred. Fragile sites are inherited in a Mendelian co-dominant fashion and can be detected by specific culture and staining methods.

fragile-X syndrome   Second most common genetic cause of mental retardation after Down syndrome. It is so named because the tip of the X chromosome tends to break off in many of those affected. The syndrome occurs in all racial and ethnic groups, in about 1 in 1,000 men and 1 in 2,500 women. It is manifested by a somewhat prominent chin, broad forehead, wide jaw, wide nose, long face, and large floppy ears. It can affect cognitive ability, behavioral characteristics, speech, and language. It is believed to be responsible for an important subgroup of autistic males. Female carriers have more schizophrenia-like disorders. Affected fetuses should be identifiable by amniocentesis. The discovery of the molecular genetic basis of the fragile X syndrome may elucidate the cause and treatment of this and perhaps other forms of mental retardation (Kremer EJ, Pritchard M, Lynch M, et al. Mapping of DNA instability at the fragile X to a trinucleotide repeat sequence p(CCG)n. *Science* 1991;252:1711–1714). An unstable CGG trinucleotide repeat sequence in the FMR1 gene at the fragile-X locus has been detected (Verkerk AJ, Pieretti M, Sutcliff JS, et al. Identification of a gene (FMR-1) containing a CGG repeat coincident with a breakpoint cluster. Region exhibiting length variation in fragile X syndrome. *Cell* 1991;65:905–914; Fu Y, Kuhl DPA, Pizzuita A. Variation of the CGG repeat at the fragile X site. Results in genetic instability: resolution of the Sherman paradox. *Cell* 1991;67:1047–1058). In normal individuals, CGG repeats range between 6 and 54 at this locus (average, 30). Individuals with no significant phenotype, but who are at high risk for having an affected child, have repeat numbers between 52 and 200. Individuals with fragile-X syndrome have 200 or more CGG repeats. This accounts for almost half of the X-linked forms of mental retardation and is now the object of increasing research on its genetic and molecular aspects (Taylor AK, Safanda JF, Majilinde Z, et al. Molecular predictors of cognitive involvement in female carriers of fragile X syndrome. *JAMA* 1994; 271:507–514). Also called "Martin-Bell syndrome" after the British investigators who first reported it in 1943.

fragmentation   See **sleep fragmentation.**

fragmented sleep See **sleep, fragmented.**

frame-shift mutation Deletion or addition of a nucleotide in the coding region of a gene that leads to an entirely different amino acid sequence on the distal site of the mutation.

"freebase" Chemically extracted alkaloid base of cocaine that does not decompensate with heat and thus has become popular for smoking. Freebase and "crack" have different production processes; crack is considered freebase in a crystalline or rock form.

"freebasing" Street term for smoking cocaine, usually through a water pipe. The activity first appeared in California as a new ritual in the drug community in 1974.

free-floating anxiety See **anxiety, free-floating.**

free fraction Proportion of total drug concentration that is not bound to protein in the blood, plasma, or serum.

free interval Period between illness episodes in patients with an affective disorder.

free running Natural, endogenous period of a rhythm when time cues (zeitgebers) are removed. It is most commonly seen as the tendency to delay some circadian rhythms, such as the sleep-wake cycle, by approximately 1 hour every day. See **zeitgeber.**

free T3 (fT3) Free triiodothyronine.

free T4 (fT4) Free thyroxine.

freezing Sudden arrest of gait in Parkinson's disease (PD) patients that often occurs when crossing doorways. This and other secondary signs of parkinsonism (e.g., micrographia, sialorrhea, loss of facial expression) may be helpful in establishing a diagnosis of PD. Subcutaneous injection of apomorphine, a rapidly acting dopamine D_1 and D_2 receptor agonist, is being tried for the treatment of freezing (Frankel JP, Lees AJ, Kempster PA, et al. Subcutaneous apomorphine in the treatment of Parkinson's disease. *J Neurosurg Psych* 1990;53:96–101).

Frenactil See **benperidol.**

freon Member of a group of liquid fluorocarbons used mainly as refrigerants, coolants, and aerosol propellants. Freons are liquid-soluble and rapidly absorbed and distributed to fatty tissues, especially the brain. When abused, they can cause sudden death from cardiac arrhythmias.

frequency Number of times a given value of an observation occurs. Also called "counts."

frequency distribution List of values that occur along with the frequency of their occurrence in a set of numerical observations. It may be set up as a frequency table.

frequency, observed Frequency that occurs in a study. Observed frequencies are generally arranged in a contingency table.

frequency polygon Line graph connecting the midpoints of the tops of the columns of a histogram. It is useful in comparing two frequency distributions.

frequency table Table showing the number or percentage of observations occurring at different values (or ranges of values) of a characteristic or variable.

Friedman Block/Treatment Test Nonparametric two-way analysis of variance.

Frisium See **clobazam.**

Froment's sign Rhythmical resistance to passive movement of a limb about a joint that is detected specifically during voluntary activity of the contralateral limb. It is seen in tremulous disorders other than Parkinson's disease (Cleeves L, Findley LJ, Koller WC. Lack of association between essential tremor and Parkinson's disease. *Ann Neurol* 1988;24:23–26).

frontal lobe syndrome Sequelae of frontal lobe injury due to trauma, stroke, brain tumor, frontal lobe degenerations (Pick's disease, frontal degeneration in association with motor neuron disease, frontal degeneration without specific histologic abnormalities), infections affecting the frontal lobe (acquired immunodeficiency syndrome [AIDS], Creutzfeldt-Jakob disease), and multiple sclerosis. *Neurological abnormalities* include deficits in olfactory function, following inferior frontal lobe injury affecting the olfactory apparatus, weakness of the arm and face with lateral frontal damage, gaze deviation with acute injury to the frontal eye fields, and leg weakness with medial frontal lesions. *Neurobehavioral disturbances* include Broca's aphasia with left inferolateral lesions, aprosodia with right inferolateral damage, and transcortical motor aphasia with left medial frontal lesions. Inattention and distractibility are common, and poor organization of material to be learned with subsequent poor recall are also frequent. Principle *neuropsychiatric disturbances* are mood and personality changes. Depression is most common with damage to the left frontal lobe; mania and euphoria occur with damage to the inferior frontal cortex, particularly on the right. Disinhibition, impulsivity, and coarsening indicate orbitofrontal dysfunction. Apathy is present with medial frontal injury. Depression associated with frontal dysfunction is treated with conventional tricyclic antidepressants; the disinhibition syndrome may respond to neuroleptics, beta-blocking agents, trazodone, or carbamazepine. Mania is treated with lithium or carbamazepine. The apathetic syndrome may improve following treatment with dopaminergic agents (levodopa/carbidopa) or bromocriptine. Frontal lobe syndromes include several of the following elements: distractibility, poor word-list generation, poor recall with variable recognition skills, impaired abstraction and judgment, abnormal motor programming abilities, and marked personality changes. A frontal lobe syndrome also can be induced by some serotonin uptake inhibitors. It is manifested by apathy, indifference, inattention, and perseveration accompanied by decreased cerebral blood flow in the frontal lobes (Hoehn-Saric R, Harris GJ, Pearlson GD, et al. A fluoxetine-induced frontal lobe syndrome in an obsessive compulsive patient. *J Clin Psychiatry* 1991;52:131–133).

frontal lobe volume loss   Possible result of severe affective disorder including hypercorticalism, malnutrition and weight loss, drug and alcohol use, neglect of physical health, and possibly the effects of previous drug treatment (e.g., benzodiazepines) (Kellner CH, Rubinow DR, Gold PW, et al. Relationship of cortisol hypersecretion to brain CT scan alterations in depressed patients. *Psychiatry Res* 1983;8:191–197; Krieg JC, Pirke KM, Lauer C, et al. Endocrine, metabolic and cranial computed tomographic findings in anorexia nervosa. *Biol Psychiatry* 1988;23:377–387; Lishman WA. Alcohol and the brain. *Br J Psychiatry* 1990;156: 635–644; Schmauss C, Krieg JC. Enlargement of cerebrospinal fluid spaces in long-term benzodiazepine abusers. *Psychol Med* 1987;17: 869–873).

frotteur   Individual who gains sexual gratification from illicitly touching others.

F test   Statistical test for comparing two variances, used in analysis of variance (ANOVA).

fugue state   Performance of bizarre acts, with or without bodily harm to another person, with subsequent amnesia for the episode. It occurs most often in patients with a history of mild or moderate head injury. The acute episode tends to be precipitated by alcohol. Fugue states lasting several hours must be differentiated from postictal automatic behavior.

functional disorder   Disorder without a physiological or anatomical cause. It can have purely psychodynamic (intrapsychic) effects and cause passing to and from pathophysiological responses without leaving definitive pathological and anatomical lesions.

functional imaging technique   Measurement of regional cerebral blood flow with cortical probes or with single photon emission computed tomography (SPECT) and positron emission tomography (PET).

functional magnetic resonance imaging   See **magnetic resonance imaging, functional.**

functional psychosis   See **psychosis, functional.**

functional tolerance   See **tolerance, functional.**

furor, epileptic   Marked confusion followed by maniacal violence or rage associated with epileptic or epileptic-equivalent attacks.

furosemide   (Lasix) Potent, anthrancillic acid derivative loop diuretic that is shorter-acting than hydrochlorothiazide. If given in excessive amounts, it can lead to profound diuresis with water and electrolyte depletion.

furosemide + chloral hydrate   See **chloral hydrate + furosemide.**

furosemide + lithium   See **lithium and furosemide.**

fusion peptide   Artificial construct containing part of a bacterial protein and part of a desired cloned segment.

fusion protein   Once a gene is cloned, it can be put into another organism that can then express the actions of this gene. Often, however, the organism must be tricked into making the new gene product because it may not have all the machinery in place to make the foreign protein. Because this is especially true in trying to get a prokaryote (e.g., bacteria) to make a eukaryote (e.g., mammalian) protein, the foreign gene is manipulated to include portions of a prokaryotic gene so that when the bacteria begin to make the foreign gene product they are actually making one of their own. The gene product eventually changes from its own to the foreign gene product, resulting in a fusion protein—one portion prokaryotic, the other eukaryotic. After it is made, the fusion is purified and can be cut with proteases to remove the bacterial portion. In this way, bacteria can be used as organic factories to produce human (or other) gene products.

Fynex   See **diphenhydramine.**

G

GABA Gamma aminobutyric acid, the most abundant and important amino acid neurotransmitter inhibitor in the central nervous system. It is involved with 30–50% of all neurons; highest concentrations are found in the substantia nigra, globus pallidus, and hypothalamus. GABA receptors are located at postsynaptic sites. GABA receptor activation increases permeability of the chloride channel in postsynaptic membranes, thus inhibiting membrane depolarization. GABA is formed from glutamic acid through the action of the enzyme glutamic acid decarboxylase (GAD) and metabolized by GABA-glutamate transaminase (GABA-T). GABA has a major neuroinhibitory influence on dopamine, serotonin, and norepinephrine. It is also associated with the sedative effects of GABA agonists (e.g., barbiturates and benzodiazepines [BZDs]). BZDs are thought to work by enhancing the effects of GABA on the transport of chloride across neuronal membranes. Drugs, normal aging, or illnesses that alter GABA binding may also affect the therapeutic potential of BZDs. With age, there is no change in the number of BZD-GABA receptors, although there may be a change in their sensitivity. GABA is implicated in several psychiatric and neurological conditions (e.g., Huntington's disease, parkinsonism, epilepsy, schizophrenia, tardive dyskinesia, senile dementia, and several behavioral disorders). See **benzodiazepine receptor.**

GABA agonist Agent (e.g., muscimol) that mimics the action of gamma aminobutyric acid (GABA) at receptors.

GABA antagonist Gamma aminobutyric acid (GABA)-inhibiting agent, of which there are two broad classes: competitive antagonists (e.g., bicuculline), which act at GABA binding sites, and noncompetitive antagonists (e.g., picrotoxin), which act at sites in the GABA-gated chloride channel. Both classes produce clinical convulsions.

GABAmimetic That which mimics the action of gamma aminobutyric acid (GABA). See **GABA agonist.**

gabapentin (Neurontin) Gamma aminobutyric acid (GABA)-related amino acid anticonvulsant marketed for the treatment of adults with refractory partial seizures with or without secondary generalized tonic-clonic seizures. On initiation of therapy, dosage should be increased over 1 week to a total of 1,200 mg/day in three divided doses. Depending on response, dosage increments to 1.8 g or 2.4 g in three divided doses per day may be needed thereafter. No adverse interactions with other antiepileptic drugs have been noted to date (Chadwick D. Gabapentin. *Lancet* 1994;343: 89–91). The CNS Advisory Committee to the U.S. Food and Drug Administration (FDA) approved gabapentin for marketing in the United States in December 1992.

GABA receptor Receptor for gamma-aminobutyric-acid (GABA) found throughout the central nervous system. These receptors generally exert an inhibitory influence on neuronal firing via their action on chloride channels. They also contain a benzodiazepine (BZD)-binding site that enhances the potency of neuronal inhibition when a BZD agonist binds to these receptors. There are two major subtypes of GABA receptors in vertebrates, $GABA_A$ and $GABA_B$. Both have been shown to have pre- and post-synaptic locations and are thought to participate independently in synaptic transmission. See **$GABA_A$ receptor; $GABA_B$ receptor.**

$GABA_A$ receptor Receptor class comprising at least four homologous but distinct membrane-spanning oligomeric protein subunits (alpha, beta, delta, and gamma) that form an intrinsic chloride ion channel. Available evidence indicates that the alpha subunit contains the benzodiazepine recognition site, and the beta subunit contains the gamma aminobutyric acid (GABA) recognition or binding site. $GABA_A$ receptors are the most abundant inhibitory neurotransmitter receptors in the brain. They contain binding sites for the primary transmitter, GABA, and other GABA agonists. See **GABA; GABA receptor.**

$GABA_B$ receptor Receptor activated by gamma aminobutyric acid (GABA) and the antispasticity agent baclofen and insensitive to benzodiazepines or barbiturates. These receptors represent the minority of the GABA sites in the vertebrate central nervous system. See **GABA; GABA receptor.**

GABOB Hydroxyl derivative of gamma aminobutyric acid (GABA) that, like GABA, is a chemical mediator with an important role in cerebral metabolism.

Gabren See **progabide.**

Gabrene See **progabide.**

gag reflex Retching caused by a foreign body coming in contact with the space between the cavity of the mouth and the pharynx. It is the most easily and commonly tested airway reflex. Response is recorded as normal (light touch), attenuated (more vigorous stimulation required), or absent. It may be compromised in an apparently conscious patient and may be significantly attenuated or absent at all levels of the Glasgow Coma Scale (Moulton C, Pennycook A, Makower R: Relation between Glasgow Coma Scale and the gag reflex. *Br Med J* 1991;303:1240–1241). Absence of the gag reflex is recognized as one of the criteria for brainstem death.

"gage"   Street name for marijuana.

galactorrhea   Secretion of milk from the breast in the absence of pregnancy. Certain psychoactive drugs, especially neuroleptics, can cause galactorrhea as a result of their influence on the endocrine system (prolactin regulation) in men and women. Neuroleptic-induced galactorrhea may occur in association with any level of prolactin and at any time during the course of neuroleptic treatment. Galactorrhea may be uncomfortable or disconcerting to the patient, but has rarely been associated with any adverse medical effect. In men, neuroleptic-induced hyperprolactinemia may lower testosterone level and cause impotence. Gynecomastia is rarely associated with neuroleptic use.

galanin   (GAL) 29-Amino acid peptide with glycine at the N-terminus and clonidine at the C-terminus. It is localized in the hypothalamus, pituitary, pancreas, and intestine. It acts as an inhibitory modulator of cholinergic functions in pathways relative to memory. It could be particularly detrimental when few cholinergic neurons remain and might block the efficacy of cholinergic drugs designed as replacement therapy. A galanin antagonist, alone or in combination with a cholinergic agonist, may provide a new approach to treating memory deficits associated with neuronal degeneration (Pramanik A, Ogren SO, Land T, Langel U. Galanin antagonists M15 and M35: differential effects on acetylcholine release in the rat striatum. *Neuropsychopharmacology* 1993;9:81S).

galanthamine   Long-acting acetylcholinesterase inhibitor that rapidly crosses the blood-brain barrier and effectively reverses a central anticholinergic syndrome. Long-term administration in Alzheimer's disease is well tolerated with no significant adverse effects (Wesnes K, Scott M, Boyle M, et al. The use of the Cognitive Drug Research Computerized Assessment System to measure the efficacy of THA and galanthamine in Alzheimer's disease. Presented at the 33rd Annual NCDEU Meeting, Boca Raton, FL, June 1993). Galanthamine also may have antimanic activity. Also called "galantamine." See **nootropic drug.**

galantamine   See **galanthamine.**

Galatur   See **iprindole.**

"galleria"   Street term for a place where substance abusers inject drugs. Also called "flash house" or "shooting gallery."

Galtonian method   One of two current, main methods for studying hereditary factors. It uses comparative studies of identical and fraternal twins and adopted children.

galvanic skin response   (GSR) Alterations in skin resistance to a weak electric current that occur as part of a physiochemical response to emotional stimuli. Changes are measured by a galvanometer. GSR is an easily measured variable widely used in experimental studies as an indicator of emotional arousal and tension. Also called "electrodermal response"; "psychogalvanic reflex."

Gamanil   See **lofepramine.**

Gamblers Anonymous   Twelve-step, self-help program similar to Alcoholics Anonymous designed to help individuals resist impulses to gamble.

gambling, pathological   Progressive disorder characterized by continuous or periodic loss of control over gambling, preoccupation with gambling and obtaining money with which to gamble, irrational thinking, and continuation of behavior despite adverse consequences (Rosenthal RJ. Pathological gambling. *Psychiatr Ann* 1992;22:72–78). It is often associated with major depression. Approximately 50% of pathological gamblers have histories of alcohol or drug abuse or dependence. Type of gambling usually depends on what is available, but preferred forms seem to be lotteries, sports betting, cards, casino gambling, and horse racing. In the hands of an experienced therapist, pathological gambling is extremely treatable. Besides participation in Gambler's Anonymous, some patients require antidepressant therapy and/or psychodynamic therapy on a group or individual basis. In some instances, family therapy is crucial.

gamete   Egg or sperm that contains exactly half the genetic information from the parent. Each gamete contributes exactly half the genetic information to the offspring.

gamma aminobutyric acid   See **GABA.**

gamma hydrate   See **gamma hydroxybutyrate.**

gamma hydroxybutyrate   (GHB) Highly toxic drug marketed illicitly in the United States since 1990 as a "steroid alternative" for body builders, for weight control, as a sleep aid, and as "replacement" for L-tryptophan. It allegedly produces a high that has led to further illicit use. It is sold nationwide in body-building gyms, fitness centers, health food stores, and through mail-order outlets. It is sold as a sodium salt (powder or granular form) that is commonly dissolved in water before use. Toxic manifestations include gastrointestinal symptoms, central nervous system and respiratory depression, and uncontrolled movements. Typically, within 15–60 minutes after ingestion, one or more of the following symptoms may occur: vomiting, drowsiness, hypnagogic state, hypotonia, and/or vertigo. Loss of consciousness, irregular and depressed respiration, tremors, or myoclonus may follow. Seizure-like activity, bradycardia, hypotension, and/or respiratory arrest also have been reported. Spontaneous resolution occurs within 2–96 hours (Dyer JE. Gamma-hydroxybutyrate: a health-food product producing coma and seizure-like activity. *Am J Emerg Med* 1991; 9:321–324; Einsprach BC, Clark SM. Near fatality results from health food store sleeping potion. *Tex Med* 1992;88:10; Galloway GP, Frederick SL, Staggers F. Physical dependence on sodium oxybate. *Lancet* 1994;343:57). Also called "gamma hydrate"; "gamma-OH"; "4-hydroxybutyrate"; "sodium oxybate"; "sodium oxybutyrate"; "Somatomax PM."

gamma-3-melanocyte stimulating hormone (Gamma-3-MSH) Cleavage product of the peptide pro-opiomelanocortin (POMC), the prohormone of adrenocorticotropic hormone (ACTH). It has been shown in both in vitro and in vivo studies to stimulate cortisone release.

gamma-OH　See **gamma hydroxybutyrate.**

gamma-vinyl-GABA　See **vigabatrin.**

ganja　Marijuana obtained from the flowering tops of leaves of carefully selected cultivated plants. It has a high quality and quantity of resin compared to bhang.

ganja psychosis　See **cannabis psychosis.**

"garbage"　Street name for heroin.

Gardenal　See **phenobarbital.**

"gas"　Street name for volatile nitrites (e.g., butyl nitrite) sold in "head," pornography, and novelty shops, and through mail order houses.

gas chromatography　(GC) Technique for separating compounds in which the compounds are volatilized to a gaseous state, eluded by a carrier gas, and passed through specifically designed filtration columns. The separated compounds are then detected and quantified by means of an electrochemical or fluorescent probe.

gas chromatography-mass spectroscopy　(GC-MS) Specific, sensitive, and accurate method of drug detection in which the gas chromatograph is linked to a mass spectrograph. It allows very small quantities of a compound to be quantified and is used to confirm an initial positive immunoassay.

gas-liquid chromatography　(GLC) Method of separating a substance's liquid phase from its gas phase. It is individualized for each compound or group of similar compounds after extraction. It is a quick and relatively simple method that provides both qualitative and quantitative results. Use of specific detectors (e.g., electron capture, nitrogen/phosphorus) gives good to excellent sensitivity and specificity. For most drugs, GLC is more specific and 100–1000 times more sensitive than thin-layer chromatography (TLC), especially when the unknown substance is analyzed on two different polarity columns.

gateway drug　Term coined by Robert DuPont for one of the three drugs that lead to abuse of other classes of drugs: alcohol, cocaine, and marijuana. These drugs are considered conducive to users' trying other illicit and usually more potent and possibly more hazardous drugs.

Gaussian distribution　See **normal distribution.**

gaze monitoring　See **joint-attention behavior.**

GBR 12909　Potent, elective dopamine uptake inhibitor with higher selectivity than other dopaminergic antidepressants such as bupropion and amineptine. Elimination half-life is estimated to be 1–2 days. Steady-state serum concentrations are attained within 1 week. Expected therapeutic dose is 25–100 mg. Higher doses result in mild to moderate side effects (e.g., difficulty concentrating, asthenia, feeling drugged, palpitations). A dose-related electrocardiographic effect has been observed, with a slight reduction of the T-wave amplitude. It is currently being tested in Europe as an antidepressant and in the treatment of Parkinson's disease (Nielsen EB, Anderson PH: GBR 12909: A new potent and selective dopamine uptake inhibitor. *In* Gessa GL, Serra G [eds], *Dopamine and Mental Depression.* Oxford: Pergamon Press, 1990, pp 77–90).

GBR-12935　Highly selective dopamine re-uptake blocker that in preclinical models showed evidence of antidepressant activity. It is in various stages of clinical trials (Nielsen EB, Anderson PH: GBR 12909: A new potent and selective dopamine uptake inhibitor. *In* Gessa GL, Serra G [eds], *Dopamine and Mental Depression.* Oxford: Pergamon Press, 1990, pp 77–90).

"geeking"　Street term for transient, compulsive foraging behavior associated with crack cocaine use. Also called "chasing ghosts." See **compulsive foraging behavior.**

gegenhalten　See **paratonia.**

Gehan's test　Statistical test of the equality of two survival curves.

gel electrophoresis　Movement of suspended particles through a fluid or gel under the action of electromotive force applied to electrodes in contact with the suspension.

Gemeril   See **melperone.**

gender dysphoria   Discomfort with anatomical gender that begins in early childhood. In transvestism, the experience is limited to the desire to wear the clothes of the opposite gender; doing so produces a calming effect and subjective experience of appropriateness, no matter how strange the appearance may be to others. Trans-sexualism is the more extreme degree of the disorder; affected individuals wish to be transformed into a member of the opposite gender. For some, the transformation improves the quality of life and relieves persisting distress. In others, it exposes the individual not only to expense and the trauma of separation from relatives, partners, and children, but to the physical dangers of the hormonal and surgical procedures required. Inadequate preparation for life in the opposite gender role and medical collusion with unattainable fantasy may precipitate a suicide attempt or requests for reversal of all procedures undertaken (Anon: Transsexualism. *Lancet* 1991;338:603–604).

gene   DNA sequence that codes for a particular protein product or that regulates other genes. Genes are the biological basis of heredity. They are arranged in a linear fashion along the chromosomes, each gene having a precise position or locus. Most genes occur in pairs; one member of each is contributed by each parent. Genes for some characteristics (dominant genes) can override effects of corresponding genes derived from the other parent (recessive genes). The entire complement of DNA arranged into chromosomes in an organism is termed the "genome." Only clones and monozygotic twins have exactly the same genome.

gene, aberrant   Defective gene that renders a person susceptible to a host of chronic and crippling diseases. Aberrant genes do not cause disease until the person comes in contact with a harmful factor. Finding aberrant genes permits avoidance of a dangerous environment or factor to which the individual is genetically susceptible.

gene action   Mechanism by which a gene carries out a biological process, usually through the production of a protein.

gene allele   Alternate form of a gene.

gene amplification   Process by which genes increase in number in a single genome.

gene, APP   Gene that encodes the major protein of plaques found in the brains of patients with Alzheimer's disease. It maps to a region of human chromosome 21 genetically linked to Alzheimer's disease (AD) in several early-onset families. It has been isolated and studied as a candidate gene for AD. Single base changes in codon 717 of the APP gene specifically associated with the Alzheimer phenotype have been identified in affected individuals. Although only a small minority of AD patients appear to have the disease as a result of mutations in the APP gene, studies of how APP mutations result in disease could result in therapies applicable to a broad range of patients with the disorder.

gene cloning   Once identified by various means, a gene can be copied with enzymes that can make DNA from RNA (reverse transcription). This cDNA ("c" for *copy* or *complementary*) will be a base-for-base copy of the gene that is made easily manipulable by inserting it into bacteria or viruses that will act as caretakers of the cDNA. The cDNA needs to be put into a larger piece of DNA (plasmid or vector) that the bacteria or virus will take up. The purified cDNA can be used as a probe to measure the mRNA specific to that gene, roughly analogous to an antibody that measures a specific protein. Such a measurement indicates the level of expression specifically for that gene. The assay of mRNA levels with cDNA is usually performed on "northern blots." Also called "DNA recombination"; "molecular genetics."

gene conversion   Changes in gene structure due to unequal pairing of strands of DNA during duplication or intragenic recombination.

gene, dominant   Member of an allele pair which, if present, determines the phenotype, whether the other member of the pair is the same or different. A dominant gene may be responsible for abnormal development and can be a cause of mental handicap (e.g., tuberous sclerosis, Apert's syndrome, Crouzon's syndrome, Hallermann-Streiff syndrome, Treacher-Collins syndrome). Some dominant genes have variable penetrance, meaning that some people are more seriously affected than others when the gene is present.

gene expression   Process by which the code present in the DNA in a gene is converted into the corresponding protein and its biological activity. It involves synthesis of an intermediate molecule (messenger RNA or mRNA) directly from the gene (and hence carrying virtually the same information as the gene) and conversion of the mRNA into the corresponding protein. Synthesis of mRNA from the gene is termed "transcription." Conversion of the mRNA into protein is called "translation." Modifications of the protein after it is synthesized are called "post-translation modifications." However, the complement of genes that are actively synthesizing RNA (i.e., "expressed") will vary from cell to cell and condition to condition in the cell.

gene family Multiple genes that control a single biological process.

gene frequency Estimate of the population prevalence of a detected major locus, given the population prevalence of the phenotype.

gene, globin Complex of genes that produce the protein portions of hemoglobin, the oxygen-carrying component of the red blood cells. Deficits in globin genes lead to a variety of inherited blood diseases, the best-known of which is sickle-cell anemia.

gene, immediate early Any of a class of genes that are transcriptionally induced by a variety of ligands acting at cell surface receptors. They are induced rapidly (within 5 minutes) and transiently in response to a stimulus. They were originally discovered in the genomes of many eukaryotic viruses. Viral immediate early genes are expressed in the initial phase of a viral life cycle. Cellular immediate early genes are inducible genes found in many types of eukaryotic cells. Many cellular immediate early genes are homologs of viral transducing genes (or oncogenes) and are thus called "proto-oncogenes." Of the cellular immediate early genes, c-fos and c-jun are perhaps the most well studied.

gene, lethal Gene whose presence brings about the death of the organism or permits survival only under certain conditions.

gene library DNA that has been produced in vitro for the purpose of molecular genetic studies.

gene locus Chromosomal site of a gene.

gene, major Gene that has a noticeable phenotypic effect.

gene mapping Determination of the relationship, order, and distance between different genes on a chromosome. It is the essential first step in the characterization of each disease locus. In 1990–1991, about 500 new genes and 1,500 other reference points were added to the human genome map.

gene, modifying Gene that has some influence on the effect of any particular gene. Modifying genes are all those other than the one under specific study.

gene mutation Change in the character of a gene that is continued in subsequent divisions of the cell in which the change occurs.

gene pool Total genes possessed by the reproductive members of a population.

gene, prion Gene that encodes for the protein that accumulates in the brains of mice infected with scrapie. Mutations in the human prion gene have been described in some families with hereditary spongiform encephalopathy. See **prion disease.**

gene product Biochemical material, either RNA or protein, made by a gene. The amount of gene product is used to measure how active a gene is; abnormal amounts can be correlated with disease-causing genes.

gene, promoter Region of DNA immediately upstream from the transcription initiation site that binds RNA polymerase. The presence of a promoter is an absolute requirement for initiation of a transcription. See **regulatory sequence.**

gene, recessive Subordinate member of a heterozygous allele pair that does not have an effect on the phenotype. A recessive gene can express itself only when another recessive gene for the same characteristic is inherited from the other parent.

gene regulation Control of expression of a gene.

gene, regulator Gene that controls the rate of production of the product of other genes by synthesis of a substance that inhibits the action of an operator.

gene, reporter Coding unit whose product is easily assayed (e.g., neomycin resistance) in transfected cells; used to evaluate transfection efficiency. See **transfection.**

gene sequencing Because the sequence of nucleotide bases differentiates genes from each other, this sequence is determined once a gene is cloned. From this sequence, the amino acid sequence of the corresponding protein can be deduced. Knowledge of the amino acid sequence facilitates understanding the biological function and metabolism of that protein.

gene splicing Any of the various techniques in which pieces of the genetic material from different species can be combined ("spliced") and inserted into living bacterial cells.

gene, suppressor Gene that deters cells from behaving abnormally. Its suppression of uncontrolled cellular behavior, for example, can prevent cancer, but if a suppressor gene is mutated, a wide rage of abnormal cellular behavior can occur.

gene therapy Insertion of normal DNA directly into cells to correct a genetic defect by altering the actions of a specific gene. Because of ethical concerns, safeguards for gene therapy have been proposed. It should be restricted to alleviation of disease in individual patients and should not be used to change normal human traits. The first candidates should be patients with a life-threatening or seriously disabling genetic disease. Severe genetic disorders that show their effects in early childhood, or even before birth, should be treated correspondingly early. Familiar ethical considerations that are likely to assume greater prominence when gene therapy is being considered include safety (because of the possibility of predicted consequences of gene insertion), the need for long-term surveillance, consent (especially regarding uncertainties about outcome), the probability that children will be among the first candidates for gene therapy, and confidentiality.

gene transfer   Introduction of a gene into a cell in which it is not usually found.

general adaptation syndrome   (GAS) Various changes in the body in response to, or as a defense against, stress. It consists of three stages: the alarm reaction, in which adaptation is not yet required; the resistance stage, in which adaptation is optimal; and the exhaustion stage, in which the acquired adaptation is lost.

general paralysis of the insane   (GPI) See **general paresis.**

general paresis   Syndrome due to cerebral syphilis secondary to the tertiary form of syphilis. It appears 15–20 years after the primary *Treponema* infection in approximately 5% of neurosyphilis patients. Symptoms include dementia, a manic-like syndrome with euphoria, and grandiose delusions associated with neurological signs (e.g., Argyll-Robertson pupils), dysarthria, myoclonic jerks, action tremors, Babinski signs, hyper-reflexia, and seizures. Blood serology is positive in nearly all cases. Depression and delusions of persecutions may also occur. Before the advent of penicillin, it was a major cause of insanity, accounting for 4–10% of psychiatric admissions; it is now a rarity. Also called "general paralysis of the insane"; "paretic neurosyphilis"; "paralytic and syphilitic meningoencephalitis."

generalized anxiety   Apprehension, tension, or uneasiness that stems from the anticipation of danger that may be internal or external.

generalized anxiety disorder   (GAD) Anxiety disorder characterized by excessive anxiety and worry (apprehensive expectation). It is manifested by motor tension (e.g., fidgeting), autonomic hyperactivity (e.g., sweaty palms), and vigilance and scanning ("keyed up"). It is largely a diagnosis of exclusion. Among factors that must be excluded are high depressive scores, phobias, panic disorder, and organic factors (e.g., hyperthyroidism, caffeinism).

generalized dystonia   Uncommon disorder that may be symptomatic or idiopathic, usually beginning in childhood or adolescence and progressing to severe disability. It is unlikely to be encountered in a primarily psychiatric setting. In many (but not all) cases it is genetic, with an autosomal dominant pattern of transmission demonstrated in many families.

generalized seizure   See **seizure, generalized.**

generalized seizure, secondary   See **seizure, secondary generalized.**

generic drug   Copy of a brand-name drug, generally made after the patent on the brand-name product expires. A generic is prescribed under its scientific name, which is officially assigned by the United States Adopted Names (USAN) Council in the United States and the World Health Organization (WHO) in other countries. It is based on the pharmacological and chemical characteristics of the drug and complies with strict criteria for naming established by both USAN and WHO. The generic name is officially adopted only after USAN, WHO, and the manufacturer agree that all criteria and safeguards outlined by USAN and WHO are met. Because of differences in quality control, a generic drug may or may not be as biologically active as the brand-name product, with differences in therapeutic effects ensuing. The U.S. Food and Drug Administration (FDA) considers a generic drug to be comparable to the brand name product if there is no more than 20% difference between them with respect to bioavailability, C_{max}, and T_{max}. This could mean a 40% higher C_{max} or a 40% decrease in bioavailability. Another drawback of prescribing by generic name is that the patient may be dispensed a different brand when the prescription is refilled. Since different preparations of a generic drug often differ in shape, size, and color, the patient may think that the wrong medication has been dispensed.

genetic   Predetermined by a gene or combination of genes. The term is synonymous with *genetical* and practically identical to *hereditary.*

genetic analysis   Determination of the mode of inheritance of a trait.

genetic code   Relationship by which a cell uses the nucleotide bases to create the sequence of amino acids of a protein.

genetic cross   Combining of different genetic traits within an offspring that results from a genetically disparate mating.

genetic counseling   Communication process dealing with human problems associated with occurrence or risk of occurrence of a genetic disorder in a family.

genetic disorder   Inherited disorder caused by the presence of one or more abnormal genes in the individual. Many such disorders are a cause of mental or emotional handicap.

genetic drift   Changes in allele frequency resulting from the accumulated sampling error in alleles transmitted from one generation to another.

genetic drift, random   Changes of gene frequency, especially in relatively small populations, due to chance preservation or extinction of particular genes.

genetic engineering   DNA manipulation and cloning and transferring genetic material from cells of one organism to cells of another organism, whether for therapeutic or industrial goals.

genetic epidemiology   Use of quantitative statistical models to understand the incidence and distribution of disease within families. It focuses on the inheritance of common diseases in humans.

genetic heterogeneity   Implication that a particular clinical phenotype can be the result of a number of distinct etiological agents, both genetic and environmental. Any one of several genes can be responsible for the same clinical disorder.

genetic linkage   See **linkage**.

genetic linkage map   See **linkage map**.

genetic marker   Physical trait (e.g., colorblindness), protein (e.g., HLA antigens), or DNA fragments whose genetic location is established and whose variation within families may be used to "map" the location of genes for unknown traits (e.g., bipolar disorder) to a known genetic locus. In psychiatry, the term is best reserved for a special subset of biological markers that have clear Mendelian modes of inheritance, are polymorphic (i.e. there are two or more alleles with a gene frequency of at least 1%), and have been assigned or are potentially assignable to specific chromosomal locations.

genetic polymorphism   See **polymorphism**.

genetic probe   Sequence of DNA or RNA used to identify genetic markers.

genetic recombination   Process by which crossing-over occurs between maternal and paternal chromatids during meiosis.

genetic redundancy   Numerous copies of the same gene repeated on a chromosome.

genetic screening   Systematic search for individuals in a population who possess certain genotypes that (a) are associated with existing disease or predisposed to future disease; (b) may lead to disease in their descendants; or (c) produce other variations of interest, but not known to be associated with disease.

genetic sequence   Order in which structures or functions determined by genes appear in development.

genetic trait   Trait determined by genes, not necessarily congenital.

genetic variance   **1.** Tendency of the genetic make-up to generate diversity within a population. **2.** Mean of the squares of the variations from the mean of a gene frequency distribution.

genetic variance, additive   Extent to which genes that influence a trait add according to gene dosage.

genetic variance, nonadditive   Dominance (interactions between alleles at a locus) and epistasis (interactions among alleles at different loci).

genetic vulnerability   Inherited predisposition to develop an illness that is continuous and chronic.

genetics   Biological science that deals with heredity and variation of individual members of a species. It was initiated by the hybridization studies of Gregor Mendel published in 1886.

genetics, behavioral   Study of the interactions of genetic and environmental influences on behavior. Some behaviors are genetically determined (nature), others are primarily influenced by environmental factors (nurture).

genetics, biometrical   Branch of population genetics originally concerned with improving domestic plants and animals using artificial selection.

genetics, clinical   Branch of genetics concerned with health and disease in individuals and their families or the science and practice (art) of diagnosis, prevention, and management of genetic disorders (McKusick VA. Medical Genetics. A 40-year perspective on the evolution of a medical specialty from a basic science. *JAMA* 1993;270:2351–2356).

genetics, community   Population-based, rather than individual family–oriented, aspects of medical genetics, particularly screening programs for genetic disorders and congenital malformations in pregnancy. The increasing number of accurate and totally age-independent tests for genetic disorders is causing expanding concern that community genetics may be misused and abused by those who believe they are acting in the best interests of the present and future populations and that these interests must override the rights and decisions of individuals.

genetics, forward   Strategy of going from the proteins to the genes.

genetics, human   Science of biological variations in humans.

genetics, medical   Science of human biological variation as it relates to health and disease. By 1983, over 3,400 single gene traits and 100 chromosome abnormalities were known; in the next 7 years, the number of single gene traits reached 4,937 and the number of chromosome abnormalities exceeded 600. In 1983, DNA probes could be used for carrier, presymptomatic, or prenatal diagnosis of hemoglobinopathies, hemophilias, and Huntington's disease. By 1990, DNA diagnosis had become the main diagnostic approach for over 40 other important single gene disorders, including cystic fibrosis, neurofibromatosis, adult polycystic kidney disease, myotonic dystrophy, spinal muscular atrophy, and Duchenne muscular dystrophy. Medical genetics is gradually extending to include psychiatric and neurological disorders of adulthood. The aims of medical genetics are (a) to ensure the maximum range of options for those at risk for genetic disease by providing accurate diagnosis and screening, empathic genetic counseling, and support; (b) to prevent genetic disease and unnecessary anxiety by facilitating personal informed choices from among these options; and (c) to aid appropriate clinical management of genetic disease and to identify preventable complications by early and accurate diagnosis (Harris R. Medical genetics. *Br Med J* 1991;303:977–979).

genetics, molecular   See **gene cloning.**

genetics, quantitative   Theory and set of methods to decompose phenotypic variance into genetic and environmental components.

genetics, reverse   Moving from linked genetic markers to the gene itself and thence to discovery of the abnormal (or necessary) gene products responsible for a disorder. The approach has produced successful results in monogenic conditions such as Duchenne's muscular dystrophy and cystic fibrosis.

genetically engineered drug   Protein manufactured through the technologies of recombinant DNA.

genogram   Graphic representation of the genealogy of a family. Also called "family tree."

genome   Complete haploid set of chromosomes derived from one parent. The human genome consists of approximately 3×10^9 base pairs and two loci that are a million base pairs apart.

genome map   Description of the position of genes on a chromosome (e.g., restriction enzyme cutting sites, genes, RFLP markers) regardless of inheritance. Distance is measured in base pairs. For the human genome, the lowest-resolution map is the banding patterns of the 23 different chromosomes; the highest-resolution map would be the complete nucleotide sequence of the chromosomes. Also called "physical map."

genome project   See **Human Genome Project.**

genomic library   Collection of clones made from a set of overlapping DNA fragments representing the entire genome of an organism.

genotype   Genetic constitution determined by an organism's alleles. In general, the term is synonymous with *genome.*

genotypical   Pertaining to the genotype.

genotyping   Identifying the hereditary constitution of one individual or organism.

geometric mean   See **mean, geometric.**

gepirone   Serotonin (5-HT)$_{1A}$ receptor agonist affecting presynaptic and postsynaptic receptors. It is a pharmacological analog of buspirone with a similar side effect profile, but with more potent serotonergic activity and less powerful noradrenergic stimulation. It is a novel, nonsedating anxiolytic. Anxiolytic effects are correlated with decrements in number and function of 5-HT$_2$ receptors. Preliminary studies suggest that unlike buspirone, gepirone may be efficacious in panic disorder. It is also reported to have antidepressant activity (Jenkins SW, Robinson DS, Fabre LF, et al: Gepirone in the treatment of major depression. *J Clin Psychopharmacol* 1990;10:77s–85s).

geriatric depression   See **depression, geriatric.**

geriatric psychiatry   See **psychogerontology.**

gerontology   Study of old age.

geropsychiatry   Term coined by Verwoerdt (1967) for the psychiatry of senescence.

Geschwind syndrome   See **interictal personality disorder.**

gesture   Body movement used as a form of silent emotional communication. Gestures range from the voluntary smile or wink to less voluntary physiognomy.

Gewacalm   See **diazepam.**

giddiness   Sense of impending faint; lightheadedness.

Gilex   See **doxepin.**

Gilles de la Tourette's syndrome   (GTS) Complex neurological disorder with a chronic, fluctuating course that afflicts children 3–5 years old, occurring 3 times as often in males as in females. Patients frequently have a family history of tics, compulsions, or GTS. Main symptoms are multiple motor and vocal tics, coprolalia (compulsive utterances of obscene words and phrases), echolalia, palilalia, and love of nonsense words. Tics are involuntary, sudden, rapid, recurrent, nonrhythmic, stereotyped motor movements or vocalizations. Although experienced as irresistible, they can be suppressed for varying lengths of time (minutes to hours). Intensity may vary over weeks to months (American Psychiatric Association. *Diagnostic and Statistical Manual of Mental Disorders. Fourth Edition* [DSM-IV]. Washington, DC: APA, 1994:101–103). GTS is genetically transmitted and probably associated with a structural or chemical diathesis; brain mechanisms involved in symptom generation remain unidentified. It also may be induced by long-term neuroleptic therapy and by stimulants (e.g., methylphenidate) used in the treatment of attention deficit hyperactivity disorder (ADHD). Although GTS is diagnosed according to arbitrarily defined clinical criteria, there is disagreement as to what constitutes the core of the syndrome and what its precise relation is to several other neurological and psychiatric conditions. These diagnostic uncertainties have hampered most research endeavors. GTS often is treated with haloperidol and pimozide. Their discontinuation, which is sometimes necessary to allow a switch to other agents, usually is benign, but in some cases there is marked short-term exacerbation of the frequency and intensity of tics and increased activity and aggressivity. Clonidine therapy also has been of some benefit.

ginkgo biloba   Tree, extracts from the leaves of which have been used therapeutically for centuries. Ginkgo is mentioned in the traditional pharmacopeia of China, where tea made from parts of the tree is used for the treatment of asthma and bronchitis. In western countries, standardized extracts from the leaves are used for other indications and administered as film-coated tablets, as a liquid, or intravenously. In Germany and France, such extracts are among the most commonly prescribed drugs. Main indications for ginkgo are peripheral vascular disease such as intermittent claudication and, more important, "cerebral insufficiency." Ginkgo biloba capsules are marketed in the United States by Solgar Vitamin and Herb Co.

"girl"   Street name for cocaine.

"girls & boys"   Street name for the injection of heroin (boys) and cocaine (girls) in a ratio of 2:1.

glabellar tap reflex   Blinking response elicited by 10 repeated taps on the glabella, which in normal subjects ceases after the first few taps.

gland   Organ that secretes substances used in the body or excreted. There are two types: endocrine or ductless glands that secrete their substances directly into the bloodstream, and exocrine or duct glands that discharge their secretions through a duct to the outside or into other organs of the body.

gland, adrenal   One of a pair of endocrine glands that overlie the kidneys and comprise two components. One is the adrenal medulla (the dark central portion), which produces epinephrine and norepinephrine, hormones important in the body's reaction to stress. The other is the adrenal cortex, which releases several hormones called "steroids" that are involved in the regulation of body metabolism and sexual functions.

gland, anterior pituitary   Portion of the pituitary gland that secretes adrenocorticotropic hormone (ACTH) and many other hormones in response to physical or emotional stress. ACTH stimulates the adrenal cortex to increase its production of hormones.

gland, pituitary   Endocrine gland, called the "master gland," comprising two parts: the anterior pituitary and the posterior pituitary. The former controls growth and the activity of other endocrine glands; the latter controls water balance.

gland, posterior pituitary   Portion of the pituitary gland derived from the embryonic brain, composed of the infundibulum and neural lobe, and concerned with the secretion of various hormones.

"glass"   Street name for methamphetamine.

glia   Brain cells that act as a physical and metabolic buffer around nerve cells.

Gliatilin   See **choline alfoscerate.**

glibenclamide   Antidiabetic drug marketed outside the United States.

glibenclamide + moclobemide   See **moclobemide + glibenclamide.**

global introspection   Unstructured mental process whereby the facts concerning a patient and his or her disease are integrated to form a diagnosis.

global rating   Assessment of overall clinical status or level of psychopathology expressed in gross units and opinions.

globin gene   See **gene, globin.**

globus hystericus   Sensation of a lump or foreign body in the throat; it must be differentiated from dysphagia. See **dysphagia.**

globus pallidus   Nucleus located within the basal ganglia.

Glorium   See **medazepam.**

glossopharyngeal contraction   Shortening and thickening of the tongue and pharynx.

glucocorticoid   Any of a group of corticoids (e.g., hydrocortisone, dexamethasone) that (a) are involved especially in carbohydrate, protein, and fat metabolism; (b) tend to increase liver glycogen and blood sugar by increasing glyconeogenesis; and (c) are anti-inflammatory and immunosuppressive. They are used widely in medicine (e.g., for symptoms of rheumatoid arthritis).

glucose-6 phosphate dehydrogenase deficiency (G-6 PD) Inheritable, sex-linked enzyme deficiency.

glue sniffing   Form of psychoactive substance abuse often practiced by children 9–12 years old who also abuse other psychoactive substances. It consists of the inhalation of the aliphatic and aromatic hydrocarbons in glue. See **solvent abuse.**

glutamate   Major excitatory amino acid neurotransmitter in the brain that accounts for about 40% of all nerve signals sent throughout the brain. It is involved in phenomena such as neuronal development, learning, and memory formation. It is normally released under close control with careful regulation of release and reuptake. In excess amounts, it is an intense excitant of nerve cells and can have toxic effects; it has been suspected as an important contributor to the pathogenesis of a number of neurodegenerative disorders, including neurolathyrism, amyotrophic lateral sclerosis, parkinsonian dementia complex of Guam, Huntington's disease, and Alzheimer's disease (Choi DW. Amyotrophic lateral sclerosis and glutamate—too much of a good thing? *N Engl J Med* 1992;326:1493–1495; Lawlor BA, Davis KL. Does modulation of glutamatergic function represent a viable therapeutic strategy in Alzheimer's disease? *Biol Psychiatry* 1992;31:337–350). Four receptor subtypes have been identified: N-methyl-D-aspartate (NMDA), kainic acid (KA), AMPA or quisqualic acid (Quis), and a metabotropic receptor for phosphatydylinositide turnover. These also behave as excitotoxants and are probably involved in the pathogenesis of certain neurodegenerative disorders, such as amyotrophic lateral sclerosis and Alzheimer's disease. Neural actions mediated via blockade of the NMDA receptor have been implicated in the pathophysiology of schizophrenia; in some patients, a glutamic acid deficiency has been implicated. Also called "excitatory amino acid."

glutamate receptor Molecular site that mediates the actions of glutamate neurotransmitters in the brain. Glutamate receptors are differentiated into N-methyl D-aspartate (NMDA) and non-NMDA types according to their agonist and antagonist affinities. Non-NMDA receptors are further divided into kainate (KA) and quisqualate (QA) receptor subtypes. The glutamate receptor system has a major influence on the development of the medial temporal lobe.

glutamatergic Neuron that releases glutamate.

glutamic acid (GLU) Precursor of gamma aminobutyric acid (GABA) and also a neurotransmitter in its own right. See **glutamate.**

glutamic acid decarboxylase (GAD) Enzyme responsible for converting glutamic acid to gamma aminobutyric acid (GABA). In general, the localization of GAD in mammalian brain correlates well with the GABA content.

glutethimide (Doriden; Doriglute) Piperidinedione derivative sedative-hypnotic. Half-life is 10–12 hours; duration of action is 4–8 hours. Usual hypnotic dose is 250–500 mg. It has been abused singly and in combination with codeine (called a "load") for its euphoriant properties. Schedule III; pregnancy risk category C.

glutethimide/breast milk Glutethimide is secreted in breast milk and may cause sedation in the neonate. Women taking it should be advised not to breast feed.

glycine Amino acid that acts as an inhibitory transmitter in the hindbrain and spinal cord. It is structurally the simplest amino acid. It may modulate the action of glutamate on the N-methyl-D-aspartate (NMDA) receptor. Trials of glycine in schizophrenia revealed no change or worsening of psychosis ratings.

glycopyrrolate (Robinul) Synthetic anticholinergic agent that can be administered (intramuscularly or intravenously) before electroconvulsive therapy (ECT) to prevent bradyarrhythmias. It has been found to have advantages over atropine for use in ECT.

Godot syndrome Repeated expression of anxiety regarding upcoming events. It is common in Alzheimer's disease. It appears related to decreased cognitive and memory abilities and inability to channel remaining thinking capacities productively. Patients repeatedly ask questions about upcoming events, sometimes so incessantly as to be intolerable to the caregiver.

"gold" Street name for marijuana.

"gold dust" Street name for cocaine.

gold standard See **criterion standard** (preferred term).

gonadal hormone Any of the hormones that contribute to individual and sex differences in brain structure and function. They promote growth and differentiation of several neural systems and sites, modulate neuronal plasticity, and influence the activity of several monoaminergic neurotransmitters. The latter may be one of the mechanisms by which gonadal hormones are involved in modulation of behavior and mood in humans.

gonadotropic hormone Pituitary hormone that stimulates growth and development of sperm and eggs in the gonads and production of androgen and estrogen.

gonadotropin-releasing hormone (GnRH) Hormone that releases luteinizing hormone into the bloodstream after a complex chain of events in the hypothalamic-pituitary axis of the brain.

"good shit" Street name for marijuana.

"goofball" Street name for central nervous system depressants, barbiturates, or glutethimide.

"goofer" Street name for barbiturates.

"goon" Street name for phencyclidine (PCP).

goosebumps Autonomic abstinence sign often considered a hallmark of opioid withdrawal. Excessive piloerection appears 1–2 days post withdrawal and may persist for as long as 2 weeks. The skin has the appearance of a plucked turkey–hence the expression "cold turkey." Goosebumps may accompany "cold flashes" and may alternate with "hot flashes" and perspiration.

G protein One of a family of guanosine triphosphate (GTP)-binding proteins that play an obligatory role in transducing extracellular, receptor-detected signals across the cell membrane to various intracellular effectors. G proteins are predominantly located close to the inner aspect of the cell membrane and constitute the nodal point between action and reaction for vast ranges of cellular processes. Understanding the mechanisms by which G proteins modulate neuronal activity may be one of the keys to understanding the functioning and complexities of the nervous system. Two main classes of G proteins are thought to be important in regulating adenylate cyclase activity—G_s, which stimulates cyclase, and G_i, which inhibits it. At present, the family of G proteins includes 12–15 already known individual proteins, as defined by their subunits: alpha, beta, and gamma. The alpha subunit contains the binding site for guanine nucleotides and possesses guanosine triphosphate (GTP)ase activity. The alpha subunit also contains the site for nicotinamide adenine nucleotide (NAD)-dependent adenosine diphosphate (ADP)-ribosylation catalyzed by bacterial toxins. The heterogeneity of alpha subunits serves to divide G proteins into the major classes (G_s, G_i, G_o, G_p, etc.) (Gilman AG. G proteins: transducers of receptor-generated signals. *Annu Rev Biochem* 1987;56:615–649). Abnormalities in the function and/or expression of G proteins have been implicated in a variety of pathophysiological states, including Alzheimer's disease, Huntington's disease, and possibly schizophrenia. There is evidence that G-proteins are "hyperfunctional" in manic patients and that lithium may alter G-protein function (Avissar S, Schreiber G: The involvement of guanine nucleotide binding proteins in the pathogenesis and treatment of affective disorders. *Biol Psychiatry* 1992;31:435–459).

G_i protein G protein that inhibits adenylate cyclase. It is activated by muscarinic cholinergic receptors and by the neurotransmitter norepinephrine through its interaction with beta-adrenergic and alpha-adrenergic receptors, respectively.

G_o protein Novel G protein that is a major constituent of bovine brain. It interacts with muscarinic receptors, but its function is unknown.

G_p protein Novel G protein that may be involved in coupling pholipase C; this generates two second messengers: inositol 1,4,5 triphosphate and diacylglycerol. G_p is activated by the neurotransmitter norepinephrine by its interaction with beta-adrenergic and alpha-adrenergic receptors, respectively. It is also activated by muscarinic cholinergic receptors.

G_s protein G protein that activates adenylate cyclase. It is activated by the neurotransmitter norepinephrine by its interaction with beta-adrenergic and alpha-adrenergic receptors, respectively.

Gradient See flunarizine.

grandiose delusion See delusion, grandiose.

grandiosity Exaggerated self-opinion and unrealistic convictions of superiority. In its mild form it is manifested by some expansiveness or boastfulness. When extreme, thinking, interactions, and behavior are dominated by multiple delusions of amazing ability, wealth, knowledge, fame, power, and/or moral stature, which may take on a bizarre quality.

grand mal seizure See seizure, tonic-clonic (preferred term). Nonfocal grand mal seizure has been reclassified as primary generalized seizure (see seizure, primary generalized). Focal-onset grand mal seizure has been reclassified as secondary generalized tonic-clonic seizure (see seizure, secondary generalized).

granisetron Serotonin (5-HT)$_3$ antagonist marketed as an antiemetic. It does not cause extrapyramidal side effects, which is important for children and young adults who are susceptible to acute dystonic reactions and akathisia. Mild headaches, constipation, and transient transaminase elevations are characteristically associated with 5-HT$_3$ antagonists, but are of little consequence. Granisetron may have antipsychotic properties and is currently being tested in schizophrenia and migraine.

granisetron + haloperidol No unwanted synergistic effects are reported (Leigh J, Link CG, Fell GJ. Effects of granisetron and haloperidol, alone and in combination, on psychometric performance and the EEG. *Br J Clin Pharmacol* 1992;34:65–70).

granulocyte-macrophage colony-stimulating factor (GM-CSF) Glycoprotein that has been shown to stimulate proliferation of precursor cells in bone marrow. It is mainly produced by T-lymphocytes, fibroblasts, endothelial cells, and keratinocytes. It is a powerful cytokine that regulates granulopoiesis and recombinant G-CSF (rG-CSF) and has been used for the treatment of neutropenia (Souza LM, Boone TC, Gabrilove J. Recombinant human granulocyte colony-stimulating factor: effects on normal and leukaemic cells. *Science* 1986; 232:61–65; Gabrilove LJ, Jakubowski A, Scher H, et al. Effect of granulocyte colony-stimulating factor on neutropenia and associated morbidity due to chemotherapy for transitional-cell carcinoma and the urothelium. *N Engl J Med* 1988;318:1414–1422). A specific GM-CSF receptor is located on neutrophils and eosinophils as well as on monocytes and leukemic blasts. Bacterially synthesized recombinant human GM-CSF has been reported to reduce the time of aplasia after cytotoxic therapy and bone marrow transplantation and to overcome primary bone marrow insufficiency. This lowers the risk of secondary infectious diseases secondary to agranulocytosis. In addition, the low incidence of severe side effects of GM-CSF enhances its usefulness for the treatment of drug-induced agranulocytosis (Morstyn G, Burgess AW. Hemopoietic growth factors: a review. *Cancer Res* 1988;48:5624–5629; Barnas C, Zwierzina H, Hummer M, Sperner-Unterweger B, Stern A, Fleishhacker WW. Granulocyte-macrophage colony-stimulating factor [GM-CSF] treatment of clozapine-induced agranulocytosis: a case report. *J Clin Psychiatry* 1992;53:245–247). GM-CSF has been shown to reduce the duration of agranulocytosis in patients with the most severe form of clozapine-induced bone marrow suppression (Gerson SL, Gullion G, Yeh HS, Masor C. Granulocyte colony-stimulating factor for clozapine-induced agranulocytosis. *Lancet* 1992;340:1097). Also called "filgrastim."

graph   Visual display of the relationship between variables.

grasp reflex   Grasping motion of the fingers or toes in response to stimulation. It can be elicited by tactile or tendon stimulation of the palm of the hand. It usually is associated with frontal lobe lesions.

"grass"   Street name for marijuana.

"grasshopper"   Street name for marijuana.

Grateful Med   System that allows access over national telecommunication networks to the MEDLINE bibliographic database. See **MEDLINE.**

"green"   Street name for phencyclidine (PCP).

"green and black"   Street term for a look-alike chlordiazepoxide.

"green and clear"   Street name for central nervous system stimulants.

"green and white"   Street name for chlordiazepoxide.

"greenie"   Street name for amphetamine/amobarbital.

grimace   Distorted facial expression or tic caused by an organic neurological disorder.

growth hormone   (GH) Vertebrate polypeptide hormone, secreted by the anterior lobe of the pituitary gland, that regulates growth. The sole approved indication is growth failure in children with inadequate endogenous GH secretion. GH is reportedly the most highly sought drug among athletes, who mistakenly believe it can produce effects similar to androgenic-anabolic steroids without causing serious adverse effects or without the potential for detection. They may take up to 20 times the recommended dose to improve athletic performance. High doses taken over the long term may cause adverse effects similar to those associated with acromegaly. Illicit users may spend up to $30,000 a year on products that may or may not be genuine; counterfeit GH is more readily available than genuine GH, which is distributed under tightly controlled procedures that require screening and documentation of need. Genuine GH may become even more difficult to obtain if the proposal that it be reclassified as a schedule II substance is enacted (Smith DA, Perry PJ. The efficacy of ergogenic agents in athletic competition. Part II: Other performance-enhancing agents. *Ann Pharmacother* 1992;26:653–659).

growth hormone releasing factor   (GRF) 44-Amino acid neuropeptide, first isolated in 1982, that releases physiologically relevant amounts of growth hormone and may have direct effects on central nervous system functioning.

growth hormone (GH) stimulation test   Neuroendocrine test that measures responsiveness of postsynaptic alpha$_2$-adrenergic receptors to various stimuli (e.g., insulin-induced hypoglycemia, L-dopa, 5-hydroxytryptamine, apomorphine, dextroamphetamine, clonidine, growth hormone releasing hormone, and thyrotropin-releasing hormone. Blood for GH estimation is collected at 90, 100, 120, and 180 minutes after the stimuli is administered. GH is assayed by double-antibody radioimmunoassay. Response is considered blunted if GH levels fail to rise at least 5 mU/L above baseline value. Blunted response may be a "trait" marker for depression (Barry S, Dinan TG. Neuroendocrine challenge test in depression: a study of growth hormone, TRH, and cortisol release. *J Affect Disord* 1990;18:229–234).

guanfacine   (Tenex) Centrally acting antihypertensive with alpha$_2$-adrenoceptor agonist properties marketed in tablet form for oral administration.

guanfacine + amitriptyline   See **amitriptyline + guanfacine.**

guanfacine + imipramine   See **imipramine + guanfacine.**

guanine   Purine base $C_5H_5NO_4$ that codes genetic information in the polynucleotide chain of DNA or RNA.

guanylate cyclase   Intracellular enzyme associated with some types of receptors that on activation produces the second messenger cyclic guanylate monophosphate (cyclic GMP).

"guerrilla"   Street name for phencyclidine (PCP).

guidance   In group therapy, imparting information and giving advice by the therapist or other group members (Bloch S, Crouch E: *Therapeutic Factors in Group Psychotherapy*. Oxford: Oxford University Press, 1985).

Guillain-Barré syndrome   Acute idiopathic polyneuritis characterized by muscular weakness and paresthesia.

guilt feelings   Sense of remorse or self-blame for real or imagined misdeeds in the past. When extreme, there are unshakable delusions of guilt that the person feels deserve drastic punishment (e.g., life imprisonment, torture, death). There may be associated suicidal thoughts or attribution of others' problems to one's past misdeeds.

gustatory hallucination   See **hallucination, gustatory.**

gyrectomy   Psychosurgical procedure in which bilateral symmetrical removals of frontal cortex are carried out to relieve certain types of mental illness. It is seldom done today.

H

"H"   Street name for heroin.

"H and H"   Street name for heroin plus hashish.

"H and stuff"   Street name for heroin.

habilitation   Training for patients with congenital and early infancy disorders.

habit   Behavior pattern acquired by frequent repetition that manifests itself in regularity and increased facility of performance.

Habitrol   See **nicotine transdermal system.**

habit spasm   See **tic.**

habitual body manipulation   Self-gratifying, compulsive, often socially offensive action (e.g., thumb-sucking, hair twiddling, nose-picking) that reflects anxiety, boredom, tiredness, or self-consciousness.

habituation   See **tolerance** (preferred term).

hair drug analysis   Detection of drug concentrations incorporated in hair. Drug molecules from blood supply to hair strands penetrate hair structure and remain there. Sections of the hair strands provide a history of the time course of drug abuse because hair grows at a rate of about 1.2 cm/month. Thus, each 1.2 cm from the root provides objective information on use or nonuse of drugs.

hair pulling   See **trichotillomania.**

halazepam   (Paxipam)   1,4-Benzodiazepine (BZD) anxiolytic that is rapidly absorbed and primarily excreted in urine. Elimination half life including metabolites is 2–4 days. It is one of the few BZDs not self-administered by primates. It is used for the same clinical indications as other BZD anxiolytics. It is claimed to be less sedative than other BZDs, but has essentially the same side effect profile. Schedule IV; pregnancy risk category D.

Halcion   See **triazolam.**

Haldol   See **haloperidol.**

Haldol Decanoas   See **haloperidol decanoate.**

Haldol Decanoate   See **haloperidol decanoate.**

half-life   (t_p) Measure of the duration of a parent drug in the body after systemic administration. It is the time required to eliminate half the amount of the plasma level of the drug in the body, assuming the distribution process has reached equilibrium. Half-life determines the time required to achieve a steady-state concentration, which occurs in about four half-lives. Half-life also determines the frequency of dosing; the shorter the half-life, the more frequently the drug has to be administered to achieve constant clinical effects. Half-life depends on the drug's volume of distribution (Vd) and clearance (Cl); if Cl is decreased, elimination half-life will be increased. A larger Vd is also associated with a longer elimination half-life. Some compounds have a short half-life because they are metabolized and eliminated very rapidly. Those that remain in the body for days or weeks have a long half-life. Knowing a drug's half-life makes it possible to predict the length of time required for the drug to be eliminated from the body. Half-life also influences termination of drug effects. Shorter half-life drugs may be associated with greater risk and intensity of withdrawal effects. Drugs with long half-lives have a built-in tapering process; when discontinued they are eliminated slowly and onset of withdrawal effects (if any) is slow. See **anxiety, breakthrough.**

half-life, alpha   Rate of decline in plasma concentration due to drug distribution from the central to the peripheral compartment(s).

half-life, beta   Rate of decline in plasma concentration due to drug elimination after metabolism to inactive conjugated forms and urinary excretion.

half-life, metabolite   Duration of a drug's metabolite(s) in the body after systemic administration. It is always equal to or longer than the half-life of the parent compound because a metabolite cannot be eliminated more quickly than it is formed.

halfway house   Residence for psychiatric patients who do not require full hospitalization, but are not well enough to function within the community without some degree of professional supervision, protection, and support.

Halidol   See **haloperidol.**

Halidol Decanòar   See **haloperidol decanoate.**

hallucination   Vivid perceptual experience that occurs in the absence of a relevant sensory stimulus (Asaad G, Shapiro B. Hallucinations. *Am J Psychiatry* 1986;143:1088–1097). Perceptions may involve any of the senses, alone or mixed.

hallucination auditory   Hallucination of sound, most commonly of voices, but sometimes of such sounds as clicks, rushing noises, and music. In drug-induced psychoses, auditory hallucinations are usually experienced as indistinct noises (DSM-IV).

hallucination, command   Auditory hallucination instructing the person to act in a certain manner that may range from grimacing to committing a suicidal or homicidal act (Hellerstein D, Frosch W, Koenigsberg HW. The clinical significance of command hallucinations. *Am J Psychiatry* 1987;144:219–221).

They are ignored 60% of the time, but are more likely to be obeyed if there is a related delusion and the voice is familiar. Most command hallucinations direct the person to commit suicide (50%+). Fewer command injury to self or others (12%). A minority command homicide (5%). Also called "imperative hallucination."

hallucination, gustatory   Hallucination of taste, usually unpleasant (DSM-IV).

hallucination, hypnagogic   Auditory, visual, or tactile hallucination at the onset of sleep.

hallucination, hypnopompic   Hallucination that occurs upon awakening in the morning.

hallucination, imperative   See **hallucination, command.**

hallucination, kinesthetic   Perception of movement of body parts that are not actually moving (e.g., phantom limb syndrome).

hallucination, olfactory   Hallucination involving smell.

hallucination, release   Amorphous visual phenomena caused by damage to occipital centers, hemispheric infarctions, or tumors. Hallucinations are more common with right-sided than with left-sided lesions. They consist of complex visual images of objects, animals, or people. They last for hours and may be influenced by manipulations such as opening, moving, or closing the eyes.

hallucination, somatic   Hallucination involving the perception of a physical experience localized within the body (DSM-IV). It can be identified with certainty only when a delusional interpretation of physical illness is present. It must be distinguished from unexplained physical sensations, hypochondriacal preoccupation with or exaggeration of normal physical sensations, and tactile hallucinations in which the sensation is usually related to the skin.

hallucination, tactile   Hallucination involving the sense of touch, often of something on or under the skin, and almost invariably associated with a delusional interpretation of the sensation (DSM-IV). A particular tactile hallucination is formication (sensation of something creeping or crawling on or under the skin). Tactile hallucinations of pain must be distinguished from somatoform pain disorder, in which there is no delusional interpretation. See **formication.**

hallucination, visual   Hallucination involving sight that may consist of formed images (e.g., people) or unformed images (e.g., flashes of light) (DSM-IV). Visual hallucinations must be distinguished from illusions, which are visual misperceptions of real external stimuli.

hallucinatory behavior   Verbal report or behavior indicating the occurrence of perceptions not generated by external stimuli. When extreme, there is almost total preoccupation with hallucinations, which virtually dominate thinking and behavior. Hallucinations may evoke a rigid delusional interpretation and may provoke verbal and behavioral responses, including obedience to command hallucinations.

hallucinogen   Substance that alters consciousness and produces auditory and/or visual hallucinations without delirium, sedation, excessive stimulation, or intellectual or memory impairment. Included are psychedelics (e.g., lysergic acid diethylamide [LSD], mescaline, psilocybin, dimethyltryptamine), hallucinogenic amphetamines (e.g., 3,4-methylenedioxymethamphetamine, 3,4-methylenedioxyamphetamine), and anticholinergics (e.g., scopolamine). Classic hallucinogens are agonists or partial agonists at several serotonin (5-HT) receptor subtypes: 5-HT_2, 5-HT_{1C}, and 5-HT_{1A} (Strassman RJ. Human hallucinogen interactions with drugs affecting serotonergic neurotransmission. *Neuropsychopharmacology* 1992;7:241–243). In a typical hallucinogenic drug intoxication, there are illusions, hallucinations (primarily visual), mood shifts ranging from euphoria to panic to bland indifference, and an investment of mundane thoughts and perceptions with a sense of novelty. A survey of college students showed that rates of hallucinogen use were similar in 1989, 1978, and 1969 (Pope H Jr, Ionescu-Pioggia M, Aizley H, Varma D. Drug use and life style among college undergraduates in 1989: a comparison with 1969 and 1978. *Am J Psychiatry* 1990;147: 998–1001). In some parts of the world, hallucinogens are called "illusionogens" or "illusionogenics" because they cause perceptual distortions of an actual stimulus in the environment. Also called "mysticimimetic"; "phantastica"; "psychedelic"; "psychotomimetic"; "psychotomystic"; "psychotoraxic." Schedule I.

hallucinosis   Persistent or recurrent hallucinations in a clear sensorium that is most commonly due to substance intoxication and/or withdrawal (especially alcohol). It has been reported in patients receiving high doses of opiates for cancer pain; hallucinations are exclusively visual and occur in patients with no impairment of cognitive status (Bruera E, Schoeller T, Montejo G. Organic hallucinosis in patients receiving high doses of opiates for cancer pain. *Pain* 1992;48:397–399).

hallucinosis, alcohol   See **alcohol hallucinosis.**

haloperidol   (Apo-Haloperidol; Haldol; Halidol; Novoperidol; Peridol; Serenace) (HAL, HPL) Potent butyrophenone (first nonphenothiazine) antipsychotic extensively used for the treatment of diverse psychiatric disorders. It can be administered orally, intravenously, intramuscularly, and in depot form. It is metabolized via a ketone reductase enzyme to reduced haloperidol (RHAL), which is biologically less active. RHAL is converted back to HAL via oxidation under the influence of the P450IID6 isozyme. HAL's plasma elimination half-life is 12–36 hours. In acute schizophrenia, optimal clinical response frequently occurs with a plasma range of 5–12 ng/ml; treatment-refractory cases may be managed at plasma levels much greater than 12 ng/ml. With fixed doses, there is a curvilinear relationship between plasma HAL and clinical response. The approximate upper and lower limits of this proposed therapeutic window are 12 and 5 ng/ml, respectively, with 2 ng/ml as a threshold level. Plasma levels beyond 12 ng/ml may worsen the patient, causing more dysphoria. Orientals generally have higher blood levels of HAL than do other ethnic groups. HAL and RHAL pharmacokinetics are correlated with their levels in the hair of patients treated with HAL (4–30 mg/day) for more than 4 months and thus represent their mean amounts in the body (Uematsu T, Matsuno H, Sato H, et al. Steady-state pharmacokinetics of haloperidol and reduced haloperidol in schizophrenic patients: analysis of factors determining their concentration in hair. *J Pharm Sci* 1992;81:1008–1011). HAL disposition is associated with the genetically determined capacity to hydroxylate debrisoquin. Pregnancy risk category C. See **reduced haloperidol.**

haloperidol/alcoholism Haloperidol (HAL) can reduce craving and impaired control following alcohol consumption, supporting the hypothesis that these phenomena are mediated by alcohol's dopaminergic effects and are consistent with the proposed etiologic role in alcoholism for nigrotegmental dopaminergic-inhibitory input to the striatoacumbens (Modell JG, Mountz JM. Effect of haloperidol on craving and impaired control following alcohol consumption in alcoholic subjects. *In* Kalivas PW, Samson HH [eds], *The Neurobiology of Drug and Alcohol Addiction.* New York: New York Academy of Sciences, 1992, pp 492–495).

haloperidol + alprazolam In a double-blind study, alprazolam (ALP) plus haloperidol (HAL) was effective in the management of 28 agitated acutely psychotic schizophrenic patients, particularly in the first 48 hours. Subjects were randomly assigned to orally receive HAL (5 mg) and ALP (1 mg) or HAL (5 mg) plus placebo. Patients treated with the combination generally require significantly less HAL to achieve similar results than do patients treated with HAL alone. The combination also may result in fewer dystonic reactions (Barbee JG, Mancuso DM, Freed CR, et al. Alprazolam as a neuroleptic adjunct in the emergency treatment of schizophrenia. *Am J Psychiatry* 1992;149:506–510).

haloperidol + benztropine Benztropine is sometimes co-prescribed with haloperidol to treat or prevent acute early onset extrapyramidal reactions. The regimen may reverse some of haloperidol's therapeutic effects (Froemming JS, Lam YW, Jann MW. Pharmacokinetics of haloperidol. *Clin Pharmacokinet* 1989;17:396–423).

haloperidol/breast milk Haloperidol has been found in small quantities in breast milk, which did not affect the infants. Long-term effects are unknown (Whalley LJ, Blain PG, Prime JK. Haloperidol secreted in breast milk. *Br Med J* 1981;282:1746–1747; Ohkubo T, Shimoyama R, Sugawara K. Measurement of haloperidol in human breast milk by high-performance liquid chromatography. *J Pharm Sci* 1992;81:947–949).

haloperidol + bromocriptine Double-blind crossover studies indicate that bromocriptine enhances therapeutic response to haloperidol in chronic schizophrenia.

haloperidol + buspirone Buspirone may increase haloperidol (HAL) serum levels 25% or more. Clinical significance of the interaction is uncertain, but it may increase HAL's antipsychotic effects. Clinicians should be aware of a possible pharmacokinetic interaction when interpreting clinical changes following addition of buspirone to neuroleptics in general (Goff DC, Midha KK, Brotman AW, et al. An open trial of buspirone added to neuroleptics in schizophrenic patients. *J Clin Psychopharmacol* 1991;11:193–197).

haloperidol + carbamazepine Carbamazepine (CBZ) powerfully induces hepatic microsomal enzymes over several weeks and increases metabolism of many drugs. It may lower haloperidol (HAL) plasma levels up to 60%, with variable clinical impact: some patients improve and have fewer extrapyramidal symptoms; others deteriorate (Arana GW, Goff DC, Friedman H, et al. Does carbamazepine-induced reduction of plasma haloperidol levels worsen psychotic symptoms? *Am J Psychiatry* 1986;143:650–651). Double-blind crossover studies indicate that adjunctive CBZ can enhance therapeutic response to HAL in chronic schizophrenia. Neurotoxicity is rare. Two cases of delirium have been reported (Kanter GL, Yerevanian BI, Ciccone JR. Case report of a possible interaction between neuroleptics and carbamazepine. *Am J Psychiatry* 1984;141:1101–1102; Yerevanian BI, Hodgman CH. A haloperidol-carbamazepine interaction in a patient with rapid-cycling bipolar disorder. *Am J Psychiatry* 1985;142:785–786). Neuroleptic malignant syndrome (NMS) developed in a 29-year-old woman with bipolar disorder 8 hours after treatment with HAL (10 mg) and CBZ (100 mg). The NMS was treated successfully with orally administered nifedipine (60 mg/day) (Hermesh H, Molcho A, Aizenburg D, Munitz H. The calcium antagonist nifedipine in recurrent neuroleptic malignant syndrome. *Clin Neuropharmacol* 1988;11:552–555). Patients whose hepatic enzymes have been induced by such factors as cigarette smoking or alcohol use may not show an additional increase in hepatic clearance of HAL when CBZ is added. This may explain why HAL levels do not fall in some patients begun on CBZ, but fall sharply in others (Belknap SM, Nelson JE. Drug interactions in psychiatry. *In* Musa MN [ed], *Pharmacokinetics and Therapeutic Monitoring of Psychiatric Drugs.* Springfield, IL: Charles C Thomas, 1993, pp 57–112).

haloperidol + clomipramine Haloperidol (HAL) may increase plasma concentration of clomipramine (CMI), augmenting its effects. CMI (75–175 mg/day) + (HAL 3–7 mg/day) has been used with benefit and good tolerance in phobic and obsessive-compulsive patients (Cassano GB, Castrogiovanni P, Mauri M, et al. A multicenter controlled trial in phobic-obsessive psychoneurosis. The effect of chlorimipramine and of its combinations with haloperidol and diazepam. *Progr Neuropsychopharmacol Biol Psychiatry* 1981;5:129–138). Co-administration produced marked improvement in delusions, hallucinations, and obsessive symptoms and completely eradicated tics in a patient with Tourette's syndrome, obsessive-compulsive disorder, and schizophrenia (Escobar R, Bernardo M. Schizophrenia, obsessive-compulsive disorder, and Tourette's syndrome: a case of triple co-morbidity. *J Clin Neuropsychiatry Clin Neurosci* 1993;5:108).

haloperidol + clonazepam In a double-blind crossover study of acute mania with adjunctive haloperidol, clonazepam (mean dose, 10.4 mg/day) was superior to lithium (mean dose, 1691 mg/day) in controlling motor overactivity and logorrhea. In addition, less total haloperidol was dose administered during clonazepam treatment (Chouinard G, Young SN, Annable L. Antimanic effect of clonazepam *Biol Psychiatry* 1983;18:451–466). In a double-blind study in schizophrenia, clonazepam (3 mg/day) added to haloperidol produced modest improvement in Brief Psychiatric Rating Scale and Extrapyramidal Side Effects Scale scores, but no changes in specific symptoms (Altamura AC, Mauri MC, Mantero M,

Brunetti M. Clonazepam/haloperidol combination therapy in schizophrenia: a double-blind study. *Acta Psychiatr Scand* 1987;76:702–706).

haloperidol + cyproheptadine Double-blind crossover studies indicate that cyproheptadine can enhance therapeutic response to haloperidol in chronic schizophrenia. It also may significantly reduce extrapyramidal symptoms. It did not reduce plasma prolactin level, but did decrease plasma cortisol level (Shick LH, Hak KJ, Moon LY, et al. Cyproheptadine augmentation of haloperidol in the chronic schizophrenic patient: a double-blind placebo-controlled study. *Neuropsychopharmacology* 1993;9:55S).

haloperidol decanoate (Haldol Decanoas; Haldol Decanoate; Halidol Decanoar; Pericate; Peridor) (HAL-D) Long-acting form of haloperidol (HAL) indicated for maintenance treatment of chronic psychoses requiring prolonged neuroleptic therapy. It is administered as an intramuscular depot injection in sesame oil. Effects are the same as those of HAL, but with longer duration of action; there is a slow and sustained release of active HAL from the injection site. Plasma concentrations rise gradually, usually peaking within the first week post injection and falling thereafter. Half-life is about 3 weeks, and the time to steady-state is about 3 months. It has a "flip-flop" pharmacokinetic model because its absorption rate constant is slower than the elimination rate constant. Whereas haloperidol decanoate (HAL-D) is labeled as to the content of active constituent, fluphenazine decanoate (FD) is labeled as to content of the salt form (1 ml of FD contains 25 mg of decanoate salt and 21.5 mg of fluphenazine). Patients unresponsive to one depot preparation are often switched to another. Since HAL-D and FD are not exactly equipotent, the difference in labeling and content of active constituent should be taken into account when switching.

haloperidol + desipramine A grand mal seizure was reported (Mahr GC, Berchou R, Balon R. A grand mal seizure associated with desipramine and haloperidol. *Can J Psychiatry* 1987;32:463–464).

haloperidol + diazepam Co-administration may lower haloperidol serum levels and impair its therapeutic efficacy.

haloperidol/dopamine receptor blockade Positron emission tomographic (PET) studies indicate a well defined curvilinear relationship between haloperidol (HAL) plasma level and dopamine receptor occupancy (Wolkin A, Brodie JD, Barouche F, Rotrosen J. Dopamine receptor occupancy and plasma haloperidol levels. *Arch Gen Psychiatry* 1989;46:482–483).

At very low plasma HAL levels, receptor blockade increased rapidly with small increases in the HAL level. The increase then tapered off at 5–15 ng/ml; above 20 ng/ml, relatively little additional increase could be measured, even with marked increases in plasma levels. This agrees with clinical experience that there is little added benefit as plasma HAL levels rise above 20 ng/ml and a strong argument for the clinical merit of measuring plasma neuroleptic drug levels. Since comparable degrees of receptor blockade are found in both responders and nonresponders, inconsistencies in clinical response at "therapeutic" plasma levels might reflect differences in biological features rather than variability in the pharmacokinetic relationship between plasma level and blockade (Beckmann H, Laux G. Guidelines for the dosage of antipsychotic drugs. *Acta Psychiatr Scand* 1990;82[suppl 358]:63–66).

haloperidol + fluoxetine   Fluoxetine (FLX) inhibits haloperidol (HAL) metabolism and raises its blood level. Addition of FLX (20 mg/day) for 7–10 days to stable HAL doses increased mean HAL concentration by 20%, but extrapyramidal symptoms (EPS) did not increase appreciably (Levinson ML, Lipsy RJ, Fuller DK. Adverse effects and drug interactions associated with fluoxetine therapy. *Drug Intell Clin Pharm* 1991;25:657–661). Examination of FLX effects on ongoing HAL treatment in eight subjects disclosed substantial increase in blood levels in three who had low initial HAL levels and who appeared to be rapid metabolizers of the drug. Slow HAL metabolizers were unaffected (Goff DC, Midha KK, Brotman AW, et al. Elevation of plasma concentrations of haloperidol after the addition of fluoxetine. *Am J Psychiatry* 1991;148:790–792). It is not clear whether these interactions have a pharmacokinetic or a pharmacodynamic basis, or both. Increased HAL levels may lead to toxicity, sometimes manifested by EPS such as akathisia and parkinsonism (Tate JL. Extrapyramidal symptoms in a patient taking haloperidol and fluoxetine. *Am J Psychiatry* 1989;146:399–400). Tardive dyskinesia also has been reported (Stein M. Tardive dyskinesia in a patient taking haloperidol and fluoxetine. *Am J Psychiatry* 1991;148:683).

haloperidol + fluvoxamine   Up to 50% of obsessive compulsive disorder (OCD) patients remain clinically unchanged after an adequate trial with serotonin uptake inhibitors. Because brain dopamine systems may also contribute to obsessive compulsive phenomena, haloperidol may potentiate response to fluvoxamine (FVX) in OCD patients resistant or partially responsive to FVX without causing any adverse interactions (Dominguez RA. Serotonergic antidepressants and their efficacy in obsessive compulsive disorder. *J Clin Psychiatry* 1992; 53[10 suppl]:56–59; McDougle CJ, Goodman WK, Price LH et al. Neuroleptic addition in fluvoxamine-refractory obsessive-compulsive disorder. *Am J Psychiatry* 1990;147:652–654).

haloperidol + granisetron   No unwanted synergistic effects are reported (Leigh J, Link CG, Fell GJ. Effects of granisetron and haloperidol, alone and in combination, on psychometric performance and the EEG. *Br J Clin Pharmacol* 1992;34:65–70).

haloperidol + indomethacin   Using haloperidol to potentiate indomethacin's analgesic effects may produce unacceptable drowsiness, due possibly to combined central nervous system effects (Bud HA, LeGallez P, Wright V. Drowsiness due to haloperidol/indomethacin in combination. *Lancet* 1983;1:830–831).

haloperidol, intravenous administration   Since 1958, thousands of patients have received one or more intravenous haloperidol (HAL) doses ranging from 2 to 350 mg+. It is the subject of or is mentioned in over 800 publications. It has been administered more often and to more patients than any other neuroleptic to achieve very rapid symptom control in the safest way possible in patients with acute delirium tremens, very severe mania (including treatment-resistant mania), or severe malignant catatonic excitement. It also may be used to control acute agitation or delirium in patients in intensive or coronary care units. Intravenously administered HAL has an impressive record for safety and effectiveness in a wide range of doses for disturbed patients with serious medical and surgical conditions. It produces its calming effect with minimal effect on alertness; repeated mental status examinations and essential physical and laboratory tests can be done to enhance the diagnostic process and to select optimal management regimens. It also can be used for those unable to take HAL orally or who have a relative contraindication for intramuscular injections such as reduced muscle mass. When warranted, a benzodiazepine such as lorazepam or alprazolam can be co-administered with intravenously administered HAL to produce additional sedation. Rarely has it reacted adversely with the many other drugs patients receive concomitantly or aggravated a medical or surgical condition. Aside from very infrequent instances of extrapyramidal reactions that are not severe or life-threatening and that quickly respond to antiparkinson drugs, transient oversedation has been the most common side effect, induced usually by serial doses at intervals of 30 minutes. There have been no reports of neuroleptic malignant syndrome or sudden death caused by intravenously administered HAL.

haloperidol/intravenous/HIV   Low-dose, intravenous haloperidol can be used safely and effectively in the treatment of acutely disturbed behavior and delirium associated with human immunodeficiency virus (HIV) and acquired immunodeficiency syndrome (AIDS).

haloperidol/intravenous infusion   Continuous intravenously administered HAL infusion has been used to treat severe refractory agitation in cancer patients. Clinical improvement has occurred despite previous unresponsiveness to bolus dosing with the same medication. It has not produced extrapyramidal side effects, which is consistent with previous experience with intravenously administered HAL (Fernandez F, Holmes VF, Adams F, Kavanaugh JJ. Treatment of severe refractory agitation with haloperidol drip. *J Clin Psychiatry* 1988;49:239–241; Menza MA, Murray GB, Holmes VF, Rafuls WA. Decreased extrapyramidal symptoms with the use of intravenous haloperidol. *J Clin Psychiatry* 1987;48:278–280).

haloperidol + levodopa   Co-administration may interfere with the therapeutic effect of levodopa.

haloperidol + lithium   Co-administration may cause severe adverse reactions, particularly during the acute manic phase. The drugs may act in an additive or synergistic fashion; toxic clinical manifestations during combined use seem to differ from the toxic reactions of either drug alone. Although lithium plus haloperidol has been reported most frequently as producing neurotoxic states, other neuroleptics (fluphenazine, thioridazine, perphenazine, chlorpromazine) combined with lithium produce identical syndromes. The higher the neuroleptic dose, the greater the risk. The elderly (age 65+) are more likely to develop neurotoxicity with neuroleptic doses considered safe when administered in the absence of other psychoactive drugs. Thus, advanced age is a relative contraindication to combined lithium-neuroleptic therapy; moderate neuroleptic dosage (400–600 chlorpromazine equivalents) can result in neurotoxicity with no proven therapeutic advantage (Batchelor DH, Lowe MR. Reported neurotoxicity with the lithium/haloperidol combination and other neuroleptics—a literature review. *Hum Psychopharmacol* 1990;5:275–280). See **lithium neurotoxicity.**

haloperidol + lorazepam   Co-administration may be effective and safe in the treatment of acute psychotic agitation, acute schizophrenia, and mania. The combination may be superior to either drug alone in terms of clinical effects and may allow use of lower doses, thus reducing risk of unwanted side effects (Garza-Trevino ES, Hollister LE, Overall JE, Alexander WF. Efficacy of combinations of intramuscular antipsychotics and sedative-hypnotics for control of psychotic agitation. *Am J Psychiatry* 1989;149:1598–1601; Stevens A, Stevens I, Mahal A, Gaertner HJ. Haloperidol and lorazepam combined: clinical effects and drug plasma levels in the treatment of acute schizophrenic psychosis. *Pharmacopsychiatry* 1992;25:273–277).

haloperidol + nicotine   Smoking can reduce haloperidol (HAL) plasma levels (Jann M, Sakalad S, Ereshefsky L, et al. Effects of smoking on haloperidol and reduced haloperidol plasma concentrations and haloperidol clearance. *Psychopharmacology* 1986;90:468–470). Open studies indicate that nicotine powerfully potentiates the action of HAL in Gilles de la Tourette's syndrome. Nicotine gum alone, however, has less effect; although it reduced tic frequency for 1 hour after being chewed, it could have had a distracting effect (McConville BJ, Fogelson H, Norman AB, et al. Nicotine potentiation of haloperidol in reducing tic frequency in Tourette's disorder. *Am J Psychiatry* 1991;148:793–794; Miller DD, Kelly MW, Perry PJ, et al. The influence of cigarette smoking on haloperidol pharmacokinetics. *Biol Psychiatry* 1990;28:529–531). Case reports suggest that transdermal nicotine may ameliorate Tourette's symptoms in nonsmoking adolescents not satisfactorily controlled with dopamine blockers (HAL) (Silver AA, Sanberg PR. Transdermal nicotine patch and potentiation of haloperidol in Tourette's syndrome. *Lancet* 1993;342:182).

haloperidol + paroxetine   Paroxetine interferes with the cytochrome P450IID6 isoenzyme, which may result in increased haloperidol (HAL) levels and increased clinical side effects. Paroxetine does not potentiate HAL's sedative or psychomotor effects, but co-administration may increase adverse central nervous system effects (Cooper SM, Jackson D, Loudon JM, et al. The psychomotor effects of paroxetine alone and in combination with haloperidol, amylobarbitone, oxazepam, or alcohol. *Acta Psychiatr Scand* 1989;80[suppl]: 53–55). There is a report of a patient being treated with paroxetine (20 mg/day) to which HAL (3 mg/day) was added. Two weeks later, she lapsed into a semistuporous state that remitted when paroxetine, but not HAL, was discontinued (Lewis J, Brazanza J, Williams T. Psychomotor retardation and semistuporous state with paroxetine. *Br Med J* 1993;306: 1169).

haloperidol + phenelzine Co-administration has been found to be efficacious in the treatment of irritability and depression in borderline personality disorder.

haloperidol + phenobarbital Co-administration can lower haloperidol plasma concentrations secondary to hepatic enzyme induction by phenobarbital (Linnoila M, Viukari M, Vaisanen K, et al. Effect of anticonvulsants on plasma haloperidol and thioridazine levels. *Am J Psychiatry* 1980;137:819–821).

haloperidol + phenytoin Phenytoin induces hepatic enzymes, significantly lowers haloperidol (HAL) plasma concentration, and may interfere with HAL's therapeutic efficacy (Linnoila M, Viukari M, Vaisanen K, et al. Effect of anticonvulsants on plasma haloperidol and thioridazine levels. *Am J Psychiatry* 1980;137: 819–821).

haloperidol + pindolol No significant interactions are reported (Greendyke RM, Gulya A. Effect of pindolol administration on serum levels of thioridazine, haloperidol, phenytoin and phenobarbital. *J Clin Psychiatry* 1988;49: 105–107).

haloperidol plasma levels/clinical efficacy Repeated studies indicate that haloperidol (HAL) plasma levels above 5 ng/ml (steady state after approximately 9 mg/day) are clinically effective, and that increased plasma levels yield no additional improvement in patients participating in research studies. Although plasma levels exceeding 12 ng/ml may be toxic, data are equivocal. Current research is focused on the clinical effectiveness of very low plasma levels; in acutely exacerbating schizophrenia, 2 ng/ml may be an adequate level for many patients, but 10 ng/ml is somewhat more effective (Hirschowitz J, Hitzemann R, Burr G, Schwartz A. A new approach to dose reduction in chronic schizophrenia. *Neuro Psychopharm* 1991;5:103–113; Volavka J, Cooper T, Czobor P, et al. Haloperidol blood levels and clinical effects. *Arch Gen Psychiatry* 1992;49:354–361; Volavka J, Cooper TB. Antipsychotic levels and optimal dosing. Presented at the 146th Annual Meeting of the American Psychiatric Association, San Francisco, May 1993).

haloperidol/pregnancy No strong data link haloperidol with birth defects in humans. It is associated with limb reduction malformation and other defects in two case reports; in both, other drugs were also taken (including diphenylhydantoin, which is known to have a teratogenic potential) (Schardein JL. Psychotropic drugs. *In Chemically Induced Birth Defects*. New York: Marcel Dekker, 1985).

haloperidol + propranolol Co-administration has no effect on haloperidol plasma levels, but may produce serious adverse cardiovascular effects including hypotension and cardiopulmonary arrest (Greendyke RM, Kanter DR. Plasma propranolol levels and their effects on plasma thioridazine and haloperidol concentrations. *J Clin Psychopharmacol* 1987;7:178–182; Alexander HE, McCarty K, Giffen MB. Hypotension and cardiopulmonary arrest associated with concurrent haloperidol and propranolol therapy. *JAMA* 1984;252:87–88).

haloperidol + psychostimulant Haloperidol (HAL), either alone or in combination with a psychostimulant, can help control aggressive symptoms of a co-morbid conduct disorder (Shekine WO. Diagnosis and treatment of attention deficit and conduct disorders in children and adolescents. *In* Simeon JG, Ferguson HB [eds], *Treatment Strategies in Child and Adolescent Psychiatry*. New York: Plenum Press, 1993). Risks due to HAL must be considered before the combination is prescribed.

haloperidol + ritanserin In preclinical studies, co-administration did not modify the effect of haloperidol (Lappalainen J, Hietala J, Koulon M, Syvalatiti E. Neurochemical effects of chronic co-administration of ritanserin and haloperidol: comparison with clozapine effects. *Eur J Pharmacol* 1990;190:403–407). In chronic, primarily type II, schizophrenia, co-administration produced improvement, especially in negative symptoms.

haloperidol therapeutic window Haloperidol is more likely to produce clinical response when plasma level is 2–12 ng/ml. Lower levels may be responsible for poor treatment outcome, and higher levels may increase side effects (e.g. akathisia, dysphoria). See **haloperidol plasma levels/clinical efficacy.**

haloperidol + valproate Co-administration may decrease valproate plasma levels and may require quite high valproate doses to obtain therapeutic serum levels (Ishizaki T, Chiba K, Saito M, et al. The effect of neuroleptics [haloperidol and chlorpromazine] on the pharmacokinetics of valproic acid in schizophrenic patients. *J Clin Psychopharmacol* 1984; 4:254–261).

haloperidol + zolpidem Co-administration does not alter the pharmacokinetics of either drug.

Halotestin See **fluoxymesterone.**

handedness Hand dominance for a given task. It should always be qualified by describing for which tasks a person is right- or left-handed.

handicap Disadvantage due to an impairment or disability that limits or prevents fulfillment of a role that is normal (depending on age, sex, and social and cultural factors) for the individual (*International Classification of Impairments, Disabilities and Handicaps*, WHO, 1980).

"hang-up activity"   Street term for compulsive foraging behavior associated with crack cocaine use. The term is being replaced by *chasing ghosts* or *geeking*. See **compulsive foraging behavior.**

hangover   Aftereffect ("morning after") syndrome following ingestion of alcohol or other sedatives (e.g., barbiturates). Symptoms include a bad taste, nausea, vomiting, polypnea, pallor, irritability, sweating, and tremor.

haphazard sample   See **sample, haphazard.**

haploid   Chromosome number of a normal gamete, which contains only one member of each chromosome pair. In humans, the haploid number is 23.

haploidy   Condition of having half the number of chromosomes present in somatic cells.

haplotype   Genetic constitution with respect to one member of a pair of allelic genes; set of genetic markers on *one* chromosome.

"happy dust"   Street name for cocaine.

"hard candy"   Street name for heroin.

"hard drug"   Street name for narcotics (heroin, morphine, opium, oxycodone).

"hard stuff"   Street name for heroin.

"hardware"   Street name for isobutyl nitrite ampules.

Hardy-Weinberg equilibrium   Stabilizing point at which all the factors of the sex ratio are present in a theoretically ideal genotype frequency.

harmaline   Reversible monoamine oxidase inhibitor that binds tightly to the enzyme so that its rate of dissociation from it is slow, resulting in longer duration of inhibitory action than that of simple reversible inhibitors.

harmful use   Pattern substance use already causing damage to health that may be either physical (liver cirrhosis from chronic drinking) or psychiatric (episodes of depression due to heavy drinking). The diagnosis is primarily for drinkers or drug users who have recently begun to experience substance abuse-related problems and for chronic users whose consequences (physical or mental) develop in the absence of marked dependence symptoms. Harmful use and alcohol abuse are distinguished by different diagnostic criteria in ICD-10 and DSM-IV. In ICD-10, harmful alcohol use is diagnosed (a) if there is clear evidence that alcohol use is responsible for causing actual psychological or physical harm to the user; and (b) if the pattern of use has persisted for at least 1 month or has occurred repeatedly over the previous 12 months. In DSM-IV, criteria for alcohol abuse are (a) maladaptive pattern of alcohol use indicated by at least one of the following: (1) continued use despite knowledge of having a persistent or recurrent social, occupational, psychological, or physical problem that is caused or exacerbated by alcohol use; or (2) recurrent use in situations in which alcohol use is physically hazardous (e.g., driving while intoxicated); and (b) some symptoms of the disturbance have persisted for at least 1 month or occurred repeatedly over a longer period.

harmine   Naturally occurring indolealkyamine derivative hallucinogen rarely used in Western societies.

harmonic mean   Measure of central tendency obtained by adding the reciprocals of the values and dividing the sum into the number of values.

Hartnup disease   Pellagra-like disorder caused by a genetic abnormality of tryptophan metabolism. Mental symptoms include anxiety, feelings of depersonalization, depression, delusions, hallucinations, delirium, confusion, irritability, apathy, emotional lability, and, in many cases, mental retardation.

"hash"   Street name for hashish.

hasheesh   See **hashish.**

Hashimoto's thyroiditis   Syndrome of thyroid enlargement without excessive thyroid hormone production. Most common cause worldwide is iodine deficiency. Also called "nontoxic goiter."

hashish   Extremely potent form of cannabis derived mostly from the resin itself.

hashish oil   Concentrated form of the resin of the cannabis plant containing high amounts of delta-9-tetrahydrocannabinol (THC).

"hawk"   Street name for lysergic acid diethylamide (LSD).

"hay"   Street name for marijuana.

hazard function   Probability that a person dies in a certain time interval, given that the person has lived until the beginning of the interval.

headache, cluster   Rare, extremely painful syndrome that affects about 1 in 10,000 people (male/female ratio is 4:1), in striking contrast to migraine, which has a prevalence of about 10%. Onset is typically in middle age. Cluster headaches are almost always nocturnal (9 PM–10 AM; most occur between 4 AM and 10 AM), but may occur during the day; such attacks can be spontaneous or provoked by sleep, or occur 20–30 minutes after drinking alcohol. Pain usually starts unilaterally behind one eye, reaches maximum intensity in 5–10 minutes, and remains excruciating for 45 minutes. The affected eye (the same eye is always involved in one bout) becomes red and waters, the ipsilateral nostril is congested or discharges a clear fluid, and the patient becomes restless (pacing around the room holding the affected site or sitting and rocking). Cluster headaches are extremely refractory to therapy, which accounts for the multiple treatments that are tried for acute attacks and prophylactically. Once an attack has started, ergot, oxygen, and sumatriptan are highly effective. Prophylaxis includes ergotamine, methysergide, pizotifen, prednisolone, calcium channel antagonists, or lithium.

head-banging Behavior of unknown etiology seen in infants and young children that consists of striking the head against a hard surface (e.g., the crib) with a rhythmic and monotonous continuity. It takes place primarily at bedtime, with the infant or child seemingly absorbed in the activity for 30–90 minutes or longer until falling asleep. It typically begins in infancy (ages 6–12 months) and ceases by age 4. Behavior of sufficient severity may meet DSM-IV criteria for stereotypy and habit disorder. It should be distinguished from the headbanging seen in the severely mentally retarded.

head injury Few injuries are as personally devastating or as costly to the medical system as head injuries. Injury to the brain may be accompanied by severe physical problems that require intensive early treatment and extended rehabilitation. Important cognitive sequelae include amnesia, disorientation, and perceptual disorder. The most troublesome long-term morbidity, however, is caused by behavioral and emotional consequences, including sexual disinhibition, aggression, apathy, anxiety, and lability of mood. Patients with these symptoms may be unable to participate in, and are often excluded from, conventional rehabilitation programs (Sumners D, Lewin J. Patients with brain injuries. A national rehabilitation service is needed to lift the burden from carers. *Br Med J* 1993;306:1220–1221).

"head shop" Street term for drug paraphernalia store that masquerades as a tobacco or variety shop and provides, among other things, kits and booklets on how to prepare free-base cocaine.

health maintenance organization (HMO) Organized system of health care that delivers comprehensive treatment services to voluntarily enrolled individuals under a qualified payment plan.

"heart" Street name for amphetamine sulfate.

"heart-on" Street name for volatile nitrites (e.g., amyl nitrite) sold in "head shops," pornography and novelty stores, and through mail order houses.

heat exhaustion Heat-related illness milder than heat stroke characterized by dizziness, weakness, and fatigue. It may develop after several days of high temperatures and inadequate or unbalanced replacement of fluids and electrolytes. It may require hospitaliza-

tion. Patients treated with neuroleptics alone or combined with anticholinergics may be at risk for heat exhaustion. See **heat stroke; hyperthermia.**

heat stroke Serious heat-related illness manifested by hyperpyrexia (body temperature >105° F [40.5° C]), confusion, tachycardia, hyperpnea, and low blood pressure. It is a medical emergency, usually occurring in places with high temperatures and high relative humidity, and among persons who overexert themselves in such environments, either at work or during recreational activities. From 1979 to 1988, 4,523 deaths in the United States were attributed to excessive heat exposure; in 1980, a year with severe heat, 1,700 heat-related deaths were reported (Anon. Heat-related deaths—United Staes 1993. *Morbid Mortal Week Rep* 1993;42:558–560). Although anyone is at risk if sufficiently exposed, those at greatest risk include young children (particularly infants), the elderly, and the immobile, who may be unable to obtain adequate fluids or avoid hot environments (Kilbourne EM, Choi K, Jones TS, Thacker SB, et al. Risk factors for heatstroke: a case-control study. *JAMA* 1982;247:3332–3336). Heatstroke also can be a complication of treatment with neuroleptic and/or anticholinergic drugs; combined use may increase risk, particularly in the elderly. Heatstroke should be considered in the differential diagnosis of neuroleptic malignant syndrome (NMS), since the etiologic agents may be the same. As in NMS, leukocytosis is common, and renal failure is a potential complication. However, unlike NMS, the skin is usually hot and dry, and in most cases sweating is not present. Although neuroleptic drug-related heatstroke and NMS have many clinical similarities and both may be fatal, distinguishing between the two is important. Both require immediate attention, but the treatment strategy in each disorder is different (Addonizio G, Susman VL. *Neuroleptic Malignant Syndrome. A Clinical Approach.* St. Louis: Mosby Year Book, 1991). See **anticholinergic toxicity; hyperthermia; neuroleptic malignant syndrome.**

"heavenly blue" Street term for change in self awareness and visual hallucinations produced by morning glory seeds, which contain a lysergic acid diethylamide [LSD]-related substance. The reaction may be very dangerous; it can produce a lethal, shock-like state. Also called "pearly gates."

hebephrenia Chronic form of schizophrenia, usually starting before age 20, characterized by marked disorders in thinking, shallow and inappropriate affect, and silly behavior and mannerisms, severe emotional disturbance, excitement alternating with tearfulness and depression, vivid hallucinations, and delusions. Delusions are often concerned with ideas of omnipotence, sex change, cosmic identity, and rebirth.

hebetude Emotional dullness or disinterest that is a common symptom of schizophrenia.

Helfergin See **meclofenoxate.**

helix, double See **double helix.**

helper T cell T cell that prompts B cells to form antibodies and that secretes interleukin-2 to facilitate cytotoxic T cell proliferation and activity.

helplessness, learned See **learned helplessness.**

hematocrit Measure of the volume of packed red cells expressed as a percentage of whole blood volume. Normal is 40–54% for men and 38–47% for women. Abnormal hematocrit warrants investigation.

hematoma, epidural Complication of head trauma usually caused by a laceration of the middle meningeal artery after a linear fracture of the temporal bone. The arterial force of the bleeding dissects the dura from the bone. Symptoms include increasingly severe headache, deterioration of consciousness, and pupillary changes. It is less common than subdural hematoma, but it is no less important, because if not recognized and treated properly, it can be responsible for permanent neurological deficits or death.

hematoma, intracerebral Consequence of intracranial hemorrhage in brain tissue damaged by head injury. The hematomas vary in size, number, and location according to where force was delivered. They may occur directly opposite the point of impact.

hematoma, subdural Hemorrhage between the inner table's dural surface and the thin, transparent leptomeninges covering the brain. Although generally of venous origin and frequently associated with contusion of the underlying cortex and white matter, subdural hematomas may also develop gradually and not produce symptoms until weeks after a head injury. They are common in alcoholics and those over age 50 who may have had seemingly trivial, quickly forgotten head injury. As the hematoma enlarges, the patient experiences increasing daily headaches, fluctuating drowsiness or confusion, and mild to moderate hemiparesis. Magnetic resonance imaging or an angiogram can help establish the diagnosis better than computed tomography (CT). Early removal improves chances of survival.

hemiballism Unilateral chorea most apparent in proximal muscles that causes the arm and leg to be thrown wildly in all directions. It is sometimes seen in children and adolescents following discontinuation of long-term neuroleptic therapy. It may be controlled with tetrabenazine or a neuroleptic drug such as haloperidol. Also called "hemichorea." See **ballismus.**

hemichorea See **hemiballism.**

hemidystonia Dystonia involving the same arm and leg and same side of the face.

hemifacial spasm Peripherally induced movement disorder involving muscles on one side of the face innervated by the ipsilateral facial nerve. It is characterized by involuntary, recurrent, episodic, paroxysmal clonic twitches or tonic contractions of the eyelids and perinasal, perioral, zygomatic, and other facial muscles. The condition may be mild and only socially embarrassing, or psychologically distressing. In some patients, it causes unilateral blepharospasm that can interfere with vision. It is now well established that hemifacial spasm is not of psychogenic origin.

Heminevrin See **chlormethiazole.**

hemiplegia Paralysis of one side of the body.

hemizygous Having unpaired genes in an otherwise diploid cell. Since males normally have only one X chromosome, they are hemizygous with respect to X-linked genes.

"hemp" Street name for marijuana.

hepatic clearance Volume of blood from which the liver removes a drug by metabolic transformation in a given unit of time.

hepatic encephalopathy Clinical syndrome characterized by abnormal psychological states and behavior that may occur in patients with severe hepatic insufficiency. It may be acute or chronic. Clinical manifestations range from slightly altered mental state to coma. Associated neuromuscular complications range from incoordination and tremor to ophthalmoplegia and incontinence. Diagnosis is based predominantly on clinical acumen. Detailed observation, psychometric testing, serial electroencephalograph (EEG) recordings, and EEG spectral analysis have been used to differentiate the stages of hepatic encephalopathy due to liver cirrhosis. Accuracy of the various testing methods increases as the severity of the encephalopathy progresses (Parsons-Smith BG, Summerskill WH, Dawson AM, Sherlock S. The EEG in liver disease. *Lancet* 1957;2:867–871; Davis MG, Rowan MJ, Feely J. Psychometrics in assessing hepatic encephalopathy—a brief review. *Ir J Psychol Med* 1991;8:144–146).

hepatic extraction See **first-pass effect.**

hepatic microsomal enzyme/drug competition Drugs that compete for microsomal sites include cimetidine, disulfiram, erythromycin, estrogens, and isoniazid. These drugs tend to promote longer functional half-lives of various drugs and their metabolites, including benzo-diazepines.

hepatic microsomal enzyme induction Acceler-ated metabolism of one drug by another drug that can result in drug interactions. Known hepatic enzyme inducers include alcohol, car-bamazepine, nicotine, phenobarbital, pheny-toin, and rifampin.

hepatic microsomal enzyme inhibition Decline in the metabolism of one drug induced by another. Like hepatic enzyme induction, it is a major cause of drug interactions. Known he-patic enzyme inhibitors include alcohol, al-lopurinol, cimetidine, disulfiram, isoniazid, metronidazole, oral contraceptives, and val-proic acid.

hepatic microsomal enzyme systems Enzyme complex responsible for the biotransforma-tion of the majority of drugs. There are two types of chemical reactions involved in hepatic metabolism: phase I and phase II. Phase I reactions usually change the parent molecule to a more polar metabolite by means of oxi-dation, reduction, or hydrolysis. The metabo-lite may be more or less active than the parent molecule, or inactive. Phase II reactions in-volve "conjugation" (coupling) of the drug or its metabolite with a polar substrate such as glucuronic acid, acetic acid, sulfuric acid, or an amino acid. Phase II reactions almost in-variably result in inactivation of the drug or its metabolite (Benet LZ, Sheiner LB. Pharmaco-kinetics: the dynamics of drug absorption, distribution and elimination. *In* Gilman AG, Goodman LS, Rall TW, Murad F [eds], *Good-man and Gilman's The Pharmacologic Basis of Therapeutics,* 7th ed. New York: Macmillan, 1985, pp 3–34).

hepatic oxidation Type of phase I hepatic metabolism that serves to metabolically inac-tivate many, but not all, drugs. Some of the phase I products (e.g., desmethyldiazepam) are pharmacologically active. Clinical effects of drugs requiring hepatic oxidation (e.g., chlordiazepoxide, chlorpromazine, diazepam, imipramine, phenytoin, prazepam) for elimi-nation are prolonged by liver disease and other medications that compete for hepatic oxidation.

hepatolenticular degeneration See **Wilson's dis-ease.**

hepatotoxin Virus or drug toxic to the liver. Hepatitis B virus, hepatitis A virus, and hepa-titis C, non A + cytomegalovirus are among the viruses that cause viral hepatitis and liver disease. Alcohol is directly hepatotoxic. Co-caine intoxications can cause hepatic necrosis. These hepatotoxins are common causes of liver disease in parenteral drug abusers.

heptylphysostigmine (L-693,487) Potent, selec-tive inhibitor of acetylcholinesterase that has a slower rate of association and dissociation than physostigmine. It has an extended dura-tion of action (pharmacodynamic half-life: 7–9 hours) and good penetration into the central nervous system. It has been tested in young and elderly volunteers and in patients with Alzheimer's disease.

heredity Inheritance by offspring of character-istics from the progenitor. It is a function of genes found in chromosomes in the nucleus of each cell. Chromosomes are made of de-oxyribonucleic acid (DNA), which contains a code determining particular characteristics of an organism. Heredity transmission is re-stricted to the action of the sex cells (sperm and ova), which fuse to form the new organ-ism. .

heredity, polygenic Heredity involving many different genes that are expressed in one phenotype.

heritability 1. Measure of the extent to which a phenotype is influenced by the genotype. 2. Proportion of liability due to additive genetic effects. 3. Measure of the proportion of the genetic component in the overall familial resemblance.

hermaphroditism Presence of both male and female sex organs. In humans, true hermaph-roditism is caused by anomalous differentia-tion of the gonads, with the presence of both ovarian and testicular tissue and ambiguous morphological criteria of sex.

heroin (diacetylmorphine) Potent, fast-acting, commonly abused opioid narcotic that is no more effective than morphine in relieving severe chronic pain. Abusers prefer intrave-nous administration because it rapidly reaches the brain to cause an orgasm-like reaction, mental alertness, and marked euphoria ("rush") followed by a state of tranquility and sleepiness ("the nod"). Most doses sold on the street are less than 25 mg, effects of which last 3–5 hours. Tolerance develops with chronic use. Like all short-acting central ner-vous system drugs, heroin must be taken sev-eral times a day to avert withdrawal symptoms in dependent users. The withdrawal syndrome begins 8–10 hours after the last dose, occur-ring in two phases. The acute phase may last 7–10 days. The secondary phase, character-ized by hypotension, bradycardia, hypother-mia, and mydriasis, lasts 24–30 weeks. Abusers also are at risk for accidental fatal overdose; hepatitis B, human immunodeficiency virus (HIV), and other infections; and acquired immunodeficiency syndrome (AIDS) and other complications from sharing contami-nated needles (e.g., meningitis, abscesses, osteomyelitis). In addition, deaths due to homicide, suicide, and accidents are common among heroin abusers. Heroin use is illegal in the United States.

heroin/acute intoxication Manifestations include euphoria, flushing, itching of the skin, miosis, drowsiness, decreased respiratory rate and depth, hypotension, bradycardia, and lowered body temperature.

heroin/breast milk Heroin enters breast milk and can prolong neonatal narcotic dependence. Heroin-dependent women should not nurse. See **heroin/pregnancy.**

heroin + fentanyl In 1991, a mixture of heroin and fentanyl was sold on the illicit market in New York, resulting in the hospitalization of 200 drug abusers and at least 22 deaths.

heroin, Persian High-purity heroin mixed with cocaine freebase.

heroin/pregnancy Chronic heroin use during pregnancy produces narcotic dependence in the fetus and neonate. Symptoms of narcotic withdrawal occur shortly after birth; severity and frequency are worse in babies whose mothers injected, rather than inhaled, heroin. Convulsions occur during neonatal heroin withdrawal, especially in newborns of mothers receiving methadone substitution therapy. Retarded growth also is associated with prenatal heroin exposure.

heroin/street names A-bomb, big H, body bag, boy, brown, brown sugar, China white, crap, deek, dirt, garbage, girls and boys (with cocaine), H, H and H (with hashish), H and stuff, hard candy, hard drug, hard stuff, horse, joy powder, junk, Mexican brown, Mexican tar, Persian heroin (with cocaine freebase), pineapple (with methylphenidate), skag, scat, shit, smack, speedball (with cocaine), tango and cash (adulterated heroin), TNT, tombstone, tootsie roll, white horse, whiz bang.

heroin + sulpiride Co-treatment may cause an acute dystonic reaction secondary to sulpiride (DeMaio D, Caponeri MA, Cicchetti V, et al. Sulpiride and extrapyramidal syndromes in chronic heroin addiction. *Neuropsychobiology* 1978;4:36–39).

heroin withdrawal Symptoms are similar to an influenza-like syndrome, along with anxiety and dysphoria. Physical manifestations include yawning, sweating, rhinorrhea, lacrimation, pupillary dilatation, piloerection, hypertension, tachycardia, restlessness, waves of gooseflesh, twitching, hyperactive bowel sounds, deep muscle and joint pain, nausea, diarrhea, vomiting, insomnia, abdominal pain, fever and hot and cold flashes, and, rarely, convulsions. These withdrawal symptoms occur within 48 hours after heroin discontinuation. Not all heroin users show the withdrawal

syndrome upon cessation of heroin. Oxytocin may be effective in the treatment of heroin withdrawal (Hruby VJ, Chow MS. Conformational and structural considerations in oxytocin-receptor binding and biological activity. *Annu Rev Pharmacol Toxicol* 1990;30:501–534).

herpes simplex Virus that causes a variety of illnesses in humans, most commonly reactivation of latent oral-labial herpes infections in about 40% of the population. Lithium carbonate may have anti–herpes simplex virus activity.

hertz (Hz) Unit of frequency (cycles per second).

heteroceptor Presynaptic receptor activated by a modulating agent that originates from a different neuron or cell. See **autoreceptor.**

heterochromatin Chromosomal material with different staining properties that shows maximal condensation in interphase nuclei. It can be divided into facultative and constitutive heterochromatins. Facultative heterochromatins contain inactivated structural genes due to developmental process (e.g., one of the X chromosomes in female somatic cells). Constitutive heterochromatin is permanent and is present in all human chromosomes with quantitative differences.

heterocyclic Chemical structure with a ring in which there is an atom different from carbon.

heterocyclic antidepressant See **antidepressant, heterocyclic.**

heterodimer Protein made up of two different polypeptides. See **homodimer.**

heterogeneity In genetics, a single phenotype being caused by any one of several genes.

heterologous desensitization See **desensitization.**

heteroplasm Cell containing two or more mitochondrial DNAs that could differ by a single nucleotide insertion, deletion, or rearrangement.

heterosexuality Sexual desire directed toward persons of the opposite sex.

heterozygousness Genetic condition of an organism whose two genes of a given factor pair are different. Having different allelic genes at one or more paired loci in homologous chromosomes.

heterozygousness, double Having both dominant and recessive alleles for two linked genes.

heuristic That which encourages discovery of solutions to problems.

heuristic paradigm Promising model or prototype for problem solving.

high expressed emotion See **expressed emotion.**

high-fiber diet/tricyclic antidepressant See **tricyclic antidepressant/high fiber diet.**

high-performance liquid chromatography (HPLC) Form of chromatography in which mobile solvent travels through a column packed with nonpolar beads while being measured at the opposite end. The substance is detected by spectrophotometer, by fluorometer, or electrochemically. It is usually less sensitive than gas liquid chromatography (GLC), but sample preparation is easier. Commercial HPLC instruments were introduced between 1970 and 1975. Since then, use has increased such that instruments are now commonplace in most neuroscience research laboratories. Since HPLC is a separation technique, it remains dependent on specific detectors with adequate sensitivity to detect very low levels of such substances as neuropeptides, catecholamines, and serotonin. The advantage of HPLC is that a single assay system can be used to measure at the same time the parent drug and active metabolites. The chief disadvantage is the need for a skilled operator and dedicated equipment.

high-potency neuroleptic See **neuroleptic, high-potency.**

high-risk situation In relapse prevention theory, set of circumstances that threaten the individual's sense of self-control and thus increase the risk of relapse.

highly protein bound See **protein, highly bound.**

hippocampus Region of the temporal lobe that is thought to play a role in learning and memory.

histamine Putative neurotransmitter in the brain where, as histamine does elsewhere in the body, it has at least two types of receptors, histamine H_1 and histamine H_2. A third histamine receptor (H_3) in the brain affects presynaptic synthesis and release of histamine, as well as other neurotransmitters.

histamine H_1 receptor H_1 receptors are involved with allergic reactions. In the brain, they may affect arousal and appetite regulation. Neuroleptics have an affinity for brain H_1 receptors; over half are more potent than the classic H_1 antagonist diphenhydramine. All tricyclic antidepressants (TCAs) are H_1 blockers, which accounts for their sedating and weight-gaining effects. Doxepin is the most antihistaminic TCA; desipramine and protriptyline are the least antihistaminic.

histamine H_2 receptor Outside the nervous system, H_2 receptors are involved with gastric acid secretion. Some tricyclic antidepressants (e.g., doxepin, trimipramine) are H_2 blockers and are probably as potent as cimetidine in the treatment of peptic ulcer disease. They also may exert their therapeutic effect in peptic ulcer disease by reducing rapid eye movement (REM) sleep, since REM sleep is associated with gastric acid production (Richelson E. Treatment of peptic ulcer with tricyclic antidepressants. *Int Drug Ther Newsl* 1985; 20:21–23; Ries R, Gilberg D, Katon W. Tricyclic antidepressant therapy for peptic ulcer disease. *Arch Intern Med* 1984;144:566–569).

Histerone See **testosterone aqueous.**

histogram Frequency distribution of a variable in the form of a bar graph. Bars are drawn so that their bases lie on a linear scale representing different intervals and their heights are proportional to the frequencies of the values in each interval.

histone Any of a family of basic proteins that bind to DNA in a way that does not depend on sequence. There are five major types of histone chains (H1, H2A, H2B, H3, and H4). Almost 150,000 activatable genes are scattered among the DNA around the histones. The amino acid sequences of the histone subfamilies have been remarkably conserved throughout evolution.

historical cohort study See **study, historical cohort.**

historical control See **control, historical.**

HMPAO-SPECT Technique for determining cerebral blood flow using the radiopharmaceutical technetium labeled HMPAO as tracer with single photon emission computed tomography (SPECT). Uptake of the tracer into the brain occurs rapidly, whereas the back diffusion is comparatively slow. Thus, a frozen picture of blood flow distribution can be obtained even several hours after the injection.

Hoffman reflex (H reflex) Electrically evoked spinal monosynaptic muscle action elicited by stimulation of sensory fibers that can be recorded electromyographically. Abnormalities have been observed in Parkinson's disease and schizophrenia.

"hog" Street name for phencyclidine (PCP).

homeobox A protein-coding sequence of 180 base pairs found in a wide variety of genes spanning a broad evolutionary spectrum from yeast to man. It is an essential element of many DNA binding proteins that most likely act as transcription factors. It was first identified as a region of homology common to several homeotic genes and to the segmentation gene *fushi tarazu* of Drosophila. Since then, it has been found in many of the genes that commit cells to follow specific pathways of development in the early embryo.

homeostasis Tendency to stability of the normal body states (internal environment) of the organism. It is achieved by a system of control mechanisms activated by negative feedback.

homicide/suicide cluster   One or more homicides with the subsequent suicide of the perpetrator. It primarily involves family members or intimates. The typical perpetrator is a man, married or living with a woman in a relationship marked by physical abuse, who has a history of alcohol and substance abuse and access to firearms. Perpetrators may be depressed and have personality disorders. Women who are ending relationships appear to be at increased risk for becoming victims. Incidence data are limited because many law enforcement agencies do not compile statistics; in the United States there are no national incidence figures.

homodimer   Protein made up of two identical polypeptides. See **heterodimer.**

homogamy   Trait similarity between husband and wife. It tends to be the rule for many demographic and personality characteristics.

homogeneity   Situation in which the standard deviation of the dependent (Y) variable is the same regardless of the value of the independent (X) variable. It is an assumption in analysis of variance and regression analysis.

homolog   One version (derived from either mother or father) of a pair of chromosomes.

homologous chromosomes   Chromosomes that pair during meiosis, have essentially the same morphology, and contain genes governing the same characteristics.

homologous desensitization   See **desensitization.**

homologous recombination   See **recombination, homologous.**

homoplasty   Cell that contains only one type of mitochondrial DNA.

homosexuality   Sexual attraction toward those of the same sex.

homovanillic acid   (HVA) Major metabolite of dopamine (DA). It is removed quickly from the brain and cerebrospinal fluid into the bloodstream and excreted primarily in urine. In plasma, it originates mainly from peripheral noradrenergic (NA) neurons and central DA neurons. Debrisoquine, a monoamine oxidase inhibitor that does not cross the blood-brain barrier, has been used to suppress the peripheral contributions of HVA to plasma and thereby enhance the degree to which plasma HVA can reflect central DA neuronal activity. In both rodents and humans, pharmacologically induced changes in brain DA activity are mirrored by parallel changes in plasma HVA (pHVA) concentrations. Thus, measurements of pHVA may be an indirect, yet practical and accessible tool to assess changes in DA turnover during administration of neuroleptic drugs in schizophrenic patients. Recent studies have shown that mean pHVA concen-trations decrease in a group of patients responsive to neuroleptic therapy, but do not change in those who do not improve. Thus, there may be a qualitative distinction between the responders and nonresponders to DA antagonists. Some studies report a positive correlation between pHVA and psychotic symptoms; others do not. After neuroleptic treatment, pHVA has been reported to correlate positively with tardive dyskinesia.

homozygous   Having genetically identical alleles at a locus on both chromosomes.

Horizon   See **diazepam.**

hormesis   Process whereby small doses of an otherwise harmful agent can result in stimulatory or beneficial effects.

hormone   Chemical substance produced by one organ and transported by the blood to another organ where it stimulates or inhibits its function by binding to cellular receptors.

hormone, adrenocortical   See **adrenocorticotropic hormone.**

hormone, adrenocorticotropic   See **adrenocorticotropic hormone.**

hormone, corticotropic   See **adrenocorticotropic hormone.**

"horse"   Street name for heroin.

hostility   Verbal and nonverbal expressions of anger and resentment, including sarcasm, passive-aggressive behavior, verbal abuse, and assaultiveness. Extreme hostility is manifested by marked anger, extreme uncooperativeness that precludes other interactions, or episodes of physical assault toward others.

"hot"   Street name for phencyclidine (PCP).

housebound   In panic disorder, refusal to leave home to avoid sparking a panic attack. It often occurs in patients who experience onset of severe panic attacks in their 20s and are told after a thorough medical evaluation that nothing is wrong with them and that their symptoms were due to stress. As a consequence, they erroneously conclude they have a medical disorder that is unrecognizable and/or untreatable. The more severe the panic disorder, the more likely is the person to stay home; some may remain housebound for 20+ years or until their panic disorder is treated effectively.

H reflex   See **Hoffman reflex.**

5-HT   See **serotonin.**

5-HT receptor   See **serotonin receptor.**

"huffing"   Street term for a method of using solvents or other inhalants that involves placing in the mouth a rag soaked with the volatile substance and then inhaling the fumes. Huffers are usually adolescents who may be violent and/or psychotic. They are also likely to be multiple substance abusers.

human gene therapy   See **gene therapy.**

human genome   See **genome.**

Human Genome Initiative   Collective name for several projects begun in 1986 to (a) create an ordered set of DNA segments from known chromosomal locations; (b) develop new computational methods for analyzing genetic map and DNA sequence data; and (c) develop new techniques and instruments for detecting and analyzing DNA.

human genome mapping   See **genome map.**

Human Genome Project   International research effort begun in 1986 to produce biological maps of human chromosomes and determine the complete sequence of human DNA. The project, which could take up to 15 years to complete, is expected to yield knowledge that will help scientists understand and eventually treat some of the more than 4,000 genetic diseases.

human granulocyte colony-stimulating factor (G-CSF; Neupogen) Hematopoietic glycoprotein that promotes proliferation of neutrophils. It is indicated for treating chemotherapy-induced neutropenia (Gabrilove JL, Jakubowski A, Scher H, et al. Effect of granulocyte colony-stimulating factor on neutropenia and associated morbidity due to chemotherapy for transitional cell carcinoma of the urothelium. *N Engl J Med* 1988;318:1414–1422; Crawford J, Ozer H, Stoller R, et al. Reduction by granulocyte colony-stimulating factor of fever and neutropenia induced by chemotherapy in patients with small-cell lung cancer. *N Engl J Med* 1991;325:164–170). It also has been used in the treatment of agranulocytosis associated with clozapine and clomipramine (Geiby CG, Marks L. Treatment of antipsychotic drug-induced agranulocytosis with human granulocyte colony-stimulating factor. Presented at ASHP Midyear Clinical Meeting, Orlando, December 1992; Hunt KA, Resnick MP. Clomipramine-induced agranulocytosis and its treatment with G-CSF. *Am J Psychiatry* 1993;150:522–523). Because of its substantial cost, it is reserved for severe neutropenia. Recommended starting dose is 5 µg/kg/day. Therapeutic response begins by the fifth day. G-CSF is continued until absolute neutrophil count remains above 500 cells/mm^3 for 48 hours and signs of infection have waned.

human growth hormone   (HGH) See **growth hormone.**

human immunodeficiency virus   (HIV) Retrovirus originally called human T-cell lymphotrophic virus type III (HTLV-III) and lymphadenopathy-associated virus (LAV). Current name (human immunodeficiency virus [HIV]) has been in use since 1986 by agreement of viral taxonomists and acquired immunodeficiency syndrome [AIDS] investigators. HIV is transmitted by sexual and parenteral contact. It causes a variety of psychiatric manifestations ranging from stress reactions associated with knowledge of having the infection to cognitive impairment to frank dementia seemingly caused by the encephalopathy common in HIV infection of the brain. It also may cause various (principally organic) psychoses.

human leucocyte antigens   (HLA) Polypeptide chains on the surface of all nucleated cells whose expression is controlled by the individual's HLA genotype. Each person has a total of eight alleles at these loci, allowing considerable polymorphism. There are five components of the human major histocompatibility complex: A, B, C, D, and DR. The molecules are potent histocompatibility antigens and can function as targets for both alloantibody and alloreactive cytotoxic T cells. There are various possible mechanisms for HLA disease associations; one is alteration or modification of HLA antigens as a result of an infectious drug or environmental agent (Pfister GM, Hanson DR, Roerig JL, et al. Clozapine-induced agranulocytosis in a Native American: HLA typing and further support for an immune-mediated mechanism. *J Clin Psychiatry* 1992;53:242–244). Several diseases occur preferentially in subjects with certain HLA genotypes (e.g., narcolepsy, in which most subjects are HLA-DR2 positive).

human lymphotropic virus—type I   (HLTV-I) Retrovirus, less infectious than human immunodeficiency virus (HIV), that has been linked with adult T-cell leukemia and myelopathy. It is rare in the United States, but endemic in parts of Japan. HTLV-I is spread via breast milk, sexual transmission (male to female), infected blood, and contaminated needles. Infection usually leads to a very slow, progressive course, although it may take a rapid, fulminant course. See **human lymphotropic virus—type I myelopathy.**

human lymphotropic virus—type I myelopathy   Chronic, adult-onset viral disorder caused by the retrovirus HLTV-I. It primarily affects women. Somatic manifestations include weakness of lower limbs, bladder and bowel disturbances, decreased libido, sensory symptoms (e.g., burning, tingling), low lumbar pain radiating to legs, arthropathy, uveitis, and optic atrophy. Deafness, cognitive impairment, and convulsions also may occur (rarely). There is no definitive treatment, but corticosteroids are palliative in about 50% of cases (Pies R. Clinical puzzles in medical psychiatry, #102. *The Psychiatric Times* 1992;10:13).

human pedigree analysis   Study of inherited disease in humans by observing the pattern of distribution in kindreds.

Humoryl   See **toloxatone**.

Huntington's disease   (HD) Relatively rare involuntary movement disorder characterized by progressive chorea and dementia and frequently complicated by major affective disorder (most commonly depression). It is transmitted by an autosomal dominant gene that lies close to the tip of the short arm of chromosome 4. HD pathology seems to be in the caudate nucleus, with symptoms due to excessive dopamine activity. There is also clinical and endocrinological evidence of abnormalities in limbic-hypothalamic brain structures. HD may occur at any age, but onset is usually between 30 and 50. Abnormal movements are indistinguishable from those induced by neuroleptics or L-dopa. Chorea and dementia may present simultaneously, or one may precede the other. In some cases, diagnosis is difficult to impossible, particularly at the extremes of life, because chorea may be absent, dementia mild, and family history negative. Juvenile cases (JHD) classically present before age 20 with akinesia, rigidity, and dystonia inherited from an affected father. In late-onset cases, there may be a very benign course and a history of elderly forebears who died before signs of the disease were recognized. HD follows a slow, progressive, downhill course and is usually fatal within 15 years. The brain becomes atrophic, especially the caudate and frontal lobes. Associated biochemical changes include gamma-aminobutyric acid (GABA) deficiency and reduction of glutamic acid decarboxylase, the enzyme that synthesizes GABA. In addition to movement disorder, Huntington's disease is almost invariably accompanied by a wide variety of psychiatric and behavioral problems. The only major palliative treatment is with neuroleptics (e.g., haloperidol); dopaminergic and anticholinergic drugs make symptoms worse (Harper HS [ed]. *Major Problems in Neurology 22. Huntington's Disease.* Philadelphia: WB Saunders, 1991; Caine ED, Shoulson I. Psychiatric syndromes in Huntington's disease. *Am J Psychiatry* 1983;140:728–733). Irritability and aggression are especially problematic. Most aggressive episodes are triggered by minor frustrations that would be disregarded by most individuals. In some patients, minor frustrations evoke fearfulness and desperation rather than aggression. Either behavior may respond favorably and quickly (within 1 week) to propranolol titrated to 120 mg/day (Stewart JR. Huntington's disease and propranolol. *Am J Psychiatry* 1993;150:166–167). Two cases of obsessive-compulsive disorder in HD patients have been reported (Cummings JL, Cummingham K. Obsessive-compulsive disorder in Hunting-ton's disease. *Biol Psychiatry* 1992;31:263–270). Also called "chronic progressive chorea."

Huntington's disease (HD)/tardive dyskinesia (TD)   Differentiating TD from HD is difficult because of the broad overlap in symptoms. Typical HD motor abnormalities consist of random choreic movements flowing from one part of the body to the other, which the person may attempt to mask by superimposing pseudopurposeful movements. The slow, repetitive choreic movements (most often in the oral region) characteristic of TD are infrequent in HD and usually appear only in the later stages. In addition, gait abnormalities (ataxia) are more frequent with HD. Characteristics favoring a diagnosis of HD include (a) positive family history of HD; (b) development of dementia; (c) progressive downhill course; and (d) progressive atrophy of the nucleus caudatus (Haag H, Ruther E, Hippius. H. *Tardive Dyskinesia.* Seattle: Hogrefe & Huber, 1992, pp 31–32).

Hybolin Decanoate   See **nandrolone decanoate**.

Hybolin Improved   See **nandrolone phenpropionate**.

hybrid   Inbred offspring of parents who differ with respect to one or more gene factors or who belong to different species.

hybridization   Formation of a double-stranded structure (DNA-DNA, DNA-RNA) by hydrogen-bonding complementary single-stranded molecules or parts of molecules.

hybridization histochemistry   Branch of histology that identifies chemical components in cells and tissues. Within molecular genetics, identification procedures involve creation of RNA-DNA hybrids by annealing a radioactively labeled RNA fraction with denatured DNA, so that the RNA becomes associated with the complementary DNA.

hybridization, in situ   Method by which RNA hybridization patterns are visualized in slices of tissue. In general, radiolabeled cDNA or RNA is incubated with a slice of tissue under conditions that favor formation of hybrid molecules between the labeled probe and RNA that has been fixed in the tissue slice. The method allows detection of RNA molecules that are endogenous to the cell types under investigation.

hybridization probe   Piece of DNA radiolabeled to allow detection of homologous DNA in a mixture.

hybridoma   Result of the fusion of two cell types using polyethylene glycol (antifreeze). The hybridoma makes antibodies to a single shape or region of a particular molecule and will live forever in culture if treated correctly. Antibodies capable of binding to a chemical or drug (e.g., cocaine) and destroying it have been isolated from hybridomas. The antibodies could be useful in treating cocaine and other addictions; a vaccine conceivably could be developed that would destroy cocaine before it reaches the brain, thereby preventing the dopamine "rush" that makes it so addictive.

hydantoin Any of a group of anticonvulsants that includes the prototype phenytoin, ethotoin, mephenytoin, and phenacemide. They are used primarily to control generalized tonic-clonic and partial seizures. Ethotoin is less toxic than phenytoin, but also less effective. It and mephenytoin are indicated for partial seizures refractory to less toxic agents. Phenacemide, which is quite toxic, is used for refractory seizures.

Hydergine See **dihydroergotoxine.**

Hydramine See **diphenhydramine.**

Hydril See **diphenhydramine.**

hydrocephalus Increased cerebrospinal fluid (CSF) volume within the skull. If CSF pressure is normal, the condition is called "compensatory hydrocephalus."

hydrocephalus, normal pressure Syndrome consisting of mild dementia, apraxia of gait, urinary incontinence, and enlarged ventricles in the presence of normal cerebrospinal fluid pressure. Some patients benefit remarkably from ventricle shunting.

hydrochlorothiazide (Aldoril) Thiazide diuretic and antihypertensive drug. Pregnancy risk category B.

hydrochlorothiazide + lithium See **lithium + diuretic.**

hydrochlorothiazide + methyldopa Combination product containing the antihypertensive methyldopa and the diuretic hydrochlorothiazide that is marketed for the treatment of hypertension. Concurrent use with alcohol, barbiturates, narcotics, analgesics, and other antihypertensive drugs increases risk of orthostatic hypotension. It should not be co-administered with lithium because it can decrease lithium clearance and cause lithium toxicity.

hydrodipsomania Episodic attacks of uncontrollable thirst that often occur in epilepsy.

hydromorphone (Dilaudid) Narcotic analgesic available in ampules, vials, and suppositories marketed for the treatment of moderate to severe pain. Adverse central nervous system effects include sedation, drowsiness, confusion, lethargy, cognitive impairment, fear, dysphoria, and mood changes. Tolerance and psychic and physical dependence may develop with prolonged use. Schedule II; and pregnancy risk category C.

hydromorphone + anticholinergic Co-administration may produce additive peripheral and central anticholinergic toxic effects. See **anticholinergic toxicity.**

hydromorphone + anxiolytic Co-administration increases central nervous system depression. Doses of one or both drugs should be reduced if used concomitantly or in close succession.

hydromorphone + monoamine oxidase inhibitor (MAOI) Therapeutic doses of hydromorphone can cause severe and possibly fatal reactions if given during MAOI administration or within 2 weeks of MAOI discontinuation.

Hydroxacen See **hydroxyzine.**

hydroxybupropion Principal active metabolite of bupropion. Concentrations exceeding 1250 mg/ml are associated with poor therapeutic response to bupropion.

4-hydroxybutyrate See **gamma hydroxybutyrate.**

hydroxyethylflurazepam Metabolite of flurazepam.

7-hydroxyfluphenazine (7OHFLU) Metabolite of fluphenazine.

hydroxyhaloperidol See **reduced haloperidol.**

2-hydroxyimipramine (2-OHIMI) Primary hydroxylated metabolite of imipramine. Animal data indicate that it may have cardiotoxic effects.

5-hydroxyindoleacetic acid (5-HIAA) Biogenic amine found in the brain and other organs that is a major metabolite of serotonin (5-HT). Functional 5-HT deficits in the central nervous system have been implicated in certain types of mood disorders. There is a suspected correlation between low cerebrospinal fluid 5-HIAA levels and violent suicidal and homicidal behavior.

hydroxynefazodone Primary metabolite of nefazodone produced through hydroxylation and dealkylation. Its pharmacological profile is similar to that of nefazodone and may contribute to therapeutic efficacy. Like the parent, it has similar affinities for serotonin $(5\text{-}HT)_2$ binding and 5-HT uptake sites, and its pharmacokinetics are nonlinear. See **nefazodone.**

hydroxynortriptyline (E-10-OHNT) Biologically active metabolite of nortriptyline (NOR) that is about half as potent as NOR in inhibiting noradrenergic uptake. It may be an effective antidepressant. It impairs cardiac conduction, and high plasma concentrations may be inversely correlated with clinical improvement (Young RC, Alexopoulos GS, Shindlevecker R, et al. Plasma 10-hydroxynortriptyline and therapeutic response in geriatric depression. *Neuropsychopharmacology* 1988;1:213–215). See **Z-10-hydroxynortriptyline.**

9-hydroxyrisperidone (9-OH risperidone) Major metabolite of risperidone formed by the hepatic cytochrome P450 isoenzyme. Its pharmacological profile and potency are similar to those of risperidone, but it is less active. In rapid acetylators, large amounts of the metabolite are formed; in slow acetylators, the parent drug undergoes only minor metabolism to 9-OH risperidone, and therefore its half-life is much longer.

hydroxytamoxifen Estrogen antagonist with mixed agonist/antagonist actions that differ from one tissue to another.

4-hydroxytriazolam One of two major metabolites of triazolam. It is rapidly glucuronated and excreted in the urine.

5-hydroxytryptamine See **serotonin.**

5-hydroxytryptophan (5-HTP) Immediate precursor of serotonin (5-HT), to which it is converted by tryptophane hydroxylase, the rate-limiting enzyme for the production of 5-HT. 5-HTP crosses the blood-brain barrier and increases central 5-HT availability after oral administration. It has been used to investigate the role of 5-HT in several neuropsychiatric disorders (e.g., depression, myoclonic epilepsy, Lesch-Nyhan syndrome, schizophrenia) and Down syndrome.

hydroxyzine (Anxanil; Atarax; Atozine; E-Vista; Hydroxacen; Hyzine-50; Multipax; Otarex; Quiess; Vistacon; Vistaject; Vistaquel; Vistaril; Vistazine) Antihistamine sedative/anxiolytic unrelated to benzodiazepine (BZD) and other non-BZD anxiolytics. It is used for symptomatic relief of anxiety and tension in nonpsychotic patients and as sedation prior to general anesthesia. It may potentiate meperidine and barbiturates, but does not produce dependence. Pregnancy risk category C.

hydroxyzine + anticholinergic Co-administration may produce severe anticholinergic symptoms or intoxication.

hydroxyzine/breast milk It is not known if hydroxyzine is excreted in human milk. For more data, consult the manufacturer.

hydroxyzine + meperidine Hydroxyzine potentiates meperidine analgesia and sedation without additional respiratory depression. It may be an advantageous addition to opioid therapy (Zsigmond EK, Flynn K, Shively JG. Effect of hydroxyzine and meperidine on arterial blood gases in healthy human volunteers. *J Clin Pharmacol* 1989;29:85–90; Maurer PM, Bartkowski RR. Drug interactions of clinical significance with opioid analgesics. *Drug Safety* 1993;8:30–48).

hydroxyzine + morphine Hydroxyzine potentiates morphine analgesia and sedation without additional respiratory depression. It may be an advantageous addition to opioid therapy (Zsigmond EK, Flynn K, Shively JG. Effect of hydroxyzine and meperidine on arterial blood gases in healthy human volunteers. *J Clin Pharmacol* 1989;29:85–90; Maurer PM, Bartkowski RR. Drug interactions of clinical significance with opioid analgesics. *Drug Safety* 1993;8:30–48).

hydroxyzine + pethidine See **hydroxyzine + meperidine.**

"hype" Street term for a substance abuser who injects drugs hypodermically.

hyperactivity 1. Increased speed of motor responses and heightened frequency and tempo of movements and speech. 2. Excessive activity in a child. Incidence depends on the way it is defined and the enthusiasm with which it is sought. The term may be used to mean physically "on the move" a great deal of the time. It also may refer to a group of symptoms (e.g., distractibility, short attention span, disturbed sleep, excitability, tantrums, low frustration tolerance) sometimes called "hyperkinetic syndrome." See **attention deficit disorder; attention-deficit hyperactivity disorder.**

hyperactive symptoms Hypervigilence, restlessness, fast or loud speech, irritability, combativeness, impatience, swearing, singing, laughing, uncooperativeness, euphoria, anger, wandering, easy startling, fast motor responses, distractibility, tangentiality, nightmares, persistent thoughts. They are often seen in mania and delirium.

hyperacusis Abnormally acute sense of hearing that may result in some sounds (especially loud noises) being experienced as painful or unpleasant. It is a frequent symptom of sedative/hypnotic (especially benzodiazepine) withdrawal. It also may occur in panic disorder.

hyperaesthesia See **compulsive sexual behavior.**

hypercapnia Elevated blood carbon dioxide level.

hypercortisolism Elevated 24-hour urinary free cortisol and dexamethasone nonsuppression. It is a normal occurrence in late pregnancy. It occurs in up to 50% of patients with Alzheimer's disease, but the exact site of dysregulation in hypothalamic-pituitary-adrenocorticotropic axis functioning is unknown. It is also a frequent neuroendocrine manifestation of endogenous depression (Sapolsky RM, Pltosky PM. Hypercortisolism and its possible neural bases. *Biol Psychiatry* 1990;27:937–952).

hypereroticism See **compulsive sexual behavior.**

hyperfrontality Increased blood flow in the medial-frontal cortex associated with heightened glucose uptake, obsessive-compulsive pathology, and other conditions. See **hypofrontality.**

hypergraphia Excessive and/or compulsive writing (notes, letters, diaries, novels, poems, hymns, autobiographies) that may occur in patients with temporal lobe epilepsy, mania, or schizophrenia. The writings are often characterized by verbosity, circumstantiality, meticulous attention to detail, and frequent religious and metaphysical allusions. They also incorporate idiosyncratic stylistic devices for emphasis (e.g., parentheses, underlining, different colored inks) (Bear D, Freeman R, Greenberg M. Behavioral alterations in patients with temporal lobe epilepsy. *In* Blumer D [ed], *Psychiatric Aspects of Epilepsy*. Washington, DC: American Psychiatric Press, 1984).

hyperhidrosis   Excessive or profuse sweating. It can be classified as thermal or emotional. Thermal perspiration is most evident on the forehead, neck, trunk, and dorsum of the hands and forearms; it may be a manifestation of a drug-induced disorder (e.g., neuroleptic malignant syndrome). Emotional perspiration is primarily on the palms, soles, and axillae; it is induced by anxiety, fear, rage, and tension. Cold, clammy hands, which are common in anxiety disorders, can be a useful sign in distinguishing an anxiety state from hyperthyroidism, in which the hands are also moist, but warm. Emotional sweating can be measured by the galvanic skin response. Persistent emotional hyperhidrosis may be responsible for a number of dermatological conditions.

hyperkalemia   Excessive blood potassium (serum K >7.5 mEq/L) that is occasionally manifested by generalized muscular weakness or by flaccid paralysis. It is usually asymptomatic until cardiac toxicity begins.

hyperkinesia   Excessive muscular movements.

hyperkinesia, axial   Symptom of tardive dyskinesia that consists of thrusting pelvic movements. Also called truncal dyskinesia.

hyperkinesis   See **attention-deficit hyperactivity disorder** (current designation).

hyperkinetic   Characterized by increased movements or activity.

hyperkinetic syndrome   See **attention-deficit hyperactivity disorder** (current designation).

hyperlibido   See **compulsive sexual behavior.**

hypermetamorphosis   Hypervigilance with short attention span.

hyperosmia   Hyperacute sense of smell that may be the result of exposure to toxic vapors (e.g., toluene). It can be very unpleasant and persistent. It can profoundly influence daily life; the person may avoid all external contact because of inability to tolerate odors from shops, markets, or food prepared by others. Cooking and cleaning may become impossible because of the hyperosmic effect of foods, household cleansers, and detergents. Because of its severity and apparent lack of causality, hyperosmia can be a prominent factor in the initiation of a depressive state.

hyperphagia   Excessive eating that is often compulsive.

hyperphilia   See **compulsive sexual behavior.**

hyperprolactinemia   Elevated plasma prolactin levels. Although normal during pregnancy and lactation, it is pathological otherwise. It results in infertility, galactorrhea, and amenorrhea. In men, impotence and azoospermia with or without lactation and gynecomastia may occur. Causes include pituitary adenoma and certain drugs (e.g., methadone, methyldopa, metoclopramide, morphine, reserpine, verapamil). Antipsychotic drugs have a marked effect on prolactin concentrations because of their dopamine receptor blocking activity at lactotrophs. Prolactin is routinely elevated in patients receiving therapeutic doses of neuroleptics, but the exact incidence of antipsychotic hyperprolactinemia and accompanying complications is unknown (Desai AG, Interzo C, Bark C, Green P. Drug induced gallium uptake in the breasts. *Clin Nucl Med* 1986;12:703–704). Severe symptoms of hyperprolactinemia should be treated first by reducing dosage of the responsible neuroleptic. Prolactin concentrations drop 2–4 days after neuroleptic discontinuation, but breast symptoms may take 3 or more weeks to resolve. The dopamine agonists bromocriptine and amantadine have been used successfully to treat galactorrhea, amenorrhea, and impotence, but they must be used judiciously to reduce the risk of side effects, especially adverse psychiatric reactions. Hyperprolactinemia also has been associated with antidepressants (amoxapine, imipramine, maprotiline, and fluoxetine). Antidepressant-induced amenorrhea, galactorrhea, and gynecomastia, which are uncommon, can be treated by reducing the dose or discontinuing the offending drug. There are conflicting data on a possible link between hyperprolactemia and depression. Men with hyperprolactinemia have a high incidence of sexual problems (loss of libido, erectile dysfunction, and ejaculatory failure occur in 50–90%).

hyperpyrexia   Extremely high fever. Core temperature above 40.6° C (105° F) may cause cardiac arrhythmias and seizures. Psychiatric drugs that may impair central thermal regulation and cause hyperpyrexia include tricyclic antidepressants (TCAs), monoamine oxidase inhibitors, and lithium. Treatment should be symptomatic (use of antipyretics such as aspirin, cooling blankets, alcohol sponging, or ice water enemas). Physostigmine (1–4 mg) administered intramuscularly or intravenously is a specific antidote for hyperpyrexia due to a TCA or an anticholinergic. See **hyperthermia.**

hypersensitivity reaction   Criteria include (a) reaction in a small proportion of exposed individuals; (b) latent period between exposure and reaction; (c) occurrence with relatively small doses; and (d) association with other known hypersensitivity phenomena (e.g., eosinophilia) (Terr AI. *Allergic disease. In* Stites DP, et al [eds], *Basic Clinical Immunology*. Los Altos: Lange Medical Publications, 1982).

hyperserotonemia   Unusually large quantity of serotonin (5-HT) in the circulating blood, commonly caused by the carcinoid syndrome. It may be manifested by nausea, vomiting, and colicky abdominal pain (5-HT, acting as a peripheral transmitter in the intestines and a central transmitter in the brain, is important to regulation of peristalsis and intestinal tone).

hypersexuality   See **compulsive sexual behavior.**

hypersomnia   Excessive sleepiness, especially during the day. It may be a symptom of depression or due to obstructive sleep apnea. It usually has a physical, not psychological, basis. Hypersomnia due to obstructive sleep apnea may respond to weight loss; avoidance of alcohol, sedatives, and hypnotics; avoidance of the supine sleeping position; and management of nasal and nasopharyngeal disease. Sedative medications administered at night may worsen sleep apnea and daytime hypersomnia. See **narcolepsy.**

Hyperstat   See **diazoxide.**

hypertensive crisis   Sudden, marked increase in blood pressure, especially systolic, in a patient on an monoamine oxidase inhibitor who ingests a tyramine-containing substance or sympathomimetic drug. The hypertension is a result of tyramine interaction, following which there may be rapid release of norepinephrine from adrenergic neurons. Manifestations are clinically similar to those seen in pheochromocytoma. Headache, often throbbing and excruciating, is a common symptom; it may or may not be associated with fever. Whenever a patient has symptoms that suggest hypertensive crisis, blood pressure should be checked immediately and phentolamine (2–5 mg) should promptly be administered intravenously to lower risk of cerebrovascular bleeding. Other immediate treatments include intravenously administered nitroprusside. Hypertensive crisis may result in intracerebral or subarachnoid hemorrhage, especially in patients with an underlying aneurysm.

hypertensive encephalopathy   See **encephalopathy, hypertensive.**

hyperthermia   Core temperature greater than 40.6° C (105° F) and anhidrosis. See **heat stroke; neuroleptic malignant syndrome.**

hyperthermia, malignant   See **malignant hyperthermia.**

hyperthermia, mild   Core temperature of 37.7–38.3° C (100–101° F).

hyperthermia, moderate   Core temperature of 39.3–40° C (101–104° F).

hyperthermia, severe   Core temperature greater than 40° C (104° F).

hyperthermic catatonia   See **catatonia, lethal.**

hyperthymia   State of overactivity less than that seen in the manic phase of manic-depressive illness, but more than average. It is a subdivision of cyclothymia probably very close to hypomania.

hyperthyroidism   Laboratory tests showing (a) raised free tri-iodothyronine (fT_3) or free thyroxine (fT_4) and suppressed thyroid-stimulating hormone (TSH); or (b) raised fT_3 and fT_4 and normal TSH. It may be manifested by a variety of psychiatric symptoms ranging from anxiety to acute delirium. Typical clinical features are anxiety and emotional over-reactivity; agitated depression, impaired cognitive function, and manic or schizophrenic-like symptoms also may occur.

hypertonia   Spasticity; having a greater degree of tension in the muscles than usual.

hyperventilation   (HV) Respiration that is excessive with respect to metabolic needs. It changes the acid-base balance in the blood by producing a fall in hydrogen ion concentrations, causing a state of respiratory alkalosis. Lowered carbon dioxide level (hypocapnia) results in vasoconstriction and, combined with alkalosis (which decreases oxygen reuptake by hemoglobin), cerebral hypoxia, symptoms of which are dizziness, faintness, and visual disturbances. Because the most obvious respiratory symptoms (dyspnea, breathlessness, and smothering sensations) also are among the most common symptoms of panic attacks, the role of hyperventilation in the etiology and treatment of panic attacks has attracted attention. Hyperventilation may also occur in anxiety attacks and is probably the most common but least recognized anxiety reaction. It may progress to tetany. Acute recurrent hypocalcemia with its neurological and psychiatric symptoms is the result, not the cause, of the hyperventilation syndrome. Drugs offer little benefit. Beta-blockers can attenuate sympathetically mediated symptoms (palpitations, tremor) but are of uncertain value. They can precipitate asthma, which in some patients is related to the hyperventilation syndrome. Benzodiazepines may reduce subjective complaints, but lasting effects have not been shown, and long-term use risks dependency. Tricyclic antidepressants and monoamine oxidase inhibitors may be useful in patients with panic attacks and multiple autonomic symptoms (Anon. Hyperventilation syndrome—not to be dismissed. *Drug Therapeutics Bull* 1991;29:83–84).

hyperventilation challenge   Test that can be used to identify a subgroup of patients for whom hyperventilation symptoms are frequently associated with panic.

hypervigilance   Excessive attention and focus on all internal and external stimuli. See **compulsive sexual behavior.**

hypnagogic   Relating to the state, or imagery that occurs during the state, between wakefulness and sleep. Hallucinations (voices speaking nonsense phrases, lights or visions, peculiar smells) may occur, but are not considered evidence of impending psychosis, although they may be associated with narcolepsy.

hypnagogic hallucination   See **hallucination, hypnagogic.**

hypnagogic imagery   Imagery occurring just before sleep onset.

hypnagogue   That which induces sleep, such as a hypnotic drug.

Hypnodorm   See **flunitrazepam.**

hypnopolygraph   See **polysomnograph.**

hypnopompic   Relating to the state, or imagery that occurs during the state, between sleep and wakefulness.

hypnopompic hallucination   See **hallucination, hypnopompic.**

hypnotic   Substance that induces drowsiness and the onset and maintenance of sleep that as far as possible resembles the natural sleep state. Although sleep induction can be produced with most sedative drugs by increasing the dosage, sedatives are not hypnotics in the true sense of the word.

hypnotic + alcohol   Co-administration of alcohol and all types of hypnotics may result in potentiation of sedative effects and decrements in performance. Patients should be cautioned to abstain from alcohol while taking a hypnotic.

hypnotic, benzodiazepine, long-acting   Compounds with elimination half-lives of more than 15 hours (e.g., flurazepam, nitrazepam). They tend to have residual and cumulative effects that may be profound and persistent, ranging in severity from psychomotor slowing and impaired judgment to excessive daytime sedation and confusional states.

hypnotic, benzodiazepine, short-acting   Compounds with elimination half-lives of less than 15 hours (e.g., temazepam). They are less likely to be associated with profound performance decrements in the elderly, particularly because residual effects are mitigated by the development of tolerance through repeated use.

hypnotic, benzodiazepine, very short-acting   Compounds with elimination half-lives of less than 6 hours, (e.g., triazolam). They may increase levels of daytime anxiety. Compared to placebo, triazolam is associated with a higher incidence of daytime anxiety, panic symptoms, depression, and in some cases, feelings of paranoia and unreality.

hypnotic jerk   See **body jerk.**

hypnotic + neuroleptic   Regular use of hypnotics that induce hepatic drug metabolizing enzymes may lower neuroleptic blood levels.

hypnotic, nonbarbiturate   See **hypnotic, nonbenzodiazepine.**

hypnotic, nonbenzodiazepine   Compounds from a variety of pharmacological classes, including barbiturates, ethchlorvynol, ethinamate, methaqualone, piperidinediones (chloral hydrate, glutethimide, methyprylon), and the cyclopyrrolone derivative zopiclone. They are quite toxic in acute overdose and when combined with alcohol. Each is associated with some degree of abuse potential. All except ethchlorvynol tend to stimulate hepatic microsomal oxidizing systems, thereby reducing the plasma levels of both inducer and any other concurrently administered drugs metabolized by the liver.

hypnotic/repeat-dose study   Investigation of the rate and extent of cumulative effects, tolerance, persistence ("carryover") effects, and rebound effects after rapid and/or gradual discontinuation.

hypnotic/single-dose study   Investigation of the time of onset, intensity, and duration of clinical action of a hypnotic.

Hypnovel   See **midazolam.**

hypoactive symptoms   Unawareness, decreased alertness, sparse or slow speech, lethargy, slow movements, staring, and apathy. They can be a manifestation of delirium, especially in the elderly.

hypocapnia   Lowered carbon dioxide level. It can be caused by hyperventilation and may cause vasoconstriction.

hypochondriasis   Learned behavior, reinforced by continued medical investigation, in which the person focuses unduly on a particular physical symptom or set of symptoms. DSM-IV criteria are (a) preoccupation with fear of having or belief that one has a serious illness, based on the interpretation of physical signs or sensations, as evidence of physical illness; (b) appropriate physical evaluation does not support the diagnosis of any physical disorder that can account for the physical signs or sensations or the person's unwarranted interpretation of them, and the symptoms are not just those of panic attacks; (c) fear of having or the belief that one has a disease that persists despite medical reassurance; (d) duration of the disturbance is at least 6 months; (e) belief in the symptoms is not of delusional intensity, as in somatic type delusional disorder (i.e., the person can acknowledge the possibility that the fear of having or the belief that he or she has a serious disease is unfounded).

hypofrontality Hypofunction of the prefrontal cortex. It is determined by measuring regional cerebral blood flow or metabolism using positron emission tomography (PET) while the subject performs various cognitive tasks such as the Wisconsin Card Sorting Test. It has been demonstrated in both medicated and nonmedicated schizophrenic patients; long-term neuroleptic treatment is not a major factor in prefrontal dysfunction in schizophrenia (Berman KF, Torrey EF, Daniel DG, Weinberger DR. Regional cerebral blood flow in monozygotic twins discordant and concordant for schizophrenia. *Arch Gen Psychiatry* 1992;49:927–934). Although the pathophysiologic importance of hypofrontality is unknown, it may be causally related to negative symptoms, neither of which is unique to schizophrenia. Hypofrontality has been reported in several PET studies of depression. Similarly, certain negative symptoms are also salient features of depression and may complicate the differential diagnosis. This raises the possibility of a common mechanism between hypofrontality and negative symptoms that is not disease-specific (Wolkin A, Sanfilipo M, Wolf AP, et al. Negative symptoms and hypofrontality in chronic schizophrenia. *Arch Gen Psychiatry* 1992;49:959–965). See **hyperfrontality.**

hypoglycemia Blood glucose level below 60 mg. It is most often induced by inappropriate doses of insulin or oral hypoglycemic agents. Onset is generally gradual, the skin is cool and moist with perspiration, and blood pressure is usually normal or slightly elevated because of the catecholamine (epinephrine-norepinephrine) response to hypoglycemia. Patients may appear to have an anxiety or depressive disorder, with symptoms including nervousness, tremor, agitation, confusion, sweating, headache, nausea and vomiting, dizziness, muscular weakness, and hunger. Hypoglycemia directly lowers the threshold for impulsive violent behavior. It may result in coma or precomatose states. It is usually counteracted by oral glucose or an ampule of 50% glucose administered by intravenous push.

hypokalemia Blood potassium (K) level of 2.0 mEq/L or less, manifested by generalized muscular weakness and at times by a confusional state. Each can be readily corrected by adding 40 mEq of K to each liter of intravenous fluid at a rate of 100 ml/hour.

hypokinesis Slow or diminished movement that may be physically or psychologically determined. It may be a symptom of depression or Parkinson's disease, or it may be drug-induced.

hypomania Milder form of mania with many of the characteristics of mania, but of lesser intensity. The patient may appear very confident, talkative, and unusually productive. Symptoms are often ego syntonic.

hypomimia Diminished facial expression with decreased rate of blinking and akinesia of the face. It is frequently seen in a wide spectrum of psychiatric and Parkinson8s disease–type disorders.

hyponatremia Common electrolyte abnormality in which serum sodium level is below 130 mEq/L. It may occur during the course of a variety of medical and psychiatric illnesses, and may be iatrogenic or noniatrogenic. It often occurs in schizophrenia and among those who smoke and/or have a history of alcohol misuse. Symptoms may include headache, lethargy, ataxia, and hypertension. In the vast majority of cases, hyponatremia is mild (serum sodium level above 120 mEq/L) and asymptomatic, and generally does not require aggressive treatment. Patients with serum sodium levels ranging from 125 to 132 mEq/L may exhibit depressed facies, emotional lability, weeping, anorexia, insomnia, and social withdrawal. It is important to distinguish between true depression and pseudo-depression in patients with hyponatremia, because in the latter, treatment with antidepressants has been associated with little reduction in depressive symptoms, worsening hyponatremia, and possible onset of neurological symptoms (MacMillan HL, Gibson JC, Steiner M. Hyponatremia and depression. *J Nerv Ment Dis* 1990;178:720–722). Severe symptomatic hyponatremia (serum sodium level less than 110 mEq/L) requires prompt correction to avert respiratory arrest with hypoxia, permanent neurological damage, or death (mortality rates are 33–86%). For severe hyponatremia, slow correction has been advocated to avoid central pontine myelinolysis (CPM). There is widespread agreement that serum sodium should be increased slowly by administration of hypertonic saline, probably by no more than 0.5 mmol/L/hour (Laureno R, Karp BI. Pontine and extrapontine myelinolysis following rapid correction of hyponatraemia. *Lancet* 1988;1:1439–1441). Severe, rapidly developed hyponatremia may lead to serious complications, including seizures, coma, and respiratory arrest; chronic hyponatremia does not generally result in brain damage. The danger of CPM with rapid treatment is greater when hyponatremia lasts longer, because of the slow osmotic adjustment of brain cells (Lundbom N, Laurila O. Central pontine myelinolysis after correction of chronic hyponatremia. *Lancet* 1993;342: 247–248).

hyponatremia/drug-induced   Drugs that increase pituitary antidiuretic hormone secretion, resulting in impaired water excretion and subsequent hyponatremia, include: acetaminophen, atypical antipsychotics (clozapine), barbiturates, carbamazepine, fluoxetine, lofepramine, monoamine oxidase inhibitors (phenelzine), narcotics, neuroleptics (fluphenazine, haloperidol, thioridazine, thiothixene, trifluoperazine), oxytocin, trazodone, tricyclic antidepressants (amitriptyline, clomipramine, desipramine), vasopressin, and vincristine.

hypophonic dysarthria   See **dysarthria, hypophonic.**

hypophrenia   See **mental retardation.**

hypophysectomy   Surgical removal of the pituitary gland.

hypophysis   See **pituitary gland.**

hypoplasia   Underdevelopment of tissue or an organ, often due to a decrease in the number of cells. It may refer to suppression of all bone marrow function. See **bone marrow.**

hypopnea   Episode of shallow breathing during sleep lasting 10 seconds or longer. It is usually associated with a fall in blood oxygen saturation value. Hypopnea technically may be defined as a decrease in airflow on thermistor channels to one-third of baseline, accompanied by decreased arterial oxygen saturation and decreased respiratory effort (Mendelson WB. *Human Sleep. Research and Clinical Care.* New York: Plenum Medical, 1987).

hypoprothrombinemia   Abnormally small amounts of prothrombin in the circulation. It can be due to liver disease, vitamin K deficiency and, infrequently, protein-binding displacement of warfarin by chloral hydrate or other chloral derivatives.

hyposomnia   Significant decrease in sleep, ranging from sleep lasting only a few hours per night to total insomnia for 24–48 hours. It is a well known feature of mania and may be a symptom of stimulant abuse.

hyposthenuria   Inability to form urine of high specific gravity.

hypotension, drug-induced   Common risk from low-potency antipsychotic and some antidepressant agents. If it occurs, patients should be kept in a supine or reverse Trendelenburg position and given intravenous fluids for hypovolemia. Only alpha-adrenergic drugs (e.g., metaraminol) should be administered.

hypotension, postural   Drop in blood pressure on changing position (rising, standing too rapidly). It may be responsible for fainting, falling, and injury. It is often induced by drugs that block alpha$_1$-adrenergic receptors (e.g., chlorpromazine, thioridazine). Initial treatment should be conservative (changing positions slowly, support hose, dosage reduction). If these measures are insufficient, more aggressive pharmacological intervention (e.g., fludrocortisone) may be warranted. See **fludrocortisone.**

hypothalamotomy   Psychosurgical procedure that produces partial ablation of the hypothalamic area. Technique is the same as in thalamotomy. It is performed after thalamotomy in patients not benefitted by the latter.

hypothalamus   Area of the diencephalon located beneath the thalamus. It comprises several nuclei wherein hormones, including oxytocin and antidiuretic hormone, are synthesized and carried via blood vessels to the pituitary. It is involved in regulating peripheral autonomic nervous system activity, some emotions, and the release of pituitary hormones. The hypothalamus seems to be the center of coordination of autonomic, endocrine, and behavioral aspects of affect and emotion.

hypothermia   Drop in core body temperature to 35° C (95° F) or less. It can be a side effect of some drugs (e.g., phenothiazines) and is more likely to occur in older patients with hypothyroidism. Treatment is symptomatic (topical or core-rewarming). All intravenous fluids, including blood, should be at room temperature before infusion is begun. See **hypothermia, drug-induced.**

hypothermia, drug-induced   Loss of thermoregulatory ability that occurs most often in elderly people being treated with phenothiazines or heterocyclic antidepressants, especially if they are malnourished and drink alcohol. Exposure to the cold in such patients may cause hypothermia, requiring prompt treatment to avert physical deterioration or death.

hypothermia, mild   Core temperature of 33–35° C (91.4–95° F).

hypothermia, moderate   Core temperature of 30–33° C (86–91.4° F).

hypothermia, severe   Core temperature below 30° C (86° F).

hypothesis   Supposition that appears to explain a group of phenomena and is assumed as a basis of reasoning and experimentation.

hypothesis, alternative   Opposite of the null hypothesis; hypothesis that is accepted if the null hypothesis is rejected.

hypothesis, falsifiable   Hypothesis stated in sufficiently precise fashion that it can be confirmed or disproved by acceptable rules of logic and empirical and statistical evidence. An unfalsifiable hypothesis is so general and/or ambiguous that all conceivable evidence can be "explained" by it.

hypothesis-generating study   Research intended to screen for previously unknown or unsuspected effects, whether adverse or beneficial. It is designed to elicit new questions (hypotheses) to be explored further in subsequent studies.

hypothesis, null   See **null hypothesis.**

hypothesis-strengthening study   Research designed to provide sufficient support for, or evidence against, an existing hypothesis to determine whether a subsequent, more definitive study should be undertaken.

hypothesis testing   Statistical technique used to determined P values. It consists of the following steps: (a) choose a test statistic; (b) choose the significance level (alpha) of the test; (c) compute the P value; and (d) if the P value is smaller than alpha, reject the null hypothesis in favor of the alternative hypothesis or hypotheses; otherwise, accept the null hypothesis. When the significance level is set at 0.05, hypothesis testing leads to rejecting the null hypothesis if the P value is less than 0.05 (Bailar JC III, Mosteller F [eds], *Medical Uses of Statistics*, 2nd ed. Boston: NEJM Books, 1992). See **P value.**

hypothesis-testing study   Investigation to evaluate in detail hypotheses raised elsewhere. It must have simultaneous comparison groups and be able to control for most known potential confounding variables.

hypothyroidism   Decrease or total absence of thyroid hormone secretion in an adult. Clinical signs and symptoms include weakness; lethargy; fatigue; memory impairment; cold intolerance; weight gain; constipation; coarse, thin hair and/or hair loss; hoarseness; deafness; dyspnea; myalgia; arthralgia; parathesia; precordial pain; menstrual irregularity; dry, coarse skin; periorbital and peripheral edema; pallor of skin; thick tongue; slow speech; decreased reflexes; hypertension; bradycardia; pleural and/or pericardial effusions; ascites; and vitiligo. Depression and/or paranoid ideas also may occur. In a middle-aged or older patient who seeks psychiatric treatment for depression, the presence of skin problems (dryness, roughness), bloating, high cholesterol, and hoarseness suggests hypothyroidism, particularly if the patient complains of feeling cold all the time, even when it is warm. Hypothyroid-associated depression usually is refractory to antidepressants and other psychotropic drugs. Appropriate endocrine therapy usually produces dramatic improvement in symptoms, including mental status.

hypothyroidism/juvenile   Spectrum of clinical presentation depends on the degree, severity, and age at onset. Myxedematous skin changes, constipation, sleepiness, and mental decline may be manifested at any age. Juvenile forms are associated with growth retardation and delayed puberty; bone age is delayed relative to chronological age. The later in life hypothyroidism occurs, the lesser the impairment of growth and development. Thyroid deficiency in a previously euthyroid child may manifest when demands on the thyroid are increased by rapid growth of the body. Hypothyroidism, and any or all of its etiologic causes, should be considered if cessation or retardation of growth occurs in a child whose growth previously had been normal.

hypothyroidism, subclinical   (SCH) Elevated basal or thyrotropin-releasing hormone stimulated by thyroid-stimulating hormone (TSH) in the presence of normal thyroid hormone concentrations. Antithyroid hormones are often present and allow the definition to be expanded to include individuals at risk for SCH. It is usually of insidious onset and affects at least 5% of the population. It is manifested by motor retardation and lethargy, with many signs and symptoms of depression. Hypothyroidism can mimic psychotic depression, paranoid schizophrenia, and manic depressive disorder. Because it is common in the elderly, they should be screened for evidence of it. Elevated TSH value usually accompanies symptoms such as psychomotor retardation, apathy, tiredness, forgetfulness, weight gain, hair loss, or increased sensitivity to cold. Lithium can cause hypothyroidism in some patients.

hypotonia   Flaccidity or reduced tension in the muscles.

hypoxia   Decreased oxygen level in inspired gases, arterial blood, or tissue.

hysteresis   Retardation of effects when forces acting upon a body are changed (as if from viscosity or internal friction). Because drugs are not instantaneously distributed into the brain, concentrations at the site of action may lag behind the plasma concentration. When plotted, a clockwise hysteresis loop is seen when at point B concentration increases, although responses begin to decline. A counterclockwise hysteresis loop is formed when plasma concentration begins to decrease at point A, although response intensity is still increasing.

hysteria   Implies laying claim to, or making an avowal of, bodily dysfunction for which the typical causes are not apparent, and in a manner that parodies the source of distress produced by organ pathology. Hysteria should not be confused with malingering.

hysterical dementia   See **pseudodementia.**

hysterical neuroses of the dissociative type   See **dissociative disorder.**

hysterical polydipsia   See **polydipsia, psychogenic.**

hysterical seizure   See **pseudoseizure.**

hysterical tremor   See **tremor, hysterical.**

hysteroid dysphoria   Subtype of atypical depression manifested by repeated depressive crashes in the face of interpersonal (particularly romantic) rejection, coupled with a constant need for approval and admiration from others to maintain feelings of normal mood and self-esteem. It occurs more often in women. Diagnostic criteria include normal state that is at least one of the following: histrionic, flamboyant, intrusive, seductive, self-centered, demanding, or greatly concerned with appearance. When depressed, patients usually overeat, oversleep, and feel extremely fatigued, yet maintain reactivity of mood. Many abuse alcohol episodically when depressed; some make suicide gestures or threats. The disorder may respond well to monoamine oxidase inhibitors (Liebowitz MR, Klein DF. Hysteroid dysphoria. *Psychiatr Clin North Am* 1979;2:555).

Hyzine-50   See **hydroxyzine.**

I

iatrogenic Producing any adverse condition as a result of any aspect of medical treatment, including hospital care. Overtreatment, complications of treatment, and unwise use of drugs are all responsible for iatrogenic illness. Inappropriate pharmacological management of serious illnesses and medication prescribing errors have been identified consistently as important causes of morbidity and mortality in hospitalized patients.

ibogaine Psychedelic derived from the root of the African plant *Tapernanthe iboga* that may be useful in the management of heroin and cocaine (COC) addiction. In morphine-dependent rats, it significantly reduces naloxone-precipitated withdrawal symptoms; in nonaddicted rats with free access to morphine, it reduces morphine intake. It also decreases dopamine increase secondary to COC administration and COC-induced hyperactivity in rats. In humans, it causes nausea and psychedelic effects, but no serious adverse reactions. Ibogaine is being used to treat addiction in the Netherlands and is being evaluated in the United States by the National Institute of Drug Abuse (NIDA).

ibuprofen (Motrin; Advil; Nuprin) Nonsteroidal anti-inflammatory agent that inhibits prostaglandin biosynthesis and has analgesic properties. Since 1984, it has been available in the United States as a nonprescription medication.

ibuprofen + lithium See **lithium + ibuprofen.**

ibuprofen + moclobemide See **moclobemide + ibuprofen.**

"ice" Street term for one of the latest illicit drugs, a smokable methamphetamine similar to crack that delivers a high concentration to the brain in a shorter time than either snorting or injection does. In contrast to crack, its effects last hours instead of minutes, making it particularly attractive to those seeking prolonged periods of energized activity. It is often smoked in "runs" (periods of continuous use) averaging 3–8 days, with 1–2 days between smoking periods spent sleeping. Marijuana and alcohol are often used to "come down" off an "ice" high. Side effects range from mild anxiety to acute hypertensive crisis. Among its more serious physical complications are increased body temperature; irreversible cardiomyopathy; pulmonary edema; and diffuse vasospasm that may result in acute myocardial infarction, cardiogenic shock, and even death. Psychiatric complications, including psychosis, occur frequently. Although smoking "ice" reduces the risk of acquired immunodeficiency syndrome (AIDS) by eliminating the use of needles, it may affect the user's judgment regarding safe sex, thus promoting potential transmission of the human immunodeficiency virus (HIV). Other problems associated with "ice" include increased violence and motor vehicle accidents.

ictal Relating to or caused by a stroke or seizure.

ictal delirium Delirium occurring as a manifestation of complex partial status epilepticus.

ictal emotions Suddenly occurring and quickly disappearing emotional reactions, especially anxiety and depression, that are most frequently associated with a seizure of temporal lobe origin.

id In psychoanalysis, one of three components of the psychic apparatus. It is in the unconscious, unorganized, the reservoir of psychic energy, and under the influence of the other two components, the ego and superego.

idazoxan Novel, experimental antidepressant that acts as a selective alpha$_2$ adrenoceptor antagonist and also blocks serotonin (5-HT)$_2$ and histamine H$_1$ receptors. In healthy volunteers, 20-mg, 40-mg, and 80-mg doses significantly increased systolic and diastolic blood pressure and produced a consistent, significant increase in plasma free 3-methoxy-4-hydroxyphenylglycol (MHPG), demonstrating that idazoxan increases norepinephrine (NE) turnover. Preliminary studies indicate that it may be an effective, sustained antidepressant for bipolar depression unresponsive to standard treatments (Osman OT, Rudorfer MV, Potter WZ. Idazoxan: a selective alpha2-antagonist and effective sustained antidepressant in two bipolar depressed patients. *Arch Gen Psychiatry* 1989;46:958–959). Long-term administration elevates NE levels in cerebrospinal fluid, plasma, and urine, accompanied by marked improvement in depressive symptoms and functioning. It has a low profile of adverse effects.

idazoxan + fluphenazine In a placebo-controlled, double-blind trial, idazoxan added to chronic fluphenazine in 12 patients with schizophrenia significantly decreased global psychosis (p < 0.03); Brief Psychiatric Rating Scale (BPRS) total symptoms (p < 0.04); and specific BPRS-positive symptoms such as suspiciousness/paranoia (p < 0.003), unusual thought (p > 0.04), and negative symptoms (p < 0.06). Improvement did not appear to be related to idazoxan-induced changes in fluphenazine plasma levels or effects on extrapyramidal symptoms (Litman RE, Hong WW, Weissman EM, et al. Idazoxan, an alpha$_2$ antagonist, augments fluphenazine in schizophrenic patients: a pilot study. *J Clin Psychopharmacol* 1993;13:264–267).

idea of reference   Idea, held less firmly than a delusion, that events, objects, or other people in the person's immediate environment have a particular and unusual meaning specifically for him or her (DSM-IV).

ideal psychotropic drug   See **psychotropic drug, ideal.**

idealization   Mechanism in which the person attributes exaggeratedly positive qualities to self or others (DSM-IV).

ideational viscosity   See **viscosity, ideational.**

identification   In group therapy, sense of psychic continuity with another group member or the therapist (Bloch S, Crouch E. Therapeutic factors in group psychotherapy. Oxford: Oxford University Press, 1985).

identity   Sense of the self that provides a unity of personality over time. Prominent disturbances in identity seen in schizophrenia, borderline personality disorder, and identity disorder (DSM-IV).

idiocy   Obsolete term for mental retardation characterized by an intelligence quotient (IQ) lower than 25.

idiogram   Diagrammatic representation of a karyotype.

idiographic measure   Measurements in the behavioral sciences and psychiatry that have no external standard; conclusions based on the magnitude of the score are invalid, but are useful as indications of direction of change. See **nomothetic measure.**

idiopathic   Disorder of unknown origin or cause.

idiopathic parkinsonism   See **parkinsonism, idiopathic.**

idiopathic recurring stupor   (IRS) Syndrome of spontaneous stupor or coma not associated with known metabolic, toxic, or structural abnormalities (Tinuper P, Montagna P, Coretlli P, et al. Idiopathic recurring stupor. A case with possible involvement of the GABAergic system. *Ann Neurol* 1992;31:503–506). A unique characteristic of all patients with IRS is rapid reversal of encephalopathy by administration of the benzodiazepine (BZD) antagonist flumazenil, which suggests that the syndrome could be caused by excess amounts of an endogenous ligand that binds to the BZD recognition site on the gamma aminobutyric acid (GABA)$_A$ receptor and has actions like those of diazepam. Endozepine-4 may contribute to or cause IRS (Rothstein JD, Guidotti A, Tinuper P, et al. Endogenous benzodiazepine

receptor ligands in idiopathic recurring stupor. *Lancet* 1992;340:1002–1004). See **endozepine.**

idiosyncrasy   See **adverse drug reaction, idiosyncratic.**

idiosyncratic drug reaction   See **adverse drug reaction, idiosyncratic.**

idiosyncratic intoxication   See **intoxication, idiosyncratic.**

Idom   See **dothiepin.**

illness behavior   Conduct or behavior in response to abnormal body signals from an illness.

illogical thinking   Thinking that contains obvious internal contradictions or in which clearly erroneous conclusions are reached, given the initial premises (DSM-IV). It may be seen in people without mental disorder, particularly in situations in which they are distracted or fatigued. It has psychopathological significance only when it is marked and not due to cultural or religious values or to an intellectual deficit. Markedly illogical thinking may lead to, or result from, a delusional belief, or it may be observed in the absence of a delusion.

illusion   Perceptual distortion of a genuine stimulus. Visual and auditory forms are the most common, but like hallucinations, illusions may involve any of the senses.

illusionogen   See **hallucinogen.**

illusionogenic   See **hallucinogen.**

imagery   Mental images used in a variety of therapeutic techniques, including behavioral conditioning and relaxation.

imagery, hypnagogic   See **hypnagogic imagery.**

imaginal flooding   See **implosive therapy.**

imaging   Making visible things hidden from or not directly perceptible to the senses. New imaging technologies not only bring into view a hidden organ, but make visible the chemical, metabolic, and physiological processes that differ so widely across its complex structure. Imaging can provide regional neuroanatomical measurement and regional functional assessment as subtyping variables. See **magnetic resonance imaging; positron emission tomography; regional cerebral blood flow; single photon emission computed tomography.**

imaging, functional   Any of the imaging techniques that allow visualization of the living brain, including (a) positron emission tomography; (b) regional cerebral blood flow; and (c) single photon emission computed tomography.

imaging, structural   Any of the imaging techniques that allow visualization of the structure of the living brain, including (a) computed tomography; and (b) magnetic resonance imaging.

Imap   See **fluspirilene.**

imazenil   Flumazenil analogue that, labeled with iodine-123, can be used to investigate benzodiazepine receptors in depression and anxiety as measured by single photon emission computed tomography.

imidazopyridine   Novel class of anxiolytic that, like benzodiazepines, bind to sites associated with the gamma aminobutyric acid (GABA) receptor complex.

Imigran   See **sumatriptan.**

imipramine   (Apo-Imipramine; Impril; Janimine; Novopramine; Presamine; Primonil; SK-Pramine; Tofranil) (IMI) Prototype tricyclic antidepressant (TCA) that is effective in the treatment of a variety of depressive disorders, panic disorders, and nocturnal enuresis in children. IMI is metabolized by cytochrome P450IID6. It takes 2–4 weeks for its antidepressant effects to become apparent. IMI should not be used for children under 6 years of age or when there is heart or liver disease. Elderly people are particularly likely to experience adverse reactions, especially anticholinergic effects and/or agitation, confusion, and hypotension. Risk of toxic effects (e.g., cardiovascular toxicity, psychotic agitation, confusion) increases at doses of 300+ mg/day. Rarely reported side effects include epileptic seizures, liver function impairment, and bone marrow depression. IMI should be withdrawn gradually to avoid cholinergic rebound. Of all the TCAs, IMI has the most quinidine-like antiarrhythmic effect, which may be an advantage in treating depressed cardiac patients, especially those with tachyarrhythmias; it is a problem, however, in the presence of A-V block, left ventricular conduction defects, or left ventricular myocardiopathies. Pregnancy risk category D.

imipramine + alcohol   Plasma concentrations of imipramine (IMI) and 2-hydroxylated IMI (2-OHIMI) are decreased, clearance is increased, and elimination half-life is unchanged in recently abstinent alcoholics. In recently abstinent alcoholics who smoke, elimination half-life is decreased and clearance is increased compared to smoking volunteers.

imipramine + alprazolam   Co-administration decreases imipramine (IMI) clearance, with continued therapeutic improvement and reduction in IMI effects after alprazolam is added (Wells BG, Evans RL, Ereshefsky L, et al. Clinical outcome and adverse effect profile associated with concurrent administration of alprazolam and imipramine. *J Clin Psychiatry* 1988;49:394–399).

imipramine + bromocriptine   Co-administration has been used effectively to augment antidepressant response to imipramine. Side effects may include nausea, dizziness, and headache (Waerens J, Gerlach J. Bromocriptine and imipramine in endogenous depression. A double-blind controlled trial in outpatients. *J Affect Disord* 1981;3:193–202).

imipramine + carbamazepine   Co-administration significantly lowers desipramine (imipramine's metabolite) mean plasma levels and summed imipramine and desipramine plasma levels. This is attributed to CBZ induction of hepatic hydroxylase enzymes (Brown CS, Wells BG, Cold JA. Possible influence of carbamazepine on plasma imipramine concentrations in children with attention deficit hyperactivity disorder. *J Clin Psychopharmacol* 1990; 10:359–362).

imipramine/children   Children can be safely treated with imipramine (IMI) if total plasma concentrations (IMI and desipramine) are in the range of 125–225 ng/ml (Naylor MW, Alessi NE. Imipramine side effects in children with disruptive behavior disorders and depressive disorders. *Biol Psychiatry* 1989;25:125a). About 75% of children treated with therapeutic doses have at least one side effect, the most common of which are cardiovascular, including lightheadedness and arrhythmia/tachycardia (20%). Autonomic side effects occur in almost 50% of treated children; most common are dry mouth (30%) and constipation (12%). About 50% have a neuropsychiatric side effect, including irritability and sedation. In up to 20%, side effects may be severe enough to warrant IMI discontinuation; however, in an otherwise responsive child, dosage reduction may lessen or abolish unwanted (especially cardiovascular) side effects, particularly if the plasma level of IMI and desipramine exceeds 225 ng/ml.

imipramine + cimetidine   Co-administration decreases N-desmethylation, resulting in reduced clearance and increased serum imipramine concentration (Henauer SA, Hollister LE. Cimetidine interaction with imipramine and nortriptyline. *Clin Pharmacol Ther* 1984;35:183–187).

imipramine + cyproheptadine   Cyproheptadine has been used successfully to treat imipramine-induced anorgasmia (Steele TE, Howell EF. Cyproheptadine for imipramine-induced anorgasmia. *J Clin Psychopharmacol* 1986;6:326–327).

imipramine + desmopressin   Co-administration for enuresis in a 10-year-old boy resulted in a hyponatremic convulsion (generalized tonic seizure) lasting 10 minutes; it was terminated by rectally administered diazepam (5 mg)

(Hamed M, Mitchell H, Clow DJ. Hyponatraemic convulsion associated with desmopressin and imipramine treatment. *Br Med J* 1993;306:1169).

imipramine + fluoxetine Elevated imipramine serum levels were reported in a patient 3 days after fluoxetine discontinuation (Hahn SM, Griffin JH. Comment: fluoxetine adverse effects and drug interactions. *Ann Pharmacother* 1991;25:1273–1274).

imipramine + fluvoxamine Co-administration markedly enhances imipramine (IMI) plasma level through inhibition of demethylation by fluvoxamine (FVX), possibly resulting in toxicity manifested by severe anticholinergic effect, tremor, and confusion. IMI also increases FVX plasma level. Serum level monitoring is indicated during co-administration (Spina E, Campo GM, Avenoso A, et al. Interaction between fluvoxamine and imipramine/desipramine in four patients. *Ther Drug Monit* 1992;42:194–196).

imipramine + guanfacine Co-administration can result in clinically significant loss of blood pressure control in hypertensive patients. When imipramine is discontinued, blood pressure may return to its former levels within 2 weeks.

imipramine + labetalol In adults taking labetalol (200 mg/day), a single dose of imipramine (IMI) (100 mg) resulted in decreased hydroxylation of IMI and its metabolite desipramine (DMI), higher plasma levels, and increased half-life of IMI and DMI. Inhibition of mephenytoin oxygenase decreases the demethylation rate of IMI to DMI, leading to an increased IMI/DMI ratio. This change is reflected in serum levels (Hermann DJ, Krol TF, Dukes GE, et al. Comparison of verapamil, diltiazem and labetalol on the bioavailability and metabolism of imipramine. *J Clin Pharmacol* 1992;32:176–183).

imipramine + lithium Lithium has been used to augment the antidepressant activity of imipramine and its antiobsessional effects in obsessive-compulsive disorder.

imipramine + methylphenidate Methylphenidate can raise imipramine plasma level and potentiate its antidepressant effects (Wharton RN, Perel JM, Dayton PG, Malitz S. A potential use for methylphenidate with tricyclic antidepressants. *Am J Psychiatry* 1976;127:1619–1625).

imipramine + moclobemide Serotonin syndrome was reported in a 39-year-old bipolar patient refractory to phenelzine, trimipramine dothiepin, lithium, and fluoxetine (FLX). A month after FLX discontinuation, moclobemide (300 mg/day) was started and increased 2 weeks later to 600 mg/day. Imipramine (IMI) (50 mg at bedtime) was added and increased gradually over 1 week to 100 mg at bedtime. After 5 days, IMI was increased to 200 mg/day and moclobemide was reduced to 300 mg/day. Five days later, the patient complained of sweating and feeling hot. She was shivering and became increasingly confused and stiff. At the hospital 2–3 hours later, her Glasgow Coma Scale score was 3/15 and she had the following signs: rapid breathing, increased salivation, flushed appearance, bilateral extensor spasms in arms and legs, jaw clamped shut, pupils fixed and dilated but eyes roving, and temperature of 39.6° C (103.2° F). No response occurred with intravenously administered benztropine (8 mg), diazepam (15 mg), and phenytoin (500 mg). Computed tomography showed no intracranial hemorrhage. Serum biochemistry was normal except for a tricyclic concentration of 1,940 microgram/L. She responded within 24 hours to intramuscularly administered chlorpromazine (100 mg every 6 hours), intravenously administered benzpenicillin, and ceftriaxone (Brodribb TR, Downey M, Gilbar PJ. Efficacy and adverse effects of moclobemide. *Lancet* 1994;343:475).

imipramine + nicotine transdermal system Because of deinduction of hepatic enzymes on smoking cessation, imipramine dosage reduction and discontinuation of the nicotine transdermal patch may be required at cessation of smoking.

imipramine/panic disorder See **panic disorder/imipramine.**

imipramine + paroxetine Co-administration may necessitate use of lower doses than usually prescribed for either drug alone. There is a report of marked elevation in imipramine (IMI) and desipramine plasma levels (IMI, 91 ng/ml; desipramine, 308 ng/ml; total, 399 ng/ml) 6 days after paroxetine (20 mg/day) was added to IMI (100 mg/day). The patient experienced worsened constipation and new-onset postural dizziness (Pittard JT. Pharmacokinetic interaction between paroxetine and tricyclic antidepressants. *Currents in Affective Illness* 1993;12:14–15).

imipramine + phenytoin Imipramine (IMI) may elevate phenytoin (PHT) plasma levels (Perucca E, Rickens A. Interaction between phenytoin and imipramine. *Br J Clin Pharmacol* 1977;4:485–486). IMI inhibits liver monooxygenase activity and may slow PHT metabolism rate, increasing plasma PHT concentration and risk of PHT toxicity (Aronson JK, Hardman M, Reynolds DJM. Phenytoin. *Br Med J* 1992;305:1215–1218).

imipramine + quinidine Co-administration increased imipramine levels 30% and desipramine levels 500% (Brosen K, Gran LF. Quinidine inhibits the 2-hydroxylation of imipramine and desipramine but not the demethylation of imipramine. *Eur J Clin Pharmacol* 1989;37:155–160).

imipramine + remoxipride   Neither drug influences the other's pharmacokinetics, nor does remoxipride influence the pharmacokinetics of the imipramine metabolites desipramine and 2-hydroxydesipramine.

imipramine + warfarin   Co-administration can increase hypothrombinemic effect.

imipramine + zolpidem   Co-administration does not alter the pharmacokinetics of either drug, although there may be increased sedation.

Imitrex   See **sumatriptan.**

immediate early gene   See **gene, immediate early.**

immune reaction   Specific reaction between antigen and antibody.

immune system   Organ system that protects against attacks by disease-producing agents (antigens). It consists predominantly of the spleen, bone marrow, lymph nodes, and lymphoid cells circulating throughout the body.

immunoassay   Laboratory test that uses specific antibodies as reagents to interact with and attach themselves to a known invading substance (e.g., a drug). Immunoassays are about 100 times more sensitive than thin-layer chromatography.

immunoblot   See **western blotting.**

immunofluorescence   Fluorescence histochemistry using antibodies to identify the compounds under investigation.

immunoglobulin   Any of a class of structurally related proteins with antibody activity. There are five major classes: IgA, IgD, IgE, IgG, and IgM. Each targets specific antigens. The whole immunoglobulin population in each person reacts with an enormous variety of antigens. A variety of immunological abnormalities, mostly nonspecific, have been reported in schizophrenia and other psychiatric disorders.

immunoglobulin A   (IgA) One of the five major classes of immunoglobulins, or antibodies, that protects outer surfaces of the body. It is found in mucous secretions of the intestinal and respiratory tract and in colostrum and milk.

immunopharmacology   Study of the regulation of the immune system by pharmacological agents and the development of methods to selectively modify immune function to treat human disease. Abused drugs and prescription drugs may be immunosuppressive agents. Alcohol, cannabinoids, and opiates have been implicated in impaired immune resistance. Independent of allergic potential, many drugs (e.g., nonsteroidal anti-inflammatory agents, antiepileptic drugs, anesthetics, tranquilizers) modulate immune responses. Although these effects are not always clinically important, physicians should be familiar with their adverse effects (Hadden JW, Smith DL. Immunopharmacology, immunomodulation and immunotherapy. *JAMA* 1992;268:2964–2969).

Imovane   See **zopiclone.**

impaired physician   The American Medical Association (AMA) defines as impaired a physician whose clinical conduct does not meet accepted standards of practice because of alcohol/drug use, psychiatric illness, and/or physical illness, or all three.

impairment   Any loss or abnormality of psychological, physiological, or anatomical structure or function (World Health Organization). It can be temporary or permanent and can be present at birth or acquired later. The description of an impairment is an objective account of the site, nature, and severity of loss of structure or function.

implicit memory   See **memory, implicit.**

implosion   Also called "flooding." See **implosive therapy.**

implosive therapy   Highly stressful behavior therapy in which the therapist causes the patient to imagine and thereby confront a phobic stimulus. Exposure is maintained until the patient's anxiety begins to decrease. It has gained increasing attention as a treatment not only for phobias and obsessive-compulsive disorder, but also for post-traumatic stress disorder. Also called "imaginal flooding."

impotence   Sexual dysfunction in which erectile capacity is impaired or absent.

impotence, organic   Impotence due to a physical disorder. The leading cause of organic impotence is diabetes. See **nocturnal penile tumescence.**

impotence, psychogenic   Sexual dysfunction in males characterized by inability to perform sexual intercourse despite the presence of sexual desire and intact genital organs. Examples include premature ejaculation; separation of the tender and sensual components of the sexual act so that intercourse is possible only with prostitutes; and the need for fixed and specific conditions to be operative before sexual intercourse can be performed.

Impril   See **imipramine.**

imprinting   In genetics, differential modification of the paternal and maternal genetic contributions to the zygote, resulting in the differential expression of parental alleles. It is most likely to occur during meiosis. During this time, genes that a female inherits from the father are redesignated as "maternal" so that they will act in a maternal manner as she passes them on to her offspring. Similarly, genes that a male inherits from the mother are changed to a "paternal" designation.

Impromen   See **bromperidol.**

improvement over chance   Measure of the level of improvement in the dependent variable compared with the average amount of improvement that would be expected from chance alone.

impulse control disorder   Disorder characterized by (a) failure to resist an impulse, drive, or temptation to perform some act that is harmful to the acting person or to others; (b) increasing sense of tension or arousal before committing the act; and (c) experience of pleasure, gratification, or release at the time of committing the act (DSM-III-R). Despite these criteria, DSM-III-R has no formal category for impulse control disorders, although it does list "impulse control disorders not elsewhere classified" (intermittent explosive disorder, kleptomania, pathological gambling, pyromania, trichotillomania) and "impulse control disorders not otherwise specified" (repetitive self-mutilation, compulsive sexual behavior, compulsive facial picking). Family history and treatment response studies suggest that intermittent explosive disorder, kleptomania, pathological gambling, pyromania, and trichotillomania may be related to mood, alcohol and psychoactive substance abuse, and anxiety (especially obsessive-compulsive) disorders. Biological studies indicate that intermittent explosive disorder and pyromania may share serotonergic abnormalities similar to those reported in mood disorders (McElroy SL, Hudson JI, Pope HG, et al: The DSM-III-R impulse control disorders not elsewhere classified: clinical characteristics and relationship to other psychiatric disorders. *Am J Psychiatry* 1992;149:318–327.)

impulse control, poor   Disordered regulation and control of action on inner urges, resulting in sudden, unmodulated, arbitrary, or misdirected discharge of tension and emotions, without concern about consequences. In its extreme form, patients exhibit homicidal attacks, sexual assaults, repeated brutality, or self-destructive behavior. It requires constant, direct supervision or external constraints.

impulsivity   **1.** Presence of behavior presumed to be impulsive in nature. **2.** Dimensional personality trait. **3.** Behavior characterized by lack of deliberation and failure to consider risks and consequences before acting. Many psychiatric disorders (e.g., substance abuse, pathological gambling, bulimia nervosa) have as their main symptom an apparent disorder of impulse control. Tests for evaluating this symptom and its response to treatment include: Ward Scales of Impulse Action; Impulsiveness Scale and Self-Report Test of Impulse Control.

impure placebo   See **placebo, impure.**

IMS America, Ltd.   One of the best known sources of drug use data in the United States. It conducts a number of different ongoing surveys of drug use, which are then sold to pharmaceutical manufacturers and regulatory agencies. IMS databases include (a) National Prescription Audit, a study of dispensed prescriptions from a panel of computerized retail pharmacies; (b) Audatrex, a longitudinal study of determinants of physicians' prescribing based on a panel of 1,000 physicians; (c) U.S. Pharmaceutical Market-Drugstores, a study of pharmaceutical purchases based on a sample of 840 representative retail pharmacies; and (d) U.S. Pharmaceutical Market-Hospitals, a study of pharmaceutical purchases based on a sample of 350 representative hospitals. See **National Disease and Therapeutic Index.**

Inapsine   See **droperidol.**

inborn error   See **inborn error of metabolism.**

inborn error of metabolism   Genetically determined biochemical disorder in which a specific enzyme defect produces a metabolic block that may have pathological consequences. Enzyme deficiency or absence may result in an accumulation of substances that would normally be broken down in the body and/or to a deficiency of substances essential to health. Many of these disorders (e.g., aminoaciduria, mucopolysaccharidosis, lipidosis) cause mental handicap that is generally progressive.

inbred   Descended from a small group of common ancestors.

inbred strain   Animals mated brother to sister for many generations, resulting in a strain in which members are near-identical genetically.

inception cohort   Group assembled at a common time early in the development of a specific clinical disorder (e.g., at first exposure to the putative cause or at initial diagnosis) and who are followed thereafter (Anon. Glossary of methodologic terms. *JAMA* 1992; 268:43–44).

incidence   Number of new cases of a disease that develop over a defined period in a defined population at risk, divided by the number of persons in that population at risk. In contrast, prevalence is the frequency of all cases, both new and old, of that disease that currently exist in a defined unit population within a given time. Measurement of incidence requires a longitudinal study design. See **prevalence.**

incoherence   Speech that, for the most part, is not understandable because of any of the following: (a) lack of logical or meaningful connection between words, phrases, or sentences; (b) excessive use of incomplete sentences; (c) excessive irrelevances or abrupt changes in subject matter; (d) idiosyncratic word usage; and (e) distorted grammar (DSM-IV). Mildly ungrammatical constructions or idiomatic usages characteristic of particular regional or ethnic backgrounds, lack of education, or low intelligence should not be considered incoherence. The term is generally not applied when there is evidence that the speech disturbance is due to aphasia. Incoherence may occur in some organic mental disorders, schizophrenia, and other psychotic disorders.

incompatibility   Host rejection of cells transplanted from a donor.

incomplete penetrance   Decreased manifestation of a genetic disease due to environmental or other factors.

incontinence   Inability to control excretory function.

incontinence, urinary   Inability to control urination. Physical disability, cognitive impairment, and diseases of the brain (e.g., frontoparietal lesions, normal pressure hydrocephalus, dementing disorders, demyelination, stroke) may lead to urinary incontinence. Among elderly nursing home residents without evidence of organic brain syndrome, incidence is about 24%; it increases to 62% in those with dementia and 63% in those with stroke (Van Nostrand JF, Zappolo A, Hing E, et al. *The National Nursing Home Survey.* Bethesda, MD: US Department of Health, Education, and Welfare, US National Center for Health Statistics; 1979. Vital and health statistics, series 13, # 43; DHEW publication # [PHS] 79-1794). There also is an association between urinary incontinence and functional psychosis, even when there are other causative factors involved. Urinary incontinence has been reported in patients with psychotic depression, mania, and schizophrenia. Overlooking the contribution of acute psychosis to urinary incontinence may result in inappropriate management. Effective treatment of the acute psychosis may improve both the psychosis and the incontinence (Williams C, Yeomans, D, Curran S, et al. An association between functional psychosis and urinary incontinence. *Ir J Psych Med* 1993;10[2];90–92).

incremental validity   Ability of a psychometric test to yield information beyond what can be acquired from informal interviewing or casual observation.

incubus   Parasomnia disorder characterized by night terrors in adults. It occurs during slow-wave sleep (Stage 4 non rapid eye movement [REM] sleep) and is thought to indicate some type of psychopathology.

IND   See **Investigational New Drug.**

indapamide   (Lozol) Nonthiazide sulfonamide diuretic with an action similar to the thiazides and having essentially the same clinical indications. Although it is claimed to alter serum lipids to a lesser degree than thiazide diuretics, this is not universally acknowledged. Like other thiazide diuretics, it can affect lithium clearance. See **lithium + indapamide.**

independent assortment   Random distribution of chromosomes (first stage of meiosis) and chromatids (second stage of meiosis) to gametes.

independent events   Events whose occurrence or outcome has no effect on the probability of each other. The probability of joint events equals the product of the separated probabilities of each event.

independent group   Comparison group treated differently than another group (e.g., treated group vs. untreated group). The idea is methodologically very sound, but often requires large samples if there is much variability among individuals.

independent observation   Observation determined by different individuals without the knowledge of each other's observations.

independent variable   See **variable, independent.**

Inderal   See **propranolol.**

index case   Statistical technique for measuring changes in groups of data.

indication   Any disease, illness, sign, or symptom for which a drug treatment is targeted.

indirect agonist   See **agonist, indirect.**

individual variation   1. Change between individuals (interindividual variation). 2. Change within the same individual (intraindividual variation).

Indocin   See **indomethacin.**

indolealkylamine   See **indole.**

indolamine   Any biogenic amine that contains an indole ring and amine group within its indole chemical structure (e.g., serotonin).

indolamine hypothesis of depression   Postulation that the indolamine serotonin (5-HT) plays a critical modulatory role in depressive disorders. The indolamine hypothesis is based in part on the following: (a) both the manic and depressive phases of bipolar illness are characterized by low central 5-HT function; and (b) treatments that may alleviate depression (electroconvulsive therapy, lithium, monoamine oxidase inhibitors, serotonin uptake inhibitors, tricyclic antidepressants) affect 5-HT in one way or another (Lapin IP, Oxenkirg GF. Intensification of the central serotonergic process as a possible determinant of the thymoleptic effect. *Lancet* 1989;1: 132–136).

indole Compound with a six-membered benzene ring joined to a five-membered ring at two different carbon atoms. Indoles are a class of biogenic amines that includes bufotenin, dimethyltryptamine, lysergic acid diethylamide (LSD), serotonin, and tryptophan. Also called "indolealkylamine."

indole-3-pyruvic acid (IPA) Ketoanalog of tryptophan widely found in vegetables and animals. It has been used to increase serotonin turnover in rat brain, melatonin turnover in the pineal gland, and kynurenic acid production in organs of treated animals. It also has been evaluated as a possible hypnotic agent for insomnia; preliminary data indicate that it has an action on human sleep similar to that of exogenous melatonin and L-tryptophan.

indomethacin (Indocin) Indole derivative, nonsteroidal anti-inflammatory agent. In the laboratory, it is the most potent of the inhibitors of prostaglandin synthesis. It is well absorbed after oral administration and highly bound to plasma proteins. It is more toxic than aspirin and causes a high incidence of dose-related adverse reactions; 20–25% of patients experience severe headaches that may be associated with dizziness, confusion, and depression. Rarely, psychosis with hallucinations has been reported. Indomethacin should be used with caution in patients with psychiatric disorders or peptic ulcer disease. A number of interactions with other drugs, including lithium, have been reported (Reimann IW, Drener U, Frolich JC. Indomethacin but not aspirin increases plasma lithium ion levels. *Arch Gen Psychiatry* 1983;40:283–286). See **lithium + indomethacin.**

indomethacin/breast milk Although indomethacin is excreted in breast milk, it is not contraindicated during nursing (Lebedevs TH, Wojnar-Horton RE, Yapp P, et al. Excretion of indomethacin in breast milk. *Br J Clin Pharmacol* 1991;32:751–754).

indomethacin + haloperidol See **haloperidol + indomethacin.**

indomethacin + lithium See **lithium + indomethacin.**

indorenate Indole that enhances central serotonergic function when given systematically. It is currently being tested as an anxiolytic.

Indormyl See **brotizolam.**

induced psychosis See **folie a deux.**

inducer Compound that increases the synthesis or activity of drug-metabolizing enzymes located in the endoplasmic reticulum of the liver.

infantile autism See **autism, infantile.**

inference Conclusion drawn about a population of observations from a sample of observations.

inference, statistical See **statistical inference.**

informatics Study of the application of computer and statistical techniques to the management of information. In genome projects, informatics includes development of methods to search databases quickly, analyze DNA sequence information, and predict protein sequence and structure from DNA sequence data.

information access Aspects of a disorder that a scale can or cannot assess. A scale constructed from behavioral items will not have access to mood; a self-assessment scale will not have access to delusional denial of illness.

information processing Identification and classification of information and its source, assessment of its significance, and comparisons of it with other incoming information or that stored in memory. As information enters the central nervous system, it passes through these processing stages. The information may or may not be retained, may or may not enter consciousness, and may or may not produce a behavioral response. To a certain extent, psychopharmacology can determine whether or not drugs affect these particular stages.

informed consent Standard consideration in medical and nursing practice that recognizes the patient's right to determine what is to happen to his or her body and mind. Its three basic elements are information, competence, and voluntariness. Informed consent by the patient for a medical procedure must be based on understanding the nature of the procedure, the risks involved, the consequences of withholding permission, and alternative procedures.

infra-additive drug effect Combined effect that is more than each drug alone but less than the sum of each drug effect.

infradian rhythm Biological rhythm or clock-driven behavior characterized by time-specific cyclical variations in biochemical and physiological functions and levels of activity (including variations in emotional state and psychomotor reactivity). Infradian rhythms last for weeks or months.

infusion 1. Product of the process of steeping a drug to extract its medicinal principles. 2. Therapeutic introduction of a fluid other than blood (e.g., saline solution) into a vein.

inhalant Any of a diverse group of volatile substances (e.g., varnish remover, gasoline, lighter fluid, airplane glue, rubber cement, cleaning fluid, nail polish remover, lighter fluid, paint thinner, spray paint) that produce psychoactive (generally short-lived) effects after their fumes are inhaled. They are relatively inexpensive, readily available, and subject to a wide variety of abuse patterns. They are quickly absorbed over the large surface of the lungs, accounting for their almost instantaneous psychoactive effects; it is estimated that abusers inhale a concentration of about 1,000–5,000 parts per million. They are central nervous system (CNS) depressants that produce euphoria, excitement, a floating sensation, and a sense of heightened power. Some produce belligerence, assaultiveness, and impaired judgment. Other effects include dizziness; slurred speech; ataxia; nystagmus; tremors; blurred vision; and irritation of the throat, lungs, and nose. Excessive inhalation can result in CNS depression (stupor and coma), cardiac arrhythmias, ventricular fibrillation, and bronchospasm. Overdoses may be fatal (Wright SP, Pottier A, Taylor J, et al. Trends in deaths associated with abuse of volatile substances. *Br Med J* 1992;305:692).

inhalant abuser   Person who inhales the fumes of volatile substances for their psychoactive effects. Clinical classifications include (a) transient social; (b) transient isolate; (c) chronic social; and (d) chronic isolate. *Transient social* characteristics include (a) short history of use; (b) use with friends; (c) petty offenses while intoxicated; (d) average intelligence; (e) possible learning disabilities; (f) age 10–16. *Transient isolate* characteristics include (a) short history of use; (b) use alone; (c) no legal offenses; (d) average or above average intelligence; (e) no learning disabilities; (f) age 10–16. *Chronic social* characteristics include (a) long history of use (5+ years); (b) daily use with friends; (c) misdemeanor offenses; (d) poor social skills; (e) 9th grade education; (f) brain damage (mental retardation prevalent); (g) age mid-20s to early 30s. *Chronic isolate* characteristics include (a) long history of use (over 5 years); (b) daily use/abuse; (c) legal offenses (assault is common); (d) poor social skills; (e) 9th grade education; (f) age mid 20s; (g) pre-use psychopathology (Sharp CW, Rosenberg HL. Volatile substances. *In* Lowenson JH, Ruiz P, Millman RB [eds], Langrod VG [assoc ed], *Substance Abuse. A Comprehensive Textbook*, 2nd ed. Baltimore: Williams & Wilkins, 1992, pp 303–327).

inhalant intoxication   Inhalant-induced organic disorder characterized by behavior changes (belligerence, assaultiveness, apathy) and central nervous system symptoms (dizziness, nystagmus, ataxia, dysarthria, tremor, psychomotor retardation, stupor, coma).

inheritance   In genetics, acquisition of characters or qualities by transmission from parent to offspring.

inheritance, dominant   Passing of a dominant gene from parent to child. Also called "autosomal dominant inheritance."

inheritance, multifactorial   Familial occurrence of disease with no obvious environmental cause or inheritance pattern; inheritance of traits affected by many genes (polygenic) and/or nongenetic factors.

inheritance, recessive   Inheritance of a trait via a recessive gene. Also called "autosomal recessive inheritance."

inhibitor   Internal or external stimulus that may produce a reduction in certain physical, psychological, or behavioral reactions.

inhibitory   Blocking or holding back physical, psychological, or behavioral reactions.

initial level effect   Conditioning of the effect of a drug by the ongoing status of the patient when the drug is taken. Hypnotics are least likely to induce sleep shortly after a person awakens from a restful, 8-hour sleep and most likely to induce sleep in a calm person at the end of the day.

initial tremor   See **tremor, movement.**

inner restlessness   Subjective feeling of psychic unrest or uneasiness. It may be associated with agitation or tension in patients who are depressed, fearful, and despondent. It also is associated with drug-induced akathisia and withdrawal from abused substances.

Innovar   See **fentanyl.**

inositol-1-phosphatase   Enzyme in the phosphoinositide cycle responsible for dephosphorylation of inositol triphosphate. Lithium inhibits the enzyme, dampens the signal of the cycle, and thus modulates neuronal and hormonal responses.

inositol phosphate   Substrate involved in the phosphoinositide system.

inositol triphosphate   Substrate of the phosphoinositide system responsible for release of calcium from endoplasmic reticulum. Intracellular calcium levels modulate the release of neurotransmitters and hormones.

inpatient family intervention   (IFI) Psychosocial intervention that can be used while the patient is in the hospital and the family is often available and interested in obtaining help.

input variable   See **variable, input.**

insert   In recombinant DNA research, that portion of DNA inserted into a plasmid. An insert can refer to cDNA, genomic DNA, or portions of either.

Insidon   See **opipramol.**

insight   Recognition by the patient that (a) symptoms of the illness are abnormalities and; (b) behaviors are maladaptive or morbid phenomena.

insight, lack of   Impaired awareness or understanding of ones own psychiatric condition and life situation. It is evidenced by failure to recognize past or present psychiatric illness or symptoms, denial of need for psychiatric hospitalization or treatment, decisions characterized by poor anticipation of consequences, and unrealistic short-term and long-range planning.

in situ hybridization   See **hybridization, in situ.**

insomnia   Difficulty initiating or maintaining sleep. It may arise from a variety of intrinsic (stress, emotional disturbance, physical disease) and/or extrinsic (noise) factors. In some diseases and conditions that cause or contribute to insomnia (e.g., congestive heart failure, hyperthyroidism, pulmonary disease, esophageal reflux, arthritis), it should be remembered that medications such as steroids and theophylline can disturb sleep, as can the timing of diuretic administration. Insomnia may also be related to circadian rhythm disorders; altered amplitude and phase relationships may occur during shift work, transmeridian travel, or changes in daily routine or sleep patterns (earlier arousal and earlier bedtime tendency), or they may occur spontaneously. Regardless of the cause, any type of sleep disorder is likely to cause impaired concentration, short-term memory problems, inability to handle minor irritations, decreased enjoyment of interpersonal relationships, and decreased ability to accomplish tasks. Some patients with a sleep disorder are at increased risk of involvement in traffic accidents. Although hypnotic medication is frequently prescribed for insomnia, it should not be the mainstay of management in most cases. Insomnia resulting from medical or psychiatric causes should be managed primarily by appropriate treatment of the underlying condition. Short-term, intermittent use of hypnotics and sedative tricyclic antidepressants may be useful for temporary problems such as bereavement, dislocation, and situational anxiety. There are no studies that demonstrate their long-term effectiveness. In addition to sedative/hypnotics, the following have been reported useful for insomnia: progressive relaxation training; electromyographic, theta, or sensorimotor rhythm biofeedback training; behavioral therapies, including stimulus control and sleep restriction therapy; and therapies for insomnia with clear organic etiologies, such as nasal continuous positive airway pressure for sleep apnea. Accumulating evidence indicates that psychological treatments (relaxation training, cognitive therapy to reduce cognitive arousal and worry about not sleeping, stimulus control procedures) can substantially affect insomnia, and that the most useful methods are not highly specialized or difficult to apply (Espie CA. *The Psychological Treatment of Insomnia.* Chichester: Wiley, 1991).

insomnia, chronic   There are at least two forms: conditioned and subjective, each of which has psychological components. In conditioned insomnia, trying to go to sleep or the setting in which the attempt occurs causes sleep dysfunction characterized by a conditioned arousal response. It may follow a traumatic experience that initially produces short-term insomnia; the patient then focuses on the sleep disturbance, which becomes persistent. In other patients, the bedroom triggers anxiety about sleeping; sleeping better away from home strongly suggests conditioned insomnia. Patients with subjective insomnia report sleeping very little or not at all, although in a sleep laboratory their sleep is relatively normal; it is unknown why there is disparity between the patient's subjective perception of sleep and objective findings.

insomnia, drug-induced   Prescription medications, over-the-counter (OTC) drugs, alcohol, caffeine, and nicotine may cause insomnia. Prescription medications that delay sleep onset or reduce sleep depth include alpha-methyldopa, antiarrhythmics, antidepressants with stimulant properties (e.g., bupropion, fluoxetine, protriptyline), beta-adrenergic agonists (e.g., isoproterenol), beta blockers (e.g., propranolol), catecholamine-blocking agents, cimetidine, diuretics, levodopa, methyldopa, phenytoin, theophylline, and thyroid hormone. Sleep-disrupting OTC preparations include nasal decongestants, those with stimulants or stimulant properties, and anoretic agents. Alcohol, caffeine, and nicotine are the most common sleep disrupters. Alcohol often causes abrupt awakenings during the night; it is a notorious producer of fragmented sleep. Caffeine lessens sleep quality and increases next-morning drowsiness. Nicotine is a stimulant that increases sleep latency and decreases sleep duration. An in-depth personal drug history (including illicit substance abuse) should be taken from every patient complaining of insomnia before a hypnotic is prescribed.

insomnia, initial   Difficulty falling asleep during the first few hours of the sleep period.

insomnia, long-term   Sleep disturbance that has lasted at least a month and has not responded to nonpharmacological therapies. It often is associated with use of medications, caffeine and alcohol consumption, and/or a medical or psychiatric disorder. A hypnotic should not be prescribed without careful evaluation to find the most likely cause of the insomnia (e.g., depression, substance and/or alcohol abuse). If a hypnotic is used, treatment should be intermittent; only if this is ineffective should continuous hypnotic therapy be prescribed with careful, regular monitoring for tolerance with dependency.

insomnia, middle Awakening after having fallen asleep and then having difficulty going back to sleep. Possible causes include depression or alcohol use.

insomnia/medical causes Almost any medical illness can affect sleep; the most common include cardiovascular diseases (e.g., coronary artery disease, angina, hypertension, especially when associated with sleep apnea and congestive heart failure with paroxysmal nocturnal dyspnea), endocrine disorders (e.g., hyperthyroidism diabetic neuropathy), gastrointestinal disturbances (e.g., hiatal hernia, esophageal acid reflux, peptic ulcer pain), and pulmonary disorders (e.g., sleep apnea, airway obstruction, hypercapnia, hypoxia). Any medical condition that causes pain, discomfort, irritation, or itching also may interfere with sleep.

insomnia, persistent Insomnia lasting longer than 1 month. It is frequently associated with depressed mood, major depression, and bereavement (where it is a persistent and debilitating symptom). It also may be due to one or more of the following: medical illness (e.g., hyperthyroidism), symptoms of medical illnesses (e.g., pain), primary sleep disorder (e.g., sleep apnea, nocturnal myoclonus), or psychophysiological conditioning. If the history, physical examination, and laboratory screening data do not clearly favor one specific diagnosis, an overnight sleep recording may be necessary before undertaking difficult treatment regimens.

insomnia, primary Insomnia lasting longer than 1 month and not associated with diagnosable mental or medical disorders.

insomnia, rebound Sleep disturbance and electroencephalographic modifications, and/or rebound anxiety following discontinuation of a daily dose of a benzodiazepine (BZD) or non-BZD hypnotic that has been administered even for a relatively short period. Rebound insomnia appears to be dose-dependent: the higher the BZD dose, the more likely it is to occur and the more severe it will be. Early morning insomnia may be a variant of rebound insomnia occurring during drug administration. Rebound is induced by BZDs with short and intermediate half-lives; BZDs with a long half-life and slow decline in plasma level are less likely to cause rebound phenomena. It has been reported with the rapidly eliminated BZDs midazolam and triazolam used nightly for several weeks. It usually is not

observed when these drugs are used in appropriate doses less than 7–10 days. Rebound insomnia can be averted or minimized by dosage tapering for a few nights before discontinuation. Marked rebound effects act as a strong stimulus (reinforcement) to continue treatment (Kales A, Soldatos CR, Bixler EO, et al. Rebound insomnia and rebound anxiety: a review. *Pharmacology* 1983;26:121–137).

insomnia, short-term Sleep disturbance evoked by situational stress that usually lasts for less than 3 weeks and occurs in individuals with no history of any form of sleep abnormality. It also occurs in normal sleepers subjected to stress of at least 2 or more weeks' duration (bereavement, marital discord, employment difficulties). Like transient insomnia, it is manifested by delayed sleep onset and difficulty maintaining sleep. If used, hypnotic drug therapy should be intermittent (i.e., avoided after 1–2 good nights' sleep).

insomnia, terminal Early morning awakening, a characteristic sleep disturbance of endogenous depression.

insomnia, transient Delayed sleep onset and difficulty maintaining sleep that occurs in normal sleepers after brief exposure to an identifiable stress (e.g., hospitalization for elective surgery) or when the individual has to rest at an unusual time of the day. When the stress is over, sleep usually returns to normal patterns. Transient insomnia is often a problem of middle age in which sleep is less restful and when the individual is still active and involved in skilled and responsible work (e.g., airline pilots). If treatment is indicated, short-term use of a benzodiazepine (BZD) hypnotic is usually all that is necessary, with careful attention paid to dosage and rate of elimination. Hypnotics used under such circumstances must be free of residual effects and accumulation on daily ingestion. Hypnotics with ultrarapid elimination (mean elimination half-life 2–3 hours) would seem to be indicated; however, relatively high doses are needed to sustain sleep over the course of the night, and the high plasma levels of the early part of the night may cause respiratory depression, alteration of sleep architecture, anterograde amnesia, and rebound insomnia on cessation of continued therapy. Clinical experience indicates that the BZD hypnotic brotizolam (mean elimination half-life 5 hours), in doses of 0.125 mg or 0.25 mg, has the potential to sustain sleep and be free of residual effects and accumulation with daily ingestion. It would be indicated when there is a need to sustain sleep in persons involved in skilled activity.

installation of hope In group therapy, patient optimism that the group can be helpful based on the patient's seeing that other members have improved or are improving (Bloch S, Crouch E. *Therapeutic Factors in Group Psychotherapy.* Oxford: Oxford University Press, 1985).

instrumental conditioning See **operant conditioning.**

insufflate To blow a substance (e.g., powder, gas) into an airway or body cavity. See **"snorting."**

insulin coma therapy (ICT) Form of shock treatment in which large amounts of insulin are given to induce profound hypoglycemia, resulting in a coma. Introduced for the treatment of schizophrenia by Manfred Sakel in 1933, its use declined dramatically after the advent of neuroleptics. It is rarely used today, although an early treatment stage called "subcoma therapy" is used occasionally.

intellectual inadequacy See **mental retardation.**

intellectualization Mechanism in which the person engages in excessive abstract thinking to avoid experiencing disturbing feelings (DSM-IV).

intensified drug use World Health Organization (WHO) classification characterized by long-term, patterned drug use of at least one episode a day. Use is motivated by a perceived need or desire to achieve relief from a persistent problem or stressful situation.

intention myoclonus See **myoclonus, intention.**

intention tremor See **tremor, intention.**

interaction Alterations in the actions of one drug produced by concurrent or recent administration of another drug or drugs. The alterations may affect attributes such as efficacy, toxicity, untoward drug effects, and may be mediated by influences on drug metabolism, elimination, binding, plasma protein, and drug receptors.

interaction, drug See **drug-drug interaction; drug-food interaction.**

interactive telemedicine See **telemedicine.**

intercept In a regression equation, the predicted value of Y when X is equal to zero.

interdose anxiety (IDA) See **anxiety, breakthrough.**

interferon Lymphokine that protects noninfected cells from viral infection and augments natural-killer-cell, cytotoxic-T-cell, and macrophage activity.

interictal In epilepsy, the period between episodes of seizure activity. During the interictal period, the person may be normal or, if there are limbic epileptic discharges in the electroencephalogram, have symptoms of the interictal behavior syndrome.

interictal aggression See **aggression, interictal.**

interictal dysphoric disorder (IDD) Newly recognized disorder in epileptic patients that is intermittent and polysymptomatic with affective and somatoform symptoms. In DSM-IV, it is listed under organic mood disorders. Its eight key symptoms, which occur in more than 50% of those with IDD, are depressive mood, anergia, irritability, euphoric mood, pain, insomnia, fear, and anxiety. It is best treated with optimal antiepileptic drug therapy plus low-dose tricyclic antidepressant drug therapy (e.g., imipramine or amitriptyline 75–125 mg/day). The lower dose should be initiated with 25 mg twice a day followed by gradual increments of 25–50 mg/day, if necessary. If there are interictal psychotic symptoms (hallucinations, paranoia, delusions), addition of small neuroleptic doses (e.g., trifluoperazine 1 mg/25–50 mg of the tricyclic) may be necessary (Blumer DP, Herman BP. *Behavioral and Emotional Adjustment in Epilepsy. Issues in Epilepsy and Quality of Life.* Landover, MD: Epilepsy Foundation of America, 1993).

interictal personality disorder Syndrome characterized by viscosity, hyper-religiousness, hypergraphia, hypermorality, and hyposexuality. Also called "Geschwind syndrome"; "temporal lobe personality syndrome."

interim analysis Test of significance done before all study data are available. Although some procedures allow for multiple looks at the data, it is increasingly common in protocols for large-scale clinical trials to specify that a single interim analysis will be undertaken halfway through the study. Special test criteria are required to ensure that the experiment-wide type I error probability associated with the interim test and a final end-of-study test, in case no interim decision to terminate the study is reached, does not exceed the specified alpha level. This is achieved by dividing the total type I error probability between the interim analysis and the subsequent end-of-study analysis, if the latter is required.

interleukin Lymphokine that regulates immune cell growth, maturation, and function.

interleukin-1 (IL-1) Inflammatory peptide hormone with potent endocrine effects. In pharmacological doses, it stimulates central nervous system production of corticotropin-releasing hormone, growth hormone, thyroid-stimulating hormone, and somatostatin, or it inhibits secretion of prolactin and luteinizing hormone. It is thought to enhance immune function and to suppress food intake.

interleukin-2 (IL-2) T cell–derived cytokine that promotes cell growth and differentiation in a variety of organs, including the brain. Its cellular effects are mediated by a receptor coupled to a glycosylphatidylinositol second-messenger system. Systemic IL-2 production is elevated in viral infections and chronic autoimmune disorders (e.g., rheumatoid arthritis, systemic lupus erythematosus, multiple sclerosis). IL-2 and IL-2 receptors have been identified in different brain regions (e.g., hippocampal formation, median-eminence-arcuate nucleus complex, cerebral cortex, lateral septum, neostriatum, cerebellum). Elevated levels of central IL-2 may contribute to increased dopaminergic neurotransmission, autoimmune phenomena, and abnormal brain morphology described in some patients with schizophrenia (Licinio J, Seibyl JP, Altemus M, et al. Elevated CSF levels of interleukin-2 in neuroleptic-free schizophrenic patients. *Am J Psychiatry* 1993;150:1408–1410).

interleukin-1 receptor   (IL-1r) Macrophage-derived polypeptide that is a key mediator of the immune response to stress, infection, and antigenic challenge. IL-1 receptor activation in the brain can cause fever, induce slow-wave sleep, and alter neuroendocrine activity, including stimulation of the hypothalamic-pituitary-adrenocortical axis and inhibition of the hypothalamic-pituitary-gonadal axis. IL-1 is produced by macrophages following antigenic challenges, such as infection.

interleukin-2 receptor   (IL-2r) Cell growth factor of the immune system thought to be of importance in the pathophysiology of schizophrenia. Cerebral asymmetry in schizophrenia may be mediated by abnormalities in central IL-2 levels.

intermediary sleep stage   See **sleep stage 2.**

intermediate care facility   Medicaid-certified health care delivery facility that provides health-related services to persons eligible for Medicaid who do not require hospital or skilled nursing facility care, but who do require institutional care above the level of room and board.

intermediate variable   See **variable, intermediate.**

intermittent   Periodic expression of symptoms of an illness with distinct periods of normalcy between episodes.

intermittent dyskinesia   See **dyskinesia, intermittent.**

intermittent explosive disorder   See **impulse control disorder.**

internal control   See **control, internal.**

internal reliability   See **reliability, internal.**

internal validity   See **consistency.**

International Classification of Diseases   (ICD-10; ICD-9) Official list of disease categories issued by the Mental Health Division of the World Health Organization (WHO) after extensive international consultation. ICD-10 is a reliable diagnostic system; ratings of its feasibility and utility by participating clinicians suggest that it will be a distinct advance over ICD-9. International Classification of Diseases, adapted for use in the United States (ICDA), prepared by the U.S. Public Health Service, is the official list of diagnostic terms to be used for each ICD category in the United States. By international treaty, the United States is committed to use ICD-10 diagnostic codes for federal medical activities, such as veterans hospitals and Medicare. Although DSM-IV is not an exact replica of ICD-10, it is as compatible as possible to facilitate "cross-walking" from one coding system to the other. Thus, DSM-IV codes could be translated into the ICD-10 numbering system in situations that require it (Liebowitz MR. Mixed anxiety and depression: should it be included in DSM-IV? *J Clin Psychiatry* 1993;54[5,suppl]:4–7).

interobserver variation   Type of misclassification that can lead to erroneous conclusions in epidemiological research (Mertens TE. Estimating the effects of misclassification. *Lancet* 1993;342:418–421).

interoception   Physiological response to a perception.

interoceptor   Any of the small sensory end organs in the viscera.

interpersonal learning/input   In group therapy, the patient learning about the nature of his or her problems through other group members sharing their perceptions of him or her (Bloch S, Crouch E. *Therapeutic Factors in Group Psychotherapy.* Oxford: Oxford University Press, 1985).

interpersonal learning/output   In group therapy, a form of "interpersonal experimentation" in which the patient learns to relate to others in a more adaptive way (Bloch S, Crouch E. *Therapeutic Factors in Group Psychotherapy.* Oxford: Oxford University Press, 1985).

interpersonal psychotherapy   See **psychotherapy, interpersonal.**

interpersonal viscosity   See **viscosity, interpersonal.**

interquartile range   See **range, interquartile.**

inter-rater reliability   See **reliability, inter-rater.**

intervening variable   See **variable, intervening.**

intervention   Interceding on behalf of an individual who is abusing or dependent on one or more psychoactive drugs, with the aim of overcoming denial, interrupting drug-taking behavior, or inducing the individual to seek and initiate treatment.

interview, amytal   See **amytal interview.**

intoxication   Organic mental disorder caused by recent ingestion of an exogenous substance that produces maladaptive behavior secondary to its effects on the central nervous system. General manifestations include disturbances of perception, wakefulness, attention, thinking, judgment, emotional control, and psychomotor behavior. The specific clinical picture depends on the nature of the substance ingested.

intoxication, idiosyncratic Profound intoxication that develops after a single drink in individuals acutely sensitive to the effects of alcohol. Altered behavior—especially aggression, delusions, hallucinations, impulsivity, and rage reactions—may occur. Sedation may be achieved with intravenously administered diazepam (10 mg) over 1–2 minutes, or intravenously administered lorazepam (1–2 mg) over 1–2 minutes; dosages can be repeated at 10-minute intervals. An alternative is intramuscularly administered haloperidol (5 mg) every hour if necessary, up to a maximum of six doses.

intoxication, inhalant See **inhalant intoxication.**

intoxication, pathological Sudden onset of marked behavior changes after consumption of a small amount of alcohol. Symptoms usually last a few hours and terminate in prolonged sleep. Later, the individual is unable to recall the episode. In some instances, there can be assaultive behavior and suicidal ideation and attempts. Also called "alcohol idiosyncratic intoxication."

intramuscular (IM) One of several options for administering drugs by injection. Rapidity of absorption of drugs in aqueous solution is enhanced by using a site well supplied with blood. The most commonly used injection sites are the deltoid muscles or the gluteus maximus (usually the latter), although any muscle area may be used. Depot IM injections of drugs dissolved in oil are used to provide a slowly absorbed reservoir of drug. Some depot neuroleptics provide significant levels of drug for several weeks after a single injection. IM drug administration may be painful depending on bulk, formulation, and site of injection. It also may be responsible for tissue damage.

intrapsychic Arising from or occurring within the psyche, mind, or personality (e.g., intrapsychic conflicts).

intrarater reliability See **reliability, intrarater.**

intravenous administration (IV) Introduction of a substance into a vein or veins by injection or infusion.

intravenously administered neuroleptic See **neuroleptic, intravenously administered.**

intrinsic activity Inherent ability of a ligand to elicit a biological response once it is bound to a receptor.

intrinsic clearance See **clearance, intrinsic.**

intrinsic sleep disorder See **sleep disorder, intrinsic.**

intron That part of every gene which is transcribed and thus present in the primary transcript. Introns are removed in the process called "RNA splicing" and are not present in the mature messenger RNA (mRNA). See **exon.**

Intropin See **dopamine HCl.**

intrusiveness 1. Degree to which a treatment technique invades one's emotional or physical self. 2. Degree of social invasiveness.

invasive treatment Therapy involving penetration of the body by injection or implantation of medicine into body tissue. Depot neuroleptics and disulfiram implants are examples of invasive treatments. Some diagnostic procedures also may be invasive.

inverse agonist See **agonist, inverse.**

Investigational New Drug (IND) 1. In the opinion of the Food and Drug Administration (FDA), any new drug, antibiotic drug, or biological drug used in a clinical investigation. 2. Application to the FDA to investigate a new compound or medication.

Investigational New Drug, emergency (emergency IND) Mechanism by which experimental drugs can be made available on an individual basis in emergency situations that do not allow time for the regular submission of an IND. The FDA may authorize shipment of an experimental drug to a sponsor for a specified use in advance of submission of all the paperwork covering the IND. Emergency use INDs are normally reserved for severe medical situations, typically when a patient is near death. An excellent overview of special IND provisions is provided in "Treatment, Compassionate Use, and Emergency INDs and Parallel Track: Understanding It All" (*US Regulatory Reporter* September, 1989;6[3]:3–6).

investigator, clinical Physician involved in the execution of a clinical trial.

investigator brochure Summary of essential drug information (e.g., chemistry, toxicology, human use, clinical safety) prepared by a pharmaceutical company to enable a clinical investigator to conduct a safe and ethical clinical trial.

in vitro exposure See **exposure in imagination.**

in vivo exposure See **exposure in practice.**

involuntary movement See **movement, involuntary.**

involuntary outpatient treatment Attempt to provide mandatory administration of psychotropic medication in the community, much like the approach to the treatment of patients with tuberculosis (Wilk RJ. Implications of involuntary outpatient commitment for community health agencies. *Am J Orthopsychiatry*

1988;58:580–591; Hiday VA, Scheid-Cook TL. A follow-up of chronic patients committed to outpatient treatment. *Hosp Community Psychiatry* 1989;40:52–59).

iodinated benzamide   Benzamide derivative (e.g., epidepride, iclopride, iodopride, ioxipride, itopride).

iomazenil   Iodinated analog of flumazenil that is a benzodiazepine (BZD) receptor antagonist and a single photon emission computed tomography (SPECT) radioligand used for imaging the BZD receptor. It has a 10-fold higher affinity for the BZD receptor than flumazenil (Innis RB. Neuroimaging with SPECT. *J Clin Psychiatry* 1992;53[suppl]:29–34).

Ionamin   See **phentermine**.

ion channel   Pore on the nerve membrane through which sodium, potassium, and other metal and nonmetal ions (e.g., chloride) pass to produce changes in the electrical activity of the nerve membrane. Ion channels are controlled by receptors located in the nerve membrane.

ionization   Removal of an electron from a neutral atom, resulting in a positively charged ion and a free, negatively charged electron.

ion pump   Metabolic mechanism responsible for moving ions through a cell membrane. For example, the sodium pump moves sodium ions out of cells, and potassium ions into them, which is one of the proposed mechanisms of lithium action.

ion selective electrode   (ISE) Analytical procedure to determine lithium concentrations in biological fluids. ISE assays have the putative advantage of small sample size requirement, short analysis time, minimal operational costs, and potential use in various biological fluids. ISE serum lithium determinations may lead to overestimation of drug clearance, and thereby overestimation of lithium maintenance dosages when pharmacokinetic prediction techniques are used.

iontophoresis   Administration of compounds through micropipettes that are released by an electric current.

iota   Opioid receptor for the enkephalins that is different from sigma receptors.

iprindole   (Galatur; Tertran) Heterocyclic agent with an indole nucleus; it resembles typical tricyclic antidepressant (TCA) drugs, but lacks monoaminergic reuptake blocking properties. In doses of 30–90 mg/day it appears to be as effective as standard TCA dosages and in some cases has fewer unwanted effects. It is marketed in England, but not in the United States.

iprindole + lithium   Lithium augmentation of iprindole has benefitted patients partially re-

sponsive or totally refractory to iprindole alone (de Montigny C, Elie R, Gaille R, et al. Rapid response to the addition of lithium in iprindole-resistant unipolar depression: a pilot study. *Am J Psychiatry* 1985;142:220–223).

iproniazid   (Formerly Marsilid) First irreversible monoamine oxidase inhibitor (MAO-A and -B) derivative of the antitubercular drug isoniazid to be recognized as an effective antidepressant. It was widely heralded when introduced to psychiatry in the late 1950s, but dropped out of use after being associated with a number of adverse reactions, including fatal hepatitis, which were responsible for its being banned in the United States.

ipsapirone   (IPSA) Azaperone derivative, novel nonbenzodiazepine anxiolytic that is a partial agonist at serotonin (5-HT)$_{1A}$ receptors, but does not affect other neurotransmitter receptors. One of its metabolites, 1-(2-pyrimidimyl) piperazine, has alpha$_2$-adrenolytic action. IPSA produces less daytime sleepiness and short-term memory impairment than benzodiazepines. Clinical trials indicate that optimal anxiolytic dose is 15 mg/day. In a multicenter, placebo-controlled comparison with lorazepam 2–6 mg/day, IPSA (10–30 mg/day) was more effective than lorazepam and caused no more side effects than lorazepam and placebo in outpatients with generalized anxiety disorder. IPSA patients had fewer withdrawal symptoms than lorazepam patients (Cutler NR, Sramek JJ, Keppel Hesselink JM, et al. Ipsapirone versus lorazepam in outpatients with generalized anxiety disorder: multicenter findings. *Biol Psychiatry* 1993;33:147a–148a). IPSA also may be effective and well tolerated in the treatment of bulimia.

irreversible dementia   See **dementia, irreversible.**

isatin   (2,3-dioxoindole) Endogenous monoamine oxidase inhibitor being studied in England as a potential anxiolytic.

isoallele   "Normal" allelic gene that can be distinguished from other isoalles only by their differing phenotypic expression when in combination with a dominant mutant allele.

isocarboxazid   (Marplan) Potent monoamine oxidase inhibitor antidepressant. Because of the risk of hypertensive crisis, it should not be co-administered with sympathomimetics (amphetamine, dopamine, epinephrine, levodopa, methyldopa, norepinephrine, tryptophan) or taken with foods containing high concentrations of tryptophan (broad beans) or tyramine (aged cheese, chicken livers, yeast extract). Pregnancy risk category C.

isocarboxazid + amitriptyline   Co-administration has precipitated mania (de la Fuente RJ, Berlanga C, Leon-Andrade C. Mania induced by tricyclic-MAOI combination therapy in bipolar treatment-resistant disorder: case reports. *J Clin Psychiatry* 1986;47:40–41).

isocarboxazid + clonazepam   Co-administration is more effective in treating panic disorder than either drug alone.

isocarboxazid + dextromethorphan   Nausea, dizziness, myoclonic jerks, choreoathetoid movements, and urinary retention developed in a patient taking isocarboxazid in less than 1 hour of taking Robitussin DMR (Sovner R, Wolf J. Interaction between dextromethorphan and monoamine oxidase inhibitor therapy with isocarboxazid. *N Engl J Med* 1988; 319:1671).

isocarboxazid + lithium   Co-administration for severe depression can be effective and safe (Zall H. Lithium carbonate and isocarboxazid. An effective drug approach in severe depression. *Am J Psychiatry* 1971; 127:1400–1403). See **lithium + monoamine oxidase inhibitor.**

isocarboxazid + pergolide   Co-administration has been used to treat patients refractory to isocarboxazid alone. Some tolerate the combination well. One patient being treated with higher dose pergolide (2 mg) + isocarboxazid (40 mg) became hypomanic; hypomania abated when pergolide was reduced to 1 mg.

isochromosome   Symmetrical chromosome with two arms of equal length, and bearing the same loci reverse sequence, formed by crosswise rather than longitudinal division of the centromere.

isodisomy   Identical chromosomes from one parent.

isoenzyme   See **isozyme.**

isogenic   Having identical genotypes, as in identical twins.

isolation   Mechanism in which the person is unable to experience simultaneously the cognitive and affective components of an experience because the affect is kept from consciousness (DSM-IV).

Isomeride   See **dexfenfluramine.**

isomerism   Existence of a molecule that possesses two or more structural forms. See **stereoisomerism.**

isomorphism   In genetics, genotypes of polyploid organisms that produce similar gametes even though the genotypes contain genes in different combinations on homologous chromosomes.

isoniazid   (Laniazid; Nydrazid) (INH) Antitubercular agent noted in 1952 to elevate mood. It is the precursor of iproniazid. It is an irreversible inhibitor of monamine oxidase A and B.

isoniazid + benzodiazepine   Isoniazid inhibits hepatic microsomal enzymes and may reduce hepatic clearance and increase plasma concentrations of benzodiazepines metabolized by oxidation (e.g., alprazolam, chlordiazepoxide, clorazepate, diazepam, estazolam, flurazepam, halazepam, prazepam, quazepam, temazepam, and triazolam).

isoniazid + carbamazepine   Isoniazid inhibits carbamazepine (CBZ) metabolism, possibly resulting in elevated CBZ plasma levels and toxicity (Block H. Carbamazepine-isoniazid interactions. *Pediatrics* 1982;69:494–495).

isoniazid + phenytoin   Co-administration may increase phenytoin (PHT) blood level and may cause PHT toxicity. Isoniazid inhibits PHT metabolism, resulting in increased steady-state concentrations. This clinically important rise in serum PHT has been observed only in slow acetylators; fast acetylators do not achieve a concentration of isoniazid in the liver sufficiently high to inhibit the microsomal enzymes (Kutt H, Brennan R, Dehejia H, et al. Diphenylhydantoin intoxication. A complication of isoniazid therapy. *Am Rev Respir Dis* 1970;101:377–384).

isoniazid + valproic acid   Co-administration has been associated with toxicity; no toxic effects occurred when each drug was used alone (Olanow CW, Finn AL, Prussak C. The effect of salicylate on the pharmacology of phenytoin. *Neurology* 1981;31:341–342).

isoproterenol   (Isuprel) Synthetic sympathomimetic amine that is structurally related to epinephrine, but acts almost exclusively on beta receptors. It has been used to induce panic attacks and other anxiety states. After treatment with tricyclic antidepressants, patients are able to tolerate a somewhat higher rate of isoproterenol and longer infusion (Pohl RB, Rainey JM Jr, Ortiz A, et al. Isoproterenol-induced anxiety states. *Psychopharmacol Bull* 1985;21:424–427).

Isoptin   See **verapamil.**

Isopulsan   See **minaprine.**

isozyme   Multiple molecular form of an enzyme within a single individual. Also called "isoenzyme."

Isuprel   See **isoproterenol.**

item   Symptom(s) and/or behavior(s) being rated (e.g., nervous, tense) on a scale.

iteration   Catatonic phenomenon in which a gesture or mannerism is repeated over a short space of time.

J

"jac aroma" Street name for abused solvents and inhalants.

Jacksonian seizures See **epilepsy, Jacksonian.**

jactation Excessive restlessness characterized by irregular and convulsive movements of the body.

Janimine See **imipramine.**

Jatrosom See **tranylcypromine + trifluoperazine.**

"jeff" Street term for ephedrine.

"jelly bean" Street name for amphetamine sulfate.

"jet" Street name for phencyclidine (PCP).

jet lag Circadian disharmony that results from crossing time zones. See **time zone change syndrome.**

jet lag syndrome See **time zone change syndrome.**

jitteriness syndrome Anxiety, restlessness, and trouble standing still that may occur in as many as 20% of patients with panic disorder and agoraphobia when treated with tricyclic antidepressants (Zitrin CM, Klein DF, Woerner MG. Treatment of agoraphobia with group exposure in vivo and imipramine. *Arch Gen Psychiatry* 1980;37:63–72).

"jittery baby" Syndrome that occurs in cocaine-addicted infants (Richards IS, Kulkarni AP, Remner WF. Cocaine-induced arrhythmia in human foetal myocardium in vitro: possible mechanism for foetal death in utero. *Pharmacol Toxicol* 1990;66:150–154). See **cocaine baby.**

"jive" Street name for cannabinoids.

"joint" Street name for a marijuana cigarette.

joint attention behavior Attempts to monitor or direct the attention of another person to an object or event (e.g., pointing, showing, gaze monitoring). Protodeclarative pointing is the use of the index finger to indicate to another person an object of interest, as an end in itself. Protoimperative pointing is the use of the index finger simply to attempt to obtain an object. Pointing for naming is to pick out an object within an array while naming it; this can be nonsocial. Joint attention behavior is normally present by 9–14 months of age; it is absent or rare in autism. Other joint attention deficits in autism include relative lack of showing objects to others, and gaze monitoring—directing one's gaze where someone else is looking (Baron-Cohen S, Allen J, Gillberg C. Can autism be detected at 18 months? The needle, the haystack and the CHAT. *Br J Psychiatry* 1992;161:839–843). See **autism; pretend play.**

joint probability Probability of two events both occurring.

joint venture in health care Any ownership, investment interest, or compensation arrangement between doctors (or any other health care professionals who make referrals) and a provider of health care goods or services, such as a pathology laboratory. It can lead to a conflict of interest.

jomazenil I-123 substituted flumazenil, a radioactively labeled benzodiazepine (BZD) antagonist. Jomazenil single photon emission computed tomography (SPECT) scan is a useful tool to investigate BZD receptor function and distribution in the brain.

"joy plant" Street name for opium.

"joy powder" Street name for cocaine or heroin.

Julodin See **estazolam.**

"junk" Street name for heroin.

junk DNA Deoxyribonucleic acid that seems to code for nothing at all; it is saved by scientists because it might be useful someday. Also called "silent DNA."

juvenile Characteristic of the period between onset of puberty and the end of adolescence.

juvenile Huntington's disease See **Huntington's disease.**

juvenile myoclonic epilepsy See **epilepsy, juvenile myoclonic.**

K

"K"   Street name for phencyclidine (PCP).

K alpha   Type of microarousal characterized by a K-complex followed by several seconds of alpha rhythm in the electroencephalogram.

K-complex   Sharp, biphasic electroencephalographic waves followed by high-voltage slow waves. The complex duration is at least 0.5 seconds and may be accompanied by a sleep spindle. They occur spontaneously during non rapid eye movement (NREM) sleep, and they begin and define stage-2 sleep. They are considered evoked responses to internal stimuli. They can also be elicited during sleep by external (particularly auditory) stimuli. See **sleep spindles.**

Kainever   See **estazolam.**

kainic acid   (KA) Glutamic analog and neurotoxin also used to define an excitatory amino acid receptor subtype.

Kantor   See **minaprine.**

Kaplan-Meier product

limit method   Technique for analyzing survival for censored observations. It uses exact survival times in the calculations.

kappa   **1.** Statistical technique for quantifying diagnostic reliability and categorical judgments, indexing agreement among clinicians, and correcting for chance agreement. Values range from 21 (total disagreement) to +1 (perfect agreement), with 0 indicating no more than chance agreement. Kappa also includes inter-rater reliability and a measure of the degree of nonrandom agreement between observers. **2.** Subset of opioid receptors that may mediate analgesia.

kappa receptor   Subtype of opioid mu receptors. Kappa receptors respond to dynorphin, ketazocine, and pentazocine. They appear to be involved in spinal anesthesia and sedation. It has been suggested that mu, delta, and kappa receptors are interchangeable forms of a single opioid receptor complex (Barnard EA, Demoliosi-Maron C. Molecular properties of opioid receptors. *Br Med Bull* 1983;39:37–46) See **opioid receptor.**

kappa statistic   Calculation devised by Cohen (1960) to correct for chance agreement by taking base rates into account to calculate what proportion of the maximum possible chance-corrected rate of agreement was obtained. Chance rate of agreement is subtracted from the observed rate of agreement, and the difference is divided by the maximum possible rate of chance-corrected agreement (i.e., 1 minus the chance rate of agreement). Studies that determine the level of diagnostic

agreement between two interviewers or two instruments use the kappa statistic (chance-corrected concordance) rather than simply reporting the percentage of agreement. In modest-sized samples, however, when a diagnosis occurs at a very low base rate, kappa has high variability; thus, many studies only calculate kappa for diagnoses occurring 5% or more of the time. Kappa values greater than approximately 0.75 are generally taken to indicate excellent agreement beyond chance; values below approximately 0.40 are generally taken to represent poor agreement beyond chance; and values in between are generally taken to represent fair to good agreement. Weighted kappa in large samples is approximately equivalent to the intraclass correlation, interpretable as a proportion of variance. Thus, a kappa value of 0.40 suggests that approximately 40% of the variance in the diagnoses made by two instruments is due to true differences in diagnosis among patients, whereas 60% is due to other things, such as instrument error (Perry JC. Problems and considerations in the valid assessment of personality disorders. *Am J Psychiatry* 1992;149:1645–1653).

karyotype   Visual representation of an individual's chromosomes that may reveal deletions, rearrangements, translocations, and other abnormalities.

karyotyping   Morphological analysis of a karyotype that allows detection of abnormal karyotypes that are the genetic basis of a disorder (e.g., Down syndrome).

Kayser-Fleischer ring   (KF) Greenish-brown pigmentation in the cornea at the sclerocorneal junction that is seen on slit-lamp examination and is pathognomonic of Wilson's disease.

"kee"   Street name for cannabinoids.

Kemadren   See **procyclidine.**

Kemadrin   See **procyclidine.**

Kemadrine   See **procyclidine.**

Kendall's terminology   System of describing particular cases in querying theory developed by D.G. Kendall (1953). It is based on initial letters of key words associated with the input, queue discipline, and service mechanism of a congestion situation. For example, D/G/K stands for a queue with deterministic (usually equally spaced arrivals), general service time distribution, and K servers.

Kendall's tau   Nonparametric measure statistic used in reliability of validity analysis, sometimes in place of Spearman's rank order correlation. Given a pair of ranks for each of several individuals, the tau statistic can be computed to express the degree of relationship between the ranks.

Kendall's W   Nonparametric measure statistic used in reliability of validity analysis.

Kerlone   See **betaxolol.**

Ketalar   See **ketamine.**

ketamine   (Ketalar) Structural analog of phencyclidine (PCP) synthesized in 1962 and available since 1969 as a surgical anesthetic. It has dose-dependent psychoactive properties similar to those of PCP; it produces psychotic phenomena in normal persons and stimulates active psychosis in schizophrenic patients even when they are taking antipsychotic medication. Although not manufactured illicitly, it has been subject to abuse, but never as widely as PCP. See **emergence phenomena.**

ketamine abuse   Once used as an adulterant in 3,4-methylenedioxymethamphetamine ("ecstasy"), ketamine is now sold on the street in pure form. It can be injected intravenously, but most abusers currently use it intranasally or orally. It can cause brief (30 minutes) psychological dissociation, hallucinations, and phenomena that may include subjective experiences of being out of the body or states similar to near-death experience. It also may cause movement disturbances (stereotypies, severe loss of coordination) and pronounced analgesia. It has been associated with "flashbacks." In some people, it may produce compulsive, repeated use; cases of self-administered injections several times daily over prolonged periods have been reported. People under the influence of ketamine are best placed in a quiet, darkened room until they recover. Diazepam may be given for unresponsive panic attacks (Jansen KLR. Nonmedical use of ketamine. *Br Med J* 1993;306: 601–602).

ketamine + tranylcypromine   There is a single case report of co-administration precipitating an adrenergic crisis. Another report described safe anesthesia induction with ketamine in a patient treated with tranylcypromine (20 mg/day for 7 weeks), although the author conceded that the absence of ill effects may have been "due more to good luck and careful anesthetic management than to the lack of interaction" (Doyle DJ. Ketamine induction and monoamine oxidase inhibitors. *J Clin Anesthesiol* 1990;2:324–325).

ketanserin   Selective serotonin (5-HT)$_2$ antagonist that distinguishes between 5-HT$_2$ and 5-HT$_{1C}$ receptors. It has anxiolytic and antidepressant properties and may be beneficial in "neuroleptic-resistant" schizophrenia.

ketazolam   (Anxon; Loftran; Unakalm) Benzodiazepine anxiolytic; major metabolite is desmethyldiazepam.

ketoconazole   (Nizoral) Cortisol biosynthesis inhibitor; 400–800 mg/day causes a transient decrease in plasma cortisol levels. Continuous use can lead to a chronic state of hypocortisolism that may be associated with psychotic symptoms, including hallucinations. It has been used with favorable results in some patients with treatment-resistant major depression. Ketoconazole-associated decreases in cortisol levels have been significantly correlated with decreases in Beck depression ratings (p = 0.01) (Wolkowitz OM, Reus VI, Manfredi F, et al. Ketoconazole administration in hypercortisolemic depression. *Am J Psychiatry* 1993;150: 810–812).

"key"   Street name for cannabinoids.

khat   Amphetamine-like compound with an active alkaloid component, cathinone, that closely resembles ephedrine and amphetamine in chemical structure. It has been commonly used for centuries in east African societies. Users chew the leaves of the khat shrub (*Catha edulis*) for its stimulating effects. It produces euphoria and increased alertness, although concentration and judgment are objectively impaired (Pantelis C, Hindler CG, Taylor JC. Use and abuse of Khat [cathedulis]: a review of the distribution, pharmacology, side effects and a description of psychosis attributed to Khat chewing. *Psychol Med* 1989;19:657–668). Users gather in rooms called *muffraji* where they normally chew 100–200 g of leaves and stems over 3–4 hours. Like amphetamine, high doses of khat can cause paranoia, psychosis, and aggression. It is unlikely that the active principle cathinone will appear in pure form on the drug market because it is difficult to extract from the leaves; amphetamine, which has practically the same effects and a more persistent action, is easier to synthesize. Nevertheless, following a World Health Organization (WHO) proposal, cathinone has been included in Schedule I of the U.N. Convention on Psychotropic Substances (Kalix P. Chewing khat, an old drug habit that is new in Europe. *Int J Risk Safety Med* 1992;3:143–156).

"kibbles and bits"   Street term for 2-pentazocine (Talwin) plus 2-methylphenidate (Ritalin) tablets, which are emulsified and injected by abusers.

"kick"   **1.** Street term for muscle jerks and contractions during opiate withdrawal. **2.** Street name for abused solvents and inhalants.

"kicking"   **1.** Street term for withdrawal from heroin, based on the central nervous system hyperexcitability and hyper-reflexia that often occurs. **2.** Street term for drawing blood from the vein back into the syringe and reinjecting it with a cocaine mixture to produce what users call a "rush."

killer T cell   See **cytotoxic T cell.**

kilobase   (kb) Unit of 1,000 bases in DNA or RNA.

kindling   Term coined by Goddard et al. (1969) to describe the consequences of repeated subthreshold electrical or chemical stimuli that progressively increase electrographic convulsive and behavioral responses and eventually culminate in a seizure. Subsequent application of a single subthreshold stimulus will again evoke a seizure. Eventually, chronic seizures can be produced without evidence of gross tissue damage. Kindling occurs most readily in limbic structures such as the amygdala. Pharmacological kindling can be induced by systematically administered metrazol, lidocaine, or cocaine. The process may explain the tendency for alcohol withdrawal symptoms to recur more rapidly and to increase in severity with repeated episodes of drinking. Kindling is associated with induction of transcription factors of immediate early genes (e.g., c-fos, fos-related antigens, zif-268) and other factors that may play a crucial role in binding to DNA and regulating transcription of transmitting receptors, neuropeptides, trophic growth factors, and enzymes involved in neurotransmitter biosynthesis and release (Post RM. Issues in the long-term management of bipolar affective illness. *Psychiatr Ann* 1993;23:86–93).

kindling, electrical   See **kindling.**

kindred   Having similar qualities.

kinesia paradoxica   Rare condition in which severely akinetic subjects respond more quickly than expected when faced with startling or threatening stimuli.

kinesthesia   Sensory perception of motion. Also called "proprioception."

kinesthetic hallucination   See **hallucination, kinesthetic.**

kinesthetic sensation   Sensation derived from muscles, joints, and inner ear responsible for the perception of body weight, position, location, and movement.

kinetic tremor   See **tremor, kinetic.**

kinetics, first order   See **pharmacokinetics, linear.**

kinetics, linear   See **pharmacokinetics, linear.**

kinetics, nonlinear   See **pharmacokinetics, nonlinear.**

kinetochore   Structure near the centromere of the chromosome that the chromosome binds to the mitotic spindle.

kleptomania   Common disorder manifested by compulsive stealing. The feature that distin-

guishes kleptomania from ordinary stealing is the conscious urge to steal which, although resisted, is in the end irresistible; kleptomaniacs steal for symptom relief rather than for personal gain. Kleptomania is more common in women. It begins by age 20 in about 50% of all cases. There are three main patient groups: those who present with kleptomania as the primary psychiatric illness; shoplifters; and patients with eating disorders. High rates of other forms of psychiatric illness, especially mood disorders, are found in all groups. There appears to be a spectrum of stealing behavior, with kleptomania occupying the severe end of the range. Reasons for impulsive stealing are unknown.

klismaphilia   Sexually motivated enema, evidence of which is frequently found among individuals who experienced fatal autoerotic asphyxia.

Klonopin   See **clonazepam.**

Kluver-Bucy syndrome   Bilateral temporal lobe loss of function manifested by visual agnosia, increased oral activity, hypermetamorphosis, lack of aggressive affect, and hypersexuality of all sorts. It can be induced by various neuroleptics. Onset is acute. Symptoms can be moderated with intramuscular antiparkinson agents (Varga E, Haher EJ, Simpson GM. Neuroleptic-induced Kluver-Bucy syndrome. *Biol Psychiatry* 1979;10:65–68).

knowledge information processing system (KIPS) System that uses "fifth-generation" computers that are expected to be capable of handling 10^8–10^9 LIPS (logical inferences per second), compared to earlier computers that handled 10^4–10^5 LIPS.

Korsakoff's psychosis   See **alcohol amnestic disorder.**

Korsakoff's syndrome   See **alcohol amnestic disorder.**

Kruskal-Wallis one-way ANOVA test   Nonparametric analysis of variance comparing mean values of more than two groups. When two parallel groups are compared for only one item, the Kruskal-Wallis test can be used.

Kruskal-Wallis test   Multisample rank randomization test for identical populations that is sensitive to unequal locations. It is a direct generalization of the two-sample Wilcoxon rank sum test to the multisample case.

"krystal"   Street name for phencyclidine (PCP).

"kw"   Street name for phencyclidine (PCP).

kynurenic acid   (KYNA) Product of the metabolism of tryptophan that is a nonspecific antagonist at glutamate/aspartate receptor sites. Brain KYNA is preferentially produced in astrocytes by enzymatic transamination of L-kynurenine.

kynurenine Neuroactive tryptophan metabolite. Plasma concentration is markedly increased at the peak of pharmacologically induced anxiety and returns to normal after anxiety has abated. It may be involved in caffeine-induced anxiety in humans, since the anxiogenic action of caffeine is associated with an increase in kynurenine plasma concentration.

L

la belle indifference   Inappropriate lack of emotion or concern for the implications of one's disability.

labetalol   (Normodyne; Trandate) Drug with beta- and alpha-adrenergic receptor blocking effects used to attenuate autonomic changes associated with electroconvulsive therapy, especially hypertension and tachycardia, and possibly arrhythmias.

labetalol + electroconvulsive therapy (ECT)   Labetalol, a beta-blocker, is commonly prescribed to modify the hypertensive/tachycardia response to an ECT-induced seizure. Since beta-blockers may increase the risk of bradycardia or asystole if a subconvulsive electrical stimulus is administered, pretreatment with an anticholinergic agent (e.g., glycopyrrolate or atropine) is indicated (Kellner CH. Labetalol and ECT. *J Clin Psychiatry* 1991;52:386–387).

labetalol + imipramine   In adults taking labetalol (200 mg/day), a single dose of imipramine (IMI) (100 mg) resulted in decreased hydroxylation of IMI and its metabolite desipramine (DMI), higher plasma levels, and increased half-life of IMI and DMI. Inhibition of mephenytoin oxygenase decreases the demethylation rate of IMI to DMI, leading to an increased IMI/DMI ratio. This change is reflected in serum levels (Hermann DJ, Krol TF, Dukes GE, et al. Comparison of verapamil, diltiazem, and labetalol on the bioavailability and metabolism of imipramine. *J Clin Pharmacol* 1992;32:176–183).

lability, emotional   See **emotional lability.**

laboratory accuracy   The production of correct test results, which depend on the calibration of the appropriate measuring instrument with reliable standards. See **laboratory precision.**

laboratory precision   Ability to reproduce results on the same or different days, and at different laboratories.

lack of insight   See **insight, lack of.**

lactate infusion test   Well established laboratory research procedure involving infusion of 0.5–1.0 M of sodium lactate dissolved in normal saline at a rate of 10 ml/kg bodyweight for 20 minutes. It provokes physiological and psychological symptoms of panic in panic disorder (PD) patients at a significantly higher rate than in normal control subjects or patients with other psychiatric disorders without co-existing PD. Imipramine greatly decreases lactate-induced anxiety, whereas placebo has no effect. The test has been used to explore a variety of questions regarding PD phenomenology.

Ladormin   See **brotizolam.**

Ladorum   See **brotizolam.**

Ladose   See **fluoxetine.**

"lady"   Street name for cocaine.

lag time   **1.** Interval between drug ingestion and its initial appearance in the systemic circulation. It is attributable to drug dissolution in gastric fluid; passage of the solution to the site of absorption in the proximal small bowel; absorption through the gastrointestinal tract mucosa into the portal circulation; and passage through hepatic circulation into systemic blood. Typical lag time is 10–20 minutes, but actual values vary from person to person and drug to drug. **2.** Interval between onset of drug therapy and appearance of its full therapeutic benefit (e.g., cyclic antidepressant drugs require 2–6 weeks' administration for occurrence of therapeutic effects). It may be due to pharmacokinetic and/or pharmacodynamic effects.

Lamictal   See **lamotrigine.**

lamotrigine   (Lamictal) New anticonvulsant chemically unrelated to other anticonvulsants. It is believed to exert its antiepileptic effect by inhibiting release of excitatory amino acid neurotransmitters. Its profile of action in an experimental model of epilepsy is similar to that of carbamazepine and phenytoin. Elimination half-life is about 24 hours; elimination is largely as the glucuronide conjugate. Advantages include infrequent impairment of cognitive function and apparent lack of effect on the metabolism of some other drugs. Lamotrigine's metabolism, however, is induced by carbamazepine, phenytoin, and phenobarbital (half-life about 15 hours) and inhibited by sodium valproate (half-life about 60 hours). Dosage in refractory epilepsy therefore depends on concomitant treatment. Results in placebo-controlled, add-on studies are encouraging, and lamotrigine is undergoing comparative trials in newly diagnosed epileptic patients in the United States. Clinical experience suggests that efficacy in patients with chronic partial epilepsies is as good as that with vigabatrin, although individual patients may do better on one drug than the other. Lamotrigine, however, may prove to be more effective than vigabatrin for primary generalized seizures. It reduces glutamate release and thus may protect nerve cells in Huntington's disease (HD); it is being investigated to determine its effectiveness in slowing the rate of progression of HD. It causes allergic rash in about 5% of patients (usually in the first 4 weeks of treatment) that disappears when treatment is stopped. Other side effects include weakness, diplopia, blurred vision, headache, drowsiness, ataxia, dizziness, nausea, and irritability. It also has been reported to cause aggressive reactions. About 8% of patients have been withdrawn from studies because of unwanted effects (Betts T. Safety of lamotrigine. Clinical update on lamotrigine: a novel antiepileptic agent. *Int Clin Pract Series* 1992;2:61–66).

lamotrigine + carbamazepine Lamotrigine increases the serum concentration of carbamazepine (CBZ) epoxide, an active metabolite of CBZ, thereby causing adverse effects such as dizziness and diplopia (Warner T, Patsalos PN, Prevett M, et al. Lamotrigine-induced carbamazepine toxicity: an interaction with carbamazepine-10,11-epoxide. *Epilepsy Res* 1992;11:147–150). CBZ, by inducing liver enzymes, can halve lamotrigine's half-life.

lamotrigine + oral contraceptive Lamotrigine does not interfere with oral contraceptive efficacy (Brodie MJ. Lamotrigine. *Lancet* 1992; 339:1397–1400).

lamotrigine overdose A case of deliberate self-poisoning (1350 mg) was reported in a 26-year-old man with a history of temporal lobe epilepsy. On hospital arrival, pulse was 96, blood pressure was 154/90, and temperature was 36° C (96.8° F). He was flushed, but bowel sounds were normal. He was alert and oriented, but had horizontal and vertical nystagmus and was hypertonic with brisk reflexes. Full blood count, electrolytes, and biochemistry were normal except for a K^+ of 3.3 mmol/L. Liver and renal function were normal. Lamotrigine levels at 3 and 17 hours after overdose were 17.4 and 6.4 µg/mL, respectively. Electrocardiogram (ECG) showed QRS width of 112 ms. The patient was treated with gastric lavage and activated charcoal. The next day he had fine nystagmus and mild ataxia, but could walk unaided; reflexes and liver and renal function were normal. At 2-month follow-up, QRS width was less than 100 ms. Because ECG changes in this case suggest a possible arrhythmogenic effect in overdose, patients with QRS prolongation due to lamotrigine poisoning should receive close ECG monitoring (Buckley NA, Whyte IM, Dawson AH. Self-poisoning with lamotrigine. *Lancet* 1993;342:1552–1553).

lamotrigine + phenobarbital Phenobarbital, by inducing liver enzymes, can reduce lamotrigine's half-life (Anon: Lamotrigine—an add-on antiepileptic. *Drug Ther Bull* 1992;30:75–76).

lamotrigine + phenytoin Phenytoin, by inducing liver enzymes, can halve lamotrigine's half-life (Anon. Lamotrigine—an add-on antiepileptic. *Drug Ther Bull* 1992;30:75–76).

lamotrigine + primidone Primidone accelerates lamotrigine elimination (Jawad S, Yuen AWC, Peck AW, et al. Lamotrigine: single dose pharmacokinetics and initial one week exposure in refractory seizures. *Epilepsy Res* 1987;1:196–201).

lamotrigine + valproate Small doses of lamotrigine combined with valproate may be useful in refractory idiopathic generalized epilepsies with typical absence seizures, potentially avoiding serious dose-related adverse effects (Panayiotopoulos CP, Ferric CD, Knott C, Robinson RO. Interaction of lamotrigine with sodium valproate. *Lancet* 1993;341:445). This combination also has benefitted children and adults with refractory partial seizures. In all cases, addition of valproate caused a striking increase in serum lamotrigine concentrations (Pisani F, DiPerri R, Perucca E, Richens A. Interaction of lamotrigine with sodium valproate. *Lancet* 1993;341:1224). Sodium valproate, which inhibits liver enzyme metabolism, may double the half-life of lamotrigine (Jawad S, Yuen WC, Peck AW, et al. Lamotrigine: single-dose pharmacokinetics and initial 1 week experience in refractory epilepsy. *Epilepsy Res* 1987;1:194–201; Yuen AWC, Land G, Weatherly BC, Peck AW. Sodium valproate acutely inhibits lamotrigine metabolism. *Br J Clin Pharmacol* 1992;33:511–513). The rise in serum lamotrigine concentrations may result in toxic symptoms (sedation, ataxia, fatigue) that remit after lamotrigine dosage reduction. Tremors also may occur, especially at higher doses (Reutens DC, Duncan JS, Patsalos PN. Disabling tremor after lamotrigine with sodium valproate. *Lancet* 1993;342:185–186).

lamotrigine + vigabatrin Co-administration has marked benefits in some patients with intractable seizures partially or fully refractory to either drug alone. Patients had clinical and electroencephalographic evidence of frequent secondary generalization that improved after lamotrigine was added to vigabatrin (Stewart J, Hughes E, Reynolds EH. Lamotrigine for generalized epilepsies. *Lancet* 1992;340:1223).

Landormin See brotizolam.

Lanexate See flumazenil.

language assessment battery Tests include (a) Peabody Picture Vocabulary Test—Revised Form (L); (b) Expressive One-Word Picture Vocabulary Test; (c) Test for Auditory Comprehension of Language Revised; (d) Test of Language Development—Intermediate; (e) Grammatic Comprehension; (f) Structured Photographic Expressive Language Test—Primary; (g) Structured Photographic Expressive Language Test—II; (h) Test of Language Development—Intermediate: Sentence Combining; (i) Rosner Test of Auditory Analysis and Segmentation; (j) Rosner Test of Auditory Analysis and Segmentation Extension; (k) Photo Articulation Test; (l) Token Test for Children; (m) McCarthy Scales—Verbal Memory; (n) Detroit Test of Learning Aptitudes—2: Word Sequences; (o) Detroit Test of Learning Aptitudes—2: Sentence Imitation (Cohen NJ, Davine M, Horodezky N, et al. Unsuspected language impairment in psychiatrically disturbed children: prevalence and language and behavioral characteristics. *J Am Acad Child Adolesc Psychiatry* 1993;32:595–603).

Laniazid   See **isoniazid.**

Lanoxin   See **digitalis.**

Lantanon   See **mianserin.**

Largactil   See **chlorpromazine.**

large sample method   Statistical method based on approximation to a normal distribution that becomes more accurate as sample size increases.

lark   In somnology, a daytime person. See **owl.**

Larodopa   See **levodopa.**

Laroxyl   See **amitriptyline.**

laryngopharyngeal dystonia   See **dystonia, laryngopharyngeal.**

laryngeal dystonia   See **dystonia, laryngeal.**

laser   Acronym for "light amplification by stimulated emission of radiation." A sample of atoms, excited to higher energy quantum states, can be induced to de-excite in a coordinated fashion, giving rise to an avalanche of photons that is monochromatic (at a single energy), intense, highly directional (i.e., can be formed into a beam of small divergence), and coherent (emissions are highly synchronized). Laser devices come in different forms with a variety of energy, power, and pulse characteristics. They are used in several surgical and diagnostic areas.

Lasix   See **furosemide.**

latchkey child   Child who comes home from school to an empty house or apartment because the parent or parents are working. There are several million such children in the United States.

latency, sleep   See **sleep latency.**

latent inhibition   (LI) Behavioral paradigm in which prior exposure to a stimulus not followed by reinforcement retards subsequent conditioning to that stimulus when it is paired with reinforcement. It is a process of learning to ignore, or tune out, irrelevant stimuli.

laterocollis   See **dystonia, cervical.**

Latin square   Square array of numbers or symbols repeated in columns and rows such that each element occurs only once in any column or row. It is used to remove from the experimental error the variation from two sources. A specimen design for a 5 × 5 square with five treatments (A, B, C, D, E) is:

A B C D E
B A E C D
C D A E B
D E B A C
E C D B A

The earliest recorded discussion of the Latin Square was given by Evler (1782), but it occurred in puzzles at a much earlier date. It was introduced into experimental design by R. A. Fisher.

"laughing gas"   Street/lay name for nitrous oxide.

laxative abuse   In some psychiatric disorders (e.g., anorexia, bulimia), excessive laxative use is common. It may cause chronic diarrhea. Constipation in bulimia can be quite uncomfortable and prolonged and associated with significant fluid retention; weight gain may be 5–15 pounds over 7–10 days after discontinuation of an abused stimulant-type laxative. This serves as a very powerful stimulus to continue taking the laxative. Abnormal laboratory findings associated with laxative abuse include hypocalcemia and other electrolyte abnormalities.

LD$_{50}$ See **median lethal dose.**

lead pipe rigidity   See **rigidity, lead pipe.**

learned helplessness   Behavioral phenomenon consisting of passivity, withdrawal, and hypoactivity after exposure to uncontrollable adverse effects. Learned helplessness is a commonly used animal model of depression wherein animals exposed to inescapable stressors exhibit decreased spontaneous activity, decreased effort to escape, and a variety of somatic changes that are reversed specifically by antidepressants (Sherman AD, Sacqurtine JL, Petty F. Specificity of the learned helplessness model of depression. *Pharmacol Biochem Behav* 1982;16:449–454). In animals with learned helplessness, dopamine depletion is in the caudate nucleus and the nucleus accumbens. Prior treatment with a dopamine agonist prevents development of the learned helplessness state. Conversely, dopamine antagonists exacerbate learned helplessness and prevent improvement with antidepressant treatment (Kapur S, Mann JJ. Role of the dopaminergic system in depression. *Biol Psychiatry* 1991;32: 1–7).

learning   Processes by which new information is acquired. Learning depends on sensory input. It is usually an incremental process that involves practice and requires some form of reinforcement.

lecithin Naturally occurring source of dietary choline found in many foods. It is used by the body to make acetylcholine. It has been used as a treatment for the cognitive impairments associated with Alzheimer's disease.

Lectopam See **bromazepam.**

Lenderm See **brotizolam.**

Lendorm See **brotizolam.**

Lendormin See **brotizolam.**

Lenitin See **bromazepam.**

Lenormin See **brotizolam.**

lentiform nucleus Part of the brain formed by the putamen and globus pallidus.

Lentizol See **amitriptyline.**

Leponex See **clonazepam.**

Lepotex See **clozapine.**

Lesch-Nyhan syndrome X-linked enzyme deficiency disorder, seen only in males, characterized by mental retardation, neuromuscular dysfunction (choreoathetosis, spasticity), and severe self-injurious behavior (SIB). Self-mutilation, not mental retardation, is the reason for most institutionalizations. The most striking characteristic is severe self-mutilation of lips, tongue, and fingers (as well as eye-gouging and head-banging). In some children self-injury is so intense that tooth extraction and constant restraint are used as last resorts. Children with Lesch-Nyhan syndrome and other self-injuring retarded children sometimes use self-restraint maneuvers to keep from hitting or injuring themselves, which suggests that there may be a compulsive component of SIB. Dopamine (DA) receptor super-sensitivity has been hypothesized in Lesch-Nyhan syndrome; low levels of DA and its metabolites have been demonstrated.

lethal catatonia See **catatonia, lethal.**

lethal gene See **gene, lethal.**

leucine-enkephalin See **enkephalin.**

leucine zipper Protein sequence in which every seventh amino acid, which would be located at every second turn of an alpha helix, is a leucine over a repeat length of 4–5 leucines.

leukoariosis Focal and bilateral periventricular lesions seen on computed tomography (hypodense lesion) and magnetic resonance imaging (hyperintense lesions on T2-weighted images). It is seen in Binswanger's disease and sometimes in normal elderly patients.

leukocytosis Increase in white blood cells that occurs normally during digestion and in pregnancy and as a pathological condition in inflammation. It also can be produced by lithium.

leukoencephalopathy Changes in brain white matter associated with aging. It can be demonstrated by imaging technologies such as computed tomography (CT) and magnetic resonance imaging (MRI). It is believed to be associated with increased water content in tissue due to cerebrovascular disease (Coffee CE, Fiegel GS, Djang WT, et al. Leukoencephalopathy in elderly depressed patients referred for ECT. *Biol Psychiatry* 1988;24:143–161).

leukopenia Reduction in the number of white blood cells (< 5000/ml). It occurs very rarely as a sensitivity reaction to some drugs (e.g., carbamazepine, thioridazine, chlorpromazine). It can be the precursor of agranulocytosis or aplastic anemia. If severe (< 500/ml), it increases susceptibility to infection and can be life-threatening.

leukotomy British term for prefrontal lobotomy. See **lobotomy.**

leuprolide acetate (Lupron) Synthetic analog of gonadotropin-releasing hormone (GnRH) that has 15 times the potency of the naturally occurring hormone. It is available by prescription for once-a-month injection. It may reduce premenstrual syndrome (PMS) symptoms, including depression, in women who meet criteria for PMS, but not in women with PMS and major depression (Freeman EW, Sondheimer SJ, Rickels K, Albert J. Gonadotropin-releasing hormone agonist in treatment of premenstrual symptoms with and without co-morbidity of depression: a pilot study. *J Clin Psychiatry* 1993;54:192–195).

leuprolide depot Long-acting luteinizing hormone releasing hormone (LHRH)-agonist being used to treat deviant sexual behavior. It has been reported to benefit a patient with multiple paraphilias resistant to medroxyprogesterone and cyproterone. He was given leuprolide depot (7.5 mg administered intramuscularly) once a month. Deviant sexual behavior stopped after 1 month. No side effects were reported (Dickey R. The management of a case of treatment-resistant paraphilia with a long-acting LHRH agonist. *Can J Psychiatry* 1992;37:567–569).

Levanxol See **temazepam.**

Levate See **amitriptyline.**

Levatol See **penbutolol.**

level of significance See **significance level.**

levodopa (Dopar; Larodopa) (L-dopa) Dopamine precursor that is the cornerstone of Parkinson's disease (PD) therapy. In the intact brain, it is produced by dopaminergic nerve terminals as an intermediary in the synthesis of dopamine from tyrosine. Oral L-dopa is absorbed rapidly from the small intestine by an active amino acid transport system. It is neither absorbed nor metabolized by the stomach. When administered alone, more than 95% is metabolized by decarboxylases during the first pass through the liver, and less than 1% reaches the brain. The dopamine produced by hepatic metabolism causes systemic toxicity. L-dopa can cause a variety of adverse reactions. Central nervous system side effects include nightmares, hallucinosis, psychosis, dyskinesia, dystonia, and "on-off" swings. Cardiovascular effects include faintness, postural hypotension, and arrhythmias. Gastrointestinal effects are nausea, vomiting, and anorexia. Other adverse reactions are increased libido, red urine, and rashes. Some of the difficulties can be circumvented by co-administration of a decarboxylase inhibitor (e.g., carbidopa, benserazide), which inhibits hepatic enzymes, but does not enter the brain. Varying ratios of L-dopa plus carbidopa (Sinemet) or L-dopa plus benserazide (Madopar) are the most frequently used formulations of L-dopa. Some patients also require supplemental administration of carbidopa alone. Patients treated with L-dopa should be monitored for muscle twitching and blepharospasm, which may be early signs of overdose. As PD progresses and L-dopa treatment continues for more than 2 years, L-dopa's duration of action shortens, producing end-of-dose akinesia (wearing off); the most common symptoms are slowness, stiffness, freezing, and falls. Pregnancy risk category C. See **akinesia, end of dose; freezing.**

levodopa/abnormal movements After 1 or 2 years of levodopa (L-dopa) therapy, some patients develop drug-induced dyskinesia manifested by athetoid, choreic, or dystonic movements that typically occur 1–3 hours after a dose, when dopamine brain levels are at their peak. Movements affecting the mouth, tongue, lips, and cheeks (oro-bucco-lingual dyskinesia) closely resemble the oro-bucco-lingual manifestations of tardive dyskinesia (TD). They include twisting, writhing, or darting (fly-catcher) tongue motions, and sucking, licking, swallowing, or protrusion of the lips and tongue. There also may be symptoms resembling spasmodic torticollis, as well as jerking, writhing, and dystonic distortions of the limbs and trunk. Dyskinesias induced by L-dopa can be disabling; they may be ameliorated by sleep and, less often, abolished by dosage reduction. They should not be confused with neuroleptic-induced TD.

levodopa + antihypertensive Co-administration may increase the hypotensive effects of each drug.

levodopa/benserazide (Madopar) Fixed-dose combination product used in the treatment of parkinsonism. It now has the generic name co-beneldopa. Marketed in England. Also called "Co-dieldopa."

levodopa/benserazide + moclobemide Studies in healthy volunteers indicate no contraindications to combination therapy (Dingemanse

J. An update of recent moclobemide interaction data. *Int Clin Psychopharmacol* 1993;7:167–180). This is in keeping with the finding that moclobemide only slightly increases brain dopamine concentration (Da Prada M, Zucher G, Wuthrich I, Haefely WE. On tyramine, food, beverages and the reversible MAO inhibitor moclobemide. *J Neural Transm* 1988; 26[suppl]:31–56). Further studies are needed in Parkinson's disease patients, since the central effects of levodopa therapy cannot be investigated easily in healthy volunteers.

levodopa + benzodiazepine Co-administration may decrease levodopa's therapeutic effects.

levodopa + bupropion In patients receiving levodopa (L-dopa), bupropion should be given cautiously, using small initial doses and small gradual dose increases. Co-administration has resulted in a high incidence of adverse reactions, including nausea, vomiting, agitation, excitement, restlessness, and tremor (Watskey EJ, Salzman C. Psychotropic drug interactions. *Hosp Community Psychiatry* 1991; 42:247–256; Goetz CG, Tanner CM, Klawans HL. Bupropion in Parkinson's disease. *Neurology* 1984;34:1092–1094).

levodopa/carbidopa (Dopicar; Sinemet; Sinemet CR) Most commonly used formulation of levodopa (L-dopa) in the United States. It is available with varying ratios of L-dopa and carbidopa. In most patients, carbidopa (75 mg/day) is sufficient to inhibit peripheral decarboxylation of L-dopa. Larger amounts can be given by using Sinemet formulations with higher ratios of carbidopa to L-dopa, or by supplemental administration of carbidopa alone. The latest formulation is a controlled release compound (Sinemet CR) containing L-dopa (200 mg) and carbidopa (50 mg) in an erodible matrix. It produces a slower rise and longer plateau in L-dopa plasma concentration when compared with standard Sinemet. Patients switched from standard Sinemet to Sinemet CR often require a 25–35% increase in total daily L-dopa dosage. Advantages of Sinemet CR include reduced frequency of dosing, more physiological dopamine replacement, increased "on" time, improved bed mobility and sleep, and improved early morning performance. In at least some patient populations, it may reduce dose-related fluctuations and side effects. Disadvantages include increased dyskinesias, delayed onset of action, lack of surge associated with standard Sinemet, less predictable fluctuations, and increased night-time hallucinations (Standaert DG, Stern MB. Update on the management of Parkinson's disease. *Med Clin North Am* 1993; 77:169–183). Also called "co-careldopa."

levodopa/carbidopa + clozapine   Some psychotic parkinsonism patients tolerate and respond well to co-administration; in others it may produce mild to marked orthostatic hypotension and obtunded sensorium (Wolk SI, Douglas CJ. Clozapine treatment of psychosis in Parkinson's disease: a report of five consecutive cases. *J Clin Psychiatry* 1992;53:373–376).

levodopa/carbidopa + fluoxetine   See **levodopa + fluoxetine.**

levodopa/carbidopa + phenelzine   Co-administration in depressed Parkinson's disease (PD) patients may produce moderate to marked improvement in both PD and depression. Co-administration of a monoamine oxidase inhibitor (MAOI) and levodopa (L-dopa) is usually avoided because of the reported risk of serious side effects, specifically hypertensive crisis. The combination with carbidopa may allow safer use of MAOIs (Hargrave R, Ashford JW. Phenelzine treatment of depression in Parkinson's disease. *Am J Psychiatry* 1992; 148:1751–1752).

levodopa + diazepam   Diazepam may inhibit the therapeutic effect of levodopa.

levodopa/fluctuations   In the early months of levodopa (L-dopa) therapy, there usually is a smooth response throughout the day. After 1–3 years, fluctuations in motor performance often develop; they occur in over 50% of patients after 5 years' treatment. They are related to Parkinson's disease severity and duration, and to duration of L-dopa treatment. They include end-of-dose wearing off; early morning wearing off; decreasing duration of "on" phase; freezing and falls; peak-dose dyskinesia in "on" phase; painful end-of-dose dystonia; diphasic dyskinesia; and a variety of ballistic, stereotyped, myoclonic movements and behavior disturbances.

levodopa + fluoxetine   Fluoxetine may be responsible for hallucinations in patients being treated with levodopa (Lauterbach EC. Dopaminergic hallucinosis with fluoxetine in Parkinson's disease. *Am J Psychiatry* 1993;150:1750).

levodopa + haloperidol   Co-administration may interfere with the therapeutic effect of levodopa.

levodopa + monoamine oxidase inhibitor (MAOI)   Levodopa (L-dopa) should not be used with nonselective or type A MAOIs because of the potential risk of appreciable rises in blood pressure or severe hypertensive crisis secondary to the release of increased amounts of catecholamine at central nervous system nerve endings or from the adrenals (Hunter KR, Boakes AJ, Lawrence DR, Stern GM. Monoamine oxidase inhibitors and l-dopa. *Br Med J* 1970;3:388). A tetracyclic antidepressant or selegiline (20–30 mg/day) may be an effective strategy for treating depression in Parkinson's disease. A nonselective or type A MAOI should be discontinued for at least 2 weeks before L-dopa is started. Co-administration of L-dopa and selective MAOI-Bs has not given rise to any adverse effects.

levodopa/"on-off"   Attacks that appear after years of levodopa (L-dopa) therapy, usually after the advent of L-dopa-induced dyskinesia and dystonia. The "on" phase occurs at peak dose when the patient is mobile and independent, but often has a variety of dyskinesias. The "off" phase consists of sudden "freezing" and immobility associated with fear and panic. Dyskinesia in the "on" phase is most evident in the limbs most affected with parkinsonian signs. Smaller, more frequent L-dopa doses may in part ease this difficult problem.

levodopa + orphenadrine   Co-administration for the treatment of parkinsonism may have a synergistic beneficial effect.

levodopa/psychiatric symptoms   Levodopa (L-dopa) may cause night-time restlessness, vivid dreams, nightmares, myoclonic jerks in the twilight state, toxic confusional states, visual hallucinations with insight, delusions, altered sleep/wake cycles, and (rarely) aggressive behavior. It may aggravate or sometimes relieve depression. Many psychiatric symptoms are dose-related and may be relieved by appropriate dosage adjustments. Chronic confusional states are infrequent and may be mistaken for dementia, which is seldom truly caused by chronic L-dopa therapy.

levodopa + reserpine   Co-administration may result in hyperexcitability, mania, or memory impairment.

levodopa + selegiline   Co-administration may reduce wearing-off phenomena and fluctuations, although the degree of improvement is modest; in some patients, selegiline may aggravate levodopa-related toxic effects such as hallucinations and dyskinesias (Standaert DG, Stern MB. Update on the management of Parkinson's disease. *Med Clin North Am* 1993; 77:169–183).

levodopa test   Test to help confirm the diagnosis of idiopathic parkinsonism. It also may have some predictive value. All therapy is discontinued for 24 hours. A clinical rating scale is completed at −30 minutes and at 0 hours. The fasting patient is given levodopa (50 mg) at 8 or 9 AM and carbidopa (50 mg) or levodopa (400 mg) and benserazide (50 mg). At the peak of improvement (usually 45–150 minutes), the clinical rating scale is again completed. Positive response is a 25% improvement (Pearce JMS. *Parkinson's Disease* and Its Management. New York: Oxford University Press, 1992).

levomepromazine (Levoprome; Minozinan; Nozinan) Aliphatic phenothiazine neuroleptic with potent antihistaminic, anticholinergic, and antiadrenergic properties, as well as potent central nervous system effects that suppress sensory impulses, reduce motor activity, and provide significant sedation. It raises pain threshold and produces amnesia; it is recommended primarily for the treatment of pain in nonambulatory patients (e.g., in obstetrical analgesia where respiratory suppression must be avoided) and for preanesthetic sedation. As a sedative, it induces calming in very agitated, anxious, combative, or otherwise overtly disturbed patients. Intramuscular administration yields a very rapid onset of action. Dosage is usually given in 10- to 20-mg increments as needed for pain and/or sedation. Side effect profile is similar to that of other sedating neuroleptics. Hypotension can be a major limiting factor with syncope or falling, especially in the elderly. Levomepromazine is available in the United States, but not listed in the current *Physician's Desk Reference*. No oral formulation is available in the United States, but it is widely used in Canada and Europe. Also called "methotrimeprazine."

levomepromazine + clomipramine Co-administration significantly increases clomipramine plasma level (Balant-Gorgia AE, Balant LP, Genet C, et al. Importance of oxidative polymorphism and levomepromazine treatment on the steady-state blood concentrations of clomipramine and its major metabolites. *Eur J Clin Pharmacol* 1986;31:449–455).

levomepromazine + fluvoxamine In a 26-year-old woman with schizotypal personality disorder and obsessive-compulsive disorder, addition of fluvoxamine (50 mg/day) to maintenance treatment (1.5 years) with levomepromazine (800 mg/day) led to development of tonic-clonic seizures (Grinspoon A, Berg Y, Mozes T, et al. Seizures induced by combined levomepromazine-fluvoxamine treatment. *Int Clin Psychopharmacol* 1993;8:61–62).

levomethadyl acetate (Orlaam) (LAAM) Synthetic opiate agonist that can produce morphine-like effects when ingested orally. In 1993, the U.S. Food and Drug Administration (FDA) approved it for the treatment of opioid dependence. LAAM (80 mg) is comparable to methadone (100 mg) with respect to safety and various measures of efficacy; it thus may be an important transitional medication for weaning patients from methadone (Greenstein RA, Fudala PJ, O'Brien CP. Alternative pharmacotherapies for opiate addiction. *In* Lowinson JH, Ruiz P, Millman RB, Langrod JG [eds], *Substance Abuse. A Comprehensive Textbook*, 2nd ed. Baltimore: Williams & Wilkins, 1992, pp 562–573). It has a slower onset and longer duration of action (average, 72 hours) than methadone because of formation of two active metabolites, noracetylmethadol and dinoracetylmethadol. Because LAAM is a prodrug, intravenous administration produces a slower onset of action than oral administration does. Abuse potential is therefore negligible. The long duration of action allows administration 3 times weekly (usually Monday-Wednesday-Friday) or every other day, reducing the need for daily clinic visits. Dosage must be carefully individualized for each patient; the slow onset of action increases risk of accidental overdosage. Like methadone, LAAM is subject to narcotic treatment regulations. It may be dispensed only by narcotic treatment programs approved by the FDA, the Drug Enforcement Administration, and the designated state methadone authority. Unlike methadone, however, LAAM dosage units may not be taken away from the clinic (Nightingale SL. Levomethadyl approved for the treatment of opiate dependence. *JAMA* 1993;270:1290).

Levophed See **norepinephrine tartrate.**

Levoprome See **levomepromazine.**

levoprotiline (LVP) Hydroxylated derivative of maprotiline and pure R(–) enantiomer of oxaprotiline that, in contrast to the (+)-enantiomer, does not inhibit noradrenaline uptake. It exhibits antidepressant properties contrary to the prediction of the catecholamine hypothesis. It enhances functional responsiveness toward 5-hydroxytryptophan and dopamine agonists, and reduces serotonin synthesis. It is comparable in antidepressant efficacy to clomipramine. Its mode of action differs from that of any known compound (Noguchi S, Okada M, Inukai T. Pharmacological profile of the new antidepressant levoprotiline. *Arzneim Forsch* 1992;42:787–794). In two trials it significantly resembled placebo in antidepressant potential, suggesting that noradrenaline uptake is not necessary for its observed therapeutic effect (Katz RJ, Lott M, Landau P, Waldmeier P. A clinical test of noradrenergic involvement in the therapeutic mode of action of an experimental antidepressant. *Biol Psychiatry* 1993;33:261–266). It is undergoing clinical trials in Europe.

levosulpiride New antidepressant that increases dopaminergic transmission by blocking presynaptic dopamine receptors. It has been compared with clomipramine in major depression and found to be an effective antidepressant.

Levothroid See **thyroxine.**

levothyroxine (Synthroid) Synthetic thyroxine (T_4) that is similar to that produced in the human thyroid gland. It is a levorotatory isomer T_4 formed by the coupling of two molecules of diiodotyrosine. It is used as replacement or supplemental therapy in patients with hypothyroidism of any etiology, except transient hypothyroidism. Dosage and rate of administration is determined by indication; it must be individualized in every case according to patient response and laboratory findings.

levothyroxine/bipolar disorder Addition of levothyroxine to the usual medication regimen of refractory rapid cycling bipolar patients has been shown to be effective in both the depressive and manic phases (Bauer MS, Whybrow PC. Rapid cycling bipolar affective disorder, II: treatment of refractory rapid cycling with high-dose levothyroxine: a preliminary study. *Arch Gen Psychiatry* 1990;47:435–440).

Lewy bodies Intracytoplasmic inclusion bodies immunoreactive to ubiquitin. They are found in nerve cells, especially in pigmented brainstem neurons. They are found in 5–10% of normal brains of people over age 60, in 10% of cases of Alzheimer's disease, and in practically every case of Lewy body dementia and parkinsonism. Their presence is not diagnostic, however, and their numbers do not correlate with the duration or the severity of the diseases in which they are found. In idiopathic Parkinson's disease, they are found in the substantia nigra, locus cerulcus, substantia innominata, hypothalamus, dorsal medulla, and sympathetic ganglia, and they are associated with disruption of melanin-containing nerve cells. Lewy body disease may cause paranoid symptoms, dementia, depression, or parkinsonism. See **dementia, Lewy body.**

Lexotan See **bromazepam.**

Lexotanil See **bromazepam.**

liaison psychiatry Specialty predominantly concerned with psychiatric disorders in the general hospital setting. It includes psychiatric management of patients who present with physical symptoms or deliberately harm themselves and treatment of psychiatric illness in physically ill patients. It involves cooperation with nonpsychiatric physicians, psychologists, nurses, and other health care workers.

Libritabs See **chlordiazepoxide.**

Librium See **chlordiazepoxide.**

"Librium rage" See **chlordiazepoxide.**

Licarbium See **lithium.**

"licorice" Street name for paregoric.

"lid" Street name for cannabinoids.

Lidanar See **mesoridazine.**

Lidanil See **mesoridazine.**

lidocaine (Xylocaine) Local anesthetic that prolongs the refractory period of the cardiac conduction system and increases the myocardial threshold to abnormal stimulation; it has been used successfully for many years to control tachyarrhythmias induced by electroconvulsive therapy.

Lidone See **molindone.**

life event Change or disruption in the pattern of living that may be associated with or produce changes in health.

life exit event Life event involving some form of permanent loss. Such events occur with significantly greater frequency in adults with depressive disorders than in control subjects. Likelihood of occurrence increases with age.

life table analysis Method for analyzing survival times for census observations that have been grouped into intervals.

lifetime prevalence Number of people who may have a disease any time during their lifetime.

ligand Diagnostic imaging agent for the central nervous system. Ligands usually are small molecules that bind to an acceptor or receptor. Several important characteristics set them apart from other pharmaceuticals or drugs; the most important is that they contain a short-lived radionucleotide or isotope. Ligands are essential to imaging techniques such as positron emission tomography (PET) and single photon emission computed tomography (SPECT). Also called "radiopharmaceutical."

ligand binding assay Use of a ligand radiolabeled to a high specific activity to detect the binding of the ligand to receptors. Such assays have been used extensively to determine the number and properties of receptors in brain and other tissues.

ligand binding study Attempt to discern the meaning of changes in receptor function by measuring receptor density and ligand affinity in tissue. To date it is not known whether observed changes in receptor number or affinity are functionally important.

ligase Enzyme that seals nicks in the sugar-phosphate chain.

ligase chain reaction (LCR) Recently (1991) developed amplification method to detect gene mutation. It uses the coupling of two adjacent synthetic oligonucleotides aligned on the template of the target DNA (Barany F. Genetic disease detection and DNA amplification using closed thermostable ligase. *Proc Natl Acad Sci U S A* 1991;88:189–193). Normal and mutant genes from individual patients can be amplified without cloning by such in vitro synthesis. LCR determines whether amplification occurs with normal or mutant pairs of oligonucleotides (Caskey CT. Molecular medicine. A spin-off from the helix. *JAMA* 1993;269:1986–1992).

light-dark cycle   Periodic pattern of light (artificial or natural) alternating with darkness.

"light drop"   Sudden lowering of the daily total solar irradiation of which visual light forms a generally fixed proportion. Light drops tend to be associated with onset of depression in some individuals. Variations in light intensity and amplitude in the autumn and spring could account for the seasonality of some affective disorders. In spring, a light drop–induced depressive phase may be arrested by the naturally improving light conditions at that time of the year (Summers L, Shur E. The relationship between onsets of depression and sudden drops in solar irradiation. *Biol Psychiatry* 1992;32:1164–1172).

light sleep   See **sleep, light.**

light therapy   See **phototherapy.**

likelihood ratio   Ratio of the joint probability under alternative hypotheses versus the joint probability under null hypotheses. Using this ratio as test statistics is called likelihood ratio test, which is widely used.

Likert scale   Commonly used measurement of attitudes. An attitudinal statement is followed by a five-choice scale (strongly disagree, disagree, uncertain, agree, strongly agree). Score usually is obtained by assigning the highest number (5) to "strongly agree." Results are factor-analyzed (Likert R. A technique for the measurement of attitudes. *In* Summers GF [ed], *Attitude Measurement*. Chicago: Rand McNally, 1970, pp 149–157).

"lilly"   Street name for amobarbital.

limbic system   Wishbone-shaped set of related brain structures associated with sense of smell, involuntary functions, emotions, and behavior. The hypothalamus is considered to be one main component of the limbic system. The limbic system comprises a heterogeneous group of functionally related structures surrounding the midbrain, including cingulate; parahippocampal; hippocampal; dentake gury; olfactory lobe, bulb, and tract; amygdaloid nucleus; anterior thalamic; systal and hippocampal nuclei; fornix; mammillothalamic tract; and stria terminals. They are closely interconnected with each other and also with the thalamus, hypothalamus, striatum, reticular activating system, and median forebrain bundle.

limbic-hypothalamic-pituitary-adrenal axis (LHPA) Axis along with the sympathetic nervous system that is activated in response to stress, major depression, and anxiety. The major input systems for this dual response are the locus ceruleus (LC) in the brainstem and the parvicellular portion of the paraventricular nucleus (PVN) of the hypothalamus.

Limbitrol   See **amitriptyline + chlordiazepoxide.**

Limovane   See **zopiclone.**

linear   Characteristic of a relationship in which the dependent and independent variables are best related by the equation $y = mx + b$, which yields a straight line in which m is the slope and b is the intercept on the y axis.

linear combination   Weighed average of a set of variables or measures (e.g., the prediction equation in multiple regression is a linear combination of the predictor variables).

linear pharmacokinetics   See **pharmacokinetics, linear.**

linear regression   See **regression, linear.**

linear relationship   Relationship indicating that x and y co-vary according to constant increments.

lingual dystonia   See **dystonia, cranial.**

linkage   Tendency of genetic variations (or alleles) at different chromosomal loci to be inherited together; two alleles close to each other on the chromosome are more likely to be inherited together than two that are further apart. Loci that are widely spaced (unlinked) assort independently because of recombination. Linkage between a disease locus and a genetic marker will only be detected if an appropriate mode of transmission is specified for the disease; otherwise, false-negative results may occur. Conversely, to exclude linkage confidently, it is necessary to show that sufficiently negative lod scores are obtained for all plausible genetic models.

linkage analysis   Search for genetic markers linked to genes. It takes advantage of genetic traits or phenotypic markers such as an enzyme deficiency occurring in individuals who also have mood disorder to demonstrate a genetic basis for the mood disorder. It seeks to show that the marker and the mood disorder are linked when they always occur together in studied families, meaning that there is a statistically high probability that the genetic marker and the disease genes are located close together on the same chromosome. Linkage analysis is a powerful technique for providing the chromosomal location of major genes that contribute to diseases with clear-cut inheritance patterns (e.g., Huntington's disease). It also may allow isolation of pathogenic proteins underlying other Mendelian disorders. In some disorders, however, linkage analysis may have limited power to detect major effects of genes that are etiological in only a small proportion of families. It has been used to study the molecular genetics of schizophrenia using (a) anonymous markers; (b) favored loci; and (c) candidate genes. To date the only positive finding is an unconfirmed linkage between chromosome 5q and schizophrenia (Kaufmann CA, Malspina D. Molecular genetics of schizophrenia. *Psychiatr Ann* 1993;23:111–112).

linkage disequilibrium Co-segregation of independent genetic markers (i.e., co-inheritance of genetic traits at a higher frequency than expected from independent segregation).

linkage map Determination of the relative positions of genetic loci on a chromosome, based on how often the loci are inherited together. Distance is measured in centimorgans.

linkage, record See **record linkage.**

linkage study Investigation of the co-segregation of genetic markers and the disease within families in which multiple members are affected. Linkage studies provide a means of identifying genetic loci that predispose to familial disorders.

Lioresal See **baclofen.**

liothyronine (Cynomel; Cytomel) Levorotary isomer of triiodothyronine (T_3). In subreplacement doses, it may potentiate the therapeutic effects of tricyclic antidepressants and convert nonresponders to responders. See **triiodothyronine.**

lipid solubility See **lipophilicity.**

lipophilicity Physiochemical property of drugs that influences the extent of drug distribution into peripheral tissue sites (e.g., adipose tissue and muscle) where the drug is pharmacologically inactive. The more lipophilic a compound, the more rapidly it crosses a lipoidal biological membrane such as the blood-brain barrier. A lipophilic drug may undergo extensive decline in plasma and brain concentrations after peak concentration is reached, which in turn may terminate its clinical action, regardless of elimination half-life. Lipophilicity also influences the equilibrium distribution ratio between brain tissue and the unbound component in plasma. All benzodiazepines are lipophilic substances, some more so or less so than others. Differences in lipophilicity may explain the apparent paradox that benzodiazepines with a long elimination half-life (e.g., diazepam) may have a shorter duration of action than agents with a short half-life. Also called "lipid solubility."

lipopigment Discrete or aggregated bodies that appear yellow or brown in unstained tissue sections. Lipopigment is present in many organs and cell types, including neurons. It is thought to be cellular debris partly derived from peroxidation of cellular constituents induced by free radicals. Volume of neuronal lipopigment has been positively correlated with advancing age, Alzheimer's dementia, and the neuronal ceroidoses, whereas various changes in neuronal lipopigment have been reported in association with chronic administration of certain drugs (e.g., alcohol, chlorpromazine).

lipoprotein High-molecular-weight (10^5–10^6 dalton) complex of lipids, cholesterol, and proteins that circulate in plasma and bind cationic drugs (e.g., propanolol, quinidine). Decreased lipoprotein concentrations have been noted in hyperthyroidism, trauma, and some liver diseases; increased concentrations occur in diabetes, hypothyroidism, and the nephrotic syndrome.

"lip popper" Street name for central nervous system stimulants.

"liquid lady" Street term for combined use of alcohol and cocaine.

liquid solubility Degree to which a chemical will dissolve in a fatty substance or tissue.

"liquid X" Street name for gamma-hydroxybutyrate.

Lisenil See **lisuride.**

lisinopril (Prinivil; Prinzide; Zestoretic; Zestril) Angiotensin-converting enzyme inhibitor used to treat hypertension. Pregnancy risk category C.

lisinopril + lithium See **lithium + lisinopril.**

Liskonum See **lithium.**

lisuride (Cuvalit; Dopergin; Dopergine; Eunal; Lisenil; Lysenyl; Lysenyl Forte; Revanil) Ergoline member of a newly developed group of dopaminergic (DA) agonists. It is the first 8-alpha-ergoline in clinical use and the first dopaminergic drug that can be used parenterally. It appears to be a partial agonist at presynaptic D_2 receptors and has some serotonergic effects. It has a higher receptor affinity and intrinsic activity than bromocriptine, antagonizes neuroleptic effects, and acts independently of endogenous DA. It is an effective treatment for severe akinetic states in Parkinson's disease. Half-life is short (about 2 hours). It has been used with success in dosages up to 0.25 mg/hour or 4.0 mg/day. High doses may produce visual hallucinations. Not available in the United States.

Litarex See **lithium citrate.**

Lithane See **lithium.**

Lithicarb See **lithium.**

Lithionet Durettes See **lithium sulfate.**

lithium (Camcolit 250; Camcolit 400; Carbolith; Duralith; Durolith; Eskalith; Eskalith CR; Licarbium; Liskonum; Litarex; Lithane; Lithicarb; Lithizine; Lithonate; Lithotabs, Manialith; Manilith; Phasal; Priadel; Quilonorm; Quilonum) Naturally occurring alkaline metal used in the treatment of mania, as a maintenance treatment for the prevention of both manias and depressions, and to augment other psychoactive drugs in treatment-resistant depression. It exerts a great variety of biochemical, biophysical, and pharmacological actions; it is uncertain which is therapeutically relevant in affective disorders. It may be used in the treatment of aggressive and self-injurious behavior, impulsivity, violence, assaultiveness, destructiveness, and antisocial personality traits. It also is effective augmentation therapy in fibromyalgia, producing prompt, marked, and sustained reduction of pain and stiffness. Episode sequence seems to play a role in bipolar patients' response to lithium: mania/hypomania-depression-interval has a response rate averaging 72%; depression-mania/hypomania-depression-interval has a response rate averaging 41%. The more complicated and severe forms of mania and the less severe forms of hypomania are less likely to respond. Other patient subgroups unlikely to respond include the elderly and those with rapid-cycling bipolar disorder, schizoaffective disorder, dysphoric or mixed mania, and organic manias from many types of central nervous system diseases (e.g., stroke, tumors, closed- and open-head injuries, infections). Lithium must be introduced carefully and blood levels monitored regularly, because the therapeutic dose is near the toxic dose. Kidney, heart, and thyroid function should be checked before and during treatment. Side effects in the therapeutic range include nausea, diarrhea, vomiting, muscle weakness, tremor, drowsiness, polyuria, and excessive thirst. Thiazide diuretics and salt and water restriction may produce increased blood levels and lithium toxicity. Lithium should be stopped immediately if there are any signs of toxicity. Hypothyroidism occurs in two cases per 100 years of lithium exposure. When a patient who has good therapeutic control on lithium begins to manifest symptom recurrence or emergence, the thyroid axis should always be investigated. Insufficient thyroid function can worsen the course of bipolar illness and make it much more resistant to treatment. Pregnancy risk category D.

lithium + acemetacin   To date, there are no data on interactions. However, acemetacin is an ester of indomethacin, which increases lithium plasma level and may cause lithium toxicity.

lithium + acetaminophen   Co-administration has not been reported to cause serious drug-drug interactions. Analgesics such as acetaminophen apparently do not interfere with lithium's reabsorption by the kidney.

lithium + acetazolamide   Acetazolamide increases glomerular filtration rate and can substantially increase lithium renal clearance, possibly interfering with lithium's therapeutic effects. If lithium doses are increased to compensate for the effect, care must be taken to readjust lithium dosage downward when acetazolamide is reduced or discontinued. Co-administration should be carefully monitored; lithium intoxication has been reported (Gay C, Plas J, Granger B, et al. Intoxication au lithium. Deux interaction inedites: l'acetazolamide et a'acide niflumique. *L'Encephale* 1985;11:261–262; Horowitz LC, Fisher GU. Acute lithium toxicity. *N Engl J Med* 1969;281: 1369).

lithium, acute self-poisoning   Although relatively rare, massive intentional or accidental overdosage with lithium has occurred with increasing frequency in recent years. This is attributable largely to the escalating prescription of lithium for bipolar and unipolar manic depressive patients who, when depressed, are at a greater risk of self-poisoning and suicide than individuals with other psychiatric illnesses. Acute self-poisoning happens most often in those on lithium prophylaxis who may or may not have adverse renal effects of prolonged lithium ingestion. The latter has important implications for the clinical features and the treatment of acute intoxication. The lithium ion is slow to cross cell membranes. It also is eliminated entirely through the kidneys, and any factor that alters fluid balance and renal function is likely to precipitate toxicity. Clinical manifestations of lithium toxicity generally evolve slowly. Patients who develop lithium toxicity during maintenance treatment usually have serum concentrations only slightly above the upper limit of the accepted therapeutic range. Infrequently, intoxication may occur with serum concentrations well within the accepted therapeutic range. By contrast, acute self-poisoning with lithium manifests itself quickly (within 24 hours or less). However, in the early phase of acute overdose-induced intoxication, clinical features are mild in comparison to those of intoxication during long-term treatment. Furthermore, acute massive overdose may produce very high serum concentrations (up to 7 mmol/L) without evidence of severe poisoning, whereas symptoms of acute intoxication in patients on prophylactic lithium are quite severe even though the serum concentration may be less than 2.5 mmol/L. This discrepancy between serum concentrations and toxicity severity reflects the distribution of lithium and its speed of movement from extracellular to intracellular water. Whenever a patient has taken a lithium overdose, the clinician should (a) measure serum lithium concentration, creatinine, electrolytes, and plasma osmolality; (b) empty the stomach by lavage; (c) initiate monitoring of fluid intake and output; (d) make every effort to obtain an accurate history of the overdose (amount and time before medical attention); and (e) do a comprehensive neurological and mental status examination along with a baseline EEG. If renal function is normal, careful monitoring of the patient's clinical status along with repeated determinations of serum lithium concentrations may be the management strategy of choice, since good renal function may result in steady, asymptomatic lithium elimination with full and uneventful recovery (Ayd FJ Jr. Acute self-poisoning with lithium. *Int Drug Ther Newsl* 1988;23:1–2).

lithium/aggressive and self-mutilating behavior For the control of aggression and self-mutilation, lithium has been found effective in 70–75% of those treated (Wickham EA, Reed JV. Lithium for the control of aggressive and self-mutilating behavior. *Int Clin Psychopharmacol* 1987;2:181–190; Craft M, Ismail IA, Krishnamorti D, et al. Lithium in the treatment of aggression in mentally handicapped patients. *Br J Psychiatry* 1987; 150:685–689). No features predictive of a positive response, however, have been identified. Serum lithium concentrations of 0.7–1.0 mmol are usually best, reducing the frequency and severity of aggressive outbursts. Difficult patients with previously uncontrollable aggression become more manageable and can have other tranquilizing medication reduced or stopped and may even become eligible for discharge from long-stay hospital units in the community. In terms of clinical effectiveness and relative infrequency of serious side effects, lithium compares favorably with neuroleptics in controlling aggressive behavior without sedating patients to such an extent that they either sleep or withdraw completely from any activity or communication. Lithium does not have a sedative or suppressive effect on other behavior despite a significant reduction in aggression. It is worth at least a 2-month trial in any patient whose repeated aggression or self-mutilation has proved difficult to control.

lithium + alcohol Alcohol has additive, occasionally synergistic, effects with lithium. Limited evidence indicates that combined use may impair driving ability (Linnoila M, Saario I, Maki M. Effects of treatment with diazepam or lithium and alcohol on psychomotor skills related to driving. *Eur J Clin Pharmacol* 1974; 7:337).

lithium/alcoholism The usefulness of lithium carbonate in treating patients with alcoholism has been debated for almost two decades. A recent double-blind trial is another addition to the list of studies casting doubt on the benefits of lithium therapy for chronic alco-holism. Results showed lithium was no better than placebo in producing total abstinence, regardless of whether patients were depressed (de-la-Fuente JR, Morse RM, Niven RG, Ilstrup DM. A controlled study of lithium carbonate in treatment of alcoholism. *Mayo Clin Proc* 1989;64:177–180).

lithium + alprazolam Therapeutic doses of alprazolam for patients on maintenance lithium therapy (900–1500 mg/day) may produce a statistically significant reduction in renal lithium clearance without any change in lithium plasma level or any adverse effects (Evans RL, Nelson MV, Melethil S, et al. Evaluation of the interaction of lithium and alprazolam. *J Clin Psychopharmacol* 1990;10: 355–359).

lithium + amiloride The diuretic amiloride is useful in treating lithium-induced diabetes insipidus. Lithium level may increase moderately over time, but less than with thiazide diuretics. Because serum lithium levels remain unchanged in some patients treated with amiloride but increase in others, serum lithium levels must be monitored closely during co-administration. Amiloride causes a greater decrease in urine values than thiazides and may need to be supplemented by thiazides for effective control of nephrogenic diabetes insipidus. See **lithium + diuretic.**

lithium + aminophylline Addition of aminophylline to lithium treatment can increase lithium excretion, possibly dropping blood levels below the minimum therapeutic threshold. If lithium dose is increased to compensate for this effect, it must be readjusted downward when aminophylline is reduced or discontinued.

lithium + amphetamine Lithium may antagonize amphetamine central stimulant effects (Van Kammen DP, Murphy D. Attenuation of the euphoriant and activating effects of d- and l-amphetamine by lithium carbonate treatment. *Psychopharmacologia* 1975;44:215).

lithium + anesthetic See **lithium + general anesthesia.**

lithium + antacid Sodium bicarbonate, the main ingredient in many over-the-counter (OTC) effervescent antacids (e.g., Alka-Seltzer), increases renal excretion of lithium, decreasing lithium serum levels. Ulcer patients are unlikely to be prescribed one of these drugs, since nonbicarbonate antacids are known to be more effective; it is possible, however, that a lithium-treated patient could use an OTC antacid for early ulcer symptoms before seeking help (Haggerty JJ, Drossman DA. Use of psychotropic drugs in patients with peptic ulcer. *Psychosomatics* 1985;26:277–284).

lithium + aspirin Aspirin has little effect on lithium renal clearance or plasma level despite a more than 60% reduction in renal prostaglandin E_2 excretion. Aspirin apparently does not interfere with lithium's reabsorption (Reimann IW, Diener U, Frolich JC. Indomethacin but not aspirin increases plasma lithium ion levels. *Arch Gen Psychiatry* 1983;40:283–286).

lithium augmentation Lithium can augment the therapeutic effects of a broad spectrum of antidepressant drugs in treatment-refractory depression. In some patients, lithium augmentation results in rapid (less than 7 days) antidepressant effects; in other patients, up to 6 weeks may be required to obtain therapeutic responses. It may cause significant neurotoxicity in elderly patients despite therapeutic doses of the antidepressant and lithium (see **lithium neurotoxicity**). Lithium augmentation is best started with 600 mg/day and adjusted to reach a plasma level of 0.5–0.8 mEq/L. It is successful in approximately 60% of cases. Available data do not offer clues as to who will respond or indicate how long treatment should be continued.

lithium + baclofen Co-administration may aggravate hyperkinetic symptoms in patients with Huntington's chorea (Anden N-E, Dalen P, Johansson B. Baclofen and lithium in Huntington's chorea. *Lancet* 1973;2:93).

lithium + benzodiazepine Co-administration may be associated with sexual dysfunction in about 50% of patients. In men, it may be associated with difficulty in achieving an erection, decreased quality of orgasm in some patients, and improved quality of orgasm in others. In women, it may be associated with absence or change in quantity of menstrual blood. Because inhibition of sexual response with benzodiazepines (BZDs) alone has been reported, it is not known if sexual dysfunction occurring with lithium plus a BZD is due to the combination or to the BZD alone. It is also possible that lithium potentiates the effects of BZDs on sexual function (Ghadirian A-M, Annable L, Belanger M-C. Lithium, benzodiazepines, and sexual function in bipolar patients. *Am J Psychiatry* 1992;149:801–805).

lithium/breast milk The American Academy of Pediatrics' Committee on Drugs considers lithium to be contraindicated during breast feeding (Anon. Transfer of drugs and other chemicals into human milk. American Academy of Pediatrics, Committee on Drugs. *Pediatrics* 1989;84:924–936). Lithium in milk can adversely affect the infant when lithium elimination is impaired, as in cases of dehydration or in neonates and premature infants. Neonates also may have lithium in their plasma

that was acquired transplacentally. Long-term effects of lithium on infants are not known; some authors do not consider lithium therapy a contraindication to breast-feeding. It can probably be used cautiously in lactating women who are carefully selected for their ability to monitor their infants. Breastfeeding should be discontinued immediately if the infant appears restless or ill. Measurement of plasma lithium concentrations in the infant can help rule out lithium toxicity (Anderson PO. Drug use during breast-feeding. *Clin Pharm* 1991;10:594–624).

lithium + brofaromine Co-administration in patients nonresponsive to brofaromine may result in therapeutic response with no serious adverse effects (Nolan WA, Haffmans J, Bouvy PF, Duivenvoorden HJ. Monoamine oxidase inhibitors in resistant major depression. A double-blind comparison of brofaromine and tranylcypromine in patients resistant to tricyclic antidepressants. *J Affective Disord* 1993;28: 189–197).

lithium + bupropion In the treatment of rapid cycling, bupropion may augment lithium or lithium and levothyroxine in patients who have also been nonresponsive to carbamazepine (Haykal RF, Akiskal HS. Bupropion as a promising approach to rapid cycling bipolar II patients. *J Clin Psychiatry* 1990;51:450–455; Apter JT, Woolfolk RL. Lithium augmentation of bupropion in refractory depression. *Ann Clin Psychiatry* 1990;2:7–10). There have been reports of changes in lithium levels and three cases of seizures (Goodnick PJ. Pharmacokinetics of second generation antidepressants: bupropion. *Psychopharmacol Bull* 1991;27:513–518).

lithium + caffeine Caffeine intake during lithium treatment can increase lithium excretion, possibly dropping blood concentrations below the minimum therapeutic threshold. If lithium dose is increased to compensate for this effect, it must be readjusted when caffeine intake is reduced or discontinued.

lithium + calcium channel blocker Co-administration occasionally is used in the treatment of psychopathology and in co-morbid cardiovascular and psychiatric disorders. It may precipitate neurotoxicity manifested by nausea, weakness, tremor, ataxia, and parkinson symptoms (Price WA, Shallet JE. Lithium-verapamil toxicity in the elderly. *J Am Geriatr Soc* 1987;35: 177–179).

lithium + captopril Co-administration may increase serum lithium level, resulting in lithium intoxication.

lithium + carbamazepine Carbamazepine (CBZ) and lithium have additive or synergistic therapeutic effects in treatment-refractory bipolar illness, particularly in patients unresponsive to either drug alone. Co-administration has been found safe and effective in rapid-cycling bipolar patients. If the combination is used, CBZ levels should be 8–12 μg/ml (DiCostanzo E, Schifano F. Lithium alone or in combination for the treatment of rapid-cycling bipolar affective disorder. *Acta Psychiatr Scand* 1991;83:456–459). Addition of lithium to depressed patients nonresponsive to CBZ monotherapy produced rapid improvement (in 4 days) in half the group. Thirteen patients were "bipolar depressives," eight of whom were also rapid cyclers (Kramlinger KG, Post RM. The addition of lithium to carbamazepine, antidepressant efficacy in treatment-resistant depression. *Arch Gen Psychiatry* 1989;46:794–800). However, some patients either do not respond or show loss of efficacy via development of tolerance during long-term prophylaxis (Post RM, Pazzaglia PJ, Ketter TA, George MS, Marangell L. Carbamazepine and nimodipine in refractory bipolar illness: efficacy and mechanisms. *Neuropsychopharmacology* 1993;9:17S). Lithium is excreted by the kidney with no hepatic metabolism. Thus, pharmacokinetic interactions do not occur, although there are several pharmacodynamic interactions. Each drug may elevate the other's serum level, leading to neurotoxicity, even when blood levels of both are in the therapeutic range (Baciewicz AM. Carbamazepine drug interactions. *Ther Drug Monit* 1986;8:305–317). Toxicity can be manifested by generalized truncal tremor, ataxia, horizontal nystagmus, hyperreflexia and muscle fasciculation, all of which usually abate within 3–7 days after CBZ discontinuation (Shukla S, Godwin CD, Long LE, Miller MG. Lithium-carbamazepine neurotoxicity and risk factors. *Am J Psychiatry* 1984;141:1604–1606). The reactions appear to be, at least in part, associated with pre-existing central nervous system abnormalities and/or rapid, large dosage increases of the drugs (Ballenger JC. The clinical use of carbamazepine in affective disorders. *J Clin Psychiatry* 1988;49[suppl]:13–19). Patients must be monitored for signs and symptoms of neurotoxicity, serum levels of each drug must be monitored, and CBZ dose may need to be decreased. Lithium's diuretic effect overrides CBZ's antidiuretic effect. CBZ does not reverse lithium-induced diabetes insipidus. Lithium may attenuate CBZ-induced hyponatremia, but its potential to do so has not been unequivocally demonstrated (Vieweg V, Glick JL, Herring S, et al. Absence of carbamazepine-induced hyponatremia among patients also given lithium. *Am J Psychiatry* 1987; 144:943–947; Kramlinger KG, Post RM. Addition of lithium carbonate to carba-

mazepine: hematological and thyroid effects. *Am J Psychiatry* 1990;147:615–620).

lithium + carbamazepine/hematological effects Lithium may reverse carbamazepine (CBZ)-induced leucopenia; however, leucopenia secondary to CBZ despite concurrent lithium treatment has been reported. There is no evidence that lithium alters the course of CBZ-induced severe bone marrow depression (Klein EM. Lithium and carbamazepine therapy in a patient with manic depressive illness: clinical effects, interactions and side effects. *Isr J Psychiatry Relat Sci* 1987;24:295–298). Neither lithium dose nor plasma level is significantly correlated with degree of change in the total white blood cell or neutrophil count.

lithium + carbamazepine/thyroid effects Co-administration produces additive antithyroidal effects, resulting in greater decreases in thyroxine and free thyroxine than with carbamazepine (CBZ) alone. Addition of lithium to CBZ can be associated with emergence of a modestly higher thyrotropin level. Regular monitoring of thyroid function during combined therapy is advisable (Kramlinger KG, Post RM. Addition of lithium carbonate to carbamazepine: hematological and thyroid effects. *Am J Psychiatry* 1990;147:615–620).

lithium/cardiac effects Serious cardiovascular toxicity resulting from lithium is rare when plasma level is well monitored and adjusted. Electrocardiographic alterations, however, appear to be very common. T-wave depression may occur in up to 20% of adequately treated patients; it appears to be benign and is probably related to partial intracellular potassium displacement. ST-segment elevation or depression, either at rest or during exercise, has not been described in lithium-treated patients without a history of cardiovascular disease, but lithium may alter cardiac conduction; reversible atrioventricular block (first degree), sinoatrial dysfunction, bradycardia, and sinus pauses have been observed, even within the therapeutic serum level range, mostly in elderly patients. Cardiomyopathy is poorly documented in lithium-treated patients; it may represent either a rare form of toxicity or be coincidental. Severe ventricular arrhythmias have been reported, but almost exclusively in acute intoxications. Cardiovascular collapse also has been reported in acute lithium intoxications with severe neurological symptoms (Perrier A, Martin P-Y, Favre H, et al. Very severe self-poisoning lithium carbonate intoxication causing a myocardial infarction. *Chest* 1991;100:863–865).

lithium/children Clinical evidence indicates that lithium is effective in reducing aggressive behavior and explosive affect in treatment-resistant children diagnosed as having aggressive conduct disorder. It may have a nonspecific effect on processes that mediate self-control, but a specific effect on aggressive explosiveness.

lithium/children/side effects Lithium has been used to treat children with manic-depressive disorder, autism, hyperactivity, and conduct disorder (aggressive type), but data on its side effects in children are scant. In one survey of children taking 500–2000 mg/day (mean, 1231.3 mg/day), there was a significant inverse relationship between age and the number of side effects. Age, however, was not related to the number of episodes of side effects that occurred at serum levels ranging from 0.32 to 1.2 mEq/L. Most children had multiple episodes of side effects (weight gain or loss, gastrointestinal disturbances, headache, tremor, enuresis, sedation, and anorexia). Autistic children had more side effects, episodes of side effects, and severe side effects than conduct disorder children (Campbell M, Silva RR, Kafantaris V, et al. Predictors of side effects associated with lithium administration in children. *Psychopharmacol Bull* 1991;27:373–380).

lithium + chlorpromazine Co-administration may cause neurotoxicity manifested by confusion, disorientation, ataxia, falls, and extrapyramidal symptoms (tremors, drooling, and akathisia). Lithium lowers plasma levels of orally administered chlorpromazine, an interaction thought to be due to altered absorption and perhaps increased gut metabolism (Rivera-Calimlin L, Kerzner B, Karch FE. Effect of lithium on plasma chlorpromazine levels. *Clin Pharmacol Ther* 1978;23:451–455).

lithium + citalopram Addition of lithium may improve affective illness in citalopram nonresponders.

lithium citrate (Litarex ; Priadel) A syrup form of lithium for oral administration that contains 8 mEq of lithium per 5 ml, equivalent to the amount in 300 mg of lithium carbonate. Generally, 10 ml of lithium citrate (2 teaspoons)—that is, 16 mEq of lithium—taken 3 times a day will produce an effective serum lithium level between 1.0 and 1.5 mEq/L.

lithium clearance Lithium excretion depends on glomerular filtration rate (GFR) and sodium balance. Since lithium is completely filtered by the glomerulus, excretion is altered by GFR fluctuations. Because most lithium and sodium reabsorption occurs in the proximal convoluted tubule, a negative sodium balance can increase proximal sodium and lithium reabsorption, potentially leading to lithium toxicity. Conditions that may alter lithium clearance and cause a negative sodium balance are medical illness, especially with diarrhea, vomiting, or anorexia; hot climate; pregnancy and delivery; advanced age; surgery; dieting; and strenuous exercise.

lithium + clometacin Co-administration may reduce renal lithium clearance and result in lithium intoxication (Edou D, Godin M, Collona L, et al. Interaction medicamenteuse: clometacin-lithium. *Presse Med* 1983;12:1551).

lithium + clomipramine Lithium does not augment antiobsessional response to clomipramine (CMI) (Pigott TA, Pato MT, L'Heureux F, et al. A controlled comparison of adjuvant lithium carbonate or thyroid hormone in clomipramine-treated patients with obsessive-compulsive disorder. *J Clin Psychopharmacol* 1991;11:242–248). High-dose CMI + lithium has been reported to be very effective in some patients with resistant endogenous depression (Hale AS, Procter AW, Bridges PK. Clomipramine, tryptophan and lithium in combination for resistant endogenous depression: seven case studies. *Br J Psychiatry* 1987; 151:213–217; Stein G, Bernadt M. Lithium augmentation therapy in tricyclic-resistant depression. A controlled trial using lithium in low and normal doses. *Br J Psychiatry* 1993;162: 634–640; Feder R. Lithium augmentation of clomipramine. *J Clin Psychiatry* 1988;49:458).

lithium + clonazepam Co-administration may be effective and safe in acute mania (Gonliaev G, Licht RW, Vestergaard P. Treatment of acute mania with lithium and clonazepam or zuclopenthixol and clonazepam. *Clin Neuropharmacol* 1992;15[suppl 1]:210B). Combined use may result in lithium toxicity secondary to a rise in serum lithium levels.

lithium + clorgyline In treatment-refractory depression, lithium may potentiate clorgyline's antidepressant effect without adverse interactions (Potter WZ, Murphy DL, Wehr TA, et al. Clorgyline, a new treatment for patients with refractory rapid-cycling disorders. *Arch Gen Psychiatry* 1983;39:505–510). See **lithium + monoamine oxidase inhibitor (MAOI)**.

lithium + clozapine Co-administration may be effective in bipolar disorder unresponsive to lithium or anticonvulsants alone. However, neurotoxicity, neuroleptic malignant syndrome, seizures, confusional states, and dyskinesias have been reported (Blake LM, Marks RC, Luchins DJ. Reversible neurologic symptoms with clozapine and lithium. *J Clin Psychopharmacol* 1992;12:297–298; Pope H, Cole J, Choras P, Fulwiller C. Apparent neuroleptic malignant syndrome with clozapine and lithium. *J Nerv Ment Dis* 1986;174:493–494). The first fatal case of agranulocytosis in the

United States occurred with clozapine (CLOZ) + lithium. Death occurred in association with lithium tapering and discontinuation, suggesting that lithium withdrawal may have played a role (Gerson SL, Lieberman JA, Friedenberg WR, et al. Polypharmacy in fatal clozapine-associated agranulocytosis. *Lancet* 1991;338:262–263). A nonfatal case of CLOZ-induced agranulocytosis during lithium treatment was reported in a 53-year-old schizoaffective woman of Ashkenazi origin. She was treated with granulocyte-macrophage colony-stimulating factor (GM-CSF) (300 mg administered subcutaneously over 3 days) without improvement. She was then treated with interleukin-3 (IL-3) (300 mg/day administered subcutaneously) for another 16 days. Agranulocytosis lasted 27 days until complete recovery. Based on these two cases, criteria for CLOZ discontinuation (white blood cell count [WBC] < 3000/mm^3 or granulocyte count > 1500/mm^3) are insufficient for detecting agranulocytosis in the presence of lithium. Consistent tendency of the WBC to decrease from baseline levels is a better indicator for CLOZ discontinuation (Valevski A, Modai I, Lahav M, Weizman A. Clozapine-lithium combined treatment and agranulocytosis. *Int Clin Psychopharmacol* 1993;8:63–65). Reports of adverse interactions suggest that lithium should be used with CLOZ only if manic symptoms are not adequately controlled with CLOZ.

lithium/dehydration   Dehydration, whether due to inadequate fluid intake, excessive sweating, severe vomiting or diarrhea, or diuretic use, may result in lithium intoxication because of a compensatory increase in proximal lithium reabsorption.

lithium + desipramine   Addition of lithium in desipramine-resistant patients may heighten therapeutic response; some responding within a week (rapid responders), others not until 1–6 weeks have passed (slow responders) (Dallal A, Fontaine R, Ontivero A, Elie R. Lithium carbonate augmentation of desipramine in refractory depression. *Can J Psychiatry* 1990;35:608–611).

lithium + desipramine + fluoxetine   Lithium augmentation may be beneficial in patients being treated with desipramine and fluoxetine for refractory depression (Fontaine R, Ontiveros A, Elie R, et al. Lithium carbonate augmentation of desipramine and fluoxetine in refractory depression. *Biol Psychiatry* 1991;29:946–948).

lithium + diclofenac   Addition of 150 mg/day of diclofenac to lithium treatment can diminish lithium's renal clearance, leading to increased lithium plasma levels and possible intoxication (Reimann IW, Frohlich JC. Effects of diclofenac on lithium kinetics. *Clin Pharmacol Ther* 1980;30:348–352).

lithium + digitalis   In a patient with elevated lithium levels, digitalis may cause serious prolonged dysrhythmias.

lithium + digoxin   Digoxin may impair the acute antimanic efficacy of lithium (Chambers CA, Smith AH, Naylor GJ. The effect of digoxin on the response to lithium therapy in mania. *Psychol Med* 1982;12:57–60).

lithium + diltiazem   Carefully monitored co-administration can be used in patients intolerant of lithium side effects. Co-administration may cause neurotoxicity, possibly due to each drug's effects on calcium metabolism. Diltiazem blocks entry of extracellular calcium into cells during depolarization. Lithium decreases calcium transport into a variety of cells. In addition, lithium may compete with calcium ions intracellularly because of the identical hydrated ion radius and similar ionic potential of both calcium and lithium. There is a report of diltiazem plus lithium causing delirium, rigidity, and cogwheeling with no change in lithium level (Binder E. Diltiazem-induced psychosis and a possible diltiazem-lithium interaction. *Arch Intern Med* 1991;151:373–374). Acute Parkinson's syndrome developed in a 58-year-old man within 4 days of adding 30 mg of diltiazem, 3 times a day, to lithium and thiothixene treatment (Valdiserri EV. A possible interaction between lithium and diltiazem: case report. *J Clin Psychiatry* 1985;46:540–541).

lithium + diuretic   Thiazide diuretics cause lithium retention at the expense of sodium loss, which may lead to lithium toxicity. They may be used to treat lithium-induced nephrogenic diabetes insipidus provided careful clinical monitoring and frequent lithium plasma level determinations are done. If co-administration is necessary, the following procedure is suggested: (a) ensure that the lithium plasma concentration is in the therapeutic range (0.6–1.2 mmol/L); (b) reduce lithium dose by 50% when starting some diuretics (loop diuretics usually do not decrease lithium clearance, whereas xanthine and osmotic diuretics increase lithium clearance); (c) use the smallest dose of diuretic needed; (d) choose a loop diuretic (furosemide, bumetanide, ethacrynic acid): (e) monitor plasma lithium concentration twice weekly; and (f) adjust lithium dose as necessary to regain the therapeutic range. The patient should be reminded of the neurological symptoms of early lithium toxicity and told to stop lithium immediately if they occur; lithium plasma concentration should be checked at the earliest opportunity. If diuretic treatment is stopped, lithium dose will need to be increased and plasma levels monitored until therapeutic range has been reached (Ramsay LE. Interactions that matter. Diuretics and antihypertensive drugs. *Prescribers' Journal* 1984;24:61–62). Using pharmacokinetic principles, it is possible to calculate the necessary adjustment in lithium dose for a given dose of thiazide diuretic: chlorothiazide (500 mg) increases lithium concentration approximately 40%; 750 mg, 60%; and 1,000 mg, 70%. Lithium dosage should be adjusted by these percentages to maintain the same serum concentration (Himmelhoch JM, Neil JF, Mallinger AG, et al. Lithium with diuretics. *Drug Ther Hosp* 1978;8:9–10). See **lithium + ethacrynic acid; lithium + furosemide.**

lithium dosage Daily maintenance doses of lithium carbonate are usually 900–1500 mg in patients under 60 years of age and 450–900 mg in older patients.

lithium + dothiepin Addition of lithium in depressed patients resistant to dothiepin therapy frequently produces a favorable clinical response.

lithium + doxepin Co-administration may augment the antiobsessional effect of chronic treatment with doxepin in patients with obsessive-compulsive disorder. Lithium also augments doxepin's antidepressant effects.

lithium + electroconvulsive therapy (ECT) Lithium levels should be carefully determined and lowered to half therapeutic levels in patients referred for ECT (American Psychiatric Association Task Force on Electroconvulsive Therapy. *The Practice of Electroconvulsive Therapy: Recommendations for Treatment, Training, and Privileging.* Washington, DC: American Psychiatric Press, 1990). It is prudent to stop lithium 1 week prior to ECT, which seems to be sufficient to prevent complications. It also is prudent not to restart lithium until 4–7 days after ECT is completed (Small JG, Milstein V. Lithium interactions: lithium and electroconvulsive therapy. *J Clin Psychopharmacol* 1990;10:346–350). Available data suggest that the higher the serum lithium concentration when ECT is administered, the greater the risk of cerebral toxicity. Even therapeutic lithium levels may be associated with organic brain syndromes, particularly in patients who become severely depressed during maintenance lithium therapy and who undergo ECT either along with lithium or within a day or two after it was discontinued. The American Psychiatric Association Task Force Report warns of the potential increased risk of delirium when ECT and lithium are given concurrently. Co-administration also has been reported to cause nonconvulsive status epilepticus 2 days after the fifth ECT treatment

(Weiner RD, Whanger AD, Ervin CW, et al. Prolonged confusional state and EEG seizure activity following concurrent ECT and lithium use. *Am J Psychiatry* 1980;137:1452–1453).

lithium + enalapril Adding enalapril to a stable lithium regimen can increase lithium plasma level and induce lithium intoxication. The mechanism for the interaction could be alteration in renal function induced by angiotensin converting enzyme inhibition and the natriuretic effect of enalapril. The more likely explanation is lithium retention related to increased sodium excretion associated with decreased aldosterone secretion induced by enalapril. Lithium serum levels should be monitored closely during co-administration (Douste-Blazy PH, Rostin M, Livarek B, et al. Angiotensin converting enzyme inhibitors and lithium treatment. *Lancet* 1986;1:448; Mahieu M, Houvenagel E, Leduc JJ, Choteau PH. Lithium inhibiteurs de conversion: Une association a eviter? *Presse Med* 1988;17:281). Elevated lithium concentrations with this combination may not be universal; they may be more likely with higher enalapril doses, higher maintenance lithium levels, or the presence of heart disease (DasGupta K, Jefferson JW, Kobak KA, Greist JH. The effect of enalapril on serum lithium levels in healthy men. *J Clin Psychiatry* 1992;53:398–400).

lithium + ethacrynic acid Co-administration may increase lithium level over time and might produce lithium toxicity. Patients should be monitored clinically for signs of lithium intoxication and lithium blood levels should be checked frequently. See **lithium + diuretic.**

lithium + fluoxetine Co-administration may augment antidepressant effects of fluoxetine (FLX) and may benefit some patients unresponsive to other antidepressants. There were no adverse interactions, possibly because patients were started on FLX, and lithium (900–1,200 mg/day) was added later (Pope HG, McElroy SL, Nixon RA. Possible synergism between fluoxetine and lithium in refractory depression. *Am J Psychiatry* 1988; 145:1292–1294). Addition of lithium to ongoing FLX treatment has been reported to improve obsessive compulsive disorder symptoms (Ruegg RG, Evans DL, Comes WS, et al. Lithium and fluoxetine treatment of obsessive compulsive disorder. *In* New Research Programs and Abstracts of the 143rd Annual Meeting of the American Psychiatric Association; May 14, 1990, New York, Abstract NR 92). Although there is evidence that FLX is unlikely to produce clinically significant changes in lithium blood concentrations (Hopwood SE, Bogle S, Wildgust HJ. The combination of fluoxetine and lithium in clinical practice. *Int Clin Psychopharmacol* 1993;8:325–327), addition of FLX may elevate serum lithium level and result in neurotoxicity (Salama AA, Shafey M. A case of severe lithium toxicity induced by combined fluoxetine and lithium carbonate. *Am J Psychiatry* 1989;146:278; Wright P, Seth R. Lithium toxicity, hypomania and leucocytosis with fluoxetine. *Ir J Psychol Med* 1992;9:59–60). Mania, seizures, and hyperpyrexia have been reported (Committee on the Safety of Medicines. Fluvoxamine and fluoxetine—interaction with monoamine oxidase inhibitors, lithium and tryptophan. *Curr Prob* 1989;26:61; Hadley A, Cason MP. Mania resulting from lithium-fluoxetine combination. *Am J Psychiatry* 1989;146:1637–1638). Toxicity has also been observed when lithium was added to FLX, although lithium serum level was well within the therapeutic range. Other adverse reactions reported with combined use include absence seizures and a toxic encephalopathy-like state (Saeristan JA, Iglesias G, Aurellano F, et al. Absence seizures induced by lithium: possible interaction with fluoxetine. *Am J Psychiatry* 1991;148:146–147; Noveske FG, Hahn KR, Flynn RJ. Possible toxicity of combined fluoxetine and lithium. *Am J Psychiatry* 1989; 146:1515). An acute confusional state was reported in a 60-year-old woman taking amitriptyline (AMI) (100 mg/day) and lithium (600 mg/day). AMI was discontinued, and FLX (20 mg/day) was started, at which time serum lithium was 0.6 mmol/L. She developed clouding of consciousness, perplexity, disorientation to time and place, reduced attention and concentration, impaired short-term memory, and visual hallucinations. Physical examination results were normal, and serum lithium was 0.5 mmol/L. FLX and lithium were stopped; within 3 days the confusional state improved and depression gradually returned. Lithium (600 mg/day) was reintroduced with no adverse cognitive effects (Shah AK, McClosky O. Case report: acute confusional state secondary to a combination of fluoxetine and lithium. *Int J Geriatr Psychiatry* 1992;7:68–69).

lithium + fluoxetine + desipramine   See **lithium + desipramine + fluoxetine.**

lithium + fluoxetine/serotonin syndrome   Symptoms of a serotonin syndrome (restlessness, increased myoclonus, hyperreflexia, shivering, tremor, diarrhea, and incoordination) appeared in a 36-year-old woman after lithium (900 mg/day) was added to a regimen of fluoxetine (40 mg/day). This is the first report of a serotonin syndrome attributed to this combination (Muly E, McDonald W, Steffens D, Book S. Serotonin syndrome produced by a

combination of fluoxetine and lithium. *Am J Psychiatry* 1993;150:1565).

lithium + fluoxetine + triiodothyronine (T₃)   Lithium may act synergistically (perhaps via separate mechanisms) with fluoxetine and T_3 to enhance mood (Geracioti TD, Loosen PT, Gold PW, Kling MA. Cortisol, thyroid hormone, and mood in atypical depression: A longitudinal case study. *Biol Psychiatry* 1992;31: 515–519). See **lithium + triiodothyronine.**

lithium + flupenthixol   Neurotoxicity has been reported (West A. Adverse effects of lithium treatment. *Br Med J* 1977;2[6087]:642).

lithium + fluphenazine   Co-administration may be associated with neurotoxicity, including extrapyramidal symptoms (Alevegor B. Toxic reactions to lithium and neuroleptics. *Br J Psychiatry* 1979;135:482; Sachdev PS. Lithium potentiation of neuroleptic-related extrapyramidal side effects. *Am J Psychiatry* 1986;143: 942).

lithium + fluvoxamine   Co-administration may be helpful in treatment-resistant depression and obsessive-compulsive disorder (OCD) partially responsive or refractory to fluvoxamine (FVX). It may rarely cause convulsions or hyperpyrexia (Committee on the Safety of Medicines. Fluvoxamine and fluoxetine—interaction with monoamine oxidase inhibitors, lithium and tryptophan. *Curr Prob* 1989;26:61; Goodman WK, Price LH, Rasmussen SA, et al. Efficacy of fluvoxamine in obsessive-compulsive disorder. *Arch Gen Psychiatry* 1989;46:36–44). Since lithium enhances FVX's serotonergic effects, the combination should be used with caution. In some bipolar patients, it has resulted in a manic episode (McDougle CJ, Price LH, Goodman WK, et al. A controlled trial of lithium augmentation in fluvoxamine-refractory obsessive-compulsive disorder: lack of efficacy. *J Clin Psychopharmacol* 1991;11:175–184; Hendricks B, Floris M. A controlled study of the combination of fluvoxamine and lithium. *Curr Therapeut Res* 1991;49:106–110).

lithium formulations   Lithium is available as tablets, capsules, or liquid, and in sustained or slow release forms. The liquid is valuable for patients who have difficulty swallowing tablets or capsules, but tablets/capsules are preferable for standard treatment. There are no significant differences between regular and sustained formulations with respect to therapeutic efficacy and side effects.

lithium + furosemide   In healthy individuals, furosemide (40 mg/day) does not significantly affect serum lithium levels and thus may be a safer and simpler approach to combining lithium and a diuretic than using hydrochlorothiazide. Nevertheless, caution should be used when co-prescribing furosemide and lithium because of the possible increased risk of lithium intoxication secondary to lithium retention. See **lithium + diuretic.**

lithium + general anesthesia There are no absolute contraindications to general anesthesia in patients on lithium. Lithium dosage should be reduced by half 2–3 days before surgery and withheld altogether 24 hours before the anesthesia. Lithium levels can be restarted to the therapeutic range as soon as the patient resumes eating and fluid and electrolyte balance is normalized. In a few case reports, lithium has been found to potentiate some anesthetics and to reduce the need for postoperative pain medications (Jefferson JW, Greist JH, Ackerman DL, Carroll JA. *Lithium Encyclopedia for Clinical Practice,* 2nd ed. Washington, DC: American Psychiatric Press, 1987). It can potentiate depolarizing and nondepolarizing classes of neuromuscular blockers, leading to delayed recovery time and resumption of spontaneous breathing.

lithium + haloperidol Co-administration may cause severe adverse reactions, particularly during the acute manic phase. The drugs may act in an additive or synergistic fashion; toxic clinical manifestations during combined use seem to differ from the toxic reactions of either drug alone. Although lithium plus haloperidol has been reported most frequently as producing neurotoxic states, other neuroleptics (fluphenazine, thioridazine, perphenazine, chlorpromazine) combined with lithium produce identical syndromes. The higher the neuroleptic dose, the greater the risk. The elderly (age 65+) are more likely to develop neurotoxicity with neuroleptic doses considered safe when administered in the absence of other psychoactive drugs. Thus, advanced age is a relative contraindication to combined lithium-neuroleptic therapy; moderate neuroleptic dosage (400–600 chlorpromazine equivalents) can result in neurotoxicity with no proven therapeutic advantage (Batchelor DH, Lowe MR. Reported neurotoxicity with the lithium/haloperidol combination and other neuroleptics—a literature review. *Hum Psychopharmacol* 1990;5:275–280). See **lithium toxicity.**

lithium/hematopoietic effects Lithium can cause neutrophilic leucocytosis, a property used in treating iatrogenic neutropenia (Lyman GH, William CC, Preston D. The use of lithium carbonate to reduce infection and leukopenia during systemic chemotherapy. *N Engl J Med* 1980;302:257–260). Aplastic and megaloblastic anemias have been reported in lithium-treated patients (Hussain MZ, Kahn AG, Chaudry ZA. Aplastic anemia associated with lithium therapy. *Can Med Assoc J* 1973;108: 724–728; Prakesh R, Sethi N, Agrawal SS, et al. A case report of megaloblastic anemia secondary to lithium. *Am J Psychiatry* 1981;138:849). The Committee on Safety of Medicines has one report of death from hemolytic anemia. Lithium effects on platelets include raised platelet count and amelioration of cytotoxic induced thrombocytopenia (Joffe RT, Kellner CH, Post RM, Uhde TW. Lithium increases platelet count. *N Engl J Med* 1984;311:674–675; Richman CM, Makii MM, Weiser PA, Herbst AL. The effect of lithium carbonate on chemotherapy induced neutropenia and thrombocytopenia. *Am J Hematol* 1984;16:313–323). Lithium enhances production of colony stimulating factor in vivo and in vitro and may protect hemopoietic stem cells against cytotoxic drugs. The mechanism for action is unclear. A single case of thrombocytopenia caused by lithium has been reported. See **lithium + carbamazepine.**

lithium holiday Temporary discontinuation (days or weeks) of lithium indicated for patients who have been stabilized for several months and have periodic or seasonal episodes, and for stabilized patients with excessive weight gain on maintenance lithium therapy. Lithium holidays may result in weight loss and decrease risk of lithium-induced kidney damage. The longer the duration of the lithium holiday, the greater the risk of recurrence of bipolar illness. Because of the risk of early recurrence of manic symptoms, some experts do not recommend lithium holidays (Faedda GL, Tondo L, Baldessarini R, et al. Outcome after rapid versus gradual discontinuation of lithium treatment in bipolar disorders. *Arch Gen Psychiatry* 1993;50:448–455).

lithium + hydrochlorothiazide See **lithium + diuretic.**

lithium + ibuprofen Ibuprofen (1200–1800 mg/day) can increase steady-state plasma lithium concentrations and decrease lithium clearance, resulting in lithium intoxication (Kristoff C, Hayes PE, Barr WH, et al. Effect of ibuprofen on lithium plasma and red blood cell levels. *Clin Pharm* 1986;1:51–55).

lithium + imipramine Lithium has been used to augment the antidepressant activity of imipramine and its antiobsessional effects in obsessive-compulsive disorder.

lithium + indapamide Therapeutic doses of indapamide may cause lithium retention, producing severe lithium toxicity (Hanna ME, Lobao CB, Stewart JT. Severe lithium toxicity associated with indapamide therapy. *J Clin Psychopharmacol* 1990;10:379–380).

lithium + indomethacin Indomethacin (150 mg/day) increases lithium plasma level and may cause lithium toxicity (Leftwich RB, Walker LA, Ragheb M, et al. Inhibition of prostaglandin synthesis increases plasma lithium levels. *Clin Res* 1978;26:291A; Herschberg SN, Sierles FS. Indomethacin-induced lithium toxicity. *Am Fam Physician* 1983;28:155–157).

lithium + iprindole Lithium augmentation of iprindole has benefitted patients partially responsive or totally refractory to iprindole alone (de Montigny C, Elie R, Gaille R, et al. Rapid response to the addition of lithium in iprindole-resistant unipolar depression: a pilot study. *Am J Psychiatry* 1985;142:220–223).

lithium + isocarboxazid Co-administration for severe depression can be effective and safe (Zall H: Lithium carbonate and isocarboxazid. An effective drug approach in severe depression. *Am J Psychiatry* 1971; 127:1400–1403) See **lithium + monoamine oxidase inhibitor.**

lithium level/plasma Recommended range for serum lithium concentration in blood samples drawn 12 hours after the last lithium intake is 0.5–0.8 mEq/L. In individual patients, lower or higher levels may be required.

lithium level/saliva Lithium concentration can be measured in saliva as an alternative to serum lithium monitoring. It is less invasive, less expensive, and allows for greater patient acceptance. There may be considerable inter-patient variability and some intrapatient variability, however.

lithium + lisinopril Lithium and sodium are not competitively reabsorbed, but are absorbed together in the proximal tubules. When lisinopril causes sodium loss, proximal reabsorption is compensatorily increased, resulting in increased reabsorption of both sodium and lithium that may produce toxic increases in serum lithium and lithium intoxication. Lithium monitoring and dose reduction are warranted during co-administration (Griffin JH, Hahn SM. Lisinopril-induced lithium toxicity. *Ann Pharmacother* 1991;25:101).

lithium/liver Lithium generally is not considered hepatotoxic, even at serum levels that may produce toxic effects on other systems. The literature on lithium intoxication uniformly makes no mention of hepatic dysfunction. Although lithium may cause alterations in certain liver enzymes, these changes do not appear to be of clinical importance and would not be reflected by changes in conventional liver function tests. Since lithium therapy and liver disease are not rare, the possibility of the two co-existing by chance must always be considered when a report of liver changes in a patient being treated with lithium is published

(Viegut V, Jefferson JW. Lithium and the liver. *Lithium* 1990;1:9–13).

lithium + lofepramine Addition of lithium in depression refractory to lofepramine may produce favorable therapeutic response (Seymour J, Wattis JP. Treatment resistant depression in the elderly: three cases. *Int Clin Psychopharmacol* 1992;7:55–57). Efficacy appears to be contingent on achieving adequate serum lithium levels (Katona CL, Robertson MM, Abou-Saleh MT, et al. Placebo controlled trial of lithium augmentation of fluoxetine and lofepramine. *Int Clin Psychopharmacol* 1993;8:323).

lithium + lorazepam Lorazepam may be useful as an adjunct in controlling agitation (Modell JG. Further experience and observations with lorazepam in the management of behavioral agitation. *J Clin Psychopharmacol* 1986;6:385–387). It also may be used in patients not fully responsive to lithium (Janicak PG, Newman RH, Davis JM. Advances in the treatment of mania and related disorders: a reappraisal. *Psychiatr Ann* 1992;22:92–103).

lithium + loxapine Co-administration can cause extrapyramidal reactions (de la Gandara J, Dominguez RA. Lithium and loxapine. A potential interaction. *J Clin Psychiatry* 1988;49:126).

lithium-7 magnetic resonance spectroscopy (Li-MRS) Method for measuring brain lithium concentrations, which correlate better with serum concentrations than with erythrocyte concentrations. Brain lithium concentration as determined by Li-MRS may be a better marker of clinical response or lithium intoxication (Kato T, Shioiri T, Inubushi T, Takahashi S. Brain lithium concentrations measured with lithium-7 magnetic resonance spectroscopy in patients with affective disorders: relationship to erythrocyte and serum concentrations. *Biol Psychiatry* 1993;33:147–152).

lithium maintenance The following ordinarily justify indefinite continuation of lithium therapy: (a) Both patient and psychiatrist conscientiously apply themselves to the program: regularity of taking medication, regular follow-up, indicated clinical inquiries and assessments, and continued mutual involvement are required. (b) Two episodes of affective disorder (one of which is mania) occur within a 5-year period. (c) Maintenance continues to be effective, with affective episodes absent or significantly attenuated. (d) Common side effects (usually a modest increase in urine volume and a slight tremor) are acceptable (Sandifer MG. Ordinary conditions for indefinite continuation of lithium therapy. *J Clin Psychiatry* 1985;46:505).

lithium + mannitol   Mannitol increases glomerular filtration rate and can substantially increase renal lithium clearance, resulting in lower serum lithium levels. Lithium dosage adjustment may be necessary when mannitol is started and discontinued.

lithium + maprotiline   Co-administration has been used to augment the treatment of depression without severe adverse effects.

lithium + marijuana   Combined use may result in lithium toxicity (Ratey JJ, Ciraulo DA, Shader RI. Lithium and marijuana. *J Clin Psychopharmacol* 1981;1:32–33).

lithium + mefenamic acid   Co-administration may cause a rise in serum lithium level with associated signs and symptoms of lithium intoxication. Serum lithium level should be obtained several days after beginning mefenamic acid (Honey J. Lithium-mefenamic Interaction. *Pharmabulletin* 1982;59:20; MacDonald J, Neale TJ. Toxic interaction of lithium carbonate and mefenamic acid. *Br Med J* 1988;297:1339).

lithium + methyldopa   Co-administration may produce lithium toxicity in patients previously stable on lithium alone (Osanloo E, Deglin JH. Interaction of lithium and methyldopa. *Ann Intern Med* 1980;92:433–434; Yassa R. Lithium-methyldopa interaction. *Can Med Assoc J* 1986;134:141–142).

lithium + methylphenidate   Lithium may augment methylphenidate in attention deficit disorder (Gammon GD. Combined medications for ADD subtypes. Presented at the 1993 Annual Meeting of the American Psychiatric Association, San Francisco, May 25, 1993).

lithium + metronidazole   Co-administration may cause lithium intoxication secondary to increased lithium serum level. Lithium level should be obtained several days after beginning metronidazole to detect any increase that may precede clinical symptoms of intoxication (Ayd FJ Jr. Metronidazole-induced lithium intoxication. *Int Drug Ther Newsl* 1982:17:15–16; Teicher MH, Altesman RI, Cole JO, Schatzberg AF. Possible neurotoxic interaction of lithium and metronidazole. *JAMA* 1987;257:3365–3366).

lithium + mianserin   Co-administration may be useful in refractory depression without severe adverse effects.

lithium + moclobemide   In 50 patients in whom moclobemide (150–675 mg/day) was added to lithium therapy for 3–52 weeks, there was no evidence of any interaction. A direct pharmacokinetic interaction appears unlikely because lithium is eliminated by the kidneys, and moclobemide is eliminated by hepatic metabolism (Amrein R, Guntert TW, Dingemanse J, et al. Interactions of moclobemide with con-comitantly administered medication: evidence from pharmacological and clinical studies. *Psychopharmacology* 1992;106:S24–S31). Addition of moclobemide in lithium-refractory depression may enhance therapeutic response.

lithium + molindone   Co-administration may produce a pharmacokinetic interaction resulting in a fourfold increase in the half-life of molindone.

lithium + monoamine oxidase inhibitor (MAOI)   The antidepressant potentiating effect of lithium in combination with MAOIs was first described in 1971. Available efficacy data indicate that co-administration is a viable option for depressed patients refractory to other antidepressant regimens, although this has not been established by rigorously controlled studies. Lithium has been co-administered with isocarboxazid, tranylcypromine, phenelzine, and clorgyline. There is no contraindication to combined use, but patients should be warned about tyramine-containing foods, diuretics, and salt-free diets. They also should be monitored regularly to detect early signs of hypomania, mania, and extrapyramidal symptoms. Although there does not appear to be substantial risk for any of these reactions, mania has been reported in patients treated with phenelzine plus lithium, and two cases of tardive dyskinesia have been reported after long-term use of lithium and tranylcypromine in patients who had not taken neuroleptics; these isolated instances of adverse reactions may be only idiosyncratic events. Response to lithium augmentation may be quite variable in onset and short-lived, necessitating at least a 3-week trial to reliably determine efficacy.

lithium + naproxen   Co-administration may interfere with lithium clearance and increase lithium plasma level, and possibly causes toxicity. Lithium dosage should be reduced, and serum lithium level should be monitored more frequently (Ragheb M, Powell AL. Lithium interaction with sulindac and naproxen. *J Clin Psychopharmacol* 1986;6:150–154).

lithium/nephrogenic diabetes insipidus (NDI)   Lithium may cause NDI by blocking the action of antidiuretic hormone on the collecting duct, producing impairment of concentrating capacity. Lithium-induced NDI occurs in 10–20% of patients, some of whom may urinate up to 8 L or more per day. Most require no specific treatment aside from adequate fluid intake to counterbalance the polyuria and avert lithium intoxication. When polyuria is severe, lithium dose reduction or discontinuation may be necessary. Some physicians co-administer a diuretic and restrict sodium intake, which can lead to lithium retention and risk of toxicity; careful monitoring of lithium levels is imperative. Also, because lithium may increase potassium excretion, most diuretics used in the treatment of any form of diabetes insipidus may precipitate hypokalemia. Amiloride, a potassium-sparing diuretic that acts on the cortical-collecting tubule and antagonizes the inhibitory effect of lithium on vasopressin-induced water transport, may be the best choice in combination with lithium. There also is evidence that amiloride may reduce polyuria.

lithium + neuroleptic   Addition of lithium to a neuroleptic may enhance dopamine metabolism (Bowers MD, Mazure CM, Nelson JC, Patlow PI. Lithium in combination with perphenazine: effect on plasma monoamine metabolites. *Biol Psychiatry* 1992;32:1102–1107). Co-administration may cause more extrapyramidal reactions than either drug alone. It also may result in toxicity manifested by confusion, disorientation, ataxia, and falling, especially with high dosages. In a comparison of patients who developed neurotoxicity with those who did not, average neuroleptic dose was 563 mg of chlorpromazine equivalents in the nontoxic group versus 1,780 mg in the toxic group; there were no differences in lithium dosages (Miller F, Menninger J. Lithium-neuroleptic neurotoxicity is dose dependent. *J Clin Psychopharmacol* 1987;7:89–91; Axelsson R, Lagerkvist-Briggs M. Clinical and neurobiological findings during treatment with neuroleptics alone and combined with lithium: comparative study of patients with bipolar disorder in acute manic phase. *Lithium* 1993;4:45–52). Neurotoxicity recedes spontaneously and without apparent sequelae after discontinuation of the drug regimen. There is some evidence that co-administration may increase the risk of neuroleptic malignant syndrome. It also has been reported to induce somnambulistic-like episodes, usually in patients on maintenance lithium following addition of a neuroleptic. Episodes occur within 2–3 hours of sleep onset; they are characterized by the patient appearing confused and walking about in a quick, detached clumsy manner. Generally, patients have no memory of the event (Charney DS, Kales A, Soldatos CR, Nelson JC. Somnambulistic-like episodes secondary to combined lithium-neuroleptic treatment. *Br J Psychiatry* 1979;135:418–424). See **lithium + tricyclic antidepressant + neuroleptic.**

lithium + nifedipine   Two doses of nifedipine had no effect on lithium clearance and glomerular filtration rate (GFR), but 6 and 12 weeks of nifedipine (40 mg/day) led to 30% reductions in lithium clearance with no effect on GFR (Bruun NE, Ibsen H, Skott P, et al.

Lithium clearance and renal tubular sodium handling during acute and long-term nifedipine treatment in essential hypertension. *Clin Sci* 1988;75:609–613).

lithium + nonsteroidal anti-inflammatory drug   Nonsteroidal anti-inflammatory drugs (NSAIDs), which decrease renal blood flow by inhibiting prostaglandin activity in the kidney, can increase serum lithium levels, diminish renal lithium clearance, and possibly induce lithium toxicity in patients with normal renal function. Indomethacin seems the most potent NSAID in this respect; sulindac and aspirin may be less likely to induce serious renal toxicity. Lithium-treated patients receiving NSAIDs should have their serum lithium levels checked every 4–5 days until the extent of the interaction is determined. Lithium dosage reduction may be needed in some patients following NSAID administration. Elderly patients seem to be more susceptible to developing lithium toxicity following NSAID administration. See **lithium + sulindac.**

lithium + nortriptyline   In a series of elderly patients on lithium augmentation for refractory depression, co-administration caused myoclonus, weakness, tremor, and neurotoxicity (Lafferman J, Solomon K, Ruskin P. Lithium augmentation for treatment resistant depression in the elderly. *J Geriatr Psychiatry Neurol* 1988;1:49–52). Caution should be used with higher doses of either drug in the elderly.

lithium + other drugs   Co-administration of lithium and many other drugs risks lithium intoxication. To minimize or avoid the risk, physicians should (a) review with the patient the early warning signs of impending lithium intoxication and instruct the patient to stop all medications if signs of toxicity emerge; and (b) check serum lithium at the start of combined therapy and at least every 5 days thereafter until it is evident that the combination is not resulting in lithium retention. The latter is especially important, since lithium retention due to other drugs usually begins within a few days of starting the interacting drug.

lithium + pancuronium   Co-administration can cause apnea during electroconvulsive therapy (Martin BA, Kramer PM. Clinical significance of the interaction between lithium and a neuromuscular blocker. *Am J Psychiatry* 1992; 139:1326).

lithium/parathyroid effects   Chronic lithium therapy increases serum parathyroid levels, resulting in increased calcium and magnesium concentrations, and possibly decreased plasma phosphate and bone mineralization.

lithium + paroxetine   Addition of paroxetine to chronic lithium therapy did not cause any clinically significant changes in vital signs or laboratory values, including plasma lithium levels. There was a high incidence of tremor (47%) and sweating (36%), but it is not known if these effects were additive (Haenen J. An interaction study of paroxetine on lithium plasma levels in depressed patients stabilized on lithium therapy. Presented at the 5th World Congress of Biological Psychiatry, Florence, June 1991). Co-administration was well tolerated in a 5-week open study (Stellamans G. A study to investigate the efficacy, adverse events, safety, and pharmacokinetic effects of co-administration of paroxetine and lithium. *Biol Psychiatry* 1991;29:354S).

lithium + phenelzine Lithium potentiation of phenelzine in refractory depression has not caused adverse effects (Nelson JC, Byck R. Rapid response to lithium in phenelzine nonresponders. *Br J Psychiatry* 1982;141:85–86). See **lithium + monoamine oxidase inhibitor.**

lithium + phenylbutazone Phenylbutazone increases serum lithium levels, reduces lithium clearance, increases tubular reabsorption of lithium, and may cause lithium intoxication (Imbs JL, Schmidt M, Mack G, et al. Baisse de la clearance renale du lithium sous l'effet de la phenylbutazone. *L'Encephale* 1978;4:33). In two cases, it may have led to onset of paranoid delusions or exacerbation of dementia (Ragheb M. The interaction of lithium with phenylbutazone in bipolar affective patients. *J Clin Psychopharmacol* 1990;10:149–150). See **lithium + nonsteroidal anti-inflammatory drug.**

lithium + phenytoin Co-administration may result in lithium toxicity (Maccallum WAG. Interaction of lithium and phenytoin. *Br Med J* 1980;280:610–611).

lithium + pimozide No interaction or additional benefit from adding lithium to pimozide has been demonstrated in clinical trials (Johnstone EC, Crow TJ, Frith CD, et al. The Northwick Park. "functional" psychosis study: diagnosis and treatment response. *Lancet* 1988;2:119–125; Braden W, Fink EB, Qualls CB, et al. Lithium and chlorpromazine in psychotic inpatients. *Psychiatry Res* 1982;7:69–81).

lithium + piroxicam Piroxicam (20 mg/day) reduces renal excretion of lithium, increases lithium plasma level, and results in lithium toxicity (Kerry RJ, Owen G, Michaelson S. Possible interaction between lithium and piroxicam. *Lancet* 1983;1:418–419; Walbridge DG, Bazire SR. An interaction between lithium carbonate and piroxicam presenting as lithium toxicity. *Br J Psychiatry* 1985;147:206–207). See **lithium + nonsteroidal anti-inflammatory drug.**

lithium/pregnancy Lithium exposure during pregnancy has been associated with both nor-

mal outcome and rare instances of cardiac malformation (especially the Ebstein anomaly). Various cardiopulmonary symptoms without cardiac or pulmonary disease have been reported in lithium babies. A 30-year-old woman taking lithium (800 mg/day) during pregnancy gave birth to a baby with fatal congenital heart defects (Youssef HA, Toal F. Case of lithium-induced cardiovascular malformations. *Adv Ther* 1992;9:338–341). There have been reports of electroencephalogram (EEG) changes (isoelectric or inverted T waves) and/or episodes of bradycardia in lithium-intoxicated newborns. Lithium frequently causes hypotonia in neonates, as well as goiter with transient hypothyroidism. Nephrogenic diabetes insipidus and hypoglycemia also have occurred in infants whose mothers took lithium while pregnant. Initial data regarding the teratogenic risk of lithium treatment were derived from biased retrospective reports. More recent epidemiological data indicate that teratogenic risk of first-trimester lithium exposure is lower than previously suggested. A controlled, prospective study of 148 women using lithium during part or all of the first trimester showed that pregnancy outcome did not differ between patients and controls (N = 48) with respect to the number of live births, frequency of major anomalies, spontaneous or therapeutic abortions, ectopic pregnancy, and prematurity. Lithium babies had a higher mean birth weight than control babies; there was no correlation between lithium dose and weight. There were no differences between groups in attainment of developmental milestones (smiling, lifting head, sitting, crawling, standing, talking, and walking). Although an association between lithium and major anomalies is not ruled out, study results suggest that the risk is lower than reported by the Danish Register of Lithium Babies. Investigators concluded that lithium is not a major human teratogen, and that lithium can be continued during pregnancy provided level II ultrasound and fetal echocardiography are done (Jacobson SJ, Jones K, et al. Prospective multicentre study of pregnancy outcome after lithium exposure during first trimester. *Lancet* 1992;339:530–533). Clinical management of women with bipolar disorder who can bear children should be modified with this revised risk estimate. Such women frequently have been counseled to avoid or terminate pregnancy. The growing number of studies indicating a more modest teratogenic risk than originally estimated with first-trimester lithium treatment gives women an opportunity for more thoughtful choices as they weigh the risk of taking lithium against the risk of untreated bipolar disorder (Cohen LS,

Friedman JM, Jefferson JW, et al. A reevaluation of risk of in utero exposure to lithium. *JAMA* 1994;271:146–150). Patients should be carefully monitored and treated with low lithium doses and serum levels below 0.8 mEq/L, especially during the first and third trimesters. See **lithium toxicity/neonate.**

lithium + propranolol Co-administration can have additive effects on the SA and AV nodes of the heart.

lithium/renal effects In 1977, a report of renal biopsy abnormalities in a small number of lithium-treated patients generated a flurry of studies evaluating renal function (Hestbech J, Hansen HE, Amdisen A, Olsen S. Chronic renal lesions following long-term treatment with lithium. *Kidney Int* 1977;12:205–213). Two reviews of these studies concluded that even chronic lithium treatment does not lead to changes in glomerular filtration rate or renal failure (Schou M. Effects of long-term lithium treatment on kidney function: an overview. *J Psychiatr Res* 1988;22:287–296; Waller DG, Edwards JG. Lithium and the kidney: an update. *Psychol Med* 1989;19:825–831). A small number of subsequent studies indicated that a small percentage of lithium-treated patients may develop rising levels of serum creatinine after a decade or more of treatment (Stancer HC, Forbath N. Hyperparathyroidism, hypothyroidism, and impaired renal function after 10 to 20 years of lithium treatment. *Arch Intern Med* 1989;149:1042–1045; Hetmar O, Povlsen UJ, Ladefoged J, Bolwig TG. Lithium: long-term effects on the kidney. A prospective follow-up study ten years after kidney biopsy. *Br J Psychiatry* 1991;158:53–58). The first well documented case of lithium-induced chronic renal failure progressing to chronic hemodialysis was published in 1990 (von Knorring L, Wahlin A, Nystrom K, Bohman SO. Uraemia induced by long-term lithium treatment. *Lithium* 1990;1:251–253). Among recently published studies, there is evidence that 0–5% of patients treated with lithium over a long period may develop signs of renal insufficiency. In the latest report, 3 of 82 bipolar patients (3.7%) were found to have developed serum creatinine levels greater than 2.0 mg/100 ml from baseline levels that were within normal limits; 1 patient progressed to chronic renal failure and hemodialysis. No common risk factor for renal disease among these patients was apparent. Previous conclusions as to the benign effects of long-term lithium treatment on renal function may need to be revised. Regular monitoring of serum creatinine levels and medical consultation if they rise and remain above 1.6 mg/100 ml have been recommended (Gitlin MJ. Lithium-induced renal insufficiency. *J Clin Psychopharmacol* 1993;13:276–279).

lithium/response predictors, favorable Clinical features associated with good response to lithium include family history of bipolar disorder and personal history of a previous episode sequence of mania-depression-euthymia (Maj M. Clinical predictors of response to lithium prophylaxis in bipolar patients: a critical update. *Lithium* 1992;3:15–21).

lithium/response predictors, poor Clinical features associated with poor response to lithium include (a) rapid cycling; (b) dysphoric or mixed mania; (c) episode sequence of depression-mania-euthymia; (d) co-morbid alcohol or drug abuse; (e) severe and/or secondary mania; (f) mania with psychosis; (g) three or more manic episodes prior to initiation of lithium treatment (Keck PE, McElroy SL. Current perspectives on treatment of bipolar disorder with lithium. *Psychiatr Ann* 1993;23:64–69; Gelenberg AJ, Kane JN, Keller MB, et al. Comparison of standard and low serum levels of lithium maintenance of bipolar disorder *N Engl J Med* 1989;321:1489–1493; O'Connell RA, Mayo JA, Flatow L, et al. Outcome of bipolar disorder on long-term treatment with lithium. *Br J Psychiatry* 1991;159:123–129). Loss of response to lithium prophylaxis also may be due to development of tolerance and tachyphylaxis and to discontinuation-induced refractoriness (Post RM. Issues in the long-term management of bipolar affective illness. *Psychiatr Ann* 1993;23:86–93; Terao T, Terao M. Refractoriness induced by lithium discontinuation. *Am J Psychiatry* 1993;150:1756).

lithium + sertraline Co-administration is safe and effective, although sertraline may increase lithium tremor, slightly decrease steady-state lithium levels, and slightly increase renal clearance of lithium (Apseloff G, Wilner KD, von Deutsch DA, et al. Sertraline does not alter steady-state concentrations or renal clearance of lithium in healthy volunteers. *J Clin Pharmacol* 1992;32:643–646; Dinan TG. Lithium augmentation in sertraline-resistant depression: a preliminary dose-response study. *Acta Psychiatr Scand* 1993;88:300–301). Sertraline may augment response to lithium in organic mood syndrome without causing any serious adverse effects (Workman EA, Harrington DP. Sertraline-augmented lithium therapy of organic mood syndrome. *Psychosomatics* 1992;33:472–473).

lithium/sodium Lithium reabsorption and excretion are bound to that of sodium. Inadequate lithium excretion is a likely consequence of restricted sodium intake, whereas reduced efficacy may follow sodium loading. Excessive sodium intake may expedite lithium excretion and lower serum blood levels below those required to alleviate symptoms of mania. Conversely, sodium depletion from salt-restricted diets or diuretics may cause lithium toxicity secondary to a rise in lithium plasma levels.

lithium + spectinomycin Co-administration decreases renal lithium clearance, increases lithium serum levels, and may produce lithium toxicity (Ayd FJ Jr. Possible adverse drug-drug interaction report. *Int Drug Ther Newsl* 1978; 13:15).

lithium + spironolactone Co-administration may moderately increase lithium level over time; lithium serum levels should be monitored (Baer L, Platman SR, Kassir S, Fieve RR. Mechanism of renal lithium handling and their relationship to mineralocorticoids: a dissociation between sodium and lithium ions. *J Psychiatr Res* 1981;8:91–105). See **lithium + diuretic.**

lithium + succinylcholine Lithium prolongs the neuromuscular blockade of succinylcholine and has been implicated as a cause of acute confusional states after electroconvulsive therapy. By contrast, 17 patients demonstrated no interaction between lithium and succinylcholine (Martin BA, Kramer PM. Clinical significance of the interaction between lithium and a neuromuscular blocker. *Am J Psychiatry* 1982;139:1326–1328).

lithium sulfate (Lithionet Durettes) Sustained release form of lithium.

lithium + sulindac There currently is no convincing evidence that sulindac (300 mg/day) can affect serum lithium levels to a clinically significant degree (Ragheb M. The clinical significance of lithium-nonsteroidal anti-inflammatory drug interactions. *J Clin Psychopharmacol* 1990;10:350–354). See **lithium + nonsteroidal anti-inflammatory drug.**

lithium + sulpiride Co-administration can evoke acute extrapyramidal reactions (Dinan TG, O'Keane V. Acute extrapyramidal reactions following lithium and sulpiride co-administration: two case reports. *Hum Psychopharmacol Clin Exp* 1991;6:67–69).

lithium + sumatriptan Co-administration may increase sumatriptan effects (Anon. Sumatriptan: a new approach to migraine. *Drug Ther Bull* 1992;30:85–87).

lithium/tardive dyskinesia Maintenance therapy with lithium and neuroleptics may increase the risk for neuroleptic-induced tardive dyskinesia (TD) (Mann SC, Greenstein RA, Eilers R. Early onset of severe dyskinesia following lithium-haloperidol treatment. *Am J Psychiatry* 1983;140:1385–1386). A significant association between length of exposure to lithium and early onset of TD was found in a prospec-

tive study (Kane JM, Woerner M, Weinhold P, et al. Incidence of tardive dyskinesia: Five-year data from a prospective study. *Psychopharmacol Bull* 1984;20:387–389). Until this association is confirmed, careful surveillance of patients on combined lithium-neuroleptic therapy is indicated. Lithium therapy for patients with TD has produced variable results, including no effect, mild improvement, and aggravation of TD. In a double-blind study, it eradicated TD in two patients, improved it in three, and worsened it in two (Rosenbaum AH, Maruta T, Duane DD, et al. Tardive dyskinesia in depressed patients: successful therapy with antidepressants and lithium. *Psychosomatics* 1980; 21:715–719).

lithium + teciptiline Co-administration may be useful for the treatment of refractory depression without serious adverse effects.

lithium + tetracycline In a single case report, co-administration resulted in increased lithium levels and toxicity due to decreased renal lithium clearance (McGennis AJ. Lithium carbonate and tetracycline interaction. *Br Med J* 1978;1:1183). A more definitive study found no interaction (Frankhauser MP, Lindon JL, Connolly B. Evaluation of lithium and tetracycline interaction. *Clin Pharm* 1988; 7:314–317).

lithium + theobromine Co-administration may increase lithium excretion and decrease lithium blood levels. Lithium dosage may have to be raised when theobromine is taken simultaneously to achieve a therapeutic lithium level or decreased when theobromine is discontinued to avert lithium toxicity.

lithium + theophylline Theophylline significantly increases renal lithium clearance, lowering serum lithium levels and possibly impairing lithium's therapeutic effects. When theophylline is added to lithium, lithium levels should be monitored every 3–4 days to assess the degree and direction of serum lithium change. Side effects should not be automatically attributed to lithium. Interactions are most important in patients previously sensitive to relapse with decreased lithium levels. When theophylline is discontinued, close monitoring of lithium levels is important, because they could rise and result in lithium toxicity (Cook BL, Smith RE, Perry PJ, et al. Theophylline-lithium interaction. *J Clin Psychiatry* 1985;46:278–279).

lithium + thiazide diuretic See **lithium + diuretic.**

lithium + thioridazine Co-administration may result in neurotoxicity (Spring G. Neurotoxicity with combined use of lithium and thioridazine. *J Clin Psychiatry* 1979;40:135–138; Bailine SH, Doft M. Neurotoxicity induced by combined lithium-thioridazine treatment. *Biol Psychiatry* 1986;21:834–837).

lithium + thiothixene   Co-administration may cause the sudden appearance of extrapyramidal side effects and neurotoxicity (Fetzer J, Kader G, Dohany S. Lithium encephalopathy: a clinical, psychiatric and EEG evaluation. *Am J Psychiatry* 1981;138:1622–1623).

lithium/thyroid effects   Lithium inhibits secretion of thyroid hormones and release of iodine from the thyroid and causes a marked increase in thyroid antibodies. Goiter and hypothyroidism are infrequent in patients on long-term lithium therapy. Abnormalities of thyroid function tests in lithium-treated patients are common. Women are more prone to develop hypothyroidism during lithium treatment. Thyroid function should be evaluated before starting lithium and monitored at regular intervals. About 38% of cases of hypothyroidism are diagnosed within the first 6 months, 55% during the first year, and 74% within the first 2 years of lithium treatment. Patients with hypothyroidism secondary to lithium therapy may show a gradation of symptoms and should be considered for thyroid replacement hormones if grade 2 or 3 changes occur. Because of the possibility of lithium-related thyroid failure, a thyrotropin-releasing hormone test should be done before adding an antidepressant to the treatment regimen.

lithium + thyroxine   High doses of thyroxine combined with lithium may decrease cycling frequency and severity in rapid cycling bipolar disorder (Bauer MS, Whybrow PC. Rapid cycling bipolar affective disorder. II. Treatment of refractory rapid cycling with high dose levothyroxine: a preliminary study. *Arch Gen Psychiatry* 1990;47:435–440).

lithium toxicity   Factors that predispose to rising serum lithium levels include (a) physical disease with fever; (b) low-salt diet; (c) vomiting and diarrhea; (d) slimming diet; (e) prolonged unconsciousness; (f) narcosis and surgery; (g) concurrent treatment with diuretics, nonsteroidal anti-inflammatory drugs, or angiotensin converting enzyme inhibitors. Initial symptoms include lethargy, poor concentration or memory, and confusion that may progress to clear disorientation, disorganization, or coma. Associated symptoms may include gastrointestinal irritability; nausea; vomiting; diarrhea; dysarthria; choreoathetoid movements; increased muscle tone; hyperreflexia and coarse tremor; seizures, including status epilepticus; urinary incontinence; and cardiovascular collapse or renal failure. Delirium is usually seen when the serum lithium level exceeds 2.0 mEq/L, but has been reported with normal or therapeutic serum

lithium levels. Predisposing factors for delirium are (a) concurrent medications; (b) age over 60; (c) pre-existing neurological disease; and (d) intercurrent medical illness.

lithium toxicity/elderly   Elderly patients treated uneventfully with lithium for many years (10+) who present with rapid onset of dementia and other new symptoms (rigidity, mutism), should be examined promptly for lithium intoxication. Serum lithium levels should be taken to confirm or rule out lithium toxicity and avoid misdiagnosis and delay of essential treatment. Lithium intoxication can become life-threatening or result in permanent neurological damage. If acute lithium intoxication is recognized early and treated promptly, however, there is usually full recovery without permanent neurological damage.

lithium toxicity, chronic   Side effects associated with long-term lithium therapy include nephrogenic diabetes insipidus, thyroid disturbances, altered renal function, blood sugar elevation, and leukocytosis.

lithium toxicity, mild   Symptoms due to slightly elevated plasma lithium levels (usually over 1 mEq/L) include anorexia, gastrointestinal discomfort, diarrhea, nausea, vomiting, thirst, polyuria, and hand tremor. Mild toxicity may occur in the early days of lithium therapy and may be related more to the steepness of the rise of the lithium level than to its height. It often disappears or moderates without dosage reduction. Appearance of signs and symptoms of mild lithium toxicity in a patient on maintenance therapy should warrant immediate plasma lithium determinations to rule out an early phase of more serious lithium intoxication. All patients should be reminded periodically of the manifestations of mild lithium toxicity and instructed to report them to their physician.

lithium toxicity/neonate   Lithium toxicity can occur in newborns at serum levels nontoxic for the mother. Symptoms may include flaccidity, cyanosis, lethargy, poor suck, and poor Moro reflexes (Woody JN, London WL, Wilbanks GB. Lithium toxicity in a newborn. *Pediatrics* 1971;47:94–96). Lithium withdrawal in a neonate may be manifested by abnormal irritability. If a neonate becomes lithium toxic, supportive management is indicated rather than exchange transfusion, peritoneal dialysis, or hemodialysis (Morrell P, Sutherland GR, Buamah PK, et al. Lithium toxicity in a neonate. *Arch Dis Child* 1983;58:538–539). Lithium may also cause reversible inhibition of thyroid function with or without goiter in the newborn, cardiac arrhythmias, and reversible diabetes insipidus (Miller LJ. Clinical strategies for the use of psychotropic drugs during pregnancy. *Psychiatr Med* 1991;9:275–298).

lithium toxicity, severe When lithium plasma level is above 1.5 mEq/L, symptoms may include muscle fasciculation and twitching, hyperactive deep tendon reflexes, ataxia, somnolence, confusion, dysarthria and, infrequently, seizures.

lithium + tranylcypromine Lithium has been co-administered with tranylcypromine to potentiate its antidepressant effects without adverse reactions in depressed patients refractory to other antidepressant regimens (Nolan WA, Håffmans J, Bouvy PF, Duivenvoorden HJ. Monoamine oxidase inhibitors in resistant major depression. A double-blind comparison of brofaromine and tranylcypromine in patients resistant to tricyclic antidepressants. *J Affect Dis* 1993;28:189–197; Price LH, Charney DS, Heninger GR. Efficacy of lithium-tranylcypromine treatment in refractory depression. *Am J Psychiatry* 1985;142:619–623). Two cases of tardive dyskinesia (bucco-lingual-masticatory type) have been reported after long-term treatment with tranylcypromine and lithium (Stancer HC. Tardive dyskinesia not associated with neuroleptics. *Am J Psychiatry* 1979; 136:727).

lithium tremor Frequently noted side effect of lithium therapy that may occur in up to 53% of patients during the first week of treatment (Schou M, Baastrup PC, Grof P, et al. Pharmacological and clinical problems of lithium prophylaxis. *Br J Psychiatry* 1970;116:615–619). Fine hand tremor is seen at rest and increases with voluntary movement and maintenance of posture. It usually decreases in intensity after 1–2 weeks of treatment. Tremor that appears during long-term lithium therapy is considered an extrapyramidal symptom that occurs most often in patients over age 60. This tremor is not correlated with serum lithium levels (Tyrer P, Alexander MS, Regan A, Lee I. An extrapyramidal syndrome after lithium therapy. *Br J Psychiatry* 1980;136:191–194).

lithium + triamterene Co-administration increases plasma lithium concentration and risk of lithium toxicity. Lithium blood levels should be checked frequently and patients should be monitored clinically for signs of lithium intoxication. See **lithium + diuretic.**

lithium + tricyclic antidepressant (TCA) Co-administration has been used successfully in treatment-resistant depression (Schou M. Lithium and treatment-resistant depression. A review. *Lithium* 1990;1:3–8). It may decrease the metabolism of each drug, resulting in increased plasma concentrations of both. Central nervous system depressant and hypotensive effects may be additive. Addition of lithium to TCAs may cause emergence or exacerbation of myoclonus (Devanand DP, Sackeim HA, Brown RP. Myoclonus during combined tricyclic antidepressant and lithium treatment. *J Clin Psychopharmacol* 1988;8:446–447). A comparison of electroconvulsive therapy (ECT) with a combination of lithium and a tricyclic antidepressant in depressed tricyclic nonresponders showed that lithium augmentation is comparable with ECT in severely depressed patients (Dinan TG, Barry S. A comparison of electroconvulsive therapy with a combined lithium and tricyclic combination among depressed tricyclic nonresponders. *Acta Psychiatr Scand* 1989;80: 97–100).

lithium + tricyclic antidepressant (TCA) + neuroleptic Several case reports indicate that lithium may potentiate response to TCA/neuroleptic treatment (Nelson JC, Maguire CM. Lithium augmentation in psychotic depression refractory to combined drug treatment. *Am J Psychiatry* 1986;143:363–366; Pai M, White AC, Deane AG. Lithium augmentation in the treatment of delusional depression. *Br J Psychiatry* 1986;148:736–738; Price LH, Yeates C, Nelson JC. Lithium augmentation of combined neuroleptic-tricyclic treatment in delusional depression. *Am J Psychiatry* 1983;140:318–322).

lithium + triiodothyronine Open and controlled studies indicate a substantial proportion of tricyclic antidepressant nonresponders may have a therapeutic response with the addition of small amounts of liothyronine (Joffe R, Singer W, Levitt AJ, MacDonald C. A placebo-controlled comparison of lithium and triiodothyronine augmentation of tricyclic antidepressants in unipolar refractory depression. *Arch Gen Psychiatry* 1993;50:387–393). See **lithium + fluoxetine + triiodothyronine.**

lithium + trimethoprim-sulfamethoxazole (TMP/SMZ) Within days of starting TMP/SMZ, two patients on chronic lithium therapy developed toxicity manifested by hand tremors, vesiculations, muscular weakness, and dysarthria, and their serum lithium levels decreased almost 50%. Symptoms resolved and lithium levels returned to normal after TMP/SMZ was discontinued (Desvilles M, Sevestre P. Effect paradoxal de l'association lithium et sulfamethoxazol-trimethoprime. *La Nouvelle Presse Medicale* 1982;11:3267–3268).

lithium + tryptophan Tryptophan may potentiate the therapeutic effects of lithium in bipolar patients partially responsive to lithium.

lithium + valproate Lithium has been shown to augment the antidepressant effect of valproate. In rapid cyclers, co-administration decreases rapid cycling, especially in patients refractory or only minimally responsive to lithium and neuroleptics (Sharma V, Persad E. Augmentation of valproate with lithium in a case of rapid cycling affective disorder. *Can J Psychiatry* 1992;37:384–385; Sharma V, Persad E, Mazmanian D, Kaarunaratne K. Treatment of rapid cycling bipolar disorder with combination therapy of valproate and lithium. *Can J Psychiatry* 1993;38:137–139).

lithium + valproic acid   Valproic acid may produce fewer central nervous system effects when combined with lithium (Calabrese JR, Delucchi GA. Phenomenology of rapid cycling manic depression and its treatment with valproate. *J Clin Psychiatry* 1989;50[suppl]:30–34).

lithium + vasopressin   Co-administration in older patients increases risk of lithium toxicity because of low plasma sodium levels. Lithium blood levels must be closely monitored and dosage must be adjusted if they increase or early signs of toxicity appear.

lithium + verapamil   With careful monitoring, co-administration can be used in patients intolerant of lithium side effects. In eight normal male volunteers, controlled-release verapamil (200 mg/day) added to lithium (600 mg/day) for 7 days did not alter previously established pharmacokinetics of lithium alone in any measure of clearance, half-life, or volume of distribution (Myers CW, Perry PJ, Kathol RG. Plasma and erythrocyte lithium concentrations before and after oral verapamil. *Lithium* 1990;1:49–53). Co-administration has been reported to cause cardiotoxicity, neurotoxic side effects, and decreased serum lithium levels (Price WA, Giannini AJ. Neurotoxicity caused by lithium-verapamil. *J Clin Pharmacol* 1986;26:717–719; Price WA, Shalley JE. Lithium-verapamil toxicity in the elderly. *J Am Geriatr Soc* 1987;35:177–179; Weinrauch LA, Belok S, D'Elia JA. Decreased serum lithium during verapamil therapy. *Am Heart J* 1984;108:1378–1379).

lithium + zidovudine   Lithium has been safely and effectively added to zidovudine for the treatment of zidovudine-induced mania (Maxwell S, Scheftner W, Kessler H, et al. Manic syndrome associated with zidovudine treatment. *JAMA* 1988;259:3406–3407). It also may decrease zidovudine-associated neutropenia, but may not be well tolerated by acquired immunodeficiency syndrome (AIDS) patients (Roberts DE, Berman SM, Nakasato S. Effect of lithium carbonate in the acquired immunodeficiency syndrome. *Am J Med* 1988;85:428–431; Parenti DM, Simon GL, Scheib RG, et al. Effect of lithium carbonate on HIV infected patients with immune dysfunction. *J Acquired Immunodefic Synd* 1988;1:119–124).

Lithizine   See **lithium**.
Lithonate   See **lithium**.
Lithotabs   See **lithium**.

litoxetine   New selective serotonin (5-HT) uptake inhibitor with potent activity in behavioral models predictive of antidepressant action. Clinical trials in Europe, in flexible daily doses of 50–100 mg/day for 4 weeks, indicate that litoxetine is an effective antidepressant. It has a 5-HT$_3$ blocking effect that may decrease side effects such as nausea.

liver enzyme induction   Increased liver enzyme activity due to chronic use of drugs such as barbiturates, glutethimide, meprobamate, or methyprylon. It can cause drug interactions when drugs that use the same enzymes for their metabolism are metabolized more quickly than normal and their therapeutic efficacy is decreased. When the drug causing enzyme induction is discontinued, enzyme induction ceases, the number of enzymes reverts to normal, and the dosage of other drugs should be reduced to avert an overdose problem.

"load"   Street name for glutethimide plus codeine used for euphoriant properties that are subjectively similar to those of parenteral opiates. Users crush and mix with water four acetaminophen + codeine (Tylenol #4) and two glutethimide (Doriden) tablets. The mixture is then injected.

lobotomy   Neurosurgical procedure introduced by Egas Moniz in which one or more nerve tracts in the frontal lobe are severed. It has been used in the treatment of certain severe mental disorders unresponsive to other treatments. Today, lobotomy is reserved almost exclusively for severe treatment-resistant depressions. Also called "leukotomy"; "prefrontal lobotomy." See **cingulotomy; tractotomy, stereotactic.**

lobotomy, Grantham   Neurosurgical procedure performed by electrocoagulation of the ventromedial quadrant of the prefrontal lobe of the brain. It is seldom done today.

lobotomy, prefrontal   See **lobotomy.**

lobotomy, transorbital   Psychosurgical procedure in which the operative instrument is inserted through the superior conjunctival sack. It is usually performed bilaterally. It is seldom done today.

locked-in syndrome   See **akinetic mutism.**

"locker room"   Street name for butyl nitrite.

locomotor skills   Skills involved in moving the body around (e.g., crawling, walking, running abilities).

"locoweed"   Street name for marijuana.

locus   1. Position that a gene occupies on a chromosome. 2. DNA region that contains the entire set of information to express the protein product encoded by the DNA.

locus ceruleus (LC) Collection of neuronal cell bodies located in the pons. It contains the largest accumulation of noradrenergic neurons (close to half) in a single identified brain region. Its neurons project their axons to virtually every region of the brain. Their activity is thought to be involved in the regulation of mood, anxiety, and attention. Overactivity of this nucleus and its ascending noradrenergic system has been causally linked to occurrence of anxiety attacks. Autopsy studies of elderly subjects have revealed a decreased number of neurons in the locus ceruleus and decreased norepinephrine content in many brain areas, suggesting an age-related decrease in noradrenergic function that may make older people more susceptible to anxiety. A relationship between the function of the locus ceruleus and psychiatric disorders, particularly depression, has been postulated. The locus ceruleus contains high concentrations of norepinephrine uptake transporters, alpha-2-adrenergic receptors, and monoamine oxidase A, all of which are sites of action of various antidepressant drugs. Depression may be associated with locus ceruleus dysfunction; modulation of locus ceruleus biochemistry may be at least one mechanism of antidepressant drug action.

Lodopin See **zotepine**.

Lodosyn See **carbidopa**.

lod score Statistical measure of linkage. A score of three or above is taken to be strongly suggestive of linkage and considered unlikely to occur by chance. A lod score of three represents odds of 1,000 to 1; it is the actual 95% confidence level used when testing one marker locus and one disease gene.

lod score method Statistical procedure based on the odds ratio (i.e., the ratio between the probability of observing the data under the hypothesis of linkage and that of there being no linkage). The ratio is commonly expressed as its logarithm, or lod score.

lofepramine (Amplit; Defton-70; Deprimil; Emdalen; Gamanil; Lopramine; Timelit; Tymelyt) Dibenzazepine derivative second generation tricyclic antidepressant structurally similar to imipramine and desipramine. Like them, it inhibits neuronal reuptake of both noradrenalin (NA) and serotonin (5-HT), thereby increasing the concentration of these neurotransmitters at their receptors. It has been shown to be as effective as amitriptyline. About 30% of lofepramine is metabolized to desipramine, its principal metabolite. It is a less potent muscarinic receptor antagonist than desipramine and less likely to produce con-

duction defects. Lofepramine may induce hyponatremia and abnormal liver function; the latter resolves after lofepramine discontinuation, but reappears with its readministration. Lofepramine is reported to be efficacious and well tolerated in the elderly (Dorman T. The management of depression: the use of lofepramine in the elderly. *Br J Clin Pract* 1988;42:459–464).

lofepramine + lithium Addition of lithium in depression refractory to lofepramine may produce favorable therapeutic response (Seymour J, Wattis JP. Treatment resistant depression in the elderly: three cases. *Int Clin Psychopharmacol* 1992;7:55–57). Efficacy appears to be contingent on achieving adequate serum lithium levels (Katona CL, Robertson MM, Abou-Saleh MT, et al. Placebo controlled trial of lithium augmentation of fluoxetine and lofepramine. *Int Clin Psychopharmacol* 1993;8:323).

lofexidine (MDL-14042) Clonidine congener and alpha-adrenergic agonist with less sedative and hypotensive effects. It has proven useful in opiate withdrawal management and detoxification. It may be effective in the treatment of alcohol withdrawal.

loflazepate Benzodiazepine (BZD) derivative. Overdose data in children indicate that it causes sleeplessness, agitation, and ataxia. Severe poisoning with this drug causes hypotonia. Thus, like the older BZDs, it has relatively low acute toxicity (Pulce C, Mollon P, Pham E, et al. Acute poisonings with ethyl loflazepate, flunitrazepam, prazepam and triazolam in children. *Vet Hum Toxicol* 1992;34:141–143).

Loftran See **ketazolam**.

logarithm Exponent indicating the power to which e (2.718) is raised to obtain a given number.

logical reasoning Measure of complex semantic processing that assesses working memory.

logistic regression Technique used when the outcome is nominal, usually dichotomous. Its major purpose is to explore the relative risk of having an event when some independent variables change, while controlling the confounding and interactional terms.

logistic regression analysis Technique that generates a prediction equation using a binary dependent variable and independent variables that may be categorical or continuous (Engleman L. Stepwise logistic regression. *In* Dixon W [ed], *BMDP Statistical Software*. Berkeley: University of California Press, 1981).

logistic regression model Model in which recorded growth rate is used to investigate the development of certain relationships in the theory of heredity. It is similar to linear regression except that it predicts a discrete outcome variable.

log-linear Linear relationship between the logarithm of the dependent variable and the independent variable.

log-linear analysis Statistical method for analyzing the relationships among three or more nominal variables. It may be used as a regression method to predict a nominal outcome from nominal independent variables.

logorrhea Speech disturbance manifested by excessive volubility that is not only copious, but coherent and logical. Transient logorrhea may be normal. Persistent logorrhea may be a symptom of a psychiatric illness. Also called "tachylogia."

log-rank test Statistical method for comparing two survival curves when there are censored observations.

Lomotil See **diphenoxylate.**

longitudinal observational study See **case series.**

longitudinal study Study in which observations on the same individuals are made at two or more different times. Most cohort and case-control studies are longitudinal.

Longopax See **perphenazine + amitriptyline.**

Longopax Mite See **perphenazine + amitriptyline.**

long-term insomnia See **insomnia, long-term.**

long-term memory See **memory, long-term.**

long-term potentiation See **potentiation, long-term.**

Lonseron See **pipotiazine.**

look-alike Inert or less potent substance intentionally formulated to look like a well known form of a more powerful, expensive, or less readily available drug. Although look-alike generics have been manufactured to compete with proprietary drugs, this has been infrequent compared to production of look-alikes for abuse purposes.

Lopramine See **lofepramine.**

loprazolam (Dormonoct) Tricyclic benzodiazepine hypnotic biotransformed by microsomal oxidation. Abrupt discontinuation results in acute withdrawal effects. Not available in the United States.

Lopressor See **metoprolol.**

Loramet See **lormetazepam.**

Loraz See **lorazepam.**

lorazepam (Alzipam; Apo-Lorazepam; Ativan; Bonton; Loraz; Lorivan; Merlit; Novolorazepam; Temesta) (LOR) Low-dose, high-potency 1,4 benzodiazepine (BZD) with a relatively short elimination half-life (including metabolites) of 12 hours. It is metabolized by glucuronide conjugation; the principal metabolite (lorazepam glucuronide) is recovered in urine. It is effective orally, intramuscularly,

and intravenously. It is the only BZD with rapid, reliable intramuscular absorption. It has been used intramuscularly and intravenously to treat extreme agitation secondary to delirium in acquired immunodeficiency syndrome (AIDS) patients. It may be especially liable to disinhibit aggressive behavior. Schedule IV; pregnancy risk category D. See **lorazepam + neuroleptic.**

lorazepam + alcohol Acute alcohol ingestion, even in chronic alcohol users, reduces elimination and thus increases the plasma level of lorazepam (Hoyumpa A, Patwardhan R, Maples M, et al. Effect of short-term ethanol administration on lorazepam metabolism. *Gastroenterology* 1980;79:1027).

lorazepam/breast milk It is not known if lorazepam is excreted in human milk. Patients taking lorazepam should be advised not to nurse. For more data consult the manufacturer.

lorazepam + clozapine Addition of low-dose lorazepam (LOR) (1 mg orally or intramuscularly, or 2 mg intramuscularly) to clozapine (CLOZ) (100–200 mg/day) produced marked sedation, excessive sialorrhea and ataxia, and unresponsiveness to verbal stimuli, suggesting a clinically significant, synergistic, pharmacodynamic interaction. Benzodiazepines should be used cautiously when initiating CLOZ (Cobb CD, Anderson CB, Seidel DR. Possible interaction between clozapine and lorazepam. *Am J Psychiatry* 1991;148:1606–1607). There are reports, however, of response to combined treatment, deterioration after LOR withdrawal, and improvement with LOR resumption (Kanofsky JF, Lindenmayer JP. Relapse in a clonazepam responder following lorazepam withdrawal. *Am J Psychiatry* 1993;150:348–349). See **clozapine + benzodiazepine.**

lorazepam + fluvoxamine Lorazepam (1–2 mg) may relieve insomnia in fluvoxamine-treated patients without adverse effects (Mallya GK, White K, Waternaux C, et al. Short- and long-term treatment of obsessive-compulsive disorders with fluvoxamine. *Ann Clin Psychiatry* 1992;4:77–80).

lorazepam + haloperidol Co-administration may be effective and safe in the treatment of acute psychotic agitation, acute schizophrenia, and mania. The combination may be superior to either drug alone in terms of clinical effects and may allow use of lower doses, thus reducing risk of unwanted side effects (Garza-Trevino ES, Hollister LE, Overall JE, Alexander WF. Efficacy of combinations of intramuscular antipsychotics and sedative-hypnotics for control of psychotic agitation. *Am J Psychiatry* 1989;149:1598–1601; Stevens A, Stevens I, Mahal A, Gaertner HJ. Haloperidol and lorazepam combined: clinical effects and drug plasma levels in the treatment of acute schizophrenic psychosis. *Pharmacopsychiatry* 1992;25:273–277).

lorazepam + lithium   Lorazepam may be useful as an adjunct in controlling agitation (Modell JG. Further experience and observations with lorazepam in the management of behavioral agitation. *J Clin Psychopharmacol* 1986;6:385–387). It also may be used in patients not fully responsive to lithium (Janicak PG, Newman RH, Davis JM. Advances in the treatment of mania and related disorders: a reappraisal. *Psychiatr Ann* 1992;22:92–103).

lorazepam + loxapine   There are three case reports of patients previously treated with loxapine without undue side effects in whom addition of lorazepam (LOR) resulted in significant respiratory depression accompanied by excessive stupor and, in one patient, hypotension. All were given the combination treatment in hospital and observed closely following occurrence of the adverse effects. There was no evidence of use of other psychotropic medications or alcohol prior to treatment. All patients made uneventful recoveries. One was subsequently given perphenazine plus LOR with no recurrence of respiratory difficulty or lethargy (Cohen S, Khan A. Respiratory distress with use of lorazepam in mania. *J Clin Psychopharmacol* 1987;7:199–200; Battaglia J, Thornton L, Young C. Loxapine-lorazepam-induced hypotension and stupor. *J Clin Psychopharmacol* 1989;9:227–228).

lorazepam + methadone   Lorazepam, diazepam, and alprazolam were much preferred over other benzodiazepines by 40 "connoisseur" methadone maintenance patients who used them to "boost" methadone effects (Iguchi MY, Griffiths RR, Bickel WR, et al. Relative abuse liability of benzodiazepines in methadone-maintained populations in three cities. *In* Harris LS [ed], *Problems of Drug Dependence.* NIDA Research Monograph No. 95, DHSS Publication [ADM] 90-1663. Washington, DC: US Government Printing Office, 1989, pp 364–365).

lorazepam + neuroleptic   Lorazepam (LOR) has been added to a variety of neuroleptics to control acutely agitated psychoses. Co-administration requires less time to control agitation, produces fewer side effects, and has a neuroleptic-sparing effect in that fewer neuroleptic doses are needed. It generally is safe, but paradoxical reactions to lorazepam do occur. Co-administration for management of acute mania has escalated because of LOR's pharmacokinetics: rapid onset of action, short half-life, relatively short duration of action, and relatively simple hepatic metabolism re-

quiring only glucuronidation for renal excretion. In addition, the likelihood of drug interactions is low. Many experts use lorazepam (3–8 mg/day) with low neuroleptic doses (Pato CN, Wolkowitz OM, Rapaport M, et al. Benzodiazepine augmentation of neuroleptic treatment in patients with schizophrenia. *Psychopharmacol Bull* 1989;25:263–266).

lorazepam/pregnancy   There are no reports of adverse fetal effects.

lordosis   Backward curvature of the spine.

Lorivan   See **lorazepam.**

lormetazepam   (Evamyl; Loramet; Minias; Noctamid; Noctaminde; Nocton; Pronoctan) 1,4-Benzodiazepine hypnotic biotransformed principally by glucuronide conjugation. Under normal clinical use, it has negligible psychomotor and amnestic effects. Not available in the United States.

loss of control   Inability to limit the use of substances (drugs, alcohol) via an internal locus of control.

Lovan   See **fluoxetine.**

"loveboat"   Street name for phencyclidine (PCP).

"love drug"   Street name for 3,4-methylenedioxyamphetamine.

"lovely"   Street name for phencyclidine (PCP).

Lou Gehrig's disease   See **amyotrophic lateral sclerosis.**

low energy emission therapy   (LEET) Nonpharmacological treatment for persistent, psychophysiological insomnia that uses intrabuccally emitted electromagnetic fields. Changes in electroencephalographic (EEG) activity and psychological test measures provide support for the hypothesis that it has physiologic activity and is effective.

lowest effective dose   Drug dosage that causes the greatest symptom reduction with the fewest adverse effects.

low expressed emotion   See **expressed emotion.**

low-potency neuroleptic   See **neuroleptic, low-potency.**

low serotonin syndrome   Impulse control disorder that afflicts a subgroup of violent offenders. It is characterized by early onset of impulsive violent behavior and alcohol abuse, increased risk of suicide, and family history of type II alcoholism. It is also associated with a constellation of psychobiological characteristics, including low cerebrospinal fluid concentrations of the monoamine metabolites 5-HIAA and possibly MHPG, and low blood glucose nadir during the glucose tolerance test. These clinical features may represent physical and behavioral manifestations of an underlying defect in serotonin (5-HT) function, specifically 5-HT regulation of the suprachiasmatic nucleus. Recognition and treatment with 5-HT medications may help reduce alcohol consumption, stabilize blood glucose levels, and prevent aggressive outbursts (Linnoila VMI, Virkkunen M. Aggressions, suicidality, and serotonin. *J Clinical Psychiatry* 1992; 53[10 suppl]:46–51).

Loxapac See **loxapine.**

loxapine (Cloxazepam; Daloxin; Daxolin; Loxapac; Loxitane; Oxilapine) Dibenzoxepine neuroleptic structurally unrelated, but pharmacologically similar to the phenothiazines, butyrophenones, thioxanthenes, diphenylbutylpiperidines, and dihydroindolones. It is an effective antipsychotic. Like all neuroleptics, it may cause extrapyramidal reactions, tardive dyskinesia, and the neuroleptic malignant syndrome. Pregnancy risk category C.

loxapine + carbamazepine Co-administration may enhance the central nervous system depressant effects of carbamazepine (CBZ), lower seizure threshold, and decrease CBZ's anticonvulsant effects. Dosage adjustments may be necessary to control seizures. Anticholinergic effects may be potentiated, leading to confusion and delirium.

loxapine + lithium Co-administration can cause extrapyramidal reactions (de la Gandara J, Dominguez RA. Lithium and loxapine. A potential interaction. *J Clin Psychiatry* 1988;49: 126).

loxapine + lorazepam There are three case reports of patients previously treated with loxapine without undue side effects in whom addition of lorazepam (LOR) resulted in significant respiratory depression accompanied by excessive stupor and, in one patient, hypotension. All were given the combination treatment in hospital and observed closely following occurrence of the adverse effects. There was no evidence of use of other psychotropic medications or alcohol prior to treatment. All patients made uneventful recoveries. One was subsequently given perphenazine plus LOR with no recurrence of respiratory difficulty or lethargy (Cohen S, Khan A. Respiratory distress with use of lorazepam in mania. *J Clin Psychopharmacol* 1987;7:199–200; Battaglia J, Thornton L, Young C. Loxapine-lorazepam-induced hypotension and stupor. *J Clin Psychopharmacol* 1989;9:227–228).

loxapine + phenytoin Loxapine has been reported to decrease serum phenytoin (PHT) levels, but there is no evidence that this is due to induction of PHT metabolism (Ryan GM, Matthews PA. Phenytoin metabolism stimulated by loxapine. *Drug Intell Clin Pharm* 1970; 11:428).

Loxitane See **loxapine.**

Lozol See **indapamide.**

L-phenylalanine See **phenylalanine.**

L-thyroxine (T_4) See **thyroxine.**

L-triiodothyronine (T_3) See **triiodothyronine.**

L-tryptophan See **tryptophan.**

L-tyrosine See **tyrosine.**

Lucidril See **meclofenoxate.**

"lude" Street name for methaqualone.

"lude out" Slang term for using methaqualone to intoxication.

Ludiomil See **maprotiline.**

Luminal See **phenobarbital.**

Lupron See **leuprolide acetate.**

Lustral See **sertraline.**

luteinizing hormone (LH) Gonadotropic hormone of the anterior pituitary that acts with the follicle-stimulating hormone to cause ovulation of mature follicles and secretion of estrogen by thecal and granulosa cells. It is also concerned with corpus luteum formation and, in the male, stimulates development and functional activity interstitial cells.

luteinizing hormone releasing hormone (LHRH) agonist Potential treatment for sexual deviant behavior that can cause complete medical castration with minimal adverse effects. LHRH agonists initially stimulate pituitary production of increased quantities of gonadotropins; with continued use, they down-regulate pituitary gonadotropic receptors, thereby decreasing follicle-stimulating hormone and luteinizing hormone secretion and secondarily decreasing testosterone production. LHRH agonists do not have steroidal activity and do not cause hormonal side effects. They may cause hypoandrogenism, potential calcium loss from bone, and possible adverse effects on lipid metabolism.

Luvox See **fluvoxamine.**

lux Measurement of the amount of light that the eye actually receives.

Lyme borreliosis See **Lyme disease.**

Lyme disease Complex, multisystem illness caused by the tick-borne spirochete, *Borrelia burgdorgeri*. Chronic neurologic manifestations, including encephalopathy, polyneuropathy, and leukoencephalopathy, usually occur late in the illness, sometimes following long periods of latent infection. Although there have been reports of severe cognitive impairment including psychosis, dementia, and vasculitic lesions, Lyme encephalopathy usually causes a subtle syndrome of memory impairment, difficulty concentrating, sleep disturbance, irritability, fatigue, or emotional lability. Encephalitic symptoms do not appear to be due to a psychological reaction to chronic illness, but to chronic central nervous system infection (Kaplan RF, Meadows ME, Vincent LC, et al: Memory impairment and depression in patients with Lyme encephalopathy. *Neurol-*

ogy 1992:42;1263–1267). Also called "Lyme borreliosis."

lymphocyte Immune system cell genetically programmed to recognize specific antigens that bind to the lymphocyte and stimulate the development of more lymphocytes that react with the antigens and produce immunoglobulins. The two main lymphocyte subpopulations are T and B cells.

lymphocyte mitogen stimulation In vitro test of immune function that measures the proliferative response of lymphocytes to a variety of stimulants (mitogens). It is used to measure the effects of stress on cell-mediated immunity. Significant alterations in mitogen-induced lymphocyte proliferation have been found to be associated with stress.

lymphokine General term including all nonantibody chemical messengers (e.g., interleukins, interferons) secreted by lymphocytes that play a major role in regulating immune reactions. Lymphokines are also produced by other cells of the body.

lyonization Process by which all X chromosomes in excess of one are made genetically inactive and heterochromatic. In the female, the decision as to which X (maternal or paternal) is inactivated is taken independently for each cell, early in embryogeny, and is permanent for all descendents of that cell.

Lysenyl See **lisuride.**

Lysenyl Forte See **lisuride.**

lysergic acid diethylamide (LSD) Potent hallucinogen discovered by Hoffmann in 1942. It is manufactured from lysergic acid, which is found in ergot, a fungus that grows on rye and other grains. Commonly referred to as "acid," it is sold on the street in tablets, capsules, or liquid. It is odorless, colorless, tasteless, and is usually taken by mouth. It is often added to absorbent paper and divided into small decorated squares or dots, each representing one dose. LSD also is sold dissolved in sugar cubes. According to the U.S. Drug Enforcement Administration, the strength of LSD samples obtained from illicit sources ranges from 20 to 80 µg/dose (considerably less than in the 1960s and early 1970s). Effects are unpredictable; they depend on the amount taken and the user's personality, mood, expectations, and surroundings. The first effects are felt 30–90 minutes after ingestion. Physical effects include dilated pupils, higher body temperature, increased heart rate and blood pressure, sweating, loss of appetite, sleeplessness, dry mouth, and tremors. Low doses produce psychotic-like symptoms and disturbed behavior (hallucinations, delusions, time-space distortions) that can be frightening and cause panic. As a hallucinogen, it is 4,000–6,000 times

more potent than mescaline and 100–200 times more potent than psilocybin. Flashbacks may occur, usually in those who use hallucinogens chronically or have an underlying personality disorder. Flashbacks and "bad trips" are only part of the risk of LSD use. Chronic users may manifest long-lasting psychoses or develop tolerance so that they require progressively higher doses to achieve the same level of intoxication, an extremely dangerous practice in view of the unpredictability of the drug's effects.

lysergic acid diethylamide (LSD) + fluoxetine Fluoxetine (FLX) (20 mg/day) may markedly decrease sensitivity to LSD; doses that had been able to elicit a full hallucinogenic effect become approximately one-half to one-third as effective in producing the desired hallucinogenic results (Strassman RJ. Human hallucinogen interactions with drugs affecting serotonergic neurotransmission. *Neuropsychopharmacology* 1992;7:241–243). Grand mal convulsions were reported in a patient taking (FLX 20 mg/day) for 1 year, who then took two doses of "blotter" LSD. The patient had taken about 30 single doses of LSD during the preceding year's treatment with FLX (Picker W, Lerman A, Hajal F. Potential interaction of LSD and fluoxetine. *Am J Psychiatry* 1992;149: 843–844).

lysergic acid diethylamide/street names acid, animal, blotter, blue dot, blue heaven, California sunshine, candy, cube, D, dot, hawk, microdot, Ousley's acid, pink wedge, sando, Stanley's stuff, sugar cube, sunshine, trip, window pane, yellow sunshine.

lysogeny 1. Ability to produce lysins or cause lysis. 2. Potential of a bacterium to produce phage. 3. Specific association of the phage genome. The prophage interacts with the bacterial genome in such a way that only a few, if any, phage genes are transcribed.

lysuride See **lisuride.**

lysergic acid diethylamide/tolerance Repeated LSD use produces a high degree of tolerance to its behavioral effects. This develops very rapidly, usually after a few days of daily consumption. Tolerance is also lost quickly after LSD use is stopped for several days. Because of tolerance development, LSD users restrict its use to once or twice weekly. Cross-tolerance develops to hallucinogens such as psilocybin and mescaline (Ungerleider JT, Pechnick RN. Hallucinogens. *In* Lowinson JH, Ruiz P, Millman RB, Langrod JG [eds], *Substance Abuse: A Comprehensive Textbook.* 2nd ed. Baltimore: Williams & Wilkins, 1992:280–289).

lytic Automolytic drug or autonomic blocking agent that produces multifocal autonomic inhibition.

lytic cocktail   Combination of small doses of synergistic drugs with different target organs or structures. Efficacy is increased or potentiated, and total toxicity is sharply reduced. Most lytic cocktails consist of an analgesic, an antihistamine, and a neuroleptic.

M

"M"   Street name for morphine.

M99   See **etorphine.**

"M & Ms"   Street name for secobarbital.

Maclamine   See **moclobemide.**

macroenvironment   Factors that may influence a person (e.g., family, close friends, work, social relations, community in which the person lives).

macrophage   Any of a class of immune cells capable of engulfing and digesting foreign or toxic matter within bodily tissues. Macrophages are secreting cytokines (inflammatory mediators) that function in immune-cell activation.

Madopar   See **levodopa/benserazide.**

magical thinking   Belief that one's thoughts, words, or actions might or will somehow cause or prevent a specific outcome in a way that defies the normal laws of cause and effect. It may be part of ideas of reference or may reach delusional proportions if the person maintains a firm conviction about the belief despite evidence to the contrary. It is seen in children, primitive cultures, schizotypal personality disorder, schizophrenia, and obsessive compulsive disorder.

"magic mushroom"   Street name for psilocybin.

Magnan's sign   See **cocaine bug.**

magnesium choline trisalicylate   (Trilisate) Nonsteroidal anti-inflammatory drug (NSAID) that is one of the least irritating to the gastrointestinal tract. It is unlikely to affect platelet function and can be used successfully in patients unable to tolerate other anti-inflammatory agents.

magnetic resonance imaging   (MRI) First in vivo brain imaging technique with sufficient resolution to permit investigations of gross structural variation in living subjects. Images are produced when mobile protons of a tissue are excited by the application of an oscillating magnetic field in the radio-frequency range. Images are displayed on a gray-scale matrix like those of computed tomography (CT). Since MRI does not use ionizing radiation, it poses no known risk to patients, who can be scanned repeatedly without hazard (unless they have metal plates or pacemakers) to observe disease progression or the effects of therapeutic intervention. MRI is superior to CT because of its multiplanar capability, high tissue contrast and resolution, ability to quantify images and identify regions of focal pathology through altered "relaxation time," and absence of ionizing radiation. It is also

better able to demonstrate brain tumors, vascular malfunctions, and focal brain atrophy. It may be useful for evaluating patients with psychiatric symptoms as a feature of neurological disease (e.g., multiple sclerosis) (Armstrong P, Keevil SF. Magnetic resonance imaging—1: basic principles of image production. *Br Med J* 1990;303:35–40; Armstrong P, Keevil SF. Magnetic resonance imaging—2: clinical uses. *Br Med J* 1991;303:105–109). MRI is the test of choice for evaluating most lesions causing epilepsy (temporal lobe glioma, mesial temporal sclerosis); periventricular white matter disease (subcortical dementia, human immunodeficiency virus [HIV]); demyelinating disease (multiple sclerosis, sarcoid); pituitary and posterior fossa lesions; axonal injury; frontal atrophy; herpes encephalitis; normal pressure hydrocephalus; and systemic lupus erythematosus, vasculitis, and sagittal sinus thrombosis. MRI advantages include (a) good resolution, excellent views of brain structure; (b) three dimensions; (c) good gray-white differentiation; (d) adjusted settings based on characteristics of the lesions; (e) good view of the posterior fossa; (f) no radiation exposure; (g) gadolinium contrast, which is relatively nontoxic; and (h) capacity for quantitative imaging, 3-D reconstruction, angiography, and spectroscopy. Disadvantages include: (a) cost; (b) some patients are ineligible because of pacemakers and other metal; (c) claustrophobia; (d) long examination time; and (e) access. Also called "nuclear magnetic resonance imaging (NMRI)."

magnetic resonance imaging, functional   Technique that images very small metabolic, blood flow, and perfusion-diffusion changes to identify functional changes in organs (usually the brain) in vivo, in real time, and with less risk to the patient. It allows "mapping" of the brain's motor and sensory functions, as well as higher functions such as emotions and thought processing (Ogawa S, Tank DW, Menon R, et al. Intrinsic signal changes accompanying sensory stimulation: functional brain mapping with magnetic resonance imaging. *Proc Natl Acad Sci U S A* 1992;89:5951–5955).

magnetic resonance spectroscopy   (MRS) Brain imaging technique that produces data on the amounts of various substances in the brain. It is the only functional imaging technique in clinical medicine that provides noninvasive access to living chemistry *in situ*. It has low sensitivity compared with other techniques such as positron emission tomography (PET) and single photon emission computed tomography (SPECT), but it can provide information on concentrations of endogenous substances that contain naturally occurring paramagnetic nuclei (e.g., hydrogen-1 and phosphorus-31). It also allows measurement of drugs that are MRS-visible (e.g., lithium, drugs containing fluorine). In vivo brain resonances have been detected in human subjects taking lithium, trifluoperazine, fluphenazine, and fluoxetine. Knowledge of brain levels of these drugs may contribute to better understanding of their therapeutic and toxic effects. Except ʻfor lithium, it has been difficult to quantitate brain drug levels or correlate values with corresponding plasma levels. In addition, many reports consist of data from a single subject taking unusually high doses of medication (e.g., trifluoperazine 120 mg/day) (Renshaw PF, Guimaraes AR, Fava M, et al. Accumulation of fluoxetine and norfluoxetine in human brain during therapeutic administration. *Am J Psychiatry* 1992;149:1592–1594). MRS advantages include noninvasiveness, no exposure to ionizing radiation, no known side effects, and quantitative regional measurements of biochemical and physiological processes in vivo. Its major weakness is insensitivity. Only certain elements or their isotopes are paramagnetic and therefore suitable for study. Molecules must be in solution and highly mobile to be examined. Localization of chemical information is difficult; areas that may not conform to specific neuroanatomic structures must be examined. Because patients must remain immobile for lengthy periods, acute response to stimulation cannot be examined. MRS requires high magnetic field strengths of great homogeneity, precluding all but the high end of currently available scanners. Absolute quantification is a challenge because of the low signal/noise ratio of data obtained, incomplete separation of spectral peaks achieved at low magnetic field strengths, and second pulse sequence selection (Guze BH. Magnetic resonance spectroscopy. *Arch Gen Psychiatry* 1991;48:572–574). Despite such drawbacks, MRS has provided new insights into brain development and aging, Alzheimer's disease, schizophrenia, and brain response to hypoxia and ischemia. It is expected to play an increasingly important role in psychopharmacology.

magnetic source imaging (MSI) Overlaying of information gained from magnetoencephalography onto anatomical images from computed tomography and magnetic resonance imaging.

magnetoencephalography (MEG) Technology whereby the origin of weak biomagnetic fields generated by synchronously active groups of neurons can be determined. It localizes the primary somatosensory cortex, sources of focal slow wave activity, sources of interictal epileptogenic activity, and abnormalities in deeper structures.

"main line" Street term for (a) the vein into which an illicit drug is injected; (b) the act of intravenous injection of a drug (e.g., heroin, cocaine) to obtain maximum effect in minimum time.

maintenance Therapeutic intervention method used with opiate addicts in which a substitute opiate drug is given orally to minimize reinforcement of drug taking, prevent a withdrawal reaction, and allow rehabilitation to be achieved. See **methadone maintenance.**

maintenance antidepressant drug therapy There are two types: continuation therapy and long-term preventive therapy. The former is continued administration of an antidepressant after remission of acute symptoms to maintain symptomatic control until the natural termination of the episode. It is based on the assumption that antidepressants suppress symptoms without altering the course of the postulated underlying disorder; medication must be continued until the underlying illness runs its natural course. If it is withdrawn before the cycle runs its course, relapse will occur. Long-term preventive therapy is administered after conclusion of an episode to prevent or attenuate new episodes. See **continuation antidepressant drug therapy; maintenance psychoactive drug therapy.**

maintenance electroconvulsive therapy (ECT) Outpatient procedure for patients who exhibit satisfactory improvement with a conventional course of ECT and for whom maintenance drug therapy has failed. The concept is similar to that of maintenance drug therapy. The goal is to maintain symptom remission by administering additional ECTs at a frequency sufficient to prevent relapse (e.g., once a month) without incurring cumulative memory loss. Continuing need for maintenance ECT should be assessed regularly. There is no recommendation for a maximum number of treatments in a year or in a lifetime.

maintenance psychoactive drug therapy Continuation of psychoactive drug therapy after improvement or recovery by acute treatment. It is used, under the assumption that acute symptoms are in remission, to prevent or delay relapse or symptom recurrence. Some patients can be maintained with progressive lowering of the effective daily drug dosage; others require continued administration of the initially effective daily dosage. Maintenance drug therapy is common for most major psychiatric disorders because, even when in remission, patients continue to have underlying neurochemical vulnerability. Examples include the use of lithium for maintenance treatment after a manic episode, neuroleptics after a schizophrenic relapse, benzodiazepines for anxiety disorders, and clomipramine for obsessive compulsive disorder.

maintenance of wakefulness test   Series of measurements of the interval from "lights out" to sleep onset used in assessing the ability to remain awake in a semireclined position in a darkened room. It is useful for assessing effects of medication on the ability to remain awake.

Majeptil   See **thioproperazine.**

major depression   See **depression, major.**

major depressive episode   (MDE) See **depression, major.**

major gene   See **gene, major.**

major sleep episode   See **sleep episode, major.**

major tranquilizer   Term for drugs now called antipsychotics. See **antipsychotic; tranquilizer.**

maladaptive behavior   Conduct disorder behavior or behaviors that are antisocial or against the normal ego defenses and/or morality of a person. It can occur in illicit drug users. In recreational cocaine users, for example, the first sign of maladaptive behavior is a pattern of oversleeping and lateness or absences from work. As the number of maladaptive behaviors increases, signs of loss of control are evident, use continues despite knowledge of negative consequences, and symptoms extend beyond a 1-month period, so that the line between abuse and dependence is crossed.

Malexil   See **femoxetine.**

malignant hyperpyrexia   Fatal, fulminant fever in patients treated with the combination of L-tryptophan, lithium, and phenelzine.

malignant hyperthermia   (MH) Rare, familial hypercatabolic reaction with core temperature higher than 41° C associated with certain potent inhalation anesthetics, muscle relaxants, tricyclic antidepressants, chlorpromazine, monoamine oxidase inhibitors (MAOIs), haloperidol, atropine, sympathomimetics, and quinidine analogs. It has significant morbidity and potentially lethal consequences, even with current treatment modalities. MAOIs have been associated with another type of hyperthermia in overdose and in adverse interaction with other drugs and tyramine-containing foods and beverages. Susceptibility to malignant hyperthermia can be ascertained by in vitro testing of tissue obtained by muscle biopsy. Although similarities between neuroleptic malignant syndrome (NMS) and MH exist, they appear to be distinct clinical entities. There is no evidence that NMS patients are at greater risk for MH

(Ellis FR, Heffron JJA. Clinical and biochemical aspects of malignant hyperthermia. *In* Atkinson RS, Adams AP [eds], *Recent Advances in Anaesthesia and Analgesia*, vol 15. Edinburgh: Churchill Livingstone, 1985:173–207). See **heatstroke; hyperthermia; neuroleptic malignant syndrome.**

malinger   To feign or protract illness with intent to deceive.

malpractice   Professional behavior contrary to established ethical codes or accepted standards of medical practice due to negligence, ignorance, or intent.

managed care   **1.** System or review mechanism that controls access to care as a cost-control measure. **2.** System that controls the selection and utilization of services and outlines benefits available to participants (e.g., health maintenance organizations [HMOs], preferred provider organizations [PPOs], individual practice associations, and direct contract agreements between employers and providers).

management, one-to-one   See **constant observation.**

management trial   See **naturalistic study.**

mandatory treatment (drug users)   Treatment as an alternative to trial or incarceration for persons arrested or convicted of crimes and found to be drug users. Failure to remain in treatment renders the person liable to criminal prosecution and penalty. Civil commitment is mandatory treatment for those who have not been accused or convicted of a crime, but who have been diagnosed as addicted and are considered incapable of self-care or potentially threatening to the public's safety because of their addiction. Also called "outpatient commitment."

Manerix   See **moclobemide.**

mania   Condition in which mood changes from normal to an overactive or hyperactive state marked by feelings of irritability, elation, expansiveness, or abnormal euphoria. The person may sleep little, talk very rapidly, take little time to eat, manifest impaired concentration, and have racing thoughts. Judgment becomes poor and impulsive behavior may have devastating results. Severe mania requires hospital care.

mania, acute/resistant   Lithium is not always effective in acute mania. Ineffectiveness is sometimes attributable to a low lithium dose that produces a serum level below 0.9 mmol/L; most acute episodes require levels of 0.9–1.3 mmol/L. When there is poor or no response to lithium in this dosage range, any of the following may be combined with lithium: carbamazepine, clonazepam, clonidine, lorazepam, neuroleptics, oxycarbamazepine, verapamil, or valproate.

mania, delirious   See **Bell's mania.**

mania, dysphoric   Mania accompanied by irritable and anxious symptoms, and sometimes by psychotic symptoms (often depressive or mood incongruent) and/or suicidal ideation. It is more common in women and those who have relatively fewer episodes of illness and no family history of mood disorders. It is estimated that about half of all manic patients have dysphoric mania sometime during an episode. Although dysphoric mania may be successfully treated with lithium alone, no study has found that it responds better to lithium than pure mania does. Dysphoric mania can be successfully treated with lithium in combination with an antipsychotic or clonazepam. In bipolar patients with dysphoric mania, psychotic features, and chronic disability, clozapine produced remarkable improvement that was sustained over a 3- to 5-year follow-up (Suppes T, McElroy SL, Gilbert J, et al. Clozapine in the treatment of dysphoric mania. *Biol Psychiatry* 1992;32:270–280). Dysphoric mania also may respond to carbamazepine, valproate, or electroconvulsive therapy. Tricyclic antidepressants may worsen it (Clothier J, Swann AC, Freeman T. Dysphoric mania. *J Clin Psychopharmacol* 1992;12:135–165; McElroy SL, Keck PE, Pope HG, et al. Clinical and research implications of the diagnosis of dysphoric or mixed mania or hypomania. *Am J Psychiatry* 1992;149:1633–1644). Also called "mixed mania."

mania/elderly   Mania is rare after age 60, even in patients with known bipolar illness. Secondary mania in the elderly, however, is increasing in incidence. Mania in the elderly warrants a thorough medical, neurological, and psychiatric evaluation. Whether mania is a recurrent bipolar episode or secondary, lithium combined with a neuroleptic is indicated. Successful therapy in the elderly requires close monitoring because of increased risk of side effects and toxicity. Starting lithium doses should be low (150–300 mg/day); higher starting doses increase the risk of lithium intoxication. For most geriatric patients, 150–300 mg/day is safe and effective. If necessary, the dose should be raised gradually with increments of 150 mg/day to a maximum of 450–600 mg/day. Since elimination half-life is prolonged in the elderly, steady-state serum levels may not be reached for 7–10 days. If more rapid symptom control is desired, low doses of neuroleptics may be co-administered. Carbamazepine (200 mg every 8 hours) also could be added to the medication regimen. Clonazepam added to lithium may take effect within 48 hours (Ayd

FJ Jr: Mania in the elderly: diagnostic and therapeutic tips. *Int Drug Ther Newsl* 1987;22: 38–39). See **mania, secondary.**

Manialith   See **lithium.**

mania, mixed   See **mania, dysphoric.**

mania, prepubertal   Once thought to be infrequent, bipolar illness in prepubertal children is being diagnosed more often each year. Patients have a manic episode with psychotic features and a family history of psychiatric, particularly affective, disorders. They usually respond very well to lithium (1,150–1,800 mg/day; average, 1,270 mg/day) and usually reach therapeutic levels (0.6–1.4 mEq/L) in 3–5 days (Alessi N, Naylor MW, Ghaziuddin M, Zubieta JK. Update on lithium carbonate therapy in children and adolescents. *J Am Acad Child Adolesc Psychiatry* 1994;33:291–304).

mania, reactive   Mania occurring in response to a particular environmental stressor. It may present with a clinical picture identical to endogenous mania, but there is a clear precipitating experience. Previous episodes of affective illness are less frequent than in endogenous mania.

mania, secondary   Manic symptoms associated with antecedent physical illness or drug use. It usually occurs in older patients with no family history of bipolar disorder. It has been reported in a variety of organic cerebral illnesses (toxic confusional state, postoperative psychosis, brain tumor, multiple sclerosis, influenza, encephalitis, syphilis, epilepsy). It also can be precipitated by stimulants and other drugs (e.g., amphetamines, antidepressants, bromocriptine, corticosteroids, cocaine, L-dopa, methylphenidate, and phencyclidine.

mania/sleep deprivation   Sleep deprivation can trigger mania in patients with bipolar affective disorder who are euthymic or depressed. A first episode of mania occurred in a previously healthy man following partial sleep deprivation for 4 nights (Wright JBD. Mania following sleep deprivation. *Br J Psychiatry* 1993;163:679–680).

mania, unipolar   Mania occurring in an individual with no evidence of prior depressive symptoms It is considered rare and is usually classified under the heading of bipolar affective disorder, even though no depressive episodes are recognized.

manic depressive cycle   Mania and depression may alternate in three types of cycles: (a) 48-hour cycles, in which mania and depression occur on alternate days; (b) rapid cycles, in which mania and depression alternate every few days or weeks; and (c) seasonal cycles, in which depression and mania recur at certain seasons.

manic depressive disorder (MDD) Affective illness manifested by severe, recurrent mood alterations. It is divided into unipolar type, characterized by episodes of either mania or depression; and bipolar or circular type, manifested by at least one episode of depression or mania and with periodic alternations between the two. MDD is designated bipolar disorder in DSM-IV.

Manilith See **lithium.**

manipulative Skillful in getting what is wanted from others, or able to control or manage others to gain what is wanted. The term is often used pejoratively.

mannerism Stereotyped involuntary or semi-voluntary movement. Mannerisms differ from most other abnormal involuntary movements in that they are less insistently repeated and are more in keeping with the subject's personality. They range from mild to extreme; when extreme, functioning is seriously impaired by virtually constant involvement in ritualistic, manneristic, or stereotyped movements, or by an unnatural fixed posture that is sustained most of the time. Mannerisms may remain constant for years or may be altered constantly. Bizarre, idiosyncratic mannerisms are characteristic of schizophrenia.

mannitol + lithium Mannitol increases glomerular filtration rate and can substantially increase renal lithium clearance, resulting in lower serum lithium levels. Lithium dosage adjustment may be necessary when mannitol is started and discontinued.

Mann-Whitney U test A nonparametric analog of the Student's t-test for testing the significance of the difference between two independent groups. Also called "rank-sum test."

Mann-Whitney-Wilcoxon test See **Wilcoxon test.**

Mantel-Haenzel method Statistical procedure commonly used in epidemiology to estimate the common relationship between two dichotomous variables and to test whether the overall relationship is statistically significant over a group of studies or a group of different samples. Each study or sample is an individual entity; the Mantel-Haenzel method allows estimating and testing of the relationship of variable A to variable B over a number of such studies, strata, or entities.

mapping See **gene mapping; chromosome mapping.**

maprotiline (Ludiomil; Melodil) (MAP) Tetracyclic antidepressant that is a specific blocker of norepinephrine (NE) reuptake with apparently no effect on serotonin uptake. It is structurally similar to the tricyclics (an additional bridge is added to the molecule) and it has a similar profile of effectiveness and ad-verse effects. It is likely to produce synaptic changes similar to those produced by tricyclics, but the effects are largely confined to NE metabolism. Its active metabolite is desmethylmaprotiline. Plasma half-life is 21–52 hours. Initial recommended dose is 75 mg/day with gradual increments to the recommended maximum daily dosage of 225 mg. Therapeutic plasma concentration is 200–300 ng/ml. Clinical efficacy is somewhat unpredictable. High doses and rapid dosage escalation have been associated with decreased seizure threshold. Pregnancy risk category B.

maprotiline + alcohol Co-administration may produce additive central nervous system depressant effects. Alcohol can precipitate maprotiline-associated seizures.

maprotiline + antiarrhythmic The concomitant use of maprotiline with the antiarrhythmics disopyramide, procainamide, and guanidine may increase the incidence of cardiac arrhythmias and conduction deficits.

maprotiline + antihypertensive Maprotiline may decrease the hypotensive effects of centrally acting antihypertensives (e.g., clonidine, guanabenz, guanadrel, guanethidine, methyldopa, reserpine).

maprotiline/breast milk Maprotiline is excreted in breast milk in concentrations equal to or greater than those in maternal serum. Its effects on nursing infants have not been studied, but it should be avoided by nursing women whenever possible (Lloyd AH. Practical considerations in the use of maprotiline [Ludiomil] in general practice. *J Int Med Res* 1977;5[suppl 4]:122–138).

maprotiline + brofaromine Brofaromine augments therapeutic response in patients refractory to maprotiline without serious drug-drug interactions.

maprotiline + carbamazepine Co-administration may enhance the central nervous system depressant effects of carbamazepine (CBZ), lower seizure threshold, and decrease CBZ's anticonvulsant effects. Dosage adjustments may be necessary to control seizures. In some patients, anticholinergic effects may be potentiated, leading to confusion and delirium.

maprotiline + citalopram Co-administration apparently produces no pharmacokinetic interactions or adverse effects (Baettig D, Bondolfi G, Montaldi S, et al. Tricyclic antidepressant plasma levels after augmentation with citalopram. A case study. *Eur J Clin Pharmacol* 1993; 44:403–405).

maprotiline + disulfiram Co-administration may cause tachycardia and delirium.

maprotiline + ethchlorvynol Co-administration may cause tachycardia and delirium.

maprotiline + fluvoxamine Co-administration has been effective in depression refractory to either drug alone.

maprotiline + lithium Co-administration has been used to augment the treatment of depression without severe adverse effects.

maprotiline + phenelzine Addition of phenelzine 15–45 mg/day to the regimen of patients only partially responsive to maprotiline may augment therapeutic response without producing more side effects than occur with maprotiline alone (Ayd FJ Jr. Combined maprotiline—MAOI therapy. *Int Drug Ther Newsl* 1982;17:4).

maprotiline + pimozide Co-administration may increase the incidence of cardiac arrhythmias and conduction defects.

maprotiline + propranolol Propranolol may increase maprotiline (MAP) bioavailability by direct (inhibition of hepatic hydrolase) and indirect interference with this substance's metabolism (reduction of hepatic blood flow) as a result of its cardiovascular effect. Delirium was reported in a patient treated with both drugs. In another patient who tolerated MAP (250 mg/day) without problems, addition of propranolol (120 mg/day) produced confusional symptoms and toxic MAP levels (Saiz-Ruiz J, Moral L. Delirium induced by association of propranolol and maprotiline. *J Clin Psychopharmacol* 1988;8:77–78; Tollefson G, Lesar T. Effect of propranolol on maprotiline clearance. *Am J Psychiatry* 1984;141:148–149).

maprotiline + sympathomimetic Co-administration may increase blood pressure.

maprotiline + tranylcypromine Tranylcypromine (10–30 mg/day) may augment therapeutic response to maprotiline (MAP) without producing any more side effects than occur with MAP alone (Ayd FJ Jr. Combined maprotiline—MAOI therapy. *Int Drug Ther Newsl* 1982;17:4).

maprotiline + warfarin Co-administration may increase prothrombin time and cause bleeding.

marche a petits pas Gait disturbance characterized by very short steps.

Marflex See **orphenadrine.**

marginal frequency Row and column frequencies in a contingency table.

marijuana Spanish-American slang term ("Mary and John") that refers to the dried leaves of male and female cannabis plants. See **cannabis sativa.**

marijuana + alcohol Combined use in variable amounts, frequencies, and settings is well established. Acute administration of tetrahydrocannabinol (THC), the primary psychoactive component of marijuana, in combination with alcohol results in additive or superadditive effects on psychomotor performance, enhanced impairment of mental performance, and marked effects such as a greater increase in pulse rate and conjunctival congestion compared to ingestion of either drug alone. Marijuana smoking reduces the peak plasma alcohol level attained after drinking a standard alcohol beverage; the attenuation parallels a delay in the time-to-peak levels but does not significantly delay the appearance of alcohol-induced intoxication. However, there is a substantial decrease in the duration of *subjective* effects consistent with a reduction of the maximum and a delay in the peak plasma alcohol levels (Lukas SE, Benedikt R, Mendelson JH, et al. Marijuana attenuates the rise in plasma ethanol levels in human subjects. *Neuropsychopharmacology* 1992;7:77–81).

marijuana/breast milk Marijuana is secreted in breast milk and absorbed by the nursing baby. Because effects on the infant of chronic exposure to THC and its metabolites are unknown, nursing mothers should abstain from marijuana use. Until further data are available, clinicians should advise their patients of the potential hazards of smoking marijuana during pregnancy and lactation (Perez-Reyes M, Wall ME. Presence of delta-9-tetrahydrocannabinol in human milk. *N Engl J Med* 1982; 307:819).

marijuana + disulfiram There is a single case report of a hypomanic-like reaction characterized by euphoria, hyperactivity, insomnia, and irritability (Lacoursiere RB, Swatek R. Adverse interaction between disulfiram and marijuana: a case report. *Am J Psychiatry* 1983;140:242–244).

marijuana + fluoxetine Combined use has been reported to cause mania, which may be due to marijuana potentiating the action of fluoxetine at central serotonergic neurons (Stoll AL, Cole JO, Lukas SE. A case of mania as a result of fluoxetine-marijuana interaction. *J Clin Psychiatry* 1991;52:280–281).

marijuana + lithium Combined use may result in lithium toxicity (Ratey JJ, Ciraulo DA, Shader RI. Lithium and marijuana. *J Clin Psychopharmacol* 1981;1:32–33).

marijuana psychosis See **cannabis psychosis.**

marijuana/street names A-bomb, Acapulco gold, ace, African black, blowing smoke, cannabis, Christmas tree, doobie, fatty, fine stuff, gage, gold, good shit, grass, grasshopper, hay, hemp, joint, locoweed, Mary Jane, MJ, morning missile, nail, pocket rocket, pot, red haired lady, reefer, rope, sativa, smoke, stick, stinkweed, stone, thai stick, tea, Texas tea, wack, weed, yesca.

marker, genetic See **genetic marker.**

Marinol See **dronabinol.**

Maronil   See **clomipramine.**

Marplan   See **isocarboxazid.**

Marsilid   See **iproniazid.**

Martin-Bell syndrome   See **fragile-X syndrome.**

"Mary Jane"   A street name for marijuana.

masked study   See **blind; blinded.**

masked tardive dyskinesia   See **tardive dyskinesia, masked.**

masking   See **blind; blinded.**

masochism   Personality trait and/or sexual deviation in which a person derives gratification from having pain inflicted on himself or herself.

mass fragmentography   Quantitative analysis of compounds by measurement of specific fragments using mass spectrometry.

mass spectrometry   (MS) Analysis of the chemical structure of a compound by measurement of the molecular weight of fragments formed by bombardment of the molecule by ions. It is inherently the most specific procedure for analyzing any organic chemical. The coupling of liquid chromatography and mass spectrometry (LC/MS) is a recent development. Developments in MS for the analysis of neuropeptides have been as significant as developments in high pressure liquid chromatography (HPLC).

matched control   See **control, matched.**

matched design   Study in which each case subject is matched with one or more deliberately chosen control subjects, who are similar to the experimental subjects in terms of variables that would be expected to influence and therefore confound results.

matching   See **matched design.**

maternal inheritance   Inheritance of genetic elements (e.g., mitochondrial DNA and X chromosomes) from one's mother.

maternity blues   See **postpartum blues.**

mating   Sexual union of two sexually dimorphic individuals that often generates offspring.

mating, assortative   Tendency for people with a given mental illness to marry others with the same illness, which may result in two-sided families with heavier loading of the disorder in parental lines. See **mating, negative assortative.**

mating, disassortative   See **mating, negative assortative.**

mating, negative assortative   Unlike individuals preferentially selecting each other. Also called "disassortative mating." See **assortative mating.**

mating, random   Selection of a mate without regard to its genotype. In a randomly mating population, the frequencies of the various matings are determined solely by the frequencies of the genes concerned.

Matulane   See **procarbazine.**

"mauve"   Street name for phencyclidine (PCP).

Maveral   See **fluvoxamine.**

"maxi"   Street name for anabolic steroids.

Maxibolan   See **ethylestrenol.**

maximum plasma concentration   (C_{max}) Maximum concentration of a drug that is affected by its physicochemical properties and formulation. It is usually inversely related to drug absorption rate (T_{max}). The faster a drug is absorbed, the higher the C_{max}, the shorter the T_{max}, and the faster the appearance of the drug's activity. C_{max} is higher after intramuscular than oral administration, and T_{max} is shifted to the left. However, drugs that crystalize in tissue (e.g., diazepam, chlordiazepoxide) are less bioavailable when administered intramuscularly, and this affects both C_{max} and T_{max}. See **drug absorption rate.**

maximum predicted effect   (E_{max}) Maximum change in effect from baseline. It is the achievement of the greatest possible predicted effect.

maximum total daily dose   The highest dose ever prescribed for a single patient for at least one day.

Maxolon   See **metoclopramide.**

Mazanor   See **mazindol.**

Mazepine   See **carbamazepine.**

Mazicon   See **flumazenil.**

mazindol   (Mazanor; Sanorex)   Isoindole anorectic with pharmacological properties similar to those of amphetamines. Preliminary data suggest that mazindol may be effective for treatment of refractory negative symptoms in otherwise stable outpatients with schizophrenia. It does not worsen positive psychotic symptoms and has minimal effects on tardive dyskinesia. Most patients have fewer extrapyramidal side effects after mazindol augmentation. Preliminary studies in schizophrenics show that mazindol may not increase positive symptoms while improving negative symptoms. It decreased cocaine craving and use in a cocaine-abusing schizophrenic patient, but whether this is a direct effect of mazindol is uncertain (Seibyl JP, Brenner L, Krystal JH, et al. Mazindol and cocaine addiction in schizophrenia. *Biol Psychiatry* 1992;31:1179–1181). It is indicated as a short-term (used for a few weeks) adjunct in a regimen of weight reduction based on caloric restriction. Schedule IV; pregnancy risk category C.

McCall's T   Specialized standard score with a mean of 50 and a standard deviation of 10.

m-chlorophenylpiperazine   (mCPP) Serotonin (5-HT) receptor agonist that readily crosses the blood-brain barrier and binds to all 5-HT receptor subtypes, most potently to 5-HT$_{1C}$ and moderately to 5-HT$_{1A}$ and 5-HT$_3$. It may have antagonistic effects at the 5-HT$_2$ receptor. It is the most extensively used probe of 5-HT function in psychiatry. Although used primarily to test the state of the 5-HT system, it can also be used to examine interactions between the 5-HT and other monoaminergic systems if peripheral markers are available. It causes a consistent, dose-dependent elevation of adrenocorticotropic hormone (ACTH), cortisol, and prolactin levels in both animals and humans, as well as increased body temperature in humans. Augmented response to mCPP indicates 5-HT receptor hypersensitivity, a blunted response of 5-HT receptor hyposensitivity. mCPP-induced ACTH release, and by inference 5-HT receptor function, may be increased in clozapine responders compared to nonresponders (Kahn RS, Davidson M, Siever L, et al. Serotonin function and treatment response to clozapine in schizophrenic patients. *Am J Psychiatry* 1993;150: 1337–1342). mCPP can exacerbate psychotic symptoms in schizophrenics, cause panic attacks, and precipitate flashbacks in patients with post-traumatic stress disorder (PTSD), suggesting that alterations in 5-HT function following psychological trauma may contribute to PTSD symptoms. See **mCPP challenge test.**

McNemar test   Chi-squared test for comparing proportions from two dependent or paired groups.

mCPP challenge test   Probe that may be useful for uncovering differences in serotonin (5-HT) receptor sensitivity between psychiatric patients and normal persons (Kahn RS, Wetzler S. m-Chlorophenylpiperazine as a probe of serotonin function. *Biol Psychiatry* 1991;30: 1139–1166; Kahn RS, Knott P, Gabriel S, et al. Effect of m-chlorophenylpiperazine on plasma homovanillic acid concentrations in healthy subjects. *Biol Psychiatry* 1992;32:1055–1061). When given intravenously (0.1 mg/kg), mCPP induces anxiety and panic in both panic disorder patients and normal control subjects. The effect appears to be dose-related. A low oral dose of mCPP (0.25 mg/kg) increases anxiety in panic patients in comparison with normal control subjects and with patients with major depression. The different effects of mCPP might be attributable to differences in 5-HT receptor sensitivity. It has been hypothesized that low oral doses of mCPP increase anxiety in panic disorder patients and not in normal control subjects because of 5-HT receptor hypersensitivity in panic disorder. High intravenous doses, in contrast, induce anxiety in both groups because of massive overstimulation of 5-HT receptors, thereby obliterating

receptor sensitivity differences. See **m-chlorophenyl piperazine.**

MDL-14042   See **lofexidine.**

"MDM"   Street name for 3,4-methylenedioxymethamphetamine.

MDMA   See **3,4-methylenedioxymethamphetamine.**

mean   Sum of the individual values or scores of a set of measurements divided by the number of individual values or scores. It is the most common measure to describe the trend of a set.

mean, arithmetic   See **mean.**

mean deviation   Variability of a frequency distribution. The amount by which each individual score differs from the mean score (considering all deviations as positive) is tabulated, and the mean is then computed. Also called "average deviation" (AD).

mean, geometric   (GM) The nth root of the product of n observations. It is used with logarithms or skewed distributions. All values must be greater than zero.

mean residence time   (MRT) Average time a drug resides within the body after rapid administration of a single intravenous dose.

mean square among groups   Summation of square of variation between group means and grand means over all groups divided by the degree of freedom associated (total number of groups minus 1). Usually it is the numerator of F-test in analysis of variation (ANOVA).

mean square within groups   Estimate of the variation in analysis of variation (ANOVA). It is used in the denominator of the F statistic. It is the summation of the square of variation between group means and the observed values within each group divided by the degree of freedom associated (subtracting the number of groups from the total number of observations).

mean total daily dose   Sum of each dose level attained by a patient, multiplied by the number of days at that level, divided by the duration of treatment in days.

measurement   Application of a standard scale to a variable or to a set of values.

measurement error   Amount by which a measurement is incorrect because of problems inherent in the measuring process.

measurement scale   Complete range of possible values for a measurement. Scales are often divided into five types: (a) dichotomous (items arranged into one of two categories); (b) nominal (unordered categories); (c) ordinal (qualitative categories); (d) interval (values assigned with distinct distances between them); and (e) ratio (interval scale with a true zero point).

measures of central tendency   Index or summary numbers that describe the middle of a distribution.

measures of dispersion   Index or summary numbers that describe the spread of observations about the mean.

mebanazine + clomipramine   Clomipramine (CMI) should not be co-administered with mebanazine or within 14 days of mebanazine's discontinuation, nor should mebanazine be given to a patient already receiving CMI. Either regimen may cause hypertension, collapse, convulsions, coma, and death.

Mebaral   See **mephobarbital.**

mechanism of action   Chemical activity by which a medication causes its therapeutic effects.

mecholyl   Drug that causes rapid drop in blood pressure.

meclizine   (Antivert) Antihistamine used in the management of nausea, vomiting, and dizziness associated with motion sickness. It is also prescribed for Ménière's disease.

meclofenoxate   (Helfergin; Lucidril) Putative acetylcholine structurally related to dimethylaminoethanol (deanol) that is marketed in Europe as a nootropic drug for the treatment of human cerebral functional disorders. It is being tested in the treatment of organic brain syndromes and tardive dyskinesia.

Meclopin   See **oxyprothepin decanoate.**

medazepam   (Glorium; Nobrium) 1,4 Benzodiazepine hypnotic that is a prodrug of desmethyldiazepam.

median   Middle value in a set of values arranged in order from highest to lowest that divides the measurements into an upper and a lower half.

median deviation   Absolute amount of deviation from the mean that is exceeded by half the measures in a distribution. It is computed by tabulating the amount by which each individual score differs from the mean score, considering all these deviations as positive, and then computing their median. Also called "probable deviation"; "probable error."

median effective dose   (ED_{50}) Dose at which 50% of individuals exhibit the specified quantal effect.

median lethal dose   (LD_{50}) Dose that produces a fatal outcome in 50% of the animals treated within a 7-day period. The LD_{50} test is a gross indication of the overall toxicity of the drug; it is provided more for historical reasons than for its scientific value.

median toxic dose   (TD_{50}) Dose required to produce a particular toxic effect in 50% of animals.

medical abuser   Individual who misuses prescription drugs. Abusers may develop toler-

ance and escalate the drug dose, putting themselves at risk for withdrawal reactions and other features of dependency. They may get all the drug from one physician or receive simultaneous supplies from a variety of medical resources. Misuse of medicines may have social, legal, medical, and vocational consequences.

medical audit   Systematic, critical analysis of the quality of medical care, including procedures used for diagnosis and treatment, use of resources, and resulting outcome for the patient.

medical decision making   Application of findings of diagnostic and laboratory procedures to the decision process in medicine.

medical genetics   See **genetics, medical.**

medical informatics   New discipline with the potential to facilitate more integrated and comprehensive use of computers in the practice of medicine. This can be attributed to (a) increasing recognition of medical informatics as a legitimate and coherent field concerned with the cognitive, information processing, and communication tasks of medical practice, education, and research; (b) merging of major national organizations concerned with this discipline into the American Medical Informatics Association; (c) attention being focused on this area in major publications (journals and books); and (d) the growing number of capable and experienced physicians who have received training in this field through fellowship programs established by the National Library of Medicine (Shortliffe EH, Perrault L, Wiederhold G, Fagen LM [eds]. *Medical Informatics: Computer Applications in Health Care.* Menlo Park, CA: Addison-Wesley, 1990).

Medical Literature Analysis and Retrieval System (MEDLARS) Continuously updated computerized database system for searching the medical literature.

medical negligence   See **negligence, medical.**

medical noncompliance   See **noncompliance with medical treatment.**

Medical Outcomes Study   (MOS) Observational study of patients in large group practice-style health maintenance organizations (HMOs); large, multi-specialty, mixed prepaid (PP) and fee-for-service (FFS) group practices; and single-specialty small group and solo practices. The MOS focuses on patients with depression, myocardial infarction, congestive heart failure, hypertension, and diabetes. Study sites are Los Angeles, Boston, and Chicago. At each site, group practices were selected and solo providers were identified who practiced in the same geographic region (Tarlov A, Ware JE Jr, Greenfield S, et al. The

Medical Outcomes Study: an application of methods for monitoring the results of medical care. *JAMA* 1989;262:925–930; Wells KB, Stewart A, Hays RD, et al. The functioning and well-being of depressed patients: results from the Medical Outcomes Study. *JAMA* 1989;262: 914–919; Wells KB, Burnam MA, Rogers W, et al. The course of depression in adult outpatients: results from the Medical Outcomes Study. *Arch Gen Psychiatry* 1992;49:788–794).

medical statistics   See **biostatistics.**

medical toxicology   Study of physical and chemical agents and their effects on subcellular structures, living cells, and organisms from dose-response and mechanistic perspectives. Medical toxicology includes clinical manifestations, differential diagnoses, and treatments of acute poisoning (including accidental, suicidal, and substance abuse), acute and chronic exposure to toxins in the workplace, and exposure to environmental toxins.

medical use (of drugs)   Taking drugs in accordance with the prescribed schedule to alleviate symptoms of a medically diagnosed disorder.

medication   See **drug.**

medication clinic   Mental health service that provides brief (15- to 30-minute) monthly appointments to check response (therapeutic and adverse) to prescribed drugs and evaluate the need for continued drug therapy, indicated dosages, and frequency of subsequent appointments.

medication compliance   See **compliance; compliance measurement.**

medication error   Order for the wrong drug, wrong patient, inappropriate dosage, inappropriate frequency, inappropriate dosage form, inappropriate route, inappropriate indication, duplicate/redundant therapy, contraindicated therapy, medication to which the patient is allergic, or missing information required for the proper administration and dispensing of the drug. It also may include an error in filling the prescription.

medication management module   Form of patient education designed at the Rehabilitation Service of the Brentwood VA Medical Center and the UCLA Clinical Research Center for Schizophrenic and Psychiatric Rehabilitation. It consists of a trainer's manual, a patient's workbook, and a demonstration video to teach four medication self-management skills: (a) obtaining information about the benefits of antipsychotic medication; (b) knowing correct self-administration and evaluation of medication; (c) identifying side effects of medication; and (d) negotiating medication issues with health-care providers (Liberman RP, Jacobs HE, Boone SE, et al. New methods for rehabilitating chronic mental patients. *In* Talbot JA [ed], *Our Patients' Future in a Changing World.* Washington, DC: American Psychiatric Press, 1986).

medications, blinded   See **blinded medications.**

medicine   See **drug.**

Meditran   See **meprobamate.**

MEDLINE   Medical literature database maintained by the National Library of Medicine. It indexes over 600,000 articles each year published in the biomedical literature. Development of the MEDLINE system is an important example of the beneficial use of information technology in medicine. A subset of the MEDLINE database available on compact disc allows access from personal computers and eliminates the need for telephone communication to a distant computer.

medroxyprogesterone   (Clinovir; Depo-Provera; Farlotal; Perluiex; Provera) (MPA) Progesterone derivative used to treat sexual offenders who have highly intrusive sexually deviant fantasies not reduced by behavioral therapy. It lowers serum testosterone levels in males and effectively reduces the degree of sexual fantasy and preoccupation. MPA (60 mg/day for an average of 15.33 months) was given in an open, nonblind trial to seven patients meeting DSM-III-R paraphilia criteria. All described significantly fewer paraphilic fantasies, and no patient reported engaging in paraphilic behaviors during treatment. There were no significant side effects (Gottesman HG, Schubert DSP. Low-dose oral medroxyprogesterone acetate in the management of the paraphilias. *J Clin Psychiatry* 1993;43:182–188). MPA has been reported to reduce aggression in temporal lobe epilepsy patients and male schizophrenic patients (Blumer D, Migeon C. Hormone and hormonal agents in the treatment of aggression. *J Nerv Ment Dis* 1975;160:127–137; O'Connor M, Baker HWG. Depo-medroxyprogesterone acetate as an adjunctive treatment in three aggressive schizophrenic patients. *Acta Psychiatr Scand* 1983;67:399–403). Its efficacy is thought to be due to its lowering of testosterone levels and to competitive inhibition of androgen action in the brain. Short-term side effects include weight gain and increased blood pressure in up to 20% of patients; long-term side effects have not been well researched. MPA is not Food and Drug Administration (FDA) approved for the treatment of sexual deviancy, but physicians may legally use any approved drug for any purpose they see fit provided they have the patient's informed written consent for the "off-label" or "nonapproved" use.

medulla oblongata   Area of brain lying below the pons.

medullary-periventricular pathway Dopaminergic system component consisting of neurons in the motor nucleus of the vagus whose projections are not well defined. It may be involved in eating behavior.

MedWatch The Food and Drug Administration's Medical Products Reporting Program, which is intended to identify and reduce serious adverse events and product problems associated with drugs, biologicals, medical devices, special nutritional products, and other medical products regulated by the Food and Drug Administration (FDA). Health professionals are asked to report only serious adverse events (death, real risk of death, significant persistence of or permanent disability, congenital anomaly, or need for medical intervention to prevent permanent impairment or damage). Even if it is not certain if a serious adverse event is related to a drug or medical device, it should be reported. The program is designed to protect both patient and physician confidentiality.

mefenamic acid (Ponstel) Nonsteroidal antiinflammatory drug.

mefenamic acid + lithium Co-administration may cause a rise in serum lithium level with associated signs and symptoms of lithium intoxication. Serum lithium level should be obtained several days after beginning mefenamic acid (Honey J. Lithium-mefenamic interaction. *Pharmabulletin* 1982;59:20; MacDonald J, Neale TJ. Toxic interaction of lithium carbonate and mefenamic acid. *Br Med J* 1988;297:1339).

megalomania Delusions of grandeur or grandiose delusions in which the individual considers himself or herself to be greater and more superior than others (e.g., believing oneself to be God).

megavitamin therapy See **orthomolecular treatment.**

Meige's syndrome Dyskinesia characterized by tonic, symmetric, nonrhythmic contractions of orofacial muscles that may be preceded or followed by brief clonic contractions. Involuntary movements of the lower face, neck, and jaw also occur. It interferes with vision and may be socially disfiguring and/or disabling. It has been associated with affective disorders (including untreated cases), but also may be caused by various medications. It can be a neuroleptic-induced, late-onset extrapyramidal reaction regarded as a form of tardive dyskinesia or tardive dystonia. It may also be caused by levo-dopa, antihistamine decongestants, and amphetamines. It has responded dramatically to injections of botulinum toxin into dystonic facial muscles. Also called "Milroy's disease." See **botulinum toxin.**

meiosis Process occurring in germinal cells (spermatozoa or ova) by which gametes containing the haploid number of chromosomes are produced from diploid cells. Homologous chromosomes originally from two parents exchange material (called "crossing-over" or "recombination"), ensuring that the chromosome number does not double with each new generation. The phenomenon allows the mapping of genetic traits.

melancholia Major depressive episode with agitation or retardation, severe mood lowering unresponsive to environmental changes, and depressive delusions.

melancholia attonita Old designation for a severe form of melancholic stupor in which cataplexy is prominent (Jackson WS. *Melancholia and Depression: From Hippocratic Times to Modern Times.* New Haven and London: Yale University Press, 1986).

melatonin (MT) Neurohormone (N-acetyl-5-methoxytryptamine) secreted by the pineal gland that is probably the only source of circulating MT. Pinealocytes, like other cells, convert tryptophan to serotonin (5-HT), and then unlike other cells, convert 5-HT to N-acetylserotonin and finally to MT. MT synthesis is stimulated by beta-adrenergic agents; darkness has a pronounced stimulatory effect not only on melatonin secretion, but on pinealocyte beta-adrenergic receptors and MT synthesis. This produces an endogenous (internally generated) circadian rhythm in MT secretion. The light-dark regulation of MT secretion is mediated by the transmission of information from the retina to the suprachiasmatic nuclei (a key circadian oscillator) in the hypothalamus and then to the reticular system, spinal cord, and cervical ganglia. From there, postganglionic sympathetic fibers reach the pineal gland in company with its arterial supply. Plasma MT concentrations are low during the day, rise in the early evening before sleep onset, peak at about midnight, and then decline regardless of whether sleep occurs. In a normal environment, the rhythm is synchronized to a 24-hour day; synchrony is achieved by the light-dark cycle acting via the retina. Duration of MT secretion depends on the duration of darkness: 24-hour MT secretion is greater during winter than summer. In northern temperate zones, there is a phase advance of the circadian rhythm in summer relative to winter (Illnerova H, Zvolsky P, Vannecek J. Circadian rhythm in plasma melatonin concentration of the urbanized man: the effect of summer and wintertime. *Brain Res* 1985;328: 186–189). In addition to setting the periodicity of the rhythm, light of suitable intensity suppresses MT production at night in a dose-dependent manner (the brighter the light, the greater the decrease in plasma MT) and in appropriate circumstances controls duration of the night-time peak. MT secretion also changes with age. Nighttime plasma concentrations are highest in children ages 1–3, lower in children and adolescents ages 8–15, and decline gradually thereafter to a low level in the elderly (Utiger RD. Melatonin—the hormone of darkness. *N Engl J Med* 1992;327: 1377–1379). MT production by the pineal gland has been used as a marker for noradrenergic function, since pineal activity is regulated primarily by the sympathetic nervous system. Controlled trials have demonstrated alleviation of jet-lag when a 7-day course of MT (8 mg) is prescribed (Nickelsen T, Lang A, Bergau L. The effects of 6-, 9- and 11-hour time shifts on circadian rhythms: adaptation of sleep parameters and hormonal patterns following the intake of melatonin or placebo. *In* Arendt J, Pevet P [eds], *Advances in Pineal Research: 5.* London: John Libbey, 1991, pp 303–306; Claustrat B, Brun J, David M, et al. Melatonin and jet lag: confirmatory result using a simplified protocol. *Biol Psychiatry* 1992;32:705–711).

melatonin hypothesis of depression   In recent years, exploration of the relationship between light-induced changes in melatonin secretion and depressive symptoms disclosed lowered nocturnal melatonin levels in some depressed patients. The melatonin hypothesis postulates that winter depression is triggered by alterations in nocturnal melatonin secretions. The demonstration that atenolol, which suppresses melatonin secretion, is not an effective therapy for seasonal affective disorder has weakened the hypothesis (Rosenthal NE, Jacobsen FM, Sach DA, et al. Atenolol in seasonal affective disorder: a test of melatonin hypothesis. *Am J Psychiatry* 1988;145:52–56).

melitracen   (Dixeran) Antidepressant not available in the United States.

melitracen + flupenthixol   (Deanxit) Combination product (antidepressant + neuroleptic) not available in the United States.

Mellaril   See **thioridazine.**

Melodil   See **maprotiline.**

melperone   (Aplacal; Bunil; Buronil; Eunerpan; Gemeril) Atypical butyrophenone neuroleptic that blocks dopamine and serotonin $(5\text{-HT})_2$ receptors. It has a well established advantage for extrapyramidal symptoms and tardive dyskinesia. There is some evidence that it is effective in treatment-resistant schizophrenia (Meltzer HY, Alphs LD, Bastani B, et al. Effect of melperone in treatment-resistant schizophrenia. *In* Stefanis CN, Soldatos CR, Rabavilis AD [eds], *Psychiatry Today, Accomplishments and Promises, VIII World Congress of Psychiatry Abstracts, Excerpta Med Int Congress Ser 899.* Amsterdam, Oxford, New York: 1990, p 502). It has been available in some European countries for decades and is in early phase II testing in the United States.

memantine   (Akatinol) Dopamine precursor and N-methyl-D-aspartate antagonist useful in the treatment of Parkinson's disease. In a placebo-controlled double-blind study in patients ages 65–80 with mild to moderate vascular dementia, memantine (10–30 mg/day) produced a highly relevant decrease in dementia-related deficits. Patients' social behavior and ability to care for themselves were considerably improved. Adverse effects included agitation, increased motor activity, sleeplessness, and restlessness (Ditzler K. Efficacy and tolerability of memantine in patients with dementia syndrome: double-blind, placebo controlled trial. *Arzneim Forsch* 1991;41: 773–780). In doses producing little or no antiparkinson effects, memantine may cause pharmacotoxic psychosis.

memory   Storage of new and old information for later use that may be dependent on learning. Memories can be stored for very short periods (seconds, milliseconds) or long periods (weeks, years, lifetime). It is hard to specify where short-term memory ends and long-term memory begins. Two types of memory are currently recognized: declarative and nondeclarative.

memory, association   Form of memory involved in learning by operant or classical conditioning that requires forming an association between two events.

memory, consolidation   Phase in which short-term memory is transferred to long-term memory. Some benzodiazepines impair memory at the consolidation phase.

memory, context-dependent   Increment of memory that occurs when the test environment is the same as the encoding environment.

memory, declarative   Memory that is consciously recognizable and can be described. Two types of amnestic problems are associated with declarative memory: in one, there is a basic defect in learning and neither recall or recognition is possible; in the second, learning occurs, but subjects cannot access information in a timely manner; spontaneous information recall is impaired, although recognition of previous relearned material is preserved.

memory enhancing drug   See **nootropic drug.**

memory, episodic   Recall of any past personal event in response to a cue word.

memory, explicit Memory revealed by conscious recollection from a previous learning episode; it is often severely impaired in depression (Graf P, Schacter DL. Implicit and explicit memory for new associations in normal and amnestic subjects. *J Exp Psychol Learn Mem Cogn* 1985;11:501–518).

memory, implicit Memory demonstrated by performance facilitation or repetition priming, without conscious recollection from a previous learning episode. It is not affected by depression. Repetition priming may be useful in differentiating between depression and dementia* (Schacter DL. Implicit memory: history and current status. *J Exp Psychol Learn Mem Cogn* 1987;13:501–518).

memory, long-term Ability to respond to a stimulus, recite a list, remember an association, etc., long after the material was presented. Its slow rate of decay and the great amount of remembered material distinguish it from short-term memory. Amnesia typically involves loss of long-term memory.

memory loss evaluation Because problems outside the realm of memory can cause patients to complain of memory loss, initial assessment of the patient's attention, concentration, distractibility, level of alertness, and mood should precede inquiry into memory function. In addition, special attention should be paid to obsessional concerns or the presence of preoccupation of thought that may interfere with evaluation of memory. Memory loss is a frequent complaint among elderly patients that may arise from a number of sources. Some may be more sensitive to minor losses associated with age; others may be perceiving the true decline that occurs in the early stages of dementia. Depressive illness has been implicated in complaints of memory loss, but the extent and nature of the change is not well documented or explained. Drugs can also contribute to memory loss, especially in the elderly.

memory, nondeclarative Memory that cannot be consciously recalled. It includes motor or procedural learning, classical conditioning, and habits. Procedural memory is mediated by the basal ganglia; learning depends on the integrity of the medial hemispheric-hippocampal system; and access to learned information depends on frontal-subcortical circuits.

memory, primary Ability to hold on to information just received. It is measured by tests that involve attention and immediate recall (Siegler IC, Poon LW. The psychology of aging. *In* Busse EW, Blazer DG [eds], *Geriatric Psychiatry*. Washington, DC: American Psychiatric Press, 1989).

memory, remote See **memory, tertiary.**

memory scanning Assessment of cognitive processes including short-term and working memory.

memory, secondary Storage of recently learned information. It is tested by serial learning, delayed recall, and delayed recognition (Siegler IC, Poon LW. The psychology of aging. *In* Busse EW, Blazer DG [eds], *Geriatric Psychiatry*. Washington, DC: American Psychiatric Press, 1989).

memory, short-term Correct recall or appropriate performance immediately or shortly after the presentation of the material. Its rapid decay and limited amount of remembered material distinguishes it from long-term memory.

memory, spatial Ability to store and retrieve spatial information.

memory, state-dependent Increment in memory that occurs when a person's physiological condition is the same during the test as it was during the encoding.

memory, tertiary Memory of items from the distant past. It is least affected by Alzheimer's disease, depression, and treatment with anticholinergic drugs (Siegler IC, Poon LW. The psychology of aging. *In* Busse EW, Blazer DG [eds], *Geriatric Psychiatry*. Washington, DC: American Psychiatric Press, 1989). Also called "remote memory."

Mendelian Characteristic of inheritance patterns that conform to the laws proposed by Gregor Mendel in 1865.

Mendelian method Study of chromosome linkage markers.

Mendelian transmission One of three recognizable forms of trait inheritance due to single gene mechanisms: (a) autosomal dominant; (b) autosomal recessive; and (c) X-linked.

Mendelism Doctrine of inheritance based on the principles that elements called *genes* are responsible for transmission of unit characters and that the genetic elements are segregated independently of each other in the reproductive processes.

Menkes' disease X-linked neurodegenerative disorder of infancy caused by a failure in copper homeostasis in the body. It results in copper accumulation in organs such as the kidney and intestinal mucosa and copper deficiency in other organs, including the brain. It is characterized by mental and growth retardation, seizures, depigmentation and peculiar steely hair, hypothermia, and failure to thrive.

menopausal affective disorder Affective and behavioral symptoms that are severe enough to interfere with some aspects of life and that appear to be specifically related to the menopausal period (during perimenopause or menopause) (Schmidt PJ, Rubinow DR. Menopause-related affective disorders: a justification for further study. *Am J Psychiatry* 1991;148: 844–852).

mensuration Measurement of areas and distances on the surface of the body.

Mentaban See **mephobarbital.**

mental age Degree of intelligence compared with others of the same age. It is based on the principle that intellectual ability can be measured and that it increases progressively with age.

mental coprolalia See **coprolalia, mental.**

mental deficiency See **mental retardation.**

mental disorder Clinically significant behavioral or psychological syndrome or pattern associated with present distress (a painful symptom) or disability (impairment in one or more important areas of functioning), or a significantly increased risk of suffering death, pain, disability, or an important loss of freedom. It must not be merely an expectable response to a particular event (e.g., the death of a loved one). Whatever its original cause, it must currently be considered a manifestation of a behavioral, psychological, or biological dysfunction in the person. Neither deviant behavior (e.g., political, religious, sexual) nor conflicts that are primarily between the individual and society are mental disorders unless the deviance or conflict is a symptom of a dysfunction in the person, as described above (DSM-IV).

mental hospital Institution, either privately, state, or federally owned, in which inpatient and outpatient diagnostic, treatment, and rehabilitative care is administered to the psychiatrically ill through various forms of therapy (e.g., psychotherapy, chemotherapy, somatotherapy, occupational therapy, rehabilitative therapy).

mental illness Disease or disorder of the brain or psyche producing symptoms of organic or nonorganic origin (e.g., disordered thinking, feeling, or behavior) and needing diagnosis and treatment when it is severe enough. The term is used interchangeably with mental, psychiatric, and behavior disorders. In the legal system it is used to distinguish psychiatric patients from the mentally retarded and chemically dependent.

mental performance 1. Ability to execute a task requiring higher cognitive functions (e.g., memory, organization, reacting to selective complex stimuli, arithmetic ability). 2. Neuropsychological measure of higher cognitive functions (IQ).

mental retardation Below-average general intellectual function originating during the developmental period and associated with impairment in adaptive behavior. It may be

classified as borderline (Weschler IQ 70–84), mild (Weschler IQ 55–69), moderate (Weschler IQ 40–54), severe (Weschler IQ 25–39), or profound (Weschler IQ below 25). Also called "feeblemindedness"; "hypophrenia"; "intellectual inadequacy"; "mental deficiency"; "oligergasia"; "oligophrenia."

mental status In clinical psychiatry, the components of the mental status examination.

mental status examination Test to determine current psychiatric status (mood, behavior, cognitive and mental functioning). Components assessed include (a) patient's attitude toward the examiner; (b) patient's appearance and grooming; (c) patient's psychomotor behavior (gait, posture, motor activity, facial expression, speech); (d) patient's mood, stream of thought, thought content; and (e) patient's sensorium (consciousness, memory, orientation, judgement, insight, ability to abstract).

Mentane See **velnacrine.**

meperidine (Demerol) Narcotic analgesic with multiple actions qualitatively similar to those of morphine but with one-tenth the potency. It is a full agonist at the mu receptor. Like morphine, it is liable to produce respiratory depression. It is contraindicated in patients taking or who have recently (within 14 days) taken monoamine oxidase inhibitors (MAOIs) because therapeutic doses occasionally have precipitated unpredictable, severe, and occasionally fatal reactions. Care also should be exercised in prescribing meperidine for patients receiving other central nervous system depressants. Schedule II. Also called "pethidine."

meperidine + anticholinergic Co-administration increases antimuscarinic effects, including the risk of paralytic ileus, and other manifestations of anticholinergic toxicity.

meperidine + cimetidine Co-administration may result in potentiated pharmacological effects and increased duration of action of meperidine (Guay DRP, Meatherall RC. Cimetidine alters pethidine disposition in man. *Br J Clin Pharmacol* 1984;18:907–914).

meperidine + hydroxyzine Hydroxyzine potentiates meperidine analgesia and sedation without additional respiratory depression. It may be an advantageous addition to opioid therapy (Zsigmond EK, Flynn K, Shively JG. Effect of hydroxyzine and meperidine on arterial blood gases in healthy human volunteers. *J Clin Pharmacol* 1989;29:85–90; Maurer PM, Bartkowski RR. Drug interactions of clinical significance with opioid analgesics. *Drug Safety* 1993;8:30–48).

meperidine + moclobemide Although moclobemide acts predominantly as a monoamine oxidase (MAO)-A inhibitor and only binds reversibly to the enzyme, animal data indicate that it may potentiate pethidine effects. Co-administration should be avoided (Amrein R, Guntert TW, Dingemanse J, et al. Interactions of moclobemide with concomitantly administered medication: evidence from pharmacological and clinical studies. *Psychopharmacology* 1992;106:S24–S31).

meperidine + monoamine oxidase inhibitor (MAOI) Co-administration has resulted in serious and potentially life-threatening reactions in some patients. Excitement, muscle rigidity, hyperpyrexia, flushing, sweating, and unconsciousness occur rapidly. Respiratory depression and hypotension may also occur. One MAOI-treated patient died after being given meperidine (Ayd FJ Jr. Drug interactions that matter: meperidine and MAOIs. *Int Drug Ther Newsl* 1991;26:16).

meperidine + phenobarbital Co-administration increases metabolism of meperidine and increases production of the less efficacious toxic metabolite, norpethidine. Debilitating lethargy and possibly seizures may develop (Maurer PM, Bartkowski RR. Drug interactions of clinical significance with opioid analgesics. *Drug Safety* 1993;8:30–48).

meperidine + phenytoin Co-administration can produce tremors, myoclonus, and seizures (Modica PA, Tempelhoff R, White PF. Pro- and anticonvulsant effects of anesthetics [part I]. *Anesth Analg* 1990;70:303–315).

meperidine + selegiline One of the most serious drug interactions with nonselective monoamine oxidase (MAO) inhibitors occurs with meperidine. It consists of rigidity, delirium, hyperthermia, convulsions, and death. Selegiline, even in low doses, may interact adversely with meperidine, documenting that such a reaction can occur with the inhibition of MAO-B alone. Delirium, stupor, severe agitation, muscular rigidity, sweating, and pyrexia (38.2 C; 100.76 F) occurred in a 56-year-old man taking various drugs (including selegiline) who was given meperidine postoperatively (Zornberg GL, Bodkin JA, Cohen BM. Severe adverse interaction between pethidine and selegiline. *Lancet* 1991;337:246). Despite selectivity and reversibility, selegiline and other similar "new" reversible MAO inhibitors are not immune to the usual interactions of "old" MAO inhibitors. However, it is difficult to determine if the adverse effects were due solely to an interaction between selegiline and meperidine.

mephentermine (Wyamine) Vasopressor marketed for the treatment of hypotension. It indirectly stimulates beta- and alpha-adrenergic receptors by releasing norepinephrine from its storage site. It may interact with phenothiazine neuroleptics, which may antagonize its pressor effects. Because monoamine oxidase inhibitors also may potentiate its pressor effects, the drugs should not be co-prescribed. Pregnancy risk category C.

mephenytoin (Mesantoin) Racemic hydantoin derivative anticonvulsant marketed for the treatment of generalized tonic-clonic and complex partial seizures. Daily dosage range for adults is 200–800 mg; for children, 50–400 mg. Mephenytoin is best administered in divided doses. Like phenytoin, it may have antiarrhythmic effects. It is metabolized in a highly stereoselective manner. In humans, it undergoes rapid and complete oxidation to a parahydroxylated product while the R-antipode is disposed of by a much slower N-demethylation pathway to form an active metabolite, 5-phenyl-5-ethylhydantoin (PEH). Mephenytoin hydroxylation capacity is an inherited trait that may be transmitted in a simple Mendelian autosomal recessive fashion. Significant inhibition of mephenytoin hydroxylation has been observed with diazepam, flurazepam, phenytoin, tranylcypromine, nialamide, papaverine, and some steroids. Mephenytoin phenotype can be determined after administration of R-mephenytoin by means of the hydroxylation index, which is a ratio of the administered dose of S-mephenytoin (half the R-dose) and the quantity of 4-hydroxy-mephenytoin excreted in the urine (Guttendorf RJ, Wedlund PJ. Genetic aspects of drug disposition and therapeutics. *J Clin Pharmacol* 1992;32:107–117). Pregnancy risk category C.

mephobarbital (Mebaral; Metaban; Mephoral) Barbiturate marketed as an anticonvulsant and nonspecific central nervous system (CNS) depressant. It is indicated for generalized tonic-clonic, absence, myoclonic, and mixed-type seizures. It also is prescribed for children with hyperexcitability states. It interacts with alcohol and other CNS depressants, increasing the degree of CNS depression. Like other barbiturates, it may be an enzyme inducer. Schedule IV; pregnancy risk category D.

Mephoral See **mephobarbital.**

Mepro See **meprobamate.**

meprobamate (Apo-Meprobamate; Equanil; Meditran; Mepro; Meprospan; Miltown; Neuramate; Novomepro; Sedabamate; SK-Bamate; Tranmep) Substituted propanediol synthesized in 1954 from mephenesin, a short-acting muscle relaxant. Its introduction began the era of "minor tranquilizers." It is rapidly absorbed from the intestinal tract, with peak effect in 2–3 hours. It also has muscle relaxant properties and may raise central nervous system seizure threshold. It crosses the placental barrier and is excreted in breast milk. Widely acclaimed and widely prescribed for over a decade, meprobamate's distinction from the barbiturates and its efficacy were questioned by the early 1970s, and its incidence of dependence/withdrawal, misuse/abuse, and lethality in overdosage, along with increased use of the benzodiazepines, led to a marked reduction in its prescription. Sudden withdrawal from high doses causes a discontinuation syndrome characteristic of barbiturate withdrawal. Schedule IV; pregnancy risk category D. •

meprobamate + benactyzine   (Deprol) Combination of meprobamate (400 mg) plus benactyzine (1 mg) formerly marketed as an antidepressant.

Meprospan   See **meprobamate.**

Merlit   See **lorazepam.**

Mesantoin   See **mephenytoin.**

"mesc"   Street name for mescaline.

"mescal"   Street name for mescaline.

mescaline   Phenylethylamine hallucinogen derived from the peyote cactus that has a slower onset of action than lysergic acid diethylamide (LSD). It is used by some Indians of the southwest United States in religious rites. Hallucinations last 1–2 hours after the usual dose. Use is frequently accompanied by unpleasant side effects (e.g., nausea, vomiting). It may cause a "bad trip" manifested by apprehension, fear, panic, perceptual distortions, hallucinations, and, less commonly, delusions and agitated delirium.

mesencephalon   Area of the brain that contains the tegmentum and the substantia nigra. Also called "the midbrain."

mesocarb   (Sidnocarb) Uniquely structured stimulant of the sydnonimine series that is marketed in Russia. Unlike amphetamine, which inhibits norepinephrine (NE) uptake, it causes few NE effects and appears to be a selective inhibitor of dopamine uptake. In vitro, it appears to inhibit synaptosomal catecholamine uptake. It has been reported to increase workload per kilogram of bodyweight, maintain work capacity, and improve cardiovascular function. Unlike other psychostimulants, it does not appear to be habit-forming.

mesocortical system   Part of the dopamine system with its cell bodies mainly in the ventral tegmental area. Its neurons project to the prefrontal cortex, accumbens, septum, and olfactory tubercles.

mesocortical tract   Pathway involving the cortex and limbic systems.

mesolimbic system   Part of the dopamine system with its cell bodies in the ventral tegmen-tal area (A10) of the midbrain and in the substantia nigra. It projects to the accumbens, olfactory tubercle, and amygdala.

mesolimbic-mesocortical pathway   One of five dopaminergic systems; it projects from cell bodies near the substantia nigra to the limbic system and neocortex.

mesoridazine   (Lidanar; Lidanil; Serentil) Piperidine phenothiazine neuroleptic. It is the side-chain sulfoxide derivative of thioridazine and its most pharmacologically active metabolite. Mesoridazine is an active neuroleptic that, milligram per milligram, is 2 to 3 times more potent than thioridazine. Clinical indications are similar to those for thioridazine and other piperidine phenothiazine neuroleptics. Like thioridazine, it tends less to evoke extrapyramidal symptoms than aliphatic and piperazine phenothiazines and other more potent non-phenothiazine neuroleptics. Unlike thioridazine, mesoridazine is available in an injectable form. Pregnancy risk category C.

mesoridazine + phenytoin   Phenytoin significantly lowers the plasma concentration of mesoridazine, thereby interfering with mesoridazine's therapeutic effects.

messenger, neural   See **neural messenger.**

messenger RNA   (mRNA) RNA molecule that carries genetic information for a particular polypeptide from the gene in the nucleus to the cytoplasm, where it combines with the ribosomes and transfer RNA (tRNA) to direct the synthesis of protein molecules. mRNA derives from the primary transcript RNA following capping, polyadenylation, and splicing.

messenger, second   See **second messenger.**

mesterolone   (Mestoranum) 1-Methyl testosterone derivative anabolic steroid. No longer available in the United States.

Mestoranum   See **mesterolone.**

meta-analysis   Statistical strategy that permits quantitative estimation of a population correlation (rho) by using sample correlations (r) from a collection of independent studies. Meta-analyses or overviews of randomized, controlled trials include observations on large numbers of patients, reduce random errors, and may detect a small treatment effect that is not clear in any individual study. It can go beyond statistical significance to estimation of effect size. In the best circumstances, meta-analysis provides an objective, noncontroversial evaluation of the results of a series of studies (Hedges LV, Olkin I. *Statistical Methods for Meta-Analysis.* Orlando: Academic Press, 1985). Meta-analysis requires the research protocol to include a clear definition of the research question, a description of the studies to be included, inclusion/exclusion criteria for selecting trials, and the method of trial selection. Misuse of bias and statistical methods and sensitivity analyses used should also be assessed. Meta-analysis, particularly of randomized trials, can provide a rigorous and sound approach to treatment evaluation and can be an integral part of any major cost-effectiveness analysis. Meta-analysis is not an exact statistical science. It can remove idiosyncrasy from the evaluation of medical issues, but it will not produce definitive simple answers to complex clinical problems. It may provide conclusions about a treatment that could not be drawn from individual trials because of small numbers. It may provide evidence about a class of drugs or treatments that allow a general qualitative conclusion to be drawn. Its results are therefore directly relevant to the formulation of broad medical policies. Meta-analysis cannot tell clinicians how to treat an individual patient, but it can provide information that helps decision-making (Thacker S. Meta-analysis: a quantitative approach to research integration. *JAMA* 1988; 259:1685–1689; Thompson SG, Pocock SJ. Can meta-analyses be trusted? *Lancet* 1991;338: 1127–1130). Meta-analysis can make it harder to move from judging whether a treatment is, in principle, efficacious, to deciding how to manage a particular patient. A comparison of meta-analysis of the literature (MAL) and meta-analysis of individual patient data (MAP) indicates that the results of MAL alone may be misleading. Hence, a meta-analysis of updated individual patient data is recommended, because this provides the least biased and most reliable means of addressing questions not satisfactorily resolved by individual clinical trials. MAPs take considerable time and resources, and usually involve worldwide collaborations (Stewart LA, Parmar MKB. Meta-analysis of the literature or of individual patient data: is there a difference? *Lancet* 1993;341:418–422).

meta-analysis, cumulative Performance of an updated meta-analysis every time a new trial appears. It is an important new development for assessing therapeutic results of randomized, controlled trials. It facilitates determination of clinical efficacy and harm and may be helpful in tracking trials, planning future trials, and making clinical recommendations for therapy. It is a response to the need for new methods to synthesize and present information from widely dispersed publications (Lau J, Antman EM, Jiminez-Silva J, et al. Cumulative meta-analysis of therapeutic trials for myocardial infarction. *N Engl J Med* 1992;327:248–254).

metabolic alkalosis See **alkalosis.**

metabolic inborn error Any of a wide range of disorders in which a genetic abnormality in a biochemical pathway causes a particular syndrome or disease (e.g., phenylketonuria and Lesch-Nyhan syndrome).

metabolic ratio Ratio of the amount of parent compound to the amount of metabolite(s).

metabolism Process involved in the removal of a drug from the systemic circulation. For many drugs, hepatic drug metabolizing enzymes play an important role. Drugs may undergo either phase I or phase II metabolism. Phase I consists of oxidation, reduction, and hydrolysis; phase II metabolism of glucuronidation and sulfation. The liver is also responsible for first-pass metabolism, which occurs when a drug is absorbed from the gastrointestinal tract into the portal circulation. Drugs are then extensively metabolized in the liver before they reach the systemic circulation. The systemic clearance of drugs that undergo extensive hepatic metabolism are sensitive to changes in hepatic blood flow (Yonkers KA, Kando JC, Cole JO, Blumenthal S. Gender differences in pharmacokinetics and pharmacodynamics of psychotropic medication. *Am J Psychiatry* 1992;149:587–595).

metabolite Breakdown product of a drug that may or may not be pharmacologically active. Many metabolites have pharmacodynamic activity and contribute to the overall pharmacodynamic response of the parent compound. Some may have a totally different effect (therapeutic or toxic) of their own until they are excreted or further metabolized. With the exception of lithium, most psychoactive drugs generate pharmacologically active metabolites. Hydroxylated or demethylated metabolites should be considered pharmacologically active until proven otherwise.

metabolite, active, type I Active metabolite with an inactive, precursor parent drug (e.g., clorazepate) (Preskorn SH. Pharmacokinetics of psychotropic agents: why and how they are relevant to treatment. *J Clin Psychiatry* 1993; 54[suppl]:3–7).

metabolite, active, type II Active metabolite with the same mechanism of action as the parent drug and contributing to the drug's duration of action (e.g., norfluoxetine) (Preskorn SH. Pharmacokinetics of psychotropic agents: why and how they are relevant to treatment. *J Clin Psychiatry* 1993;54[suppl]:3–7).

metabolite, active, type III Active metabolite with mechanism of action different from that of the parent drug (e.g., desmethylclomipramine and clomipramine) (Preskorn SH. Pharmacokinetics of psychotropic agents: why and how they are relevant to treatment. *J Clin Psychiatry* 1993;54[suppl]:3–7).

metabolite, active, type IV   Active metabolite with mechanism of action antagonistic to that of the parent drug (e.g., m-chlorophenylpiperazine and trazodone) (Preskorn SH. Pharmacokinetics of psychotropic agents: why and how they are relevant to treatment. *J Clin Psychiatry* 1993;54[suppl]:3–7).

metabolizer, extensive   See **acetylator, rapid.**

metabolizer, poor   See **acetylator, slow.**

metabotropic receptor   Receptor that, in response to specific membrane proteins, is activated by a protein kinase by cyclic adenosine monophosphate (cAMP) and then opens an ion channel to cause efflux of potassium and influx of sodium ions. Many neurotransmitters are now thought to work by this receptor-linked second messenger system.

metacentric   Chromosome with a centrally located centromere.

metachlorophenylpiperazine   (mCPP) Major metabolite of trazodone and the second metabolite formed from nefazodone. It is a potent and specific serotonin (5- HT)$_{1A}$, 5-HT$_{1B}$, and 5-HT$_{1C}$ receptor agonist that has affinity for 5-HT$_1$ and 5-HT$_2$ binding sites in the human brain. Binding affinity is highest at the 5-HT$_{1C}$ receptor. It also has an effect on alpha$_2$ receptors, and to a lesser extent, alpha$_1$, dopamine, and muscarinic receptors (Hamik A, Peroutka S. 1-m-chlorophenylpiperazine (mCPP) interactions with neurotransmitter receptors in human brain. *Biol Psychiatry* 1989;25:569–575). It stimulates secretion of prolactin and cortisol, which is presumably dose-related. It is widely used as a pharmacological probe of the 5-HT system in humans. It provokes obsessional behavior, dysphoria, anxiety attacks, and panic attacks. It decreases slow-wave sleep in humans, suggesting that 5-HT$_{1C}$ receptors may regulate slow-wave sleep (Katsuda Y, Walsh AES, Ware CJ, et al. Meta-chlorophenylpiperazine decreases slow-wave sleep in humans. *Biol Psychiatry* 1993;33:49–51). In obsessive-compulsive disorder patients, it significantly blunts cortisol responses, but has no significant potentiation of prolactin. Recent research indicates that mCPP blood level may be gender-dependent, being almost twice as high in males as in females.

metachromatic leukodystrophy   (MLD) Rare metabolic disorder of aryl sulfatase that is associated neuropathologically with early subprefrontal dysmyelination. If onset is in adolescence or early adulthood, psychosis occurs in the majority of cases (Hyde TM, Ziegler JC, Weinberger DR. Psychiatric disturbances in metachromatic leukodystrophy: insights into the neurobiology of psychosis. *Arch Neurol* 1992;49:401–406).

metamemory   Memory complaints (rather than memory disturbance) demonstrated by memory performance tests.

Metandren   See **methyltestosterone.**

metanopirone   Azaspirone derivative nonbenzodiazepine anxiolytic currently undergoing clinical trials for use in treating anxiety and depression. It is related to gepirone and ipsapirone.

metaphase   Stage of meiosis or mitosis when the chromosomes move about within the spindle and arrange themselves on the equatorial plate.

metaraminol   (Aramine) Potent sympathomimetic amine that increases both systolic and diastolic blood pressures. Use with a monoamine oxidase inhibitor (MAOI) or tricyclic antidepressant may result in potentiation of the pressor effect. Metaraminol should not be administered until 14 days after an MAOI has been discontinued.

met-ENK   See **methionine-enkephalin.**

met-enkephalin   See **methionine-enkephalin.**

metergoline   Nonselective serotonin (5-HT) antagonist that blocks both 5-HT$_1$ and 5-HT$_2$ receptor subtypes. It also possesses significant dopaminergic agonist properties. It effectively blocks the pharmacological probe meta-chlorophenylpiperazine (mCPP) when it is administered orally to patients with obsessive-compulsive disorder.

"meth"   Street name for methamphetamine.

methadone   (Dolophine; Physeptine) Synthetic, relatively long-acting opioid analgesic developed in Germany during World War II that yields a very stable level of active metabolite. It is effective when administered orally, rectally, and parenterally. When administered orally its effects are reliable. Withdrawal signs and symptoms are milder but more prolonged than those of morphine, making methadone a useful drug for detoxification and maintenance of heroin addicts. Its long duration of action is believed responsible for the more prolonged and less severe withdrawal syndrome that makes substitution of methadone for the abused opioid advantageous in detoxification. Methadone does not produce euphoric effects when given orally to highly tolerant patients and has long been the mainstay of treatment for heroin addiction because of its efficacy and acceptability to addicts. It curbs heroin use by several mechanisms: (a) long action prevents the addict from needing more heroin to avoid withdrawal; (b) tolerance to methadone induces cross-tolerance to other opiates, making heroin less euphorigenic; and (c) methadone program structure can be used to facilitate addict enrollment in other psychosocial treatments. Methadone addicts report more severe withdrawal responses than heroin addicts during an inpatient gradual methadone reduction program. Methadone is also used for the treatment of pain, but its use is limited by its long and unpredictable half-life. Schedule II; pregnancy risk category C. See **methadone maintenance.**

methadone/alcoholism Many methadone-maintained patients need to be treated simultaneously for alcoholism. In addition to the benefits that all alcoholics derive from treatment, 'methadone-maintained patients, because of their high rate of chronic liver disease, receive an extra benefit: prevention of further damage to the liver. There is no justifiable reason to deny treatment for alcoholism to alcoholics who are well stabilized on a program of methadone maintenance. Methadone, as used in a methadone-maintenance program, is pharmacologically different from heroin and alcohol. It eliminates physical craving for heroin without producing abnormal euphoria, allowing former heroin users to stabilize their lives and return to normal patterns of living. There also is little adverse interaction between methadone and other chemotherapeutic agents (i.e., disulfiram) used in alcoholism treatment. Methadone maintenance does not interfere in the successful utilization of long-term alcoholism treatment, including participation in Alcoholics Anonymous (AA).

methadone + alprazolam Since its introduction in 1983, alprazolam has become more popular than diazepam (Valium) among methadone maintenance patients who use a benzodiazepine to "boost" methadone effects. They take 20–40 mg after ingesting methadone to produce a "high" without sedation (Weddington WW, Carney AC. Alprazolam abuse during methadone maintenance therapy. *JAMA* 1987; 257:3363). Many patients typically take a large dose in the morning prior to receiving their methadone, then engage in sporadic use throughout the day. Alprazolam's greater addiction liability, shorter half-life, and more intense withdrawal symptoms make addiction to it more likely and its management in methadone patients more complicated (McDuff DR, Schwartz RP, Tommasello A, et al. Outpatient benzodiazepine detoxification procedure for methadone patients. *J Subst Abuse Treat* 1993; 10:297–302).

methadone + amitriptyline Amitriptyline potentiates opioid-associated respiratory depression and sedation (Hasten PD, Horn JR. *Drug Interactions,* 6th ed. Philadelphia: Lea & Febiger, 1990).

methadone + amoxapine Amoxapine prolongs and potentiates methadone's analgesic effects, and potentiates methadone-induced respiratory depression (Hasten PD, Horn JR. *Drug Interactions,* 6th ed. Philadelphia: Lea & Febiger, 1990).

methadone/breast milk Although methadone is secreted in breast milk, breastfeeding during methadone maintenance is permissible. If the mother stops methadone or breast feeding abruptly, signs of opiate withdrawal may occur in the infant. See **methadone/pregnancy; methadone withdrawal/neonate.**

methadone + carbamazepine Addition of carbamazepine during methadone maintenance results in mild opiate withdrawal symptoms and a 60% decrease in plasma methadone trough levels (Bell J, Seres V, Bowron P, et al. The use of serum methadone levels in patients receiving methadone maintenance. *Clin Pharmacol Ther* 1988;43:623–629).

methadone + cimetidine Cimetidine inhibits the clearance of methadone.

methadone + cocaine Methadone may increase or prolong cocaine euphoria ("speedball" effects) or attenuate the anxiety and dysphoria associated with cocaine use (Schottenfeld RS, Pakes J, Ziedonis D, Kosten TR. Buprenorphine: dose-related effects on cocaine and opioid use in cocaine-abusing opioid-dependent humans. *Biol Psychiatry* 1993;34:66–74).

methadone + desipramine After 2 weeks of co-administration, desipramine levels increased between 73% and 169% (Maany I, Dhopesh V, Arndt IO, et al. Increase in desipramine serum levels associated with methadone treatment. *Am J Psychiatry* 1989;146: 1611–1613; Kosten TR, Gawin FH, Morgan C, et al. Desipramine and its 2-hydroxy metabolite in patients taking or not taking methadone. *Am J Psychiatry* 1990;147:1379–1380).

methadone detoxification One of the most widely used methods of withdrawal for opiate addicts. It consists of substituting methadone for heroin before withdrawal followed by gradually reducing doses of oral methadone, usually over 10–21 days. In an inpatient setting, more than 80% of opiate addicts complete the program. Many addicts, however, report residual withdrawal symptoms well beyond the last day of methadone administration. Many also believe that withdrawal from methadone is more severe than withdrawal from heroin. Bone pains and muscular aches are prominent adverse effects that addicts attribute to methadone. Some addicts prefer an unmodified withdrawal from heroin to a short-term methadone detoxification.

methadone + diazepam Co-use by some methadone maintenance patients occurred frequently in the late 1970s and early 1980s. Diazepam (DZ) was generally taken within an hour of the methadone dose; its desired effect was to "boost" methadone (Budd RD, Walkin E, Jain NC, et al. Frequency of use of diazepam in individuals on probation and in methadone maintenance programs. *Am J Drug Alcohol Abuse* 1979;6:511–514). In two methadone clinics, the urine samples of 65–70% of patients showed traces of benzodiazepines in a 1-month period; the majority used DZ in a single daily dose, often in excess of 100 mg and up to 300 mg (Stitzer ML, Griffiths RR, McLellàn AT, et al. Diazepam use among methadone maintenance patients: patterns and dosages. *Drug Alcohol Dependence* 1981;8: 189–199). By the late 1980s, alprazolam became more popular than DZ among methadone patients (Weddington WW, Carney AC. Alprazolam abuse during methadone maintenance therapy. *JAMA* 1987;257:3363). Although DZ has been reported not to alter methadone metabolism, in one case it inhibited hepatic metabolism of methadone, resulting in elevated plasma methadone concentrations (Pond SM, Benowitz NL, Jacob P, Rigod J. Lack of effect of diazepam on methadone metabolism in methadone-maintained addicts. *Clin Pharmacol Ther* 1982;31:139–143; Preston KL, Griffiths RR, Stitzer ML, et al. Diazepam and methadone interactions in methadone maintenance. *Clin Pharmacol Ther* 1984;36: 534–541; Stimmel B. Prescribing psychotropic agents in opiate dependency: the need for caution. *Adv Alcohol Subst Abuse* 1986;5:121–133). See **alprazolam + methadone.**

methadone + disulfiram   Disulfiram inhibits clearance of methadone, possibly resulting in methadone toxicity.

methadone + fluoxetine   Co-administration is associated with ·increased plasma methadone concentrations. Prescription of fluoxetine (FLX) for patients in a methadone-maintenance treatment program has had positive results in reducing cocaine (COC) use (Pollack MH, Rosenbaum JF. Fluoxetine treatment of cocaine abuse in heroin addicts. *J Clin Psychiatry* 1991;52:31–33). In an open prospective study, 16 COC-dependent methadone maintenance patients took FLX (mean dose, 45 mg/day) for 9 weeks. It was well tolerated and did not appear to alter methadone plasma concentrations. Few adverse effects were noted; none required FLX discontinuation (Batki SL, Manfredi LB, Jacob P, Jones RT. Fluoxetine for cocaine dependence in methadone maintenance: quantitative plasma and urine cocaine/benzoylecgonine concentrations. *J Clin Psychopharmacol* 1993;13:243–250).

methadone + lorazepam   Lorazepam, diazepam, and alprazolam were much preferred over other benzodiazepines by 40 "connoisseur" methadone maintenance patients who used them to "boost" methadone effects (Iguchi MY, Griffiths RR, Bickel WR, et al. Relative abuse liability of benzodiazepines in methadone-maintained populations in three cities. *In* Harris LS [ed], *Problems of Drug Dependence.* NIDA Research Monograph No. 95, DHSS Publication [ADM] 90-1663. Washington, DC: US Government Printing Office, 1989, pp 364–365).

methadone maintenance   Ambulatory treatment for opiate dependence. Once tolerance has developed, orally administered methadone (30–100 mg/day) produces neither subjective intoxication nor clinically detectable behavioral impairment. Toxic side effects are extremely rare, and general health improves as compared with daily heroin regimens. Methadone maintenance keeps the patient in a "normal" state, without euphoria or withdrawal, and can even block the euphoric effect of injected heroin, thereby helping extinguish the mystique of the needle. By establishing a new stable setpoint for the opioid receptor system, methadone restores adrenal, immune, and sexual function. Patients become more amenable to counseling, environmental changes, and support services that can help shift their orientation and behavior away from seeking illicit drugs. Methadone maintenance is frequently complicated by continued drug abuse and associated human immunodeficiency virus (HIV) high-risk behaviors. Some patients may have an affective disorder and use illicit drugs to "self-medicate." Studies of tricyclic antidepressant treatment in depressed methadone patients indicate some improvement in mood but little evidence of reduced drug abuse. Methadone maintenance treatment of opioid dependence has been studied more thoroughly than any other therapeutic approach. The literature has been reviewed by independent scholars, the Institute of Medicine of the National Academy of Sciences, the Office of Technology Assessment of the U.S. Congress, and the General Accounting Office. All conclude that methadone treatment, given in appropriate doses and with adequate psychological counseling, is cost-effective and results in a sharp and substantial decrease in illicit opioid use (Johnson RE, Jaffe JH, Fudala PJ. [Letter to the editor]. *JAMA* 1992;268:2376–2377).

methadone + naloxone   Naloxone causes methadone withdrawal symptoms that last until the naloxone is metabolized (about 20–30 minutes).

methadone + neuroleptic Co-administration may produce a superior antipsychotic effect compared to that of the neuroleptic alone, although this has not been conclusively established. Methadone in narcotic-abusing schizophrenic patients sometimes alters patients' neuroleptic requirements.

methadone + pentazocine Pentazocine may exert antagonist effects and possibly cause methadone withdrawal symptoms.

methadone + phenobarbital Co-administration may precipitate opioid withdrawal in methadone maintenance patients (Liu SJ, Wang RIH. Case report of barbiturate-induced enhancement of methadone metabolism and withdrawal syndrome. *Am J Psychiatry* 1984;141:1287–1288).

methadone + phenytoin Phenytoin can cause methadone abstinence symptoms in previously stable patients because of increased methadone clearance (Tony TG, Pond SM, Kruk MJ, et al. Phenytoin-induced methadone withdrawal. *Ann Intern Med* 1981;94:349–351).

methadone/pregnancy Oral methadone is sometimes used during pregnancy to keep patients from resorting to heroin. Except for risk of neonatal dependence and withdrawal, the effects of methadone on the fetus and the neonate are not fully known. Although methadone maintenance is probably safer than continued heroin use, methadone should be avoided during pregnancy whenever possible. The fetus is adversely affected by opioid withdrawal, and great care must be exercised in withdrawing the mother. See **methadone/breast milk; methadone withdrawal/neonate.**

methadone + rifampin Co-administration may significantly lower methadone plasma levels and necessitate increasing the methadone dose to avert narcotic withdrawal symptoms (Kreck MJ, Gatjahr CL, Garfield JW, et al. Drug interactions with methadone. *Ann N Y Acad Sci* 1976;281:350–371).

methadone toxicity Methadone is highly toxic to anyone who is not tolerant of opioids. As methadone maintenance therapy continues to grow, partly because of its inclusion in the harm reduction approach to opioid use in the context of the acquired immunodeficiency syndrome (AIDS) epidemic, there has been an increase in reports of methadone poisonings and deaths shortly (2–6 days) after initiation of methadone maintenance therapy, especially in nontolerant adults and in children of mothers receiving maintenance therapy. The main toxic effects are respiratory depression with pulmonary edema and/or aspiration pneumonia. They may occur during induction of methadone maintenance, when tolerance is incorrectly assessed, or during drug maintenance if several days' doses are combined. Accidental ingestion also may cause death (Harding-Pink D. Methadone: one person's maintenance dose is another's poison. *Lancet* 1993;341:665–666).

methadone withdrawal/neonate Withdrawal symptoms similar to those of opiate withdrawal occur in newborns of methadone-maintenanced women who took methadone during the last trimester of pregnancy. As a rule, symptoms might not appear until 3–7 days after birth. To prevent withdrawal, pregnant women being maintained on methadone should have the dosage reduced to 20 mg/day or less during the last 6 weeks before delivery. The newborn should be carefully evaluated regarding symptom severity before any treatment is started. As few as 25% of these infants may require active treatment, usually for less than 2 weeks. Pharmacotherapy for these infants is well covered by Finnegan (Finnegan LP. Neonatal abstinence syndrome: assessment and pharmacotherapy. *In* Rubaltelli FF, Granati B [eds], *Neonatal Therapy: An Update.* New York: Elsevier, 1986). It is also possible to treat withdrawal symptoms, at least initially, by having the infant breast-feed while the mother continues on methadone.

methadone + zidovudine Zidovudine (AZT) does not affect methadone serum levels, but some patients on methadone maintenance treatment show a potentially toxic increase in serum levels of AZT. The pharmacokinetic disposition of methadone is not changed by AZT, nor does AZT cause methadone withdrawal symptoms. Methadone may affect the pharmacokinetics of AZT, resulting in higher AZT blood levels even though neither AZT metabolism nor excretion is altered by methadone. These interactions do not necessarily warrant making changes in AZT dosage, but they do indicate that careful monitoring for symptoms of dose-related AZT toxicity is prudent (Schwartz EL, Brechbuhl AB, Kahl P, et al. Pharmacokinetic interactions of zidovudine and methadone in intravenous drug-using patients with HIV infection. *J Acquired Immunodeficiency Syndrome* 1992;5:619–626).

methamphetamine (Desoxyn; Methedrine) (MAP) Increasingly abused psychostimulant that is metabolized to amphetamine and toxic to dopaminergic neurons of the nigrostriatal system. Typical abusers are 20–35 years old, white, and high-school educated. About one-third are women of childbearing age. Oral or intravenous routes of administration are most common, but smoking is becoming popular among young drug abusers, because MAP can be synthesized into a crystalline smokable form ("ice") that allegedly produces a sensation of euphoria similar to that of crack cocaine. MAP misuse during pregnancy can result in prematurity and low birth weight because it crosses the placenta and concentrates in fetal tissues. In any abuser, it can cause cardiomyopathy, acute myocardial infarction, cardiogenic shock, and death. It also can cause psychosis with characteristic features very similar to those of paranoid schizophrenia. There are two types of clinical course in MAP psychosis after abstinence. Type A is a psychotic state that begins to improve with disappearance of the acute central action of MAP. The type B psychotic state continues for up to a month, even though MAP is metabolized and excreted rapidly. Chronic MAP use results in a lasting change in both dopaminergic and nondopaminergic systems that relate to the paranoid psychotic state. Schedule II; pregnancy risk category C.

methamphetamine + fluoxetine   An 11-year-old child with obsessive-compulsive disorder, major depression, and attention deficit hyperactivity disorder was successfully treated with fluoxetine (mean 30 mg/day) and methamphetamine (sustained release 10 mg/day). Methamphetamine was selected to avoid stimulations with commercial formulations containing food dyes because this child was sensitive to tartrazine. There did not appear to be any significant adverse effects (Bussing R, Levin GM. Methamphetamine and fluoxetine treatment of a child with attention-deficit hyperactivity disorder and obsessive-compulsive disorder. *J Child Adolesc Psychopharmacol* 1993; 3:53–58).

methandienone   Androgenic anabolic steroid.

methandriol   Commonly abused anabolic steroid.

Methandroid   See **methandrostenolone.**

methandrostenolone   (Diabanol; Methandroid) Oral anabolic steroid that is a 17-alpha-methyl testosterone derivative.

methaqualone   (formerly Quaalude; Optimil; Parest; Somnafec) Nonbarbiturate, nonbenzodiazepine sedative-hypnotic that has become a favorite of illicit drug users who take it for its intoxicating effects. It frequently produces peripheral numbness and paresthesias, described as a "buzz." Like cocaine, it is extremely lipid-soluble, but its half-life is 20–60 hours. Because it is biotransformed slowly, both blood or urine tests can effectively detect the parent compound. It may produce delirious states that may include hallucinations and nightmares. Street names include "ludes," "sopor," and "Q." No longer marketed in the United States.

Methedrine   See **methamphetamine.**

methimazole   Antithyroid compound widely used in the treatment of hyperthyroidism. It decreases thyroid function tests by complex intrathyroidal and extrathyroidal mechanisms. Usual dose range is 20–60 mg/day, although 15–20 mg/day, often administered as a single dose, significantly decrease but maintain thyroid function tests within the normal range. Some preliminary evidence suggests that methimazole may have some antidepressant efficacy in major depression (Joffe RT, Singer W, Levitt AJ. Methimazole in treatment-resistant depression. *Biol Psychiatry* 1992;31:1235–1237).

methionine-enkephalin   (met-ENK; Met-enkephalin) Endogenous opioid peptide found in the brain that stimulates PHA (a T helper cell antigen)-induced blastogenesis in mice and markedly stimulates OKT 4 (T helper cell) production in normal volunteers. Similar elevation of T helper cells has occurred in acquired immunodeficiency syndrome (AIDS) patients with Kaposi's sarcoma. It also stimulates production of interleukin-2. See **enkephalin.**

methixene   Anticholinergic drug used in the treatment of parkinsonism.

method comparison study   Experiment to assess the reproducibility of two well-defined methods (e.g., A and B). If the difference between measurements obtained with methods A and B is X for one subject and X for another, the resulting mean difference to be considered should be zero in a method comparison study (Bland JM, Altiman DG. Statistical methods for assessing agreement between two methods of clinical measurement. *Lancet* 1986;1:307–310).

methodology   **1.** Scientific study of methods, usually for scientific research. **2.** Overall strategy of a scientific research project (e.g., double-blind methodology). It should not be confused with "methods."

methohexital   (Brevital) Ultrashort-acting barbiturate commonly used for electroconvulsive therapy anesthesia. It also can be used to partially block acute onset of withdrawal symptoms induced by naloxone in opiate addicts. Schedule IV.

Methosarb   See **calusterone.**

methotrimeprazine   See **levomepromazine.**

3-methoxy-4-hydroxy-phenylglycol   (MHPG) Main metabolite of central norepinephrine formed by the actions of monoamine oxidase (MAO) and catechol-O-methyl transferase (COMT). It is the most reliable indicator of MAO inhibition in vivo. Smaller amounts generally are found in the urine of depressed bipolar patients compared to normal subjects. Altered excretion rates of MHPG may predict response to treatment with certain types of antidepressants (e.g., maprotiline) (Rosenbaum AH, Schatzberg AF, Maruta T, et al. MHPG as a predictor of antidepressant response to imipramine and maprotiline. *Am J Psychiatry* 1980;37:1090–1092).

methscopolamine   (Pamine) Anticholinergic drug that can be used as an antidote for tricyclic antidepressant withdrawal in which peripheral autonomic manifestations predominate.

methsuximide   (Celontin) Succinimide derivative anticonvulsant used for the treatment of absence (petit mal) seizures refractory to other drugs. It suppresses the paroxysmal 3-Hz spike and wave activity associated with lapses in consciousness. It is available in 150-mg and 300-mg capsules. Maximum daily dose for children and adults is 1.2 g. Abrupt withdrawal may precipitate absence seizures. Pregnancy risk category C.

methylation   Addition of a methyl (-CH$_3$) moiety to the nucleoside cytosine of a DNA molecule; methylated cytosine mimics thymine and becomes a potential site for mutation. Methylation likely has a role in gene regulation and may produce some instances of imprinting.

methyl-2,5-dimethoxyamphetamine   See **dimethoxymethylamphetamine.**

methyldopa   (Aldomet) Antihypertensive that reduces the tissue concentration of serotonin, dopamine, and especially norepinephrine and epinephrine by competitive inhibition of levodopa decarboxylase. It has been reported to cause depression with agoraphobia and agitation by creating false neurotransmitters (alpha methylnorepinephrine and alpha methyldopamine).

methyldopa + hydrochlorothiazide   Combination product containing the antihypertensive methyldopa and the diuretic hydrochlorothiazide that is marketed for the treatment of hypertension. Concurrent use with alcohol, barbiturates, narcotics, analgesics, and other antihypertensive drugs increases risk of orthostatic hypotension. It should not be co-administered with lithium because it can decrease lithium clearance and cause lithium toxicity.

methyldopa + lithium   Co-administration may produce lithium toxicity in patients previously stable on lithium alone (Yassa R. Lithium-methyldopa interaction. *Can Med Assoc J* 1986; 134:141–142).

methyldopa + paroxetine   No interactions have been demonstrated (Bannister SJ, Houser VP, Hulse JD, et al. Evaluation of the potential for interactions of paroxetine with diazepam, cimetidine, warfarin and digoxin. *Acta Psychiatr Scand* 1989;80[350 suppl]:102–106).

3,4-methylenedioxyamphetamine   (MDA) Mildly hallucinogenic phenethylamine derivative amphetamine called the "love drug." It has been described as producing a "warm glow," increased aesthetic sense, increased spirituality and sense of "oneness," and heightened tactile sensation. It has also been described as producing increased desire for interpersonal contact, increased sense of well-being, increased insight, heightened self-awareness, and diminished anxiety and defensiveness. Besides having a mild amphetamine-like stimulant effect, it induces a feeling of euphoria and although it tends to enhance perception, its hallucinogenic potential is low. Schedule I. See **3,4-methylenedioxymethamphetamine.**

3,4-methylenedioxyethamphetamine   (MDEA, "Eve") Unrestricted N-ethyl-derivative of 3,4-methylenedioxymethamphetamine (MDMA). It has not yet (1989) been classified as a Schedule I drug, even though it has become popular on the streets (Beck J. The public health implications of MDMA use. *In* Peroutka SJ [ed], *Ecstasy: The Clinical, Pharmacological and Neurotoxicological Effects of the Drug MDMA.* Boston: Kluwer Academic Publishers, 1989, pp 77–103). Electroencephalographic studies indicate stimulant, amphetamine-like properties (Gouzoulis E, Steiger A, Ensslin M, et al. Sleep EEG effects of 3,4-methylenedioxyethamphetamine [MDEA; "Eve"] in healthy volunteers. *Biol Psychiatry* 1992;32:1108–1117). It has been reported to induce a toxic psychosis (Gouzoulis E, Borchardt D, Hermle L. A case of toxic psychosis induced by "Eve" [3,4-methylenedioxyethylamphetamine]. *Arch Gen Psychiatry* 1993;50:75). See **entactogen.**

3,4-methylenedioxymethamphetamine   (MDMA, "ecstasy," "MDM," "XTC") Potent, potentially neurotoxic "designer drug" that combines the effects of amphetamines and lysergic acid diethylamide (LSD). In addition to psychomotor stimulant effects, MDMA shares with amphetamines the ability to deplete brain monoamines when given in high doses. Serotonin (5-HT) depletion produced by MDMA may last for months and appears to be due to degeneration of 5-HT axon terminals. It has been advocated as an adjunct to psychotherapy and has become increasingly popular as a recreational drug. Effects are usually euphorigenic; it typically produces a heightened sense of self-awareness and insight and greater feelings of closeness to others. "Ecstasy" is also a trance-like state in which religious ideation and complete surrender occupy almost the entire field of consciousness. These effects are thought to be mediated through the 5-HT neurotransmitter system, because MDMA is a potent releaser of serotonin that also has dopaminergic actions. High doses in animals may be irreversibly toxic to serotonergic neurons: experiments on primates suggest that this can occur at doses comparable with those taken by some drug misusers. Regular users develop tolerance and increase their intake, increasing the likelihood of adverse effects. MDMA misuse has been associated with flashbacks, anxiety, confusion, insomnia, panic, dysphoria, and de novo chronic paranoid psychosis (Creighton FJ, Black DL, Hyde CE. "Ecstasy" psychosis and flashbacks. *Br J Psychiatry* 1991;159:713–715; McGuire P, Fahy T. Chronic paranoid psychosis following use of MDMA ["Ecstasy"]. *Br Med J* 1991;302:697; Mc Guire P, Fahy T. Flashbacks following MDMA. *Br J Psychiatry* 1992;160:276; Peroutka SJ [ed]. *Ecstasy: The Clinical, Pharmacological and Neurotoxicological Effects*. Dordrecht, The Netherlands: Kluwer Academic, 1989; McCann UD, Ricaurte GA. MDMA ["Ecstasy"] and panic disorder: induction by a single dose. *Biol Psychiatry* 1992;32:950–953). A single tablet in a previously physically fit 16-year-old produced visual hallucinations, widely dilated pupils, agitation, hyperthermia (40° C; 104° F), tachycardia (pulse 190), hypotension (80/50 mm Hg), coagulopathy, and death (Chadwick IS, Curry PD, Linsley A, et al. Ecstasy, 3,4-methylenedioxymethamphetamine [MDMA], fatality associated with coagulopathy and hyperthermia. *J R Soc Med* 1991;84:371). Two patients became mute and catatonic for 48 hours after taking MDMA. One developed hyponatremia. One also had a prolonged QTc interval, a cardiac effect not previously reported. It is a risk factor for ventricular tachycardia, ventricular fibrillation, and sudden death that may explain some of the reported deaths with MDMA. Electrocardiographic monitoring is warranted in cases of toxicity (Maxwell DL, Polkey MI, Henry JA. Hyponatraemia and catatonic stupor after taking "ecstasy." *Br Med J* 1993;307:1399). Other reported effects include recurrent acute hepatitis, acute renal failure, convulsions, acute rhabdomyolysis, and spontaneous intracerebral hemorrhage (Shearman JD, Chapman RWG, Satsangi J, et al. Misuse of ecstasy. *Br Med J* 1992;305:309; Screaton GR, Singer M, Cairns HS, et al. Hyperpyrexia and rhabdomyolysis after MDMA ["ecstasy"] abuse. *Lancet* 1992;339:677–678; Campkin NT, Davies UM. Another death from ecstasy. *J R Soc Med* 1992;85:61; Fahal IF, Sallomi DF, Yaqoob M, et al. Acute renal failure after ecstasy. *Br Med J* 1992;305:29; Sawyer J, Stephens WP. Misuse of ecstasy. *Br Med J* 1992;305:310; DeSilva RN, Harries DP.

Misuse of ecstasy. *Br Med J* 1992;305-310). Schedule I. See **entactogen**.

3,4-methylenedioxymethamphetamine (MDMA) + monoamine oxidase inhibitor (MAOI)   Co-administration has been reported to produce a marked hypertensive reaction with diaphoresis, altered mental status, and hypertonicity (Smilkstein MJ, Smolimske SC, Rumack BH. A case of MAO inhibitor/MDMA interaction: agony after ecstasy. *Clin Toxicol* 1987;25:149–159).

3,4-methylenedioxymethamphetamine (MDMA) overdose   MDMA overdose causes manifestations similar to those of severe hyperthermia: muscle rigidity, trismus, sinus tachycardia, sweating, cardiac arrhythmias, cardiac arrest, tachypnea, cyanosis, metabolic acidoses, rhabdomyolysis, myoglobinuria, and disseminated intravascular coagulation. These signs and symptoms can develop several hours after drug ingestion. An incorrect diagnosis of severe hyperthermia will result in a fatal outcome. When the above signs and symptoms develop in a young adult, MDMA intoxication should be suspected and MDMA serum concentrations should be measured promptly (Rittos DB, Rittos D. Complications of "ecstasy" misuse. *Lancet* 1992;340:725–726).

3,4-methylenedioxymethamphetamine (MDMA) + phenelzine   There are two reports of serotonin syndrome associated with combined use (Smilkstein MJ, Smolinske SC, Rumack BH. A case of MAO inhibitor/MDMA interaction: agony after ecstasy. *J Toxicol Clin Toxicol* 1987; 25:149–159; Kaskey GB. Possible interaction between an MAOI and "Ecstasy." *Am J Psychiatry* 1992;149:411–412).

3,4-methylenedioxymethamphetamine/(MDMA) toxicity   Certain features of the serotonin syndrome and the neuroleptic malignant syndrome are similar to the toxic effects of MDMA, causing speculation that toxicity may be due to MDMA's combined effects on the serotonin and dopaminergic systems. The serotonin syndrome has been reported in patients taking a combination of medications (e.g., tryptophan, monoamine oxidase inhibitors, and other antidepressants) that enhance central nervous system serotonin function. The most frequently reported symptoms of this syndrome are mental status changes, restlessness, myoclonus, hyperreflexia, diaphoresis, shivering, and tremor. In some patients, MDMA toxic effects appear to be similar to certain features of the serotonin syndrome (e.g., hyperthermia, tachycardia, disseminated intravascular coagulation, rhabdomyolysis, acute renal failure (Ames D, Wirshing W. Ecstasy, the serotonin syndrome, and neuroleptic malignant syndrome—a possible link.

JAMA 1993;269:869; Friedman R. Ecstasy, the serotonin syndrome, and neuroleptic malignant syndrome—a possible link. *JAMA* 1993; 269:869–870).

3-methylfentanyl (TMF, "China white") Designer opiate and homolog of fentanyl that is approximately 1,000 times as potent as morphine. Fentanyl and its homologs reach peak effectiveness within 4 minutes of intravenous injection and can be recovered from urine 4–72 hours thereafter. TMF overdose resembles that of other narcotics, presenting with loss of consciousness and shallow, infrequent respirations. Other symptoms include decreased heart rate and blood pressure, depressed mental status, coma, hypokalemia, hyperacute T waves, pulmonary edema, seizures, and atrial fibrillation. Like other opiates, TMF may cause death by blocking respiratory drive. Its actions can be blocked by naloxone.

methylfolate Substance used for the enhancement of recovery from psychiatric illnesses in patients who may have a folate deficiency. Its main effect is on mood. Among both depressed and schizophrenic patients, it has significantly improved clinical and social recovery. These findings add to the evidence implicating disturbances of methylation in the nervous system in the biology of some forms of mental illness.

methylphenidate (Ritalin) Piperidine derivative structurally related to amphetamine. It is an indirect dopamine agonist used in the treatment of hyperkinetic children and in attention-deficit disorders in children and adults. It is readily absorbed after oral administration, crosses the blood-brain barrier, and reaches peak plasma levels in about 2 hours. Half-life is 1–2 hours. In attention deficit hyperactivity disorder (ADHD), it improved the percentage of correct responses in reading series; methylphenidate-treated children attempted more reading and math problems than when treated with placebo. Higher doses are advised for boys with ADHD who also have anxiety or depression. Methylphenidate has been reported to have growth-suppressant effects in children. It may potentiate the antidepressant effects of a tricyclic antidepressant (Wharton RN, Perel JM, Dayton PG, Malitz S. A potential use for methylphenidate with tricyclic antidepressants. *Am J Psychiatry* 1976; 127:1619–1625). It can be used as an antidepressant in noncognitively impaired, depressed human immunodeficiency virus (HIV)-infected patients. There are reports of methylphenidate being abused, especially by known drug abusers (Leong G, Shaner A, Silva J. Narcolepsy, paranoid psychosis and analeptic abuse. *Psychia-*

try Journal of the University of Ottawa 1989;14: 481–483). Schedule II; pregnancy risk category C.

methylphenidate + clomipramine Co-administration increases the plasma level of clomipramine (CMI) and risk of CMI toxicity.

methylphenidate + clonidine In children and adolescents with attention deficit hyperactivity disorder whose attentional capacity improved with stimulant treatment, behavioral problems improved with adjunctive clonidine administration (Huessy H, Cohen S, Blair C, Rood P. Clinical explorations in adult minimal brain dysfunction. *In* Bellak L [ed], *Psychiatric Aspects of Minimal Brain Dysfunction in Adults.* New York: Grune & Stratton, 1979; Hunt RD, Minderaa MD, Cohen DJ. Clonidine benefits children with attention deficit hyperactivity: report of a double-blind placebo-crossover therapeutic trial. *J Am Acad Child Adolesc Psychiatry* 1985;24:617–629; Gammon GD. Combined medications for ADD subtypes. Presented at the 1993 Annual Meeting of the American Psychiatric Association, San Francisco, May 25, 1993). Co-administration has been shown to have a greater effect on physical aggression and verbal oppositionality than either medication alone.

methylphenidate + clozapine Methylphenidate (up to 80 mg/day) has been used with therapeutic doses of clozapine (CLOZ) to alleviate CLOZ-induced sedation with no adverse interactions or aggravation of psychosis.

methylphenidate + desipramine In a double-blind, placebo-controlled crossover study, nausea, dry mouth, and tremor occurred in at least twice as many children on combined therapy than on any other treatment regimen. Nausea/vomiting, headaches, other aches, food refusal, and feeling "tired" were significantly more frequent during combined treatment compared with methylphenidate alone or baseline conditions. Significantly higher ventricular heart rate was found on combined therapy compared with baseline conditions or desipramine (DMI) or methylphenidate alone. Side effects during combined therapy appeared to be similar to and no more serious than those associated with DMI alone. No side effects were severe enough to require medication discontinuation during combined treatment. It is possible that more serious side effects did not occur because some subjects never reached the desired DMI level (125–225 ng/mL). Careful monitoring is warranted for children being treated with the combination (Pataki CS, Carlson GA, Kelly KL, et al. Side effects of methylphenidate and desipramine alone and in combination in children. *J Am Acad Child Adolesc Psychiatry* 1993;32:1065–1072).

methylphenidate/elderly   Methylphenidate has been used successfully in treating elderly depressed patients, especially those who are withdrawn and apathetic, or those who have concomitant medical disorders. Starting dose is usually 2.5 mg twice a day, with a gradual increase to 20–40 mg/day, usually given in the morning and at noon. Response generally occurs within 5 days of initiating therapy in patients for whom the drug is effective. Side effects include decreased appetite, anxiety, agitation, and insomnia. There may be a minor increase in blood pressure and sinus tachycardia. Methylphenidate can be used in conjunction with tricyclic antidepressants for refractory cases; in some cases the combination may elevate tricyclic plasma level (Blake LM. Somatic therapies in geriatric psychiatry. *Psychiatric Med* 1991;9:263–273).

methylphenidate + fluoxetine   Addition of methylphenidate (10–40 mg/day) to fluoxetine (FLX) (20–80 mg/day) produced definite and sustained (6 months) antidepressant response in patients refractory to FLX alone (Zajecka JM, Fawcett J. Antidepressant combination and potentiation. *Psychiatric Med* 1991;9:55–75). Some attention deficit disorder patients unresponsive to methylphenidate may benefit from FLX augmentation (Gammon GD, Brown TE. Fluoxetine and methylphenidate in combination for treatment of attention deficit disorder and co-morbid depressive disorder. *J Child Adolesc Psychopharmacol* 1993;3:1–10).

methylphenidate + imipramine   Methylphenidate can raise imipramine plasma level and potentiate its antidepressant effects (Wharton RN, Perel JM, Dayton PG, Malitz S. A potential use for methylphenidate with tricyclic antidepressants. *Am J Psychiatry* 1976;127:1619–1625).

methylphenidate + lithium   Lithium may augment methylphenidate in attention deficit disorder (Gammon GD. Combined medications for ADD subtypes. Presented at the 1993 Annual Meeting of the American Psychiatric Association, San Francisco, May 25, 1993).

methylphenidate + monoamine oxidase inhibitor (MAOI)   Co-administration is safe and effective in treatment-resistant depressions without the drawback of habituation. In some patients, this combination may cause orthostatic hypotension, anxiety, restlessness, agitation or irritability, and hypomania (Feighner JP, Herbstein J, Damlouji N. Combined MAOI, TCA and direct stimulant therapy of treatment resistant depression. *J Clin Psychiatry* 1985;46:206–209).

methylphenidate + morphine   Methylphenidate may potentiate morphine analgesia, but it also antagonizes morphine-associated respiratory depression and sedation (Bruera E, Chadnick S, Brennels C, et al. Methylphenidate associated with narcotics for the treatment of cancer pain. *Cancer Treatment Reports* 1987;71:67–70).

methylphenidate + nadolol   Nadolol (20–40 mg/day) added to the drug regimen of adults with attention deficit hyperactivity disorder responsive to methylphenidate may alleviate persistent feelings of inner tenseness, anxiety, and temper outbursts, resulting in a marked improvement (Ratey JJ, Greenberg MS, Linden KJ. Combination of treatments for attention deficit hyperactivity disorder in adults. *J Nerv Ment Dis* 1991;179:699–701; Gammon GD. Combined medications for ADD subtypes. Presented at the 1993 Annual Meeting of the American Psychiatric Association, San Francisco, May 25, 1993).

methylphenidate + nortriptyline   Methylphenidate can raise the plasma level of nortriptyline and potentiate its antidepressant effects (Wharton RN, Perel JM, Dayton PG, Malitz S. A potential use for methylphenidate with tricyclic antidepressants. *Am J Psychiatry* 1971;127:1619–1625).

methylphenidate SR   (Ritalin-SR) Sustained-release formulation with a longer duration of action. It may be the drug of choice for the treatment of children with attention deficit hyperactivity disorder who require sustained behavioral effects because of after-school social problems or participation in organized recreational activities (Pelham WE, Greenslade KE, Vodde-Hamilton M, et al. Relative efficacy of long-acting stimulants on children with attention-deficit hyperactivity disorder: a comparison of standard methylphenidate, sustained-release methylphenidate, sustained-release dextroamphetamine, and pemoline. *Pediatrics* 1990;86:226–237). Children should not chew the methylphenidate SR tablet, since unpredictably high blood levels and toxic effects can result (Rosse RB, Licamele WL. Slow-release methylphenidate: problems when children chew tablets. *J Clin Psychiatry* 1984;45:525).

methylphenidate test   (MPT) Test in which immediate mood response to a single dose of methylphenidate is used as a guide for differentiating organic and primary mood disturbances. It also has been used to predict relapse in schizophrenia.

methylphenidate + warfarin   Co-administration may increase prothrombin-time (PT) response. It also may decrease metabolism of methylphenidate, resulting in increased methylphenidate plasma levels. When methylphenidate is added to warfarin, PT should be monitored more frequently.

1-methyl-4-phenyl-1,2,3,6-tetrahydropyridine (MPTP) Chemical discovered by chance as a contaminant of illicit drugs. It produces a rapidly progressive parkinsonian syndrome that is clinically and neuropathologically similar to idiopathic Parkinson's disease (PD). This is attributed to the fact that selective destruction of dopaminergic neurons requires the conversion of MPTP to the 1-methyl-4-phenylpyridinium ion (MPP+) by monoamine oxidase within the substantia nigra, and inhibitors of monoamine oxidase block the neurotoxic effect of MPTP. MPTP has been responsible for more research into the etiology of PD (Langston JW, Ballard P, Tetrud JW, et al. Chronic parkinsonism in humans due to a product of meperidine analog. *Science* 1983; 219:979–980; Ballard PA, Tetrud JW, Langston JW. Permanent human parkinsonism due to 1-methyl-4-phenyl-1,2,3,6-tetrahydropyridine (MPTP): seven cases. *Neurology* 1985;35:949–956).

methylprednisolone + carbamazepine See **carbamazepine + methylprednisolone.**

methyltestosterone (Android; Metandren; Oreton Methyl; Testred; Vigorex; Virilon) (MT) 17-Alpha-methyl testosterone derivative anabolic steroid used by athletes and body builders. High doses (240 mg/day) in normal volunteers produce marked irritability and aggressiveness; one subject asked to be placed in seclusion. Motor activity and mood lability increased inconsistently during high-dose treatment. Libido increased during low-dose (40 mg/day) MT administration, but decreased with higher doses. Volunteer studies provide striking but inconsistent evidence of neuropsychiatric changes induced by even brief exposure to MT. Schedule III.

methyltetrahydrofolate (MTHF) Naturally occurring substance involved in synthesis of s-adenosyl-l-methionine (SAMe). It is a major source of methyl groups in the brain. When given in supraphysiological doses (15 mg/day), MTHF enhances antidepressant response in depressed patients with borderline or definite folate deficiency as compared with placebo (Godfrey PSA, Toone BK, Carney MWP, et al. Enhancement of recovery from psychiatric illness by methylfolate. *Lancet* 1990; 336:392–395). In the treatment of depression accompanying senile or organic mental disorders in normal folatemic patients, MTHF was found to be as effective as trazodone (Passeri M, Ventura S, Abate G, et al. Oral 5-methyltetrahydrofolate [MTHF] in depression associated with senile organic mental disorders [OMDs]: a double-blind, multicenter study vs

trazodone [TRZ]. *Eur J Clin Invest* 1991;21:24). In a 6-week trial, MTHF (50 mg/day) was given to 20 elderly patients with a DSM-III-R diagnosis of depressive disorder and a HAM-D-21 score higher than 18. Sixteen patients completed at least 4 weeks of treatment and showed markedly significant improvement in depressive symptoms at endpoint; 81% were considered responders. There were no clinically relevant changes in routine laboratory tests, and no adverse events definitely drug-related were reported (Guaraldi GP, Fava M, Mazzi F, la Greca P. An open trial of methyltetrahydrofolate in elderly depressed patients. *Ann Clin Psychiatry* 1993;5:101–105).

methyprylon (Noludar) Piperidine derivative, nonbarbiturate hypnotic pharmacologically very similar to glutethimide and barbiturates. Half-life is approximately 4 hours. It is effective for at least 7 consecutive nights. Usual adult dosage is one capsule (300 mg) or one or two tablets of 200 mg (200–400 mg). Dosage above 400 mg/day does not significantly increase hypnotic effects. Methyprylon suppresses rapid eye movement (REM) sleep, which rebounds on drug discontinuation. It is cross-tolerant with other sedative hypnotic drugs. Tolerance and physical and psychological dependence can occur with chronic use. Abrupt discontinuation is followed within 24 hours by a withdrawal syndrome manifested by insomnia, confusion, agitation, hallucinations, and convulsions. Acute overdose symptoms are similar to those with barbiturates. Concomitant use with alcohol or other central nervous system (CNS) depressants may produce additive CNS depressant effects. Methyprylon is contraindicated in patients with acute intermittent porphyria. Schedule III; pregnancy risk category B.

methysergide (Sansert) Methylated derivative of lysergic acid diethylamide (LSD) effective for prophylaxis of migraine. It is a nonselective serotonin receptor antagonist that can prevent the rise in serum prolactin that occurs during sleep. It has fallen into disfavor because of complications such as retroperitoneal fibrosis and because safer migraine treatments are available.

metoclopramide (Emperal; Maxolon; Paspertin; Primperan; Reglan) (MCP) Benzamide derivative, non-neuroleptic marketed as an antiemetic. It is presumed to be a selective dopamine (DA) D_2 receptor antagonist. Low doses significantly decrease the number of DA neurons spontaneously active in the DA striatal or A-9 system. Low doses do not have antipsychotic effects, but may cause acute and tardive extrapyramidal reactions. Tardive dyskinesia in elderly patients treated with long-term MCP has been reported (Stewart RB, Cerda JJ, Moore MT, Hale WE. Metoclopramide: analysis of inappropriate long-term use in the elderly. *Ann Pharmacother* 1992;26:977–979). Its superior efficacy in high doses suggests that other receptors are also involved, because occupancy of DA receptors should be maximal at lower doses. Preclinical studies indicate that it blocks serotonin (5-HT$_3$) receptors. Thus, efficacy may be mediated via 5-HT$_3$ receptors, whereas toxicity may be due to interaction with DA receptors. MCP can stimulate prolactin secretion through DA mechanisms. Like neuroleptics, MCP can cause the full range of extrapyramidal reactions. It also has caused neuroleptic malignant syndrome. Dose-limiting adverse effects such as dystonic reactions, akathisia, and diarrhea cause some patients to refuse further treatment, resulting in even more difficult control of nausea and vomiting. These side effects can be circumvented by combining MCP with other antiemetic regimens (Kris MG, Gralla RJ, Tyson LB, et al. Improved control of cisplatin-induced emesis with high dose metoclopramide with combination metoclopramide and dexamethasone and diphenhydramine. Results of consecutive trials in 225 patients. *Cancer* 1985;55:527).

metoclopramide + alcohol Metoclopramide may increase the sedative effects of alcohol (Bateman D, Kahn C, Mashiter K, Davies DS. Pharmacokinetic and concentration-effect studies with IV metoclopramide. *Br J Clin Pharmacol* 1978;6:401–405).

metoclopramide + carbamazepine Co-administration of therapeutic doses may cause acute neurotoxicity (Saudyk R. Carbamazepine and metoclopramide interaction: possible neurotoxicity. *Br Med J* 1984;288:830).

metoclopramide + chlorpromazine Co-administration may evoke very severe extrapyramidal reactions. Fatal acute dystonia has been reported (Schou H, Kongstad LL. Acute dystonia with fatal outcome. A possible adverse drug reaction in the simultaneous administration of chlorpromazine and metoclopramide. *Ugeskr Laeger* 1986;148:2357–2358).

metoclopramide + fluoxetine Co-administration may increase risk of extrapyramidal side effects. This may be caused indirectly by increased plasma level of either drug or more directly by an interactive effect on the extrapyramidal system.

metoclopramide + morphine Metoclopramide increases the rate of absorption of oral morphine and increases its sedative effects (Manara AR, Shelley MP, Quinn K, Park GR. The effect of metoclopramide on the absorption of oral controlled release morphine. *Br J Clin Pharmacol* 1988;25:518–521).

metoclopramide + succinylcholine Co-administration may increase and prolong succinylcholine's neuromuscular blocking effects (Kao YJ, Turner DR. Prolongation of succinylcholine blockade by metoclopramide. *Anesthesiology* 1989;70:905–908).

metoclopramide + zopiclone Co-administration may decrease zopiclone plasma levels (O'Toole DP, Carlisle RJT, Howard PJ, Dunkee JW. Effects of altered gastric motility on the pharmacokinetics of orally administered zopiclone. *Ir J Med Sci* 1986;155:136).

Metopirone See **metyrapone.**

metoprolol (Lopressor) Nonlipophilic, nonselective beta-blocker that has greater peripheral than central activity. When dose selectivity is maintained, metoprolol does not ameliorate neuroleptic-induced akathisia; higher nonselective doses do (more than 200 mg/day). It may produce mild reduction in the intensity of tardive akathisia. It has been used for the treatment of aggression in dementia patients with variable results (Adler LA, Angrist B, Rotrosen J. Metoprolol versus propranolol. *Biol Psychiatry* 1990;27:673–675). Pregnancy risk category C.

metoprolol + fluoxetine Profound lethargy and bradycardia (36 beats/min) occurred in a 54-year-old man 2 days after fluoxetine (FLX) (20 mg/day) was started. He had taken metoprolol (100 mg/day) for 1 month when FLX was added. FLX was discontinued; over the next 5 days, heart rate returned to its previous rate. Metoprolol was withdrawn and replaced with sotalol (160 mg/day). FLX was reintroduced a week later with no recurrence of bradycardia. FLX may have inhibited the oxidative metabolism of metoprolol, leading to higher metoprolol concentrations and symptomatic bradycardia (Walley T, Pirmohamed M, Proudlove C, Maxwell D. Interaction of metoprolol and fluoxetine. *Lancet* 1993;341:967–968).

metoprolol + moclobemide Co-administration may lower blood pressure more than during metoprolol treatment alone. Moclobemide enhancement of the blood-pressure-lowering effect of metoprolol may be beneficial provided blood pressure is not reduced too far and no orthostatic hypotension occurs (Amrein R, Guntert TW, Dingemanse J, et al. Interactions of moclobemide with concomitantly administered medication: evidence from pharmacological and clinical studies. *Psychopharmacology* 1992;106:S24–S31).

metoprolol + phenelzine Sinus bradycardia occurred in two elderly depressed patients when phenelzine was added to their metoprolol therapy. Metoprolol dosage reduction or discontinuation ameliorated the bradycardia (Reggev A, Vollhardt BR. Bradycardia induced by an interaction between phenelzine and beta blockers. *Psychosomatics* 1989;30:106–108).

metrifonate Organophosphorase cholinesterase (CI*e*) inhibitor being considered for the treatment of memory and cognitive impairment of Alzheimer's disease. Duration of inhibition of brain ChE is 4 times longer than physostigmine. Active metabolite is 1-desamino-8-D-argine vasopressin.

metronidazole + lithium See **lithium + metronidazole.**

metyrapone (Metopirone) Inhibitor of endogenous adrenal corticosteroid synthesis marketed in 250-mg tablets used to test hypothalamic-pituitary adrenocorticotropic hormone function. It also inhibits the effects of dexamethasone on both homovanillic acid and 3-methoxy-4-hydroxyphenylglycol plasma levels. There is some evidence that it is involved in the maintenance of major depression and that its suppression may lead to readjustment of the hypothalamic-pituitary-adrenal axis with remission of the depression. It had a significant antidepressant effect compared to placebo (Checkley S, Capstick C, O'Dwyer AM, et al. Neuroendocrine studies of the mechanism of action of antidepressant treatments. *Neuropsychopharmacology* 1993;9:23S). It has been used in treatment-resistant major depression with improvement in some, but not all, patients.

Meval See **diazepam.**

Mevaril See **amitriptyline.**

"Mexican brown" Street name for heroin.

"Mexican tar" Dark, gummy version of relatively high-potency heroin. Also called "tootsie roll."

mianserin (Bolvidon; Bonserin; Lantanon; Norval; Tolvin; Tolvon) (MIA) Tetracyclic, second-generation antidepressant structurally and pharmacologically distinct from tricyclic antidepressants (TCAs). It has little or no effect on norepinephrine and serotonin (5-HT) reuptake in vivo, but has at least moderate affinity for $alpha_2$, $alpha_1$, and postsynaptic 5-HT receptors. It is the most powerful $alpha_2$ adrenoceptor antagonist of all the antidepressants, but has no affinity for beta-adrenergic receptors. It has strong antihistaminic activity and a weak effect on the cholinergic system. Mechanisms underlying its antidepressant activity are unknown, but a prevalent belief is that it enhances noradrenergic transmission by inhibiting the presynaptic $alpha_2$-adrenoceptors that control the release of noradrenaline by negative feedback. Chronic administration produces down-regulation of both the $alpha_2$-adrenoceptors and $5HT_2$, thus suggesting a possible role for serotonin in its antidepressant action. It causes sedation and has a low propensity for anticholinergic side effects. In contrast to TCAs, cardiac side effects after intoxication with MIA are rare, even in patients with cardiovascular disorders. The mortality rate from MIA overdose is much lower than with TCAs. Only very few cases of electroencephalographic changes or rhythm disturbances during MIA treatment have been reported. After excessive doses, however, MIA may induce potentially fatal ventricular arrhythmia, and close monitoring for at least 48 hours is advisable. Marketed in several European countries and Australia, but not the United States.

mianserin + carbamazepine Carbamazepine decreases mianserin serum concentration and may interfere with its therapeutic efficacy. Mianserin dosage may have to be increased and its serum levels carefully monitored (Leinonen E, Lillsunde P, Laukkanen V, Ylitalo P. Effects of carbamazepine on serum antidepressant concentration in psychiatric patients. *J Clin Psychopharmacol* 1991;11:313–318).

mianserin + lithium Co-administration may be useful in refractory depression without severe adverse effects.

microcephaly Abnormal smallness of the head.

"microdot" Street name for lysergic acid diethylamide (LSD).

microenvironment Patient's family.

micrographia Reduction in size of the lettering of writing compared with the person's normal script. It is often a sign of idiopathic or drug-induced parkinsonism (Haase HJ. Extrapyramidal modifications of fine-movements—a "condition sine qua non" of fundamental therapeutic action of neuroleptic drugs. *Rev Can Biol* 1961;20:425–449).

micromania Delusion or conviction that an individual's body, or some part of it, has become abnormally small.

micromolar Very low concentrations in receptor binding assays and blood levels for most psychotropics.

micron One millionth of a meter. Also called "micrometer."

microorganism Microscopic or submicroscopic organism (e.g., bacterium, virus).

microphthalmia Abnormal smallness of the eyes.

microsleep Period lasting up to 30 seconds during which the polysomnogram suddenly shifts from waking characteristics to sleep and external stimuli are not perceived. It is associated with excessive daytime sleepiness and automatic behavior.

microsomal enzyme oxidase system   (MEOS) Hepatic enzyme system involved in the two phases of drug metabolism: (a) detoxification through oxidation, hydroxylation, sulfoxidation, and demethylation; and (b) conjugation of the metabolite so it can be eliminated. Also called "cytochrome P450."

microsomal ethanol oxidizing system   Enzyme complex in the liver that metabolizes alcohol and other compounds.

microsome   Subcellular particle, found in most types of cells, involved in the metabolism of drugs and natural substances.

microtubule   Cytoplasmic element formed in the nucleus of a neuron by a class of fibrous proteins. Microtubules transport material between the nucleus and the end of the axon.

Midamor   See **amiloride**.

midazolam   (Dormicum; Hypnovel; Versed) (MID)   Ultra-short-acting benzodiazepine (BZD). Mean elimination half-life is 2 hours. MID is very lipophilic, has a large volume of distribution (V_2), and is rapidly metabolized; thus, both clearance and distribution contribute to the cessation of its therapeutic effect. Low orally administered doses (7.5–15 mg) are effective for transient insomnia and inducing sleep onset. However, relatively high doses are needed to sustain sleep over the night; the high plasma levels of the early part of the night may unduly depress the central nervous system, resulting in respiratory depression, alteration of sleep architecture, anterograde amnesia, and rebound insomnia on cessation of continued therapy. MID can be administered intramuscularly or intravenously to produce sedation before surgery or diagnostic procedures. It is used in emergency rooms to control acute agitation. It also has been found to reverse catatonia. It has caused acute oral dystonia that was reversed by flumazenil. In 1989, the 26th Expert Committee on Drug Dependence of the World Health Organization (WHO) rated the abuse liability of MID as moderate and the therapeutic usefulness as moderate to high. MID has anxiolytic and amnestic properties similar to those of other BZDs. Schedule IV.

midazolam + amiodarone   A patient treated with erythromycin (4 g daily), amiodarone (1.7 g over 3 days), and an estimated dose of intravenous midazolam (MID) (300 mg over 14 hours) slept for 6 days; flumazenil twice produced brief awakening. Amiodarone, a known enzyme inhibitor, may have increased MID concentration, and there may have been competitive inhibition between MID and erythromycin, the biotransformation of which

is mediated by the same cytochrome P450IIIA (Gascon MP, Dayer P. In vitro forecasting of drugs which may interfere with biotransformation of midazolam. *Eur J Clin Pharmacol* 1991; 41:573–578).

midazolam + erythromycin   Co-administration may markedly elevate peak plasma concentration of midazolam (MID), resulting in profound sedation (Aranko K, Olkkola KT, Hiller A, Saarvinaara L. Clinically important interaction between erythromycin and midazolam. *Br J Clin Pharmacol* 1992;33:217–218). In adult volunteers, erythromycin increased the area under the MID concentration-time curve more than 4 times after oral intake and reduced clearance of intravenous MID by 54%. Oral MID plus erythromycin produced severe, long-lasting hypnotic effects and amnesia lasting several hours. Co-administration should be avoided, or MID dosage should be reduced 50–75% (Olkkola KT, Aranko K, Luurila H, et al. A potentially hazardous interaction between erythromycin and midazolam. *Clin Pharmacol Ther* 1992;53:298–305).

midazolam/hallucinations   Hallucinations and confusion occurred in a woman with no previous psychiatric history who received midazolam (2 mg) intravenously before surgery (Cross JL, Plattenburg PD, Egbunike IG, Jackson DM. Hallucinations and confusion following midazolam administration. ASHP Midyear Clinical Meeting 28:P-426[d]).

midbrain   See **mesencephalon**.

middle insomnia   See **insomnia, middle**.

migraine   Episodic attacks of unilateral, severe headaches with pulsating, throbbing pain; photophobia; nausea; vomiting; sensitivity to sound; seeing shimmering lights, circles, or other shapes or colors; and various prodromata (e.g., numbness of the lips, tongue, fingers, or legs). The syndrome is thought to involve serotonin (5-HT). It is estimated that 8.7 million women and 2.6 million men suffer from migraine headache, with moderate to severe disability, in the United States. Of these, 3.4 million women and 1.1 million men experience one or more attacks per month. Women ages 30–49 from lower-income households are at especially high risk and are more likely than other groups to use emergency care services for their acute condition (Stewart WF, Lipton RB, Celentano DD, Reed ML. Prevalence of migraine headache in the United States. Relation to age, income, race, and other sociodemographic factors. *JAMA* 1992;267:64–69).

milacemide   Type B monoamine oxidase inhibitor that readily crosses the blood-brain barrier and is converted to glycine in the brain. It is being tested in Alzheimer's disease and is believed to have neuroprotective actions in stroke models. It was not effective or well tolerated in schizophrenia. See **nootropic drug.**

milieu In psychiatry, the patient's social setting, the most important of which is the home.

milieu therapy Psychiatric treatment based on the assumption that the total environment is itself a treatment agent and needs to be considered in planning programs and establishing therapeutic regimens (Coons DH. Milieu Therapy. *In* Reichel W [ed], *Topics in Aging and Long Term Care.* Baltimore: Williams & Wilkins, 1981, pp 53–65).

milnacipran Antidepressant that inhibits both noradrenaline and serotonin reuptake. In clinical trials in Europe, it has been well tolerated; therapeutic efficacy has been rated comparable to that of fluvoxamine.

Milroy's disease See **Meige's syndrome.**

Miltown See **meprobamate.**

minaprine (Brantur; Cantor; Isopulsan; Kantor) Aminophenylpyridazine atypical antidepressant that facilitates serotonergic, dopaminergic, and cholinergic transmission. It is reported to be relatively free of anticholinergic effects, cardiotoxicity, drowsiness, and weight gain. It has psychostimulant properties and improves mood in depressed patients with senile or multi-infarct dementia at a dosage of 200 mg/day. It also improves behavioral impairment and some aspects of cognitive function with few side effects (Wheatley D. Minaprine in depression. A controlled trial with amitriptyline. *Br J Psychiatry* 1992;161:113–115). Overdose, however, can be fatal.

Minias See **lormetazepam.**

minimal brain dysfunction (MBD) See **attention-deficit hyperactivity disorder** (preferred term).

minimal effective concentration (MEC) Plasma concentration below which clinical effects are negligible. See **minimal effective plasma concentration.**

minimal effective dose Least amount of a drug needed to obtain the desired therapeutic effect.

minimal effective plasma concentration (C_{min}) Level below which plasma concentrations exert no clinical effects. It may vary with the clinical effect being measured and the method used to measure it. See **minimal effective concentration.**

minor tranquilizer Term introduced after the advent of meprobamate and the early benzodiazepines to distinguish their effects from the barbiturates and the "major tranquilizers" or antipsychotics. See **anxiolytic.**

Minozinan See **levomepromazine.**

miosis Constriction of the pupil of the eye. It is a characteristic symptom of opiate use due to an excitatory action of the opiate on the autonomic segment of the nucleus of the oculomotor nerve that may be due to stimulation of mu receptors. Tolerance to opiate miotic effects develop, but slowly.

mirtazapine (Org 3770) Tetracyclic piperazinoazepine compound structurally and pharmacologically similar to mianserin. It is an antagonist of both alpha$_2$ and serotonin (5-HT)$_2$ and 5-HT$_3$. It is as effective an antidepressant as amitriptyline, with a rapid onset of action (1 week) and a minimum propensity to cause side effects, especially drowsiness (Freeman AM, Stankovic SMI, Bradley RJ, et al. Tritiated platelet imipramine binding and treatment response in depressed outpatients. *Depression* 1993;1:20–23).

misclassification Error in measurement that biases estimates of variables of interest.

misclassification, differential Measurement that can be influenced by disease or exposure status. To minimize misclassification, measurement on which the classification is based must be as accurate as possible. Differential misclassification of disease or exposure may lead to bias in either direction and often to overestimation of the association. To avoid differential misclassification, observers and study participants must be kept as blind to the study hypothesis as possible (Mertens TE. Estimating the effects of misclassification. *Lancet* 1993; 342:418–421).

misclassification, nondifferential Error in categorization of disease that is unrelated to exposure status, or misclassification of exposure unrelated to the individual's disease status. With a dichotomous exposure, nondifferential misclassification underestimates the association. When the exposure has more than two levels, nondifferential misclassification may overestimate or underestimate the association (Mertens TE. Estimating the effects of misclassification. *Lancet* 1993;342:418–421).

misidentification False statement thought to be related to visuospatial impairment and to reflect the presence of agnosia. It is often made by patients with Alzheimer's disease. It may include (a) inability to recognize oneself in the mirror and belief that the reflection is someone else; (b) belief that strangers are living in the house; (c) belief that one's caretaker is someone else; or (d) belief that one needs to "go home" despite the fact that one is home. Misidentifications are significantly associated with hallucinations. See **Capgras syndrome.**

"Miss Emma" Street name for morphine.

"mist"   Street name for phencyclidine (PCP).

misuse   Use of legitimately obtained drugs, in a manner or amount other than prescribed, to produce a certain psychological state. The quality of misuse is not equal to abuse. Misuse covers the use of substances that result in, or may lead to, physical, psychological, and social problems. See **substances, misused.**

mitgehen   Motor sign manifested by a tendency to overly cooperate with passive movements during the motoric part of a physical examination (e.g., "anglepoise lamp" arm raising in response to light pressure). See **paratonia**

mitmachen   Neurologic sign manifested by immediate return to a resting or initial limb position after manipulation by the examiner (e.g., palm turned up by the examiner is returned to its prior pronated position). It is most commonly seen in schizophrenia.

mitochondria   Rod-shaped subcellular particles involved in energy production (e.g., adenosine triphosphate [ATP]) and metabolism.

mitochondrial inheritance   Transmission of a phenotype-producing (disease-causing) mutation of a mitochondrial chromosome.

mitochondrial myopathy   Variant that presents with psychiatric symptoms and/or mental retardation.

mitochondrial receptor   See **benzodiazepine receptor, peripheral type.**

mitogen   Substance foreign to the body that induces lymphocytes to proliferate. Different mitogens stimulate different subpopulations of lymphocytes.

mitosis   Somatic cell division resulting in the formation of two cells, each with the same chromosome complement as the parent cell.

mitten pattern   Electroencephalographic recording that consists of a slow spike-and-wave resembling the thumb and hand portion of a mitten. It is found more often in psychotic than in nonpsychotic patients.

mixed mania   See **mania, dysphoric.**

"MJ"   A street name for marijuana.

MK-212   (6-Chloro-2[1-Piperazinyl]-Pyrazine) Serotonin (5-HT) agonist being tested as an antidepressant. It appears to act mainly by stimulating 5-HT_{1C}, or possibly 5-HT_2, receptors. It significantly elevates temperature in normal controls, but not in unmedicated schizophrenic patients. In the latter, it produces significant increases in nausea, feeling "strange," and arousal, but does not exacerbate psychosis.

MK-458   See **naxagolide.**

MK-801   See **dizocilpine.**

Moban   See **molindone.**

Moclobamine   See **moclobemide.**

moclobemide   (Aurorix; Maclamine; Manerix; Moclobamine) Benzamide derivative that is a short-acting reversible inhibitor of monoamine oxidase type A (RIMA). It appears to act as a prodrug, having active metabolites in vivo that have a greater affinity for monoamine oxidase type A (MAO-A) than the parent compound. It influences turnover of noradrenaline, serotonin (5-HT), and, to a lesser degree, dopamine, at least in higher doses. It is as effective as amitriptyline, imipramine, clomipramine, and desipramine. It is effective in depression associated with anxiety or psychomotor retardation, in neurotic and agitated depression, in first episodes of depression and recurrent and chronic depression, and in young and older patients. When administered to depressed elderly demented patients, it noticeably improves dementia and depression. It has been used to effectively treat depression in Alzheimer's patients, with some improvement in cognitive performance. It has been reported effective in the treatment of panic disorder with or without agoraphobia. It is as effective as phenelzine in the treatment of social phobia. Long-term treatment (up to 5.5 years) has been reported to be safe and effective. The recommended initial dosage is 300 mg daily, usually administered in three divided doses. Dosage range is 300–600 mg/day. Dosing is not affected by age or renal function, but patients with liver impairment may require lower doses. There is generally no need to begin treatment with low doses and gradually increase to the effective dose; the full therapeutic dose can be given from the start, leading to a somewhat earlier onset of action compared to fluoxetine and fluvoxamine. Onset of clinical effect is rapid and readily controlled through dose adjustment. Moclobemide should be taken after meals to minimize any tyramine-related reactions (e.g., headaches). With dosages of up to 600 mg/day, a tyramine-restricted diet is not required with moclobemide (Gieschke R, Schmid-Burgk W, Amrein R. Interaction of moclobemide, a new reversible monoamine oxidase inhibitor with oral tyramine. *J Neural Transm* 1987;26:97–104). In contrast to the nonselective and irreversible monoamine oxidase inhibitors (MAOIs), moclobemide is devoid of hepatic toxicity. Unlike the irreversible MAOIs, it has a half-life of only 2 hours, and MAO activity recovers completely in 24 hours. Since there are no long-lasting carryover effects on stopping treatment, patients can switch from treatment with reversible MAOIs to another antidepressant and vice versa without the need for a drug-free interval. Moclobemide appears to be a well-tolerated antidepressant without the liability of producing significant postural hypotension or impairment of car driving performance. It has not been reported to induce weight gain, edema, and sexual dysfunction. In animals, moclobemide, followed by 5-HT blockers (clomipramine, fluoxetine) showed less pronounced adverse effects than the irreversible MAOI phenelzine. The most frequent adverse reactions to moclobemide in descending order are dry mouth, dizziness, nausea, insomnia, diarrhea, agitation, anxiety, blurred vision, anorexia, irritability, and excitability. The side effect profile of moclobemide has been comparable with that of placebo in double-blind, placebo-controlled trials. Moclobemide is the 'first RIMA antidepressant marketed. Not available in the United States.

moclobemide + alcohol   No clinically relevant interactions have been reported (Priest R. Therapy-resistant depression. *Int Clin Psychopharmacol* 1993;7:201–202).

moclobemide + amitriptyline   Possible interactions were investigated in 21 female inpatients. After 2 weeks' treatment with moclobemide (300 mg/day), amitriptyline (up to 150 mg/day) was given to 7 patients after a treatment-free interval of 0–3 days. In 4 patients, AMI was added to current moclobemide treatment after 2 weeks, and in 10 patients combined moclobemide and AMI therapy was given from the beginning. In all three groups, tolerance was excellent and there were no signs of incompatibility (Amrein R, Guntert TW, Dingemanse J, et al. Interactions of moclobemide with concomitantly administered medication: evidence from pharmacological and clinical studies. *Psychopharmacology* 1992;106:S24–S31). No clinically relevant interactions have been reported (Priest R. Therapy-resistant depression. *Int Clin Psychopharmacol* 1993;7:201–202).

moclobemide + antidiabetic drug   During co-administration with different antidiabetic drugs (glibenclamide, gliclazide, metformin, chlorpropamide), there were no unusual adverse events; neither general tolerance nor fasting blood glucose level showed any evidence of an interaction (Amrein R, Guntert TW, Dingemanse J, et al. Interactions of moclobemide with concomitantly administered medication: evidence from pharmacological and clinical studies. *Psychopharmacology* 1992;106:S24–S31).

moclobemide + antihypertensive   Co-administration did not lead to orthostatic hypotension or increased incidence of other side effects, suggesting that moclobemide can be safely prescribed to patients undergoing antihypertensive therapy (Amrein R, Guntert TW, Dingemanse J, et al. Interactions of moclobemide with concomitantly administered medication: evidence from pharmacological and

clinical studies. *Psychopharmacology* 1992;106: S24–S31).

moclobemide + benzodiazepine   In a meta-analysis, 467 patients received one or several benzodiazepines (BZDs) with moclobemide. Tolerance was rated as very good or good in over 83%, and there was no evidence of any relevant pharmacokinetic or pharmacological interactions (Amrein R, Guntert TW, Dingemanse J, et al. Interactions of moclobemide with concomitantly administered medication: evidence from pharmacological and clinical studies. *Psychopharmacology* 1992;106:S24–S31).

moclobemide/breast milk   Moclobemide is lipophilic and extensively distributed in the body. Although it appears in breast milk, infants receive less than 1% of the maternal dose.

moclobemide + buspirone   Currently (1994) there are no data on co-administration.

moclobemide + carbamazepine   Co-administration in three patients for at least 4 weeks produced no adverse interactions (Amrein R, Guntert TW, Dingemanse J, et al. Interactions of moclobemide with concomitantly administered medication: evidence from pharmacological and clinical studies. *Psychopharmacology* 1992;106:S24–S31).

moclobemide + cimetidine   Cimetidine prolongs elimination half-life of moclobemide, increasing its maximal plasma concentration and area under the curve by about 100%. Moclobemide should be started with a low dose in cimetidine-treated patients and adapted to clinical response. If cimetidine is added to moclobemide, moclobemide dose initially should be reduced by 50% and then adjusted according to clinical need (Amrein R, Guntert TW, Dingemanse J, et al. Interactions of moclobemide with concomitantly administered medication: evidence from pharmacological and clinical studies. *Psychopharmacology* 1992;106:S24–S31).

moclobemide + citalopram   Three cases of fatal serotonin syndrome were reported in patients who took overdoses of moclobemide and citalopram. Death occurred rapidly (3–16 hours) (Neuvonen PJ, Pohjola-Sintonen S, Tacke U, Vuori E. Five fatal cases of serotonin syndrome after moclobemide-citalopram or moclobemide-clomipramine overdoses. *Lancet* 1993; 342:1419).

moclobemide + clomipramine   The serotonin syndrome occurred in a 76-year-old woman switched to moclobemide (300 mg/day) the day after several months of treatment with clomipramine (50 mg/day). After a few days, she recovered fully. She also was taking levodopa-benserazide, bromocriptine, triazolam, diflunisal, dextropropoxyphene, estradiol, and lactulose (Spigest O, Mjorndal T,

Lovheim O. Serotonin syndrome caused by a moclobemide-clomipramine interaction. *Br Med J* 1993;306:248). Fatal serotonin syndrome was reported in two patients who took an overdose of moclobemide and clomipramine (Neuvonen PJ, Pohjola-Sintonen S, Tacke U, Vuori E. Five fatal cases of serotonin syndrome after moclobemide-citalopram or moclobemide-clomipramine overdoses. *Lancet* 1993;342:1419). Data from a patient who overdosed with moclobemide and clomipramine along with 20 mg of flunitrazepam and a bottle of wine suggest a possible interaction with an additive effect that may lead to serious toxicity (Myrenfors PG, Eriksson T, Sandstedt CS, Sjoeberg G. Moclobemide overdose. *J Intern Med* 1993;233:113–115).

moclobemide + cyclic antidepressant   Co-administration seems to be safe if the drugs are gradually initiated together. A direct change can be made from moclobemide to a tricyclic antidepressant or second-generation antidepressant (e.g., maprotiline, mianserin) without an intervening wash-out period (Amrein R, Guntert TW, Dingemanse J, et al. Interactions of moclobemide with concomitantly administered medication: evidence from pharmacological and clinical studies. *Psychopharmacology* 1992;106:S24–S31). See **moclobemide + tricyclic antidepressant.**

moclobemide + desipramine   Co-administration may benefit treatment-resistant depressed patients without causing serious adverse reactions (Priest R. Therapy-resistant depression. *Int Clin Psychopharmacol* 1993;7:201–202). In a pharmacodynamic study involving healthy volunteers, tyramine sensitivity was measured with each drug alone and with combined treatment to determine if tricyclic antidepressants prevent tyramine reactions by inhibiting reuptake of sympathomimetic substances by the adrenergic neuron. Desipramine treatment decreased tyramine reactivity, which was not affected by concomitant administration of moclobemide. Co-administration was well tolerated, with no adverse events (Amrein R, Guntert TW, Dingemanse J, et al. Interactions of moclobemide with concomitantly administered medication: evidence from pharmacological and clinical studies. *Psychopharmacology* 1992;106:S24–S31).

moclobemide + dextromethorphan   Animal data indicate that co-administration may cause a serious adverse interaction (Amrein R, Guntert TW, Dingemanse J, et al. Interactions of moclobemide with concomitantly administered medication: evidence from pharmacological and clinical studies. *Psychopharmacology* 1992;106:S24–S31).

moclobemide + dextropropoxyphene   Animal data indicate that moclobemide may potentiate the effects of dextropropoxyphene and that co-administration should be avoided (Amrein R, Guntert TW, Dingemanse J, et al. Interactions of moclobemide with concomitantly administered medication: evidence from pharmacological and clinical studies. *Psychopharmacology* 1992;106:S24–S31).

moclobemide + digoxin   There is no evidence of interactions (Amrein R, Guntert TW, Dingemanse J, et al. Interactions of moclobemide with concomitantly administered medication: evidence from pharmacological and clinical studies. *Psychopharmacology* 1992;106:S24–S31).

moclobemide + ephedrine   Complete lack of interaction with moclobemide has been demonstrated for directly acting pressor amines (Zimmer R, Gieschke R, Fischbach R, Gasic S. Interaction studies with moclobemide. *Acta Psychiatr Scand* 1990;360[suppl]:84–86). In interaction studies, however, high doses of ephedrine added to steady-state conditions produced by high therapeutic doses of moclobemide resulted in significant potentiation of the cardiovascular effects of ephedrine; adverse events included palpitations and lightheadedness. If patients on moclobemide take low doses of indirectly acting sympathomimetic amines, risk of a hypertensive crisis is low, although high doses or overdoses should be avoided. Under normal circumstances, potentiation of sympathomimetic amine effects is unlikely to be of clinical relevance (Dingemanse J. An update of recent moclobemide interaction data. *Int Clin Psychopharmacol* 1993;7:167–180).

moclobemide + fluoxetine   Adverse events during co-administration are similar to those seen when each drug is given separately (Dingemanse J. An update of recent moclobemide interaction data. *Int Clin Psychopharmacol* 1993;7:167–180).

moclobemide + fluvoxamine   In 25 healthy volunteers, fluvoxamine (FVX) (100 mg) plus moclobemide caused adverse effects similar to those of FVX monotherapy. High FVX doses were not tested, because they are poorly tolerated by healthy volunteers. There was no indication of the serotonin syndrome during combined treatment (Dingemanse J. An update of recent moclobemide interaction data. *Int Clin Psychopharmacol* 1993;7:167–180). See **moclobemide + serotonin uptake inhibitor.**

moclobemide + glibenclamide   In healthy volunteers, co-administration had no effect on glucose and insulin concentrations in serum after oral glucose tolerance tests. C-peptide concentrations were higher after the drug combination, but not significantly different from levels after glibenclamide alone (Amrein R, Guntert TW, Dingemanse J, et al. Interactions of moclobemide with concomitantly administered medication: evidence from pharmacological and clinical studies. *Psychopharmacology* 1992;106:S24–S31).

moclobemide + ibuprofen   In animals, moclobemide potentiated ibuprofen. In healthy volunteers, however, investigation of moclobemide influence on ibuprofen-induced fecal blood loss showed no statistically significant change in the indices of absorption and disposition of ibuprofen, including protein binding (Amrein R, Guntert TW, Dingemanse J, et al. Interactions of moclobemide with concomitantly administered medication: evidence from pharmacological and clinical studies. *Psychopharmacology* 1992;106:S24–S31).

moclobemide + imipramine   Serotonin syndrome was reported in a 39-year-old bipolar patient refractory to phenelzine, trimipramine dothiepin, lithium, and fluoxetine (FLX). A month after FLX discontinuation, moclobemide was started at 300 mg/day and increased 2 weeks later to 600 mg/day. Imipramine (IMI) (50 mg at bedtime) was added and increased gradually over 1 week to 100 mg at bedtime. After 5 days, IMI was increased to 200 mg/day, and moclobemide was reduced to 300 mg/day. Five days later, the patient complained of sweating and feeling hot. She was shivering and became increasingly confused and stiff. At the hospital 2–3 hours later, her Glasgow Coma Scale score was 3/15 and she had rapid breathing, increased salivation, flushed appearance, bilateral extensor spasms in arms and legs, jaw clamped shut, pupils fixed and dilated but eyes roving, and temperature of 39.6° C (103.2° F). No response occurred with intravenously administered benztropine (8 mg), diazepam (15 mg), and phenytoin (500 mg). Computed tomography showed no intracranial hemorrhage. Serum biochemistry was normal except for tricyclic concentration of 1,940 µg/L. She responded within 24 hours to intramuscularly administered chlorpromazine (100 mg every 6 hours), intravenously administered benzpenicillin, and ceftriaxone (Brodribb TR, Downey M, Gilbar PJ. Efficacy and adverse effects of moclobemide. *Lancet* 1994;343:475).

moclobemide + lithium   In 50 patients in whom moclobemide (150–675 mg/day) was added to lithium therapy for 3–52 weeks, there was no evidence of any interaction. A direct pharmacokinetic interaction appears unlikely, because lithium is eliminated by the kidneys and moclobemide is eliminated by hepatic metabolism (Amrein R, Guntert TW, Dingemanse J, et al. Interactions of moclobemide with con-

comitantly administered medication: evidence from pharmacological and clinical studies. *Psychopharmacology* 1992;106:S24–S31). Addition of moclobemide in lithium-refractory depression may enhance therapeutic response.

moclobemide + levodopa/benserazide   Studies in healthy volunteers indicate no contraindications to combination therapy (Dingemanse J. An update of recent moclobemide interaction data. *Int Clin Psychopharmacol* 1993;7:167–180). This is in keeping with the finding that moclobemide only slightly increases brain dopamine concentration (Da Prada M, Zucher G, Wuthrich I, Haefely WE. On tyramine, food, beverages and the reversible MAO inhibitor moclobemide. *J Neural Transm* 1988; 26[suppl]:31–56). Further studies are needed in Parkinson's disease patients, since the central effects of levodopa therapy cannot be investigated easily in healthy volunteers.

moclobemide + meperidine   Although moclobemide acts predominantly as an monoamine oxidase type A (MAO-A) inhibitor and only binds reversibly to the enzyme, animal data indicate that it may potentiate pethidine effects. Co-administration should be avoided (Amrein R, Guntert TW, Dingemanse J, et al. Interactions of moclobemide with concomitantly administered medication: evidence from pharmacological and clinical studies. *Psychopharmacology* 1992;106:S24–S31).

moclobemide + metoprolol   Co-administration may lower blood pressure more than during metoprolol treatment alone. Moclobemide enhancement of the blood-pressure-lowering effect of metoprolol may be beneficial, provided blood pressure is not reduced too far and no orthostatic hypotension occurs (Amrein R, Guntert TW, Dingemanse J, et al. Interactions of moclobemide with concomitantly administered medication: evidence from pharmacological and clinical studies. *Psychopharmacology* 1992;106:S24–S31).

moclobemide + neuroleptic   Moclobemide (150–450 mg/day) has been co-prescribed with one or more neuroleptics in over 110 patients taking low-potency neuroleptics (methotrimeprazine, thioridazine, clozapine, pipamperone, prothipendyl, chlorpromazine, sulpiride, clopenthixol, chlorprothixene, cyamemazine), in 8 taking high-potency neuroleptics (haloperidol, fluspirilene, fluphenazine, penfluridol, bromperidol, flupenthixol), and in 7 taking both low- and high-potency neuroleptics. Tolerability was rated very good or good in 84% and moderate (n = 10) or poor (n = 7) in 16%. Co-administration does not lead to clinically relevant interactions, although some adverse events may occur more frequently because of synergism (Amrein R,

Guntert TW, Dingemanse J, et al. Interactions of moclobemide with concomitantly administered medication: evidence from pharmacological and clinical studies. *Psychopharmacology* 1992;106:S24–S31).

moclobemide + opioid   Data are available on two patients who received moclobemide plus codeine and on one who received moclobemide plus dextropropoxyphene. Moderate agitation occurred as an adverse event in one patient; no other adverse events or changes in vital signs indicating a relevant interaction were recorded. Co-administration should be undertaken with caution until a larger data base is available (Amrein R, Guntert TW, Dingemanse J, et al. Interactions of moclobemide with concomitantly administered medication: evidence from pharmacological and clinical studies. *Psychopharmacology* 1992;106:S24–S31).

moclobemide + oral contraceptive   Co-administration does not appear to interfere with oral contraceptive efficacy (Amrein R, Guntert TW, Dingemanse J, et al. Interactions of moclobemide with concomitantly administered medication: evidence from pharmacological and clinical studies. *Psychopharmacology* 1992;106:S24–S31).

moclobemide + other drugs   Co-administration with the following does not appear to be hazardous: amitriptyline, antipsychotics, benzodiazepines, carbamazepine, chlorpropamide, codeine, desipramine, dextropropoxyphene, digoxin, glibenclamide, gliclazide, hydrochlorothiazide, ibuprofen, lithium, metformin, metoprolol, nifedipine, oral contraceptives, and phenprocoumon (Amrein R, Guntert TW, Dingemanse J, et al. Interactions of moclobemide with concomitantly administered medication: evidence from pharmacological and clinical studies. *Psychopharmacology* 1992;106:S24–S31).

moclobemide overdose   Available data include 24 cases of overdose (3–20 g). The highest ingested dose was 20 g, corresponding to 137 tablets of 150 mg each (the dose amount for 2 months); the patient was discharged after 1 night without any sequelae. No deaths have been reported, and there is no evidence of an increase of the usual toxicity of tricyclic antidepressants or neuroleptics when taken with moclobemide (Amrein R, Hetzel W, Stabl M, Schmid-Burgk, RIMA—a new concept in the treatment of depression with moclobemide. *Int Clin Psychopharmacol* 1993;7:123–132). Overdoses of moclobemide and citalopram or moclobemide and clomipramine have been fatal (Neuvonen PJ, Pohjola-Sintonen S, Tacke U, Vuori E. Five fatal cases of serotonin syndrome after moclobemide-citalopram or

moclobemide-clomipramine overdoses. *Lancet* 1993;342:1419).

moclobemide + selegiline   Co-administration leads to a supra-additive tyramine effect on sensitivity to intravenously administered tyramine. It should only be considered when accompanied by dietary restrictions with respect to tyramine-containing foods. When switching from selegiline to moclobemide, a washout period of about 2 weeks should be sufficient. When switching from moclobemide to selegiline, a washout period of 1–2 days is sufficient (Dingemanse J. An update of recent moclobemide interaction data. *Int Clin Psychopharmacol* 1993;7:167–180).

moclobemide + serotonin uptake inhibitor (SUI) Interaction studies with moclobemide have confirmed its relative safety compared to classic irreversible inhibitors of isoenzymes A and B. Moclobemide does not interact adversely with SUIs, and when switching from an SUI to moclobemide, no wash-out period is necessary. This does not apply to clomipramine, which inhibits both serotonin and noradrenaline reuptake and also exerts activity at central dopamine D_2, histamine H_1, and alpha-adrenergic receptors (Dingemanse J. An update of recent moclobemide interaction data. *Int Clin Psychopharmacol* 1993;7:167–180).

moclobemide + tricyclic antidepressant   Co-administration is associated with minimal risk of adverse drug-drug interactions (Korn A, Eichler HG, Fischbach R, Gasic S. Moclobemide, a new reversible MAO inhibitor—interaction with tyramine and tricyclic antidepressants in healthy volunteers and depressive patients. *Psychopharmacology* 1986;88:153–157; Carl G, Laux G. Moclobemide in long-term treatment of depression. *Psychiatr Prac* 1990; 17:26–29).

moclobemide + tyramine   Co-administration poses minimal risk of adverse drug-drug interactions (Korn A, Da Prada M, Raffesberg W, et al. Tyramine absorption and pressure response after MAO-inhibition with moclobemide. The Second Amine Oxidase Workshop, Uppsala, August 1986. *Pharmacol Toxicol* 1987; 60:30; Gieschke R, Schmid-Burgk W, Amrein R. Interaction of moclobemide, a new reversible monoamine oxidase inhibitor, with oral tyramine. *In* Youdin MBH, Da Prada M, Amrein R [eds], The cheese-effect and new reversible MAO-A inhibitors. *J Neural Transm* 1988;26[suppl]:97–104; Schmid-Burgk W, Gieschke R, Allen SR, Amrein R. Moclobemide, a new reversible monoamine oxidase inhibitor, and tyramine interaction studies. *Curr Ther Res* 1988;42:5; Burkard WP, Bonetti EP, Da Prada M, et al. Pharmacological profile of moclobemide, a short-acting and reversible inhibitor of monoamine oxidase type A. *J Pharmacol Exp Ther* 1989;248:391–399; Simpson GM, Gratz SS. Comparison of the pressor effect on tyramine after treatment with phenelzine and moclobemide in healthy male volunteers. *Clin Pharmacol Ther* 1992;52:286–291).

Modal   See **sulpiride.**

modality   Method or technique of treatment.

modal total daily dose   Most common of the daily doses that are maintained during a patient's participation in a drug trial.

mode   Most frequently occurring value in a set of observations or measurements.

Modecate   See **fluphenazine decanoate.**

model   Statistical statement of the relationship among variables.

model class   Interval that contains the highest frequency of observations.

model-fitting   Statistical technique used in quantitative genetic analysis to test the fit between a genetic model and observed data.

moderate drinking   See **drinking, moderate.**

modifiable risk factor   Symptom that can respond to early intervention.

modification   1. Any change in structure, function, or behavior. 2. Any change in the phenotype due to environmental influences without a corresponding change in the genotypic configuration.

modifier   Factor that appears to modify the effect of other factors, having little or no effect when the main factor is not present.

modifying gene   See **gene, modifying.**

Moditen   See **fluphenazine.**

Moditen Enanthate   See **fluphenazine enanthate.**

Mogadon   See **nitrazepam.**

molar   Large-scale units of analysis.

molecular cloning   See **cloning, molecular.**

molecular diagnostics   Study of DNA or RNA within the context of clinical testing. Applications span a wide range of human disease, including hereditary, neoplastic, and infectious diseases (e.g., cystic fibrosis). Also called "diagnostic molecular biology."

molecular genetics   See **gene cloning.**

molindone   (Lidone; Moban)   Oxygenated indole not structurally related to other known neuroleptics, but with pharmacological properties similar to those of established neuroleptics. Like piperazine phenothiazines, it causes fewer side effects, except extrapyramidal reactions, than piperidine and aliphatic phenothiazine derivatives. Milligram per milligram, it is less potent than trifluoperazine, fluphenazine, haloperidol, and thiothixene; somewhat higher doses of molindone may be required to achieve the same therapeutic response. It has

less effect on seizure threshold than other neuroleptics. Pregnancy risk category C.

molindone + benztropine   A patient receiving both drugs developed difficulty swallowing solids and liquids 1 month after they were begun. Esophageal manometry revealed increased upper esophageal sphincter pressure and a poorly contractile esophagus that reversed 5 days after the medications were stopped (Moss HB, Green H. Neuroleptic-associated dysphagia confirmed by esophageal manometry. *Am J Psychiatry* 1982;139:515–516).

molindone + carbamazepine   Co-administration may enhance the central nervous system depressant effects of carbamazepine (CBZ), lower seizure threshold, and decrease CBZ's anticonvulsant effects. Dosage adjustments may be necessary to control seizures. In some patients, anticholinergic effects may be potentiated, leading to confusion and delirium.

molindone + lithium   Co-administration may produce a pharmacokinetic interaction resulting in a fourfold increase in the half-life of molindone.

Molipaxin   See **trazodone.**

mongolism   See **Down syndrome** (preferred term).

"monkey"   Street name for morphine.

monoamine   Biogenic amine or class of neurotransmitters that includes three catecholamines (dopamine, norepinephrine, and epinephrine), an indoleamine (serotonin), a quaternary amine (acetylcholine), and an ethylamine (histamine).

monoamine hypothesis of depression   Postulation that depression is caused by decreased availability and diminished function of the monoaminergic system and that antidepressants exert therapeutic action by increasing synaptic monoamine availability and neurotransmission. With advances in molecular research strategies, the hypothesis has been modified to focus on the function of specific norepinephrine receptors. Evidence also exists for the serotonin (5-HT) hypofunction hypothesis, which postulates that 5-HT neurotransmission is diminished in depression, possibly as a consequence of hypersensitive postsynaptic 5-HT_2 receptors.

monoamine oxidase   (MAO) Enzyme that catalyzes the oxidative deamination of biogenic and xenobiotic amines (e.g., noradrenaline, adrenaline, dopamine, phenylethylamine, serotonin), the aldehyde products of which are subsequently converted by aldehyde dehydrogenases to pharmacologically inactive acidic derivatives. MAO also regulates the concentration of these amines in the brain and in peripheral tissues. It exists as two isoenzymes. Type A predominantly deaminates serotonin and norepinephrine. Type B deaminates phenylethylamine. Tyramine and dopamine are substrates for both forms of the enzyme. MAO must be at least 80% inhibited to achieve an antidepressant effect.

monoamine oxidase inhibitor (MAOI) Drug that inhibits the enzyme monoamine oxidase, thereby permitting an increase in neurotransmitters such as norepinephrine and serotonin at brain synapses. MAOIs are excellent antidepressants and antipanic drugs. Controlled studies also have shown them effective in the treatment of patients with social phobia, mixed anxiety and depression, bulimia, posttraumatic stress disorder, and borderline personality. Their clinical efficacy is at least equal to that of tricyclic antidepressants for both "atypical" depressions and those meeting standard diagnostic criteria. Uncontrolled studies have shown MAOI efficacy in obsessive-compulsive disorder, trichotillomania, dysmorphophobia, and avoidant personality disorder. MAOIs are generally without anticholinergic, cardiotoxic, or sedative side effects. They are often the drug of choice for atypical depression (hypersomnia and hyperphagia); depression associated with anxiety, agitation, or phobias; patients intolerant of anticholinergic side effects; the elderly; and the medically compromised. Although they lack anticholinergic activity, MAOIs do have autonomic side effects such as dry mouth and bowel and bladder dysfunction, possibly due to an adrenergic-cholinergic imbalance. Previously they were divided into hydrazines (tranylcypromine and pargyline) and nonhydrazines (phenelzine and isocarboxazid). These are known as the older, first-generation MAOIs, which shared two properties: they are nonselective, inhibiting both type A and type B monoamine oxidase; and their actions are relatively long-lasting and irreversible. These MAOIs can interact adversely with certain foodstuffs (mainly those with high tyramine content) and medications including meperidine, sympathomimetic decongestants, and antihistamines (particularly long-acting preparations and those containing sympathomimetics), as well as local anesthetics containing sympathomimetics to cause hypertensive crisis. Interactions due to the peripheral effects of norepinephrine release (the hypertensive crisis) and the central effects of serotonin release (the central excitatory syndrome) are due to the fact that these older MAOIs inhibit both isoenzymes. See **monamine oxidase inhibitor/ "cheese reaction"; reversible inhibitor of monoamine oxidase, type A.**

monoamine oxidase inhibitor (MAOI)/alcohol-free beer For over a quarter of a century, it has been known that ethyl alcohol and MAOIs may potentiate each other's action, because certain alcoholic drinks (e.g., beer, some liquors, fortified wine) contain substantial quantities of tyramine, which can cause hypertensive crises in the presence of MAOIs. In 1984, the first report of an adverse interaction between the MAOI tranylcypromine and non-alcoholic beer was published (Draper R, Sandler M, Walker PL. Clinical crisis: monamine oxidase inhibitors and non-alcoholic beer. *Br Med J* 1984;289:308). The tyramine content of dealcoholized beer is similar to that in regular beer. There have been reports of severe vascular headaches and of an acute generalized headache followed by a right hemiplegia and expressive dysphagia in tranylcypromine-treated patients who drank alcohol-free beer (Murray JA, Walker JP, Doyle JS. Tyramine in alcohol-free beer. *Lancet* 1988;1:1167–1168). Until the free-tyramine content has been measured in the various alcohol-free beers, they should be included in the list of prohibited substances for patients taking an MAOI.

monoamine oxidase inhibitor (MAOI) + amitriptyline Amitriptyline may help protect against tyramine-induced hypertensive reactions associated with MAOI therapy (Pare CMB, Kline N, Hallstrom C, et al. Will amitriptyline prevent the "cheese" reaction of monoamine-oxidase inhibitors? *Lancet* 1982;2: 183–186; Kline NS, Pare M, Hallstrom C, Cooper TB. Amitriptyline protects patients on MAOI from tyramine reactions. *J Clin Psychopharmacol* 1982;2:434–435).

monoamine oxidase inhibitor (MAOI) + amoxapine Co-administration may cause hyperpyrexia, excitability, convulsions, coma, and death.

monoamine oxidase inhibitor (MAOI) + amphetamine The psychostimulant dextroamphetamine combined with an MAOI can be safe and effective in depressed patients. However, concurrent use of amphetamine with an MAOI, including furazolidone, procarbazine, and selegiline, may prolong and intensify amphetamine's cardiac stimulant and vasopressor effects and produce symptoms such as headaches, cardiac arrhythmias, vomiting, and sudden and severe hypertensive and hyperpyretic crises. Recreational drug users, especially those who abuse amphetamines, risk hypertensive crises if they abuse these drugs while being treated with an MAOI or within several weeks of discontinuation of MAOI therapy (Devabhaktuni RV, Jampala VC. Using street drugs while on MAOI therapy. *J Clin*

Psychopharmacol 1987;7:60–61). See **monoamine oxidase inhibitor + dextroamphetamine.**

monoamine oxidase inhibitor (MAOI)/anesthesia
Because of a few case reports published in the 1960s suggesting that long-term MAOI therapy may be associated with seizures, hyperpyrexia, hypertension, hypotension, and prolongation of the effects of narcotics and barbiturates, for many years it was recommended that an MAOI be discontinued 2 weeks before surgery. During the 1980s, however, a number of publications presented data attesting that discontinuation of chronic MAOI therapy prior to surgery and electroconvulsive therapy is unnecessary. These findings have some support from studies in animals. The latest data on this subject should allay the many concerns that have been expressed in the anesthetic and psychiatric literature (Michael I, Serrins M, Shier NQ, Barach PG. Anesthesia for cardiac surgery in patients receiving monoamine oxidase inhibitors. *Anesth Analg* 1984;63:1041–1044; El-Ganzouri AR, Ivankovich AD, Braverman B, Land PC. Should MAOI be discontinued preoperatively? *Anesthesiology* 1983;59:A384; El-Ganzouri AR, Ivankovich AD, Braverman B, McCarthy R. Monoamine oxidase inhibitors: should they be discontinued preoperatively? *Anesth Analg* 1986;64:592–596; Remick RA, Jewesson P, Ford RWJ. Monoamine oxidase inhibitors in general anesthesia: a re-evaluation. *Convul Ther* 1987;3:196–203; Janowski EC, Jonawski DS. What precautions should be taken if a patient on an MAOI is scheduled to undergo anesthesia? *J Clin Psychopharmacol* 1985;5:128–129).

monoamine oxidase inhibitor (MAOI)/breast milk
There are no data on the amounts of MAOIs excreted into breast milk, possibly because these drugs reportedly inhibit lactation. Because of potential toxicity, MAOIs should be avoided during nursing (Buist A, Norman TR, Dennerstein L. Breastfeeding and the use of psychotropic medication: a review. *J Affect Disord* 1990;19:197–206).

monoamine oxidase inhibitor (MAOI) + bromocriptine Bromocriptine may be used safely with monoamine oxidase type A inhibitors. Although their strength is less than that occurring with optimal doses of levodopa, parkinsonian disabilities may improve substantially.

monoamine oxidase inhibitor (MAOI) + bupropion Animal data indicate that the acute toxicity of bupropion (BUP) is enhanced by phenelzine. BUP's manufacturer advises that concurrent administration of BUP and an MAOI is contraindicated. At least 14 days should elapse between MAOI discontinuation and BUP initiation. This recommendation is made not because of any specific known problem, but because of a lack of data (Settle EC Jr. Bupropion: general side effects. *J Clin Psychiatry Monogr* 1993;11:33–39).

monoamine oxidase inhibitor (MAOI) + buspirone Limited clinical experience is restricted to buspirone combined with phenelzine or tranylcypromine. Several patients have been treated safely and effectively; in a few, the combination has produced a slight elevation of blood pressure. At this time there are no data warranting total prohibition of combined use (Gelenberg AJ. Buspirone-MAOI interaction. *Biol Ther Psychiatry Newsl* 1990;13:36).

monoamine oxidase inhibitor (MAOI) + carbamazepine With the exception of isoniazid, MAOIs and carbamazepine (CBZ) may be used together when required to maximize antidepressant effects. Isoniazid has been shown to inhibit the metabolism of CBZ and substantially increase blood levels producing toxicity manifested by disorientation, extreme drowsiness, and aggression. An interval of 14 days is recommended between discontinuation of isoniazid therapy and the start of CBZ therapy, or vice versa (Wright JM, Stokes EF, Sweeney VP. Isoniazid-induced carbamazepine toxicity and vice versa. *N Engl J Med* 1982;18:1325–1327). Several reports suggest that MAOIs do not alter CBZ plasma levels. On the other hand, there is a report that four patients taking phenelzine required a mean daily dose of 450 mg of CBZ (range 300–700 mg/day) to attain CBZ levels of 8.6–10.9 µg/ml. By contrast, five patients taking tranylcypromine required a mean daily dose of CBZ of 1,040 mg (range 800–1,600 mg/daily) to produce CBZ plasma levels of 8.0–11.1 µg/ml. Thus, tranylcypromine patients needed a 2.3 times higher dose of CBZ to reach similar levels (Barklage NE, Jefferson JW, Margolis D. Do monoamine oxidase inhibitors alter carbamazepine blood levels? *J Clin Psychiatry* 1992;53:258).

monoamine oxidase inhibitor (MAOI)/"cheese reaction" Reaction between an irreversible MAOI and foods or drugs containing tyramine. It is manifested by sweating, cardiac palpitations, severe headache, and elevated blood pressure that may result in subarachnoid hemorrhage. It can be treated with intravenously administered phentolamine (5 mg). It does not occur with MAO-B inhibition. The adrenergic neuron solely contains monoamine oxidase type A (MAO-A), the enzyme form responsible for oxidase deamination of noradrenaline and serotonin, the neurotransmitters implicated in the pathogenesis of depressive illness. Although irreversible selective MAO-A inhibitors possess antidepressant activity and down-regulate pre- and post-synaptic alpha- and beta-adrenoreceptors and continue to exhibit the "cheese effect," reversible selective MAO-A inhibitors are less likely to induce it. This can be explained partly by the possible ability of tyramine (a substrate for both MAO forms) to displace the reversible inhibitor from its binding site on the enzyme in the small intestine when ingested and in the adrenergic neuron. There is now sufficient evidence to support this hypothesis as well as the antidepressant property of reversible MAO-A inhibitors that can selectively increase brain noradrenaline and serotonin (Youdim MBH, Fenberg JPM. Monoamine oxidase A and B inhibitors and substrates as antidepressants. *In* Leonard B, Spencer P [eds], *Antidepressants: Thirty Years On.* London: CNS Publishers, 1990). See **phentolamine.**

monoamine oxidase inhibitor (MAOI) + clomipramine Co-administration may induce hyperpyrexia, muscle spasms, convulsions, coma, and death. It should be reserved for highly refractory depression.

monoamine oxidase inhibitor (MAOI) + cocaine Recreational drug use, especially cocaine use, increases risk of hypertensive crises during or within several weeks of discontinuation of MAOI therapy (Devabhaktuni RV, Jampala VC. Using street drugs while on MAOI therapy. *J Clin Psychopharmacol* 1987;7:60–61).

monoamine oxidase inhibitor (MAOI) + codeine Co-administration may increase the pharmacological effects of MAOIs.

monoamine oxidase inhibitor (MAOI) + dextroamphetamine Co-administration is generally considered contraindicated because of the risk of hypertensive crisis or hyperthermia. However, some investigators have suggested that co-administration could be a safe and effective intervention for treatment-resistant depression (Sovner R. Amphetamine and tranylcypromine in treatment-resistant depression. *Biol Psychiatry* 1990;28:1011–1013). Dextroamphetamine (D-AMPH) (5–40 mg/day) has been given to patients partially responsive to an MAOI without significantly serious adverse interactions and with robust therapeutic effects (Fawcett J, Kravitz HM, Zajecka JM, et al. CNS stimulant potentiation of monoamine oxidase inhibitors in treatment-refractory depression. *J Clin Psychopharmacol* 1991;11:127–132). However, since norepinephrine accumulates during MAOI therapy, addition of D-AMPH can liberate large amounts of intraneuronal norepinephrine, resulting in elevations in blood pressure, hyperpyrexia, and headache. Hypertensive emergency with intracerebral hemorrhage may ensue if hypertension is not quickly controlled with an alpha-

adrenergic blocking agent such as phentolamine. In recent years, nifedipine has been shown to be an effective treatment for MAOI-induced hypertensive crisis (Stockley I. Chewing nifedipine to treat MAOI-cheese reaction. *Pharm J* 1991;247:784). See **nifedipine.**

monoamine oxidase inhibitor (MAOI) + dextromethorphan Co-administration can result in agitation, cardiovascular irritability, hyperpyrexia, and death.

monoamine oxidase inhibitor (MAOI)/diet Fear of interactions between MAOIs and food and drink or other drugs has discouraged their use in many patients who might benefit from them. Long, complicated diets and lists of food and drinks to be avoided have served as an obstacle to the ready use of MAOIs. It is likely that some potential dangers have been exaggerated and may be erroneous. Many foods have been restricted on dubious grounds, largely because of excessive anxiety concerning potential hypertensive crises. It is questionable whether liver and canned or freshly cured meats should be restricted. Sour cream and yogurt appear to be perfectly safe. Freshness is extremely important, but as long as foods are purchased from reputable shops, stored properly, and eaten promptly, there should be no real danger of a hypertensive crisis. Serious interactions are unlikely if patients do not eat matured cheese in any form; avoid "Marmite," "Borvil," or any similar meat or yeast extract; take alcoholic drinks in *true* moderation (1–2 drinks/day); avoid broad bean pods and banana skins; eat only *fresh* food (or freshly prepared foods that have been frozen or canned), particularly meat, fish, poultry, game, and offal; do not eat pickled herrings; and avoid any food that has previously produced unpleasant symptoms (Stewart MM. MAOIs and food—fact and fiction. *Adverse Drug Reaction Bull* 1976;58:200–203). Clinicians must determine that necessary restrictions are feasible in any given patient. The risks of adverse reactions with tyramine-containing food must also be balanced against the morbidity and suffering of chronic intractable depressive illness, a condition for which MAOIs may be particularly suitable (Sullivan EA, Shulman KI. Diet and monoamine oxidase inhibitors: a re-examination. *Can J Psychiatry* 1984;29:707–711).

monoamine oxidase inhibitor (MAOI) + diphenhydramine MAOIs prolong diphenhydramine's central depressant and anticholinergic effects.

monoamine oxidase inhibitor (MAOI) + doxepin Co-administration can be safe and effective for treatment-resistant depression (White K, Simpson G. Combined monoamine oxidase inhibitor-tricyclic antidepressant treatment: a reevaluation. *J Clin Psychopharmacol* 1981;1: 264–281).

monoamine oxidase inhibitors (MAOIs) + electroconvulsive therapy (ECT) ECT administration to patients receiving *chronic* MAOI therapy has been safe and effective. Little data are available to indicate whether co-administration enhances ECT's antidepressant effect. Concerns about adverse interactions between ECT anesthesia and an MAOI have prompted many authors to recommend that the MAOI be discontinued up to 2 weeks prior to ECT.

monoamine oxidase inhibitor (MAOI) + fluoxetine Co-administration reportedly helped two treatment-resistant patients (Peterson G. Strategies for fluoxetine-MAOI combination therapy. *J Clin Psychiatry* 1991;52:87). Administration, either together or in close succession, generally should be avoided because of the very high incidence of adverse effects, especially the serotonin syndrome. Because of the long duration of action of norfluoxetine, it has been recommended that an MAOI not be taken for at least 4–5 weeks after fluoxetine (FLX) has been discontinued (Feighner JP, Boyer WF, Tyler DL, Neborsky RJ. Adverse consequences of fluoxetine-MAOI combination therapy. *J Clin Psychiatry* 1990;51:222–225). A longer period may be necessary, however. A serotonin syndrome developed after tranylcypromine was started in a patient who had discontinued FLX for over 5 weeks. Thus, if FLX is discontinued 5 weeks before an MAOI is started, the level of FLX and norfluoxetine should be determined, or the MAOI should be started with caution (Doplan JK, Gorman JM. Detectable levels of fluoxetine metabolites after discontinuation: an unexpected serotonin syndrome. *Am J Psychiatry* 1993;150:837). See **serotonin syndrome.**

monoamine oxidase inhibitor (MAOI) + fluvoxamine Because the serotonin syndrome has occurred with fluoxetine plus an MAOI, a similar reaction could occur with fluvoxamine. Co-administration is not recommended.

monoamine oxidase inhibitor (MAOI) + hydromorphone Therapeutic doses of hydromorphone can cause severe and possibly fatal reactions if given during MAOI administration or within 2 weeks of MAOI discontinuation.

monoamine oxidase inhibitor (MAOI)/hypertensive crisis Sharp rise in systolic blood pressure with diastolic pressure above 120 mm Hg that can be precipitated in MAOI-treated patients who eat food with a high tyramine content or ingest a sympathomimetic drug, a tricyclic antidepressant, or an antihistamine. Within 30–120 minutes, the patient also devel-

ops a throbbing occipital headache that radiates frontally and laterally, accompanied by anxiety, sweating, nausea, and vomiting. Attacks can terminate spontaneously in a few hours or progress to very severe hypertension, chest pain, intracranial bleeding, or death. Lifesaving blood pressure reduction and headache relief may be obtained in minutes with cautious intravenous administration of phentolamine (5 mg). If phentolamine is not available, chlorpromazine (50 mg) can be given intramuscularly. If symptoms persist, phentolamine (0.25–0.5 mg) may be given intravenously 4–6 hours later, or chlorpromazine (25 mg administered intramuscularly) may be repeated within an hour or two of the first injection. Meperidine (pethidine) or similar preparations and parenteral reserpine should not be given. Injudicious treatment can be more hazardous than the hypertensive crisis. MAOI-treated outpatients are sometimes given a 20-mg capsule of nifedipine to use in case of severe headache, but they should be warned of the risk of nifedipine-induced hypotension (Stockley I. Chewing nifedipine to treat the MAOI-cheese reaction. *Pharm J* 1991;247:784). See **monoamine oxidase inhibitor + nifedipine.**

monoamine oxidase inhibitor (MAOI) + levodopa Levodopa (L-dopa) should not be used with nonselective or type A MAOIs because of the potential risk of appreciable rises in blood pressure or severe hypertensive crisis secondary to the release of increased amounts of catecholamine at central nervous system nerve endings or from the adrenals (Hunter KR, Boakes AJ, Lawrence DR, Stern GM. Monoamine oxidase inhibitors and l-dopa. *Br Med J* 1970;3:388). A tetracyclic antidepressant or selegiline (20–30 mg/day) may be an effective strategy for treating depression in Parkinson's disease. A nonselective or type A MAOI should be discontinued for at least 2 weeks before L-dopa is started. Co-administration of L-dopa and selective MAOI-Bs has not given rise to any adverse effects.

monoamine oxidase inhibitor (MAOI) + lithium The antidepressant potentiating effect of lithium in combination with MAOIs was first described in 1971. Available efficacy data indicate that co-administration is a viable option for depressed patients refractory to other antidepressant regimens, although this has not been established by rigorously controlled studies. Lithium has been co-administered with isocarboxazid, tranylcypromine, phenelzine, and clorgyline. There is no contraindication to combined use, but patients should be warned about tyramine-containing foods, diuretics, and salt-free diets. They also should be monitored regularly to detect early signs of hypomania, mania, and extrapyramidal symptoms. Although there does not appear to be substantial risk of any of these reactions, mania has been reported in patients treated with phenelzine plus lithium, and two cases of tardive dyskinesia have been reported after long-term use of lithium and tranylcypromine in patients who had not taken neuroleptics; these isolated instances of adverse reactions may be only idiosyncratic events. Response to lithium augmentation may be quite variable in onset and short-lived, necessitating at least a 3-week trial to reliably determine efficacy.

monoamine oxidase inhibitor (MAOI) + meperidine Co-administration has resulted in serious and potentially life-threatening reactions in some patients. Excitement, muscle rigidity, hyperpyrexia, flushing, sweating, and unconsciousness occur rapidly. Respiratory depression and hypotension may also occur. One MAOI-treated patient died after being given meperidine (Ayd FJ Jr. Drug interactions that matter: meperidine and MAOIs. *Int Drug Ther Newsl* 1991;26:16).

monoamine oxidase inhibitor (MAOI) + 3,4-methylenedioxymethamphetamine Co-administration has been reported to produce a marked hypertensive reaction with diaphoresis, altered mental status, and hypertonicity (Smilkstein MJ, Smolimske SC, Rumack BH. A case of MAO inhibitor/MDMA interaction: agony after ecstasy. *Clin Toxicol* 1987;25:149–159).

monoamine oxidase inhibitor (MAOI) + methylphenidate Co-administration is safe and effective in treatment-resistant depressions without the drawback of habituation. In some patients, this combination may cause orthostatic hypotension, anxiety, restlessness, agitation or irritability, and hypomania (Feighner JP, Herbstein J, Damlouji N. Combined MAOI, TCA and direct stimulant therapy of treatment resistant depression. *J Clin Psychiatry* 1985;46:206–209).

monoamine oxidase inhibitor (MAOI) + morphine MAOIs may exaggerate and prolong morphine's central nervous system depressant effects.

monoamine oxidase inhibitor (MAOI) + nifedipine Nifedipine is an effective treatment for MAOI hypertensive crisis (Clary C, Schweiger E. Treatment of MAO hypertensive crisis with sublingual nifedipine. *J Clin Psychiatry* 1987;48:249–250; Gonzalez-Carmone VM, Ibara-Perez C, Jerjies-Sanchez C. Single-dose sublingual nifedipine as the only treatment in hypertensive urgencies and emergencies. *Angiology* 1991;42:908–913). See **nifedipine.**

monoamine oxidase inhibitor (MAOI) overdose Overdose can result in agitation, delirium, hyperpyrexia, convulsions, and hypertension. Symptoms may take up to 12 hours to develop and may appear similar to some manifestations of neuroleptic malignant syndrome (NMS). Unlike NMS, however, rigidity and creatine kinase elevation do not occur (Guze BH, Baxter LR. Neuroleptic malignant syndrome. *N Engl J Med* 1985;313:163–166; Lazarus A. Neuroleptic malignant syndrome: detection and management. *Psychiatr Ann* 1985; 15:706–712).

monoamine oxidase inhibitor (MAOI) + paroxetine Animal data indicate that co-administration can cause symptoms of the serotonin syndrome. In the only human data available to date (1992), single paroxetine doses (30 mg) increased the maximum plasma concentration of single tranylcypromine doses (20 mg) by 15% in healthy volunteers (data on File, SmithKline Beecham). The manufacturer recommends waiting at least 2 weeks after paroxetine is stopped before an MAOI is initiated.

monoamine oxidase inhibitor (MAOI) + pemoline Clinical trials indicate that co-administration is safe and effective in treatment-resistant depression without the drawback of habituation or any significantly serious adverse interaction (Fawcett J, Kravitz HM, Zajecka JM, et al. CNS stimulant potentiation of monoamine oxidase inhibitors in treatment-refractory depression. *J Clin Psychopharmacol* 1991;11:127–132).

monoamine oxidase inhibitor (MAOI) + pergolide Pergolide may be used safely with inhibitors of MAO type A. Although less effective than optimal doses of levodopa, co-administration may substantially improve parkinsonian disabilities.

monoamine oxidase inhibitor (MAOI)/peripheral neuropathy Complication of long-term therapy that occurs most often in the elderly. It begins with gradual weakness of the legs, paresthesias, and sensations of pain and vibration in the hands and feet; it may result in gait disturbance and falls. It can be detected early by monitoring for its manifestations. Vitamin B_6 can prevent or reduce symptoms.

monoamine oxidase inhibitor (MAOI) + phentermine Co-administration may cause hypertensive crisis.

monoamine oxidase inhibitor (MAOI) platelet inhibition Platelet MAO activity may be decreased in depression and schizophrenia. Phenelzine studies show a fairly good correlation between degree of inhibition of the platelet enzyme and magnitude of antidepressant response. Since the platelet contains the B form of the enzyme, MAOIs that inhibit only the A form of the enzyme (e.g., moclobemide) do not cause platelet MAO inhibition.

monoamine oxidase inhibitor (MAOI) + reserpine Co-administration may result in hyperexcitability, mania, or memory impairment.

monoamine oxidase inhibitor (MAOI), selective MAOI that specifically inhibits either the isoenzyme MAO-A or MAO-B. Clorgyline and moclobemide are inhibitors of MAO-A; selegiline is a relative inhibitor of MAO-B.

monoamine oxidase inhibitor (MAOI)/sleep High MAOI dosages for depression completely obliterate rapid eye movement (REM) sleep for long periods. When the drug is discontinued, there may be marked REM rebound, often associated with vivid dreaming or nightmares for 1–2 weeks.

monoamine oxidase inhibitor (MAOI) + street drug Recreational drug users, especially those who abuse amphetamine or cocaine, risk hypertensive crises if they abuse these drugs while being treated with an MAOI or within several weeks of discontinuing MAOI therapy. Although MAOI-treated patients regularly are told to avoid certain medications and food containing tyramine to prevent hypertensive crisis, they may not be warned about the risks of using street drugs. The risk that a patient who takes an MAOI will also ingest a street drug is likely to increase, especially as more and more young patients are being prescribed MAOIs for depression, anxiety, and panic disorders. For this reason, MAOI prescribers should specifically caution their patients against using street drugs (Devabhaktuni RV, Chowdary Jampala VO. Using street drugs while on MAOI therapy. *J Clin Psychopharmacol* 1987;7:60–61).

monoamine oxidase inhibitor (MAOI) + sumatriptan Co-administration increases sumatriptan effects (Anon. Sumatriptan: a new approach to migraine. *Drug Ther Bull* 1992;30: 85–87).

monoamine oxidase inhibitor (MAOI)/teratogenicity MAOI are known animal teratogens, but human data are too scant to permit valid conclusions.

monoamine oxidase inhibitor (MAOI) + thiazide diuretic Co-administration increases risk and degree of hypotension; this is a potentially significant interaction.

monoamine oxidase inhibitor (MAOI) + trazodone It is not known if interactions occur. If an MAOI is discontinued shortly before trazodone use or is given with trazodone, therapy should be initiated cautiously with gradual dosage increases until optional response is achieved.

monoamine oxidase inhibitor (MAOI) + tricyclic antidepressant (TCA) Since 1966, several thousand patients with mixed depression, anxiety, phobic, and somatic symptoms not relieved by other therapies have been treated successfully with combined TCA-MAOI therapy. Candidates are depressed/anxious patients of good previous personality who, regardless of age, sex, or severity and duration of illness, are not and never have been psychotic; do not have symptoms of a classic endogenous depression; have never had a hypomanic or manic episode; have not responded to or possibly have been made worse by separate, adequate trials of a TCA, MAOI, or electroconvulsive therapy (ECT); refuse or have a physical contraindication to ECT or to very high doses of a TCA or an MAOI; have not benefitted from prophylactic lithium therapy for depression; have considerable overt anxiety not relieved substantially by a benzodiazepine alone or in combination with an MAOI or beta blocker; are not a serious suicidal risk; and are likely to adhere faithfully to dietary and other precautions while taking an MAOI. Most side effects are mild and usually can be relieved by dosage reduction of one or both drugs. Speed of improvement and individual dosage requirements are unpredictable; some patients respond in a few days to low doses, but most require weeks of the usual therapeutic dosages; some may require even higher dosages to achieve benefit. Medications should not be stopped as soon as improvement occurs; they should be continued for some weeks thereafter and then gradually withdrawn. Some patients relapse unless kept on maintenance therapy. Before treatment is started, patients and responsible relatives should receive clear, firm instructions about dietary and other precautions, which should be explicit but not too stringent (Stewart MM. MAOIs and food: fact and fiction. *Adverse Drug Reaction Bull* 1976;58:200–203). Patients and responsible relatives should be told to inform any physician, dentist, or pharmacist whose services may be required that the patient is taking an MAOI to obviate any potential adverse drug-drug interaction. They should receive an explanation of expected and infrequent side effects and what should be done if they occur.

monoamine oxidase inhibitor (MAOI) + tryptophan Co-administration potentiates the antidepressant effect of an MAOI and may induce hypomania. In normal subjects it induces a lysergic acid diethylamide (LSD)-like syndrome and worsens psychotic symptoms among schizophrenic patients (van Praag HM. Serotonergic mechanisms in the pathogenesis of schizophrenia. *In* Lindenmayer JP, Kay SR [eds], *New Biological Vistas on Schizophrenia.* New York: Brunner/Mazel 1992, pp 187–206). It can result in the serotonin syndrome, manifested by myoclonus, hyperreflexia, ataxia, ocular muscle oscillation, and drowsiness. See **serotonin syndrome.**

monoamine oxidase inhibitor (MAOI), type A Drugs include amiflamine, belfoxatone, brofaromine, cimoxatone, clorgyline, FLA-314, FLA-405, and moclobemide. Prolonged inhibition of MAO-A (but not MAO-B) may result in enhanced serotonin neurotransmission. MAO-A' and MAO-B are found in the human brain.

monoamine oxidase inhibitor (MAOI), type B These drugs (e.g., selegiline) have a low propensity to cause the "cheese reaction" and thus may play an increasingly important role in the future management of parkinsonism. MAO-A and MAO-B are found in the human brain. MAO-B is also found in platelets, but there is no connection between platelet and brain MAO-B.

monoamine oxidase inhibitor (MAOI), types A and B Drugs include tranylcypromine, phenelzine, isocarboxazid, nialamide, and pargyline. Each is equally potent at inhibiting both forms of MAO. Their inhibition of the MAO enzyme is irreversible, prolonged, and only relieved with synthesis of new enzyme. Inhibition of MAO-A is important for antidepressant action.

monoamine oxidase inhibitor (MAOI) + warfarin Co-administration may increase prothrombin-time (PT) response. When an MAOI is added to warfarin, PT should be monitored more frequently.

monoamine oxidase, type A (MAO-A) Enzyme found in the lining of the intestines that is relevant to depression through deamination of neurotransmitters. It deaminates serotonin and noradrenaline; dopamine and tyramine are common substrates for MAO-A. See **monoamine oxidase inhibitor, type A.**

monoamine oxidase, type B (MAO-B) Enzyme that acts on phenylethylamine and benzylamine. Dopamine and tyramine are common substrates for MAO-B. See **monoamine oxidase inhibitor, type B.**

monoaminergic compound Any of the biogenic amines widely distributed within the central nervous system (serotonin, norepinephrine, dopamine, epinephrine, acetylcholine).

monogenic trait Major effect from a single gene.

monomer Protein made of a single polypeptide. A protein made of a series of different amino acids is called a polypeptide.

monosodium glutamate (MSG) Analog of glutamic acid commonly used in cooking to enhance flavor. At high concentrations, it can produce neurotoxicity ("Chinese restaurant syndrome").

monosomy Condition in which one chromosome of a pair is missing (e.g., in Turner's syndrome there is a single X chromosome instead of the normal female double X complement).

monosymptomatic hypochondriacal psychosis (MHP) Single hypochondriacal delusion that may be sustained for years. Personality remains well preserved, although way of life may be affected adversely. It can be part of other psychiatric conditions (e.g., schizophrenia, affective disorder). In its pure form, MHP is not as rare as had been thought in the past, and the literature on it is growing. Many subvarieties have been described, but only three are commonly encountered in clinical practice: delusion of skin infestations, delusion of body odor, delusion of physical defect. Differential diagnoses include schizophrenia and obsessive compulsive disorder. Some specialists believe that MHP is particularly responsive to pimozide.

monotherapy Use of a single drug to treat acute symptoms or for maintenance therapy. In most cases it is considered superior to multiple-drug therapy.

monozygotic Derived from the division and autonomous development of a single zygote. Monozygotic twins are genetically identical.

montage Simultaneous display of a number of derivations in an electrophysiological recording.

mood Degree of well-being experienced more or less habitually. It is influenced by affects, which are discrete, strong, transient emotions not synonymous with mood. By way of analogy, *mood* refers to climate and *affect* to the actual weather. Although *mood* can be used to indicate the entire gamut of affects and emotions, this usage creates confusion and should be avoided. See **affect.**

mood, congruent Symptoms and behavior consistent with the patient's expressed or prevailing mood.

mood-congruent psychotic feature Delusion or hallucination consistent with the mood of the individual.

mood disorder See **affective disorder.**

mood-incongruent psychotic feature Delusion or hallucination inconsistent with depressed or manic mood. In the case of depression, content of the delusion or hallucination does not involve themes of personal inadequacy, guilt, disease, death, nihilism, or deserved punishment; in the case of mania, it does not involve themes of inflated worth, power, knowledge, or identity with or special relationship to a deity or a famous person. Examples include persecutory delusions, thought insertion, thought broadcasting, and delusions of being controlled in which content has no apparent relationship to any of the themes listed above (DSM-IV).

mood swing   See **cyclothymia.**

morbidity   Any departure from a state of physiological or psychological well-being. According to the World Health Organization (WHO), it can be measured in terms of three units: persons who are ill, the illnesses these persons experience, and the duration of their illnesses.

morbidity rate   Number of individuals in a defined population who develop a morbid condition over a specified period. See **incidence.**

morbidity risk   Likelihood that an individual will develop a particular disorder between specified ages.

morbid obesity   See **obesity, morbid.**

morbid risk   Individual lifetime risk of having a first episode of illness.

moricizine   (Ethmozine) Class I antiarrhythmic phenothiazine.

moricizine + fluoxetine   No interactions are reported.

"morning missile"   Street name for marijuana.

morphine   (Duramorph) Alkaloid, discovered in 1803, that gives opium its analgesic actions. It remains the standard against which new analgesics are measured. In man, morphine's narcotic action is manifested by analgesia, drowsiness, mood changes, and alterations in cognitive function. Repeated use characteristically produces tolerance and physical dependence. Schedule II.

morphine + amitriptyline   Co-administration increases morphine bioavailability and degree of analgesia. Although a useful interaction, it also may increase morphine toxicity (Ventafridda V, Ripamonti C, DeConno F, et al. Antidepressants increase bioavailability of morphine in cancer patients. *Lancet* 1987;1:1204). Amitriptyline also potentiates opioid-associated respiratory depression and sedation (Hasten PD, Horn JR. *Drug Interactions,* 6th ed. Philadelphia: Lea & Febiger, 1990).

morphine + amoxapine   Amoxapine prolongs and potentiates morphine's analgesic effects, and potentiates morphine-induced respiratory depression (Hasten PD, Horn JR. *Drug Interactions,* 6th ed. Philadelphia: Lea & Febiger, 1990).

morphine + amphetamine   Co-administration is synergistic in producing analgesia and euphoria, but not additive side effects or toxicity. It

produces fewer unwanted adverse effects than morphine alone (Jasinski DR, Preston K. Evaluation of mixtures of morphine and D-amphetamine for subjective and physiological effects. *Drug Alcohol Depend* 1986;17:1–13).

morphine + cimetidine   Oral cimetidine (900 mg/day) and intramuscular morphine (15 mg every 4 hours) produced apnea, confusion, and disorientation that remitted with multiple intravenous doses of naloxone (0.4 mg) (Fine A, Churchill DN. Potentially lethal interaction of cimetidine and morphine. *Can Med Assoc J* 1981;124:1434–1435). Cimetidine (600 mg) also potentiated morphine-induced ventilatory depression in eight healthy volunteers (Lam AB, Clement JL. Effect of cimetidine premedication on morphine-induced ventilatory depression. *Can Anaesth Soc J* 1984;31:36–43). Pharmacokinetics of morphine (10 mg) did not change significantly in a crossover study of seven healthy male volunteers following 4 days' pretreatment with cimetidine (1,200 mg/day) or placebo (Mojaverian P, Fedder IL, Vlasses PH, et al. Cimetidine does not alter morphine disposition in man. *Br J Clin Pharmacol* 1982;14:809–813; Maurer PM, Bartkowski RR. Drug interactions of clinical significance with opioid analgesics. *Drug Safety* 1993;8:30–48).

morphine + clomipramine   Co-administration increases morphine's bioavailability and degree of analgesia. Although the interaction is useful, morphine toxicity also may be increased (Ventafridda V, Ripamonti C, DeConno F, et al. Antidepressants increase bioavailability of morphine in cancer patients. *Lancet* 1987;1:1204).

morphine + desipramine   Co-administration requires caution. Desipramine (DMI) prolongs and potentiates morphine's analgesic and respiratory depression effects. Morphine increases DMI plasma concentration, which should be monitored whenever the combination is prescribed. It is possible that these clinical effects are observed with all opioids (Hasten PD, Horn JR. *Drug Interactions,* 6th ed. Philadelphia: Lea & Febiger, 1990).

morphine + dextroamphetamine   Dextroamphetamine antagonizes morphine-associated respiratory depression and sedation and may potentiate morphine analgesia (Bourke DL, Allan PD, Rosenberg M, et al. Dextroamphetamine with morphine: respiratory effects. *J Clin Pharmacol* 1983;23:65–70).

morphine + fluoxetine   Fluoxetine increases morphine blood level and may result in toxicity.

morphine + hydroxyzine   Hydroxyzine potentiates morphine analgesia and sedation without additional respiratory depression. It may be an advantageous addition to opioid therapy (Zsigmond EK, Flynn K, Shively JG. Effect of hydroxyzine and meperidine on arterial blood gases in healthy human volunteers. *J Clin Pharmacol* 1989;29:85–90; Maurer PM, Bartkowski RR. Drug interactions of clinical significance with opioid analgesics. *Drug Safety* 1993;8:30–48).

morphine + methylphenidate Methylphenidate may potentiate morphine analgesia, but it also antagonizes morphine-associated respiratory depression and sedation (Bruera E, Chadnick S, Brennels C, et al. Methylphenidate associated with narcotics for the treatment of cancer pain. *Cancer Treatment Reports* 1987;71:67–70).

morphine + metoclopramide Metoclopramide increases the rate of absorption of oral morphine and increases its sedative effects (Manara AR, Shelley MP, Quinn K, Park GR. The effect of metoclopramide on the absorption of oral controlled release morphine. *Br J Clin Pharmacol* 1988;25:518–521).

morphine + monoamine oxidase inhibitor (MAOI) MAOIs may exaggerate and prolong morphine's central nervous system depressant effects.

morphine + naloxone Naloxone can antagonize opioid overdose and precipitate opioid withdrawal. In addition, cardiac arrhythmias, severe hypertension, and pulmonary edema have occurred following naloxone administration to antagonize opioid effects. Naloxone use with morphine and other opioids should be restricted to life-threatening circumstances (Maurer PM, Bartkowski RR. Drug interactions of clinical significance with opioid analgesics. *Drug Safety* 1993;8:30–48).

morphine + phenothiazine Co-administration results in additive and prolonged central nervous system depressant effects. Some phenothiazines (e.g., chlorpromazine) can enhance morphine's analgesic effects, an effect that may be valuable in the treatment of severe, chronic pain (Thompson JW. Opioid peptides. *Br Med J* 1984; 288:259–261).

morphine + tricyclic antidepressant (TCA) Tricyclic antidepressants may exaggerate and prolong morphine's central nervous system depressant effects.

"morpho" Street name for morphine.

"mort" Street name for morphine.

mortality rate Number of deaths in a defined population over a specified period divided by the number of people at risk during the period.

mosaic Individual or tissue with at least two cell lines differing in genotype or karyotype, derived from a single zygote.

Motilium See **domperidone.**

motor neuron disease See **amyotrophic lateral sclerosis.**

motor retardation Slowing or lessening of movements and speech, diminished responsiveness to stimuli, and reduced body tone. When extreme, the patient is almost completely immobile and unresponsive to external stimuli.

Motrin See **ibuprofen.**

mourning Normal grief as contrasted with pathological sadness or depression.

movement arousal Body movement associated with an electroencephalograph pattern of arousal or a full awakening.

movement, involuntary Forced or unwilled movement resulting from adventitious contractions of muscles or muscle groups. Most frequent forms are athetosis, chorea, myoclonus, tic, and tremor.

movement time In sleep record scoring, the time when electroencephalography and electro-oculography tracings are obscured for more than half the scoring epoch because of movement. It is only scored when the preceding and subsequent epochs are in sleep (Thorpy MJ. *Handbook of Sleep Disorders.* New York: Marcel Dekker, 1990).

movement tremor See **tremor, movement.**

Moxadil See **amoxapine.**

"muggles" Street name for cannabinoids.

"mule" Street term for a low-level, illicit drug smuggler who swallows cocaine wrapped in a condom, plastic bag, or aluminum foil. Also called "body stuffer."

multiaxial diagnosis Diagnostic approach used in the Diagnostic and Statistical Manual (DSM) published by the American Psychiatric Association. Each axis incorporates various parameters of a clinical condition, including psychiatric and somatic disorders associated with the primary diagnosis, effects of psychosocial stressors, and measures of social functioning. Axis I usually refers to major psychiatric disorders (e.g., psychoses); axis II to personality disorders; and axis III to physical diagnoses.

multicenter trial Study conducted simultaneously or consecutively at several geographically separated centers. Each center has a principal experienced investigator and several trained collaborators. Multicenter trials are often used to achieve adequate numbers of patients or subjects and are used with increasing frequency to evaluate psychoactive drugs. They may avoid the bias of a single investigator, but error variance between centers may be considerable. This can only be avoided by adequate planning, appropriate selection of participating investigators, and joint rater training sessions before and during the trial.

Training sessions should focus on rating symptoms, global clinical judgment of syndrome severity, clinical judgment of improvement, assessment of side effects, and clinical diagnosis.

multicompartmental model   Pharmacokinetic model that takes into account the behavior of a drug in several body compartments or spaces.

multidimensional scaling   Use of more than one dimension of a study within the scaling process.

multidimensional study   Investigation in which findings are based on more than one dimension of the study.

multidisciplinary team   People from different professional disciplines working together as a team to assess, treat, train, rehabilitate, or support patients or clients. The community mental health team is an example.

multifactorial   Determination of a phenotype by genetic and nongenetic inheritance factors.

multifactorial disorder   In genetics, disease that is partly genetic, due to the effects of many genes, and partly environmental in causation.

multifactorial etiology   See **multiple causation.**

multifactorial inheritance   See **inheritance, multifactorial.**

multi-infarct dementia   (MID) Dementia involving multiple ischemic brain lesions without other changes known to cause dementia. It can be divided into cortical and subcortical types based on computed tomography or magnetic resonance imaging findings of multiple small or large infarcts. MID is most often caused by hypertension or extracerebral vascular disease. MID should be considered in those with signs of dementia who also are at high risk for vascular disorders (diabetes, hypertension).

Multipax   See **hydroxyzine.**

multiple abstract   Abstract that has more than one purpose or aspect for its proposal.

multiple abstract multiple allele   See **allele, multiple.**

multiple causation   Concept that a given disease or other outcome may have more than one cause. Also called "multifactorial etiology."

multiple chemical sensitivity syndrome   (MCS) Chronic syndrome characterized by patterns of multiple somatic, cognitive, and affective symptoms with no consistently abnormal findings on routine laboratory testing. It is presumed to be triggered by low levels of common indoor and outdoor environmental chemicals (e.g., pesticides, solvents). Some researchers believe that foods may perpetuate the problem and that chronic exposure in-

duces adaptation and blunted symptoms, whereas removal from exposure followed by re-exposure produces de-adaptation and heightened symptoms. Skeptics suggest that MCS is simply a manifestation of traditional psychiatric disorders, especially depression, anxiety, and somatization disorders, in combination with a misattributed, projective belief in an environmental chemical etiology. Data from large bodies of research in neurotoxicology, occupational medicine, and biological psychiatry suggest that MCS and affective spectrum disorder phenomenology overlap in that both involve limbic pathway dysfunction (Bell IR, Miller CS, Schwartz GE. An olfactory-limbic model of multiple chemical sensitivity syndrome: possible relationships to kindling and affective spectrum disorders. *Biol Psychiatry* 1992;32:218–242; Haller E. Successful management of patients with "multiple chemical sensitivities" on an inpatient psychiatric unit. *J Clin Psychiatry* 1993;54:196–199). See **ecologic illness.**

multiple comparison   Comparison resulting from many statistical tests performed on the same observations. If a set of subjects is divided into more than two groups, comparisons of common measure(s) on those subjects are called multiple comparisons, usually the alpha level adjusted by the number of comparisons.

multiple dependence   See **dependence, multiple.**

multiple-dose study   Investigation in which subjects are randomly assigned to various fixed drug doses, generally with the intention of determining a dose-response relationship. The abscissa x represents a series of doses administered to groups. The ordinate y represents the percentage of each of the groups responding to the doses. Relationship between the doses and the responses is determined by fitting a linear regression line of logit response on a logit dose.

multiple monitored electroconvulsive therapy (ECT)   See **electroconvulsive therapy, multiple monitored.**

multiple personality disorder   Dissociative disorder in which two or more personalities exist independently, with amnestic barriers between them. It can be associated with temporal lobe epilepsy. See **dissociative disorder.**

multiple regression   Method for determining a statistical regression or prediction equation to predict the dependent variable "y" from a set of independent variables, x_1, x_2, etc.

multiple sclerosis   (MS) Chronic inflammatory disease characterized by loss of myelin sheath and gliosis in the central nervous system that typically results in progressive neurological disability beginning in early adulthood. Pathological and immunological evidence indicates that demyelination is secondary to an immune response, and epidemiological evidence suggests that patients were exposed to an infectious agent at a young age. Genetic factors also have been implicated. Although genes conferring susceptibility have not been identified, a promising candidate is an allele at the myelin basic protein locus on chromosome 18 (Tierari PJ, Wikstrom J, Sajantila A, et al. Genetic susceptibility to multiple sclerosis linked to myelin basic protein gene. *Lancet* 1992;340:987–991). In young patients, MS is more common in females. It may run one of two courses: the first is remittent or remittent and progressive, with onset at ages 20–40; the second is relentlessly progressive, with onset at ages 30–35 (Bundey S. Demyelinating disorders. *In* Emery AEH, Rimoin DL [eds], *Principles and Practice of Medical Genetics*, volume 1, 2nd ed. New York: Churchill Livingston, 1990). Psychopathological abnormalities are primarily related to extent of periventricular demyelinization (Reischies FM, Baum K, Nehrig C, Schorner W. Psychopathological symptoms and magnetic resonance imaging findings in multiple sclerosis. *Biol Psychiatry* 1993; 33:676–678). There is no correlation between psychiatric morbidity (especially depression) and magnetic resonance imaging findings (Ron MA, Callanan MM, Warrington EK. Cognitive abnormalities in multiple sclerosis: a psychometric and MRI study. *Psychol Med* 1991; 21:59–68).

multiple sleep latency test (MSLT) Polysomnographic procedure that quantitatively assesses daytime sleepiness. The technique was developed in the mid-1970s at the Stanford University Sleep Research Center in an effort to overcome the lack of sensitivity demonstrated by psychomotor performance testing and subjective questionnaires used to assess the level of daytime sleepiness. The MSLT has been validated in a wide variety of psychopharmacological studies. It determines the time it takes to fall asleep 4–5 times over the course of a single day in a sleep-inducing environment (i.e., without competing stimuli such as noise, excessive light, uncomfortable room temperature). Subjects lie on a bed in a darkened sleep laboratory for 20 minutes at 2-hour intervals and attempt to fall asleep. Sleep onset is recorded polysomnographically; if no sleep occurs after 20 minutes, the test terminates for that interval. In a normal adult control subject, typical sleep latency score is 10–20 minutes (Dement WC: Introduction: clinical considerations. Overview of the efficacy and safety of benzodiazepine hypnotics

using objective methods. *J Clin Psychiatry* 1991; 52:27–30).

multiple somatization disorder (MSD) Disorder included in the new edition of the International Classification of Diseases (ICD-10) that is similar to somatization disorder (SD) in DSM-IV. MSD diagnosis requires the presence for at least 2 years of unexplained somatic symptoms unrelated to organic pathology that do not respond to reassurance. By contrast, SD diagnosis requires onset by age 30 and the presence of at least 13 of 35 specific symptoms. Before a symptom can be considered present in SD, the patient must have consulted a doctor, taken medicine, or changed his or her lifestyle. Evidence for the validity of SD cannot be used to support the validity of MSD (Stern J, Murphy M, Bass C. Attitudes of British psychiatrists to the diagnosis of somatization disorder. A questionnaire survey. *Br J Psychiatry* 1993;162:463–466).

multiple stepwise linear regression Method to chain persistent variables in a linear regression.

multiple stepwise logistic regression model Model in which a multiple regression equation is developed to represent the combined relationship of the set of X variables with the Y variables by adding one variable at a time to the subset until the addition of a variable no longer results in a significant increment in explanatory power. It is similar to a linear model, but applied to dichotomous outcome data.

multiple system atrophy (MSA) Degenerative disease of the central nervous system that produces various combinations of extrapyramidal, pyramidal, cerebellar, and autonomic signs and symptoms. It is characterized pathologically by neuronal degeneration involving the putamen, substantia nigra, pons, cerebellar cortex, and Onuf's nucleus. The distribution of cell loss and absence of Lewy bodies distinguish MSA from idiopathic Parkinson's disease (IPD). The two conditions can be difficult to distinguish clinically; in different series, 5–22% of patients diagnosed as having IPD show the pathological changes of MSA at autopsy (Davie CA, Wenning GK, Barker GJ, et al. MRS to differentiate multiple system atrophy from idiopathic Parkinson's disease. *Lancet* 1993;342:681–682).

multiplex DNA sequencing Technique in which many DNA samples are sequenced simultaneously. It is expected to enhance the search for disease-causing genes (Church GM, Kieffer-Higgins S. Multiple DNA sequencing. *Science* 1988;240:185–188).

multi-state sampling Sampling from a hierarchical structure of a population (e.g., taking a random sample of schools and then a random sample of children from each school).

multivariance analysis design   (MAVA) Study design for discovering relative proportions of environmental versus hereditary determination for personality traits (nature/nurture ratio).

multivariate   Study or analysis involving multiple independent or dependent variables.

multivariate analysis   Analytic statistical method that allows simultaneous study of two or more dependent variables.

multivariate analysis of variance   (MANOVA) Multivariate technique that uses analysis of variance (ANOVA) design, but that includes multiple dependent variables.

"mumm dust"   Street name for phencyclidine (PCP).

mu receptor   One of at least three subtypes of opioid receptors. Mu receptors are found in the corpus striatum, but are not associated with dopaminergic terminals. Mu receptors are the main sites of action of narcotic analgesics. Their selective agonist is DAMGO; their classic agonist is morphine. Naloxone and nalorphine also are antagonists. The analgesic action of morphine results from stimulation of mu receptors at several levels in the central nervous system. Mu_1 subtypes are high-affinity receptors that mediate supraspinal analgesia; mu_2 subtypes are relatively low-affinity receptors involved in respiratory depression, sedation, and bradycardia, and in the gastrointestinal effects of the agonists.

muscarinic   Any postganglionic parasympathetic receptor stimulant. See **muscarinic receptor.**

muscarinic antagonist   Antiparkinson agents, tricyclic antidepressants, and piperidine phenothiazines. They may elevate body temperature through inhibition of cholinergic effects on central thermoregulatory mechanisms or through inhibition of sweating.

muscarinic radioreceptor assay   Assay for anticholinergic substances that has been used to demonstrate a significant inverse relationship between anticholinergic levels and drug-induced extrapyramidal side effects. It also has been used to demonstrate an inverse correlation between serum and anticholinergic levels and performance on a memory task.

muscarinic receptor   Cholinergic receptor with a selective preference for muscarinic drugs. Many psychoactive drugs produce peripheral side effects by antagonizing muscarinic receptors. Muscarinic receptor blockade can produce blurred vision, dry mouth, sinus tachycardia, constipation, and urinary retention, and can affect short-term memory function.

muscarinic receptor subtypes   Five have been identified (M_1, M_2, M_3, M_4 and M_5) according to their differential affinity for pirenzepine. All are present in the brain, but their precise physiological function is unknown. M_1, M_3, and M_5 activate a G protein that activates phospholipase. M_2 and M_4 are linked to another group of G proteins (G_s and G_i) that inhibit adenylate cyclase activity.

muscle tone   Resting muscle potential or resting muscle activity.

Mutabase-2-10   See **perphenazine + amitriptyline.**

Mutabon-A   See **perphenazine + amitriptyline.**

Mutabon Ansiolittico   See **perphenazine + amitriptyline.**

Mutabon Antidepressivo   See **perphenazine + amitriptyline.**

Mutabon-D   See **perphenazine + amitriptyline.**

Mutabon-F   See **perphenazine + amitriptyline.**

Mutabon-M   See **perphenazine + amitriptyline.**

Mutabon Mite   See **perphenazine + amitriptyline.**

mutagenesis   Origin of a particular mutation of a gene or DNA econ.

mutation   Permanent change in genetic material not caused by genetic segregation or recombination. It can be passed on to future generations in the usual way. Cause usually is not known, although certain factors such as radiation are known to increase the mutation rate.

mutation rate   Rate at which mutations occur per gene or generation in a particular population.

mutism   Absence of sound production in a patient capable of phonation without evidence for aphasia or laryngeal or labial dysfunction. It suggests psychosis or severe depression. Mutism accompanied by akinesia suggests the possibility of structural damage within the brain.

mutism, akinetic   State of disturbed consciousness and severe apathy in which the patient is alert, conscious of surroundings, and able to see and hear, but is completely paralyzed and unable to communicate, except through eye blinks. It may be due to a third ventricle tumor, lesions of the thalamic nuclei or cingulate gyrus, occlusion involving the midpontine level of the brain, certain acute brain syndromes, and Guillain-Barré syndrome. It also may be produced as an extreme form of the extrapyramidal effects of potent neuroleptics and can be secondary to central pontine myelinolysis developing as a complication of too rapid correction of hyponatremia. Prognosis is poor, since damage to the central basal pons is permanent and systemic complications may intervene. Amantadine, bromocriptine, or levodopa/carbidopa may have beneficial effects in some patients with or without structural abnormalities. Also called "coma vigil"; "locked-in syndrome"; "pseudocoma."

mutism, elective Childhood condition characterized by persistent refusal to talk in one or more major social situations despite the ability to speak and comprehend spoken language (DSM-IV). The most common manifestation is refusal to speak in school and to adults outside the home, although the child will speak at home to siblings and at least one parent; in a few cases, the reverse may occur. Onset is usually between ages 3 and 8, but onset after age 12 has been reported. Onset is usually insidious, with varying degrees of improvement to no improvement thereafter (Klin A, Volkmar FR. Elective mutism and mental retardation. *J Am Acad Child Adolesc Psychiatry* 1993;32:860–864).

muton In molecular genetics, unit of mutation. It may be as small as one nucleotide pair.

myasthenia Weakness of the muscles and/or fatiguability.

myasthenia gravis Chronic, progressive muscular weakness not accompanied by atrophy. The characteristic symptom is muscular fatiguability that begins in the ocular muscles, producing ptosis and diplopia. It eventually results in a snarling smile, nasal speech, and difficulty in swallowing and articulation. Upper limbs are more affected than the lower. Permanent paralysis of the affected muscles ultimately develops.

mydriasis Dilation of the pupil. It sometimes occurs as an anticholinergic side effect of phenothiazines and tricyclic antidepressants.

Myidone See **primidone.**

myoclonic epilepsy, juvenile See **epilepsy, juvenile myoclonic.**

myoclonic seizure See **seizure, myoclonic.**

myoclonus Sudden, brief, shock-like, repetitive contractions of muscle groups that may be caused by active muscle contraction (positive myoclonus) or inhibition of ongoing muscle activity (negative myoclonus), an example of which is asterixis. Although myoclonus may be seen in the body and face, it occurs most frequently in the limbs. Myoclonic jerks may be irregular or rhythmic and often occur repetitively in the same muscles. In this respect, myoclonus differs from chorea, which is random in time and distribution, but the distinction is not always clear. Myoclonus can be a sign of tardive dyskinesia. Tricyclic antidepressants, lithium, and monoamine oxidase inhibitors may cause myoclonus. There are four main pathophysiological categories. In cortical myoclonus, the abnormal activity originates in the sensorimotor cortex and is transmitted down the spinal cord via the pyramidal tract. Subcortical myoclonus includes forms that arise in structures located between the cerebral cortex and the spinal cord (e.g., reticular reflex myoclonus originates in the brain stem; jerks are generalized and produced by external stimuli). Cortical-subcortical myoclonus is due to abnormal cortical discharge spreading via cortico-reticulo-spinal pathways or a subcortical focus producing its effect via the motor cortex-pyramidal tract. Spinal myoclonus is due to abnormal discharges of spinal neurons; lesions affecting spinal roots, plexi, or nerves may produce myoclonus by inducing abnormal firing of spinal or supraspinal neurons (Obeso JA, Artieda J, Martinez-Lage JM. The physiology of myoclonus in man. *In* Quinn NP, Jenner PG [eds], *Disorders of Movement. Clinical, Pharmacological and Physiological Aspects.* London: Academic Press, 1989). In contrast to other extrapyramidal disorders, some types of myoclonus (e.g., palatal myoclonus) persist during sleep.

myoclonus, intention Highly specific syndrome that occurs after severe hypoxia. It is characterized by myoclonus associated with volitional activity. Preliminary, unconfirmed evidence indicates that 5-hydroxytryptophan may benefit some patients.

myoclonus, neuroleptic-induced Arrhythmic, rapid, shock-like muscle contractions after long-term neuroleptic treatment that occur in about 38% of patients (significantly more often in men). Patients with myoclonus have been treated with significantly higher cumulative neuroleptic doses than have patients without myoclonus. It appears to be an independent side effect, as there is no correlation between myoclonus and parkinsonian side effects or tardive dyskinesia (Fukuzako H, Tominaga H, Izumi K, et al. Postural myoclonus associated with long-term administration of neuroleptics in schizophrenic patients. *Biol Psychiatry* 1990;27:1116–1126).

myoclonus, nocturnal See **periodic movements in sleep.**

Myolin See **orphenadrine.**

myonecrosis See **rhabdomyolysis.**

myotonia Delay in relaxation of muscles after voluntary contraction. It is most evident in muscles of the hand, face, and tongue. Repetitive movements lessen myotonia, and exposure to cold aggravates it. It occurs in a number of genetic conditions.

myristicin Psychoactive substance found in the seed coat and oil of nutmeg. Overuse or abuse can cause visual hallucinations, alterations in time and space perception, and agitation.

Severe poisoning may result in fatal hepatic degeneration.

Mysoline   See **primidone.**

mysophobia   Excessive fear or dread of filth or contamination.

mysticimimetic   See **hallucinogen.**

N

nabilone (Cesamet) Cannabis preparation that is a homolog of dronabinol. It is marketed for the treatment of nausea and vomiting associated with cancer chemotherapy.

N-acetylaspartyl glutamate (NAAG) Dipeptide not concentrated in putative glutamatergic neurons, but co-localized to several aminergic systems and motor neurons. It may play a dual role in mediating glutamatergic neurotransmission and in alternating excessive stimulation of N-methyl-D-aspartate (NMDA) receptors during periods of high glutamatergic neuronal activity (Coyle JT, Puttfarken P, Berger U, et al. N-acetyl glutamate: dual role as synaptic glutamate precursor and NMDA antagonist. *Neuropsychopharmacology* 1993;9:37S–38S). See **N-methyl-D-aspartate (NMDA) receptors.**

nadolol (Corgard) Nonselective, water-soluble beta-blocker with low lipophilicity. It undergoes renal metabolism; half-life is 14–24 hours. Dosage range is 40–240 mg once daily. In patients with renal disease, dosage must be adjusted downward. Placebo-controlled, double-blind studies document that nadolol is useful in the treatment of aggression in chronic psychiatric inpatients. Since it does not penetrate the brain over time and its primary locus of action is peripheral, its efficacy suggests that it may have a role in affecting the central nervous system and the soma in the management of aggression (Ratey JJ, Sorgi P, O'Driscoll GA, et al. Nadolol to treat aggression and psychiatric symptomatology in chronic psychiatric inpatients: a double-blind, placebo-controlled study. *J Clin Psychiatry* 1992; 53:41–46). Nadolol increases plasma neuroleptic levels, which might explain an indirect antiaggressive action via potentiation of neuroleptic action. Pregnancy risk category C. See **beta-blocker/psychiatric uses.**

nadolol/akathisia Nadolol has been reported to exert some control of neuroleptic-induced akathisia (Adler LA, Angrist B, Weinreb H, Rotrosen J. Studies on the time course and efficacy of beta-blockers in neuroleptic-induced akathisia and the akathisia of idiopathic Parkinson's disease. *Psychopharmacol Bull* 1991; 27:107–111; Ratey JJ, Sorgi P, Polakoff S. Nadolol as a treatment for akathisia. *Am J Psychiatry* 1985;142:640–642). A double-blind, placebo-controlled trial in 20 patients treated with 40–80 mg/day, however, did not support the efficacy of nadolol in the treatment of neuroleptic-induced akathisia and did not support the notion of a peripheral site of action for beta-blockers in the treatment of this condition (Wells BG, Cold JA, Marken PA, et al. A placebo-controlled trial of nadolol in the treatment of neuroleptic-induced akathisia. *J Clin Psychiatry* 1991;52:255–260).

nadolol + methylphenidate Nadolol (20–40 mg/day) added to the drug regimen of adults with attention-deficit hyperactivity disorder responsive to methylphenidate may alleviate persistent feelings of inner tenseness, anxiety, and temper outbursts, resulting in a marked improvement (Ratey JJ, Greenberg MS, Linden KJ. Combination of treatments for attention deficit hyperactivity disorder in adults. *J Nerv Ment Dis* 1991;179:699–701; Gammon GD. Combined medications for ADD subtypes. Presented at the 1993 Annual Meeting of the American Psychiatric Association, San Francisco, May 25, 1993).

nadolol + neuroleptic Co-administration increases neuroleptic plasma levels and may enhance a neuroleptic's therapeutic or toxic effects.

nadolol + phenelzine Sinus bradycardia occurred in two elderly depressed patients when phenelzine was added to their nadolol therapy. Nadolol dosage reduction or discontinuation ameliorated the bradycardia (Reggev A, Vollhardt BR. Bradycardia induced by an interaction between phenelzine and beta blockers. *Psychosomatics* 1989;30:106–108).

"nail" Street name for a marijuana cigarette.

nalbuphine (Nubain) Synthetic narcotic agonist/antagonist analgesic of the phenanthrene series. It is chemically related to the narcotic antagonist naloxone and the narcotic analgesic oxymorphone. It is indicated for the relief of moderate to severe pain and as a supplement to anesthesia. It has low abuse potential, but should be prescribed cautiously for individuals with a history of narcotic abuse. Pregnancy risk category C.

nalbuphine + central nervous system (CNS) depressant Phenothiazines and other tranquilizers, sedative-hypnotics, alcohol, and other CNS depressants produce additive effects when co-administered with nalbuphine. If combined therapy is contemplated, dosage of one or both agents should be reduced.

nalmefene Long acting opiate antagonist that blocks kappa, delta, and mu receptors. It has a much longer half-life (8–9 hours) and is approximately 50 times more potent than naloxone. It is active orally and parenterally. Single oral doses of 50 mg block physiological and subjective effects of intravenously administered fentanyl for up to 48 hours. Nalmefene may be useful as an adjunctive treatment to assist detoxified opiate addicts to maintain abstinence. It also may be useful for the treatment of opiate overdose and to reverse opiate-induced respiratory depression or sedation. It may have a role in reducing alcohol consumption and preventing relapse; a placebo-controlled, double-blind trial indicates that it is safe and well tolerated (Mason BJ, Ritvo EC, Salvato F, et al. Nalmefene modification of alcohol dependence: a pilot study. Presented at the 146th Annual Meeting of the American Psychiatric Association, San Francisco, May 1993). Preliminary data support the hypothesis that nalmefene augments response in neuroleptic-stabilized schizophrenia (Rapaport MH, Wolkowitz O, Kelsoe JR, et al. Beneficial effects of nalmefene augmentation in neuroleptic-stabilized schizophrenic patients. *Neuropsychopharmacology* 1993;9:111–115). Side effects include dizziness, lightheadedness, fatigue, and lassitude. Higher doses (100 mg) induce agitation/irritability and muscle tension, which may not be truly dose-related. Nalmefene has no apparent abuse potential (Fudala PF, Hershman SJ, Henningfield JE, et al. Human pharmacology and abuse potential of nalmefene. *Clin Pharmacol Ther* 1991;49:300–306).

nalmefene + fluphenazine Co-administration successfully augmented effects of fluphenazine (mean dose, 28 mg/day) (Rapaport MH, Wolkowitz O, Kelsoe JR, et al. Beneficial effects of nalmefene augmentation in neuroleptic-stabilized schizophrenic patients. *Neuropsychopharmacology* 1993;9:111–115).

nalmefene + neuroleptic Nalmefene augmentation of neuroleptics successfully decreases residual positive symptoms in neuroleptic-stabilized schizophrenia (Rapaport MH, Wolkowitz O, Kelsoe JR, et al. Beneficial effects of nalmefene augmentation in neuroleptic-stabilized schizophrenic patients. *Neuropsychopharmacology* 1993;9:111–115).

nalmefene + thioridazine Nalmefene plus thioridazine (300 mg/day) successfully augmented the effects of thioridazine (Rapaport MH, Wolkowitz O, Kelsoe JR, et al. Beneficial effects of nalmefene augmentation in neuroleptic-stabilized schizophrenic patients. *Neuropsychopharmacology* 1993;9:111–115).

naloxone (Narcan) Specific, short-acting opioid receptor antagonist that has been shown to be anxiogenic. It can block the analgesic effect of placebo, suggesting that release of endogenous opioids may explain some placebo effects. In opioid-dependent persons, small naloxone doses may precipitate moderate to severe withdrawal symptoms, an effect that can be used to diagnose physical dependence on narcotic drugs. The most important use of naloxone is treatment of narcotic overdosage, although its short duration of action (2–4 hours) limits its usefulness for chronic treatment of narcotic addiction. Large doses have been used to produce narcotic blockade for up to 18 hours in addicts involved in day-treatment programs. Using naloxone to treat respiratory depression in opiate overdose may cause serious side effects, including precipitation of withdrawal symptoms, intense pressor responses, tachycardia, and pulmonary edema. Deaths have been reported in patients immediately after receiving naloxone, probably because of release of catecholamines. Animal data indicate that naloxone decreases alcohol drinking (Samson HH, Doyle TF. Oral ethanol self-administration in the rat: effect of naloxone. *Pharmacol Biochem Behav* 1985;22:91–99). Pregnancy risk category B.

naloxone challenge test Test in which naloxone (up to 0.8 mg) is injected subcutaneously to detect opiate abuse. If the person is opiate-dependent, opiate withdrawal signs and symptoms will occur about 3 minutes after the injection. The test should not be attempted when medical risk would be increased by abrupt induction of a state of withdrawal or intoxication (e.g., pregnancy, hypertension, acute medical conditions) (Jacobsen LK, Kosten TR. Naloxone challenge as a biological predictor of treatment outcome in opiate addicts. *Am J Drug Alcohol Abuse* 1989;15:355–366). Nasal administration of naloxone is as effective as the parenteral route. In addition to identifying physically dependent opiate users, naloxone may be useful in emergency medicine and for withdrawal treatment.

naloxone + methadone Naloxone causes methadone withdrawal symptoms that last until the naloxone is metabolized (about 20–30 minutes).

naloxone + morphine Naloxone can antagonize opioid overdose and precipitate opioid withdrawal. In addition, cardiac arrhythmias, severe hypertension, and pulmonary edema have occurred following naloxone administration to antagonize opioid effects. Naloxone use with morphine and other opioids should be restricted to life-threatening circumstances (Maurer PM, Bartkowski RR. Drug interactions of clinical significance with opioid analgesics. *Drug Safety* 1993;8:30–48).

naloxone + neuroleptic Naloxone (100 mg/day) added to neuroleptics for the treatment of negative schizophrenic symptoms produced clinical improvement and improvement in Brief Psychiatric Rating Scale and Clinical

Global Impression Scale scores. No adverse interactions occurred.

naloxone + nifedipine   Co-administration is relatively well tolerated (Fudala PJ, Berkow LC, Fralich JL, Johnson RE. Use of naloxone in the assessment of opiate dependence. *Life Sci* 1991;49:1809–1814; Kanof PD, Handelsman L, Aronson MJ, et al. Clinical characteristics of naloxone-precipitated withdrawal in human opioid-dependent subjects. *J Pharm Exp Ther* 1992;260:355–363).

naloxone/opioid-induced constipation   Orally administered naloxone (0.5–16 mg/day) may ameliorate opioid-induced constipation. To avoid adverse reactions, one must titrate the dosage to a maximum of 12 mg administered at intervals of at least 6 hours (Culpepper-Morgan JA, Inturrisi CE, Portenoy RK, et al. Treatment of opioid-induced constipation with oral naloxone: pilot study. *Clin Pharmacol Ther* 1992;52:90–95).

naltrexone   (Trexan) Long-acting opioid antagonist that binds to opiate receptors more potently than heroin or morphine. It is a structural analog of naloxone that is a competitive antagonist at the mu-opioid receptor. It is capable of remaining in plasma up to 72 hours after a single dose. It is used to maintain abstinence in detoxified opioid addicts in a manner different from that of methadone. Naltrexone is usually initiated after withdrawal is completed to avoid exacerbation or further precipitation of signs of abstinence. Patients maintained on naltrexone will not get high from an injection of heroin because opiate receptors are blocked. Clinical use of naltrexone requires caution to avoid precipitating narcotic withdrawal. It should be reserved for healthy patients who have been free of opiates for at least 5 days. Even at very low doses (1 mg), it will precipitate substantial withdrawal symptoms in patients discontinued from methadone 18 hours earlier; 10–14 days must pass between the last methadone dose and the first naltrexone dose to avoid precipitating withdrawal. To be certain that patients can tolerate naltrexone, they should be challenged with 0.8 mg. If this dose evokes few or no withdrawal symptoms, naltrexone can be started with 10 mg. Over the next 10 days, daily dose is increased to 100 mg for 2–3 days and then raised to 150 mg. The main difficulty with naltrexone is convincing addicts to take it, as it does little for craving and has no reinforcing properties. Successful utilization generally requires highly motivated patients; it is a meaningful alternative to methadone for those whose occupations do not permit them to work while in a methadone maintenance program. It has been found to be most effective for those who enter treatment with good jobs to protect, career and family supports, and histories of adequate or above-adequate functioning. Naltrexone treatment linked with probation is effective in reducing crime related to heroin (Tilly J, Cornish J, Metzger DS, et al. Naltrexone and the treatment of federal probationers. *NIDA Res Monogr* 1991;199:458). Naltrexone has few side effects (relatively mild gastrointestinal distress, anxiety, and insomnia that subsides in a few days). Since it is free of agonistic properties, there are no withdrawal symptoms on abrupt discontinuation. It may be a safe and effective adjunct to treatment in alcohol-dependent subjects, particularly in preventing alcohol relapse (Volpicelli JR, Davis MA, Olgin JE. Naltrexone blocks the post-shock increase of ethanol consumption. *Life Sci* 1986;30:841–847; Volpicelli JR, Alterman AI, Hayashida M, et al. Naltrexone in the treatment of alcohol dependence. *Arch Gen Psychiatry* 1992;49:876–880; O'Malley SS, Jaffee AJ, Chang G et al. Naltrexone and coping skills therapy for alcohol dependence. *Arch Gen Psychiatry* 1992;49:881–887). In alcohol-dependent patients, the most frequent side effects are nausea, weight loss, and dizziness. Pregnancy risk category C.

naltrexone + clonidine   Co-administration in opioid-dependent patients shortens the opioid withdrawal syndrome significantly without substantially increasing patient discomfort (Kleber HD, Topazian M, Gaspari J, et al. Clonidine and naltrexone in outpatient treatment of heroin withdrawal. *Am J Drug Alcohol Abuse* 1987;13:1–17). The combination can reduce methadone detoxification to 3–5 days.

naltrexone + clonidine + diazepam   Co-administration has been shown to significantly reduce average opioid withdrawal time from 3.3 to 2.3 days, despite lower clonidine dosage and significantly lower diazepam dosage on the second day.

naltrexone + fluoxetine   In open trials, fluoxetine (FLX) has been effective as an "anti-craving" drug in heroin patients on naltrexone (Maremmani I, Castrogiovanni P, Daini L, Zolesi O. Use of fluoxetine in heroin addiction. *Br J Psychiatry* 1992;160:570–571). Co-administration also was used to treat a 9-year-old boy with Prader-Willi syndrome manifested by compulsive eating, severe skin picking, mild mental retardation, and behavioral problems who had been refractory to various pharmacotherapies, including FLX (60 mg/day) for a year. Naltrexone (12.5–50 mg/day) was added to FLX, and the patient was placed on a strict behavioral program, a 900 kcal American Diabetic Association (ADA) diet, wound care, and treatment with bactroban. At 9-month follow-up, there was continued improvement in behavior and social interactions, decreased self-mutilation, continued weight control, and continued academic progress in school (Benjamin E, Buot-Smith T. Naltrexone and fluoxetine in Prader-Willi syndrome. *J Am Acad Child Adolesc Psychiatry* 1993; 32:870–873).

naltrexone + nifedipine   Co-administration may precipitate delirium (Silverstone PH, Attenburrow MJ, Robson P. The calcium channel antagonist nifedipine causes confusion when used to treat opiate withdrawal in morphine-dependent patients. *Int Clin Psychopharmacol* 1992;7:87–90).

Nandrobolic   See **nandrolone phenpropionate.**

Nandrobolic LA   See **nandrolone decanoate.**

nandrolone decanoate   (Anabolin LA 100; Androlone D 100; Deca-Durabolin; Decolone; Hybolin Decanoate; Nandrobolic LA; Neo-Durabolic) 19-Nortestosterone ester derivative anabolic steroid. It is a long-acting preparation that should be injected deeply into the gluteal muscle. Schedule III; pregnancy risk category X.

nandrolone phenpropionate   (Anabolin IM; Androlone; Durabolin; Hybolin Improved; Nandrobolic) 19-Nortestosterone ester derivative anabolic steroid. It is a long-acting preparation that should be injected deeply into the gluteal muscle. Schedule III; pregnancy risk category X.

nanogram   (ng) One billionth (10^{-9}) of a gram.

nanometer   (nm) One billionth (10^{-9}) of a mole, expressed as concentration. Preferred term for "millimicron."

nanomolar 10^{-9} molar concentration.

nap   Short period of sleep taken intentionally or unintentionally during the period of habitual wakefulness. It may be a symptom of narcolepsy.

Naprosyn   See **naproxen.**

naproxen   (Anaprox; Naprosyn) Orally or rectally administered nonsteroidal anti-inflammatory drug with analgesic and antipyretic properties. It inhibits prostaglandin synthesis. Pregnancy risk category B.

naproxen + lithium   See **lithium + naproxen.**

NARANON   Twelve-step self-help group for co-dependents and adult children in recovery.

Narcan   See **naloxone.**

narcoanalysis   See **narcotherapy.**

narcocatharsis   See **narcotherapy.**

narcolepsy   Rare, disabling sleep disorder of unknown origin characterized by sudden attacks of flaccid paralysis (cataplexy), excessive daytime sleepiness, sleep paralysis, hypnagogic hallucinations, and the appearance of rapid eye movement (REM) sleep within 10 minutes of sleep onset (sleep-onset REM, or "SOREM")

(Dahlitz M, Parkes JD. Sleep paralysis. *Lancet* 1993;341:406–407; ASDA—American Sleep Disorder Association. *In* Thorpy MJ [ed], *International Classification of Sleep Disorders, Diagnostic and Coding Manual.* Lawrence, KS: Allen Press, 1990). Narcolepsy symptoms also include REM-sleep intrusion hallucinations during the day. Some patients may be so hallucinated that they become delusional and are diagnosed as schizophrenic (Douglass AB, Shipley JE, Haines RF, et al. Schizophrenia, narcolepsy, and HLA-DR15, DQ6. *Biol Psychiatry* 1993;34:773–780). Motor dyscontrol during sleep is common in narcolepsy. It takes the form of periodic limb movements during non-REM and REM sleep and persistence of electromyographic (EMG) tone throughout REM sleep and/or excessive, aperiodic EMG twitching during REM sleep. REM sleep behavior disorder also can be associated with narcolepsy (Schenck CH, Mahowold MW. Motor dyscontrol in narcolepsy: rapid-eye-movement [REM] sleep without atonia and REM sleep behavior disorder. *Ann Neurol* 1992;32:3–10). The prevalence of narcolepsy in the United States is 1:5,000. In Japan, it is 1:600. It occurs equally in men and women, most often by age 30, and shows marked familial incidence. Diagnosis excludes other hypersomnia disorders (e.g., sleep apnea syndrome, nocturnal myoclonus, depression, drug and alcohol abuse, idiopathic central nervous system hypersomnolence). Treatment with stimulants such as pemoline, methylphenidate, and dextroamphetamine has been successful; tricyclic antidepressants or, in some cases, monoamine oxidase inhibitors also have been useful. Also called "sleep seizure." See **cataplexy; REM sleep behavior disorder; sleep paralysis.**

narcomania   Seldom-used term that in the late 19th and early 20th centuries was used to indicate abuse of narcotics or anesthetics (often ether or chloroform) (McBridge CA. *The Modern Treatment of Alcoholism and Drug Narcotism.* London: Rebman, 1910, pp 299–324).

narcosis   Generalized, nonspecific, reversible central nervous system depression produced by any of a number of sedative/narcotic agents.

narcosuggestion   See **narcotherapy.**

narcosynthesis   See **narcotherapy.**

narcotherapy   Form of psychotherapy in which a slow intravenous injection of amobarbital (Amytal) or sodium pentothal is given to induce a state of complete relaxation to allow subjects to express themselves freely. It was used extensively for "war neuroses" during World War II. It also is used to attempt to extract confessions from criminals ("truth serum"). Also called "Amytal interview";

"narcoanalysis"; "narcocatharsis"; "narcosug-gestion"; "narcosynthesis"; "pentothal inter-view."

narcotic   Drug derived from opium or opium-like substances that has a potent analgesic effect; may affect mood and behavior; and may produce dependence, tolerance, and ab-stinence symptoms after abrupt discontinua-tion. Cocaine is not a narcotic, although some legal definitions incorrectly define it as such. The greatest liability of narcotics is abuse potential.

narcotic agonist   Agent structurally similar to opiates that probably occupies the same recep-tor sites in the central nervous system. In sufficient doses, it blocks the effects of opiates by competing for their receptor sites. If given to an opiate-dependent person, it precipitates an acute abstinence syndrome.

narcotic analgesic   Agent that acts on endog-enous opioid receptors to produce naloxone-reversible analgesia.

narcotic analgesic + neuroleptic   Co-administra-tion may increase blood level and enhance the toxic effects of narcotic analgesics.

narcotic blockade   **1.** Inhibition of the eu-phoric effects of opioids (e.g., heroin) by drugs such as methadone. **2.** Inhibition of all opiate actions at their respective receptors; antagonism of receptor actions of these types of drugs.

Narcotics Anonymous   (NA) Twelve-step, self-help group that may be useful as a primary or adjunctive treatment modality for opioid de-pendence. Like Alcoholics Anonymous (AA), it stresses total abstinence. In 1982, there were 2,000 active groups in 50 U.S. states; in 1990, there were an estimated 14,000 groups in the United States and 2,000 groups in 50 other countries. Crack cocaine (CA) dependence accounts for the majority of drug abusers at NA meetings (even though CA is not a nar-cotic). See **narcotic.**

narcotic treatment regulations   In the United States, there are standards for narcotic addic-tion treatment and rules governing treatment program organization and structure, approval requirements, minimum standards for patient evaluation and admission, minimum medical and rehabilitative support services, and pro-gram sanctions. Drugs used in treatment (e.g., methadone) may be dispensed only by nar-cotic treatment programs approved by the U.S. Food and Drug Administration (FDA), Drug Enforcement Administration (DEA), and the designated state methadone author-ity.

Nardelcine   See **phenelzine.**

Nardil   See **phenelzine.**

Narphen   See **phenazocine.**

nasopharyngeal electroencephalogram   Electro-encephalographic (EEG) technique in which specialized recording electrodes placed in the nasopharynx reflect activity from the mesial and basal portions of the temporal lobe. It is used to discover underlying temporal lobe seizures that otherwise are missed in routine EEG recordings. It is often done when pa-tients are drowsy after sleep deprivation.

Natalin   See **procarbazine.**

National Alliance for the Mentally Ill   (NAMI) Advocacy organization devoted to improving the lives of persons with serious mental ill-nesses (e.g., schizophrenia, major depression, bipolar disorder). Founded in 1979, it has more than 150,000 members in 1,000 affiliate groups and coalitions operating in all 50 U.S. states. Members include those with mental disorders as well as their relatives and friends. NAMI services include a toll-free number for information about mental illnesses, affiliate groups, and self-help meetings; public educa-tion to reduce the stigma of and ignorance about mental illness; and federal, state, and local advocacy to increase research funding and improve services for people with serious mental illnesses.

National Alliance for Research on Schizophrenia And Depression   (NARSAD) Private U.S. organization formed in 1986, when the Schizo-phrenia Foundation, a local group in Ken-tucky, realized its ambition for better research could be achieved only with national support. NARSAD is dedicated to funding and support-ing mental illness research.

National Council On Alcoholism   (NCA) Volun-tary agency specializing in education and in-creasing public awareness about alcoholism.

National Depressive and Manic Depressive Asso-ciation   (NDMDA) Nonprofit organization established to educate patients, families, pro-fessionals, and the public about the nature and management of depression and manic depressive disorders; to foster self-help for patients and families; to eliminate discrimina-tion and stigma associated with these illnesses; to improve access to care; and to advocate for research toward elimination of these illnesses. There are 35,000 members, a 23-member na-tional Board of Directors, and a 55-member Scientific Advisory Board composed of highly qualified, recognized experts on these ill-nesses.

National Disease and Therapeutic Index   (NDTI) Rotating panel of over 2,100 of the approxi-mately 200,000 office-based U.S. physicians that reports to IMS America 4 times each year on all contacts with patients during a 48-hour period. Data are collected on the drug pre-scribed and its quantity, diagnosis for which it was prescribed, action desired, concomitant drugs, concomitant diagnoses, and whether the prescription in question was the first time the patient received the drug or whether it was for continuing therapy. Demographic data about the patient and the prescriber are also collected. Periodic reports are prepared, including reports organized by drug and by diagnosis. In addition, special analyses can be performed (National Disease and Therapeutic Index, IMS America, Ltd., Ambler, PA 19002). See **IMS America Ltd.; National Prescription Audit.**

National Institute on Drug Abuse   (NIDA) Federally supported institution that sponsors and formulates policies on issues of drug abuse, drug addiction, and treatment issues.

National Institute of Mental Health   (NIMH) One of several agencies of the U.S. government that is a component of the National Institute of Health (NIH) within the Department of Health and Human Services. It administers grant programs supporting research, training, and service programs in mental health.

National Institute for Neurological and Communicative Disorders and Stroke   (NINCDS) In conjunction with the Alzheimer's Disease and Related Disorders Association, NINCDS has established criteria for probable Alzheimer's disease. This group divided the diagnosis of dementia of the Alzheimer's type into definite, probable, and possible. See **dementia of the Alzheimer type.**

National Practitioner Databank   Database established by the U.S. government to track malpractice actions and disciplinary proceedings against doctors, dentists, and other licensed health care practitioners and to prevent them from concealing a damaging history by moving to a different state. It began operation in 1990.

National Prescription Audit   (NPA) One of two major data sources on prescriptions in the United States. It is a database of dispensed prescriptions from a panel of computerized retail pharmacies, conducted on an ongoing basis by IMS America, Inc.

natural killer (NK) cell   Any of a class of cells that can spontaneously recognize and kill tumor- and virus-infected cells without previous exposure to the antigen. They are critical to initial defense against infections, especially viral. NK cell cytotoxicity is decreased in depressives and alcoholics and further reduced in patients with co-existing depression and alcoholism (Petitto JM, Folds JD, Ozer H, et al. Abnormal diurnal variation in circulating natural killer cell phenotypes and cytotoxic

activity in major depression. *Am J Psychiatry* 1992;149:694–696).

natural selection   Theory of evolutionary change suggested simultaneously by Darwin and Wallace in 1858. It asserts that evolution occurs because individuals of a species whose characteristics best fit them for survival contribute more offspring to the next generation. The offspring will tend to have the characteristics by virtue of which their parents survived, and in this way the adaptation of the species to the environment will gradually be improved (Bullock A, Stallybrass O [eds], *Fontana Dictionary of Modern Thought.* London: Collins, 1977).

naturalistic study   Longitudinal study in which treatment is based on the clinical decision of the treating physician and is not under the control of the investigator, who simply observes and evaluates the results of ongoing medical care. Study designs (e.g., case reports, analyses of secular trends, case-control studies, cohort studies) do not involve randomization. Naturalistic studies may represent the course of patients under typical clinical conditions and so yield valuable information from a public health and health policy perspective. Also called "management trial."

Navane   See **thiothixene.**

naxagolide   (MK-458; (+)-PHNO) Potent dopamine agonist with affinity for the D_2 receptor. Limited clinical trials indicate that it may be effective in reversing parkinsonian rigidity, tremor, and gait in moderately and severely affected patients (Grandas-Perez FJ, Jenner PG, Nomoto M, et al. [+]-4-Tropyl-9-hydroxynaphthoxazine in Parkinson's disease. *Lancet* 1986;1:906; Cutler NR, Reines SA, McLean LF, et al. Pharmacokinetics and dose proportionality of D2-agonist MK-458 [HPMc]. *Clin Pharmacokinet* 1992;22:223–230).

N-desalkylflurazepam   Active flurazepam metabolite. Half-life is 37–89 hours.

N-desmethyladinazolam   (NDMAD) Active metabolite of adinazolam. Approximately 95% of an adinazolam dose is converted to NDMAD, which accounts for approximately 50% of the dose recovered in urine. Both adinazolam and NDMAD exhibit in vitro binding to central benzodiazepine (BZD) receptors, but the affinity of NDMAD is approximately 25 times greater. In humans, NDMAD is apparently responsible for the BZD-like effects (sedative and psychomotor effects) observed following administration of adinazolam that, at therapeutic doses, does not contribute significantly to these effects. NDMAD plasma concentrations and half-life are increased approximately 40% in the elderly because of reduced clearance; this is responsible for increased decrements in psychomotor performance, even with administration of slow-release adinazolam, which produces minimal effects on performance in young subjects. A lower starting dose or increased patient monitoring may be necessary when initiating adinazolam treatment in elderly subjects (Fleishaker JC, Hulst LA, Ekernas S-A, Grahnen A. Pharmacokinetics and pharmacodynamics of adinazolam and N-desmethyladinazolam after oral and intravenous dosing in healthy young and elderly volunteers. *J Clin Psychopharmacol* 1992;12:403–414). See **adinazolam.**

N-desmethylclomipramine   Metabolite of clomipramine. Unlike the parent compound, which is a potent serotonin (5-HT) uptake inhibitor, the metabolite is primarily a noradrenergic uptake inhibitor.

N-desmethyldiazepam   (Nordiazepam; DMDZ) Metabolite of diazepam.

N-desmethylflurazepam   Metabolite of flurazepam.

N-desmethylsertraline   Major metabolite of sertraline. It has a similar profile, but is less potent and may be clinically inactive. See **sertraline.**

"nebbie"   Street name for pentobarbital.

nefazodone   (NEF) Nontricyclic triazolo structure compound that is a member of the phenylpiperazine class of antidepressants. It is chemically related to but lacks the alpha$_1$-adrenoceptor antagonist properties of trazodone. Pharmacological profile is distinct from that of tricyclic antidepressants (TCAs), monoamine oxidase inhibitors, serotonin (5-HT) or norepinephrine uptake inhibitors, or 5-HT$_{1A}$ partial agonists. NEF acts as a 5-HT antagonist and inhibits neuronal uptake of 5-HT. It is inactive at most receptor binding sites including muscarinic, cholinergic, histamine (H$_1$), dopamine (D$_2$), benzodiazepine, gamma aminobutyric acid (GABA)$_A$, and the calcium channel. Primary metabolite is hydroxynefazodone, the pharmacological properties of which resemble the parent compound. A second metabolite is m-chlorophenylpiperazine (mCPP), a nonselective 5-HT receptor agonist that provokes anxiety (Eison AS, Eison MS, Torrente JR, et al. Nefazodone: preclinical pharmacology of a new antidepressant. *Psychopharmacol Bull* 1990;26:311–315). NEF is rapidly and completely absorbed, but because of extensive first-pass metabolism, absolute bioavailability is about 20%. Antidepressant efficacy is comparable to that of imipramine. Dosage must be individualized according to therapeutic response. Antidepressant dose range is 200–600 mg/day; optimal therapeutic dose range is 300–500 mg/day. A dose of 50 mg has no therapeutic efficacy, and

degree of improvement diminishes at 600 mg/day. Compared to most other antidepressants, NEF is devoid of anticholinergic activity and has no cardiac toxicity. NEF (600 mg/day) has benign side effects and few troubling adverse effects. It has decreased anticholinergic, antihistaminic, alpha-adrenolytic, and sedative activity relative to TCAs and is less likely to potentiate sedative/hypnotic agents, including alcohol. A single-blind crossover study in healthy volunteers showed a dose-related increase in plasma prolactin without significant alteration in plasma concentrations of adrenocorticotropic hormone (ACTH) and only marginal effects on plasma cortisol. NEF also raised oral temperature. These results are consistent with an acute facilitatory effect of some aspects of 5-HT neurotransmission, perhaps mediated through the mCPP metabolite (Walsh AES, Hockney RA, Campling G, et al. Neuroendocrine and temperature effects of nefazodone in healthy volunteers. *Biol Psychiatry* 1993;33:115–119).

nefazodone + alcohol   Nefazodone is a less potent alpha blocker than trazodone and may be less likely to potentiate alcohol and sedatives/hypnotics (Tillar JW. Antidepressants, alcohol and psychomotor performance. *Acta Psychiatr Scand* 1990;460[suppl]:13–17). In normal subjects it does not potentiate the sedative-hypnotic (depressant) effect of alcohol (Frewer LJ, Lader M. The effects of nefazodone, imipramine and placebo, alone and combined with alcohol, in normal subjects. *Int Clin Psychopharmacol* 1993;8:13–20).

nefiracetam   (DM-9384) (NEF) Nootropic, pyrrolidone derivative (N-[2,6-dimethylphenol]-2-[2-oxo-1-pyrrolidinyl]acetamide) that is a cyclic derivative of gamma aminobutyric acid (GABA). In animals, it has a protective action against scopolamine-induced amnesia that is attributed to its ability to reverse acetylcholine (ACh) depletion. In pharmacological studies, it exhibits antiamnestic and antihypoxic effects, and has potentiated learning acquisition by activating cholinergic and GABAergic neuronal systems (Nabeshima T. Nootropic effects of nefiracetam, a pyrrolidone derivative. *Neuropsychopharmacology* 1993;9:51S). It is in phase II and phase III clinical trials for senile dementia of the Alzheimer type and cerebrovascular disease, respectively. In a phase II cerebrovascular disease trial, NEF showed objective effects on parameters such as initiative, hypobulia, emotional deficits, behavior problems, and subjective disorders. There was a significant correlation between dose and efficacy; the most effective dosage was 450 mg/day.

negative assortative mating   See **mating, negative assortative.**

negative correlation See **correlation, inverse.**

negative eugenics See **eugenics, negative.**

negative predictive power See **predictive power, negative.**

negative reinforcement See **reinforcement, negative.**

negative symptoms See **schizophrenia/negative symptoms.**

negligence, medical In tort law, failure to meet the standard of practice of an average qualified physician practicing in the specialty in question. Negligence occurs not merely when there is error, but when the degree of error exceeds an accepted norm. Error is a necessary, but not sufficient, condition for the determination of negligence. Perfection cannot be the standard of practice, since the vagaries of biology and human behavior make it unattainable. Thus, standards of practice must include acceptance of some degree of error (Leaps LL, Brennan TA, Laird N, et al. The nature of adverse events in hospitalized patients. Results of the Harvard Medical Practice Study II. *N Engl J Med* 1991;324:377–384).

"nembie" Street name for pentobarbital (Nembutal).

Nembutal See **pentobarbital.**

Neocyten See **orphenadrine.**

Neo-Durabolic See **nandrolone decanoate.**

neologism New word invented by the subject, distorted word, or standard word to which the subject has given new, highly idiosyncratic meaning. The judgment that the subject uses neologisms should be made cautiously, taking into account his or her educational and cultural background (DSM-IV).

neonatal Any event or condition directly affecting a newborn during the first month after birth.

"neopterin" Only product of activated macrophages that is significantly elevated in symptomatic human immunodeficiency virus (HIV)-seropositive patients. Levels are up in the cerebrospinal fluid and especially in the serum of patients who have meningitis or other neurological opportunistic infections.

Neostigmin See **neostigmine.**

neostigmine (Neostigmin; Prostigmin) Quaternary ammonium anticholinesterase compound that can be used in the treatment of anticholinergic delirium caused by muscarinic receptor blockers. It is considered peripherally active, but it can cause a cholinergic crisis in overdosage. It has been proposed as an antidote for sexual dysfunction caused by monoamine oxidase inhibitors; 7.5–15 mg 30 minutes before sexual intercourse may help alleviate impaired ejaculation.

neostriatum Area of the brain that contains the caudate nucleus and the putamen. It balances the inhibitory dopaminergic and the excitatory cholinergic components of the basal ganglia.

nephentin Large polypeptide that is a putative endogenous ligand for the benzodiazepine (BZD) receptor, although distribution in the brain does not coincide with that of the BZD receptors. It may be a precursor of the lower-molecular-weight peptide that can block the BZD receptor. It has no effect on other neurotransmitter receptors.

nephrogenic diabetes insipidus (NDI) Diabetes insipidus due to a failure of the kidney to react to vasopressin. It can lead to dehydration, compensatory thirst, and polydipsia. Lithium may cause NDI by blocking the action of antidiuretic hormone (ADH) on the collecting duct, producing impairment of concentrating capacity. See **lithium/nephrogenic diabetes insipidus.**

"nephrotic range" proteinuria Occurrence of proteinuria (i.e., greater than 3.5 g) in some lithium-treated patients.

nerve growth factor (NGF) Member of a class of proteins, the neurotrophins, that plays an important role in regulating neuronal cell death during development, maintaining the differentiated state of these neurons and aiding in their recovery from injury or aging. Two members of this family are EDNF and NT-3.

nervine Over-the-counter bromide preparation implicated in causing symptoms of an organic brain disorder.

nervous system, autonomic System of nerves controlling many internal involuntary processes such as heart rate, digestion, and pupil diameter.

nervous system, central (CNS) Neurons and glia of the brain and spinal cord.

nervous system, parasympathetic Part of the autonomic nervous system that controls the life-sustaining organs of the body (heart, lungs) and uses acetylcholine as the neurotransmitter, resulting in effects opposite from those of the sympathetic nervous system. See **nervous system, sympathetic.**

nervous system, sympathetic Component of the autonomic nervous system that centers about two chains of ganglia running along the sides of the spinal cord and connects with many sympathetic ganglia, facilitating widespread discharge. Stimulation usually results in an effect opposite from the effects of stimulation of the parasympathetic nervous system.

Neulactil See **pericyazine.**

Neuleptil See **pericyazine.**

Neupan See **oxiracetam.**

Neupogen   See **human granulocyte colony-stimulating factor.**

neural messenger   Chemical substance (neuroregulator, neuromodulator, neurotransmitter, neurohormone) that conveys impulses or information from one cell to another.

Neuramate   See **meprobamate.**

neurasthenia   Neurotic disorder characterized by fatigue, irritability, headache, depression, insomnia, difficulty concentrating, and anhedonia. It may follow or accompany infection or exhaustion or arise from continued emotional stress. The term is rarely used today; preferred descriptions are postviral fatigue syndrome, chronic fatigue syndrome, and myalgic encephalomyelitis ("malaise of the 80s") (Wessely S. Old wine in new bottles: neurasthenia and "ME." *Psychol Med* 1990;20:35–53).

neuroacanthocytosis   Disorder manifested by chorea, tics, and caudate atrophy that has been associated with compulsive lip and finger biting and head banging (Wyzinski B, Merriam A, Medalia A, Lawrence C. Choreoacanthocytosis. *Neuropsychiatry Neuropsychol Behav Neurol* 1989;2:137–144).

Neuractiv   See **oxiracetam.**

neuritic plaque   Characteristic pathological occurrence in the brains of Alzheimer disease patients. Plaques occur throughout the neocortex and hippocampus; density is correlated with the degree of cognitive impairment manifested at the time of death.

neuroactive steroid   Any natural or synthetic steroid that rapidly alters the excitability of neurons and selectively augments the inhibitory properties of gamma aminobutyric acid (GABA) by binding to sites distinct from those used by barbiturates and benzodiazepines. Some neuroactive steroids are also neurosteroids in that they are synthesized de novo within the central nervous system (Paul S. Neuroactive steroids. *Biol Psychiatry* 1993;33: 70A).

neuroadaptation   Physical dependence manifested by a withdrawal syndrome of varying intensity upon abrupt discontinuation or dosage reduction of the causative drug or substance. Characteristics of the syndrome are generally typical for specific classes of psychoactive agents (e.g., alcohol, amphetamines, barbiturates, benzodiazepines, opiates).

neurobehavioral probe   See **probe, neurobehavioral.**

neurochemistry   Branch of chemistry dealing with phenomena occurring within the nervous system.

neurocognitive disorder, mild   Syndrome that is frequently the harbinger of early dementia. Two probable causes of the disorder are cerebrovascular disease and Alzheimer's disease.

Symptoms are subtle and include decreased performance capacities (e.g., forgetting names and important appointments), concentration and calculation deficits, memory deficits manifested by a tendency to be repetitive, remote memory deficits, and praxis deficits. Patients complain of anxiety and apprehension; some become agitated and have sudden verbal outbursts of anger; others may become transiently tearful and pessimistic but not overtly depressed. Symptoms usually do not warrant treatment with anxiolytics or antidepressants. Low doses of a monoamine oxidase inhibitor may relieve moderate or severe depression. See **age-associated memory impairment.**

neurodevelopmental brain changes   Disruption of brain development resulting in structural brain abnormalities that can be detected by computed tomography (CT) and magnetic resonance imaging (MRI). They include lateral and third ventricular enlargement, medial temporal lobe hyperplasia, reduced total cerebral volume, cortical sulcal and fissure widening, and cerebellar atrophy. They have been found in patients with schizophrenia and bipolar disorder and have been considered an integral part of the evidence for a neurodevelopmental etiological process in these disorders.

neurodynamics   Interactions of large numbers of neurons that transform information derived from their environments into meaningful outputs and use this information to alter their own architectures. The concept may be useful in framing and investigating research questions that could advance understanding of the nature, course, and treatment of schizophrenia (Hoffman RE, McGlashen TH. Neurodynamics and schizophrenia research: editors' introduction. *Schizophrenia Bull* 1993;19: 15–19).

neuroendocrine   Relating to the shared influence of and interactions between the nervous and endocrine systems, including the production of hormones.

neuroendocrine challenge paradigm   Administration of a drug with selective action on a particular neurotransmitter and observing resultant changes in plasma concentrations of hormones, the release of which is regulated by the neurotransmitter. Such paradigms allow evaluation of the functional activity of neurotransmitter systems.

neuroendocrine challenge test   Any of the various tests that examine the functional integrity of the monoamine pathways that control the secretion of pituitary hormones. They were developed during the quest for an objective biological marker for clinical depression that could facilitate accurate diagnosis and effective treatment planning. Included are the buspirone challenge test, clonidine challenge test, desipramine/growth hormone stimulation test, dexamethasone suppression test, growth hormone stimulation test, protirelin tests, and thyrotropin-releasing hormone test.

neuroendocrine serotonin challenge tests Use of intravenous L-tryptophan or oral fenfluramine to stimulate prolactin response in depressed patients (Heninger GR, Charney DS, Sternberg DE. Serotonergic function in depression. Prolactin response to intravenous tryptophan in depressed patients and healthy subjects. *Arch Gen Psychiatry* 1984;41:398–402; Coccaro EF, Siever LJ, Klar HM, et al. Serotonergic studies in patients with affective and personality disorders. *Arch Gen Psychiatry* 1989; 46:587–599).

neuroendocrinology Study of the neural mechanisms involved in hormone secretion. Of particular importance is the action of the hypothalamus, which stimulates or inhibits the pituitary secretion of hormones.

neurofibrillary tangle (NFT) One of the principal histopathological changes observed in Alzheimer's disease. NFTs occur in a wide range of neurological disorders apparently unrelated to Alzheimer's disease, suggesting that they may be a nonspecific marker of neuronal degeneration.

neurohormone Hypothalamus-produced chemical messenger carried to the pituitary and then to other cells within the central nervous system (CNS). Neurohormones are similar to neurotransmitters except that they interact with a variety of cells, including neurotransmitters (e.g., peptides), whereas neurotransmitters interact only with other neurons. Neurohormones include corticotropin-releasing hormone, vasopressin, taurine, antidiuretic hormone, and cholecystokinin. They produce slight changes in brain neurochemistry. They may be safer than most current drugs and may have potential as pharmacotherapeutic agents for CNS disorders. Also called "neuromodulator"; "neuroregulator."

neuroimaging Techniques that provide data on regional brain activity and function. Regional brain physiology can be measured with topographic electroencephalography and evoked potentials, positron emission tomography (PET), single photon emission computed tomography (SPECT), and the noninvasive isotropic method xenon-133 clearance measures of cerebral blood flow. In addition, there are ligands for assessing density and affinity of neurotransmitter receptors with PET and SPECT.

neuroimmunology Study of the interaction between the nervous system and the immune system. For example, alterations in the nervous system due to the shock of an illness and/or a person's general mood, outlook, and life view may influence the number and activity level of various immune cell lines. Such changes can affect survival in illnesses such as cancer and human immunodeficiency virus (HIV) infection.

neurokinin A (NKA) Tachykinin peptide that activates some dopaminergic neurons. It may be associated with negative schizophrenic symptoms (Deutch AY, Maggio JE, Bannon MJ, et al. Substance K and substance P differentially modulate mesolimbic and mesocortical systems. *Peptides* 1985;6[suppl]:113–122). See **tachykinin peptide.**

neuroleptanalgesia Use of a neuroleptic to potentiate anesthesia (e.g., droperidol in connection with a narcotic). Formerly called "potentiated anesthesia." See **droperidol.**

neuroleptic (NL) Term coined by Delay (1955) meaning "to take the neuron" (the suffix *-leptic* is derived from the Greek *leptomai* meaning "to hold or capture") because chlorpromazine reduced nervous tension rather than paralysis (neuroplegia). At the Second International Congress of Psychiatry (1955), *neuroleptic* was chosen by vote over *tranquilizer* and *ataraxic.* The term, referring to dual drug actions on psychoses and motor function, replaced the term *major tranquilizer.* Although still used, it is being gradually replaced by the term *antipsychotic.* The advent of clozapine and other atypical neuroleptics, which are antipsychotic but seldom cause extrapyramidal reactions, has demonstrated that antipsychotic effects can be achieved without affecting motor function. Thus, *neuroleptic* and *antipsychotic* are no longer interchangeable terms. *Neuroleptic* is used for all psychoactive compounds that produce both antipsychotic and extrapyramidal effects. Neuroleptics are antipsychotic agents of proven benefit in the acute and long-term treatment of psychotic states, particularly schizophrenia. In 1957, Delay and Deniker suggested the following five-point definition of the characteristics of a neuroleptic: (a) induction of a state of psychomotor indifference quite different from sedation produced by barbiturates; (b) efficacy with respect to agitation, excitation, and aggression; (c) efficacy in acute and chronic psychotic disorders; (d) distinctive pattern of neurological (extrapyramidal) and vegetative (e.g., cardiovascular, gastrointestinal, endocrine) side effects; and (e) predominantly subcortical action. Neuroleptics are known to affect the following neurotransmitter systems:

dopaminergic, alpha-adrenergic, muscarinic-anticholinergic, serotonergic, histaminergic, gamma aminobutyric acid (GABA)-ergic, and peptidergic. By antagonizing dopamine receptors in the pituitary, neuroleptics can cause elevated serum levels of prolactin, which, in turn, can cause galactorrhea and menstrual and sexual dysfunction.

neuroleptic + alprazolam   Neuroleptic augmentation with alprazolam has been reported to be effective and safe (Donyon R, Angrist B, Peselow E, et al. Neuroleptic augmentation with alprazolam: clinical effects and pharmacokinetic correlates. *Am J Psychiatry* 1989;146: 231–234).

neuroleptic + antacid   Antacid ingestion 1–2 hours before neuroleptic administration reduces neuroleptic absorption and may affect therapeutic response to it.

neuroleptic + anticonvulsant   Anticonvulsants that induce hepatic drug metabolizing enzymes may reduce neuroleptic blood levels and neuroleptic therapeutic efficacy.

neuroleptic, atypical   Term coined in the 1970s to identify newly developed antipsychotics (e.g., clozapine, melperone, piquindone, risperidone, remoxipride) that differ from their predecessors by reduced or absent propensity to evoke extrapyramidal reactions. They are anatomically more selective in their effects on mesolimbic and mesocorticol dopamine neuronal firing than typical neuroleptics in that they induce depolarization in A10 (the central tegmental area of the midbrain) only. They generally cause no elevation of serum prolactin levels following repeated administrations. Putative mechanisms of action include: (a) antagonism of D_1 as well as, or rather than, D_2 receptors; (b) antagonism of sigma and D_2 receptors; and (c) antagonism of serotonin and D_2 receptors (Meltzer HY. Clozapine: mechanisms of action in relation to its clinical advantages. *In* Kales A, Stefanis CN, Talbott JA [eds], *Recent Advances in Schizophrenia.* New York: Springer-Verlag, 1990, pp 237–256).

neuroleptic, atypical, type A   Compound more potent against serotonin $(5-HT)_2$ than dopamine D_2 binding sites by about 1.2 log units. Included are amperozide, clozapine, fluperlapine, melperone, perlapine, risperidone, ritanserin, and tiospirone.

neuroleptic, atypical, type B   Compound more potent at dopamine D_2 than serotonin $(5-HT)_2$ binding sites by about 0.3 log units. Included are cis-flupenthixol, chlorpromazine, fluphenazine, haloperidol, loxapine, raclopride, remoxipride, and thioridazine.

neuroleptic + benzodiazepine   Co-administration is currently used as an adjunct in the treatment of partially unresponsive or nonre-sponsive schizophrenia and in acutely agitated, psychotic patients; as a substitute for neuroleptics alone in the acute treatment of mania; and as acute treatment for catatonia. There is no evidence that one benzodiazepine (BZD) is more effective than another, but many experienced clinicians recommend higher-potency BZDs (e.g., lorazepam, clonazepam, alprazolam). Although there is evidence that BZDs are efficacious in the treatment of acute mania, there is no evidence that they are equal or superior alternatives to neuroleptics alone or that co-administration of a BZD and a neuroleptic is more effective than a neuroleptic alone. There is some evidence that co-administration may allow use of a lower neuroleptic dose (Arana GW, Ornsteen ML, Kanter F, et al. The use of benzodiazepines for psychotic disorders: a literature review and preliminary clinical findings. *Psychopharmacol Bull* 1986;22:77–87; Salzman C, Green AI, Rodriquez-Villa F, et al. Benzodiazepines combined with neuroleptics for management of severe disruptive behavior. *Psychosomatics* 1986;27:17–21; Garza-Trevino ES, Hollister LE, Overall JE, et al. Efficacy of combinations of intramuscular antipsychotics and sedative-hypnotics for control of psychotic agitation. *Am J Psychiatry* 1989;146:1598–1601). Parenterally administered (i.e., intramuscularly or intravenously administered) BZD has been found to be effective in the treatment of catatonia. The majority of patients have been treated with intramuscularly administered lorazepam or intravenously administered diazepam. If results are not seen quickly with lorazepam, aggressive treatment with a high-potency neuroleptic should be started (Easton MS, Janicak PG. Benzodiazepines for the management of psychosis. *Psychiatr Med* 1991;9:25–36). Of 16 double-blind studies assessing adjunctive BZD treatment in schizophrenia, 7 reported positive results and 4 reported mixed or transiently positive results. Overall response rate of patients is 30–50% (Wolkowitz OM, Pickar D. Benzodiazepines in the treatment of schizophrenia: a review and reappraisal. *Am J Psychiatry* 1991;148:714–726; Arana GW, Ornsteen ML, Kanter F, et al. The use of benzodiazepines for psychotic disorders: a literature review and preliminary clinical findings. *Psychopharmacol Bull* 1986;22:77–87). Therapeutic response to adjunctive BZDs usually occurs within hours or within 2–3 weeks. If it does not, BZDs should be withdrawn. In some cases, BZDs lose efficacy after several weeks as tolerance develops. New data suggest that severely refractory patients show little response other than sedation to BZD augmentation. In some patients, high doses are needed to achieve a therapeutic response.

Close monitoring during dosage titration is necessary to avert behavioral disinhibition, a side effect that occurs in approximately 10% of patients and responds to dosage lowering (Wolkowitz OM. Rational polypharmacy in schizophrenia. *Ann Clin Psychiatry* 1993;5:79–90). See **benzodiazepine/adjunctive therapy; neuroleptic + alprazolam; neuroleptic + clonazepam; neuroleptic + diazepam; neuroleptic + lorazepam.**

neuroleptic + benzodiazepine + valproate Combination frequently used when manic patients have psychotic symptoms such as hallucinations, threats to others, and insomnia not responsive to benzodiazepines (BZDs). Concomitant use of valproate, a neuroleptic, and a BZD (clonazepam, lorazepam) as clinically indicated is safe and effective and reduces drop-outs. Furthermore, a BZD can enhance sedation and reduce the amount of neuroleptic needed. As the manic episode comes under control, dosage of the neuroleptic and the BZD is reduced gradually until total discontinuation. See **benzodiazepine/adjunctive therapy; neuroleptic + benzodiazepine.**

neuroleptic + benztropine Prophylactic benztropine effectively reduces occurrence of neuroleptic-induced dystonia in young patients receiving high-potency neuroleptic therapy for acute psychosis. However, not all patients require anticholinergics, and these drugs can produce cognitive deficits. Co-administration of benztropine with piperidine or aliphatic phenothiazines, which are anticholinergic, can lead to additive anticholinergic effects, including fecal compaction. The effect of benztropine on neuroleptic plasma levels is unresolved; some studies report lowering of plasma levels; one, an increase; most, no effect.

neuroleptic + bromocriptine Adjunctive, low-dose bromocriptine has been reported to improve psychotic symptoms in neuroleptic-resistant schizophrenia without producing adverse drug-drug interactions. It has been co-administered with chlorpromazine, flupenthixol, fluphenazine, and haloperidol (Wolf M-A, Diener J-M, Lajeunnesse C, et al. Low-dose bromocriptine in neuroleptic-resistant schizophrenia. A pilot study. *Biol Psychiatry* 1992;31:1166–1168).

neuroleptic + carbamazepine Carbamazepine (CBZ), a potent inducer of hepatic microsomal enzymes, may cause a significant (50% or higher) decrease in the level of co-administered neuroleptics (Fast DK, Jones BD, Kusalic M, Erickson M. Effect of carbamazepine on neuroleptic plasma level and efficacy. *Am J Psychiatry* 1986;143:117–118; Jann M, Ereshefsky L, Sakalad S. Effects of carbamazepine on

plasma haloperidol levels. *J Clin Psychopharm* 1985;5:106–109). This can result in loss of efficacy in neuroleptic-responsive patients. Neuroleptic plasma levels should be checked if patients fail to respond to standard doses during combined therapy with CBZ. Also, abrupt CBZ discontinuation can markedly increase neuroleptic plasma levels, possibly resulting in serious side effects. In patients with affective and schizoaffective disorders, combined use is more likely to cause hyponatremia than CBZ alone. See **carbamazepine + haloperidol.**

neuroleptic/catatonia See **catatonia, neuroleptic-induced.**

neuroleptic + cimetidine Co-administration reduces steady-state neuroleptic level and may affect neuroleptic therapeutic efficacy.

neuroleptic + clomipramine Addition of clomipramine (CMI) to ongoing neuroleptic treatment in schizophrenic patients with obsessive-compulsive symptoms has been associated with specific reduction of those symptoms. CMI has been co-administered with chlorpromazine, haloperidol, and fluphenazine decanoate (Zohar J, Kaplan Z, Benjamin J. Clomipramine treatment of obsessive-compulsive symptomatology in schizophrenic patients. *J Clin Psychiatry* 1993;45:385–388).

neuroleptic + clonazepam In a double-blind crossover study of acute mania with adjunctive haloperidol, clonazepam (mean dose, 10.4 mg/day) was superior to lithium (mean dose, 1691 mg/day) in controlling motor overactivity and logorrhea. In addition, total haloperidol dose administered was lower during clonazepam treatment (Chouinard G, Young SN, Anarable L. Antimanic effect of clonazepam. *Biol Psychiatry* 1983;18:451–466). In a double-blind study in schizophrenia, clonazepam (3 mg/day) added to haloperidol produced modest improvement in Brief Psychiatric Rating Scale and Extrapyramidal Side Effects Scale scores, but no changes in specific symptoms (Altamura AC, Mauri MC, Mantero M, Brunetti M. Clonazepam/haloperidol combination therapy in schizophrenia: a double-blind study. *Acta Psychiatr Scand* 1987;76:702–706).

neuroleptic, depot Long-acting injectable formulation that eliminates or reduces many of the disadvantages of oral preparations because it is administered directly into skeletal muscles. Absorption into circulation depends on local muscle factors and the physiochemical nature of the preparation. Depot formulations are often preferred for maintenance treatment in chronic schizophrenia, both for the convenience of patients and to ensure compliance because of their long duration of action (1–4 weeks). Effective administration requires a 2-inch needle; 0.1 ml of air in the syringe; allowing the alcohol on the skin to dry before injecting; and sliding the skin to the side and then back after the injection (z-track technique), which prevents drug leakage. The injection site should not be massaged. Fluphenazine and haloperidol are marketed in depot forms in the United States.

neuroleptic + desipramine   Co-administration may increase plasma levels of both drugs (Craig Nelson J, Jatlow PI. Neuroleptic effect on desipramine steady-state plasma concentrations. *Am J Psychiatry* 1980;137:1232–1234).

neuroleptic + diazepam   Co-administration of high doses of diazepam to patients with neuroleptic-resistant chronic schizophrenia may augment therapeutic response (Nestoros JN, Nair NPV, Pulman JR, et al. High doses of diazepam improve neuroleptic-resistant chronic schizophrenia patients. *Psychopharmacology* 1983;18:42–47).

neuroleptic + disulfiram   Disulfiram inhibits clearance of neuroleptic, possibly resulting in neuroleptic toxicity.

neuroleptic efficacy   Numerous studies have documented that all neuroleptics produce consistent changes in the same symptoms and that no neuroleptic is consistently superior to another. Neuroleptics differ primarily only in their side effect profiles.

neuroleptic + electroconvulsive therapy (ECT) Co-administration may be effective in the treatment of psychotic symptoms in drug-resistant schizophrenia.

neuroleptic + fenfluramine   Co-administration has no effect on the steady-state plasma concentrations of fenfluramine, neuroleptics, and metabolites (Hubbard JW, Marshall BD, Srinivas NR, et al. Pharmacokinetics of fenfluramine and neuroleptics in the treatment of refractory schizophrenia. *Drug Invest* 1992;4:99–111).

neuroleptic + fluoxetine   In neuroleptic-resistant schizophrenia, addition of fluoxetine (FLX) (20 mg/day) to ongoing neuroleptic therapy may improve both positive and negative schizophrenic symptoms and depressive symptoms (Goff DC, Brotman AW, Waites M, et al. Trial of fluoxetine added to neuroleptics for treatment-resistant schizophrenic patients. *Am J Psychiatry* 1990;147:492–494). Co-administration may exacerbate any neuroleptic-induced extrapyramidal symptoms (EPS) and may potentiate FLX's ability to cause extrapyramidal disorders such as akathisia (Chouinard G. Fluoxetine and preoccupation with suicide. *Am J Psychiatry* 1991;148:1258–1259). Some evidence suggests that FLX precipitation of EPS may be more likely during the early stages of neuroleptic treatment, when serotonergic modulation of dopamine activity may be greatest and when dopamine levels are elevated above resting conditions (Goff DC, Baldessarini RJ. Drug interactions with antipsychotic agents. *J Clin Psychopharmacol* 1993;13:57–65).

neuroleptic + fluvoxamine   Co-administration has been used with some success in obsessive-compulsive disorder refractory to fluvoxamine alone.

neuroleptic/high-dose   There is no general agreement as to what constitutes high or very high neuroleptic dosage. Present data suggest that doses over 100 mg of haloperidol have no advantage over more moderate doses. There is, however, a greater margin of safety with low and moderate doses of haloperidol and other neuroleptics.

neuroleptic, high-potency   Neuroleptic with high potency on a milligram-per-milligram basis (e.g., fluphenazine, haloperidol, thiothixene, trifluoperazine). These neuroleptics are the least sedating and have a high propensity to evoke extrapyramidal reactions and a low propensity to elicit anticholinergic effects.

neuroleptic + hypnotic   Regular use of hypnotics that induce hepatic drug metabolizing enzymes may lower neuroleptic blood levels.

neuroleptic/intermittent   Intermittent neuroleptic prophylaxis was introduced because of concern about adverse effects of long-term continuous treatment, especially the risk of tardive dyskinesia. It requires careful patient selection, medication tapering, careful monitoring for prodromal signs of exacerbation, and medication resumption with early signs of relapse. It is based on the assumption that, since relapse usually occurs in stages, it can be aborted before a florid psychotic state develops. The regimen does substantially reduce neuroleptic use in a large proportion of patients (Carpenter WT Jr, Heinrichs DW, Hanlon TE. A comparative trial of pharmacologic strategies in schizophrenia. *Am J Psychiatry* 1987;144:1466–1470). It may have no advantage for the majority of stable outpatients if they are taking moderate antipsychotic doses as maintenance therapy. Relapse and rehospitalization rates have been worse with intermittent treatment than with continuous treatment. Continuous oral and depot neuroleptic prophylaxis is superior to intermittent prophylaxis in preventing both psychotic and neurotic or dysphoric morbidity in schizophrenia. It is recommended that clinicians seek the minimum effective maintenance dose for a particular patient combined with an early intervention strategy. Also called "targeted pharmacotherapy."

neuroleptic, intramuscular/microdose Elderly or debilitated patients who become hyper-aroused, agitated, or combative may benefit from very small doses of a neuroleptic given intramuscularly (e.g., haloperidol 0.5 mg twice a day or 3 times a day). Although measuring less than 1 ml (5 mg haloperidol) is difficult with most syringes, U-100 insulin syringes make it possible to divide 1 ml into 50 parts. Thus, 0.5 mg of haloperidol given intramuscularly would be converted to 10 units (0.5/5 ml) of haloperidol. When symptom control is achieved, the patient can be switched to appropriate oral dosages (Granacher RP, Jr. Titrating intramuscular dosages for elderly patients. *Am J Psychiatry* 1979;136:997).

neuroleptic, intravenous Intravenous administration of high-potency neuroleptics (especially haloperidol) has increased steadily in recent years. It can be safe and effective, with side effects generally no greater than those with other routes of administration. A lower incidence of extrapyramidal side effects has been reported with intravenous administration compared to oral administration. See **haloperidol, intravenous administration.**

neuroleptic + lithium Addition of lithium to a neuroleptic may enhance dopamine metabolism (Bowers MD, Mazure CM, Nelson JC, Patlow PI. Lithium in combination with perphenazine: effect on plasma monoamine metabolites. *Biol Psychiatry* 1992;32:1102–1107). Co-administration may cause more extrapyramidal reactions than either drug alone. It also may result in toxicity manifested by confusion, disorientation, ataxia, and falling, especially with high dosages. In a comparison of patients who developed neurotoxicity with those who did not, average neuroleptic dose was 563 mg of chlorpromazine equivalents in the non-toxic group versus 1,780 mg in the toxic group; there were no differences in lithium dosages (Miller F, Menninger J. Lithium-neuroleptic neurotoxicity is dose dependent. *J Clin Psychopharmacol* 1987;7:89–91; Axelsson R, Lagerkvist-Briggs M. Clinical and neurobiological findings during treatment with neuroleptics alone and combined with lithium: comparative study of patients with bipolar disorder in acute manic phase. *Lithium* 1993;4:45–52). Neurotoxicity recedes spontaneously and without apparent sequelae after discontinuation of the drug regimen. There is some evidence that co-administration may increase the risk of neuroleptic malignant syndrome. It also has been reported to induce somnambulistic-like episodes, usually in patients on maintenance lithium following addition of a neuroleptic. Episodes occur within 2–3 hours of sleep onset; they are characterized by the patient appearing confused and walking about in a quick, detached clumsy manner. Generally, patients have no memory of the event (Charney DS, Kales A, Soldatos CR, Nelson JC. Somnambulistic-like episodes secondary to combined lithium-neuroleptic treatment. *Br J Psychiatry* 1979;135:418–424). See **lithium + haloperidol.**

neuroleptic + lithium + tricyclic antidepressant Several case reports indicate that lithium may potentiate response to tricyclic antidepressant/neuroleptic treatment (Nelson JC, Maguire CM. Lithium augmentation in psychotic depression refractory to combined drug treatment. *Am J Psychiatry* 1986;143:363–366; Pai M, White AC, Deane AG. Lithium augmentation in the treatment of delusional depression. *Br J Psychiatry* 1986;148:736–738; Price LH, Yeates C, Nelson JC. Lithium augmentation of combined neuroleptic-tricyclic treatment in delusional depression. *Am J Psychiatry* 1983;140:318–322).

neuroleptic + lorazepam Lorazepam (LOR) has been added to a variety of neuroleptics to control acutely agitated psychoses. Co-administration requires less time to control agitation, produces fewer side effects, and has a neuroleptic-sparing effect in that fewer neuroleptic doses are needed. It generally is safe, but paradoxical reactions to lorazepam do occur. Co-administration for management of acute mania has escalated because of LOR's pharmacokinetics: rapid onset of action, short half-life, relatively short duration of action, and relatively simple hepatic metabolism requiring only glucuronidation for renal excretion. In addition, the likelihood of drug interactions is low. Many experts use lorazepam (3–8 mg/day) with low neuroleptic doses (Pato CN, Wolkowitz OM, Rapaport M, et al. Benzodiazepine augmentation of neuroleptic treatment in patients with schizophrenia. *Psychopharmacol Bull* 1989;25:263–266).

neuroleptic, low-potency Neuroleptic with low potency on a milligram-per-milligram basis (e.g., chlorpromazine, chlorprothixene, levopromazine, mesoridazine, sulpiride, thioridazine). These neuroleptics are less likely to evoke extrapyramidal reactions, but are more likely to cause anticholinergic and sedative effects than are high-potency neuroleptics.

neuroleptic malignant syndrome (NMS) Syndrome attributed to neuroleptics, non-neuroleptic dopamine-blockers (metoclopramide), some tricyclic antidepressants, and withdrawal of dopamine-agonist antiparkinson drugs (e.g., amantadine). It is characterized by acute onset of fever, altered state of consciousness (delirium, stupor, or coma), autonomic imbalance (tachycardia, hypertension, hypotension, diaphoresis), and severe extrapyramidal signs ("lead-pipe" rigidity, dystonic/dyskinetic movements). Laboratory findings include moderate leukocytosis and moderately abnormal liver function tests. There is a substantial rise in serum creatine phosphokinase that stems from muscle fiber breakdown (rhabdomyolysis) in the highly contracted state of skeletal muscles. Temperature may rise to 107° F (41.6° C). Mortality rate has been estimated to be as high as 30%. Major causes of mortality and morbidity are respiratory failure, thromboembolism, aspiration pneumonia, cardiovascular collapse, arrhythmias, and acute renal failure. NMS is thought to result from a severe hypodopaminergic state. It affects patients of all ages across a broad range of psychiatric disorders. More than 20 different neuroleptics have been associated with it. Symptoms may appear within the first few days of neuroleptic administration and develop quickly into the full syndrome. Use of PRN neuroleptics may increase the risk of NMS by increasing the severity of extrapyramidal symptoms. Bromocriptine mesylate, a dopamine agonist, has effectively reversed NMS symptoms in some patients. Common recommendations for management of patients with a history of NMS include alternative drugs such as lithium or carbamazepine, electroconvulsive therapy, or low-potency neuroleptics and careful monitoring for adverse effects. Clozapine also can be used with little risk of recurrence in a patient with a history of NMS (Weller M, Kornhuber J. Clozapine rechallenge after an episode of "neuroleptic malignant syndrome." *Br J Psychiatry* 1992;161:855–856).

neuroleptic malignant syndrome (NMS)/diagnostic criteria NMS is diagnosed only when the following stringent criteria are met: Altered mental status (confusion, mutism, delirium, or coma); pyrexia (> 99° F; 37.2° C) without other cause; lead-pipe muscular rigidity; and autonomic dysfunction (tachycardia > 100/minute; blood pressure fluctuations > 30 mmHg systolic or 15 mmHg diastolic; hypertension > 140/90 mmHg, or lability > 19 mmHg variation of both systolic and diastolic within a 24-hour period; excessive sweating; tachypnea > 20 respirations/minute; or incontinence). Other proposed major criteria include severe extrapyramidal symptoms (EPS) and elevated creatine kinase (CK > 250 IU/L). Proposed minor criteria include leukocytosis (> 11 K/mm^3), incontinence, and minor EPS (Gelinas JG, Cullen S, Riba M. Polymyositis and neuroleptic malignant syndrome. Presented at the 146th Annual Meeting of the American Psychiatric Association, San Francisco, May 1993).

neuroleptic malignant syndrome (NMS)/risk factors Proposed risk factors include dosage, potency, and rate of increase of neuroleptics; adjuvant lithium therapy; psychomotor agitation; dehydration; medical or neurological illness; recent history of alcohol or other substance abuse or dependence; electrolyte imbalance; thyrotoxicosis; elevated ambient temperature; and history of prior NMS (Caroff SN, Mann SC, Lazarus A, et al. Neuroleptic malignant syndrome: diagnostic issues. *Psychiatr Ann* 1991;21:130–147; Keck PE. Epidemiology of neuroleptic malignant syndrome. *Psychiatr Ann* 1991;21:148–151).

neuroleptic/mania Since the mid-1950s, neuroleptics have been used to treat acute mania. Efficacy has been variable; in some studies, neuroleptics are less effective than lithium, and in other studies, they are more effective. In all studies, neuroleptics are more effective than placebo. They appear to be effective in 50–70% of acutely ill manic patients, especially those who are very hyperactive and need prompt sedation. In the past, however, many acute patients were given high neuroleptic doses that often caused extrapyramidal side effects, especially acute dystonic reactions. Over the years, many clinicians restricted neuroleptic therapy for acute mania for fear of causing tardive dyskinesia or neuroleptic malignant syndrome. Others, however, persisted, and by the late 1980s in Scandinavia, neuroleptics had become the preferred first-line drugs for acute mania (Vestergaard P. Treatment and prevention of mania: a Scandinavian perspective. *Neuropsychopharmacology* 1992; 7:249–259). Also by the late 1980s, clinicians again acknowledged that high doses (e.g., haloperidol, 30–80 mg/day) are no more effective than low doses (e.g., haloperidol, 10 mg/day) (Rifkin A, Karajgio B, Doddi S, Cooper T. Dose and blood levels of haloperidol in treatment of mania. *Psychopharmacol Bull* 1990; 26:144–146). In addition to being an alternative to lithium, neuroleptics are being used as adjuncts to lithium for prophylactic treatment of bipolar illness. Atypical neuroleptics (e.g., clozapine, remoxipride) have a low propensity to evoke acute extrapyramidal reactions and have antipsychotic properties comparable to those of conventional neuroleptics; they may prove to be effective in the treatment of acute mania (McElroy SL, Dessain EC, Pope HG, et al. Clozapine in the treatment of psychotic mood disorders, schizoaffective disorders and schizophrenia. *J Clin Psychiatry* 1991;52:411–414). See **neuroleptic + lithium.**

neuroleptic/megadose Technique in which patients are given larger-than-standard doses of a neuroleptic (over 1,000 mg of chlorpromazine equivalents). It is used primarily for patients refractory to standard neuroleptic doses who are actively psychotic and chronically ill. It is only effective for a small portion of refractory patients.

neuroleptic + methadone Co-administration may produce a superior antipsychotic effect compared to that of the neuroleptic alone, although this has not been conclusively established. Methadone in narcotic-abusing schizophrenic patients sometimes alters patients' neuroleptic requirements.

neuroleptic + moclobemide Moclobemide (150–450 mg/day) has been co-prescribed with one or more neuroleptic(s) in over 110 patients taking low-potency neuroleptics (methotrimeprazine, thioridazine, clozapine, pipamperone, prothipendyl, chlorpromazine, sulpiride, clopenthixol, chlorprothixene, cyamemazine), in 8 taking high-potency neuroleptics (haloperidol, fluspirilene, fluphenazine, penfluridol, bromperidol, flupenthixol), and in 7 taking both low- and high-potency neuroleptics. Tolerability was rated very good or good in 84% and moderate (n = 10) or poor (n = 7) in 16%. Co-administration does not lead to clinically relevant interactions, although some adverse events may occur more frequently because of synergism (Amrein R, Guntert TW, Dingemanse J, et al. Interactions of moclobemide with concomitantly administered medication: evidence from pharmacological and clinical studies. *Psychopharmacology* 1992;106:S24–S31).

neuroleptic + nadolol Co-administration increases neuroleptic plasma levels and may enhance a neuroleptic's therapeutic or toxic effects.

neuroleptic + nalmefene Nalmefene augmentation of neuroleptics successfully decreases residual positive symptoms in neuroleptic-stabilized schizophrenia (Rapaport MH, Wolkowitz O, Kelsoe JR, et al. Beneficial effects of nalmefene augmentation in neuroleptic-stabilized schizophrenic patients. *Neuropsychopharmacology* 1993;9:111–115).

neuroleptic + naloxone Naloxone (100 mg/day) added to neuroleptics for the treatment of negative schizophrenic symptoms produced clinical improvement and improvement in Brief Psychiatric Rating Scale and Clinical Global Impression Scale scores. No adverse interactions occurred.

neuroleptic + narcotic analgesic Co-administration may increase narcotic blood level and enhance the toxic effects of narcotic analgesics.

neuroleptic + neuroleptic Co-administration has not been shown to be more efficacious than treatment with a single neuroleptic. Con-

comitantly administered antipsychotics have been shown to affect each other's plasma concentrations; because of possible pharmacokinetic and pharmacodynamic interactions, plasma level monitoring has been questioned (Dahl SG. Plasma level monitoring of antipsychotic drugs. Clinical utility. *Clin Pharmacokinet* 1986;11:36–61; McCreadie RG, Mackie M, Wiles DH, et al. Within-individual variation in steady state plasma levels of different neuroleptics and prolactin. *Br J Psychiatry* 1984;144: 625–629).

neuroleptic + nicotine Nicotine significantly lowers neuroleptic plasma levels; smokers have less sedation, sleepiness, and hypotension compared to nonsmokers (Kim YJ. Tobacco smoking and psychotropic drug therapy. *Pharm News* 1992;21:1–11). Smoking cessation by patients taking neuroleptics may increase neuroleptic serum levels, placing them at greater risk for neuroleptic side effects (Blumberg D, Safran M. Effects of smoking cessation on serum neuroleptic levels. *Am J Psychiatry* 1991;148:1269).

neuroleptic + nifedipine Addition of nifedipine results in small but statistically significant improvements in schizophrenic symptoms and tardive dyskinesia. Nifedipine may significantly increase neuroleptic plasma concentrations, which could be due to inhibition of the liver metabolism of the neuroleptic by cytochrome P450 (De Beaurepaire R. Treatment of neuroleptic-resistant mania and schizoaffective disorders. *Am J Psychiatry* 1992;149:1614).

neuroleptic nonresponse Refractoriness to a trial of one or more neuroleptics given in adequate doses for 6–8 weeks. About 25% of schizophrenic patients do not respond to neuroleptic treatment. Most have serum neuroleptic and prolactin levels as high or higher than those of responsive patients, so poor response is not accounted for by inadequate dose. In some cases, "mega" doses can be beneficial. It is very difficult to identify nonresponders in advance, especially with a first episode of schizophrenia. Serum neuroleptic and prolactin measures may help identify those who are "nonresponsive" because of inadequate dose and who require unusually high doses (Brown WA, Farone S. Serum neuroleptic and prolactin levels as predictors of schizophrenic relapse. *In* Lieberman JA, Kane JM [eds], *Predictors of Relapse in Schizophrenia.* Washington, DC: American Psychiatric Press, 1986). In some studies, poor or no response has been associated with significantly enlarged ventricles (Luchins DJ, Lewine RRJ, Meltzer HY. Lateral ventricular size, psychopathology and medication response in psychosis. *Biol Psychiatry* 1984;19:29–44; Weinberger DR,

Bigelow LB, Kleinman JE et al. Cerebral ventricular enlargement in chronic schizophrenia. *Arch Gen Psychiatry* 1980;37:11–13). In others, nonresponders have been found to have higher neurological soft sign scores and lower Mini Mental State scores than responders do (Schulz SC, Conley RR, Kahn M, Alexander J. Nonresponders to neuroleptics: a distinct subtype. *In* Schulz SC, Tamminga CA [eds], *Schizophrenia: Scientific Progress.* New York: Oxford University Press, 1987, pp 341–350).

neuroleptic, oral   In clinical practice, an oral neuroleptic has practical disadvantages, including a high rate of patient noncompliance, erratic absorption from the gastrointestinal tract, and high first-pass metabolism in the liver.

neuroleptic/persistence   Neuroleptics may remain in plasma and body tissues for prolonged periods after drug discontinuation (Campbell A, Baldessarini RJ. Prolonged pharmacologic activity of neuroleptics. *Arch Gen Psychiatry* 1985;42:637; Hubbard JW, Ganes D, Midha KK. Prolonged pharmacologic activity of neuroleptic drugs. *Arch Gen Psychiatry* 1987; 44:99–100). In a study of plasma levels after abrupt neuroleptic discontinuation, average levels decreased to 21.8% of steady-state baselines by week 3, but rebounded to 119% in week 5 and remained at 35.8% in patients studied for 7 weeks (Sramek J, Herrera J, Costa J, Heh C. Persistence of plasma neuroleptic levels after drug discontinuation. *J Clin Psychopharmacol* 1987;7:436–437). Fluphenazine decanoate has been reported to persist for 6 months to 2 years after discontinuation (Wistedt B, Jorgenzon A, Wiles D. A depot neuroleptic withdrawal study: plasma concentrations of fluphenazine and flupenthixol and relapse frequency. *Psychopharmacology* 1982;78: 301–304; Pajari KL. Persistence of neuroleptic drugs in plasma and body tissues. *J Clin Psychopharmacol* 1988;8:446). This phenomenon has significance for clinical studies, especially with regard to drug-free washout periods.

neuroleptic + phenytoin   Co-administration may elevate phenytoin blood levels and increase risk of phenytoin toxicity.

neuroleptic plasma level/therapeutic   Range in which good antipsychotic effect occurs without undue side effects. Therapeutic levels have been tentatively identified for haloperidol, perphenazine, fluphenazine, and chlorpromazine.

neuroleptic/pregnancy   The closer to delivery a neuroleptic is taken, the greater the risk of extrapyramidal symptoms in the newborn. Risk can be minimized by lowering antipsy-

chotic dose or discontinuing it completely 2–3 weeks before delivery.

neuroleptic + propranolol   By competing for the same drug metabolizing enzymes, propranolol and a neuroleptic may increase each other's blood levels.

neuroleptic radioreceptor assay   (NRRA) Assay using a radiolabeled neuroleptic (usually spiroperidol) to measure levels of neuroleptics during treatment. The patient's serum or plasma (usually serum) is added to a test tube containing the radiolabeled neuroleptic; the amount of displacement from serum determines the blood level of the neuroleptic. The assay is useful with neuroleptics that block dopamine D_2 receptors.

neuroleptic relapse prevention therapy (NRPT) Phase of drug therapy for schizophrenia that follows neuroleptic-induced alleviation of acute psychotic symptoms (usually positive symptoms) and drug continuation for another 6 months. In relapse prevention therapy, an oral or depot neuroleptic is continued for 2–5 years (in some cases, indefinitely) to prevent relapse. For first-episode patients, relapse prevention therapy is recommended for 2 years because of the paucity of controlled studies lasting for longer periods. For multi-episode patients with a history of suicide attempts or aggressive behavior, such therapy may be indicated for 5 years or more. The goal is to use the minimum effective prophylactic dose, to manage side effects, especially extrapyramidal ones, and to gradually reduce neuroleptic dosage to the point at which intermittent therapy can be used with psychosocial therapies.

neuroleptic + sedative   Sedatives that induce hepatic drug metabolizing enzymes may reduce neuroleptic blood levels.

neuroleptic/seizures   Almost every neuroleptic may cause seizures. Neither the incidence of seizure associated with each of the available neuroleptics nor the mechanism of seizure production is known. Relative seizure risk may be related to the electroencephalographic (EEG) effects of various neuroleptics. All neuroleptics useful in the treatment of schizophrenia increase slow waves and decrease fast activity in the EEG. All can produce epileptic potentials in the EEG that vary according to neuroleptic dose, route, and rate of administration and the baseline EEG of the subject. Clozapine has the highest seizure risk, followed by chlorpromazine. Fluphenazine, molindone, haloperidol, and pimozide appear to have low epileptogenic properties. Seizures are more likely to occur when neuroleptic treatment is initiated or when doses are increased abruptly. The more drugs co-prescribed with a neuroleptic, the greater the risk of seizure occurrence. High blood levels, at least with some neuroleptics (e.g., clozapine) have been reported concomitantly with seizure occurrence. Seizure-proneness (e.g., epilepsy, history of seizures, organic brain disorder, abnormal EEG) also may increase risk. If seizures occur during treatment and lower neuroleptic doses are not feasible, concomitant anticonvulsant use is indicated. If this is done, the patient should be monitored for adverse drug interactions and, since these drugs may alter each other's plasma levels, monitoring of both neuroleptic and anticonvulsant plasma levels may be useful (Marks RC, Luchim, DJ. Anti-psychotic medications and seizures. *Psychiatr Med* 1991;9:37–52).

neuroleptic threshold theory   Postulation that the minimum effective antipsychotic dose of a neuroleptic ("threshold dose") correlates with the appearance of "fine motor" symptoms (micrography) as opposed to the appearance of manifest "coarse motor" extrapyramidal side effects (Haase HJ. Extrapyramidal modification of fine movements—a "conditio sine qua non" of the fundamental therapeutic action of neuroleptic drugs. *In* Bordelau JM [ed], *Extrapyramidal System and Neuroleptics.* Montreal: Editions Psychiatriques, 1961, pp 329–353). About 50% of acutely exacerbated schizophrenic patients respond to threshold doses, but no predictors are known to characterize responders. Neuroleptic threshold doses were found to be low, and the low-dose treatment strategy is supported by results of positron emission tomography (PET) and neuroleptic plasma level studies (Bitter I, Volavka J, Schrurer J. The concept of the neuroleptic threshold: an update. *J Clin Psychopharmacol* 1991;11:28–33). The concept of a neuroleptic threshold offers clinicians psychomotor and psychometric indicators for the operational definition of minimum effective dose. The concept, however, is limited to conventional neuroleptics and is not valid for atypical antipsychotics (e.g., clozapine, sulpiride, remoxipride, ritanserin, risperidone).

neuroleptic + tricyclic antidepressant (TCA)   Coadministration may decrease the metabolism of each drug, resulting in increased plasma concentrations of both. Anticholinergic, central nervous system depressant, and hypotensive effects of the drugs may be additive (Gram LF, Overo KF, Kirk L. Influence of neuroleptics and benzodiazepines on metabolism of tricyclic antidepressants in man. *Am J Psychiatry* 1974;131:863–866).

neuroleptic + tricyclic antidepressant (TCA) + lithium   See **neuroleptic + lithium + tricyclic antidepressant.**

neuroleptic + valproate + benzodiazepine   See **neuroleptic + benzodiazepine + valproate.**

neuroleptic + warfarin   Neuroleptics decrease the blood concentration of warfarin, resulting in decreased bleeding time.

neuroleptization   See **rapid tranquilization.**

Neurolite   See **technetium-99m-ethylcysteinate dimer (^{99m}Tc ECD).**

neurological soft sign   (NSS) Abnormal performance on testing such as dysdiadochokinesia, astereognosis, mirror phenomena, choreiform movements, primitive reflexes, diminished dexterity, sensory extinction, and cortical sensory loss. NSSs are often seen in schizophrenia. None by itself indicates a clearly localizable central nervous system lesion. A condensed neurological examination for NSSs has been published by Rossi and co-workers (Rossi A, De Cataldo S, Di Michele A, et al. Neurological soft signs in schizophrenia. *Br J Psychiatry* 1990;157:735–739).

neurological "watch"   Counterpart of constant observation for psychiatric patients that encompasses monitoring of the level of consciousness and notation of neurological abnormalities that are critical for the diagnosis of cerebral compression and other brain disorders.

neurology   Study of the etiology, diagnosis, and treatment of organic diseases of the nervous system. In some respects, it overlaps psychiatry and clinical psychology in dealing with behavior disorders related to diseases of the brain.

Neuromet   See **oxiracetam.**

neurometrics   Method to estimate the probability that quantitative data derived from qualitative features of brain electrical activity reflect dysfunction. Recordings of the resting electroencephalogram and various sensory-evoked potentials are obtained by computer under standardized testing conditions. Computer algorithms extract quantitative features from the recordings, which are then compared with a normative database using multivariate statistical procedures. The real-time value of any feature is replaced with an estimate of the probability that the value in an individual patient might be found in a healthy, normally functioning person of the same age. Such methods lend themselves readily to the creation of electrophysiological profiles for clinically identifiable disease states. Neurometrics form the basis of brain mapping.

neuromodulator   See **neurohormone.**

neuromorphometry   Art and science of measuring the shape and size of the central nervous system (CNS). It is used mainly for measuring ventricular size and CNS structures with magnetic resonance imaging (MRI) and computed tomography (CT).

neuron Nerve cell consisting of a cell body or soma with several extensions called the axon and dendrites. Axons carry signals from the soma to their terminals, where the signal is transmitted to other neurons across gaps between cells (synapses). At the synapse, neurotransmitter substances are released from the axon terminal. The neurotransmitter then binds to receptors on the receiving cells, resulting in electrochemical changes at the receptor sites that are then carried as a messenger from the dendrites to the soma and then possibly on to other cells.

Neurontin' See **gabapentin.**

neuropathy 1. Organic disease of any segment of the nervous system. 2. Disease involving cranial or spinal nerves.

neuropeptide Substance that translates emotions into bodily events. Originally defined as hormone-like substances produced by nerve cells, they include endorphins and substances studied in other contexts (e.g., lymphokines, growth factors) that carry messages to the brain and throughout the body to control a wide variety of bodily functions. Neuropeptides pass messages by attaching themselves to receptors on cell walls. They are produced by neurons, lymphocytes, and other cells of the body. Behavioral effects of neuropeptides came to light when De Vied (1971) discovered that vasopressin delays extinction of active shock avoidance in rats, leading to the hypothesis that vasopressin modulates processes underlying memory consolidation. In 1975, Hughes isolated two endogenous opioid peptides that are ligands for the morphine receptor (methionine- and leucine-enkephaline), suggesting that peptides are a class of synaptic agents. Neuropeptides are used as neurotransmitters by a large number of neurons in the central nervous system. At least 200 neuropeptides have been identified in the brain. They have been implicated in a diverse set of functions including endocrine secretion, various behaviors, pain perception, memory, blood pressure regulation, temperature regulation, cell growth and differentiation, appetite control, and immune function. Neuropeptides such as adrenocorticotropic hormone, thyrotropin-releasing hormone, and arginine vasopressin are believed to have important roles in maintaining cholinergic and monoaminergic transmission in the brain. Continued discovery of neuropeptides has produced a wave of interest in their possible roles in mental illness. Neuropeptides have been implicated as etiologic factors in different neuropsychiatric diseases on the basis of alteration in brain neuropeptide content or changes in plasma neuropeptide levels.

neuropeptide Y A 36-amino-acid residue found in human and other mammal species. It is found in neurons and frequently with catecholamines.

neurophysin Neuroendocrine peptide.

neuroplasticity Ability of the central nervous system to modify its structure in response to a variety of intrinsic and extrinsic factors.

neuroplegia Inhibition by a drug such as chlorpromazine of the entire autonomic nervous system.

neuroprotective therapy (NPT) Interventions that preserve the integrity and function of vulnerable neurons of the basal ganglia and thereby slow or halt clinical decline of degenerative disorders. The only established NPT is decoppering therapy for Wilson's disease, which forestalls decline and may reverse deficits and prevent illness onset in presymptomatic homozygotes.

neuropsychiatry Medical specialty combining neurology and psychiatry. It emphasizes the somatic substructure on which emotions are based and the organic disturbances of the central nervous system that give rise to psychiatric disorders. It bridges conventional boundaries imposed between mind and matter and intention and function.

neuropsychological sequelae Aftermath or results remaining after some insult, injury, or psychic trauma that affects psychological functioning.

neuropsychological tests (NPT) Indicators of cerebral integrity that are more sensitive than the clinical neurological examination or the electroencephalogram (EEG). They include the Weschler Adult Intelligence Scale—Revised, Benton Visual Retention Test, Rey Auditory Verbal Learning Test, and Lauria-Nebraska Neuropsychological Battery. In the early stages of dementing disease, NPTs probably exceed the diagnostic sensitivity of neuroradiological procedures, wherein gross morphological injury may not be present or detectable upon visual inspection. NPTs are especially informative for rehabilitation purposes, because data obtained describe functional cerebral integrity. NPTs characterize the person according to commonly recognized psychological processes (e.g., attention, memory, language, learning, concentration) that are generally understood to be important for educational, vocational, and social adjustment.

neuropsychology Study of the relationship between brain structure and function. It attempts to understand patterns and variations of cognition, emotion, and behavior in the context of cortical and subcortical neuroanatomical organization. Neuropsychology's main aim is to contribute to the diagnosis of neurological disease, monitoring severity and change in function. It also plays a major role in differentiating between organic and nonorganic disorders.

neuropsychometric testing Evaluation of memory, reasoning, coordination, writing, and the ability to express one's self and understand instructions. General indications include clarifying a differential diagnosis; presence of language disorder or emotional problems that hamper clinical assessment; need for a quantitative, detailed baseline picture to assess change in the patient; and assessment of strengths and weaknesses for detailed treatment planning.

neuroreceptor Central nervous system binding site for neurotransmitters. Neuroreceptors may be located on the neuron releasing the transmitter (presynaptic) or more commonly, on the neuron receiving the information (postsynaptic) transmitted by the neurotransmitter. The receptor usually is a protein molecule located on the cell membrane. Many psychoactive drugs (e.g., neuroleptics) act on the neuroreceptor or indirectly affect neuroreceptor functioning.

neuroregulator See **neurohormone.**

neuroscience Multidisciplinary science that includes molecular biology, cell biology, biochemistry/neurochemistry, neuropharmacology, clinical psychopharmacology, and many other disciplines.

Neurosine See **buspirone.**

neurosis Originally, any type of emotional disorder or disturbance other than a psychosis. Today the term may mean (a) psychoneurosis; (b) neurotic disorder in general; (c) specific types of neurotic disorders.

neurosteroid 3-Alpha-hydroxy-5-alpha-pregnan-20-one (allopregnilone or 3-alpha-OH-DHP) and 3-alpha,21-dihydroxy-5-alpha-pregnan-20-one (allotetrahydrodioxycortisone or THDOC). They potentiate the gamma aminobutyric acid (GABA) response in all possible forms of the $GABA_A$ receptor.

neurosyphilis Syphilitic infection of the central nervous system. Incidence declined markedly after the advent of antibiotic therapy, but it has not been eliminated and presents most frequently in attenuated and/or atypical forms. It may manifest itself in a number of distinct forms, including lues cerebri, syphilitic meningomyelitis, tabes dorsalis, and general paralysis of the insane. It has been called "the great imitator" because of its ability to mimic a great variety of medical, neurological, and psychological conditions.

neurotensin (NT) Endogenous peptide containing 13 amino acids (tridecapeptide) with several behavioral and pharmacological properties similar to those of antipsychotic drugs. It is found in the central nervous system (CNS) with highest concentrations in the hypothalamus, substantia nigra, periaqueductal gray matter, and limbic system, including the nucleus accumbens, septum, and amygdala. High-affinity binding sites (putative NT receptors) have been identified; they are also distributed heterogeneously in the mammalian CNS. NT is thought to be one of the central neurotransmitters or neuromodulators. Changes in transmission have been observed in schizophrenia. When administered centrally, NT appears to have effects similar to those of classic neuroleptic drugs. Low NT levels in cerebrospinal fluid may be associated with a delayed but significant response to treatment with an antipsychotic drug.

neurotic depression See **depression, neurotic.**

neurotoxicity Quality or action of a neurotoxin. See **neurotoxin.**

neurotoxin Agent (e.g., antibody) that destroys nerve cells and nervous tissue. See **1-methyl-4-phenyl-1,2,3,6-tetrahydropyridine.**

neurotransmission Transmission of an electrically mediated impulse along the nerve fiber and from one neuron to another across the synapse. It involves synthesis and storage of the neurotransmitter (NT) in the prejunctional nerve structure, release of the NT from the nerve terminal, interaction of the NT with a specific postjunctional receptor, rapid termination of the NT-receptor interaction, destruction of the NT, or reuptake into the terminal.

neurotransmitter (NT) Chemicals in the brain (e.g., dopamine, noradrenaline, serotonin) produced and released by nerve cells that stimulate activity in target cells (e.g., nerve cells, organ cells) interact with a specific receptor on an adjacent structure and elicit a specific physiological response. NTs are available for release from the nerve terminal as needed. They have a very short life after release (less than a millisecond) because they are either metabolized by enzymes into inactive products or taken back into the nerve terminal by an active reuptake process. Psychotropic drugs affect the rate of release of neurotransmitters and/or their destruction once released, or the activity state of the neuroreceptors. The list of NTs has grown from acetylcholine, norepinephrine, dopamine, serotonin, glycine, and gamma aminobutyric acid (GABA) to more than 60 possible NTs. According to Coyle, a substance can be considered an NT if it is contained by neurons, synthesized by neurons, released by neurons upon depolarization, and physiologically active on neurons, and if its postsynaptic physiological response is identical to that of the NT released by neurons (Coyle JT. Neuroscience and psychiatry. *In* Talbott JA, Hales RE, Yudofsky SC [eds], *Textbook of Psychiatry.* Washington, DC: American Psychiatric Press, 1988). Substances that meet most of these criteria are called "putative" NTs.

neurotransmitter, amine Fast-acting molecule rapidly inactivated following synaptic secretion via presynaptic reuptake systems. Included are epinephrine, norepinephrine, dopamine, histamine, and acetylcholine.

neurotransmitter, amino acid Fast-acting molecule rapidly inactivated following synaptic secretions via presynaptic reuptake systems. Amino acid neurotransmitters are present in numerous metabolic pools in the brain and are not restricted to one particular type of neuron. Included are aspartic acid, glutamic acid, gamma aminobutyric acid (GABA), and glycine.

neurotransmitter receptor There are two classes, fast and slow. Fast (class I) receptors are directly linked to an ion channel and mediate millisecond responses when activated by a transmitter (e.g., nicotine acetyl choline [ACh] receptor, gamma aminobutyric acid [GABA]$_A$ receptor, glycine receptor). Slow (class II) receptors mediate responses that are generally medullary, either dampening or enhancing the signal that acts on class I receptors (e.g., all subtypes of adrenergic receptors, muscarinic cholinergic [M_1 and M_2] receptors, dopaminergic [D_1 and D_2] receptors, serotonergic [5-HT$_{1A}$ and 5-HT$_2$] receptors, and opiate [omega and mu] receptors.

neurotransmitter system Organized tracts and nuclei (e.g., noradrenergic, serotonergic, dopaminergic) that use a neurotransmitter.

neurotransmitter transporter Molecule responsible for packaging transmitter into storage vesicles prior to release and for terminating signaling by removing transmitter from the synapse. Three major families of neurotransmitter transporters have been identified by amino acid homology from cloned cDNAs. Plasma membrane transporters can be divided into two distinct families, the Na$^+$/Cl-dependent transporters, including those for monoamines and inhibitory amino acids, and the Na$^+$/K$^+$-dependent transporters for glutamate. Within the Na$^+$/Cl-dependent transporter family, amino acid transporters form a subgroup distinguishable from the monoamine transporters. The third family comprises two vesicular monamine transporters. They are antiporters and require an H$^+$ electrochemical gradient. Neurotransmitter transporters may play a role in regulating the amount and duration of neurotransmitter availability to interact with pre- and postsynaptic receptors. Transporter function may be altered at the transcriptional or the posttranslational level (Hoffman BJ. Molecular biology of monoamine and glycine transporters: mechanisms of regulating neurotransmission. *Neuropsychopharmacology* 1993;9:33S).

neurotrophin Gene family of neurotrophic factors that includes nerve growth factor (NGF), brain-derived neurotrophic factor, neurotrophin-3 (NT-3), and neurotrophin-4 (NT-4). Preliminary research indicates that neurotrophins may have some therapeutic potential in Parkinson's disease, Alzheimer's disease, amyotrophic lateral sclerosis, and various types of peripheral neuropathy.

neutropenia Decreased amount of neutrophils in relationship to white blood count. It is a consequence of some drug treatments (e.g., clozapine, carbamazepine, chlorpromazine). See **agranulocytosis; aplastic anemia; blood dyscrasia; bone marrow.**

Newcastle cocktail Lithium, clomipramine, and tryptophan (2–3 g/day). It is used for treatment-resistant depression. Its effect should become apparent within 3 weeks; if not, the treatment should be discontinued. Tryptophan, which is considered the least important component, has been withdrawn from the market.

new chemical entity (NCE) Any new drug in development.

New Clinical Drug Evaluation Unit (NCDEU) Title of an annual meeting organized by the Clinical Research Division of the National Institute of Mental Health (NIMH). It is a good forum for the major components of psychopharmacological research (the NIMH, the Food and Drug Administration [FDA], the pharmaceutical industry, investigators) to present findings and informally discuss developments in psychopharmacology. Formerly called Early Clinical Drug Evaluation Unit (ECDEU).

New Drug Application (NDA) Submission to the Food and Drug Administration (FDA) by a pharmaceutical company for marketing approval for a new drug following completion of phase 1, 2, and 3 trials. It provides extensive details on the drug's development history; early studies; results of clinical trials; the nature of the drug; how it behaves in the body; and how it is manufactured, processed, packaged, and labeled.

Newman-Keuls procedure Method for making pairwise comparisons between means following a significant F test in analysis of variance.

nialamide (Niamid) Irreversible inhibitor of monoamine oxidase A and B no longer marketed in the United States.

Niamid   See **nialamide.**

Nicoderm   See **nicotine transdermal system.**

Nicorette   See **nicotine polacrilex gum.**

nicotinamide   Nonpeptide with low affinity for the benzodiazepine (BZD) receptor that may have mixed agonist-antagonist properties.

nicotinamide + carbamazepine   Nicotinamide can increase plasma carbamazepine (CBZ) levels and may cause CBZ toxicity (Bourgeois BF, Dodson WE, Ferrendelli JA. Interactions between primidone, carbamazepine and nicotinamide. *Neurology* 1982;32:1122–1126).

nicotine   Tertiary amine composed of a pyridine and pyrrolidine ring. It is the psychoactive drug primarily responsible for the addictive nature of tobacco use. It is a weakly water-soluble base that is rapidly absorbed through the lungs, skin, and buccal mucosa, depending on the pH of the tissue and the pH of the nicotine-delivery vehicle (e.g., smoke). Concentrations of nicotine in blood rise quickly during cigarette smoking and peak at its completion. Nicotine is also deposited in the lungs, spleen, liver, and brain, where concentrations are typically twice those of measurable blood concentrations. Only about 5–10% of nicotine is excreted; the majority of circulating nicotine is metabolized in the liver. Cigarette smoking, because it contains polycyclic aromatic hydrocarbons, is a potent inducer of cytochrome P450-mediated drug metabolism. Nicotine readily crosses the blood-brain barrier, leading to the release of acetylcholine, norepinephrine, dopamine, serotonin, vasopressin, growth hormone, cortisol, prolactin, neurophysin I, and adrenocorticotropic hormone, which eventually causes various pharmacological effects. Thus, nicotine is known to strongly affect both central acetylcholine and catecholamine systems, which may play a role in the etiology of major depression (Siever LJ. Role of noradrenergic mechanisms in the etiology of the affective disorders. *In* Meltzer HY, Coyle JT, Kopin IJ, et al [eds], *Psychopharmacology: The Third Generation of Progress.* New York: Raven Press, 1987, pp 493–504; Janowsky DS, Risch SC. Role of acetylcholine mechanisms in the affective disorders. *In* Meltzer HY, Coyle JT, Kopin IJ, et al [eds], *Psychopharmacology: The Third Generation of Progress.* New York: Raven Press, 1987, pp 527–533). It has been suggested that the association between smoking and depression results from shared predisposition, either genetic or environmental (Breslau N, Kilbey MM, Andreski P. Nicotine dependence and major depression: new evidence from a prospective investigation. *Arch Gen Psychiatry* 1993; 50:31–35). Nicotine and other constituents in cigarette smoke elevate blood pressure; cause tachycardia, arrhythmia, and vasoconstriction in cutaneous tissue and skin; lower body temperature; stimulate the central nervous system; inhibit diuresis; increase gastrointestinal tone; antagonize ulcer healing; and decrease pain threshold. Humans readily develop tolerance to the effects of nicotine. Cigarette smoking by women is associated with a dose-related reduction in fecundity and fertility and with early menopause (Baron JA, LaVecchia C, Levi F. The antiestrogenic effect of cigarette smoking in women. *Am J Obstet Gynecol* 1990;162: 502–514). Infertile women should be advised to stop or reduce smoking generally and especially before treatment by in-vitro fertilization (Rosevear SK, Holt DW, Lee TD, et al. Smoking and decreased fertilization rates in vitro. *Lancet* 1992;340:1195–1196). Smoking a pack of cigarettes a day yields sufficient amounts of nicotine (about 20–50 mg) to alter the pharmacological or physiological effects of medications.

nicotine + benzodiazepine   Data are conflicting. Smokers treated with benzodiazepines are reported to experience less drowsiness from their medication. Smokers showed a significantly shorter half-life and lower C_{max} (peak plasma concentration) of the active metabolites of clorazepate and desmethyldiazepam. Oxazepam clearance also has been found to be higher in smokers than in nonsmokers. However, no significant differences in clearance, volume of distribution, and half-life of diazepam, midazolam, lorazepam, and triazolam have been demonstrated between smokers and nonsmokers (Kim YJ. Tobacco smoking and psychotropic drug therapy. *Pharm News* 1992;21:1–11).

nicotine + chlorpromazine   Nicotine lowers chlorpromazine (CPZ) plasma level. Unless CPZ dosage is reduced after smoking cessation, CPZ plasma level may increase markedly and result in sedation (Stimmel GL, Falloon IRH. Chlorpromazine plasma levels, adverse effects and tobacco smoking: case report. *J Clin Psychiatry* 1983;44:420–422).

nicotine + clomipramine   Nicotine increases metabolism of clomipramine (CMI), resulting in lower levels of CMI and its active metabolite desmethylclomipramine and possibly interfering with CMI's therapeutic effects (Peters MD, Davis SK, Austin LS. Clomipramine: an antiobsessional tricyclic antidepressant. *Clin Pharm* 1990;9:165–178).

nicotine + clozapine   Nicotine reduces the average plasma level of clozapine (CLOZ) in smokers compared to nonsmokers. Patients should be monitored closely after smoking cessation since this may increase CLOZ serum level and side effects (Haring C, Fleischhacker

W, Schett P, et al. Influence of patient-related variables on clozapine plasma levels. *Am J Psychiatry* 1990;147:1471–1475).

nicotine dependence, mild   Presence of three or four dependence symptoms. It does not include interference in social, occupational, or recreational functioning.

nicotine dependence, moderate   Presence of five or six dependence symptoms, or three symptoms if one is interference in functioning.

nicotine dependence, severe   Presence of all seven dependence symptoms that apply to nicotine dependence.

nicotine + fluphenazine   Smoking significantly increases fluphenazine (oral and decanoate) clearance and decreases plasma level and shortens half-life (Ereshefsky L, Jann MW, Faklad SR, et al. Effects of smoking on fluphenazine clearance in psychiatric inpatients. *Biol Psychiatry* 1985;20:329–332).

nicotine + haloperidol   Smoking can reduce haloperidol (HAL) plasma levels (Jann M, Sakalad S, Ereshefsky L, et al. Effects of smoking on haloperidol and reduced haloperidol plasma concentrations and haloperidol clearance. *Psychopharmacology* 1986;90:468–470). Open studies indicate that nicotine powerfully potentiates the action of HAL in Gilles de la Tourette's syndrome. Nicotine gum alone, however, has less effect; although it reduced tic frequency for 1 hour after being chewed, it could have had a distracting effect (McConville BJ, Fogelson H, Norman AB, et al. Nicotine potentiation of haloperidol in reducing tic frequency in Tourette's disorder. *Am J Psychiatry* 1991;148:793–794; Miller DD, Kelly MW, Perry PJ, et al. The influence of cigarette smoking on haloperidol pharmacokinetics. *Biol Psychiatry* 1990;28:529–531). Case reports suggest that transdermally administered nicotine may ameliorate Tourette's syndrome symptoms in nonsmoking adolescents not satisfactorily controlled with dopamine blockers (HAL) (Silver AA, Sanberg PR. Transdermal nicotine patch and potentiation of haloperidol in Tourette's syndrome. *Lancet* 1993;342:182).

nicotine nasal spray   (NNS) Because nicotine absorption from the nasal mucous membranes is second only to absorption from inhalation, a nasal spray for smoking cessation has been devised. Preliminary testing demonstrated that plasma nicotine concentrations peaked 5 minutes after a 2-mg dose and that concentrations in the smoking range were easily obtained after repeated doses. In a 1-year, double-blind, placebo-controlled trial, NNS as an adjunct to group treatment was an effective aid to smoking cessation. Tobacco-withdrawal symptoms, craving for cigarettes, and weight gain in abstinent subjects were reduced by the active spray. Minor irritant side effects were frequent in both active and placebo sprays. No serious adverse effects were encountered (Sutherland G, Stapleton JA, Russell MAH, et al. Randomised controlled trial of nasal nicotine spray in smoking cessation. *Lancet* 1992;340:324–329). In two other studies, NNS significantly repressed the self-reported desire to smoke and the number of cigarettes smoked during short-term treatment (Perkins KA, Grobe JE, Stiller RL, et al. Nasal spray nicotine replacement suppresses cigarette smoking desire and behavior. *Clin Pharmacol Ther* 1992;52:627–634).

nicotine + neuroleptic   Nicotine significantly lowers neuroleptic plasma levels; smokers have less sedation, sleepiness, and hypotension compared to nonsmokers (Kim YJ. Tobacco smoking and psychotropic drug therapy. *Pharm News* 1992;21:1–11). Smoking cessation by patients taking neuroleptics may increase neuroleptic serum levels, placing them at greater risk for neuroleptic side effects (Blumberg D, Safran M. Effects of smoking cessation on serum neuroleptic levels. *Am J Psychiatry* 1991;148:1269).

nicotine/panic attacks   There have been reports that nicotine may have antipanic properties and that nicotine gum may be useful to treat panic attack patients (Brodsky L. Can nicotine control panic attacks? *Am J Psychiatry* 1985;142:524; Hughes JR. Nicotine gum to treat panic attacks? *Am J Psychiatry* 1986;143:271). Nicotine may suppress locus ceruleus firing and nicotine withdrawal may activate it. In high enough doses, nicotine may decrease anxiety because of its sedative effects. On the other hand, it may make panic attacks worse in some patients. The antipanic effect of nicotine should be interpreted with caution; more studies should be done with nonsmokers (Yeragani VK, Pohl R, Balon R, Jankowski W. Nicotine and panic attacks. *Biol Psychiatry* 1988;24:365–366).

nicotine polacrilex gum   (Nicorette) Nicotine bound to an ion exchange resin in a sugar-free unflavored chewing gum base. Chewing releases nicotine, which is absorbed through the buccal mucosa. Each piece of gum contains nicotine polacrilex equivalent to 2 mg of nicotine. Efficacy is greater when the gum is incorporated into a comprehensive behavioral treatment program. In a double-blind study of 315 medical patients who received either nicotine or placebo gum, use of the gum beyond the recommended 4-month period was prevalent but rarely persisted; investigators concluded that treatment for nicotine-gum dependence (beyond a recommendation to stop) is probably not needed unless use continues for more than 1 year. In the same study, when physicians did advise subjects to taper gum use, they did not have withdrawal symptoms, problems stopping, increased probability of smoking relapse, or weight gain. Patients should stop smoking completely before beginning to chew the gum. The gum may be addictive.

nicotine + psychotropic drug   Smoking can significantly modify the pharmacokinetics and pharmacodynamics of many psychotropic drugs. Physicians should attempt to determine the true extent of a patient's smoking since the number of cigarettes smoked per day affects the extent of these changes. Knowledge of the pharmacokinetic and pharmacodynamic changes produced by smoking may explain the therapeutic failure of a psychotropic medication and provide direction for dosage modification or substitution of one medication with another (Shoaf SE, Linnoila M. Interaction of ethanol and smoking on the pharmacokinetics and pharmacodynamics of psychotropic medications. *Psychopharmacol Bull* 1991;27:577–594).

nicotine replacement system   Method to systematically reduce nicotine plasma levels to enable smokers to quit. Four types have been clinically tested for efficacy and safety: nicotine polacrilex gum, nicotine transdermal patches, nicotine nasal spray, and a nicotine inhaler. Nicotine gum and nasal sprays are "fast acting," whereas patches provide slow steady-state administration and produce a gradual and better tolerated withdrawal.

nicotine/schizophrenia   Patients with schizophrenia are prone to smoke cigarettes, often quite heavily; smoking rates of 74–92% have been reported (Gopalaswamy AK, Morgan R. Smoking in chronic schizophrenia. *Br J Psychiatry* 1986;149:523). Smoking may decrease antipsychotic drug side effects through a pharmacokinetic interaction. It also may affect schizophrenic symptoms and antipsychotic actions through modulation of dopamine activity, and it is associated with a significant reduction in levels of parkinsonism. It is a significant factor that should be considered in assessing neuroleptic dose requirements, efficacy, and side effects. Physicians should be cautious in abruptly subjecting schizophrenic smokers to smoke-free therapeutic environments because nicotine abstinence symptoms may cloud the picture. Alternative methods for delivering nicotine to schizophrenics also should be investigated (Goff DC, Henderson DC, Amico E. Cigarette smoking in schizophrenia: relationship to psychopathology and medication side effects. *Am J Psychiatry* 1992;149:1189–1194).

nicotine/tardive dyskinesia   Smoking appears to be a risk factor for developing tardive dyskinesia (TD) in patients taking neuroleptics, although a cause-effect relationship is controversial. Because nicotine triggers dopamine (DA) release in the nigrostriatal and mesolimbic systems, worsening of TD by cigarette smoking is attributed to nigrostriatal supersensitivity to DA (Yassa R, Lol S, Korpassi A, Ally J. Nicotine exposure and tardive dyskinesia. *Biol Psychiatry* 1987;22:267–272).

nicotine transdermal system   (NTS) (Habitrol; Nicoderm; Nicotrol; Prostep) Patch that delivers nicotine through the skin over a 16-hour period as a part of a comprehensive smoking cessation program. It is worn during waking hours and removed at bedtime. Nicotine is administered initially at a dosage of 15 mg/day for 4–12 weeks, and then 10 mg/day for 2–4 weeks, followed by 5 mg/day for 2–4 weeks. The most common adverse effects are mild, transient erythema, pruritus, or burning at the application site. NTS should not be used for periods longer than 5 months. NTS has been a major breakthrough in the treatment of nicotine addiction. Patient acceptance and compliance is quite good. One-year success rates are reported to be 29–35% (Anon. Nicotine patches. *Med Lett Drugs Ther* 1992;34:37–38). Pregnancy risk category C.

nicotine transdermal system + acetaminophen   Because of the deinduction of hepatic enzymes on smoking cessation, a reduced dose of acetaminophen may be required at cessation of smoking and discontinuation of the nicotine transdermal patch.

nicotine transdermal system + imipramine   Because of deinduction of hepatic enzymes on smoking cessation, imipramine dosage reduction and discontinuation of the nicotine transdermal patch may be required at cessation of smoking.

nicotine transdermal system + oxazepam   Because of the deinduction of hepatic enzymes on smoking cessation, a reduced dose of oxazepam may be required at cessation of smoking and discontinuation of the nicotine transdermal patch.

nicotine transdermal system/pregnancy   Nicotine patches are not recommended during pregnancy or nursing because there is some positive evidence of fetal risk. Some experts, however, contend that nicotine replacement therapy during pregnancy is less hazardous than continued smoking, particularly for heavy smokers (Bercowitz NL. Nicotine replacement therapy during pregnancy. *JAMA* 1991;266:3174–3177).

nicotine transdermal system + propranolol Because of the deinduction of hepatic enzymes on smoking cessation, a reduced dose of propranolol may be required at cessation of smoking and discontinuation of the nicotine transdermal patch.

nicotine withdrawal Abstinence from smoking is associated with craving for cigarettes or other tobacco products, dysphoria, irritability, nervousness, decreased concentration, restlessness, increased appetite, headache, drowsiness, disturbed sleep, upset stomach, and tremor. Other symptoms include changes in the electroencephalogram (EEG), cognitive impairment, and decreases in psychomotor performance, heart rate, blood pressure, and plasma epinephrine levels. Symptoms typically peak during the first week or two of abstinence and are reported by more than half of those who discontinue smoking. Severity of withdrawal is associated with nicotine intake level prior to quitting, but the relationship is weak and unreliable (Fiore MC, Joremby DE, Baker TB, Kenford SL. Tobacco dependence and the nicotine patch. Clinical guidelines for effective use. *JAMA* 1992;268:2687–2694). Symptoms are more severe in white than in black smokers and in those with histories of major depression or anxiety disorders.

nicotinic receptor Cholinergic receptor located in autonomic ganglia, skeletal muscle neuromuscular end-plate, and spinal cord. It is a basic type of neurotransmitter receptor. Nicotinic receptors are classified as N-n or N-m receptors. N-m receptors are located in the neuromuscular junction, and N-n receptors are located in the autonomic ganglia, adrenal medulla, and brain. Tubocurarine and related neuromuscular blockers inhibit the N-m receptor, and the antihypertensive trimetaphan blocks the N-n receptor. The nicotinic acetylcholine receptor consists of five different proteins aggregated to form the receptor complex. The proteins are arranged so that the ion channel traverses the membrane. The neurotransmitter acetylcholine binds to the receptor complex, which results in the opening of the ion channel. Loss of central nicotinic receptors is a neurochemical hallmark of several degenerative brain disorders (e.g., Alzheimer's and Parkinson's diseases). See **muscarinic receptor.**

Nicotrol See **nicotine transdermal system.**

nifedipine (Adalat; Procardia) Calcium channel blocker that in recent years has been shown to be an effective treatment of hypertensive crisis associated with monoamine oxidase inhibitors (MAOIs) (Clary C, Schweizer E. Treatment of MAO hypertensive crisis with sublingual nifedipine. *J Clin Psychiatry* 1987;48: 249–250). It is rapidly absorbed through the mucous membrane under the tongue and normally begins to alleviate symptoms within 5–10 minutes without causing serious side effects. Sublingual and buccal administration techniques include biting the capsule and holding it under the tongue for 10–20 minutes, puncturing the capsule and squeezing the liquid under the tongue, and withdrawing the contents of the capsule with a syringe and administering them under the tongue. Some clinicians co-prescribe nifedipine along with MAOIs to decrease the risk of intracerebral bleeding (Stockley I. Chewing nifedipine to treat the MAOI-cheese reaction. *Pharm J* 1991; 247:784). Nifedipine may be effective for hypertensive emergencies of all causes. A single dose (10–20 mg) controlled hypertensive emergencies in all 118 patients tested with it. Patients with complications, including hypertensive encephalopathy, renal dysfunction, and/or angina, responded slower than did those without complications. One patient died as a result of cerebral hemorrhage (Gonzalez-Carmone VM, Ibara-Perez C, Jerjies-Sanchez C. Single-dose sublingual nifedipine as the only treatment in hypertensive urgencies and emergencies. *Angiology* 1991;42:908–913). Nifedipine also can be used to treat hypomania, but has been reported to cause serious depressive reactions and refractoriness to the therapeutic effects of electroconvulsive therapy and antidepressant drug therapy. In patients with depressive disorders, particularly if they arise without antecedent or obvious cause or are refractory to antidepressant treatment, consideration should be given to discontinuing nifedipine. In view of the widespread use of nifedipine, particularly in the elderly, physicians should be alert to the possibility of depression occurring as an adverse effect. Nifedipine has been shown to produce a statistically significant decrease in tardive dyskinesia following treatment with dosages up to 60 mg/day, without producing hypotension or bradycardia.

nifedipine + alcohol In healthy volunteers, the area under the plasma concentration-time profile of nifedipine increased 54% in the presence of alcohol. The maximum pulse rate was achieved more rapidly in the presence of alcohol, but neither increase in pulse rate nor change in blood pressure index reached significance between treatments. Patients should be warned of the potential consequences of alcohol consumption during nifedipine treatment (Qureshi S, Langaniere S, McGilveray IJ, et al. Nifedipine-alcohol interaction. *JAMA* 1990;264:1660–1661).

nifedipine + lithium Two doses of nifedipine had no effect on lithium clearance and glomerular filtration rate (GFR), but 6 and 12 weeks of nifedipine (40 mg/day) led to 30% reductions in lithium clearance with no effect on GFR (Bruun NE, Ibsen H, Skott P, et al. Lithium clearance and renal tubular sodium handling during acute and long-term nifedipine treatment in essential hypertension. *Clin Sci* 1988;75:609–613).

nifedipine + monoamine oxidase inhibitor (MAOI) Nifedipine is an effective treatment for MAOI hypertensive crisis (Clary C, Schweiger E. Treatment of MAO hypertensive crisis with sublingual nifedipine. *J Clin Psychiatry* 1987;48:249–250; Gonzalez-Carmone VM, Ibara-Perez C, Jerjies-Sanchez C. Single-dose sublingual nifedipine as the only treatment in hypertensive urgencies and emergencies. *Angiology* 1991;42:908–913). See **nifedipine.**

nifedipine + naloxone Co-administration is relatively well tolerated (Fudala PJ, Berkow LC, Fralich JL, Johnson RE. Use of naloxone in the assessment of opiate dependence. *Life Sci* 1991;49:1809–1814; Kanof PD, Handelsman L, Aronson MJ, et al. Clinical characteristics of naloxone-precipitated withdrawal in human opioid-dependent subjects. *J Pharm Exp Ther* 1992;260:355–363).

nifedipine + naltrexone Co-administration may precipitate delirium (Silverstone PH, Attenburrow MJ, Robson P. The calcium channel antagonist nifedipine causes confusion when used to treat opiate withdrawal in morphine-dependent patients. *Int Clin Psychopharmacol* 1992;7:87–90).

nifedipine + neuroleptic Addition of nifedipine results in small but statistically significant improvements in schizophrenic symptoms and tardive dyskinesia. Nifedipine may significantly increase neuroleptic plasma concentrations, which could be because of inhibition of the liver metabolism of the neuroleptic by cytochrome P450 (De Beaurepaire R. Treatment of neuroleptic-resistant mania and schizoaffective disorders. *Am J Psychiatry* 1992;149:1614).

nifedipine/opiate withdrawal Nifedipine is ineffective in the clinical treatment of opiate withdrawal. If combined with naltrexone, it may precipitate delirium (Silverstone PH, Attenburrow MJ, Robson P. The calcium channel antagonist nifedipine causes confusion when used to treat opiate withdrawal in morphine-dependent patients. *Int Clin Psychopharmacol* 1992;7:87–90).

nightmare Frightening or bad dream that must be differentiated from night terror (pavor nocturnus). In nightmares there is vivid and detailed dream recall, whereas in night terrors there is no recall or just a vague perception of a frightening dream-like experience. See **pavor nocturnus.**

night terror See **pavor nocturnus; nightmare.**

nigrostriatal system Part of the dopamine (DA) system that projects from the substantia nigra to the neostriatum (i.e., putamen and caudate). It controls complex muscular movements and posture and is involved in the coordination of voluntary movement. Reduced DA concentrations in this tract cause the stiffness, tremor, and muscular discoordination associated with Parkinson's disease.

nihilistic delusion See **delusion, nihilistic.**

nimetazepam Benzodiazepine currently available only in Japan.

nimodipine (Admon; Nimotop; Periplum) (NMD) 1,4 Dihydropyridine derivative and calcium channel blocker that has been marketed as a nootropic drug for the treatment of human cerebral function disorder. It readily crosses the blood-brain barrier and acts on cerebral neurons to limit influx of calcium ions, which is the putative mechanism by which it lessens ischemic damage after subarachnoid hemorrhage and stroke and slows the progression of some organic dementias. NMD has a wider spectrum of anticonvulsant action than verapamil. It has been found effective in the treatment of pure manic states and manic episodes in schizoaffective disorder. In preclinical studies, it attenuated opiate withdrawal. It effectively blocks cocaine-induced hyperactivity and dopamine overflow and normalizes the electroencephalogram (EEG) in cocaine users, even more effectively than carbamazepine. It has not been found effective in the treatment of the alcohol withdrawal syndrome. It is well tolerated and has minimal sedative and other side effects. Pregnancy risk category C.

nimodipine + carbamazepine Preliminary data indicate that nimodipine does not substantially influence carbamazepine (CBZ) pharmacokinetics (Ketter TA, Post RM, Worthington K. Principles of clinically important drug interactions with carbamazepine. Part II. *J Clin Psychopharmacol* 1991;11:306–313). Co-administration has been shown to be efficacious in a subgroup of patients with ultra-ultra rapid (ultradian) cycling (Post RM, Pazzaglia PJ, Ketter TA, et al. Carbamazepine and nimodipine in refractory bipolar illness: efficacy and mechanisms. *Neuropsychopharmacology* 1993;9:17S). Co-administration may decrease plasma nimodipine concentrations, necessitating increased doses to achieve adequate therapeutic levels (Tartara A, Galimberti CA, Manni R, et al. Differential effects of valproic acid and enzyme-inducing anticonvulsants on nimodipine pharmacokinetics in epileptic patients. *Br J Clin Pharmacol* 1991;32:335–340).

nimodipine + phenobarbital Co-administration may decrease plasma nimodipine concentrations and necessitate increased nimodipine dosage to achieve adequate therapeutic levels (Tartara A, Galimberti CA, Manni R, et al. Differential effects of valproic acid and enzyme-inducing anticonvulsants on nimodipine pharmacokinetics in epileptic patients. *Br J Clin Pharmacol* 1991;32:335–340).

nimodipine + phenytoin Co-administration may decrease plasma nimodipine concentrations and necessitate increased nimodipine dosage to achieve adequate therapeutic levels (Tartara A, Galimberti CA, Manni R, et al. Differential effects of valproic acid and enzyme-inducing anticonvulsants on nimodipine pharmacokinetics in epileptic patients. *Br J Clin Pharmacol* 1991;32:335–340).

nimodipine + valproic acid Co-administration may decrease plasma nimodipine concentrations and necessitate increased nimodipine dosage to achieve adequate therapeutic levels (Tartara A, Galimberti CA, Manni R, et al. Differential effects of valproic acid and enzyme-inducing anticonvulsants on nimodipine pharmacokinetics in epileptic patients. *Br J Clin Pharmacol* 1991 32:335–340).

Nimotop See **nimodipine.**

Niotal See **zolpidem.**

Nipolept See **zotepine.**

Nitan See **pemoline.**

Nitoman See **tetrabenazine.**

Nitrador See **nitrazepam.**

nitrazepam (Benzaline; Mogadon; Nitrador; Numbon) (NZP) 1,4 Benzodiazepine hypnotic biotransformed mainly by nitroreduction. Side effects include drowsiness and impaired performance the next day. It may cause confusion in the elderly and withdrawal effects if stopped suddenly after prolonged use. Mild to moderate renal insufficiency does not alter its kinetics. A case of depersonalization that began 9 days after the last dose of NZP and dramatically disappeared with reinstitution has been reported (Terao T, Yoshimura R, Terao M, Abe K. Depersonalization following nitrazepam withdrawal. *Biol Psychiatry* 1992;31:212–213). NZP is widely used in Europe but is not available in the United States.

nitrendipine Calcium channel blocker that has been used in the treatment of alcohol withdrawal syndrome to reduce the incidence of tremor and seizures.

nitric oxide Free radical that occurs in the brain and is thought to be the prime member of an entirely new class of neurotransmitters. When psychiatrist/neuroscientist Solomon Snyder's laboratory discovered that it is a crucial carrier of messages between brain cells, *Science* magazine in 1992 declared it the "molecule of the year." Discovery of its function in the brain established gases as an entirely new class of neural messengers and created a whole new way of thinking about biological signaling. In the brain, the enzyme that synthesizes nitric oxide is localized in discrete populations of neurons that are selectively resistant to neurotoxic damage as a result of stroke and Huntington's disease. In the peripheral autonomic nervous system, the enzyme occurs also in neurons to the adrenal medulla and posterior pituitary and in neurons that regulate peristalsis in the intestine. In all of these systems, nitric oxide operates as a neurotransmitter, released as a consequence of new stimulation (Dixon B. Nitric oxide goes center stage. *Br Med J* 1992;305:779). It is the messenger through which the white cells known as macrophages attack and destroy cancer cells and invading bacteria. It also is the substance that, released from endothelium in response to acetylcholine and other vasodilators, makes blood vessels relax. It also mediates penile erection. It is difficult to measure because its half-life is only a few seconds. It should not be confused with nitrous oxide.

nitrocellulose paper Paper-like sheet that very tightly binds RNA or DNA.

"nitrous" Street name for nitrous oxide.

nitrous oxide (N_2O) Gas that produces analgesic effects when inhaled and in high concentrations can produce anesthesia. Its principal application is as an adjuvant to anesthesia in dentistry or surgery. Abuse tends to occur chiefly among professionals. When self-administered, it produces impaired concentration, dreaminess, euphoria, numbness and tingling, unsteadiness, and visual and auditory disturbances. It is usually inhaled as 35% N_2O mixed with oxygen; inhalation of 100% N_2O may be fatal. It is available in tanks and cartridges that can be purchased in hardware, gourmet, restaurant supply, and drug paraphernalia stores. The cartridge is placed in a special "charger" (purchased in a drug paraphernalia store). It is inhaled by placing the mouth over the dispensing spout and pushing down the dispensing lever, which punctures the opening to the ampule and releases its contents. Daily use of N_2O for several months can result in a paranoid reaction with confusion. Also called "laughing gas."

Nizoral See **ketoconazole.**

N-methyl-D-aspartate (NMDA) Synthetic amino acid that activates a subclass of glutamate receptors.

N-methyl-D-aspartate (NMDA) receptor One of the three subclasses of glutamate (excitatory amino acid) receptors. It is an integral membrane protein that comprises recognition domains for glutamate and several endogenous co-agonist and modulatory substances (e.g., glycine, polyamines). NMDA receptors are widespread in the brain (cortex, amygdala, basal ganglia) and far more prevalent than noradrenergic and serotonergic receptors. They are expressed widely throughout the vertebrate central nervous system and may participate in neurotransmission at many, if not the majority, of excitatory synapses in the brain and spinal cord (Rogawski MA. The NMDA receptor, NMDA antagonists and epilepsy therapy. *Drugs* 1992;44:279–292). Because NMDA receptor activation induces a form of neuronal plasticity known as long-term potentiation, it is important in learning and memory. Alcohol inhibition of the receptor may be involved in the neural and cognitive impairments of alcohol intoxication (e.g., learning and memory). Prolonged receptor stimulation due to ischemia (heart attack, stroke), hypoglycemia, or trauma is thought to mediate injury and/or death of neurons. The receptors also are important in neurodegenerative disorders (e.g., parkinsonism, Alzheimer's disease, Huntington's disease); there is vigorous activity to develop antagonists to suppress their activity in degenerative conditions. Their action can be modulated by the amino acid neurotransmitter glycine. Phencyclidine (PCP) antagonizes their excitatory effects. NMDA agonists can induce seizures.

Nobesine-75 See **diethylpropion.**

Nobrium See **medazepam.**

"nocebo" effect Adverse effect of a placebo.

nociceptive Impulses that give rise to pain sensations.

Noctamid See **lormetazepam.**

Noctamide See **lormetazepam.**

Noctec See **chloral hydrate.**

Nocton See **lormetazepam.**

nocturia Need to urinate during the night. It is extremely common in the elderly and is probably related to various factors (diabetes, use of diuretics, decreased bladder capacity, decreased renal concentrating ability). Surveys indicate that nocturia disturbs sleep 3 or more times a week in almost 60% of persons 65 years of age and older.

nocturnal confusion Episodes of delirium and disorientation close to or during night-time sleep. It is often seen in the elderly and may indicate organic central nervous system deterioration.

nocturnal encopresis See **encopresis.**

nocturnal enuresis See **enuresis.**

nocturnal epilepsy See **epilepsy, nocturnal.**

nocturnal leg cramps Painful sensations of muscular tightness or tension in the calf or foot that occur during sleep. They may be associated with prior vigorous exercise, pregnancy, diabetes, metabolic and neuromuscular disorders, arthritis, or Parkinson's disease. They may occur for the first time in the elderly.

nocturnal myoclonus See **nocturnal movements in sleep.**

nocturnal penile tumescence (NPT) Natural periodic cycle of penile erections that occur during sleep and typically are associated with rapid eye movement (REM) sleep. It can be used as the basis for diagnosis of organic versus psychogenic erectile dysfunction. NPT is monitored by two mercury-filled strain gauges, one placed at the base and one at the tip of the penis to measure circumference changes. An NPT episode is defined as an abrupt increase in base circumference (3 mm or greater) during a 60-second period that is maintained at least 5 minutes. Full tumescence is a 15-mm or greater increase in tip and base circumference. Partial tumescence is tip and base change of 3–15 mm (Karacan I, Salis PJ, Williams RL. The role of the sleep laboratory in the diagnosis and treatment of impotence. *In* Williams RL, Karacan I [eds], *Sleep Disorders: Diagnosis and Treatment.* New York: John Wiley & Sons, 1989, pp 353–382). Abnormally diminished NPT time and rigidity is found in one-fourth to one-third of depressed men (Thase ME, Reynolds CF, Jennings JR, et al. Diminished nocturnal penile tumescence in depression: a replication study. *Biol Psychiatry* 1992;31:1136–1142). NPT is largely unaffected by changes in depression or sexual attitudes and behavior in early remission. NPT appears to be relatively stable during the acute course of a depressive episode (Nofzinger EA, Thase ME, Reynolds CF III, et al. Sexual function in depressed men: assessment by self-report, behavioral and nocturnal penile tumescence measures before and after treatment with cognitive behavior therapy. *Arch Gen Psychiatry* 1993;50:24–30).

nocturnal sleep See **sleep, nocturnal.**

"(the) nod" Street term for state of tranquility and sleepiness that follows a "rush" induced by intravenous heroin.

n of 1 design See **single-patient design.**

Noludar See **methyprylon.**

nomenclature List or catalog of approved terms for describing and recording clinical observations. It provides the basis for a classification system and meaningful communication among scientists and practitioners in a given field.

nominal scale   Simplest scale of measurement. It is used for characteristics that have no numerical values.

nomogram   Graph on which a number of variables are plotted to form a computation chart for the solution of complex numerical formulae. It represents an equation containing three variables by means of three scales so that a straight line cuts the scales in values of three variables, satisfying the equation. Also called "ABAC"; "alignment chart"; "nomograph."

nomograph   See **nomogram.**

nomothetic measure   In the behavior sciences and in psychiatry, measurement using an instrument that has been standardized against the disorder it presumes to measure; scores for those with the index disorder and normal populations should be available. See **idiographic measure.**

nonadditive genetic variance   See **genetic variance, nonadditive.**

nonapproved drug use   See **"off label" drug use.**

nonbarbiturate hypnotic   See **hypnotic, nonbenzodiazepine.**

nonbenzodiazepine anxiolytic   See **anxiolytic, nonbenzodiazepine.**

nonbenzodiazepine hypnotic   See **hypnotic, nonbenzodiazepine.**

noncomparative trial   Trial in which the investigational drug is compared only to placebo and not to another active drug. In comparison trials, a conventional marketed drug is used as a comparator.

noncompliance with medical treatment   DSM-III-R category for a patient's lack of cooperation with the physician in the prescribed medical care. It may be due to denial of illness, phobias, religious beliefs, and personal value judgments about the advantages and disadvantages of treatment. Estimates of noncompliance range from 4% to 92% (average, 30–35%). Partial or full noncompliance with a medical regimen is an important cause of ineffective pharmacotherapy. Factors that affect compliance include the number of daily drug doses to be taken (compliance is better with fewer doses); the number of drugs to be taken (the more drugs, the less compliance); and age (the elderly are often treated with multiple drugs, many of which have to be taken in divided daily doses and which may cause some impairment in reading and memory).

noncontact paraphilia   See **paraphilia, noncontact.**

nonconvulsive seizure   See **seizure, nonconvulsive.**

nonconvulsive status   See **status, nonconvulsive.**

nondeclarative memory   See **memory, nondeclarative.**

nondifferential misclassification   See **misclassification, nondifferential.**

nondisjunction   Failure of the two members of a chromosome pair to separate during cell division, resulting in one daughter cell receiving both and the other none of the chromosomes in question, causing the presence of an extra chromosome in that cell. It is the most common cause of the extra-chromosome Down syndrome.

nonfearful panic disorder   See **panic disorder, nonfearful.**

nonfocal grand mal seizure   See **seizure, primary generalized.**

nonlinear pharmacokinetics   See **pharmacokinetics, nonlinear.**

nonmedical drug use   1. Use of a medically sanctioned drug for a different purpose (e.g., use of a sleeping pill to produce a drunken state). 2. Use of a drug (e.g., mescaline) that has no currently recognized medical purpose. Nonmedical drug use often involves use of multiple drugs, including alcohol.

nonmutually exclusive tests   Two or more events for which the occurrence of one event does not preclude occurrence of the others.

nonparametric method   Statistical test that makes no assumptions regarding distribution of the observations.

nonparametric test of significance   Statistical procedure that does not require assumption of normality and that often is based on analysis of ranks other than the distribution of the actual scores themselves. Widely used examples are the chi-squared, Spearman rank order correlation, and Mann-Whitney U tests.

nonprobability sample   See **sample, nonprobability.**

nonrandomized trial   Clinical trial in which subjects are assigned to treatment other than on a randomized basis. It is subject to several biases.

non-REM sleep   See **sleep stage non-REM.**

non-REM sleep intrusion   See **sleep intrusion, non-REM.**

nonresponsive psychosis   See **psychosis, nonresponsive.**

nonselective monoamine oxidase inhibitor (MAOI) + levodopa   See **monoamine oxidase inhibitor + levodopa.**

nonsense codon   See **codon, nonsense.**

nonsituational aggression   See **aggression, nonsituational.**

nonsteroidal anti-inflammatory drug   (NSAID) Any of a heterogeneous group of compounds, mostly organic acids, that have anti-inflammatory, analgesic, and antipyretic actions. NSAIDs appear to owe their therapeutic efficacy to inhibition of prostaglandin biosynthesis. Prostaglandins have a variety of biological effects, including mediation of the inflammatory response. They also are important in renal physiological function, including maintenance of renal blood flow and glomerular filtration. When this prostaglandin-mediated compensatory mechanism is suppressed by NSAID therapy, impairment in renal function can result.

nonsteroidal anti-inflammatory drug + lithium See **lithium + nonsteroidal anti-inflammatory drug.**

nontoxic goiter See **Hashimoto's thyroiditis.**

nonulcer dyspepsia Common functional gastrointestinal disorder manifested by postprandial fullness or bloating, early satiety, excessive flatulence, upper abdominal pain, excessive belching, and nausea or vomiting. Symptoms can be persistent and occasionally disabling. Although pathogenesis is unclear, it may be due to hypersensitive central serotonin (5-HT) receptors resulting in abnormalities in gastric motility. Serotonin uptake inhibitors (e.g., fluoxetine, fluvoxamine) produce a similar syndrome (Silverstone T, Tinner P. *Drug Treatment in Psychiatry.* London: Routledge and Kegan Paul, 1988; Dinan TG, Yatham LN, Barry S, et al. Serotonin supersensitivity: the pathophysiologic basis of non-ulcer dyspepsia? *Scand J Gastroenterol* 1990;25:541–544; Chua A, Keating J, Hamilton D, et al. Central serotonin receptors and delayed gastric emptying in non-ulcer dyspepsia. *Br Med J* 1992;305:280–282). Nonulcer dyspepsia has been diagnosed as dysmotility-like dyspepsia, gastroesophageal reflux-like dyspepsia, aerophagia, and essential dyspepsia.

Nootrop See **piracetam.**

nootropic drug Psychotropic compound that acts directly on the higher integrative brain mechanisms, enhancing their efficacy and resulting in a positive, direct impact on mental functions (Guirgea C. The pharmacology of nootropic drugs: geropsychiatric implications. *In* Deniker P, Radouco-Thomas C, Villeneuve A [eds], *Proceedings of the 10th Congress of the Collegium Internationale Neuro-Psychopharmacologicum, 1976.* Oxford: Pergamon Press, 1978, pp 67–72). The term *nootropic* is used in different ways. In central Europe, it means all drugs used to improve cognitive impairment. In Scandinavia, nootropic drugs are used to favor brain metabolism and protect the brain from toxic effects. Nootropics are analogs of gamma aminobutyric acid (GABA) that are believed to enhance higher cerebral functions selectively and to have no effects on the limbic and reticular activating systems. They have no sedative, analeptic, analgesic, neuroleptic, or tranquilizing properties, and do not act as agonists or antagonists of receptors of any known neurotransmitter. They are thought to have beneficial effects on cognitive functioning, particularly in the elderly. The most widely studied nootropic is piracetam. Potential nootropics include aniracetam, 3OH-aniracetam, CAS 493, D-cycloserine, etiracetam, galantamine, HOE 427, idebenone, milacemide, oxiracetam, pramiracetam, rolziracetam, S-12024-2, tacrine, tanakan, tenilsetam, trandolapril, and velnacrine. Sometimes other drugs are classified as nootropics, including fipexide, hydergine, meclofenoxate, and vinpocetine. To date, most nootropics have failed to ameliorate cognitive decline in dementia of the Alzheimer type.

Nootropil See **piracetam.**

Noradex See **orphenadrine.**

noradrenaline (NA) See **norepinephrine.**

noradrenaline hypothesis of depression Postulation that enhancement of noradrenergic transmission is involved in at least some of the observed therapeutic effects of antidepressant drugs in the treatment of depressive states. Now entering its third decade, this hypothesis has been progressively expanded to accommodate involvement of other transmitter systems as well as changes in receptor sensitivity, cellular performance or output, or second-messenger function observed after repeated antidepressant treatment. Supporting evidence is largely indirect. It includes preclinical findings of central nervous system changes in noradrenaline (norepinephrine) levels or receptor activity, most typically in rodents, clinical probes of adrenergically mediated neuroendocrine function in depressive states, and acute challenge studies with catecholamine-releasing agents (Katz RJ, Lott M, Landau P, Waldmeier P. A clinical test of noradrenergic involvement in the therapeutic mode of action of an experimental antidepressant. *Biol Psychiatry* 1993;33:261–266).

noradrenaline hypothesis of schizophrenia Postulation that the lack of goal-directed behavior in schizophrenia may be related to degeneration of the cortical noradrenaline (norepinephrine) reward system. There has been little evidence to support the hypothesis.

noradrenergic Of or relating to neurons that use noradrenaline (norepinephrine) as a neurotransmitter. See **adrenergic receptor.**

noradrenergic receptor See **adrenergic receptor.**

norclozapine (NOR) N-desmethylated metabolite of clozapine. It is not clearly established whether it is pharmacologically active.

norcocaine Only known pharmacologically active metabolite of cocaine (COC). It is produced by N-desmethylation of COC in hepatic microsomes. Kinetics are believed to be similar to those of COC. It is hepatotoxic and capable of inducing hepatic necrosis (Ranckman Ed, Rosen GM Cavagnars J. Norcocaine nitroxide—a potential hepatotoxic metabolite of cocaine. *Mol Pharmacol* 1982;21:458–463).

nordiazepam   See **desmethyldiazepam.**

norepinephrine   (NE) Principal neurotransmitter released from nerve endings of the sympathetic nervous system. It is synthesized from dopamine in the adrenergic neurons and is related to epinephrine, which has one more methyl group. Major metabolic products are dihydroxyphenylglycol (DHPG), 3-methoxy-4-hydroxyphenylglycol (MHPG), and vanillylmandelic acid (VMA). Plasma levels of NE and its metabolites are determined by a variety of competing factors, including level of sympathetic nervous system activity, rates of intraneuronal NE synthesis and release, rates of intraneuronal reuptake and diffusion into extraneuronal tissues, and site and methodology of sampling (Eisenhofer G, Goldstein DS, Ropchak TG, et al. Source and physiological significance of plasma 3,4-dihydroxyphenylglycol and 3-methoxy-4-hydroxyphenylglycol. *J Autonom Nerv Syst* 1988;24:1–14). NE in the brain is correlated with mood. It also participates in regulating arousal and memory. Functional excesses in the brain have been implicated in the pathogenesis of manic states; deficits have been implicated in certain depressive states. Cocaine's euphorigenic action may be due to provocation of a temporary functional excess of NE. Presynaptic metabolism of NE results from the activity of monoamine oxidase (MAO). Because MAO activity in presynaptic nerve endings increases with age, NE metabolism also increases, leading to decreased amounts of NE neurotransmission in the elderly. Also called "noradrenaline."

norepinephrine blockade   Can be produced by some antidepressants. It may result in diaphoresis, jitteriness, tremors, tachycardia, and erectile and ejaculatory dysfunction.

norepinephrine tartrate   (Levophed) Primary amine that differs from epinephrine by the absence of a methyl group on the nitrogen atom. It functions as a powerful peripheral vasoconstrictor, inotropic stimulator of the heart, and dilator of coronary arteries. It is used to restore blood pressure in certain acute hypotensive states. It does not cross the blood-brain barrier.

norethandrolone   Anabolic steroid that in men produces decreased libido, decreased sexual potency, diminished testicular size, and azoospermia, with recovery several months after treatment is discontinued. It may cause permanent testicular damage.

Norflex   See **orphenadrine.**

norfluoxetine   Demethylated metabolite of fluoxetine (FLX) that is as potent as the parent drug in terms of serotonin uptake inhibition. Elimination half-life may be as long as 330 hours, resulting in a delay of several weeks before steady-state plasma concentration is established and a lengthy washout period when FLX is discontinued; pharmacologically active compounds are present in the body up to 7 weeks following an FLX dose, and the full pharmacological effects of FLX and norfluoxetine following an increase or decrease in daily dose may not occur for several days or weeks.

Normabrain   See **piracetam.**

normal control   (NC) Subject that does not have the symptom(s) or illness being studied. Effects of an experimental treatment on the "ill" population are compared with those in normal control subjects.

normal distribution   Symmetrical, bell-shaped probability distribution. Also called "gaussian distribution."

normal pressure hydrocephalus   See **hydrocephalus, normal pressure.**

normal sleep   See **sleep, normal.**

normal-weight bulimia   See **bulimia, normal-weight.**

norm database   Database of values collected from a normal population.

normeperidine   Meperidine metabolite that may produce dysphoria, tremulousness, hyperreflexia, and seizures (Karko RF, Foley KM, Grabinoski PY, et al. Central nervous system excitatory effects of meperidine in cancer patients. *Am Neurol* 1983;13:180–185).

Normison   See **temazepam.**

Normodyne   See **labetalol.**

normorphine   Demethylated morphine metabolite.

Normoson   See **ethchlorvynol.**

Norpace   See **disopyramide.**

Norpramin   See **desipramine.**

19-nortestosterone   Testosterone in which the 19-methyl group is deleted (e.g., nandrolone). These compounds act directly on androgen receptors, but with greater affinity than testosterone. They have a direct effect on the testes that results in incomplete recovery of testicular function after prolonged use (Bijlsma JWJ, Dunrsma, SA, Phijssen JKK, et al. Influence of nandrolone decanoate on the pituitary gonadal axis in males. *Acta Endocrinol* 1982;101:108–112).

northern blotting   See **Southern blotting.**

nortriptyline   (Aventyl; Pamelor) (NOR; NTL) Secondary amine tricyclic antidepressant

(TCA) comparable in efficacy and overall safety to other TCAs. Its major metabolite is E-10-hydroxynortriptyline. NOR is a demethylated metabolite of amitriptyline with fewer anticholinergic effects and was considered by many clinicians to be a first-line choice for depressed elderly patients before the advent of selective antidepressants (e.g., bupropion, fluoxetine). It is among the most studied TCAs. It is the only heterocyclic antidepressant in which therapeutic response increases with the plasma level up to a maximum point (50–150 ng/ml), beyond which response tends 'to diminish (therapeutic window). Plasma level monitoring may be necessary to achieve optimal therapeutic response. When similar doses are given, plasma levels vary extensively among individual patients because of the great variation in the liver cytochrome P450 enzyme, which hydroxylates NOR. NOR has been found effective in the treatment of emotional lability following stroke (Robinson RG, Parikh RM, Lipsey JR, et al. Pathological laughing and crying following stroke: validation of a measurement scale and a double-blind treatment study. *Am J Psychiatry* 1993; 150:286–293). Pregnancy risk category D.

nortriptyline + alcohol   Intermittent ingestion of low levels of alcohol has no effect on steady-state nortriptyline concentrations.

nortriptyline/breast milk   No detectable levels have been found in the serum of nursing mothers and their infants. Although some infants developed low concentrations of 10-hydroxynortriptyline, no adverse effects were attributed to it (Wisner KL, Perel JM. Serum nortriptyline levels in nursing mothers and their infants. *Am J Psychiatry* 1991;148:1234–1236).

nortriptyline + carbamazepine   Carbamazepine (CBZ) may enhance hepatic hydroxylation of nortriptyline, producing relatively low levels of the parent compound and elevated ratios of the metabolite 10-hydroxynortriptyline to nortriptyline (Baldessarini RJ, Teicher MH, Cassidy JW. Anticonvulsant cotreatment may increase metabolites of antidepressants and other psychotropic drugs. *J Clin Psychopharmacol* 1988;8:381–382). In another study, CBZ reduced nortriptyline concentrations by 67% (Brosen K, Kragh-Sorensen P. Concomitant intake of nortriptyline and carbamazepine. *Ther Drug Monit* 1993;15:258–260).

nortriptyline + clozapine   Co-administration can be effective and safe for depression occurring during clozapine treatment for chronic schizophrenia.

nortriptyline + cyclosporine   In depressed cardiac transplant patients being treated with cyclosporine immunosuppressive therapy, addition of nortriptyline does not cause adverse effects. However, its precise effect on cyclosporine levels needs further evaluation.

nortriptyline + fluconazole   In a 65-year-old woman taking nortriptyline (NOR) (75 mg/day), bumetanide, cyclosporine, metoclopramide, and morphine, the addition of fluconazole (initial dose 200 mg, followed by 100 mg/day) raised NOR serum drug concentration from 140 to 252 ng/ml (Gannon RH, Anderson ML. Fluconazole-nortriptyline drug interaction. *Ann Pharmacother* 1992;26:1456–1457).

nortriptyline + fluoxetine   Co-administration may be effective in patients resistant to a standard antidepressant and a full course of electroconvulsive therapy (Seth R, Jennings AL, Bindman J, et al. Combination treatment with noradrenaline and serotonin reuptake inhibitors in resistant depression. *Br J Psychiatry* 1991;161:562–569). Fluoxetine (FLX) can markedly elevate nortriptyline plasma level at steady state (2–11 times), apparently through inhibition of the P450 enzyme system. The interaction may result in hypotension, adverse cardiovascular effects (prolongation of PR, QRS, and QT intervals), a grand mal seizure, and anticholinergic delirium. Thus, nortriptyline plasma levels should be monitored during co-administration (Vaughan DA. Interaction of fluoxetine with tricyclic antidepressants. *Am J Psychiatry* 1988;145:1478; Kahn DG. Increased plasma nortriptyline concentration in a patient cotreated with fluoxetine. *J Clin Psychiatry* 1990;51:36).

nortriptyline + fluvoxamine   Fluvoxamine increases nortriptyline plasma concentration. This may potentiate antidepressant effects, but also may cause adverse reactions (Bertschy G, Vandel S, Vandel B, et al. Fluvoxamine-tricyclic antidepressant interaction. *Eur J Clin Pharmacol* 1991;40:119–120).

nortriptyline + lithium   In a series of elderly patients on lithium augmentation for refractory depression, co-administration caused myoclonus, weakness, tremor, and neurotoxicity (Lafferman J, Solomon K, Ruskin P. Lithium augmentation for treatment resistant depression in the elderly. *J Geriatr Psychiatry Neurol* 1988;1:49–52). Caution should be used with higher doses of either drug in the elderly.

nortriptyline + methylphenidate   Methylphenidate can raise the plasma level of nortriptyline and potentiate its antidepressant effects (Wharton RN, Perel JM, Dayton PG, Malitz S. A potential use for methylphenidate with tricyclic antidepressants. *Am J Psychiatry* 1971; 127:1619–1625).

nortriptyline + paroxetine   Co-administration may require lower doses of each drug.

nortriptyline + pergolide Co-administration has been used to treat patients refractory to nortriptyline alone. Response is usually rapid (within a week), but without incremental improvement over the next month. Some patients tolerate the combination well; others develop nausea and vomiting that may or may not respond to pergolide dose reduction (Bouckoms A, Mangini L. Pergolide: an antidepressant adjuvant for mood disorders. *Psychopharmacol Bull* 1993;29:207–211).

nortriptyline + sertraline Co-administration can be effective in patients resistant to a standard antidepressant and a full course of electroconvulsive therapy (Seth R, Jennings AL, Bindman J, et al. Combination therapy with noradrenaline and serotonin reuptake inhibitors in resistant depression. *Br J Psychiatry* 1992;161:562–565).

Norval See **mianserin.**

"nose candy" Street name for cocaine.

"nose powder" Street name for cocaine.

nosology Identification and classification in medicine. Psychiatric nosology is a way of looking at behavioral disorders as distinct, clearly separable entities, each with its own symptomatology, causation, outcome, and treatment.

"no-suicide" contract Agreement between patient and physician that the patient will refrain from suicidal actions and notify the physician if suicidal thoughts or plans are contemplated and that the physician or designated replacement will be available at all times to consult with the patient. Some clinicians find the "contract" helpful, others do not. No substantive data from scientific studies support its efficacy.

Noveril See **dibenzepin.**

Novocain See **procaine.**

Novo-Chlorhydrate See **chloral hydrate.**

Novo-Chlorpromazine See **chlorpromazine.**

Novoclopate See **clorazepate.**

Novodipam See **diazepam.**

Novodorm See **triazolam.**

Novoflupam See **flurazepam.**

Novo-Flurazine See **trifluoperazine.**

Novohexidyl See **trihexyphenidyl.**

Novolorazepam See **lorazepam.**

Novomepro See **meprobamate.**

Novoperidol See **haloperidol.**

Novopramine See **imipramine.**

Novo-Ridazine See **thioridazine.**

Novosecobarb See **secobarbital.**

Novotriptyn See **amitriptyline.**

Novoxapam See **oxazepam.**

Nozinan See **levomepromazine.**

n-terminal pro-opiomelanocortin (N-POMC) Peptide of 76 amino acids. Plasma N-POMC shows a pattern of secretion similar to that of adrenocorticotropic hormone (ACTH), with circadian variation, suppression by dexamethasone, and elevation in response to insulin hypoglycemia and intravenous administration of corticotrophin-releasing hormone (CRH) (Leake A, Charlton BG, Lowry PJ, et al. Plasma N-POMC, ACTH and cortisol concentrations in a psychogeriatric population. *Br J Psychiatry* 1990;156:676–679).

Nubain See **nalbuphine.**

nuclear magnetic resonance imaging See **magnetic resonance imaging.**

nuclear medicine Medical speciality that uses radioactive pharmaceuticals for imaging or other diagnostic studies.

nuclear schizophrenia See **schizophrenia, nuclear.**

nucleolus RNA-rich granular structure associated with specific chromosomal sites called the nucleolus organizer regions, which are located at the short arms of acrocentric chromosomes in humans.

nucleosome Repeating nucleoprotein unit of chromatin consisting of a core of eight histone molecules wrapped by a DNA segment about 146 base pairs in length.

nucleotide Subunit that makes up the informational content of DNA and RNA. It consists of a nitrogenous base (adenine, guanine, thymine, or cytosine in DNA; adenine, guanine, uracil, or cytosine in RNA), a phosphate molecule, and a sugar molecule (deoxyribose in DNA and ribose in RNA). Thousands of nucleotides are linked to form the DNA or RNA molecule. Also called "base."

nucleus Control center of a cell that contains the chromosomes.

nucleus accumbens Central nervous system nucleus that is part of the limbic system, which controls mood and emotions. It may be involved in schizophrenia and other conditions.

Nuctalon See **estazolam.**

Nu-Dispoz See **diethylpropion.**

null hypothesis Assumption that there is no significant difference between two random samples of a population. It also states that observed differences or variations in scores can be attributed to random sources. When the null hypothesis is rejected, observed differences between groups are deemed to be improbable by chance alone. Testing the null hypothesis has been the cornerstone of much statistical theory and practice over the last few decades. It requires a computation to determine the limits within which two groups may differ in their results (e.g., an experimental and a control group), even though no difference would be found if the experiment were often repeated or the groups were larger. The probability that the obtained difference would be found if no true difference existed is commonly expressed as a p-value (e.g., p < .05, that the null hypothesis is true). See **error, alpha; error, beta.**

Numbon   See **nitrazepam.**

numerical scale   Highest level of measurement. It is used for characteristics that can be given numerical values.

Numorphan   See **oxymorphone.**

Nuprin   See **ibuprofen.**

nurse practitioner   Registered nurse empowered to provide primary care or special services after special training in an approved graduate education program. Nurse practitioners usually work under the supervision of a physician.

nutmeg   See **myristicin.**

Nydrazid   See **isoniazid.**

nymphomania   See **compulsive sexual behavior.**

nystagmus   Oscillatory movement of the eyeballs that usually occurs from side to side but may follow an up-and-down or rotary pattern.

Nytol   Nonprescription, proprietary hypnotic that contains small quantities of scopolamine. It can cause delirium if taken in accidental or deliberate overdose.

O

Obedial   See **dexfenfluramine.**

Obe-Nix   See **phentermine.**

Obephen   See **phentermine.**

Obermine   See **phentermine.**

obesity, morbid   Weight at least 100% or 100 pounds over ideal body weight. It is a risk factor for life-threatening conditions including cardiovascular, metabolic, neoplastic, and orthopedic disorders. It is often resistant to conventional regimens for weight loss. Most morbidly obese persons are women of low socioeconomic status who have been obese for years. They have higher rates of mood disorders, anxiety disorders, bulimia, tobacco dependence, and personality disorders than do nonobese individuals.

objective probability   See **probability, objective.**

observation variance   Different judges having different perceptions of the same data.

observational study   Study in which the investigator observes a process or disease without intending to alter it during the study (e.g., case report, case series, analysis of secular trends, case-control study, cohort study).

observed frequency   See **frequency, observed.**

observer rating scale   See **rating scale, observer.**

observer reliability   See **reliability, observer.**

observer variation   See **variation, observer.**

obsession   Recurrent, persistent idea, thought, image, or impulse that is ego-dystonic (i.e., not experienced as voluntarily produced, but as senseless or repugnant and invading consciousness) (DSM-IV). Common obsessions are fear of causing harm to oneself or others, bizarre sexual ideation, matching imagery, and doubting.

obsessional depression   See **depression, obsessional.**

obsessional slowness   Uncommon but disabling variant of obsessive-compulsive disorder characterized by meticulous concern for orderliness. The patient takes hours to carry out daily tasks of self-care (washing, shaving, getting dressed). The activities are not rituals and there is no reduction in anxiety or dysphoria before or after the activity. The slowness may be a form of avoidance used to ensure that an activity is done "correctly" and that no part of a sequence is left out, thus obviating the need to start all over again. Basal-ganglia dysfunction may be important in the pathophysiology of obsessional slowness because of the slowness of thinking (Veale D. Classification and treatment of obsessional slowness. *Br J Psychiatry* 1993;162:198–203).

obsessive-compulsive disorder   (OCD) Illness characterized by recurrent, intrusive thoughts and compulsive, stereotyped, repetitive behaviors or cognitions. Patients may fear that some potential danger has been left unchecked or that they are about to perform an act that is harmful to themselves or others. Behaviors such as handwashing, hoarding, or counting may be conducted to forestall the imagined danger and to relieve anxiety. Functioning is impaired because patients are so focused on obsessive thoughts and compulsive rituals that they ignore many ordinary concerns of daily living. The obsessions and compulsions seem irrational to the patients, but when they attempt to resist them, they experience increased anxiety that can be relieved only by returning to the compulsive behaviors and preoccupations. OCD afflicts 2% of the population and appears to be transmitted genetically, although no clear biochemical abnormalities have been elucidated (Altemus M, Pigott T, Kalogeras KT, et al. Abnormalities in the regulation of vasopressin and corticotropin releasing factor secretion in obsessive-compulsive disorder. *Arch Gen Psychiatry* 1992; 49:9–20). Neuroimaging studies and the occurrence of obsessive-compulsive symptoms in several neurological conditions (e.g., Gilles de la Tourette's syndrome, postencephalitic Parkinson's disease, Huntington's chorea, temporal lobe epilepsy) support the idea of underlying brain dysfunction. In addition, more than 90% of OCD patients have "soft signs" consistent with subtle neurological disorder. Investigations of the neurochemistry, neuropathology, and neurophysiology of neurological disorders all suggest that the frontal-caudate-pallidal circuit plays a vital role in OCD (Cummings JL, Cunningham K. Obsessive-compulsive disorder in Huntington's disease. *Biol Psychiatry* 1992;31:263–270). There may be a link between OCD and Tourette's syndrome, since many patients with Tourette's syndrome have obsessions and compulsions, and patients with OCD frequently have tics. However, there are phenomenological differences between OCD and OCD with co-morbid Tourette's syndrome that may reflect differential involvement of neurochemical and neuroanatomical pathways (George MS, Trimble MR, Ring HA, et al. Obsessions in obsessive-compulsive disorder with and without Gilles de la Tourette's syndrome. *Am J Psychiatry* 1993;150:93–97). OCD occurs with apparently greater frequency than panic disorder, schizophrenia, or mania. Idiopathic OCD typically begins in adolescence and exhibits a waxing and waning lifelong course. There is ample evidence that serotonin uptake inhibitors and behavioral therapies that use exposure and response-prevention are quite effective in reducing OCD symptoms; the latter may be more effective for compulsions than for obsessions.

obsessive-compulsive disorder (OCD), serotonin hypothesis of   Postulation that serotonin (5-HT) plays a role in the modulation of OCD. Formerly viewed as a manifestation of psychodynamic conflict, OCD now is widely considered a neuropsychiatric illness. That dysregulation in 5-HT function may attend OCD is supported by response to 5-HT uptake inhibitors (e.g., clomipramine), peripheral markers of 5-HT function, and pharmacological challenge studies (Barr LC, Goodman WK, Price LH, et al. The serotonin hypothesis of obsessive compulsive disorder: implications of pharmacologic challenge studies. *J Clin Psychiatry* 1992;53:17–28).

obstipation   Severe constipation or intestinal blockage by very hard stools or feces.

obstructive sleep apnea   See **sleep apnea, obstructive.**

obtunded   Moderate to severe suppression of consciousness (e.g., comatose).

ocular pigmentation   Pigmentary changes in the skin and eyes induced by long-term administration of moderate to high doses of certain phenothiazine neuroleptics. Chlorpromazine in particular may cause a pigmentation of light-exposed skin (face, neck, hands), sclera and conjunctiva, and/or granular deposits in the lens and cornea, producing opacities. In rare cases, retinal pigmentation may occur. Some patients with a history of prolonged, high-dose therapy have experienced reduced visual acuity due to cataract formation. These ocular reactions should not be confused with pigmentary retinopathy or the central chorioretinopathy produced by high doses of thioridazine. See **thioridazine.**

Oculinum   See **botulinum toxin.**

oculogyric crisis   Form of dystonia that begins with a fixed stare for a few moments, followed by the eyes rotating upwards and to the side and remaining fixed in that position. At the same time, the head tilts backward and laterally, the mouth opens wide, the tongue protrudes, and the facial expression suggests pain. Spasms can be tonic or clonic and are often associated with retrocollis. They may last from minutes to hours. The most common cause today is treatment with a neuroleptic or other antidopaminergic drug. Carbamazepine, lithium, and pentazocine have evoked acute ocu-

logyric crises secondary to their dopamine-receptor blocking effects (Henry E. Oculogyric crisis and carbamazepine. *Arch Neurol* 1980;37:326; Sandyk R. Oculogyric crisis induced by lithium carbonate. *Eur Neurol* 1984;23:92–94; Burstein AH, Fullerton T. Oculogyric crisis possibly related to pentazocine. *Ann Pharmacother* 1993;27:874–876). See **dystonia.**

odds   Ratio of the probability of occurrence of an event to that of nonoccurrence, or the ratio of the probability that something is so to the probability that it is not so. Odds vary from 0 to infinity, often being expressed as 1:2 (that is, 1 case per 2 noncases), 3:2, 7:4, etc.

odds ratio   (OR) Statistical parameter for expressing the degree of association between two binary (dichotomous) variables. In epidemiology, two dichotomous variables are frequently used to express the relationship between those exposed or not exposed with those who have the disease or do not have the disease. OR measures the strength of association between diagnostic subgroup ("disease") and primary interested outcome variable ("exposure").

odds ratio/matched design   Each control subject is selected by being identical to an experimental subject or a by embodying a variable that may influence the result. When one control subject is matched with one experimental subject, the odds ratio is the ratio of the discordant pairs. It is the number of pairs in which the case subject is exposed and control subjects are not exposed, divided by the number of pairs in which the control subjects are exposed and the case subject is not exposed.

"off-label" drug use   Use of approved drugs for indications that have not been approved by the Food and Drug Administration (FDA) (e.g., desipramine for the treatment of cocaine addiction and carbamazepine for treatment of affective disorders). Off-label use is generally based on drug studies published in medical journals or presented at conferences. Although the FDA may deem a drug safe for one use because potential benefits outweigh potential risks, if the drug is used for another indication, potential benefits may be significantly lower and the risk would not warrant FDA approval. According to the FDA, physicians prescribing off-label must be well informed about the drug, base use on a firm scientific rationale and sound medical evidence, and maintain records of use and effects. Physicians who prescribe drugs off-label may wish to use measures similar to those used in clinical drug investigations: writing a treatment protocol, having the protocol reviewed and approved by an institutional review board, and using informed consent procedures that state to prospective patients that the drug is so far unproven for the intended indication. If sued for malpractice, physicians who prescribe off label may have to justify their decision to the satisfaction of a jury (journal articles, evidence of widespread use, expert testimony that the prescription had a rational medical basis). They also should check their malpractice insurance policies: some may not cover liabilities incurred as a result of "experimental" treatments (Appler WD, McMann GL. View from the nation's capitol. "Off-label" uses of approved drugs; limits on physicians' prescribing behavior. *J Clin Psychopharmacol* 1989;9:368–370). Also called "nonapproved drug use."

olanzapine (LY170053) New antipsychotic that in preclinical studies appeared to be an atypical antipsychotic. European and U.S. clinical trials indicate that 5–30 mg/day may be effective in patients filling DSM-IV criteria for schizophrenia or schizoaffective disorder. Olanzapine also appears to be less likely to evoke extrapyramidal reactions than typical neuroleptics are.

olanzapine + diazepam To date no adverse reactions have been reported.

olanzapine + procyclidine Co-administration in a patient with a tremor that existed prior to olanzapine therapy was well tolerated.

olanzapine + propranolol Co-administration in a patient who had been receiving propranolol for over a year produced no adverse interactions.

olanzapine + temazepam Co-administration in patients who had been taking temazepam produced no adverse interactions.

Olcadil See **cloxazolam.**

olfactory hallucination See **hallucination, olfactory.**

oligergasia See **mental retardation.**

oligonucleotide Short (generally less than 30 nucleotides) piece of DNA. Once a gene's nucleotide sequence is determined, it can be made artificially by a molecular biologist. Instead of making the entire gene (which would be thousands of nucleotides long), a relatively small portion of the sequence (usually a stretch unique to the gene or shared by a few genes of interest) is made using a chemical synthesizer. This oligonucleotide is then hybridized to a Southern or northern blot or library to determine if there are other genes or messages that also contain the oligonucleotide. Genes that share key nucleotide sequences generally share some functional similarities.

oligonucleotide probe Synthetic DNA molecule radiolabeled to detect either RNA or DNA in a wide variety of techniques. It is usually a short molecule (from 10 to 50 bases in length) generated with a specific sequence according to the particular needs of the researcher.

oligophrenia See **mental retardation.**

omeprazole + benzodiazepine See **benzodiazepine + omeprazole.**

Omnipress See **amoxapine.**

oncogene Gene that normally has important functions in development and differentiation, but that causes cancer when mutated. Oncogenes are created by spontaneous mutation of normal genes in somatic cells, not the germ cells, and therefore are not inherited. They cause cancer when stimulated by a cancer gene and must be active before a cell can turn malignant. They are named by a three-letter code derived from their associated neoplastic disease, sometimes with prefixes *v* and *c* (viral or cellular); other prefixes (e.g., H-ras) distinguish oncogene subtypes.

oncogenesis Production of cancer by biological, chemical, or physical agents.

ondansetron (Ramesin; Zamanol; Zofran; Zophran; Zophren; Zopran) (OND) Serotonin $(5-HT)_3$ antagonist marketed as an antiemetic. Its greatest advantage over metoclopramide appears to be a lack of important adverse effects; it may become the antiemetic of choice in selected patients in whom the risk of adverse effects from high-dose metoclopramide outweighs the added cost of OND (Chaffee BJ, Tankanow RM. Ondansetron—the first of a new class of antiemetic agents. *Clin Pharm* 1991;10:430–446). Controlled studies indicating that OND reduces alcohol consumption provide the first clinical evidence that a $5-HT_3$ antagonist may modify substance abuse. Open clinical trials indicate that OND may offer a therapeutic alternative to dopamine receptor antagonists in the treatment of schizophrenia (Truckleband MD. Interactions between dopamine and $5-HT_3$ receptors suggest new treatments for psychosis and drug addiction. *Trends Pharmacol Sci* 1989;10:127–128). Because it is a $5-HT_3$ antagonist, OND is less likely to cause extrapyramidal symptoms (EPS), although there are anecdotal reports of OND-caused EPS (Halperin JR, Murphy B. Extrapyramidal reaction to ondansetron. *Cancer* 1992;69:1275). Mild headaches, constipation, and transient transaminase elevations are characteristically associated with the $5-HT_3$ antagonists, but are of little consequence. OND (8 mg) does not produce acute effects on sleep in healthy subjects. OND (12–20 mg/day) has been shown to be well tolerated and effective for hallucinosis in advanced Parkinson's disease (PD) without worsening the basic severity of PD or counteracting the efficacy of levodopa (Zoldan J, Friedberg G, Goldberg-Stern H, Melamed E. Ondansetron for hallucinosis in advanced Parkinson's disease. *Lancet* 1993;341:562–563).

one-compartment model   View of the body as a single large compartment in which absorbed drug is distributed to the various organs, tissues, and fluids instantaneously. In this model, distribution is completed before a measurable fraction of the drug is eliminated. See **compartment.**

oneiric behavior   Behavior during rapid eye movement (REM) sleep that includes hitting, kicking, moving arms and legs rapidly, getting up on the bed, walking or jumping out of the bed, and/or striking the body against the wall or furniture. It usually is accompanied by "noisy" sleeping, talking, and vivid dreams. It differs from somnambulism. Clonazepam treatment may be effective.

oneiric stupor   Spontaneous lapses from quiet wakefulness into a sleep state with enacted dreams.

one-side test   See **one-tail test.**

one-tail test   Statistical significance test for the hypothesis that the parameter(s) is/are smaller or larger than a certain value. The name comes from the fact that the statistic needs to be compared with only one side of the probability distribution. Also called "one-side test."

one-to-one management   See **constant observation.**

on-off   Phenomenon that occurs in Parkinson's disease patients after long-term treatment with levodopa or other dopaminergic agents. The "on" phase (choreoathetotic dyskinesia) occurs at peak dose effect; patients are mobile and independent, but also have distressing abnormal dyskinetic movements. In the "off" phase (akinesia), patients suddenly freeze, feel that their feet are immobile and sticking to the floor, and may be fearful and panic-stricken. Patients may suddenly switch from one phase to the other. Such vacillations are disconcerting and may erroneously be thought to be psychological in origin, whereas they may be due to pharmacokinetic factors secondary to altered levodopa absorption and metabolism to irregular dopamine storage, release, and reuptake.

onychophagia   Habitual fingernail biting. It is a widespread behavior among children and adults of all ages, degrees of intelligence, and socioeconomic status. It is more common in females than in males (1.5:1). Prevalence in childhood has been estimated to be approximately 50%. Starting as early as age 4, it peaks at ages 10–18. By ages 17–18, it decreases somewhat. Although most childhood nail bit-

ers probably discontinue the behavior sometime during adulthood, up to 4.5% of people in their 60s retain the habit. Twins studies suggest that it may be familial. Severe, morbid onychophagia may cause both medical and dental problems.

onychotillomania   Compulsive picking or tearing at the fingernails. It may be a variation of severe onychophagia.

operant behavior   Behavior governed by its consequences (i.e., the organism must first do something before reinforcement occurs).

operant conditioning   Response to a stimulus that increases the probability that the operant or response to the environment that immediately preceded presentation of the reinforcer will occur again. Cocaine (COC)-induced euphoria, for example, acts to strengthen behavior that preceded its delivery. Since euphoria serves as a reward that follows the behavioral response or operant of COC self-administration, COC euphoria effectively strengthens the behavior of self-administration. The reward or positive reinforcement of COC euphoria thus increases the frequency of those behaviors that preceded the reward. Also called "instrumental conditioning."

operant techniques   Behavioral procedures requiring that subjects operate specific instruments (e.g., levers, press-plates) in response to specific environmental conditions or stimuli. Environmental conditions in a given operant situation can be organized such that the responses or behaviors emitted by subjects are thought to depend on rather specific (albeit often poorly defined) functions of the brain. Examples of such functions include learning; short- and long-term memory; attention or vigilance; sensory perception (color, sound, and position discrimination); temporal or time perception; reproduction; and motivation. Because operant techniques allow the design of experiments that generate behaviors thought to indicate the status of specific brain functions, such techniques are of interest to those studying the functional integrity of the brain.

operational definition   Meaning of a concept when it is translated into terms amenable to systematic observation and measurement (e.g., temperature defined by a thermometer reading under standard conditions).

operator   That which produces effects (e.g., operator gene).

operons   System of adjacent genes on a chromosome with an operator gene controlling the activity of the system.

opiate   Product derived from opium, usually morphine derivatives (e.g., heroin). Opiates act on endogenous opioid receptors.

opiate addiction Chronic relapsing disorder for which there are four major forms of treatment: methadone maintenance, antagonistic drug treatment, residential therapeutic community, and outpatient drug-free treatment. All may be effective, but only for some patients. Detoxification should be considered only as a first step in a comprehensive rehabilitation program.

opiate withdrawal/gamma-hydroxybutyric acid (GHB) Because oral GHB was found to be highly effective in suppressing withdrawal symptoms in alcoholics, a double-blind, placebo-controlled trial (25 mg/kg) was conducted in 14 heroin addicts and 13 methadone-maintained subjects. GHB effect occurred within 15 minutes and persisted for 2–3 hours. In an open study, the same subjects subsequently received GHB every 2–4 hours for 2 days and then every 4–6 hours for the following 6 days. Most abstinence signs and symptoms remained suppressed, and subjects reported feeling well. Urinalysis failed to detect any presence of opiate metabolites. No withdrawal symptoms recurred when treatment was suspended after 8 days and patients were challenged with an intravenous injection of naloxone (0.4 mg) (Gallimberti L, Cibin M, Pagnin P, et al. Gamma-hydroxybutyric acid for treatment of opiate withdrawal syndrome. *Neuropsychopharmacology* 1993;9:77–81). The mechanism by which GHB suppresses opiate withdrawal syndrome is unknown.

opiate withdrawal/neonate Syndrome that occurs in 50–70% of children born to women who abuse opiates during the latter part of pregnancy. Mortality rate may be as high as 30%. It usually begins 1–2 days after birth in a child of low birth weight and is likely to increase the length of hospital stay. Symptoms include irritability, crying, tremor, hyper-reflexia, increased respiratory rate, diarrhea, hyperactivity, vomiting, and sneezing/yawning/hiccupping (Hoder EL, Leckman JF, Ehrenkranz R, et al. Clonidine in neonatal narcotic-abstinent syndrome. *N Engl J Med* 1981;305:1284).

opioid Any of a group of compounds with pharmacological effects resembling those of morphine. Opioids are commonly used for pain relief, prevention of an abstinence syndrome, cough suppression, and sedation in an agitated patient, and as an adjunct to anesthesia. They are frequently abused for their intoxicating effects. Medical complications of opioid abuse are many and diverse, and are due most often to (a) failure to use aseptic techniques during injection; (b) the presence of particulate contaminants in the injected solution; and (c) the direct pharmacological actions of the drug. Opioid toxicity or overdose should be suspected in any undiagnosed coma patient or in patients with respiratory depression, pulmonary edema, hypothermia, pupillary constriction, and needle marks. Opioid overdose should be treated immediately by the opioid antagonists naltrexone (long-acting) and naloxone (short-acting). See **naloxone; naltrexone.**

opioid abstinence syndrome, protracted Protracted syndrome that occurs in an indeterminate number of formerly physically dependent individuals after the more obvious manifestations of opioid withdrawal have subsided. Symptoms may range from not feeling normal to depression and abnormal responses to stressful situations. There also may be psychological disturbances such as decreased self-esteem and anxiety. The syndrome may contribute to relapse following withdrawal. Many patients in methadone maintenance programs often complain of protracted abstinence symptoms even when withdrawal has been carried out quite slowly. In many cases there is also a return of thoughts about opioid use (drug hunger). The biological basis for protracted opioid abstinence is largely unexplored, and study of the phenomenon is complicated by the high prevalence of other psychiatric disorders (e.g., affective disorders, antisocial personality) among those who become dependent on opioids (Jaffee JH. Opiates: clinical aspects. *In* Lowenson JH, Ruiz P, Millman RB, Langrod JG [eds], *Substance Abuse. A Comprehensive Textbook*, 2nd ed. Baltimore: Williams & Wilkins, 1992). See **benzodiazepine postwithdrawal syndrome.**

opioid agonist These include codeine, diphenoxylate, dextromoramide, dextropropoxyphene, dihydrocodeine, fentanyl, heroin, hydromorphone, levorphanol, methadone, meperidine, morphine, oxycodone, and oxymorphone.

opioid agonist/antagonist, mixed Included are buprenorphine, butorphanol, nalbuphine, nalorphine, and pentazocine.

opioid analgesic Any of the opiate/opioid drugs used for pain relief. Those usually administered for moderate pain include codeine, hydrocodone, meperidine, oxycodone, pentazocine, and propoxyphene. Those usually administered for severe pain are morphine agonists (e.g., fentanyl, hydromorphone, levorphanol, methadone, morphine, oxycodone, oxymorphone) or mixed agonist-antagonists (e.g., buprenorphine, butorphanol, nalbuphine, pentazocine).

opioid analgesic + benzodiazepine Co-administration results in various and often contradictory pharmacological effects that depend principally on the pharmacodynamic action studied (i.e., sedation-hypnosis, respiratory depression, analgesia, hemodynamics), the interacting agents, and the route of administration. Different benzodiazepines can alter opioid-associated respiratory mechanics differently (Maurer PM, Bartkowski RR. Drug interactions of clinical significance with opioid analgesics. *Drug Safety* 1993;8:30–48).

opioid antagonist　　Substance (e.g., levallorphan, nalorphine, nalorone, naltrexone) that binds to opioid receptors, but does not produce effects. When an antagonist is present in sufficient quantity to occupy all or most opioid receptors, opiate agonists (e.g., morphine) cannot reach and bind to the receptors. As a result, an injection of heroin will have little or no agonist effect, and the pattern of addiction or readdiction may be interrupted.

opioid, endogenous　　Polypeptide similar in structure to morphine that binds to the same receptors in the central nervous system (CNS). Included are the dynorphins, endorphins, and enkephalins. Although the three families are derived from different prehormone molecules and have different affinity profiles for receptors, there are structural similarities among them. Methionine, enkephalin, and beta-endorphin have been shown to produce physical dependence in rats. The CNS effects of both endogenous opioids and exogenous opiates (morphine and heroin) are blocked by the opioid antagonists naloxone and naltrexone because of their affinity for the opioid receptors in the brain. Endogenous opioids may play a role in the maintenance of self-injurious behavior; parenteral naloxone (half-life, 30–80 minutes) and oral naltrexone (half-life, 12–96 hours) may prove to be effective treatment. Also called "opioid neuropeptide"; "opiopeptin." See **self-injurious behavior.**

opioid hypothesis　　Postulation that self-injurious behavior (SIB) is due to either a pathologically altered pain threshold or the behavior's supplying a "fix" for an addicted endogenous opioid system. The finding that opioid antagonists attenuate SIB is the strongest evidence for the hypothesis.

opioid + moclobemide　　Data are available on two patients who received moclobemide plus codeine and on one who received moclobemide plus dextropropoxyphene. Moderate agitation occurred as an adverse event in one patient; no other adverse events or changes in vital signs indicative of a relevant interaction were recorded. Co-administration should be undertaken with caution until a larger database is available (Amrein R, Guntert TW, Dingemanse J, et al. Interactions of moclobemide with concomitantly administered medi-

cation: evidence from pharmacological and clinical studies. *Psychopharmacology* 1992;106: S24–S31).

opioid neuropeptide　　See **opioid, endogenous.**

opioid receptor　　Specific neuronal cell site that interacts with opioid drugs and determines their pharmacological actions. The demonstration of highly selective receptors led to the discovery of endogenous opioid substances (enkephalins, endorphins), the physiological functions of which are presumably mediated by the opioid receptor. Opioid receptors can be divided into mu_1 (supraspinal analgesia), mu_2 (respiratory depression, sedation, bradycardia); kappa (spinal analgesia, sedation); delta (analgesia); epsilon (analgesia); and sigma (dysphoria, psychomotor stimulation, tachycardia) (Boucher BA, Phelps SJ. Acute management of the head injury patient. *In* DiPiro JT, Talbert RL, Hayes PE, Yee GC, Matzke GR, Posey LM [eds], *Pharmacotherapy: A Pathophysiologic Approach*, 2nd ed. New York: Elsevier, 1992, p 926).

opioid withdrawal　　Syndrome precipitated by abrupt cessation of opioid administration after continuous use for 1–2 weeks or longer. It also can be precipitated by administration of an opioid antagonist such as naloxone. Therapeutic discontinuation is generally a comparatively lengthy process: 2–3 weeks for inpatients and 8 weeks or more for outpatients is the rule for methadone substitution and withdrawal programs. Drop-out rate can be high (20–25%). Clonidine plus an opioid antagonist accelerates withdrawal without increasing the overall severity of withdrawal symptoms compared with clonidine treatment alone. The rationale is that antagonists compress withdrawal symptoms into 2–3 days, enabling them to be treated energetically with appropriate medication and psychological support. Clonidine plus naltrexone, aided by moderate doses of sedatives, can reduce methadone detoxification to 3–5 days. If clonidine is not used, patients must usually wait until 7–10 days after their last dose of methadone and 5–7 days after their last dose of heroin before starting naltrexone. A combination of clonidine, naltrexone, and diazepam significantly reduces the average withdrawal time from 3.3 days to 2.3 days, despite lower clonidine dosage and significantly lower diazepam dosage on the second day. See **clonidine.**

opioid withdrawal/intensive care (ICU)　　Withdrawal from opioids and sedative hypnotic drugs is commonly encountered during weaning from the ventilator in intensive care patients. Pharmacological management includes use of droperidol or clonidine. Methadone has been used for iatrogenic narcotic dependency in pediatric ICU patients (Tobias JD, Schleien CL, Haun SE. Methadone as treatment for iatrogenic narcotic dependency in pediatric intensive care unit patients. *Crit Care Med* 1990;18:1292–1293). Adult ICU patients with iatrogenic narcotic dependency can be treated safely and effectively with subcutaneous injections of methadone, starting with 5 mg every 3 hours for 1 day. The dose is tapered over several days in accordance with individual patient needs (Bohrer H, Schmidt H, Bach A, et al. Methadone treatment of opioid withdrawal in intensive care patients. *Lancet* 1993;341:636–637).

opioid withdrawal, neonate Infants of heroin-dependent mothers manifest withdrawal within hours after birth, but this may be delayed for days in babies who have been exposed in utero to methadone.

opiopeptin See **opioid, endogenous.**

opipramol (Insidon) Tricyclic antidepressant with a nucleus almost identical to that of imipramine and a side chain identical to that of the piperazine phenothiazine neuroleptic perphenazine. It is as therapeutically effective as imipramine. Not marketed in the United States.

Opiran See **pimozide.**

opisthotonus Form of dystonia in which the spine and extremities are bent forward in such a way that the body rests on the head and heels. See **dystonia.**

opium Narcotic/analgesic obtained from the juice of poppy plant seeds that have been air-dried into a milky exudation and then powdered commercially to produce opium products.

opportunistic infection Infection with organisms when the body's immunological defenses are compromised. Common in acquired immunodeficiency syndrome (AIDS).

oppositional disorder (OPD) Pervasive opposition to all in authority regardless of self-interest, continuous argumentativeness, and unwillingness to respond to reasonable persuasion (DSM-IV).

opsoclonus Irregular, fine eye movements interrupted by rapid and unequal larger movements, usually side to side. When the person attempts to change the position of the eyes, the abnormal movements become more evident.

optimal dosage Drug dosage that produces maximum therapeutic benefit with minimal unwanted side effects. It varies from individual to individual.

Optimil See **methaqualone.**

optional sleep See **sleep, optional.**

oral contraceptive + alprazolam See **alprazolam + oral contraceptive.**

oral contraceptive + benzodiazepine See **benzodiazepine + oral contraceptive.**

oral contraceptive + carbamazepine See **carbamazepine + oral contraceptive.**

oral contraceptive + clomipramine See **clomipramine + oral contraceptive.**

oral contraceptive + diazepam See **diazepam + oral contraceptive.**

oral contraceptive + lamotrigine See **lamotrigine + oral contraceptive.**

oral contraceptive + moclobemide See **moclobemide + oral contraceptive.**

oral contraceptive + paroxetine See **paroxetine + oral contraceptive.**

Oralep Forte See **pimozide.**

Oraleptin See **penfluridol.**

Oranabol See **oxymesterone.**

"orange" Street name for central nervous system stimulants.

Orap See **pimozide.**

Ora Testryl See **fluoxymesterone.**

ordinal scale See **ranking scale.**

ordinate Distance of a point from the horizontal (*x*) axis of a graph, measured along the vertical (*y*) axis.

Oreton See **testosterone.**

Oreton Methyl See **methyltestosterone.**

Oreton Propionate See **testosterone propionate.**

Orflagen See **orphenadrine.**

organic affective syndrome See **organic mood disorder.**

organic brain syndrome (OBS) Confusion, disorientation, decreased intellectual function, and stable vital signs in the absence of signs of withdrawal.

organic crying Condition due to interruption of the corticobulbar tract, which inhibits limbic input to the brainstem nuclei that control the motor aspect of crying. It is distinguished by its lability, dissociation from stimuli normally associated with crying, and propensity for being stereotyped with facial grimacing. It may occur in dementia, multiple sclerosis, pseudobulbar palsy, and other neurological illnesses.

organic disorder Illness characterized by alteration in the structure or metabolism of tissues or organs.

organic hallucinosis See **hallucinosis.**

organic mental disorder Psychiatric disturbances resulting from transient or permanent central nervous system dysfunction attributable to specific organic factors (aging, drugs, toxins, infection, trauma, tumors, metabolic disorders). Also called "cognitive impairment disorder."

organic mood disorder Disorder characterized by absence of cognitive impairment in patients with a history of depression. It follows accentuation of psychosocial stressors and has an insidious onset. Causes include endocrinopathies (hypothyroidism), infectious diseases, renal or hepatic failure, parkinsonism, chronic obstructive pulmonary disease, viral infections, malignancies, and neurological diseases. It also can be induced by drugs (e.g., reserpine, corticosteroids, methyldopa, amphetamines, hallucinogens, and over-the-counter and illicit drugs). Formerly called "organic affective syndrome."

organic psychosyndrome Organic mental disorder in the elderly. Characteristic symptoms are transient or permanent impairment of cognitive performance and, depending on course and severity, change in the whole personality. Toward the end, the clinical picture is that of severe dementia with almost complete loss of cognitive and communicative abilities. Causes include primary degenerative processes or pathological vascular changes.

orientation 1. Awareness of where one is in relation to time, place, and person (DSM-IV). 2. Bias inherent in a rating scale.

Orlaam See **levomethadyl acetate.**

Ormazine See **chlorpromazine.**

orofacial dyskinesia See **dyskinesia, orofacial.**

oromandibular dystonia See **dystonia, oromandibular.**

orphan drug Drug made hesitantly by a pharmaceutical company because it cannot be patented or is used only in rare conditions by very few people. In such cases, the federal government collaborates with manufacturers to help make the drugs available to those who need them. The U.S. Orphan Drug Act (Public Law 97-414), passed in 1983, gives 7-year exclusive marketing rights and tax incentives to manufacturers that develop and sell drugs for rare diseases. The law defines an orphan drug as any product used to treat diseases that afflict fewer than 200,000 people at the time of Food and Drug Administration (FDA) approval. In the first 7 years that the law was in effect, 39 of 42 orphan products were marketed. In addition, 301 experimental products were given orphan designation.

orphenadrine (Banflex; Biorphen; Brocadisipal; Disipal; Flexoject; Flexon; Marflex; Myolin; Neocyten; Noradex; Norflex; Orflagen; Orphenate) Diphenhydramine analog marketed as an anticholinergic and antiparkinsonian drug for the treatment of idiopathic and drug-induced early-onset extrapyramidal reactions. It can be administered orally, intramuscularly, or intravenously. It is useful for treating early tremor and rigidity, but is less potent than levodopa in treating akinesia and bradykinesia and their associated slowness,

stooping, and falls. It helps to control hypersalivation and drooling, but may cause an annoying dry mouth with its associated adverse effects. This and other anticholinergic and antihistaminic side effects limit its usefulness in treating moderate and advanced stages of parkinsonism. Pregnancy risk category C.

orphenadrine + alcohol Alcohol should be avoided during orphenadrine administration because it enhances hepatic metabolism of orphenadrine, lowers its blood concentration, and decreases its therapeutic effect.

orphenadrine + anticholinergic Co-administration may increase anticholinergic effects and risk of anticholinergic toxicity.

orphenadrine + chlorpromazine Orphenadrine induces microsomal oxidizing enzymes that reduce chlorpromazine plasma concentration and may interfere with its therapeutic effects (Loga S, Curry S, Lader M. Interactions of orphenadrine and phenobarbitone with chlorpromazine: plasma concentration and effects in man. *Br J Clin Pharmacol* 1985;2:197–208).

orphenadrine + central nervous system (CNS) depressant Co-administration may produce additive CNS depressant effects and necessitate reduction of the dosage of both drugs.

orphenadrine + dextropropoxyphene Co-administration may produce additive central nervous system effects and necessitate reduction of the dosage of both drugs.

orphenadrine + levodopa Co-administration for the treatment of parkinsonism may have a synergistic beneficial effect.

Orphenate See **orphenadrine.**

orthomolecular psychiatry Branch of psychiatry that uses very high doses of vitamins and/or amino acids to treat psychoses.

orthomolecular treatment Therapy based on the theory that psychiatric and perhaps other illnesses are due to vitamin deficiencies. Treatment consists of high doses of vitamins, especially niacin, vitamin C, and vitamin B_6. The scientific basis of this therapy is not on firm ground; it is currently practiced by only a few psychiatrists. Also called "megavitamin therapy."

orthopsychiatry Cross-disciplinary science combining child psychiatry, developmental psychology, pediatrics, social work, and family care. It is devoted to discovery, prevention, and treatment of mental disorders in childhood and adolescence.

orthostatic hypotension (OH) Elevation of pulse rate, drop in systolic (at least 20 mm Hg) and diastolic blood pressures, and occurrence of postural symptoms (lightheadedness or faintness after moving from a supine to a standing position). It can be a troublesome side effect of many drugs (aliphatic phenothiazine neuroleptics, clozapine, tricyclic antidepressants, monoamine oxidase inhibitors) in terms of morbidity and a factor-limiting adequate drug dosage. Major consequences of OH include myocardial infarction and falls resulting in fractures and lacerations. Extra care should be exercised when prescribing OH-inducing drugs for patients who have cardiac disorders (in particular, cardiac conduction disease or congestive heart failure) or who take medication that can lower blood pressure, especially if they are older than 40. Antidepressants are not contraindicated in these patients, but the risk of developing significant OH is greater in these patient subgroups. Medications such as flurinef (Apothecon) can sometimes control this side effect.

orthostatic tremor   See **tremor, orthostatic.**

osmotic demyelination syndrome   See **central pontine myelinolysis.**

Osnervan   See **procyclidine.**

Ospolat   See **sulthiame.**

Otarex   See **hydroxyzine.**

"Ousley's acid"   Street term used in the mid-1960s for a lysergic acid diethylamide (LSD) street product of high quality that many believed matched the quality of legitimately manufactured LSD by Sandoz Laboratories.

outcome   All possible changes in health status that may occur in following subjects or that may stem from exposure to a causal factor or from preventive or therapeutic interventions. *End-point* is a narrower term referring to an event that leads to completion or termination of follow-up of a subject (e.g., death or major morbidity) (Anon: Glossary of methodologic terms. *JAMA* 1993;269:154–155).

outcome variable   See **variable, outcome.**

outpatient commitment   See **mandatory treatment.**

outpatient psychiatric treatment   All forms of accepted therapy for behavioral or emotional disorders for which there are no "in-residence" requirements (e.g., outpatient hospital clinics, office visits to private practitioners, child guidance clinics, community mental health clinics).

overdose   Inadvertent or deliberate consumption of a much larger dose than that habitually used by the individual. Depending on the dose taken and toxic potential of the substance, it may result in serious toxic reactions, including death in some cases.

Overeaters Anonymous   Twelve-step program similar to that of Alcoholics Anonymous that can be a helpful adjunct to initial treatment of bulimia nervosa and subsequent relapse prevention.

overmedicated society   Mid-1960s term used to raise public concern over what critics perceived as growing overuse of antianxiety medications, especially benzodiazepines and particularly diazepam.

over-read   Re-evaluation of automatically generated test results by an expert doctor.

over-the-counter drug   Drug available without a prescription. Physicians should routinely inquire about use of over-the-counter (OTC) drugs, especially by elderly patients. Many patients take a number of OTC drugs, but do not spontaneously report such use to physicians because they do not consider these preparations as medicines that might be responsible for their symptoms or that might interact adversely with prescription drugs.

overuse, drug   Excessive use of a drug (in terms of length of use or severity of the disorder treated), but within the framework of use for diseases in which there is medically accepted evidence of therapeutic effect (WHO: Expert Committee on Drug Dependence, Sixteenth Report. World Health Organization Technical Report, Series No. 407, Geneva, WHO, 1969).

overvalued idea   Unreasonable, sustained belief or idea that is maintained with less than delusional intensity. It differs from an obsessional thought in that the person holding the overvalued idea does not recognize its absurdity and thus does not struggle against it. As with a delusion, the idea or belief is not one ordinarily accepted by other members of the person's culture or subculture (DSM-IV).

owl   In somnology, a night-time person. See **lark.**

oxandrolone   (Anavar) 17-Alpha-methyl testosterone derivative anabolic steroid.

Oxanid   See **oxazepam.**

oxatomide H_1 antihistaminic, anti-allergy agent that has caused acute dystonic reactions in children followed by 2–3 days of impaired consciousness (Casteels-Van-Daele M, Eggermost E, Caesar P, et al. Acute dystonic reactions and long-lasting impaired consciousness associated with oxatomide in children. *Lancet* 1986;1:1204–1205).

oxazepam   (Anxiolit; Apo-oxazepam; Novoxapam; Oxanid; Ox-Pam; Persumbran; Praxiten; Serax; Sobril; Vaben; Zapex) 1,4 Benzodiazepine anxiolytic that is an active metabolite of diazepam, but has no metabolites of its own. Metabolism is by glucuronide conjugation. Elimination half-life is 8 hours. Despite its widespread use, there have been infrequent reports of dependency, abuse, and withdrawal. Schedule IV; pregnancy risk category D.

oxazepam + alcohol   Alcohol can delay absorption of oxazepam (Greenblatt DJ, Shader RI,

Weinberger DR, et al. Effect of cocktail on diazepam absorption. *Psychopharmacology* 1978; 57:199–203).

oxazepam/breast milk Oxazepam is secreted in human milk and should be discontinued during lactation and breast feeding.

oxazepam + disulfiram Co-administration minimally alters oxazepam disposition. Oxazepam may be the drug of choice if benzodiazepine therapy is used for patients taking disulfiram (MacLeod SM, Sellers EM, Giles HG, et al. Interaction of disulfiram with benzodiazepines. *Clin Pharmacol Ther* 1978;24:583–589).

oxazepam + nicotine transdermal system Because of the deinduction of hepatic enzymes on smoking cessation, a reduced dose of oxazepam may be required at cessation of smoking and discontinuation of the nicotine transdermal patch.

oxazepam + paroxetine Paroxetine does not potentiate oxazepam's sedative effects. No clinically important interactions have been reported (Boyer WF, Feighner JP. An overview of paroxetine. *J Clin Psychiatry* 1992;53[suppl]: 3–6).

oxazepam/pregnancy Oxazepam should be avoided during the last trimester and labor. Like other benzodiazepines (BZDs), it may cause hypotonia, poor sucking, and hypotension in the neonate. Mobius's (Moebius) syndrome was reported in a female infant whose mother had taken diazepam (20 mg/day) from week 25 until delivery and oxazepam (20 mg/day) from the 7th month of gestation. The infant's serum diazepam concentration on day 13 was greatly elevated. It has been suggested that because of the teratogenic potential of BZDs, in utero exposure to them should be excluded in each case of Mobius's syndrome and that electromyography of the facial muscles be performed in infants whose mothers took BZDs during pregnancy (Courtens W, Vamos E, Hainaut M, Vergauwen P. Moebius syndrome in an infant exposed in utero to benzodiazepines. *J Pediatr* 1992;121:833–834).

oxazolam Benzodiazepine currently available only in Germany and Japan.

oxazolidinedione Any of a major group of anticonvulsants (prototype, trimethadione). They are structurally similar to the hydantoins and are used primarily to treat absence seizures. Advent of the equi-effective and less toxic succinimides resulted in decreased use of oxazolidinediones.

oxcarbazepine (Trileptal) (OXC) 10-Keto analog of carbamazepine (CBZ) with similar anticonvulsant efficacy, both as monotherapy and adjuvant treatment, with fewer central nervous system side effects and allergic reactions. Its main metabolite is hydroxycarbamazepine, which leads to less induction of hepatic enzymes (especially microsomal cytochrome P450) and is responsible for its anticonvulsant effect. Unlike CBZ, OXC does not appear to be an enzyme inducer in humans or to have an active epoxide metabolite. Because of these pharmacological differences, it may have more predictable dose-concentration-effect relations, better tolerability, and fewer physiological and drug interactions than CBZ. It can exert antimanic effects in up to 70% of manic patients about as rapidly as neuroleptics can (Emrich HM. Studies with oxcarbazepine [Trileptal] in acute mania. *Int Clin Psychopharmacol* 1990;5[suppl]:83–88; O'Shea B. Non-lithium pharmacological treatment of manic depression: a review. *Ir J Psychol Med* 1993;10:114–120).

oxcarbazepine + felodipine Steady-state pharmacokinetic parameters of felodipine and its pyridine metabolite were not influenced by a single dose of oxcarbazepine. Repeated co-administration significantly reduced the area under the concentration-time curve of felodipine by 28% and reduced the felodipine maximum plasma concentration by 34% (Zaccara G, Gangemi PF, Bendoni L, et al. Influence of single and repeated doses of oxcarbazepine on the pharmacokinetic profile of felodipine. *Ther Drug Monit* 1993;15:39–42).

oxcarbazepine + valproic acid Oxcarbazepine (OXC) may decrease valproic acid (VPA) serum levels. When OXC is discontinued, there is an average 30% increase in the level/dose ratio of total VPA at the end of a study, preceded by an average 50% increase in the level/dose ratio of free VPA. This leads to VPA-related side effects, requiring retitration of VPA daily doses (Battino D, Croci D, Granata T, et al. Changes in unbound and total valproic acid concentrations after replacement of carbamazepine with oxcarbazepine. *Ther Drug Monit* 1992;14:376–379).

oxidation, hepatic See **hepatic oxidation.**

Oxilapine See **loxapine.**

oxiracetam (Neupan; Neuractiv; Neuromet) Putative nootropic drug structurally related to piracetam. It has been shown to enhance new learning and to protect against cerebral hypoxia. It is being tested in the treatment of the cognitive symptoms of Alzheimer's disease and multi-infarct dementia (Smirne S, Truci G, Piero E, et al. Efficacy and tolerability of oxiracetam in Alzheimer's disease: a double blind, six month study. *Clin Neurol Neurosurg* 1987;89:19).

oxiracetam + carbamazepine Carbamazepine (CBZ) influences the half-life of oxiracetam, necessitating its more frequent administration. No adverse interactions have been reported.

oxiracetam + clobazam   Clobazam influences the half-life of oxiracetam, necessitating its more frequent administration. No adverse interactions have been reported.

oxicaretam + valproic acid   Valproic acid lowers the half-life of oxiracetam, necessitating its frequent administration. No adverse interactions have been reported.

Ox-Pam   See **oxazepam.**

oxprenolol + clomipramine   See **clomipramine + oxprenolol.**

oxycodone   Semisynthetic narcotic analgesic/sedative with multiple actions qualitatively similar to those of morphine; the most prominent involve the central nervous system and organs composed of smooth muscles. It is similar to codeine and methadone in that it retains at least half of its analgesic activity when administered orally. Oral potency is high: 50 mg administered orally is equipotent to 10 mg of intramuscularly administered morphine. Oxycodone can produce drug dependence of the morphine type and has abuse potential. Psychic dependence, physical dependence, and tolerance may develop with repeated use. Schedule II; pregnancy risk category C.

oxycodone + aspirin   (Percodan) Semisynthetic combination narcotic analgesic, the principal ingredient of which is oxycodone. Schedule II.

oxycodone + acetaminophen   (Percocet) Semisynthetic combination narcotic analgesic, the principal ingredient of which is oxycodone. Schedule II.

oxycodone + fluoxetine   No serious adverse interactions have been reported.

Oxydess II   See **dextroamphetamine.**

oxymesterone   (Oranabol) Androgenic anabolic steroid.

oxymetholone   (Adroyd; Anadrol-50; Androl-50) 17-Alpha-methyl testosterone derivative anabolic steroid. No longer available in the United States. Schedule III.

oxymorphone   (Numorphan) Narcoleptic available in ampuls, vials, and suppositories. Schedule II.

oxypertine   Indole derivative based on the serotonin molecule. Addition of a phenylpiperazine side chain confers lipid-solubility that enables it to cross the blood-brain barrier and enhances its effect on brain amines. It is more potent at depleting brain noradrenaline than at depleting brain dopamine. Antipsychotic effect is approximately equal to that of chlorpromazine. Oxypertine has been shown to be significantly superior to placebo in the treatment of tardive dyskinesia.

oxyprothepin decanoate   (Meclopin) Long-acting depot neuroleptic that has been found comparable in efficacy and safety with haloperidol decanoate. Available in Europe.

oxytocin   (Syntocinon) (OT) Endogenous or synthetic neuropeptide that plays an important role in integrated hypothalamic function. It may be effective in the treatment of heroin withdrawal (Hruby VJ, Chow MS. Conformational and structural considerations in oxytocin-receptor binding and biological activity. *Ann Rev Pharmacol Toxicol* 1990;30:501–534).

P

P50 Early component (about 50 ms) of mid-latency auditory event-related responses (MLAERs). These are a series of positive and negative waves recorded at the scalp 10–200 ms following an auditory stimulus (click or tone). A characteristic of MLAERs is a tendency to decrease in amplitude with fast stimulation rates. In normal subjects, the response to the second of paired clicks is much reduced. In subjects with schizophrenia, little or no reduction occurs (impaired habituation), which has been interpreted as an impaired ability to selectively filter incoming information. A disorder of P50 habituation is also present among relatives of schizophrenic subjects.

P200 Auditory event-related potential some 200 ms after a single stimulus, which is of lower amplitude in subjects with schizophrenia than in control subjects.

P300 Late positive component of event-related potentials that has been established as a manifestation of neural activity related to cognitive processes. It is generated during performance of a task that requires resolution of uncertainty. During this task, the subject is exposed to two different stimuli (e.g., a high-pitched and a low-pitched tone), one of which occurs relatively infrequently and is designated as a target. When the subject's attention is directed to the target by counting or pressing a button, a positive potential is generated some 300 ms after the signal. This response occurs with auditory, visual, and somatosensory stimuli. It is relatively independent of the physical characteristics of the stimulus itself. It is a reflection of mental activity and not merely a response to the stimulus itself. The latency of P300 increases with the difficulty of the task required. The amplitude of P300 increases with the unexpectedness of the target tone. P300 may be useful in studying dementias, depression, and schizophrenia.

paired helical filaments (PHFS) Abnormal filaments that dominate in ultrastructural images of neurofibrillary tangles, neuropil threads, and dystrophic neurites surrounding senile plaques in Alzheimer's disease.

pairing See **matched design.**

palilalia Pathological repetition of one's own last words or phrases. It is sometimes associated with Gilles de la Tourette's syndrome.

palindrome In genetics, a sequence of nucleotides that read the same forward and backward (e.g., APCPA).

palinopsia Persistence or reappearance of a recently viewed scene. It has been reported in trazodone therapy for depression (Hughes MS, Lessell S. Trazodone-induced palinopsia. *Arch Ophthalmol* 1990;108:399–400).

palliative treatment Therapy administered to delay an inescapable outcome (e.g., death). Results of palliative treatment can be defined by the incidence with which the outcome occurs as a function of time or within a given time (e.g., 5 years' survival) or by the mean or median interval that elapses between the start of treatment and the outcome's occurrence (e.g., median duration of survival).

palm-chin reflex See **palmomental reflex.**

palmomental reflex Drawing up of the muscles on one side of the chin in response to irritation of the thenar eminence of the same-side palm by rapidly and vigorously stroking it with a needle. Also called "palm-chin reflex."

Pamelor See **nortriptyline.**

Pamine See **methscopolamine.**

"pancakes and syrup" Street term for a combination of 15 ml of Tussionex cough medicine (hydrocodone) and four 7.5-mg Lortab (hydrocodone + acetaminophen) tablets. It is said to provide a "mellow high."

pancuronium (Pavulon) Nondepolarizing curariform neuromuscular-blocking agent used to control muscle rigidity.

pancuronium + carbamazepine See **carbamazepine + pancuronium.**

pancuronium + diazepam See **diazepam + pancuronium.**

pancuronium + lithium See **lithium + pancuronium.**

pancytopenia Reduction in the numbers of all types of cells in the blood. It is rare but potentially very serious, especially if due to aplasia of the bone marrow (aplastic anemia). If severe, infection and bleeding are the most troublesome complications. It may be a very rare sensitivity reaction to certain drugs including carbamazepine, clozapine, and chlorpromazine.

panhibin See **somatostatin.**

panic Acute episode of overwhelming anxiety. It can be a symptom of panic disorder, depression, and other major psychiatric illnesses. See **panic attack.**

panic attack Sudden attack of fear or anxiety associated with one or more of 12 autonomic symptoms (e.g., shortness of breath, dizziness, palpitation or accelerated heart rate, trembling or shaking, sweating). There may be two types of panic attacks (cardiac and psychological); people tend to experience one or the other. Attacks may be spontaneous or situational. Nocturnal panic attacks occur in 30% of panic disorder patients. Nocturnal attacks occur during non–rapid eye movement (NREM) sleep and are not secondary to dreaming. Panic attacks in the elderly may be divided into early onset and late onset. The former are characterized by avoidance behaviors similar to those occurring in younger people. The latter are characterized by fewer avoidance behaviors. See **panic attack, cardiac; panic attack, psychological.**

panic attack, cardiac   Panic attack in which cardiac or cardiorespiratory symptoms are felt more strongly than they are during attacks characterized by psychological symptoms.

panic attack, psychological   Panic attack characterized by psychological symptoms rather than by physical symptoms.

panic control treatment   (PCT) New treatment for panic disorder developed at the Center for Stress and Anxiety Disorders at the University of Albany (NY) using systematic, structured exposure to feared internal sensations. Fear patterns are assessed by having patients engage in a variety of exercises designed to produce different physiological symptoms.

panic disorder   (PD) Series of severe and unexplained panic attacks accompanied by four or more autonomic symptoms that occur at least once without phobic stimulus. The most significant neurochemical theories about pathophysiology involve serotonergic, noradrenergic, and benzodiazepine systems. Abnormal dopaminergic function also has been hypothesized (Pitchot W, Ansseau M, Gonzalez Moreno A, et al. Dopaminergic function in panic disorder: comparison with major and minor depression. *Biol Psychiatry* 1992;32: 1004–1011). PD patients have blunted growth hormone (GH) responses to clonidine and to growth-related hormone relative to normal control subjects, indicating possible abnormalities in the noradrenergic control of GH release. The lifetime rate of all panic disorders is about 1%. The frequency of attacks characteristically changes over time and varies highly from individual to individual. The overwhelming majority of PD patients have abnormal, catastrophic cognitions (e.g., fear that they are dying during a panic attack) that are present during and between panic attacks. Other common cognitions are fear of a serious medical disorder, going crazy, or loss of control. Suicide attempts are associated with both uncomplicated and co-morbid PD; risk magnitude is comparable to that associated with uncomplicated and co-morbid major de-

pression. Gastrointestinal and cardiorespiratory symptoms are common; a greater proportion of PD patients have irritable bowel symptoms than do individuals without anxiety disorders. Treating PD effectively also reduces gastrointestinal symptoms. PD is often accompanied by serious alcohol abuse. The DSM-IV diagnostic criteria for PD emphasize recurrent unexpected panic attacks in which at least one attack is followed by a month or more of one of three conditions: persistent concern about having additional attacks, worry about the implications of the attack or its consequences, or a significant change in behavior related to the attacks (Ballenger JC, Fyer AJ. DSM-IV In Progress. Examining criteria for panic disorder. *Hosp Comm Psychiatry* 1993;44:226–228).

panic disorder/assessment   Instruments include Acute Panic Inventory, Cornell-Yale Panic Anxiety Scale, Hamilton Anxiety Rating Scale, Panic Associated Symptoms Scale, Panic Attack Cognitions Questionnaire, Panic Attack Symptoms Questionnaire, Sheehan's Panic and Anticipatory Anxiety Scale, and Westergaard Assessment Scale for Panic Attacks.

panic disorder (PD)/cardiac disease   PD patients often complain of chest pain. Since some may be experiencing coronary artery spasm and cardiac ischemia during panic episodes, ambulatory monitoring of the electrocardiogram (ECG) to detect ST segment depression has been done, using the Monitor One Star device; analysis of over 70 panic attacks detected no cases in which ST depression occurred (Clark DB, Taylor CB, Hayward C. Naturalistic assessment of the physiology of panic. *In* Ballenger JC [ed], *Clinical Aspects of Panic Disorder*. New York: Wiley-Liss, 1990).

panic disorder (PD)/flumazenil   Flumazenil, a benzodiazepine (BZD) receptor antagonist, displaces BZDs from the receptor. It has little clinical effect in normal volunteers not taking BZDs, but produces anxiety and panic in PD patients, suggesting that PD may be associated with an abnormality in BZD receptor function.

panic disorder (PD)/growth hormone blunting   Administration of clonidine or growth hormone releasing hormone causes a substantial increase in growth hormone (GH) release by the pituitary gland in normal subjects, but the GH response to these agents is remarkably and consistently blunted in PD patients. The blunting may be a trait of PD that endures even when the patient is in clinical remission.

panic disorder (PD)/imipramine   Imipramine (IMI) is the standard nonbenzodiazepine pharmacotherapy for PD with agoraphobia, producing a marked response rate of approximately 75% when it is the sole or main treatment (Mavissakalian M. Sequential combination of imipramine and behavioral instructions in the treatment of panic disorder with agoraphobia. *J Clin Psychiatry* 1990;51: 184–188). Relapse is likely, however, when pharmacotherapy with IMI or other antidepressants is discontinued (Noyes R Jr, Perry P. Maintenance treatment with antidepressants in panic disorder. *J Clin Psychiatry* 1990;51 [suppl A]:24–30). In one study, approximately 75% of PD patients with agoraphobia who had shown marked and stable response to 6 months of acute IMI treatment relapsed within 6 months of its discontinuation, whereas IMI responders who had received maintenance IMI treatment for 12 additional months did not relapse or sustain worsening of panic or phobic symptoms throughout the 1-year maintenance period (Mavissakalian M, Perel JM. Clinical experiments in maintenance and discontinuation of imipramine therapy in panic disorder with agoraphobia. *Arch Gen Psychiatry* 1992;49:318–323; Mavissakalin M, Perel JM. Protective effects of imipramine maintenance treatment in panic disorder with agoraphobia. *Am J Psychiatry* 1992;149:1053–1057).

panic disorder (PD)/maintenance treatment Although controlled research has yet to establish the optimal duration of pharmacotherapy for PD, in many patients PD is a chronic or recurrent condition that frequently recurs after short-term drug therapy with antidepressants or benzodiazepines. Consequently, maintenance drug therapy is frequently used. In a prospective, placebo-controlled, 32-week comparison of alprazolam (ALP) and imipramine (IMI), significantly more ALP-treated patients than IMI- or placebo-treated patients remained in therapy and experienced panic attack and phobia relief during the acute treatment phase. During the maintenance phase, neither tolerance nor daily dose increase was observed. All patients who completed the maintenance phase (ALP, 27; IMI, 11; placebo, 10) were panic-free at the end of 8 months of study treatment. ALP was effective and well tolerated (mean dose, 5.7 mg/day). IMI (175 mg/day) also produced significant panic relief, but was associated with poor patient acceptance (Schweizer E, Rickels K, Weiss S, Zavodnick S. Maintenance drug treatment of panic disorder. I. Results of a prospective, placebo-controlled comparison of alprazolam and imipramine. *Arch Gen Psychiatry* 1993;50:51–60). The same 48 patients in the above study who completed 8 months' maintenance treatment underwent gradual medication taper over a 4-week period. A withdrawal syndrome was observed in almost all ALP-treated patients, but only in a few IMI- or placebo-treated patients. Clinical worsening of withdrawal symptoms tended to subside over the course of 3 medication–free weeks, but 33% of ALP-treated patients were unable to discontinue their medication regimen successfully. Severity of panic attacks at baseline but not daily ALP dose appeared to be a significant independent predictor of taper difficulty. Of the total study population, 49% continue to receive drug therapy: 82% ALP and 18% IMI (Rickels K, Schweizer E, Weiss S, Zavodnick S. Maintenance drug treatment for panic disorder. II. Short and long-term outcome after drug taper. *Arch Gen Psychiatry* 1993;50: 61–68).

panic disorder (PD), nonfearful Disorder that meets criteria for PD, but is not associated with subjective fear and anxiety. Lactate infusion causes the same cluster of symptoms that prompted patients to seek medical help. Many of these patients initially are referred to neurologists instead of psychiatrists because primary complaints are of "dizzy spells," pseudoseizures, or paresthesias. Nonfearful panic responds favorably to treatment with antipanic medication (alprazolam, clonazepam, imipramine).

panicogen Substance or physical state that can provoke panic attacks in panic disorder patients. Substances include benzodiazepine (BZD) receptor inverse agonists and antagonists, caffeine, cholecystokinin-tetrapeptide (CCK-4), carbon dioxide, clomipramine, fenfluramine, flumazenil, isoprenaline, isoproterenol, procaine, lactate, noradrenaline, sodium bicarbonate, tricyclic antidepressants, and yohimbine. Panicogenic physical states include hypercapnia, hyperventilation, and hypoglycemia. Cocaine-induced panic disorder may persist for months or years after cocaine use has ceased. The BZD receptor antagonist flumazenil is markedly anxiogenic; an intravenous dose of 2 mg produces a panic attack in 80% of PD patients (Nutt DJ, Glue P, Lawson CW, et al. Flumazenil provocation of panic attacks: evidence for altered BZD receptor sensitivity in panic disorder. *Arch Gen Psychiatry* 1990;47: 917–925).

panmixis In genetics, equal and unrestricted mating conditions of organisms with different racial characteristics in a mixed population group (random mating).

panmyelopathy See **aplastic anemia.**

Panwarfin See **warfarin.**

papaverine (Cerespan) Smooth-muscle relaxant frequently used in the treatment of conditions associated with vascular or visceral spasms. Because it has dopamine antagonist actions, it has been tried in tardive dyskinesia with modest improvement in some patients.

paper chromatography   Separation of a mixture of compounds on filter paper according to their relative solubility in organic solvents that diffuse through the paper by capillary action.

papilledema   Choked disks or edema of the optic disks. It usually indicates increased intracranial pressure and is usually bilateral. It also may be a manifestation of diffuse retinal edema.

paracetamol + clomipramine   See **clomipramine + paracetamol.**

parachlorophenylalanine   (pCPA) Tryptophan hydroxylase inhibitor enzyme involved in the first and rate-limiting step of serotonin (5-HT) synthesis. It causes a significant decrease in central 5-HT and 5-hydroxyindoleacetic acid (5-HIAA). When it is given to tricyclic antidepressant (TCA)-remitted patients, depression relapse occurs. Discontinuation of pCPA rapidly reinstates therapeutic remission, suggesting that TCAs may exert their effect via the 5-HT system.

paradigm   Pattern or model that illustrates all the possible functions or forms.

"paradise"   Street name for cocaine.

paradoxical excitation   See **benzodiazepine disinhibition.**

paradoxical pain   Episode in which pain ceases to be relieved or is actually worsened by morphine. Increasing doses of morphine produce toxicity. Some forms of paradoxical pain may be due to abnormal morphine metabolism (Morley JS, Miles JB, Wells JC, Bowshear D. Paradoxical pain. *Lancet* 1992;340:1045).

paradoxical rage reaction   Manifestation of drug-induced disinhibition that usually occurs in patients with a history of aggressive behavior or poor impulse control. Since disinhibition is probably mediated through the limbic system, a paradoxical rage reaction must be differentiated from an underlying limbic ictal disorder. A number of benzodiazepines (e.g., alprazolam) can cause paradoxical rage reactions. See **behavioral dyscontrol; paradoxical reaction.**

paradoxical reaction   Behavioral response to a drug that differs from normally evoked responses and is not a more intense expression of the drug's usual pharmacological effects. Paradoxical reactions are opposite to clinical expectations and are exemplified by behavioral dyscontrol symptoms such as increased hostility, aggressiveness, or suicidality. They have been attributed to drugs with gamma aminobutyric acid (GABA), noradrenergic, serotonergic, or mixed effects, including benzodiazepines (chlordiazepoxide, alprazolam), tricyclic antidepressants (imipramine, amitriptyline, desipramine, nortriptyline), second-

generation antidepressants (amoxapine, trazodone, maprotiline), and the serotonin uptake inhibitor fluoxetine. Reactions occur most often in children and the elderly who have been given hypnotics or anxiolytics. See **paradoxical rage reaction.**

paradoxical sleep   See **sleep-stage rapid eye movement (REM).**

Paral   See **paraldehyde.**

paraldehyde   (Paral) Acetaldehyde polymer anticonvulsant and sedative/hypnotic used primarily for the management of seizures, status epilepticus, and the alcohol withdrawal syndrome. It must always be administered fresh (not as a brown solution or with a vinegary odor) and diluted with iced juice or milk to mask its unpleasant taste and odor and to minimize gastrointestinal distress. It also can be given by deep intramuscular injection or as a retention enema diluted 2:1 in olive or cottonseed oil. It is rapidly absorbed after oral administration, reaching maximum serum levels within 1 hour and producing rapid sleep onset. It does not possess analgesic properties. Disadvantages include possible development of sterile abscesses with intramuscular injection, pulmonary edema after intravenous injection, and difficulty in adjusting dosage with rectal administration. The unpleasant smell lingers on the patient's breath because of pulmonary excretion. Paraldehyde can cause dependence and severe withdrawal symptoms and is potentially toxic; since many safer alternatives are available, it is seldom used. Schedule IV; pregnancy risk category C.

parallel study   Study designed to compare treatments given to different patients in a single clinical trial.

parallel track drug study   New type of study conducted in parallel with the principal controlled investigation, but without the existence of concurrent control groups.

paralysis agitans   See **Parkinson's disease.**

paralysis, sleep   See **sleep paralysis.**

paralytic and syphilitic meningoencephalitis See **general paresis.**

parameter   Quantitative value that characterizes a certain probability distribution.

paramethoxyamphetamine   (PMA) Methoxylated amphetamine-like variant of methylenedioxymethamphetamine (MDMA). It is a potent hallucinogen that also has sympathomimetic effects. It may provoke serious hypertensive reactions. A number of fatalities in men ages 17–30 have been attributed to it; all suffered from agitation, seizures, and hyperthermia. PMA has been classified as a restricted drug.

paramnesia   Falsification of memory by distortion of recall.

paranoia   Term used by Kraepelin to describe an uncommon but striking group of patients with extensive delusional symptoms, but no hallucinations. It originally was regarded as a separate and stable condition, but follow-up studies showed that many paranoid patients developed typical schizophrenic symptoms in subsequent years. Some patients, however, do remain stable and show little deterioration.

paranoid ideation   Suspiciousness or belief, of less than delusional proportions, that one is harassed, persecuted, or unfairly treated. Some clinicians may use the term when they are unsure whether the disturbances are actually delusional. Ideas of references often involve paranoid ideation.

paranoid personality disorder   Disorder characterized by a pervasive distrust and suspiciousness of others such that their motives are interpreted as malevolent.

paranoid state   Temporary descriptive label for patients with prominent delusions of persecution who have neither first-rank symptoms of schizophrenia nor prominent affective symptoms; many such patients may develop more obvious schizophrenic or affective symptoms as the illness progresses.

paraphasia   Loss of ability to speak correctly characterized by misnaming and inappropriate substitution of words. It raises the suspicion of an underlying neurological process. It can be one of multiple speech abnormalities that occur during delirium.

paraphilia   Any of a group of sexual disorders whose essential features are recurrent, intense sexual urges and sexually arousing fantasies generally involving either nonhuman objects, suffering or humiliation of self or partner (not merely simulated), or children or other nonconsenting persons. Unusual sexual interest, rather than excessive sexual drive, is characteristic. Victims of paraphilic acts include 37% by exhibitionists, 29% by frotteurs, 14% by pedophiles, and 14% by voyeurs; rape victims constitute less than 1% of all victims of paraphiliacs. Because sexually deviant fantasies, desires, and behavior are pleasurable and reduce anxieties, paraphiliacs seldom seek treatment. Those who want and need treatment often stay away because they fear legal consequences or social stigma (Abel GG, Becker JV, Cunningham-Rathner J, et al. Multiple paraphilic diagnoses among sex offenders. *Bull Am Acad Psychiatr Law* 1989;16:153–168).

paraphilia, contact   Pedophilia, rape, sexual sadism, and zoophilia.

paraphilia/drug therapy   Medroxyprogesterone or cyproterone acetate are used in some countries to treat paraphilias. The drugs do not change sexual interest, but reduce sexual drive and improve control. Although medroxyprogesterone acetate and similar drugs can have significant side effects, in clinical experience they occur relatively infrequently. Less invasive medication intervention involves fluoxetine, which appears to reduce sexual drive as a drug side effect (Abel GG, Osborn C. Stopping sexual violence. *Psychiatr Ann* 1992; 22:301–306).

paraphilia, noncontact   Compulsive masturbation, exhibitionism, sexual masochism, telephone scatologia, transvestic fetishism, and voyeurism.

paraphrenia   Onset of schizophrenic symptoms after age 45. There is no consensus about the meaning of this term. See **schizophrenia, late-onset.**

paraplegia   Paralysis of the lower half of the body, often including the bladder and bowel. It can be caused by disease of or injury to the spinal cord or by some parasagittal brain tumors.

parasomnia   Sleep disorder category that includes abnormal behaviors during sleep (e.g., enuresis, somnambulism, nocturnal epilepsy, nightmares, pavor nocturnus) or some adventitious movements that are not part of normal sleep. Also included are sleep starts, nocturnal leg cramps, sleep-related painful erections, sleep behavior disorders, and sleep-related abnormal swallowing syndrome. Benzodiazepines may be used to treat some parasomnia disorders and, at times, may paradoxically produce some of these behaviors in susceptible individuals.

parasuicide   Deliberately nonfatal self-poisoning or injury.

parasuicidal behavior   Behavior that includes self-mutilation and other intentional self-injurious behavior (SIB). It has been called the behavioral specialty of those with borderline personality disorder that can be viewed as a form of communication or way of relating. Linehan (1987) developed a behavioral treatment that, viewing SIB as problem-solving behavior used to cope with or ameliorate psychic distress, teaches alternative problem-solving techniques.

parathyroid disease/cognitive deficits   Cognitive deficits occur in both hyper- and hypoparathyroidism. In the former, a toxic confusional syndrome is common; in the latter, cataracts, seizures, parkinsonism, and dementia (even in the absence of tetany) may occur. Even with treatment, irreversible intellectual deficits are not uncommon.

paratonia   Variable resistance to all passive movement that reflects bihemispheric dysfunction. It occurs in a wide range of disorders (e.g., Alzheimer's, multi-infarct dementia, metabolic encephalopathy). It is the opposite of mitgehen. Formerly called "gegenhalten."

parens patriae English law term based on the concept that the king is the parent to the country and, as such, has a parental responsibility for subjects unable to care for themselves. When applied to involuntary commitment, parens patriae is used to justify a protective mechanism for citizens in need of protection. It makes the state protector of patients from their inability to survive unaided.

paresis Partial loss of motor function in limbs and facial muscles due to a neurological disease.

paresis, general See **general paresis.**

Parest See **methaqualone.**

paresthesia Abnormal sensation (e.g., tingling).

paretic neurosyphilis See **general paresis.**

pargyline (Eutonyl) Nonhydrazine, irreversible monoamine oxidase inhibitor with antihypertensive activity. It is rarely used for the treatment of depression.

Paritrel See **amantadine.**

Parkinson's disease (PD) Neurological disorder, first described by James Parkinson (1817), associated with degeneration of the nigrostriatal dopaminergic system and loss of the midbrain, limbic, and cortical projections. It is associated with dopamine depletion in the basal ganglia. Cerebrospinal fluid levels of homovanillic acid (the major dopamine metabolite), the dopamine-synthesizing enzyme tyrosine hydroxylase, and the co-factor tetrahydrobiopterin are lower than normal. The cause of PD is unknown, but may be related to environmental toxins (e.g., 1-methyl-4-phenyl-1,2,3,6-tetrahydropyridine [MPTP]). PD is characterized by rapid, coarse resting tremor, pill-rolling movements, cogwheel rigidity, drooling, masklike facies, akinesia, bradykinesia, gait disturbances, postural abnormalities, and dementia. PD patients develop stooped posture with trunk flexion. They have difficulty taking initial steps in walking and take small, shuffling steps (*marche a petit pas*). Once patients start walking, festination (a gradual increase in walking speed) occurs. Retropulsion, in which the patient falls backward rapidly with minimal ability to regain balance, also may occur. Other characteristics are reduced arm, trunk, or body movements; impaired postural reflexes; stiffness; and cogwheel rigidity, in which there is a slight catch with each movement. Rigidity and bradykinesia affect handwriting, initially manifested by micrographia; as PD progresses, handwriting deteriorates to the point of illegibility. During

sleep there is a marked diminution in tremor and muscular rigidity, but sleep fragmentation and respiratory disorders during sleep are common. Pain (cramps of the neck and spine; radicular, neuritic, or joint pains; and the diffuse discomfort of akathisia and dystonia) occurs with a reported frequency of 12–46% (Goetz CG, Wilson RS, Tanner CM, Garron DC. Relationships among pain, depression, and sleep alterations in Parkinson's disease. *Adv Neurol* 1986;45:345–347). Pain assessment should be included in the evaluation of PD patients. Although depression is no more common among patients with pain than among those without pain, depression rating scale scores are significantly higher in patients experiencing pain, suggesting that depression is more severe in those with painful disorder (Cummings JL. Pain in depression and Parkinson's disease. *Am J Psychiatry* 1993;150:354). Also called "paralysis agitans."

Parkinson's disease (PD)/dementia Dementia is very common among PD patients; incidence estimates vary from 10% to 20%. The association between PD and Alzheimer's disease remains controversial because many believe that concurrent Alzheimer's disease does not account for all of the cognitive deficits observed in PD. It is important to consider the possible contribution of medications in the evaluation of a PD patient who develops dementia. Anticholinergic agents are frequent offenders, as are benzodiazepines, which are often prescribed because of sleep disturbance (Standaert DG, Stern MB. Update on the management of Parkinson's disease. *Med Clin North Am* 1993;77:169–183).

Parkinson's disease (PD)/depression Depression is the most common affective disturbance reported in PD patients. Incidence is about 40–50%, but its characteristics, course, treatment responsiveness, and neurobiological substrates are at best only partially established. Diagnosis can be difficult because many of the characteristic features of depression (psychomotor retardation, anorexia, insomnia, poor concentration) are also common features of PD (Marder K, Mayeux R. Recognition and management of major behavior problems in Parkinson's disease. *In* Stern MB, Hurtig HH [eds], *The Comprehensive Management of Parkinson's Disease.* New York: PMA, 1988, pp 171–186). It has been suggested that the increased incidence of depression in PD can be attributed solely to the disabling effects of chronic illness (Gotham AM, Brown RG, Marsden CD. Depression in Parkinson's disease: a quantitative and qualitative analysis. *J Neurol Neurosurg Psychiatry* 1986;49:381–389). However, factors that argue against a reactive etiology include the emergence of depression before the onset of PD motor symptoms, the lack of relation between PD severity and depression, and the higher incidence of depression in PD patients even when compared with patients with equally disabling illnesses (Mayeux R. Parkinson's disease. *J Clin Psychiatry* 1990;51[suppl]: 20–23). Depressed PD patients can be divided into three distinct groups: those in whom depression is an integral part of PD; those in whom it is not an integral component of PD, but an affective reaction to its occurrence; and those with a history of bipolar or (more often) unipolar illness in whom depression is an independent affective disorder co-existing with PD (Cummings JL. Depression and Parkinson's disease: a review. *Am J Psychiatry* 1993; 149:443–454). Before antidepressant drugs, patients in the third group often were treated with electroconvulsive therapy (ECT), particularly if they were suicidal and/or psychotic. In some, but not all, patients, ECT not only relieved depression, but seemed to secondarily improve PD. L-dopa, by contrast, treats the motor components of PD, but does not always alleviate depression. When the first of the tricyclic antidepressants became available, they were prescribed for depressed PD patients, alleviating the depression and some PD symptoms as well. Imipramine, nortriptyline, desipramine, and bupropion effectively treat depression in PD. Selegiline, an monoamine oxidase B (MAO-B) inhibitor, may have some mild antidepressant properties. Experience with serotonin (5-HT) uptake inhibitor (SUI) antidepressants in PD currently is limited; however, alteration in 5-HT function is becoming increasingly evident in depressed patients with PD. Sleep deprivation has been reported to be effective in the treatment of depression in an elderly patient with Parkinson's disease (Perry W, Benbow C, West L, et al. Sleep deprivation in an elderly man with Parkinson's disease. *Am J Psychiatry* 1993;150:350). See **selegiline.**

Parkinson's disease (PD)/depression/dopamine
Evidence supporting the role of dopamine (DA) in depression and PD includes: (a) DA neurons of the ventral tegmental area are more involved in depressed than in nondepressed PD patients; (b) depression is more prevalent in patients with DA-mediated deficits in intellectual function; (c) depression frequently occurs in the off state when there is marked DA deficiency; (d) positron emission tomography (PET) shows disproportionate hypometabolism in brain regions with prominent DA function (frontal lobe, caudate nucleus) in depressed compared to nondepressed PD patients; and (e) DA is critical in reward mediation, stress responses, and anticipation functions likely to be involved in mood and emotion (Cummings JL. Serotonin and Parkinson's disease. *Am J Psychiatry* 1993;150: 844).

Parkinson's disease (PD)/hallucinations   Hallucinations in PD may consist of well-formed visual images of people or animals; auditory hallucinations occur less frequently. They are most often a complication of levodopa therapy, but also may result from dopamine (DA) agonists or anticholinergics. The first treatment should be dosage reduction. In some cases, redistribution of the daily levodopa dose in the evening may alleviate night-time hallucinations and nightmares. Dosage reduction, in some patients, may lead to unacceptable reduction in motility. Typical neuroleptics should not be prescribed because they may markedly worsen PD, but the atypical neuroleptic clozapine is usually well tolerated (Standaert DG, Stern MB. Update on the management of Parkinson's disease. *Med Clin North Am* 1993;77:169–183). Ondansetron, a serotonin (5-HT)$_3$ antagonist, may be an effective and safe therapy to control PD hallucinosis without causing deterioration of the motor signs and symptoms or suppression of levodopa-induced clinical benefit. It also may allow an increase in the levodopa dosage or use of other methods of central DA stimulation to improve patients' mobility and quality of life (Zoldan J, Friedberg G, Goldberg-Stern H, Melamed E. Ondansetron for hallucinosis in advanced Parkinson's disease. *Lancet* 1993;341:562–563).

Parkinson's disease (PD)/panic attacks   During levodopa therapy, the "on-off" periods are associated with intense autonomic symptoms (e.g., tachycardia, sweating) and fear. As an off period begins, panic attacks may occur (Marsden CD, Parkes JD. "On-off" effects in patients with Parkinson's disease on chronic levodopa therapy. *Lancet* 1976;1:292–296; Wise MG, Rieck SO. Diagnostic considerations and treatment approaches to underlying anxiety in the medically ill. *J Clin Psychiatry* 1993; 54[suppl 5]:22–26).

parkinsonian tremor   See **tremor, parkinsonian.**

parkinsonism   Presence of resting tremor, rigidity, bradykinesia, or postural instability. Its most common cause is Parkinson's disease (PD), although other etiologies include infectious, vascular, pharmacological, toxic, metabolic, structural, and degenerative disorders. Differential diagnosis is important, because treatments and prognoses differ.

parkinsonism, drug-induced   Reversible syndrome resembling Parkinson's disease (PD) that results from the dopamine-blocking action of neuroleptic drugs and metoclopramide. In state residential child psychiatric centers, approximately 34% of child/adolescent inpatients have drug-induced parkinsonism, which is significantly associated with longer neuroleptic treatment periods. Women are more susceptible than men; incidence is higher over age 60. Symptoms develop slowly and are noticed by others before the patient complains about them. They are generally bilateral, but may be asymmetrical. Pill-rolling movements are less common than in the naturally occurring disorder. Symptoms are quite similar to those of idiopathic PD and frequently interfere with age-appropriate activities; they are often cited as a reason for outpatient noncompliance. If the responsible drug is discontinued as early as possible, symptoms usually (not always) disappear slowly (average, 3 months) (Stern MB. The clinical characteristics of Parkinson's disease and parkinson syndromes: diagnosis and assessment. *In* Stern MB, Hurtig HH [eds], *The Comprehensive Management of Parkinson's Disease.* New York: PMA, 1988, pp 3–50). Also called "pseudoparkinsonism." See **extrapyramidal side effects.**

parkinsonism/electroconvulsive therapy (ECT) ECT is effective in reducing motor symptoms (particularly rigidity) and affective mood disorders in patients with severe Parkinson's disease (PD). Although there is a risk of delirium, especially in patients receiving dopaminergic (DA) drug treatment (usually Sinemet) for PD symptoms, it can be minimized if DA treatment is reduced before beginning ECT.

parkinsonism/falls Frequent falls are a common source of embarrassment and injury in parkinsonian patients. When postural dizziness, fainting, and tripping are excluded, many falls are caused by akinetic freezing (inability to move the leading foot forward when the trunk starts in motion.) Physiologically, there is a failure to select the right agonist muscles in advance of rapid and precise movement, a delay in switching from one movement to another, and a defect in simultaneously activating different parts of the body (Pearce JMS. *Parkinson's Disease and Its Management.* Oxford: Oxford University Press, 1992, pp 30–32).

parkinsonism, idiopathic Most common of all forms of Parkinson's disease (PD), accounting for 90% of cases of PD. PD is a disorder of middle or late life, typically with a gradual progression and prolonged course. In patients with idiopathic parkinsonism, dopamine (DA) deficiency causes substantia nigra depigmentation. The most common physical signs in-

clude akinesia, hypokinesia, bradykinesia, micrographia, slow starting movements, poverty of spontaneous actions, lead pipe and cogwheel rigidity, slow rhythmic "pill-rolling" tremor, lack of normal automatic movements (e.g., fidgeting), unnatural stillness, flexed "simian" posture of the trunk and limbs, short shuffling steps, feet "frozen" to the ground, masked facies, lack of expression, infrequent blinking, staring, dribbling, reduced swallowing, hoarseness, dysarthria, and positive glabella tap sign (Pearce JMS. *Parkinson's Disease and Its Management.* New York: Oxford University Press, 1992, pp 26–36). Idiopathic parkinsonism should be separated from symptomatic neuronal degeneration and from other cerebral lesions, including pseudoparkinsonism.

parkinsonism, idiopathic/diagnostic criteria, revised Three or more of the following features: (a) at onset: slow, 4- to 6-Hz, resting tremor in one or more limbs; (b) predominantly unilateral distribution at onset; (c) rigidity (lead-pipe or cogwheel in axial muscles or limbs), plus hypokinesia or bradykinesia of face, trunk, or limb movement, including gait; postural abnormalities; (d) substantial and unequivocal clinical response (33–100% reduction of clinical rating scales) to levodopa treatment within 2 months (Gibbs WRG, Lees AJ. The relevance of Lewy body disease to the pathogenesis of idiopathic Parkinson's disease. UK Parkinson's Disease Society brain bank clinical diagnostic criteria. *J Neurol Neurosurg Psychiatry* 1988;51:745–752).

parkinsonism, idiopathic/diagnostic criteria, traditional Bradykinesia, plus one of the following: (a) resting tremor (4–6 Hz); (b) rigidity (usually lead-pipe or cogwheel) in limbs, neck or trunk; and (c) postural instability not of visual, vestibular, cerebellar, or proprioceptive origin.

parkinsonism/MPTP See **1-methyl-4-phenyl-1,2,-3,6-tetrahydropyridine (MPTP).**

parkinsonism/neuroprotective therapy Treatment for early parkinsonism can be divided into symptomatic therapy and neuroprotective therapy. Neuroprotective therapy is believed to slow the rate of disease progression. Selegiline and pergolide are thought to have a neuroprotective action.

parkinsonism, postencephalitic Parkinsonism that develops in patients with "sleeping sickness" or encephalitis lethargica. It is characterized by abnormal sleep-wake cycles that may be the result of the loss of dopaminergic neurons in the substantia nigra.

Parlodel See **bromocriptine.**
Parmine See **phentermine.**
Parnate See **tranylcypromine.**

paroxetine (Apropax; Aropax; Paxil; Seroxat) Novel, phenylpiperidine serotonin (5-HT) uptake inhibitor (SUI). In vitro data indicate that it is more selective and more potent than other available SUIs. It effectively relieves depression and associated symptoms of anxiety. Initial adult dose is 20 mg/day (less in the elderly). If necessary, dosage may be increased by increments of 10 mg/day up to 40 mg/day according to response. Elderly patients have tolerated paroxetine, although there is a report of hyponatremia associated with it in a 69-year-old woman (Goddard C, Paton C. Hyponatraemia associated with paroxetine. *Br Med J* 1992;305:1332). Available data indicate that paroxetine is free from serious cardiovascular side effects. No electrocardiographic changes have been recorded in paroxetine-treated patients. In double-blind studies comparing paroxetine and fluoxetine, both drugs were equally effective, with paroxetine causing fewer and less severe adverse effects than fluoxetine. The most common side effects in paroxetine-treated patients are nausea, headaches, and diarrhea. It may interact with warfarin and other oral anticoagulants. It should not be co-administered with a monoamine oxidase inhibitor (MAOI) or used within 2 weeks before or after MAOI therapy. To date (1994), overdoses of paroxetine alone or with other drugs have not resulted in death attributable to paroxetine. Pregnancy risk category B.

paroxetine + alcohol Paroxetine with or without alcohol produces no significant impairment compared with placebo on any tests (critical flicker fusion threshold, choice reaction time, simulated car steering, memory scanning, memory reaction, peripheral attention, and subjective ratings of sedation). Although paroxetine does not potentiate the sedative or psychomotor effects of alcohol, co-administration may increase central nervous system adverse effects (Cooper SM, Jackson D, Loudon JM, et al. The psychomotor effects of paroxetine alone and in combination with haloperidol, amylobarbitone, oxazepam, or alcohol. *Acta Psychiatr Scand* 1989; 80[suppl 350]:53–55; Hindmarch I, Harrison C. The effects of paroxetine and other antidepressants in combination with alcohol on psychomotor activity related to car driving. *Hum Psychopharmacol* 1988;3:13–20).

paroxetine + aluminum hydroxide Co-administration did not affect paroxetine plasma concentrations (Greb WH, Brett MA, Buscher G, et al. Absorption of paroxetine under various dietary conditions and following antacid intake. *Acta Psychiatr Scand* 1989;80[suppl 350]: 99–101).

paroxetine + amitriptyline Co-administration may necessitate use of lower doses than usually prescribed for either drug, since each inhibits the other's metabolism, raising the plasma level of each.

paroxetine + amobarbital Paroxetine does not potentiate the sedative effects of amobarbital. No clinically significant interactions have been reported (Boyer WF, Feighner JP. An overview of paroxetine. *J Clin Psychiatry* 1192;53[suppl]: 3–6).

paroxetine + barbiturate Although paroxetine does not potentiate the sedative or psychomotor effects of barbiturates, co-administration may increase adverse central nervous system effects (Cooper SM, Jackson D, Loudon JM, et al. The psychomotor effects of paroxetine alone and in combination with haloperidol, amylobarbitone, oxazepam or alcohol. *Acta Psychiatr Scand* 1989;80[suppl 350]:53–55).

paroxetine + benzodiazepine Paroxetine does not potentiate the sedative or psychomotor effects of benzodiazepines, but co-administration may increase central nervous system adverse effects (Cooper SM, Jackson D, Loudon JM, et al. The psychomotor effects of paroxetine alone and in combination with haloperidol, amylobarbitone, oxazepam, or alcohol. *Acta Psychiatr Scand* 1989;80[suppl 350]:53–55).

paroxetine/breast milk Paroxetine appears in breast milk in quantities that may be pharmacologically significant (Kaye CM, Haddock RE, Langley PF, et al. A review of the metabolism and pharmacokinetics of paroxetine in man. *Acta Psychiatr Scand* 1989;80[suppl 350]: 60–75) It should not be administered during breastfeeding.

paroxetine + carbamazepine Co-administration in well-controlled epileptics was well tolerated in a single-blind, placebo-controlled study. No seizures or clinically relevant changes in carbamazepine plasma concentrations occurred (Mikkelsen M, Anderson BB, Dam M, et al. Paroxetine: no interaction with anti-epileptic drugs. *Psychopharmacology* 1991; 103:B13).

paroxetine + charcoal Co-administration effectively prevented paroxetine absorption (Greb WH, Buscher G, Dierdorf H-D, et al. Ability of charcoal to prevent absorption of paroxetine. *Acta Psychiatr Scand* 1989;80[suppl 350]:156–157).

paroxetine + cimetidine Cimetidine may impair first-pass metabolism of paroxetine, resulting in paroxetine plasma levels about 50% higher (clinical significance is unknown). During co-administration, dosage adjustment of paroxetine after the starting dose should be guided by clinical effect (Bannister SJ, Houser

VP, Hulse JD, et al. Evaluation of the potential for interactions of paroxetine with diazepam, cimetidine, warfarin and digoxin. *Acta Psychiatr Scand* 1989;80[suppl 350]:102–106; Greb WH, Buscher G, Dierdorf HD, et al. The effect of liver enzyme inhibition by cimetidine and enzyme induction by phenobarbitone and the pharmacokinetics of paroxetine. *Acta Psychiatr Scand* 1989;80[suppl 350]:95–98).

paroxetine + desipramine   Paroxetine (30 mg/day) causes a threefold increase in half-life and a fivefold decrease in the clearance of serum desipramine (DMI), which is metabolized by cytochrome P450IID6 (Brosen K, Graham LF, Sindroup S. Pharmacokinetics of tricyclic antidepressants and novel antidepressants: recent developments. *Clin Neuropharmacol* 1992;15:80A–81A). Co-administration may necessitate use of lower doses than usually prescribed for either drug. In an 18-year-old man with major depression partially responsive to DMI, addition of paroxetine (20 mg/day) resulted in rapid elevation of DMI level to 503 ng/ml. Depressive symptoms improved markedly, and he experienced mild anticholinergic side effects (Pittard JT. Pharmacokinetic interaction between paroxetine and tricyclic antidepressants. *Curr Affect Ill* 1993;12:14–15).

paroxetine + diazepam   No interactions have been demonstrated. Paroxetine concentrations were not increased by multiple-dose co-administration of diazepam (Bannister SJ, Houser VP, Hulse JD, et al. Evaluation of the potential for interactions of paroxetine with diazepam, cimetidine, warfarin and digoxin. *Acta Psychiatr Scand* 1989;80[suppl 350]:102–106).

paroxetine + digoxin   No interactions have been demonstrated (Bannister SJ, Houser VP, Hulse JD, et al. Evaluation of the potential for interactions of paroxetine with diazepam, cimetidine, warfarin and digoxin. *Acta Psychiatr Scand* 1989;80[suppl 350]:102–106).

paroxetine + electroconvulsive therapy (ECT)   Some interactions may occur. At steady-state concentrations, paroxetine can inhibit and saturate the high-affinity components of the hepatic P450 enzyme system, resulting in potentially higher plasma levels of compounds metabolized by these pathways and possible interference with the metabolism of anesthetics used during ECT. Because paroxetine is a selective inhibitor of serotonin uptake, there is a theoretical possibility of its provoking a serotonin syndrome with ECT-induced elevations of brain serotonin. Paroxetine should be discontinued prior to ECT (Jarvix MR, Goevert AJ, Zorumski CF. Novel antidepressants

and maintenance electroconvulsive therapy. A review. *Ann Clin Psychiatry* 1992;4:275–284).

paroxetine/extrapyramidal reactions   Extrapyramidal reactions have been reported no more frequently than with fluvoxamine and fluoxetine (estimated incidence, 1 per 1,000 patients). They occur early in treatment and may be due to pre-existing Parkinson's disease or to concurrent medication (Anon. *Current Problems in Pharmacovigilance* 1993;19:1).

paroxetine + fluoxetine   Co-administration may require doses lower than usually prescribed for either drug alone.

paroxetine + haloperidol   Paroxetine interferes with the cytochrome P450IID6 isoenzyme, which may result in increased haloperidol (HAL) levels and increased clinical side effects. Paroxetine does not potentiate HAL's sedative or psychomotor effects, but co-administration may increase adverse central nervous system effects (Cooper SM, Jackson D, Loudon JM, et al. The psychomotor effects of paroxetine alone and in combination with haloperidol, amylobarbitone, oxazepam, or alcohol. *Acta Psychiatr Scand* 1989;80[suppl 350]:53–55). There is a report of a patient being treated with paroxetine (20 mg/day) to which HAL 3 mg/day was added. Two weeks later, she relapsed into a semistuporous state that remitted when paroxetine, but not HAL, was discontinued (Lewis J, Brazanza J, Williams T. Psychomotor retardation and semistuporous state with paroxetine. *Br Med J* 1993;306:1169).

paroxetine + imipramine   Co-administration may necessitate use of lower doses than usually prescribed for either drug alone. There is a report of marked elevation in imipramine (IMI) and desipramine plasma levels (IMI, 91 ng/ml; desipramine, 308 ng/ml; total, 399 ng/ml) 6 days after paroxetine (20 mg/day) was added to IMI (100 mg/day). The patient experienced worsened constipation and new-onset postural dizziness (Pittard JT. Pharmacokinetic interaction between paroxetine and tricyclic antidepressants. *Curr Affect Ill* 1993;12:14–15).

paroxetine + lithium   Addition of paroxetine to chronic lithium therapy did not cause any clinically significant changes in vital signs or laboratory values, including plasma lithium levels. There was a high incidence of tremor (47%) and sweating (36%), but it is not known if these effects were additive (Haenen J. An interaction study of paroxetine on lithium plasma levels in depressed patients stabilized on lithium therapy. Presented at the 5th World Congress of Biological Psychiatry, Florence, June 1991). Co-administration was well tolerated in a 5-week open study (Stellamans G. A study to investigate the efficacy, adverse events, safety, and pharmacokinetic effects of co-administration of paroxetine and lithium. *Biol Psychiatry* 1991;29:354S).

paroxetine/mania Like all antidepressants, paroxetine may induce mania. In clinical evaluations, patients with a history of mania included 134 given paroxetine; of these, 3 paroxetine-treated patients (2%) and 10 control subjects (11%) had a manic reaction, a statistically significant difference (p < 0.05). In the paroxetine-treated patients, onset ranged from 63–133 days; in the control subjects, 10–90 days. Incidence of mania in unipolar patients during short- and long-term treatment was 0.9% with paroxetine, 0.5% with active control, and 0.4% with placebo.

paroxetine + methyldopa No interactions have been demonstrated (Bannister SJ, Houser VP, Hulse JD, et al. Evaluation of the potential for interactions of paroxetine with diazepam, cimetidine, warfarin and digoxin. *Acta Psychiatr Scand* 1989;80[suppl 350]:102–106).

paroxetine + monoamine oxidase inhibitor (MAOI) Animal data indicate that co-administration can cause symptoms of the serotonin syndrome. In the only human data available to date (1992), single paroxetine doses (30 mg) increased the maximum plasma concentration of single tranylcypromine doses (20 mg) by 15% in healthy volunteers (data on file, SmithKline Beecham). The manufacturer recommends waiting at least 2 weeks after paroxetine is stopped before an MAOI is initiated.

paroxetine + nortriptyline Co-administration may require use of lower doses of each drug.

paroxetine + oral contraceptive No interactions have been demonstrated (Bannister SJ, Houser VP, Hulse JD, et al. Evaluation of the potential for interactions of paroxetine with diazepam, cimetidine, warfarin and digoxin. *Acta Psychiatr Scand* 1989;80[suppl 350]:102–106).

paroxetine overdose Animal data indicate that, like other serotonin uptake inhibitors, paroxetine is considerably safer than tricyclic antidepressants in overdose (Kelvin AS, Hakansson S. Comparative acute toxicity of paroxetine and other antidepressants. *Acta Psychiatr Scand* 1989;80[suppl 350]:31–33). In humans, 30 overdose cases (up to 850 mg) occurred by the end of 1992, alone or in combination with other substances. No loss of consciousness, cardiovascular complications, or seizures occurred. All patients recovered fully with supportive care. Prompt administration of charcoal may help reduce paroxetine plasma levels (Greb WH, Buscher G, Dierdorf HD, et al. Ability of charcoal to prevent absorption of paroxetine. *Acta Psychiatr Scand* 1989;80[suppl 350]:156–157).

paroxetine + oxazepam Paroxetine does not potentiate oxazepam's sedative effects. No clinically important interactions have been reported (Boyer WF, Feighner JP. An overview of paroxetine. *J Clin Psychiatry* 1992;53[suppl]:3–6).

paroxetine + phenobarbital No significant interactions have been reported. In some studies, phenobarbital caused a 25% decrease in paroxetine plasma concentrations, most likely due to accelerated metabolism as a result of enzyme induction (Kaye CM, Haddock RE, Langley PF, et al. A review of the metabolism and pharmacokinetics of paroxetine in man. *Acta Psychiatr Scand* 1989;80[suppl 350]:60–75; Greb WH, Buscher G, Dierdorf H-D, et al. The effect of liver enzyme inhibition by cimetidine and enzyme induction by phenobarbitone on the pharmacokinetics of paroxetine. *Acta Psychiatr Scand* 1989;80[suppl 350]:95–98).

paroxetine + phenytoin A single oral dose of paroxetine, administered to a patient whose phenytoin plasma level was in steady-state, reduced paroxetine's area under the curve (AUC) and half-life ($T_{1/2}$) by an average of 50% and 35%, respectively, compared to paroxetine administered alone. When a single oral dose of phenytoin (300 mg) was administered at paroxetine steady-state (30 mg every day for 14 days), phenytoin's AUC was slightly reduced (average, 12%) compared to the AUC of phenytoin administered alone. No initial dosage adjustments are considered necessary when these drugs are co-administered; subsequent adjustments should be guided by clinical effect (Kaye CM, Haddock RE, Langley PF, et al. A review of the metabolism and pharmacokinetics of paroxetine in man. *Acta Psychiatr Scand* 1989;80[suppl 350]:60–75; Mikkelsen M, Anderson BB, Dam M, et al: Paroxetine: no interaction with anti-epileptic drugs. *Psychopharmacology* 1991;103:B13).

paroxetine/pregnancy In animals, paroxetine was associated with teratogenic or selective embryotoxic effects only at doses toxic to the mother (Baldwin JA, Davidson EJ, Pritchard AL, et al. The reproductive toxicology of paroxetine. *Acta Psychiatr Scand* 1989;80[suppl 350]:37–39). In full-term human pregnancies during which paroxetine was taken, babies were reported healthy. Paroxetine's safety during pregnancy, however, has not been established, and its use should be avoided until more is known about its safety for the mother and fetus.

paroxetine + procyclidine Paroxetine (30 mg/day) increases procyclidine's (5 mg every day) steady-state area under the curve (AUC) 0–24 by 35%, C_{max} by 37%, and C_{min} by 67% compared to procyclidine given alone at steady state. If anticholinergic effects occur, procyclidine dose should be reduced.

paroxetine + propranolol No interactions have been demonstrated (Bannister SJ, Houser VP, Hulse JD, et al. Evaluation of the potential for interactions of paroxetine with diazepam, cimetidine, warfarin and digoxin. *Acta Psychiatr Scand* 1989;80[suppl 350]:102–106).

paroxetine/seizure Paroxetine does not alter seizure threshold in animals. Neither a single dose nor 30 mg/day for 4 weeks altered the electroencephalogram (EEG) or produced epileptiform changes in normal subjects (Sedgwick EM, Cilasun J, Edwards JG. Paroxetine and the electroencephalogram. *J Psychopharmacol* 1987;1:31–34).

paroxetine/stupor As of July 1993, four reports of paroxetine-associated stupor had been received by the Committee on Safety of Medicines in England. None of the patients took concurrent neuroleptics or was elderly. See **paroxetine + haloperidol; paroxetine + thioridazine.**

paroxetine + thioridazine Concomitant use of paroxetine with thioridazine, which is metabolized by cytochrome P450IID6, may require use of lower doses than usually prescribed for either drug alone. A patient treated with paroxetine (up to 40 mg/day), thioridazine (30 mg/day), and trifluoperazine (10 mg/day) became oversedated, withdrawn, immobile, and unresponsive. Cessation of the neuroleptics produced no significant change. Two weeks later, paroxetine was discontinued; within 5 days, psychomotor function returned (Lewis J, Braganza J, Williams T, et al. Psychomotor retardation and semistuporous state with paroxetine. *Br Med J* 1993;306:1169).

paroxetine + tranylcypromine Animal data indicate that co-administration can cause symptoms of the serotonin syndrome. In healthy volunteers, single paroxetine doses (30 mg) increased the maximum plasma concentration of single tranylcypromine doses (20 mg) by 15% (data on File, SmithKline Beecham). The manufacturer recommends waiting at least 2 weeks after paroxetine therapy is stopped before a monoamine oxidase inhibitor is initiated.

paroxetine + tricyclic antidepressant Paroxetine, a potent inhibitor of the cytochrome P450IID6 isoenzyme in the liver responsible for metabolism of drugs such as tricyclic antidepressants (TCAs), may increase TCA plasma concentrations (van Harten J. Clinical pharmacokinetics of selective serotonin reuptake inhibitors. *Clin Pharmacokinet* 1991;24:203–220).

paroxetine + trifluoperazine See **trifluoperazine + paroxetine.**

paroxetine + tryptophan Co-administration may produce increased agitation, restlessness, gastrointestinal effects, and other manifestations of the serotonin syndrome.

paroxetine + valproate Co-administration in patients with well-controlled epilepsy was well tolerated in one single-blind, placebo-controlled study. No clinically relevant changes in valproate plasma concentration were noted (Mikkelsen M, Anderson BB, Dam M, et al. Paroxetine: no interaction with anti-epileptic drugs. *Psychopharmacology* 1991;103:B13).

paroxetine + warfarin Co-administration may increase bleeding tendency. Despite paroxetine's lack of significant effect on prothrombin time, mild but clinically significant bleeding occurred in 5 of 27 healthy volunteers given both drugs; 3 were withdrawn from the study (Bannister SJ, Houser VP, Hulse JD, et al. Evaluation of the potential for interactions of paroxetine with diazepam, cimetidine, warfarin and digoxin. *Acta Psychiatr Scand* 1989; 80[suppl 350]:102–106; *British National Formulary Number 24*. London: British Medical Association and the Royal Pharmaceutical Society of Great Britain, 1992; 5-Hydroxytryptamine reuptake inhibitors. *MeReC Bull* 1991;2:29–32). Careful monitoring of prothrombin time is advisable when warfarin and paroxetine are co-prescribed.

paroxetine/withdrawal Paroxetine discontinuation may be associated with dizziness, sweating, nausea, insomnia, tremor, and confusion. Symptoms are mild and transient, but seem to be somewhat more common than with other serotonin uptake inhibitors (Anon. *Current Problems in Pharmacovigilance* 1993;19:1). In a double-blind study of withdrawal effects following abrupt discontinuation of paroxetine (20–40 mg/day) or imipramine (150 mg/day) in patients with major depression, at least one adverse event occurred in 42% of the 20 mg paroxetine group, 38% of the 40 mg group, and 34% of the imipramine group. There was no significant difference between either low- or high-dose paroxetine and imipramine (Stoker MJ. A comparison of withdrawal effects following discontinuation of paroxetine and imipramine. Presented at the 146th Annual Meeting of the American Psychiatric Association, San Francisco, May 1993).

paroxysm Epileptiform discharge on the electroencephalogram (EEG) that occurs abruptly, peaks rapidly, and terminates suddenly.

paroxysmal hypnogenic dystonia See **dystonia, paroxysmal hypnogenic.**

paroxysmal nocturnal dyspnea (PND) See **dyspnea, paroxysmal nocturnal.**

Parsidol See **ethopropazine.**

Parstelin See **tranylcypromine + trifluoperazine.**

Partane See **trihexyphenidyl.**

partial agonist See **agonist, partial.**

partial hospitalization Alternative to inpatient treatment based on the premise that most patients with serious mental disorders can be successfully treated in a less restrictive and less costly environment. It includes major diagnostic, medical, psychiatric, psychosocial, and prevocational treatments for patients who require coordinated, intensive, comprehensive, and multidisciplinary treatment not provided in an outpatient clinic setting (American Psychiatric Association, New York County District Branch, Task Force on Partial Hospitalization. *Guidelines for Standards for Partial Hospitalization.* New York: APA New York County District Branch, January 1980). Although the experience of mental health professionals supports the validity of partial hospitalization as a treatment approach, traditional in- and out-patient modalities are used more often and receive better third-party reimbursement in the United States. Also called "day-hospital care"; "day treatment."

partial inverse agonist See **agonist, partial inverse.**

partial seizure See **seizure, partial.**

partial sleep deprivation See **sleep deprivation, partial.**

partial status See **status, partial.**

partial trisomy See **trisomy, partial.**

particle concentration fluorescent polarization See **fluorescent polarization, particle concentration.**

particulate fraction Fraction of a tissue homogenate that contains subcellular particles.

paruresis Functional disorder characterized by inability to urinate in the presence of others. It is listed in DSM-IV under *Social phobia, situational type.* Also called "bashful bladder syndrome"; "psychogenic urinary retention."

Pasaden See **etizolam.**

Paspertin See **metoclopramide.**

passive aggression See **aggression, passive.**

passivity phenomenon Feeling of being under the control or will of an outside agency. It is one of several Schneiderian first rank symptoms of schizophrenia.

"pasta" Coca paste, smoked by some cocaine abusers, that is an intermediate product in the processing of cocaine hydrochloride. It is a gray-white or dull brown powder with a lightly sweet smell which is 40–85% cocaine sulfate. Also called "bazooka."

pathognomonic One or more typical symptoms, findings, or pattern of abnormalities specific for a disease or pathological condition.

pathological gambling See **gambling, pathological.**

pathological intoxication See **intoxication, pathological.**

pathoplasticity Idiosyncratic description or manifestation of a symptom largely influenced by the patient's personality overlay.

patient guidance leaflet (PGL) Consumer information sheet provided by pharmaceutical companies in the United Kingdom that is comparable to the patient package insert used by pharmaceutical companies in the United States.

pavor nocturnus Parasomnia disorder that occurs chiefly in preschool children, often, but not always, after psychological trauma. The child awakens in the middle of the night panic-stricken, agitated, and sometimes hallucinating, then falls back into sleep with complete amnesia. Other reported features include vocalizations, motor movements, fear-related behaviors, heightened autonomic activity, and nonreactivity to external stimuli. Pavor nocturnus has been found to be familial and associated with other parasomnias. It occurs in stage 4 sleep and therefore differs from a nightmare that occurs during stage 1 (rapid eye movement, or REM) sleep. It may be a dose-dependent side effect of antidepressant drugs or benzodiazepine hypnotics that usually resolves with dosage reduction or discontinuation. Pavor nocturnus is usually outgrown by adulthood, but it may occur in adults (Llorente MD, Currier MB, Norman SE, Mellman TA. Night terrors in adults: phenomenology and relationship to psychopathology. *J Clin Psychiatry* 1992;53:392–394). Also called "night terror."

Pavulon See **pancuronium.**

Paxil See **paroxetine.**

Paxipam See **halazepam.**

PCE Street name for an analog of phencyclidine.

p-chloroamphetamine Drug that releases serotonin (5-HT) and produces effects in laboratory animals secondary to activation of brain 5-HT receptors by the released 5-HT.

p-chlorophenylalanine (PCPA) Inhibitor of serotonin (5-HT) synthesis that increases aggressive and filicidal behavior in rats, suggesting that aggression or self-injurious behavior may be linked to 5-HT depletion. It produces long-lasting inhibition of tryptophan hydroxylation and depletion of brain 5-HT in vivo, despite being a relatively weak inhibitor of tryptophan hydroxylase in vivo.

PCP See **phencyclidine.**

p-dope Designer drug that is a fentanyl/opiate derivative.

"peace" Street name for dimethoxymethylamphetamine.

"PeaCePill"   Street name for phencyclidine (PCP).

"peach"   Street name for amphetamine.

"peanut"   Street name for barbiturates.

"pear"   Street name for amyl nitrite.

"pearly gates"   Street term for change in self awareness and visual hallucinations produced by morning glory seeds, which contain a lysergic acid diethylamide (LSD)-related substance. The reaction can produce a lethal, shock-like state. Also called "heavenly blue."

Pearson's coefficient of correlations   See **Pearson's correlation.**

Pearson's correlation   Correlation coefficient used with interval- or ratio-scaled variables. Correlation is the appropriate method for describing the relationship between two mutually dependent variables. The coefficient of correlation describes the degree of relationship between x and y. Also called "Pearson's coefficient of correlations." See **coefficient of correlation; Spearman rank order correlation.**

pedigree   Diagram of the ancestral relationships and transmission of genetic traits over several generations of a family. See **human pedigree analysis.**

pedophile   Adult who turns to prepubescent youths for sexual gratification and who has been unable to attain any degree of psychosexual maturity. DSM-IV criteria include (a) over a period of at least 6 months, recurrent intense sexual urges and sexually arousing fantasies involving sexual activity with a prepubescent child or children (generally age 13 or younger); (b) the person has acted on these urges, or is markedly distressed by them; and (c) the person is at least 16 years old and at least 5 years older than the child or children. Hormonal research suggests that pedophilia has more chemically related abnormalities than other paraphilias. Whether homosexual, heterosexual, or bisexual, pedophiles appear to have a smaller left frontal-temporal area of the brain, which is asymmetrical. They have some language dysfunction (Broca's and Wernicke's areas are in that hemisphere) and hypersecrete luteinizing hormone in response to gonadotropic-releasing hormone from the pituitary gland. Thus, the whole left frontal-temporal area of the cortex may have suffered some insult or may be abnormal for other reasons that can be associated with pedophilic behavior per se (Langevin R. Biological factors contributing to paraphilic behavior. *Psychiatr Ann* 1992;22:307–314) There are two main categories of pedophilia, preferential and situational, each with several subtypes. Also called "child molester."

pedophile, fixated   Person who has an exclusive sexual preference for children.

pedophile, preferential   Individual with a defined sexual preference for children. Subtypes include seductive (exclusive sexual interest in children and tries to court and seduce them); introverted (fixated interest in children but does not have the social skills to seduce them; typically molests strangers or very young children or marries women with children of the preferred age); and sadistic (sexual preference for children and needs to inflict pain to obtain sexual gratification).

pedophile, regressed   Individual who deviates from a pattern of normal sexual adjustment and molests a child or children, usually during a period of stress.

pedophile, situational   Individual who does not have a defined sexual preference for children. Subtypes include regressed (immature, socially inept individuals who relate to children as peers; they may have experienced a brief period of low self-esteem and turned to their own children or to others for sexual satisfaction); morally indiscriminate (antisocial individuals who use and abuse everything they touch; they choose victims on the basis of vulnerability and opportunity and only coincidentally because they are children); sexually indiscriminate (those with vaguely defined sexual preferences who experiment with almost any type of sexual behavior); and inadequate (developmentally disabled, psychotic, senile, or organically dysfunctional).

pedophilia   Type of paraphilia in which the preferred route to sexual excitement is fantasized or enacted sex with prepubescent children. It can include exposure of genitals, manual manipulation of the child or penetration, and self-masturbation with or without the child's awareness or participation. It has been reported in heterosexual and homosexual males, most frequently among heterosexuals. See **pedophile.**

"peep"   Street name for phencyclidine (PCP).

peer review   Review by other scientists or clinicians in the same field of research protocols, manuscripts, abstracts, clinical work, etc., to determine scientific and technical merit.

pellagra   Disorder often characterized by mental abnormalities such as anxiety, irritability, and depression. Its classic symptoms are known as the "4 D's": dementia, diarrhea, dermatitis, and death. Inflammation of mucosal surfaces, weakness, anorexia, and other gastrointestinal disturbances also occur.

pemoline   (Cylert; Nitan) Psychostimulant used in the treatment of hyperkinetic and attention-deficit disorders (ADD) in children. Like other psychostimulants, it works predominantly by releasing biogenic amines from their storage sites in presynaptic nerve terminals and blocking their reuptake. Its pharmacological activity is similar to that of methylphenidate and dextroamphetamine, but it is structurally dissimilar and has minimal sympathomimetic effects (hyperexcitability, tachycardia, and hypertension). It has little or no effect on sleep. Because of its longer onset and duration of action, it is less likely to be abused than amphetamine and is preferred over methylphenidate by some therapists for ADD. Delayed onset of therapeutic action may require continued treatment before results are apparent. It has been used to counteract neuroleptic-induced parkinsonian side effects. It has also been used to treat memory difficulties and fatigue. Dependence has been reported only rarely (Metz A, Shader RI. Combination of fluoxetine with pemoline in the treatment of major depressive disorder. *Int Clin Psychopharmacol* 1991;6:93–96). Schedule IV; pregnancy risk category B.

pemoline + fluoxetine Co-administration has been used successfully to treat depressed patients partially responsive or unresponsive to fluoxetine (FLX) alone. Potential side effects include agitation, anxiety, insomnia, anorexia, and weight loss (Metz A, Shader R. Combination of fluoxetine with pemoline in the treatment of major depressive disorder. *Int Clin Psychopharmacol* 1991;6:93–96). FLX (80 mg/day) was reported to potentiate therapeutic response to pemoline (75 mg/day) without causing adverse effects (Zajecka JM, Fawcett J. Antidepressant combination and potentiation. *Psychiatr Med* 1991;9:55–75).

pemoline + monoamine oxidase inhibitor (MAOI) Clinical trials indicate that co-administration is safe and effective in treatment-resistant depression without the drawback of habituation or any significantly serious adverse interaction (Fawcett J, Kravitz HM, Zajecka JM, et al. CNS stimulant potentiation of monoamine oxidase inhibitors in treatment-refractory depression. *J Clin Psychopharmacol* 1991;11:127–132).

pemoline + warfarin Co-administration decreases pemoline metabolism, resulting in increased pemoline plasma levels.

penbutolol (Levatol) Beta-adrenergic blocking agent used for the treatment of hypertension. Psychiatric uses are being investigated.

penetrance Extent to which a genetically determined condition is expressed in an individual. It determines the frequency with which a genetic effect occurs in a population. Penetrance of the single genetic mechanism in schizophrenia is calculated to be 60–70% in twin-family studies. When the frequency of expression of a genotype is less than 100%, the trait exhibits incomplete penetrance. In an individual who has a genotype that characteristically produces an abnormal phenotype but who is phenotypically normal, the trait is nonpenetrant.

penetrance, reduced Less than 100% chance of manifesting an illness in an individual carrying the gene for that illness.

penfluridol (Cyperon; Flupidol; Oraleptin; Semap) Diphenylpiperidine derivative neuroleptic that may have specific dopamine-blocking effects without blocking norepinephrine or serotonin. Duration of action is 5–7 days. Like pimozide, it can be an effective treatment for Gilles de la Tourette's syndrome.

penile buckling pressure Amount of force applied to the glans of the penis sufficient to produce at least a 30-degree bend in the shaft.

penile plethysmograph Gauge or transducer that is attached to the penis to measure changes in penile circumference in response to sexual stimuli (audiotapes or slides depicting sexually explicit scenes). Changes are recorded on a strip chart, giving the clinician a record of the individual's response to each stimulus. It may be used to distinguish psychological from organic impotency by measuring sleep erection phenomenon. It is the most common method of assessing both deviant and appropriate sexual arousal.

penile rigidity Firmness of the penis. Normally, the fully erect penis has maximum rigidity.

pentagastrin Pentapeptide that has an active-site structure identical to the terminal amino acid sequences of gastrin and cholecystokinin (CCK). It is a centrally active CCK agonist that is anxiogenic in healthy subjects and patients with panic disorder (Abelson JL, Nesse RM. Cholecystokinin-4 and panic. *Arch Gen Psychiatry* 1990;47:395).

pentazocine (Fortral; Talacen; Talwin) Member of the benzazocine series that exerts competitive antagonism at mu opiate receptors and agonism at kappa and sigma receptors. Unique to pentazocine is its propensity for sigma receptor binding, an interaction thought to provoke many of its deleterious effects (e.g., dysphoria, autonomic stimulation, hallucinations). Given orally, its analgesic potency is approximately equivalent on a milligram-per-milligram basis to that of codeine. It can decrease the effect of other narcotics and has dependence and abuse potential. Schedule IV; pregnancy risk category C.

pentazocine + fluoxetine Co-administration may cause excitatory toxicity resembling the serotonin syndrome (Hansen TE, Dieter K, Keepers GA. Interaction of fluoxetine and pentazocine. *Am J Psychiatry* 1990;147:949–950).

pentazocine + methadone   Pentazocine may exert antagonist effects and possibly cause methadone withdrawal symptoms.

pentazocine/oculogyric crisis   Acute oculogyric crisis was reported in a 39-year-old woman following administration of Talacen (pentazocine plus acetaminophen) for pain relief, possibly due to pentazocine agonism of sigma opiate receptors and subsequent modulation of dopamine receptors. It resolved after discontinuation of the drug and administration of intravenous diphenhydramine (50 mg) (Burstein AH, Fullerton T. Oculogyric crisis possibly related to pentazocine. *Ann Pharmacother* 1993;27:874–876).

pentobarbital   (Nembutal) Short-acting barbiturate with a rapid onset of action. It is available in tablets for oral use as a sedative/hypnotic or preanesthetic, and in an injectable form for intramuscular or intravenous administration that can be used as an anticonvulsant. As with all barbiturates, tolerance and dependence may occur with continued use. Schedule II; pregnancy risk category D.

pentobarbital challenge test   Test used to confirm the presence of tolerance to sedative/hypnotics, which is a sign of physiological dependency. In a nontolerant, nondependent person, oral pentobarbital (200 mg) will produce sleep or signs of intoxication (slurred speech, ataxia, nystagmus, Romberg's sign [unsteadiness while standing with eyes closed]) within 1 hour of administration.

pentobarbital substitution withdrawal technique   Detoxification method for patients who have been abusing barbiturates and nonbarbiturate sedative/hypnotics. Pentobarbital (200 mg) is given orally at 6:00 P.M.; changes in the neurological examination are assessed after 1 hour. If there is no drowsiness, dysarthria, and ataxia, abuse level is probably above that of 1,200 mg/day of pentobarbital. Three to four hours later, pentobarbital (300 mg) is given; no response suggests a habit above 1,600 mg/day. Daily pentobarbital use is estimated, divided into four equal doses, and administered orally every 6 hours; then it is reduced at a rate of one-tenth the starting dose per day. Reduction should be made from the morning and afternoon doses initially to assist the patient with sleep.

Pentothal   See **thiopental.**

Pentothal interview   See **narcotherapy.**

pentoxifylline   (Trental) Drug used in the treatment of moderate and peripheral vascular dementia.

"pepap"   Street name for an analog of 1-methyl-4-phenyl-1,2,3,6-tetrahydropyridine (MPTP).

Pepcid   See **famotidine.**

"pep pill"   Street name for central nervous system stimulants.

peptidase   Substance that rapidly inactivates peptides by cleaving specific amino acyl bonds within the peptide structure.

peptide   Compounds made from strings of amino acids linked covalently, like proteins, but much smaller. Peptides are found in the brain and periphery of all mammals. In most instances, they co-exist with classic transmitters such as noradrenaline, dopamine, acetylcholine, and gamma aminobutyric acid (GABA); frequently, more than one peptide is found in the same cell. Although the peptides are released together with transmitters, the conditions and time course vary. Peptides also act on specific receptors and affect second messengers. Peptides, their fragments, and recently developed peptide antagonists exhibit distinct physiological and pharmacological effects. On the basis of these findings and documented peptide changes in affective disorders, dementias, and schizophrenia, it is suggested that drugs modifying the peptide systems should be useful in treating major psychiatric and other central nervous system disorders (Mathe AA, Hokfelt T. Neuropeptides-neurotransmitter coexistence: an opportunity for drug development. *Neuropsychopharmacology* 1993;9:7S). Peptides may function as neurotransmitters or neuromodulators. Neurotensin, a neuropeptide consisting of 13 amino acids, appears to be important in the pharmacology of neuroleptics.

peptidergic   Characteristic of nerve cells or fibers that use small peptide molecules as their neurotransmitter.

peptide YY   (PYY) Recently discovered neuropeptide that is a potent stimulant of feeding in experimental animals. Cerebrospinal fluid PYY concentrations are elevated in normal-weight bulimic patients who have abstained from pathological eating for a month. It has been suggested that increased brain PYY activity contributes to bulimic patients' powerful and uncontrollable urge to binge.

peptoid   Nonpeptide that blocks or mimics the actions of peptides at their receptor sites. The archetypal peptoid is morphine, which was the only major example of this drug class until the peptoid antagonists to angiotensin, substance P and cholecystokinin, were developed. It is theorized that many neuropeptides exert a mainly modulatory action on ongoing neuronal processes, and that this influence is principally exerted through the process of "co-transmission."

perazine   (Psytomin; Taxilan) Antipsychotic used in the treatment of schizophrenia. Its main (inactive) metabolite is desmethylperazine. Acute neuropathy after lengthy sun exposure was reported in five patients (ages 23–68 years) with chronic schizophrenia taking 50–400 mg/day for over 1–24 months (Roelke U, Hornstein C, Hund E, et al. Acute neuropathy in perazine-treated patients after sun exposure. *Lancet* 1992;340:729–730).

perazine + clozapine   Agranulocytosis has been reported (Grohmann R, Schmidt LG, Spiess-Kiefer C, Ruther E. Agranulocytosis and significant leukopenia with neuroleptic drugs. Results from the AMUP program. *Psychopharmacology* 1989;[suppl]:109S–112S).

"perc"   Street name for oxycodone.

perception   Active process of extracting information from the environment and one's body, interpreting it, and integrating it in a meaningful way.

perceptual distorter   Controversial designation for a group of drugs (e.g., lysergic acid diethylamide, phencyclidine, psilocybin, mescaline) that are chemically different and have different physical and perceptual effects. Many experts prefer the terms *hallucinogen, psychotomimetic,* and *psychedelic.*

Percocet   See **oxycodone + acetaminophen.**

Percodan   See **oxycodone + aspirin.**

percutaneous endoscopic gastrostomy   (PEG) Method for obtaining access to the stomach in patients requiring long-term tube feeding (Gauderer MWL, Ponsky JL, Izant RJ. Gastrostomy without laparotomy: a percutaneous endoscopic technique for feeding gastrostomy, *J Pediatr Surg* 1992;15:872–875). The tube is inserted using a gastroscope while the patient is sedated. It has become one of the favorite techniques of feeding patients with persistent swallowing difficulty due to neurological or oropharyngeal disorders. It has been used to feed a patient with severe endogenous depression with secondary anorexia and weight loss and should be considered a safe alternative to nasogastric and intravenous feeding for patients with treatable depressive disorders complicated by cachexia (Hussain A, Cox JGC, Proctor SE. Percutaneous endoscopic gastrostomy and severe endogenous depression. *Br J Psychiatry* 1993;163:699–700).

Perenum   See **toloxatone.**

performance anxiety   See **anxiety, performance.**

performance test   Any of various tests used to evaluate drug effects on the various stages of information processing. Tests range from ability to tap a stylus rapidly to simulated car driving. Many are computerized, enabling all aspects of test performance to be measured. As a result, it is now possible to identify drug effects that previously were masked by the insensitivity of the test available.

pergolide   (Celance; Permak; Permax; Pharkan) Synthetic ergoline dopamine (DA) receptor agonist at D_1, D_2, and D_3 receptor sites. It is indicated as adjunctive treatment to levodopa-carbidopa in the management of the signs and symptoms of advanced Parkinson's disease (PD). It does not require the release of presynaptic DA. It is rapidly absorbed and reaches peak concentrations in 60–120 minutes. Half-life is about 27 hours. Antiparkinson action lasts 5–9 hours. It allows reduction of levodopa dosage by one-third to one-half and lessens disability and "off" time. Recent data also indicate that pergolide may retard progression of PD. It has a longer duration of action and is 10–100 times more potent than bromocriptine. It is usually administered 2 or 3 times daily; average dose range is 1–4 mg/day. It also may be used as an adjuvant medication (0.25–2 mg range; 0.5–1 mg average) in patients with treatment-resistant depression being treated with heterocyclic antidepressants or monamine oxidase inhibitors. Early experimental work indicates that it may be effective in treating cocaine withdrawal. Side effects are similar to those of other DA agonists (nausea, sedation, dyskinesia, postural hypotension). Nausea/vomiting is a common and sometimes treatment-limiting side effect that is unpredictable (not dose-related) and may last for 12 hours. Pregnancy risk category B.

pergolide + amoxapine   Co-administration has been used to treat patients refractory to amoxapine alone. Response is usually rapid (within a week), but without incremental improvement over the next month. Some patients tolerate the combination well; others develop nausea and vomiting that may or may not respond to lowering pergolide dosage.

pergolide + clozapine   Co-administration in the treatment of co-morbid psychosis in patients with Parkinson's disease produced clearing of psychotic illness, with no serious adverse interactions or worsening of parkinsonism (Wolk SI, Douglas CJ. Clozapine treatment of psychosis in Parkinson's disease: a report of five consecutive cases. *J Clin Psychiatry* 1992;53:373–376).

pergolide + desipramine   Co-administration has been used to treat patients refractory to desipramine (DMI). Response is usually rapid (within 1 week), but without incremental improvement over the next month. Some patients tolerate the combination well; others develop nausea and vomiting which may or may not respond to lowering pergolide dose (Bouckoms A, Mangini L. Pergolide: an antidepressant adjuvant for mood disorders. *Psychopharmacol Bull* 1993;29:207–211).

pergolide + doxepin Co-administration has been used in patients refractory to doxepin alone. Response is usually rapid, within a week, and without incremental improvement over the next month. Some patients tolerate the combination well; others develop nausea and vomiting that may or may not respond to lowering pergolide dose (Bouckoms A, Mangini L. Pergolide: an antidepressant adjuvant for mood disorders. *Psychopharmacol Bull* 1993;29:207–211).

pergolide + fluoxetine Co-administration has been used to treat patients refractory to fluoxetine (FLX) alone. Response is usually rapid (within a week), but without incremental improvement over the next month. Some patients tolerate the combination well; others develop nausea and vomiting that may or may not respond to lowered pergolide dose (Bouckoms A, Mangini L. Pergolide: an antidepressant adjuvant for mood disorders. *Psychopharmacol Bull* 1993;29:207–211). No adverse interaction in depressed Parkinson's disease patients has been reported.

pergolide + isocarboxazid Co-administration has been used to treat patients refractory to isocarboxazid alone. Some tolerate the combination well. One patient being treated with higher-dose pergolide (2 mg) + isocarboxazid (40 mg) became hypomanic; hypomania abated when pergolide was reduced to 1 mg.

pergolide + monoamine oxidase inhibitor (MAOI) Pergolide may be used safely with inhibitors of MAO type A. Although less effective than optimal doses of levodopa, co-administration may substantially improve parkinsonian disabilities.

pergolide + nortriptyline Co-administration has been used to treat patients refractory to nortriptyline alone. Response is usually rapid (within a week), but without incremental improvement over the next month. Some patients tolerate the combination well; others develop nausea and vomiting that may or may not respond to pergolide dose reduction (Bouckoms A, Mangini L. Pergolide: an antidepressant adjuvant for mood disorders. *Psychopharmacol Bull* 1993;29:207–211).

pergolide + trazodone Co-administration has been used to treat patients refractory to trazodone alone. Response is usually rapid (within a week) and without incremental improvement over the next month. Some patients tolerate the combination well; others develop nausea and vomiting that may or may not respond to lowering pergolide dose (Bouckoms A, Mangini L. Pergolide: an antidepressant adjuvant for mood disorders. *Psychopharmacol Bull* 1993;29:207–211).

Periactin See **cyproheptadine.**

Pericate See **haloperidol decanoate.**

pericyazine (Neulactil; Neuleptil) Piperidine phenothiazine neuroleptic similar to chlorpromazine, but more sedating. It is used in the treatment of aggression in dosages up to 120 mg/day.

Peridol See **haloperidol.**

Peridor See **haloperidol decanoate.**

"period effect" Changes in rates of illnesses associated with the period in which the onset of illness occurred (e.g., impact of unemployment on suicide rates) (Cormier HJ, Klerman GL. Unemployment and male/female labor force participation as determinants of changing suicide rates of males and females in Quebec. *Soc Psychiatry* 1985;20:109–114).

periodic leg movements in sleep See **periodic movements in sleep.**

periodic movements in sleep (PMS) Disorder characterized by repetitive stereotyped movements of the lower extremities occurring every 10–120 seconds during sleep. Most characteristically, movements resemble the Babinski response and may include flexion of the great toe, ankle, and knee. The movements may occur in either or both lower extremities simultaneously. In extreme cases, the hip and upper extremities are also involved. Movements may occur several hundred times per night. Electromyographic manifestations may last from 0.5 to 5.0 seconds and may be scored when there are at least four serial phenomena separated by 4–90 seconds. The phenomena may resemble a brief jerk sometimes so slight as to only be perceptible electromyographically, or they may involve definite clonic movements. Some diagnose PMS when there are at least five characteristic movements per hour of sleep. Criteria of the Association of Sleep Disorders Centers (ASDC) (1979) require at least three episodes of at least 30 leg jerks each. More rapid myoclonic movements or slower, prolonged dystonic-like movements of the feet and legs also may be present when subjects are awake. Movements are responsible for complaints of an unsatisfactory night's sleep, insomnia, and/or daytime sleepiness when sleep has been disrupted over a prolonged period. PMS is common in the elderly. It may be caused by monoamine oxidase inhibitors (MAOIs) and may be associated with some neurological and metabolic conditions, sleep apnea, and narcolepsy. Short-term controlled studies have demonstrated that benzodiazepines (clonazepam and temazepam), mild opiates, and L-dopa are successful in suppressing subjective and objective manifestations of PMS. No treatment for PMS has been adequately studied in the elderly. Also called "nocturnal myoclonus"; "periodic leg movements in sleep (PLMS)."

period prevalence   Measure that expresses the total number of cases of a disease known to have existed during a specified period (e.g., January 1 to December 31, 1993).

peripheral-type benzodiazepine receptor   See **benzodiazepine receptor, peripheral type.**

Periplum   See **nimodipine.**

peristasis   In genetics, state in which the environment of any genetic factor includes all the biophysiological processes in the organism itself that are essential to the phenotypical development of the given genotype.

periventricular lucency   White-matter change in the computed tomography (CT) scans of demented patients and normal elderly subjects. It seems to be related to cognitive decline and motor abnormalities and may reflect underlying amyloid angiopathy.

perlapine   See **neuroleptic, atypical, type A.**

Perluiex   See **medroxyprogesterone**

Permak   See **pergolide.**

Permax   See **pergolide.**

Permitil   See **fluphenazine.**

Perphenan   See **perphenazine.**

perphenazine   (Apo-Perphenazine; Phenazine; Perphenan; Trilafon) Piperazine phenothiazine neuroleptic used in the treatment of schizophrenia, mania, anxiety, and violent or dangerously impulsive behavior. It can be given by mouth or by injection. It often causes acute extrapyramidal reactions. Like all neuroleptics, it also may cause tardive dyskinesia and the neuroleptic malignant syndrome. Pregnancy risk category C.

perphenazine + amitriptyline   (Etrafon; Etrafon-A; Etrafon-D; Etrafon-F; Etrafon-M; Etrafon-2-10; Longopax; Longopox Mite; Mutabase-2-10; Mutabon-A; Mutabon Ansiolittico; Mutabon Antidepressivo; Mutabon-D; Mutabon-F; Mutabon-M; Mutabon Mite; Triavil) Combination product composed of the piperazine phenothiazine neuroleptic perphenazine and the tricyclic antidepressant amitriptyline (AMI). Each inhibits the other's metabolism. AMI may block the extrapyramidal effects of perphenazine; combined therapeutic effects are greater than those of either component alone. It is prescribed for moderate to severe anxiety/depression, agitation and depression, and psychotic depression.

perphenazine + carbamazepine   Carbamazepine (CBZ) can substantially reduce perphenazine plasma levels, making it difficult to achieve effective antipsychotic drug levels (Nelson JC. Combined treatment strategies in psychiatry. *J Clin Psychiatry* 1993;54[suppl 9]:42–49).

perphenazine + disulfiram   Co-administration may reduce perphenazine plasma levels (Hansen L, Larsen N. Metabolic interaction between perphenazine and disulfiram. *Lancet* 1982;2:1472).

perphenazine enanthate   (Trilafon Enanthate) Long-acting depot form of perphenazine used for maintenance therapy of schizophrenia. Not available in the United States.

perphenazine + fluoxetine   Co-administration has been found effective in depression with psychotic features (Rothschild AJ, Samson JA, Bessette MP, Carter-Campbell J. Efficacy of the combination of fluoxetine and perphenazine in the treatment of psychotic depression. *J Clin Psychiatry* 1993;54:338–342). Increased extrapyramidal symptoms have been reported (Lock JD, Gwirtsman HE, Targ EF. Possible adverse drug interactions between fluoxetine and other psychotropics. *J Clin Psychopharmacol* 1990;10:383–384). It is not clear whether the interactions have a pharmacokinetic or pharmacodynamic basis, or both.

perphenazine + valproic acid   Addition of valproic acid to perphenazine has been reported to substantially reduce the number of aggressive outbursts per month, with no adverse interactive effects, in mentally retarded patients with nonaffective aggression (assaultive behavior not necessarily associated with dysphoria, anger, or a specific precipitant) (Mattes J. Valproic acid for nonaffective aggression in the mentally retarded. *J Nerv Ment Dis* 1992;180:601–602). Valproic acid has no effect on perphenazine plasma levels (Ellenore GL, Kodsi AB. Drug interactions: case report of carbamazepine vs valproic acid with perphenazine. *ASHP Midyear Clinical Meeting* 1993;28:169).

persecutory delusion   See **delusion, persecutory.**

perseveration   Continuation of a response after it is no longer appropriate. It is a common feature of frontal lobe dysfunction that may be tested by asking the patient to copy and maintain alternating letters or repetitive sequential patterns of hand movements. It should be suspected if a patient spontaneously repeats certain words, phrases or gestures.

Persian heroin   See **heroin, Persian.**

persistent dyskinesia   See **dyskinesia, persistent.**

persistent insomnia   See **insomnia, persistent.**

personality   Deeply ingrained patterns of behavior that include the way one relates to, perceives, and thinks about the environment and the self. Personality traits are prominent aspects of personality and do not imply pathology.

personality disorder   (PD) Inflexible, stylized, maladaptive behavior patterns of sufficient severity to cause significant impairment in adaptive functioning and/or subjective distress. The characteristic maladjustment patterns are evident from childhood and throughout much of the life span. DSM-IV PDs are antisocial, avoidant, borderline, compulsive, cyclothymic, dependent, histrionic, narcissistic, paranoid, passive-aggressive, schizoid, and schizotypal. They are medically and psychiatrically important because individuals with these disorders are at high risk for drug and/or alcohol abuse, self-destructive behavior, and clashing with society and its mores.

personality disorder/tests/questionnaires Structured Interview for Personality Disorders; Personality Disorders Questionnaire.

Persumbran See **oxazepam.**

Pertofrane See **desipramine.**

perversion See **compulsive sexual behavior.**

"Peter" Street name for chloral hydrate.

pethidine See **meperidine (U.S. designation).**

petit mal absence See **seizure, absence** (preferred term).

petit mal status See **absence status.**

peyote Hallucinogenic drug derived from a cactus that causes psychedelic effects such as mood changes, delusions, and hallucinations. See **mescaline.**

peyotism Intoxication with the psychedelic peyote or mescaline. It is manifested by visual and sometimes auditory hallucinations, a sense of timelessness, and a complete withdrawal from reality. Southwest American Indians use peyote to produce ecstasies as a part of a religious ritual. See **mescaline.**

"PG" Street name for paregoric.

phage Virus that infects bacteria and that can be genetically engineered to carry and express genes (cloning vector).

phalometric test See **penile plethysmograph.**

phantastica See **hallucinogen.**

Pharkan See **pergolide.**

pharmaceutical alternates Different formulations of the same drug, including enteric-coated products, different dosage forms (tablet, capsule, liquids), derivatives of the same active ingredient (ester, salt, acid, base), sustained-release formulations that use different technologies to achieve controlled release, physicochemical variants (micronized vs. macronized or crystalline vs. amorphous particle sizes), and products of natural versus synthetic origin. They may differ substantially in efficacy, required dose, bioavailability, pharmacokinetic profile, or incidence of side effects.

pharmaceutical equivalents Product in which the active agents have the same chemical structure, but differ in some aspect of formulation and so have different bioavailabilities.

pharmacoanthropology Medical science dealing with interethnic differences of pharmacology or toxicology. It is concerned with both genetic and nongenetic factors that may affect response to drugs. See **pharmacogenetics.**

pharmacodynamic drug-drug interaction Co-administration of drugs with the same or opposing pharmacological actions resulting in alteration of the sensitivity or responsiveness of the tissues to one drug by another. Knowledge of the pharmacology of each drug may allow prediction of these interactions. Careful monitoring of patients being treated with two drugs may lead to quick detection of unexpected interactions and appropriate medication or dosage adjustments.

pharmacodynamic interaction Potentiation or antagonism of drug effects at the site of action (e.g., enhancement of alcohol's central nervous system–depressant activity by barbiturates and other sedative/hypnotics).

pharmacodynamics All drug effects, beneficial and undesired, as well as the body's compensatory homeostatic adjustments to the presence of a drug. Pharmacodynamics affects the response elicited by the drug at the receptor site. It depends on the concentration of a drug reaching the site of action, which is linked with pharmacokinetics. See **pharmacokinetics.**

pharmacodynamic "sensitivity" Intensity of drug response at any specific plasma concentration, brain concentration, or receptor occupancy. Emotional and medical illness can alter pharmacodynamic sensitivity.

pharmacodynamic "sensitivity," enhanced Increased intensity of drug action despite similar plasma or brain concentrations of a drug. Pharmacodynamic "sensitivity" to psychoactive drugs (e.g., benzodiazepines) may be enhanced in the elderly, regardless of an age-related change in pharmacokinetics. Emotional and medical illness may potentially alter pharmacodynamic sensitivity.

pharmacoepidemiology Use of epidemiological techniques to study drug use and effects (beneficial and adverse) in large numbers of people. It also examines the rates at which drugs are prescribed in the general population.

pharmacogenetic reaction Variation in drug response due to an hereditary factor. Many of these reactions are unexpected and can be adverse. They may be either direct (secondary to genetic alterations in the function of a particular tissue or receptor site) or indirect (due to an altered rate of biotransformation or an abnormally low enzyme level, which is a major mechanism for pharmacogenetic responses).

pharmacogenetics Study of the inter-relations of hereditary constitution and response to drugs. All elements of pharmacogenetics are or may be parts of pharmacoanthropology. Objectives include identification of differences in drug effects that have a genetic basis and the development of simple methods by which susceptible individuals can be identified before the drug is administered.

pharmacogenic depression See **depression, postpsychotic.**

pharmacogeriatrics Study of the use and effects of pharmacological agents in the elderly. It is becoming an increasingly important medical subspecialty.

pharmacokinetic depression Depression putatively attributed to depot neuroleptics.

pharmacokinetic interaction 1. Additive effects of two drugs on target organs (e.g., enhancement of central nervous system depression when substances with sedative effects are co-administered). Alcohol can potentiate the sedative effects of benzodiazepines by as much as 50%. 2. Effect of one drug on the plasma concentration of another drug. For example, fluoxetine can increase plasma concentrations of tricyclic antidepressants, and haloperidol blood levels may drop substantially in the presence of carbamazepine. 3. Alteration of the absorption, distribution, metabolism, or excretion of one drug by another. For example, cigarette smoking lowers serum neuroleptic levels by stimulating hepatic microsomal enzyme activity.

pharmacokinetics Term coined by Dost (1955) for quantitative analysis between drug and organism. It is the study of the biochemical and physiological effects of drugs and how the body processes them (mechanisms of action, absorption, distribution, biotransformation, and excretion). It is concerned with the nature of a drug's form (e.g., ester, salt, complex); the physical state, including particle size and surface area; presence or absence of adjuncts with the active drug; dosage form in which the drug is administered; and pharmaceutical processes used to prepare the dosage form. Pharmacokinetic factors affect the quantity of administered drug that reaches its receptor sites and in large part how quickly a drug's onset of action occurs and how long it persists. They also determine how frequently a drug should be administered and its therapeutic and toxic doses. Pharmacokinetics can be an important factor in drug dependency, misuse, abuse, and onset and severity of a withdrawal syndrome. Diseases and aging can change a drug's pharmacokinetics. There has been an explosion of knowledge of pharmacokinetics due largely to advances in analytical

chemistry, such as radioimmunoassay, gas chromatography, and high-performance liquid chromatography, that allow very small amounts of drugs and metabolites to be quantified in body fluids and tissues. Pharmacokinetics are often divided into four major processes: absorption, distribution, metabolism, and elimination. Also called "biopharmaceutics." See **pharmacodynamics.**

pharmacokinetics, first-order Rate of a drug's metabolism and elimination independent of its concentration, because all the liver enzymes have not been saturated. Hence, there is a proportional change in the plasma level with a change in drug dose; if dosage is increased, there is a predictable proportional increase in serum concentration that will persist until the liver enzymes are saturated.

pharmacokinetics, "flip-flop" Drug in which absorption rate constant is slower than the elimination rate constant.

pharmacokinetics, linear Rate of metabolism of a drug proportional to the amount of drug present. When concentration versus time is plotted on a log-linear graph paper, it produces a straight line. Also called "first-order kinetics."

pharmacokinetics, nonlinear Rate of metabolism of a drug that is not proportional to the amount of drug present. When dose and plasma levels have a nonlinear relationship, differences in bioavailability among brand-name and generic preparations may be exaggerated and make the issue of generic equivalence more complicated than it might be with other drugs.

pharmacokinetics, population Statistical analysis of a limited number of measurements from many individuals that can then be used to "individualize" a patient's pharmacokinetics or pharmacodynamics.

pharmacokinetics, postmortem/tricyclic antidepressant (TCA) Postmortem blood values of some drugs may be affected by a phenomenon called "postmortem release" or "redistribution" of drugs. Tricyclic antidepressants (TCAs) have a high protein binding affinity and are stored in specific binding sites in the body. At death, these drugs are released from their antemortem sites because of a variety of mechanisms, including (a) decompensation of circulating proteins and membrane macromolecules that bind drugs and (b) destruction of biological membranes that delineate drug compartments in the body. Postmortem release can lead to massive increases (to 150,000 ng/ml or higher) in TCA blood levels during the hours following death, especially if there has been a delay between death and the autopsy. TCA levels rise 2 to 8 times over the first 15 postmortem hours and continue to rise over at least another 15 hours. The longer the postmortem interval, the greater the difference in the heart/femoral drug concentration ratio (Popper C, Elliott GR. Postmortem pharmacokinetics of tricyclic antidepressants. Are some deaths during treatment misattributed to overdose? *J Child Adolesc Psychopharmacol* 1993;3:x–xii; Apple FS, Brandt CM. Liver and blood postmortem TCA concentrations. *Am J Clin Pathol* 1988;89:794–796; Prouty RW, Anderson WH. The forensic science implications of site and temporal influences on postmortem blood-drug concentrations. *J Forens Sci* 1990;35:243–270). Thus, postmortem drug redistribution can create difficulties in the interpretation of how much drug the decedent took (Hilberg T, Bugge A, Beylich KM, et al. An animal model of postmortem amitriptyline redistribution. *J Forens Sci* 1993;38:81–90). Although postmortem levels greater than 1,000 ng/ml may be viewed as consistent with death secondary to TCA ingestion, pathologists now emphasize that high postmortem blood levels *cannot* be assumed to indicate overdose or even intoxication (Hebb JH, Caplan YH, Crooks CR, Mergner WJ. Blood and tissue concentrations of TCAs in post-mortem cases: literature survey and a study of 40 deaths. *J Anal Toxicol* 1982;6:209–216; Hanzlick RL. Postmortem blood concentrations of parent tricyclic antidepressant [TCA] drugs in 11 cases of suicide. *Am J Forens Med Pathol* 1984;5:11–13; Hanzlick RL. Postmortem tricyclic antidepressant concentrations: lethal vs. nonlethal levels. *Am J Forens Med Pathol* 1989; 10:326–329). Following fatal TCA overdose, there are significant differences in TCA levels in the body (Bailey DN, Shaw RF. Tricyclic antidepressants: interpretation of blood and tissue levels in fatal overdose. *J Anal Toxicol* 1979;3:43–46). Release of drug from drug-rich tissue (heart, lung, liver) increases drug concentration in the blood adjacent to the tissue. Blood concentrations in the central vessels (abdominal and thoracic) are much higher (50–760%) than in the peripheral vessels (femoral and subclavial veins); highest concentration is in blood from the pulmonary vein and artery. Drugs with the widest concentration in blood are most highly concentrated in organ tissues, particularly the lungs and liver. This is probably due to (a) postmortem release of drugs from tissue sites of high concentration into blood contained within those tissues or in connecting vessels; (b) drugs concentrated in the lungs being released from organ parenchyma into the pulmonary arterial and venous blood and ultimately to the heart; (c) drugs concentrated in the liver being diffused into the hepatic

venous blood and then only a few centimeters into the inferior vena cava in the right atrium of the heart; (d) blood within the aorta having high TCA concentrations because of its intimate relationship to the heart and lungs; and (e) arterial venous differences in drug concentration if death occurs before steady-state has been reached (Jones GR, Pounder DJ. Site dependence of drug concentrations in postmortem blood—a case study. *J Anal Toxicol* 1987;11:186–190). Recent data on postmortem TCA levels and ratios in adults suggest that samples obtained from the liver are more reliable than blood samples for differentiating acute overdose from therapeutic usage (Apple FS. Post-mortem TCA concentration: assessing cause of death using parent drug to metabolite ratio. *J Anal Toxicol* 1989;13:197–198). The assumption that postmortem blood concentrations mirror blood concentrations at the time of death cannot be considered valid. Findings of postmortem pharmacokinetics document that there is a risk of attributing the cause of death to overdose (whether acute or chronic, medical or self-inflicted, intentional or accidental) when the culprit may be the toxicity of the drug itself.

pharmacokinetics, quantitative   Study of the relationship between drug concentration and biological effects (physiological, behavioral, and biochemical).

pharmacokinetics, regional   Study of factors that influence drug concentrations in specific regions of the body. Its physiological basis is a function of the interactions of the drug between the cells and proteins in blood, the blood flow supplying a region, the structure of the capillaries of the region, and the types of specific and nonspecific binding within the region. Its physicochemical basis is a function of the factors influencing the rate and extent of diffusion of a drug through aqueous and lipid medium (e.g., molecular weight, ionization, charge, lipophilicity).

pharmacokinetic screen   Means of identifying subgroups of patients in whom a drug has unusual pharmacokinetic characteristics, even if no such subgroups are suspected. In Phases 2 and 3 of a clinical investigation, a small number (one to several) of steady-state blood level determinations are obtained for all or most patients to determine the variability of blood concentrations of a drug under defined dosing conditions. A pharmacokinetic screen may help determine whether concomitant diseases affect blood levels of the test drug, and clinical observations should permit detection of specific adverse effects associated with the other diseases. A screen also should help evaluate whether concomitant medications affect the kinetics of the test drug.

pharmacokinetics, single-dose absorption phase Phase during which plasma levels rise as the drug is absorbed into the circulation.

pharmacokinetics, single-dose distribution phase Phase during which there is usually a steep drop in plasma levels as the drug leaves the circulation to enter peripheral tissues (e.g., fat, skeletal muscle, liver).

pharmacokinetics, single-dose elimination phase Distribution equilibrium during which the drug disappears from all body compartments at a rate determined solely by the elimination rate.

pharmacokinetics, systemic Study of the relationships among drug dose, systemic blood concentrations, and time. Concentrations of the test drug and/or metabolite(s) are measured in blood or plasma or serum.

pharmacokinetics, zero-order Elimination of only a fixed amount of a drug for every time interval because the enzymes for biotransformation and elimination are saturated. Since output of a drug is fixed, even slight dosage increases result in a large increase in plasma concentration that is going to be higher than just a proportional increase, but how much higher cannot be predicted.

pharmacological challenge test Use of a drug to uncover an abnormality that may otherwise remain hidden (e.g., use of naloxone to precipitate withdrawal symptoms in a narcotic abuser who denies substance abuse).

pharmacological interaction Drug interaction that occurs at the central or peripheral receptor site, resulting in additive, synergistic, antagonistic, or no effects. An additive effect (potentiation) would be increased sedation caused by co-administration of two or more central nervous system depressants. A synergistic effect would be increased efficacy due to co-administration of a neuroleptic and antidepressant in the treatment of psychotic depression. An antagonist effect is illustrated by treatment with a neuroleptic (dopamine antagonist) that produces effects requiring administration of L-dopa (dopamine agonist). Another antagonistic action is negation of the therapeutic activity of guanethidine by desipramine (blockade of uptake of guanethidine into noradrenergic neurons). No effect occurs with co-administration of lithium and a benzodiazepine anxiolytic.

pharmacological model for depression Classic studies in which reserpine was found to induce depression generated the various biogenic amine theories. Drugs are more likely to induce depression in patients who are susceptible by virtue of past history or genetic predisposition, whereas head injury can induce depression in nonsusceptible individuals. See **biogenic amine hypothesis of depression.**

pharmacological probe See **probe, pharmacological.**

pharmacological receptor See **receptor, pharmacological.**

pharmacology Study of the effects of drugs on the body.

pharmacotherapeutics Use of drugs in the treatment and prevention of disease or illness.

pharmacotherapy See **drug therapy.**

Phasal See **lithium.**

phase advance Movement of a sleep or wake episode to an earlier position in the 24-hour sleep-wake cycle (e.g., sleep phase shift from 11 P.M.—7 A.M. to 8 P.M.—4 A.M.). See **circadian phase sleep disorder; phase delay.**

phase advanced rhythm In chronobiology, rhythm established when a person retires and arises early.

phase delay Movement of a sleep or wake episode to a later position in the 24-hour sleep-wake cycle. It is the exact opposite of phase advance. See **circadian phase sleep disorder; phase advance.**

phase delayed rhythm In chronobiology, rhythm established when a person retires and arises late.

phase transition One of the two junctures of the major sleep and wake phases in the 24-hour sleep-wake cycle.

phase 1 (I) trial First of three stages of clinical trials of a new drug required by the Food and Drug Administration (FDA). It generally includes under 100 subjects, most often healthy volunteers, given single, fixed, and chronic doses. Focus is on drug safety (how much drug to use, how use is to be phased, and precautions needed to ensure safe use). Phase 1 trials usually require 6 months to 1 year to be completed.

phase 2 (II) trial Second of three stages of clinical trials of a new drug required by the Food and Drug Administration (FDA). It usually involves randomized, controlled, blinded trials in several hundred patients, including those suffering from the target disorder. The goal is to demonstrate whether the drug effectively treats the disease or condition for which it is intended. Some short-term safety issues are also answered. Phase 2 trials take somewhat longer than phase 1 studies to complete. About one-third of drugs involved in phase 2 trials move on to phase 3 trials.

phase 3 (III) trial Third of three stages of clinical trials of a new drug required by the Food and Drug Administration (FDA). It generally does not begin without formal consultation with the FDA regarding protocol. It generally involves large-scale testing in several thousand patients with the target disorder and extends over 3–4 years. The goal is to develop a full range of information regarding safety, effectiveness, and dosage that will allow the drug to be marketed and used safely.

phase 4 (IV) trial   Clinical study conducted after a drug has been marketed. Because it is a postmarketing activity, some consider postmarketing surveillance a type of phase 4 study.

phasic event   Brain, muscle, or autonomic event (e.g., eye movements, muscle twitches) of a brief (milliseconds to 1–2 seconds), episodic nature that occurs during sleep. Phasic events are characteristic of rapid eye movement (REM) sleep.

phenacemide   (Phenurone) Hydantoin derivative anticonvulsant marketed for the treatment of refractory complex-partial, generalized tonic-clonic, absence, and atypical absence seizures. Effective adult dosage ranges from 1,500 mg (500 mg orally 3 times a day) up to 5 g/day; in children ages 5–10, the effective dosage ranges from 250 mg 3 times a day up to 1.5 g/day. Because phenacemide can be extremely toxic, it is usually reserved for severe, treatment-resistant epilepsy. Pregnancy risk category D.

Phenazine   See **perphenazine.**

phenazocine   (Narphen) Structural analog of pentazocine with a qualitatively similar profile.

phencyclidine   (PCP) Widely abused psychotomimetic street drug that is an N-methyl-D-aspartate (NMDA)-receptor antagonist. It can be taken orally or intravenously, smoked or inhaled. It also is misused as an adulterant of other, more expensive illicit drugs. It can be detected in urine for several days after use, and its effects may last for several days. PCP-induced psychosis incorporates both positive (e.g., hallucinations, paranoia) and negative (e.g., emotional withdrawal, motor retardation) schizophrenic symptoms as well as the formal thought disorder and neuropsychological deficits associated with schizophrenia. It has caused status epilepticus that may be fatal. There are about 30 known chemical analogs of PCP; a new drug with a strange name that profoundly alters perception in a bizarre way is likely to be PCP unless proven otherwise. Schedule II.

phencyclidine/neonate   Phencyclidine (PCP) crosses the placental barrier and enters the fetal circulation. Infants exposed to PCP in utero may be apathetic, jittery, and irritable and show abnormalities in muscle tone and reflexes. Behavioral measurements at 6 and 15 months by the Gesell Developmental Examination indicate language impoverishment and

a significantly lower developmental quotient. Qualitative analysis of PCP-exposed children at play indicates some ataxia; poor abduction and extension of fingers, hands, and arms; and some intentional tremor. In a study of neonates born to mothers who regularly used PCP during pregnancy, wherein PCP was found in the urine of both mother and newborn, birthweight for gestational age was below the 25th percentile in 42%; birth height for gestational age was below the 25th percentile in 37.3%; and head circumferences was below the 25th percentile in 45.7% and below the 10th percentile in 12% (Rahbar F, Fomufod A, White D, Westney LS. Impact of intrauterine exposure to phencyclidine [PCP] and cocaine on neonates. *J Natl Med Assoc* 1993;85: 349–352).

phencyclidine/N-methyl-D-aspartate (NMDA) hypothesis of schizophrenia   Postulation based on the observation that phencyclidine (PCP) and related agents potently and acutely induce a schizophrenia-like psychosis in normal subjects and prolonged symptom-specific exacerbations of illness in schizophrenic subjects. In contrast to other drugs that induce psychoses, PCP reproduces positive symptoms, negative symptoms, and the cognitive dysfunction and thought disorder of schizophrenia. Schizophrenic patients manifest prominent deficits in learning and memory function that are related to glutamatergic pathways in hippocampus and cortex. In model systems, PCP-like drugs create electrophysiological deficits in event-related potentials similar to those observed in schizophrenic patients. PCP effects are initiated by its binding to a unique site within the ion channel gated by the NMDA class of glutamate receptors. PCP thus blocks ion flux through this channel noncompetitively, leading to a decrease in NMDA receptor–mediated neurotransmission. If schizophrenia involves an endogenous deficiency of NMDA receptor activity, then treatment strategies aimed at enhancement of NMDA receptor function would be expected to lead to clinical improvement by a nondopaminergic mechanism. The degree of NMDA receptor activation at a given agonist concentration depends on the local concentration of glycine, which is a co-agonist with glutamate (Zukin SR, Javitt DC, Zylberman I, Heresco-Levy U. Glutamatergic dysfunction in psychiatric disorders. *Neuropsychopharmacology* 1993;9:38S).

phencyclidine psychosis   Schizophreniform psychosis following phencyclidine (PCP) use that may persist for days or weeks with no additional PCP use. It can be divided into three phases, based on time course: acute, prolonged, and recurrent. The acute phase can be correlated with the presence of high PCP plasma levels (usually 4–6 hours). The prolonged phase can last beyond the plasma half-life of PCP and produce psychotic symptoms for up to 4 weeks. The recurrent or delayed psychotic effects that are symptomatically identical to mania and schizophrenia may not be related to significant PCP levels in plasma and brain. They can last 2–4 weeks. Other than a history of recent PCP use, features that differentiate PCP psychosis from functional schizophrenia are a higher incidence of violent behavior and clouded sensorium. Clinical evidence indicates that PCP psychosis, if it persists, may be indistinguishable from a functional psychotic reaction. The acute psychosis can be treated by leaving patients alone and avoiding any interpersonal stimulation. If this is ineffective, treatment options include oral diazepam (10–30 mg); intramuscularly administered lorazepam (2–4 mg); haloperidol (5 mg administered intramuscularly or 10 mg given as an oral concentrate); or thiothixene (10 mg administered intramuscularly or 20 mg given as an oral concentrate). Intravenously administered haloperidol also may be effective. Acidification of the urine is often necessary for at least 1 week to expedite PCP excretion.

phencyclidine/street names   angel dust, angel hair, angel mist, aurora, aurora borealis, bust bee, cheap cocaine, cosmos, crystal, dummy mist, dust, flakes, goon, green, guerrilla, hog, hot, jet, K, kw, krystal, loveboat, lovely, mauve, mist, mumm dust, PCP, PeaCePill, peep, purple, rocket fuel, sheets, sherm, sherman, special L.A. coke, superacid, supercoke, supergrass, superjoint, tac, the pits, tac, tranq, wack, whack.

phencyclidine withdrawal   Syndrome similar to withdrawal from marijuana and cocaine, with a more protracted and more pronounced subjective component. Symptoms include anxiety, depression, suicidality, restlessness, agitation, suspiciousness, and at times combativeness. Vital signs usually return to normal within a few hours or days following intoxication. The patient may remain intermittently confused, with periods of disorientation, anxiety, and depression that may take days to weeks to clear. Occasionally, a toxic delirium persists for months or indefinitely in some heavy users (Miller SN. Special problems of the alcohol and multiple-drug dependent: clinical interactions and detoxification. *In* Frances RJ, Miller SI [eds], *Clinical Textbook of Addictive Disorders*. New York: Guilford Press, 1991).

phencyclidine withdrawal/neonate   Using a specially designed score sheet for recording neonatal drug withdrawal symptoms, researchers showed that in neonates exposed only to PCP and whose urine toxicology screen demonstrated only PCP, symptoms were primarily neurobehavioral (high-pitched cry, poor tracking, decreased attention) (Rahbar F, Fomufod A, White D, Westney LS. Impact of intrauterine exposure to phencyclidine [PCP] and cocaine on neonates. *J Natl Med Assoc* 1993;85: 349–352).

phendimetrazine   (Adipost; Bacarate; Phenzine; Prelu-2; Statobex) Amphetamine congener that is a short-acting sympathomimetic amine marketed for short-term anorexigenic effects. It is considered a second-line drug for weight control because it causes euphoria, has a high abuse potential, and often causes undesirable central nervous system stimulation. Schedule III; pregnancy risk category C.

phenelzine   (Nardelcine; Nardil) (PHE) Hydrazine, irreversible and nonselective monoamine oxidase inhibitor (MAOI) antidepressant that may be an effective therapy for severe depression, atypical depression, neurotic depression, and depression accompanied by anxiety. It also is used for migraine prophylaxis, bulimia nervosa, panic disorder, and post-traumatic stress disorder. Of the original irreversible and nonselective MAOIs, phenelzine has become the most widely prescribed. Side effects and disadvantages (e.g., tyramine interaction) are the same as those of other MAOIs in its class. Pregnancy risk category C.

phenelzine + alprazolam   Alprazolam enhances the therapeutic effect of phenelzine with no significant adverse effects and no effect on phenelzine's platelet monoamine oxidase activity (Fawcett J. Targeting treatment in patients with mixed symptoms of anxiety and depression. *J Clin Psychiatry* 1990;51[suppl 11]: 40–43).

phenelzine + amantadine   A patient taking amantadine, haloperidol, and flurazepam developed hypertension after taking four doses of phenelzine (Jack RA, Daniel DG. Possible interaction between phenelzine and amantadine. *Arch Gen Psychiatry* 1984;41:726).

phenelzine/breast milk   Although there are no data on phenelzine in breast milk or its effects on nursing newborns, phenelzine-treated women should be advised not to breastfeed.

phenelzine + bupropion   See **bupropion + monoamine oxidase inhibitor**.

phenelzine + buspirone   See **buspirone + monoamine oxidase inhibitor**.

phenelzine + clomipramine   Addition of phenelzine (60 mg/day) to clomipramine

(CMI) at a reduced dose of 150 mg/day resulted in almost complete disappearance of avoidance behavior and agoraphobia within 2 weeks in a patient who remained completely symptom-free for about 2 years. Low maintenance doses of the drugs produced no significant side effects (Klein E, Metz L. Differential drug response of panic and agoraphobic avoidance in a case of panic disorder. *Acta Psychiatr Scand* 1990;82:86–87). Catastrophic illness manifested by hyperpyrexia (110 F), blood pressure lability, tachycardia, renal failure, and coma occurred in a patient treated with clomipramine, phenelzine, and chlorpromazine (Stern TA, Schwartz JH, Shuster JL. Catastrophic illness associated with the combination of clomipramine, phenelzine and chlorpromazine. *Ann Clin Psychiatry* 1992;4: 81–85). The serotonin syndrome, resulting from an interaction between phenelzine (which reduces serotonin metabolism within neurons) and clomipramine (which inhibits serotonin uptake at synapses), has been reported (Nierenberg DW, Semprebon M. The central nervous system serotonin syndrome. *Clin Pharmacol Ther* 1993;53:84–88). Thus, addition of clomipramine to phenelzine should be considered potentially dangerous and probably should be avoided.

phenelzine + clonazepam   Two cases of facial flushing have been reported. The mechanism for the interaction is unknown, but has been attributed to additive or synergistic serotonergic effects (Karagianis JL, March H. Flushing reaction associated with the interaction of phenelzine and clonazepam. *Can J Psychiatry* 1991;36:389). After taking clonazepam (0.5 mg at bedtime), a patient stabilized for 9 years on phenelzine (45 mg/day) experienced severe occipital headache (Eppel AB. Interaction between clonazepam and phenelzine. *Can J Psychiatry* 1990;35:647).

phenelzine + cyproheptadine   Addition of cyproheptadine to the therapeutic regimen of a depressed patient responsive to phenelzine caused rapid recurrence (a few hours to 4 days) of depressive symptoms (Zubieta JK, Demitrack MA. Depression after cyproheptadine: MAO treatment. *Biol Psychiatry* 1992;31: 1177–1178).

phenelzine + dextromethorphan   Co-administration has been associated with hyperpyrexia, hypotension, and fatal cardiac arrest (Rivers N, Horner B. Possible lethal reaction between Nardil and dextromethorphan. *Can Med Assoc J* 1970;103:85).

phenelzine + dextropropoxyphene   A patient taking phenelzine, estrogen replacement therapy, and propranolol became sedated and complained of a groggy feeling within 2 hours of ingesting dextropropoxyphene (100 mg) and acetaminophen (650 mg). The reaction recurred with rechallenge, but not with acetaminophen alone (Garbutt JC. Potentiation of propoxyphene by phenelzine. *Am J Psychiatry* 1987;144:251–252). A 63-year-old woman with bipolar disorder was stabilized on a regimen of valproate (250 mg 3 times a day), lithium (450 mg/day), phenelzine (15 mg 3 times a day), and trazodone (100–200 mg at bedtime) for 9 months. Twelve hours after taking oral propoxyphene (100 mg) and acetaminophen (650 mg), she experienced leg shaking and weakness in general. On admission to the hospital she was anxious, confused, and intensely diaphoretic. She also demonstrated impaired coordination and ataxia on tandem gait testing. On the second hospital day she became hypotensive, requiring treatment. She recovered after 4 days with no residual neurological deficits (Zornberg GI, Hegarty JD. Adverse interaction between propoxyphene and phenelzine. *Am J Psychiatry* 1993;150: 1270–1271).

phenelzine + fluoxetine   Co-administration may cause symptoms of the serotonin syndrome and should always be avoided. See **fluoxetine + monoamine oxidase inhibitor; serotonin syndrome.**

phenelzine + haloperidol   Co-administration has been found efficacious in the treatment of irritability and depression in borderline personality disorder.

phenelzine + levodopa/carbidopa   Co-administration in depressed Parkinson's disease (PD) patients may produce moderate to marked improvement in both PD and depression Hargrave R, Ashfold JW. Phenelzine treatment of depression in Parkinson's disease. *Am J Psychiatry* 1992;149:1751–1752). Co-administration of a monoamine oxidase inhibitor (MAOI) and levodopa (L-dopa) is usually avoided because of the reported risk of serious side effects, specifically hypertensive crisis. The combination with carbidopa may allow safer use of MAOIs (Hargrave R, Ashford JW. Phenelzine treatment of depression in Parkinson's disease. *Am J Psychiatry* 1992;148:1751–1752).

phenelzine + lithium   Lithium potentiation of phenelzine in refractory depression has not caused adverse effects (Nelson JC, Byck R. Rapid response to lithium in phenelzine nonresponders. *Br J Psychiatry* 1982;141:85–86). See **lithium + monoamine oxidase inhibitor.**

phenelzine + maprotiline   Addition of phenelzine (15–45 mg/day) to the regimen of patients only partially responsive to maprotiline may augment therapeutic response without producing more side effects than occur with maprotiline alone (Ayd FJ Jr. Combined maprotiline-MAOI therapy. *Int Drug Ther Newsl* 1982;17:4).

phenelzine + metoprolol Sinus bradycardia occurred in two elderly depressed patients when phenelzine was added to their metoprolol therapy. Metoprolol dosage reduction or discontinuation ameliorated the bradycardia (Reggev A, Vollhardt BR. Bradycardia induced by an interaction between phenelzine and beta blockers. *Psychosomatics* 1989;30:106–108).

phenelzine + 3,4-methylenedioxymethamphetamine (MDMA) There are two reports of serotonin syndrome associated with combined use (Smilkstein MJ, Smolinske SC, Rumack BH. A case of MAO inhibitor/MDMA interaction: agony after ecstasy. *J Toxicol Clin Toxicol* 1987;25:149–159; Kaskey GB. Possible interaction between an MAOI and "Ecstasy." *Am J Psychiatry* 1992;149:411–412)

phenelzine + nadolol Sinus bradycardia occurred in two elderly depressed patients when phenelzine was added to their nadolol therapy. Nadolol dosage reduction or discontinuation ameliorated the bradycardia (Reggev A, Vollhardt BR. Bradycardia induced by an interaction between phenelzine and beta blockers. *Psychosomatics* 1989;30:106–108).

phenelzine/pregnancy Although there are no data documenting that phenelzine has any teratogenic effects, it should be avoided during pregnancy.

phenelzine + succinylcholine Co-administration may enhance succinylcholine effects (Bleaden FA, Czekanska G. New drugs for depression. *Br Med J* 1960:1:200; Bodley PO, Halwax K, Potts L. Low serum pseudocholinesterase levels complicating treatment with phenelzine. *Br Med J* 1969;3:510).

phenelzine + tryptophan Several cases of myoclonus have developed after the serotonin precursor tryptophan was added to phenelzine. Symptoms included ataxia, ocular movements, dysarthria, hyperreflexia, and spontaneous jerking movements of the legs. They usually disappeared within 24 hours after stopping tryptophan (Levy AB, Bucher P, Votolato N. Myoclonus, hyperreflexia and diaphoresis in patients on phenelzine-tryptophan combination therapy. *Can J Psychiatry* 1985;30:434–436).

Phenergan See **promethazine.**

Phenibut See **beta-phenyl-GABA.**

phenmetrazine (Adipost; Anorex; Bontril; Preludin) Sympathomimetic amine with pharmacological activity similar to that of amphetamines that is marketed as an anorectic drug. Like all amphetamine products, it is subject to abuse. Schedule II; pregnancy risk category C.

"phennie" Street name for phenobarbital.

phenobarbital (Barbita; Barbital; Gardenal; Luminal; Solfoton) Barbiturate sedative-hypnotic and anticonvulsant used in the treatment of epilepsy and febrile convulsions. Dosage is adjusted carefully in small amounts until seizures are controlled or side effects occur. Blood levels can be measured to determine the therapeutic dose. Side effects include drowsiness, sedation, unsteadiness, dizziness, and poor coordination, especially in the first week. In children and the elderly, excitement, restlessness, and confusion are more likely to occur. Overdosage has been used in suicide attempts. Withdrawal seizures are a serious problem, especially if phenobarbital is stopped suddenly. Although other drugs such as carbamazepine and sodium valproate have taken its place in the treatment of epilepsy, phenobarbital may be better than these drugs for generalized epilepsy. Schedule IV; pregnancy risk category D.

phenobarbital + benzodiazepine Higher benzodiazepine doses may be required for anxiolysis (Stoudemire A, Moran MG. Psychopharmacologic treatment of anxiety in the medically ill elderly patient: special considerations. *J Clin Psychiatry* 1993;54[suppl 5]:27–33).

phenobarbital + bupropion Because phenobarbital may affect hepatic drug-metabolizing enzyme systems, care should be exercised in co-prescribing it with bupropion.

phenobarbital + carbamazepine Phenobarbital can adversely affect carbamazepine (CBZ) metabolism, doubling CBZ epoxide plasma levels. When drugs that stimulate epoxide formation are co-administered with CBZ, serum levels may remain relatively normal, but intoxication can occur from high metabolite concentrations.

phenobarbital + chlorpromazine Phenobarbital reduces chlorpromazine (CPZ) plasma concentration by inducing microsomal oxidizing enzymes and may interfere with CPZ's therapeutic effects (Loga S, Curry S, Lader M. Interactions of orphenadrine and phenobarbitone with chlorpromazine: plasma concentration and effects in man. *Br J Clin Pharmacol* 1985;2:197–208).

phenobarbital + clobazam Clobazam (CLB) has been reported to have no significant effect on the blood level/dose ratio (LDR) of phenobarbital (PB). However, PB significantly decreased the LDR of the CLB metabolite N-desmethylclobazam (NCLB), thereby increasing the NCLB/CLB ratio (Sennome S, Mesduian E. Interactions between clobazam and standard antiepileptic drugs in patients with epilepsy. *Ther Drug Monit* 1992;14:269–274).

phenobarbital + clomipramine Co-administration can decrease steady-state plasma concentrations of clomipramine and its desmethyl metabolite compared with such concentrations in control subjects (Luscombe DK, Jones RB. Effects of concomitantly administered drugs on plasma levels of clomipramine and desmethylclomipramine in depressive patients receiving clomipramine therapy. *Postgrad Med J* 1977;53[suppl 4]:77–78).

phenobarbital + haloperidol Co-administration can lower haloperidol plasma concentrations secondary to hepatic enzyme induction by phenobarbital (Linnoila M, Viukari M, Vaisanen K, et al. Effect of anticonvulsants on plasma haloperidol and thioridazine levels. *Am J Psychiatry* 1980;137:819–821).

phenobarbital + lamotrigine Phenobarbital, by inducing liver enzymes, can reduce lamotrigine's half-life (Anon. Lamotrigine—An add-on antiepileptic. *Drug Ther Bull* 1992;30:75–76).

phenobarbital + meperidine Co-administration increases metabolism of meperidine and increases production of the less efficacious toxic metabolite, norpethidine. Debilitating lethargy and possibly seizures may develop (Maurer PM, Bartkowski RR. Drug interactions of clinical significance with opioid analgesics. *Drug Safety* 1993;8:30–48).

phenobarbital + methadone Co-administration may precipitate opioid withdrawal in methadone maintenance patients (Liu SJ, Wang RIH. Case report of barbiturate-induced enhancement of methadone metabolism and withdrawal syndrome. *Am J Psychiatry* 1984;141:1287–1288).

phenobarbital + nimodipine Co-administration may decrease plasma nimodipine concentrations and necessitate increased nimodipine dosage to achieve adequate therapeutic levels (Tartara A, Galimberti CA, Manni R, et al. Differential effects of valproic acid and enzyme-inducing anticonvulsants on nimodipine pharmacokinetics in epileptic patients. *Br J Clin Pharmacol* 1991;32:335–340).

phenobarbital + paroxetine No significant interactions have been reported. In some studies, phenobarbital caused a 25% decrease in paroxetine plasma concentrations, most likely because of accelerated metabolism as a result of enzyme induction (Kaye CM, Haddock RE, Langley PF, et al. A review of the metabolism and pharmacokinetics of paroxetine in man. *Acta Psychiatr Scand* 1989;80[suppl 350]:60–75; Greb WH, Buscher G, Dierdorf H-D, et al. The effect of liver enzyme inhibition by cimetidine and enzyme induction by phenobarbitone on the pharmacokinetics of paroxetine. *Acta Psychiatr Scand* 1989;80[suppl 350]:95–98).

phenobarbital + phenytoin Serum phenobarbital levels require monitoring when phenytoin (PHT) is added to avoid overdosing or underdosing during the early or later course of combination therapy, respectively (Encinas MP, Santos Buelga D, Alonso Gonzalez AC, et al. Influence of length of treatment on the interaction between phenobarbital and phenytoin. *J Clin Pharm Ther* 1992;17:49–50). Phenobarbital may reduce PHT steady-state plasma concentrations through inductions of hepatic microsomal enzymes.

phenobarbital + pindolol Co-administration increases phenobarbital serum level (Greendyke RM, Gulya A. Effect of pindolol administration on serum levels of thioridazine, haloperidol, phenytoin and phenobarbital. *J Clin Psychiatry* 1988;49:105–107).

phenobarbital substitution technique Method of withdrawing patients from a benzodiazepine (BZD) that is preferred because it is unlikely to precipitate withdrawal seizures and because in treating drug dependence, it is preferable not to administer the drug of dependence to the patient during treatment. Phenobarbital is chosen over other sedatives with approximately the same half-life (e.g., diazepam) because it rarely produces a "high." Daily BZD use in the month before treatment is used to compute the initial detoxification dose of phenobarbital, which is given daily in three or four doses (regardless of the total computed conversion, the maximum phenobarbital dose is 500 mg/day). After 2 days of stabilization, phenobarbital dosage is decreased by 30 mg daily. Before each dose, the patient is checked for sustained horizontal nystagmus, slurred speech, and ataxia. If sustained nystagmus and sedation are present, the scheduled dose is withheld. If all three signs are present, the next two doses are withheld and the total daily dose for the next day is cut in half (Smith DE, Wesson DR. Phenobarbital technique for treatment of barbiturate dependence. *Arch Gen Psychiatry* 1971;24:56–60). See **phenobarbital substitution technique.**

phenobarbital + thioridazine Thioridazine may depress phenobarbital levels (Gay PE, Madsem JA. Interaction between phenobarbital and thioridazine. *Neurology* 1983;33:1631–1632).

phenobarbital + valproate Co-administration may lower valproate blood level (Heinemeyer G, Nau H, Hildebrandt AG, Roots I. Oxidation and glucuronidation of valproic acid in male rats—influence of phenobarbital, 3-methylcholanthrene, beta-naphthofarone and clofibrate. *Biochem Pharmacol* 1985;34:133–139). See **valproate/polypharmacy.**

phenobarbital + valproic acid   Valproic acid may impair phenobarbital metabolism and increase its plasma levels. In 20 epileptic patients receiving 900 mg/day of valproate sodium plus 100 mg/day of phenobarbital, valproate plasma levels were significantly lower during concomitant phenobarbital therapy. Maximum plasma concentrations after a single dose of valproate alone were 61–98 mg/L, compared with 45.5–79 mg/L in patients on combined therapy. Area under the concentration-time curve, plasma clearance, and elimination rate constant were significantly higher in patients on combined therapy, whereas the elimination half-life was significantly lower. Phenobarbital may have a clinically significant effect on the pharmacokinetics of valproate (Pokrajac M, Miljkovic B, Varagic VM, Levic Z. Pharmacokinetic interaction between valproic acid and phenobarbital. *Biopharm Drug Dispos* 1993;14:81–86).

phenobarbital withdrawal dosage equivalents/non-benzodiazepine   Phenobarbital (30 mg) is estimated to equal secobarbital (100 mg), pentobarbital (100 mg), amobarbital (100 mg), butabarbital (100 mg), chloral hydrate (250 mg), glutethimide (250 mg), meprobamate (200 mg), and methaqualone (300 mg).

phenobarbital withdrawal dosage equivalents/benzodiazepine   Phenobarbital (30 mg) is estimated to equal alprazolam (1 mg), chlordiazepoxide (25 mg), clorazepate (15 mg), diazepam (10 mg), flurazepam (15 mg), halazepam (40 mg), oxazepam (10 mg), prazepam (10 mg), and temazepam (15 mg). Phenobarbital (15 mg) is estimated to equal clonazepam (2 mg) and lorazepam (1 mg).

phenocopy   Person who does not carry the genotype but who manifests the trait, a phenomenon often attributed to other genetic or nongenetic causes.

phenothiazine   Any of a group of neuroleptics (aliphatic, piperazine, and piperidine derivatives) that differ in milligram potency and in the propensity to cause certain side effects. Phenothiazines are among the most widely used neuroleptics, even though they cause a number of adverse effects, including early-onset extrapyramidal reactions, tardive dyskinesia and other tardive extrapyramidal disorders, and the neuroleptic malignant syndrome. See **phenothiazine, aliphatic; phenothiazine, piperazine; phenothiazine, piperidine.**

phenothiazine + alcohol   Combined used may precipitate an acute dystonic reaction, especially with piperazine phenothiazines (e.g., trifluoperazine, fluphenazine), that may be due to either alcohol-lowered neurological threshold or altered absorption that increases phenothiazine plasma level and risk of side effects. Alcohol plus a phenothiazine, especially piperidines and aliphatics, may cause pronounced sedation.

phenothiazine, aliphatic   Any of a group of phenothiazine derivative neuroleptics with an aliphatic side chain, antipsychotic effects, and moderate milligram potency. Included are chlorpromazine, promazine, and triflupromazine. Aliphatics are slightly more potent on a milligram-per-milligram basis than piperidines. The pharmacological effects of the aliphatics are more similar to those of piperidine than to those of piperazine phenothiazines. Aliphatics produce more sedation, anticholinergic side effects, hypotension, dermatitis, convulsions, and agranulocytosis, but fewer extrapyramidal reactions, than piperazines. Because of the propensity of aliphatics to sedate, many psychiatrists favor aliphatics (orally or intramuscularly administered) for the treatment of acute toxic and functional psychoses (schizophrenia, schizoaffective disorder, mania) characterized by excitedness, combativeness, and assaultiveness.

phenothiazine derivative   Any of a group of psychotropic drugs that have a phenothiazine chemical configuration, but differ from each other through variations in other components of the molecule (e.g., the side chain and the halogen attached to the phenothiazine nucleus). Most are antipsychotic drugs or neuroleptics (e.g., chlorpromazine), although some are primarily antiemetics or antipiuretics (e.g., prochlorperazine; trimeprazine).

phenothiazine + morphine   Co-administration results in additive and prolonged central nervous system depressant effects. Some phenothiazines (e.g., chlorpromazine) can enhance morphine's analgesic effects, an effect that may be valuable in the treatment of severe, chronic pain (Thompson JW. Opioid peptides. *Br Med J* 1984; 288:259–261).

phenothiazine + pimozide   Because both drugs prolong the QT interval, an additive effect may occur with co-administration.

phenothiazine/ocular changes   Pigmentary changes with long-term phenothiazine use is well documented. Ocular changes have been more frequently reported with the aliphatic and piperidine than with piperazine phenothiazines. Cataracts may develop, but their incidence does not appear to be greater than the incidence in patients not taking phenothiazine drugs. Although routine ocular monitoring during long-term phenothiazine drug treatment has not been considered mandatory, it may be desirable in developmentally disabled patients whose life-time cumulative dosage may place them more at risk, particularly if they have metabolic conditions (e.g., phenylketonuria) wherein the likelihood of cataract development is higher (Anon. Ocular damage from long-term use of phenothiazines. News and notes. *The Royal Australian and New Zealand College of Psychiatrists*, April 1990, p 9).

phenothiazine, piperazine Any of a group of phenothiazine derivative neuroleptics with antipsychotic effects and high milligram potency. Included are acetophenazine, fluphenazine, perphenazine, prochlorperazine, and trifluoperazine. Piperazines are less sedative and anticholinergic; less likely to cause cardiovascular side effects (especially hypotension), seizures, agranulocytosis, and dermatitis; but more likely to evoke extrapyramidal reactions than aliphatic or piperidine phenothiazines.

phenothiazine, piperidine Any of a group of phenothiazine derivative neuroleptics with antipsychotic effects and a low milligram potency. Included are mesoridazine, pericyazine, pipotiazine, and thioridazine. Milligram per milligram, piperidines are the least potent. They are less likely than piperazines and aliphatics to cause extrapyramidal reactions, but more likely to cause cardiovascular side effects (conduction disturbances, arrhythmias, sudden death), retinal toxicity, and sexual dysfunction (ejaculatory inhibition, anorgasmia). Piperidines also are sedative and anticholinergic.

phenotype Observable physical, biochemical, and physiological characteristics of an individual (e.g., the mutation of gene coding for hemoglobin is the genotype, whereas sickle cell anemia is a phenotype).

phentermine (Adipex-P; Anoxine-AM; Dapex-37.5; Duromine; Fastin; Ionamin; Obe-Nix; Obephen; Obermine; Parmine; Phentrol 2; Phentrol 4; Phentrol 5; Wilpowr) Anorectic drug with a spectrum of pharmacological effects similar to that of amphetamines, but with weaker central nervous system stimulation effects. It can cause psychosis, often·with paranoid features. Schedule IV; pregnancy risk category C.

phentermine + fenfluramine Co-administration in 150 obese patients produced significant weight loss, minimal side effects, and a dropout rate of less than 20%. In 11 of 12 consecutive alcoholics, fenfluramine (80 mg) + phentermine (30 mg) produced marked or total decrease in alcohol craving and consumption, usually in less than 24 hours (Hitzig P. Combined dopamine and serotonin agonist: a synergistic approach to alcoholism and other addictive behaviors. *Maryland Med J* 1993;42: 153–157).

phentermine + monoamine oxidase inhibitor (MAOI) Co-administration may cause hypertensive crisis.

phentolamine (Regitine) Short-acting alpha$_1$-adrenergic blocker marketed as an antihypertensive. It is used intravenously for the treatment of hypertensive crises in patients receiving monoamine oxidase inhibitors. It is also self-administered in combination with papaverine for the treatment of erectile impotence. See **monoamine oxidase inhibitor/hypertensive crisis.**

Phentrol 2 See **phentermine.**

Phentrol 4 See **phentermine.**

Phentrol 5 See **phentermine.**

Phenurone See **phenacemide.**

phenylalanine Essential amino acid that cannot be synthesized de novo by the human body, but has to be obtained from an external source. It is a precursor of monoamines and phenylethylamine. It is converted by the liver into tyrosine through the action of the enzyme phenylalanine hydroxylase. Accumulation due to reduced phenylalanine hydroxylase activity causes phenylketonuria in children.

phenylalanine + selegiline Combination that can be used effectively in patients with treatment-resistant major depressive disorder. Effects are rapid and often without side effects.

phenylbutazone (Butazolidin) Nonsteroidal anti-inflammatory drug.

phenylbutazone + lithium See **lithium + phenylbutazone.**

phenylephrine (Neo-Synephrine) (PE) Synthetic sympathomimetic structurally similar to epinephrine and ephedrine. It is available as a prescription medication for use as a vasoconstrictor and is also an ingredient in a number of over-the-counter nasal decongestants.

phenylephrine + brofaromine See **brofaromine + phenylephrine.**

phenylephrine + terbutaline + toloxatone See **toloxatone + terbutaline + phenylephrine.**

phenylethylamine (PEA) Endogenous monoamine presumably produced from phenylalanine via decarboxylation and mainly metabolized by monoamine oxidase type B. It is a relatively potent inhibitor of the reuptake and stimulator of the release of dopamine and noradrenaline from nerve terminals. It has amphetamine-like effects. Abnormal urinary excretion of PEA has been reported in a variety of psychiatric and neurological disorders, including affective disorders. Also called "beta-phenylethylamine."

phenylketonuria (PKU) Disease characterized by mental deficiency that is associated with the presence of phenylpyruvic acid in the urine and elevated phenylalanine levels. It is due to a hereditary (autosomal recessive) deficiency of phenylalanine hydroxylase, which converts phenylalanine to tyrosine.

phenylpiperidine Group of opioid analgesics, the most widely used of which are meperidine and fentanyl. See **fentanyl; meperidine.**

phenylpropanolamine (Acutrim) (PPA) Sympathomimetic structurally similar to amphetamines that may directly stimulate adrenergic receptors, but probably indirectly stimulates both alpha- and beta-adrenergic receptors by releasing norepinephrine from its storage sites. It has long been used as a nasal decongestant (it is an ingredient in many over-the-counter decongestant and cough medicines) and more recently as an anorexiant. It may cause a psychotic reaction with mixed affective symptoms or a hypertensive reaction in patients treated with some monoamine oxidase inhibitors.

phenylpropanolamine + brofaromine See **brofaromine + phenylpropanolamine.**

phenytoin (Dilantin) (PHT) Sodium salt of 5,5-diphenyl derivative of hydantoin, marketed as an anticonvulsant effective in the treatment of generalized tonic-clonic seizures and certain partial seizures. On the basis of many clinical trials, it is considered to have a very good overall combination of efficacy and freedom from adverse effects during treatment of partial epilepsy. PHT given intravenously is the first drug of choice for the treatment of status epilepticus of the major motor type unless the patient previously was treated with another anticonvulsant. Although half-life is long enough to make once-daily dosage feasible, twice-daily dosing is necessary because of individual variability; it is seldom administered 3 or 4 times daily. If PHT is ineffective at a dose of 18–25 mg/kg, it should be replaced with another drug (e.g., phenobarbital, paraldehyde). PHT is a well known inducer of the cytochrome P450 enzyme system of the liver responsible for the metabolism of many drugs. It is one of the few commonly used drugs that have substantially nonlinear elimination characteristics at therapeutic doses. Therefore, the time to steady-state concentration may be considerably longer than would be suggested by rough estimates based on a dose-independent half-life. In addition, steady-state concentration at one dose does not directly predict steady-state concentration at another dose. Attempts to increase or decrease the steady-state concentration by simple linear extrapolation from a known plasma level may often result in an unexpectedly high and possibly toxic or low and subtherapeutic concentration. In any individual patient with toxic serum levels, one cannot reliably predict the time that will be required for PHT concentration to fall to the therapeutic range. Severe side effects include hepatitis, neuropathy, cerebellar ataxia, lymphoma, pseudolymphoma, and osteomalacia. Toxic levels can evoke typical signs of acute dystonia that resolve when blood levels return to the therapeutic range (Chadwick D, Reynolds EH, Marsden CD. Anticonvulsant-induced dyskinesias: a comparison with dyskinesias induced by neuroleptics. *J Neurol Neurosurg Psychiatry* 1976;39:1210–1218). PHT may aggravate neuroleptic-induced tardive dyskinesia (DeVeaugh-Geiss J: Aggravation of tardive dyskinesia by phenytoin. *N Engl J Med* 1978;298:457). Pregnancy risk category D.

phenytoin + acetophenazine Acetophenazine may inhibit metabolism of phenytoin, increasing risk of phenytoin toxicity.

phenytoin + alcohol Acute alcohol intake may increase serum phenytoin levels, whereas chronic alcohol use may decrease them. The former may result in phenytoin toxicity; the latter may result in loss of seizure control. In chronic drinkers, a period of abstinence leads to an enhanced rate of phenytoin clearance (Rall TW. Hypnotics and sedatives: ethanol. *In* Gilman AG, Rall TW, Nigs AS, et al [eds], *Goodman and Gilman's The Pharmacological Basis of Therapeutics*, 8th ed. New York: Pergamon Press, 1990, pp 345–382).

phenytoin + benzodiazepine Patients taking phenytoin require higher benzodiazepine (BZD) doses for anxiolysis than other patients (Stoudemire A, Moran MG. Psychopharmacologic treatment of anxiety in the medically ill elderly patient: special considerations. *J Clin Psychiatry* 1993;54[suppl 5]:27–33). Data on BZD effects on phenytoin metabolism are scanty and conflicting; in general, BZDs have no important effects (Pisani F, Perucca E, Di Perri R. Clinically relevant anti-epileptic drug interactions. *J Int Med Res* 1990;18:1–15).

phenytoin + bupropion Co-administration for 2 weeks resulted in delayed gastrointestinal absorption, significantly prolonged terminal elimination half-life, and delayed clearance of phenytoin (PHT) as manifested by an increase in the area under the curve. This has been attributed to the inhibition of hepatic microsomal enzymes that metabolize PHT (Tekle A, Al-Khamis KI. Phenytoin-bupropion interaction: effect on plasma phenytoin concentrations in the rat. *J Pharm Pharmacol* 1990;42:799–801).

phenytoin + carbamazepine Each drug may lower the other's plasma level, resulting in reduced therapeutic efficacy. Through induction of hepatic microsomal enzymes, each may decrease the other's steady-state concentrations (Hansen J, Siersbaek-Nielsen K, Skovsted L. Carbamazepine-induced acceleration of diphenylhydantoin and warfarin metabolism in man. *Clin Pharmacol Ther* 1971;12:539–543; Zielinski JJ, Haidukewych D, Lehata BJ. Carbamazepine-phenytoin interaction: elevation of plasma phenytoin concentrations due to carbamazepine comedication. *Ther Drug Monit* 1983;7:51–53). Altered mental status occurred in a patient treated with phenytoin (450 mg/day) and carbamazepine (600 mg/day) (Browne TR, Feldman RG, Mikati MA, et al. Nineteen-year-old man with altered mental status. *J Clin Pharmacol* 1992;32:511–519).

phenytoin + chloral hydrate   Co-administration can significantly reduce phenytoin levels (up to 70%).

phenytoin + chlorpromazine   Chlorpromazine (CPZ) may increase phenytoin levels, but generally its effects are not significant (Kuth H. Interactions between anticonvulsants and other commonly prescribed drugs. *Epilepsia* 1984;25[suppl 2]:118–131). CPZ's inhibition of hepatic mono-oxygenase activity may reduce the rate of phenytoin metabolism, resulting in a rise in plasma phenytoin concentration with increased risk of toxicity (Aronson JK, Hardman M, Reynolds DJM. Phenytoin. *Br Med J* 1992;305:1215–1218).

phenytoin + cimetidine   Co-administration results in increased phenytoin serum concentration (Frigo GM, Lecchini S, Caravaggi M, et al. Reduction in phenytoin clearance caused by cimetidine. *Eur J Clin Pharmacol* 1983;25:135–137).

phenytoin + clobazam   Clobazam (CLB) has been reported to have no significant effect on the blood level/dose ratio (LDR) of phenytoin (PHT). However, PHT significantly decreased the LDR of the CLB metabolite N-desmethylclobazam (NCLB), thereby increasing the NCLB/CLB ratio (Sennome S, Mesdjian E. Interactions between clobazam and standard antiepileptic drugs in patients with epilepsy. *Ther Drug Monit* 1992;14:269–274).

phenytoin + clomipramine   Co-administration can decrease steady-state plasma concentrations of clomipramine and its desmethyl metabolite compared with those of control subjects (Luscombe DK, Jones RB. Effects of concomitantly administered drugs on plasma levels of clomipramine and desmethylclomipramine in depressive patients receiving clomipramine therapy. *Postgrad Med J* 1977; 53[suppl 4]:77–78).

phenytoin + clonazepam   In an epileptic patient, phenytoin (300 mg/day) and clonazepam (CNP) (1.5 mg/day) resulted in decreased phenytoin plasma levels (from 22 to 16 µg/ml) and increased seizures. CNP dos-

age was gradually reduced by 0.5 mg/week and finally discontinued; phenytoin was maintained at 375 mg/day. Signs of intoxication resolved.

phenytoin + clozapine   Addition of phenytoin (PHT) to clozapine (CLOZ) may increase CLOZ clearance by inducing hepatic cytochrome P450 oxidase enzymes, significantly decrease (65–85%) CLOZ steady-state plasma concentrations, and produce clinical deterioration requiring increased CLOZ dosage (Miller DD. Effect of phenytoin on plasma clozapine concentrations in two patients. *J Clin Psychiatry* 1991;52:23–25).

phenytoin + disulfiram   Co-administration decreases phenytoin (PHT) clearance and markedly increases its serum levels. PHT toxicity has occurred when disulfiram was added to an anticonvulsant regimen (Kiorboe E. Phenytoin intoxication during treatment with Antabuse. *Epilepsia* 1966;7:246; Svendsen TL, Kristensen MB, Hansen JM, Skovsted L. The influence of disulfiram on the half-life and metabolic clearance rate of diphenylhydantoin and tolbutamide in man. *Eur J Clin Pharmacol* 1976;9:439).

phenytoin + felbamate   Co-administration increases phenytoin (PHT) plasma concentrations; PHT dosage may have to be reduced 10–30% to maintain stable PHT levels. Felbamate (FBM) is a competitive inhibitor of PHT metabolism, since PHT concentrations increase primarily at higher (> 20 mg/kg) FBM doses (Graves RM, Holmes GB, Fuerst GP, Leppik IE. Effect of felbamate on phenytoin and carbamazepine serum concentrations. *Epilepsia* 1989;30:225–229; Leppik IE, Dreifuss FE, Pledger GW, et al. Felbamate for partial seizures: results of a controlled clinical trial. *Neurology* 1991;41:785–789). PHT induces FBM metabolism to give lower-than-expected steady-state concentrations (Wagner ML, Leppik IE, Graves NM, et al. Felbamate serum concentrations: effect of valproate, carbamazepine, phenytoin and phenobarbital. *Epilepsia* 1990;31:642).

phenytoin + fluoxetine   Signs and symptoms of phenytoin intoxication occurred in two patients 5 and 10 days, respectively, after fluoxetine (20 mg/day) was started. Symptoms included gait ataxia, vertigo, diplopia, altered consciousness, vomiting, difficulty in getting up, and increased serum phenytoin concentrations (Jalil P. Toxic reaction following the combined administration of fluoxetine and phenytoin: two case reports. *J Neurol Neurosurg Psychiatry* 1992;55:412–413).

phenytoin + haloperidol   Phenytoin induces hepatic enzymes, significantly lowers haloperidol (HAL) plasma concentration, and may interfere with HAL's therapeutic efficacy (Linnoila M, Viukari M, Vaisanen K, et al. Effect of anticonvulsants on plasma haloperidol and thioridazine levels. *Am J Psychiatry* 1980;137: 819–821).

phenytoin + imipramine Imipramine (IMI) may elevate phenytoin (PHT) plasma levels (Perucca E, Rickens A. Interaction between phenytoin and imipramine. *Br J Clin Pharmacol* 1977;4:485–486). IMI inhibits liver monooxygenase activity and may slow PHT metabolism rate, increasing plasma PHT concentration and risk of PHT toxicity (Aronson JK, Hardman M, Reynolds DJM. Phenytoin. *Br Med J* 1992;305:1215–1218).

phenytoin intoxication Following an acute rise in phenytoin blood level, symptoms may include ataxia and inability to walk due to balance impairment, diplopia, and horizontal and vertical nystagmus, with little or no impairment of consciousness.

phenytoin + isoniazid Co-administration may increase phenytoin (PHT) blood level and may cause PHT toxicity. Isoniazid inhibits PHT metabolism, resulting in increased steady-state concentrations. This clinically important rise in serum PHT has been observed only in slow acetylators; fast acetylators do not achieve a concentration of isoniazid in the liver sufficiently high to inhibit the microsomal enzymes (Kutt H, Brennan R, Dehejia H, et al. Diphenylhydantoin intoxication. A complication of isoniazid therapy. *Am Rev Respir Dis* 1970;101:377–384).

phenytoin + lamotrigine Phenytoin, by inducing liver enzymes, can halve lamotrigine's half-life (Anon: Lamotrigine—an add-on antiepileptic. *Drug Ther Bull* 1992;30:75–76).

phenytoin/liquid food concentrate A 67-year-old man taking an oral suspension or intravenous doses of phenytoin (PHT) experienced gross fluctuations in serum drug levels that appeared to be related to the intake of liquid food concentrates and therapy with the suspension form. Serum PHT concentrations recovered only after resumption of solid food intake (day 34) and change to PHT tablets (day 40) (Taylor DM, Massey CA, Willson WG, Dhillon S. Lowered serum phenytoin concentrations during therapy with liquid food concentrates. *Ann Pharmacother* 1993;27:369).

phenytoin + lithium Co-administration may result in lithium toxicity (MacCallum WAG: Interaction of lithium and phenytoin. *Br Med J* 1980;280:610–611).

phenytoin + loxapine Loxapine has been reported to decrease serum phenytoin (PHT) levels, but there is no evidence that this is due to induction of PHT metabolism (Ryan GM, Matthews PA. Phenytoin metabolism stimu-

lated by loxapine. *Drug Intell Clin Pharm* 1970; 11:428).

phenytoin + meperidine Co-administration can produce tremors, myoclonus, and seizures (Modica PA, Tempelhoff R, White PF. Pro- and anticonvulsant effects of anesthetics [part I]. *Anesth Analg* 1990;70:303–315).

phenytoin + mesoridazine Phenytoin significantly lowers mesoridazine plasma concentration and interferes with its therapeutic effects.

phenytoin + methadone Phenytoin can cause methadone abstinence symptoms in previously stable patients because of increased methadone clearance (Tony TG, Pond SM, Kruk MJ, et al. Phenytoin-induced methadone withdrawal. *Ann Intern Med* 1981;94:349–351).

phenytoin + neuroleptic Co-administration may elevate phenytoin blood levels and increase risk of phenytoin toxicity.

phenytoin + nimodipine Co-administration may decrease plasma nimodipine concentrations and necessitate increased nimodipine dosage to achieve adequate therapeutic levels (Tartara A, Galimberti CA, Manni R, et al. Differential effects of valproic acid and enzyme-inducing anticonvulsants on nimodipine pharmacokinetics in epileptic patients. *Br J Clin Pharmacol* 1991;32:335–340).

phenytoin + paroxetine A single oral dose of paroxetine administered to a patient whose phenytoin plasma level was in steady state reduced paroxetine's area under the curve (AUC) and half-life ($T_{1/2}$) by an average of 50% and 35%, respectively, compared to paroxetine administered alone. When a single oral dose of phenytoin (300 mg) was administered with paroxetine in a steady state (30 mg daily for 14 days), phenytoin AUC was slightly reduced (average, 12%) compared to these values for phenytoin administered alone. No initial dosage adjustments are considered necessary when these drugs are co-administered; subsequent adjustments should be guided by clinical effect (Kaye CM, Haddock RE, Langley PF, et al. A review of the metabolism and pharmacokinetics of paroxetine in man. *Acta Psychiatr Scand* 1989;80[suppl 350]:60–75; Mikkelsen M, Anderson BB, Dam M, et al. Paroxetine: no interaction with antiepileptic drugs. *Psychopharmacology* 1991;103: B13).

phenytoin + phenobarbital Serum phenobarbital levels require monitoring when phenytoin (PHT) is added to avoid overdosing or underdosing during the early or later course of combination therapy, respectively (Encinas MP, Santos Buelga D, Alonso Gonzalez AC, et al. Influence of length of treatment on the interaction between phenobarbital and phenytoin. *J Clin Pharm Ther* 1992;17:49–50). Phenobarbital may reduce PHT steady-state plasma concentrations through inductions of hepatic microsomal enzymes.

phenytoin + pindolol In phenytoin (PHT)-treated patients, addition of pindolol produces no significant interactions. However, in a patient receiving haloperidol, PHT, and phenobarbital, addition of pindolol significantly increased PHT plasma level (up to 35–41%) (Greendyke RM, Gulya A. Effect of pindolol administration on serum levels of thioridazine, haloperidol, phenytoin and phenobarbital. *J Clin Psychiatry* 1988;49:105–107).

phenytoin + primidone Phenytoin may decrease the effects of primidone and increase its conversion to phenobarbital. Primidone's plasma level should be monitored to prevent toxicity.

phenytoin + prochlorperazine Prochlorperazine may increase phenytoin plasma levels, but effects generally are insignificant (Kuth H. Interactions between anticonvulsants and other commonly prescribed drugs. *Epilepsia* 1984; 25[suppl 2]:118–131).

phenytoin + remoxipride Pharmacokinetic studies indicate no interaction.

phenytoin + thioridazine Thioridazine may increase phenytoin plasma levels. Effects are generally not significant, but there may be an increased risk of phenytoin toxicity (Kuth H. Interactions between anticonvulsants and other commonly prescribed drugs. *Epilepsia* 1984;25[suppl 2]:118–131; Aronson JK, Hardman M, Reynolds DJ. ABC of monitoring drug therapy. Phenytoin. *Br Med J* 1992;305:1215–1218).

phenytoin + trazodone Co-administration may raise phenytoin serum levels by as much as 50%, increasing the risk of adverse phenytoin effects (Dorn JM. A case of phenytoin toxicity precipitated by trazodone. *J Clin Psychiatry* 1986;47:89–90).

phenytoin + valproate Co-administration may decrease valproate blood level and possibly its therapeutic efficacy.

phenytoin + valproic acid Valproic acid may increase phenytoin (PHT) metabolism and decrease serum PHT levels. Co-administration may require PHT dosage adjustment according to the clinical situation (Pisani F, Perucca E, Di Perri R. Clinically relevant anti-epileptic drug interactions. *J Int Med Res* 1990;18:1–15).

phenytoin + verapamil Phenytoin, an inducer of hepatic drug metabolizing enzymes, can interfere with verapamil absorption and markedly reduce its steady-state concentration (Woodcock BG, Kirsten R, Nelson K, et al. A reduction in verapamil concentrations with phenytoin. *N Engl J Med* 1991;325:1179).

phenytoin + vigabatrin Vigabatrin may reduce phenytoin's (PHT) steady state by 20–40%, possibly reducing PHT efficacy. Vigabatrin discontinuation may increase PHT serum level and risk of PHT intoxication (Rimmer RM, Richens A. Interaction between vigabatrin and phenytoin. *Br J Clin Pharmacol* 1989;27:27S–33S). During co-administration, PHT plasma levels should be monitored and dosage should be adjusted to assure therapeutic levels and maintenance of seizure control.

phenytoin + viloxazine Co-administration may increase phenytoin (PHT) serum levels and risk of PHT intoxication. PHT plasma levels should be monitored and its dosage should be adjusted to avoid toxicity.

phenytoin + warfarin Co-administration may increase phenytoin (PHT) blood levels and risk of PHT toxicity.

Phenzine See **phendimetrazine.**

phobia Irrational, involuntary, and inappropriate fear associated with certain objects or situations. It may involve a feeling of intense dread. Basic types include simple phobia, social phobia, and agoraphobia.

phobia, simple Unreasonable fear of a specific object or situation, such as snakes, heights, or thunderstorms. Most childhood phobias of animals are examples of simple phobias. These are often triggered by an actual frightening experience and generally disappear as the child gets older.

phobia, social (SP) Disorder characterized by fear of being judged by others and embarrassing oneself in public. SP patients fear and avoid situations in which they believe they may be subject to scrutiny while performing a specific task or interacting with other people (e.g., public speaking, eating in restaurants, using public restrooms). SP is formally recognized in DSM-IV as a discrete diagnostic entity. To be a true SP, the persistently feared situation must cause its avoidance or its dreaded endurance. Fears must impair occupational functioning and usual social activities or relationships as well as produce marked distress over having the fear. In anticipation of or actually in social phobic situations, SP patients complain of tachycardia, tremor, and blushing. Because SP is the least studied of the major psychiatric disorders, there are gaps in knowledge concerning definition, prevalence, etiology, pathophysiology, assessment, and treatment. However, it is amenable to one or more specific treatments including pharmacotherapy with monoamine oxidase inhibitors (MAOIs), beta-blockers plus MAOIs, and cognitive behavior therapy. The most studied drug is the MAOI phenelzine. Alprazolam and clonazepam have also been found to be effective. Beta-blockers are effective for stage fright and performance anxiety. Treatment approaches that ignore cognitive, behavioral, or social skills training or appropriate drug therapy are unlikely to be helpful in alleviating core symptoms (Liebowitz MR, Schneier FR, Hollander E, et al. Treatment of social phobia with drugs other than benzodiazepines. *J Clin Psychiatry* 1991;52:10–15; Davidson JRT, Ford SM, Smith RD, Potts NLS. Long-term treatment of social phobia with clonazepam. *J Clin Psychiatry* 1991;52:16–20).

phobia, social/rating scales Hamilton Anxiety Scale (HAS); Social Phobia Scale; Leibowitz Social Phobia Scale.

phocomelia Defective development of an extremity or extremities in which the hands or feet are attached close to the body, resembling the flippers of a seal. It has been caused by teratogenic drugs, notably thalidomide.

phosphatidylinositol cycle Second messenger system linked to the intracellular calcium signal and protein kinase C that mediates actions of numerous hormones, neurotransmitters (e.g., norepinephrine, serotonin, acetylcholine, histamine), and peptides.

phosphatidylinositol system (PI system) G protein–linked secondary messenger system that, by controlling the concentration of intracellular calcium, modulates the actions of some transmitters. It may mediate lithium action.

phosphoinositide system Cascade of enzymatic reactions that serves as an intracellular second messenger system.

phospholipase A$_2$ (PLA$_2$) Ubiquitous enzyme that cleaves fatty acids from the sn2 position of phospholipids. In brain it is present in cell membranes, microsomes, and cytosol. It plays an important role in signal transduction by generating lipid second messengers (e.g., arichnidonic acid). It also affects neuronal function by altering receptor sensitivity. Elevated PLA$_2$ activity has been reported in plasma and serum from schizophrenic patients and may underlie previously described alterations in phospholipid and prostaglandin metabolism in schizophrenia (Noponen M, Sanfilipo M, Samanich K, et al. Elevated PLA$_2$ activity in schizophrenics and other psychiatric patients. *Biol Psychiatry* 1993;34:641–649).

phospholipase C Major enzyme for activating one of the two major second messenger systems (the other being adenylate cyclase) that come into play following stimulation or blockade of receptors embedded in the cell membrane. Generally, the adenylate cyclase system modulates cyclic adenosine monophosphate, and the phospholipase C system modulates phosphatidylinositol metabolism in the two second messengers formed (diacylglycerol and IP$_3$).

phospholipid (PL) Phosphorus-containing lipid that is a major structural component of the cell membrane. PLs interact with membrane enzymes and transport molecules.

photoaffinity labeling Method of studying and isolating specific benzodiazepine (BZD) binding sites in which tritiated BZDs with a nitro group in position 7 (e.g., flunitrazepam, clonazepam) are used as photoaffinity labels. Under the influence of ultraviolet light, their reversible binding is changed into a covalent binding (Muhler H, Battersby MK, Richards JG. Benzodiazepine receptor protein identified and visualized in brain tissue by a photoaffinity label. *Proc Natl Acad Sci U S A* 1980;77: 1666–1670).

photoallergic reaction Formation of antigen(s) due to light energy acting on or altering drug and skin proteins. Previous exposure to the offending drug is necessary, but dose does not play a role. Lesions may be eczematous, papular, or urticarial, or they may resemble a sunburn. They may extend beyond areas exposed to light.

photon, single See **single photon.**

photoperiod Duration of light in a light-dark cycle.

photosensitivity Sensitivity to the sun and its phototoxic effects manifested by an increased tendency to sunburn after relatively brief exposure to direct or indirect sunlight, especially in the spring and summer. Phenothiazine neuroleptics, particularly chlorpromazine, may enhance photosensitivity. Patients should be warned to avoid overexposure to the sun, wear protective clothing (broad-brimmed hats), and use sun screens (e.g., lotions) that block ultraviolet rays.

phototherapy Use of bright light (2,500–2,800 lux) for the treatment of seasonal affective disorder and premenstrual syndrome. It was initially inspired by the finding that bright light can suppress nocturnal melatonin secretion, whereas ordinary room light cannot. Treatment with 10,000 lux is significantly superior to 2,500 lux and is effective when used for only 30 min/day; 2,500 lux is significantly superior to dim light treatment (300 lux or less). Phototherapy can reset the biological clock in symptoms of jet lag, shift work, and certain sleep disorders. Also called "bright light therapy"; "light therapy." See **seasonal affective disorder.**

phototherapy + fluoxetine Combined treatment may be helpful in otherwise refractory bulimia nervosa patients (Schwitzer J, Neudorfer C, Fleishhacker WW. Seasonal bulimia treated with fluoxetine and phototherapy. *Am J Psychiatry* 1993;150:1752).

phototherapy/ocular effects   Although there have been no reports of either short- or long-term ocular damage, light intensities of about 2,000 lux, if viewed directly for sustained periods, may damage the susceptible eye. A case of perimacular vertical-pigment epithelial scar, resembling a healed central serous retinopathy, has been reported. Ophthalmological examination is advisable before phototherapy is initiated, even when there is no history of eye complaint, because bright artificial light could exacerbate existing retinopathy, and eye damage discovered subsequent to light therapy could be wrongly attributed to the treatment (Vanselow W, Dennerstein L, Armstrong S, Lockie P. Retinopathy and bright light therapy. *Am J Psychiatry* 1991;148:1266–1267).

phototoxic reaction   See **photoallergic reaction.**

physical aggression   See **aggression, physical.**

physical dependence   See **drug dependence.**

physical disability   Difficulty performing one or more activities generally accepted as essential components of daily living (e.g, self-care, social relations, economic activity) (World Health Organization. Disability prevention and rehabilitation: reports of specific technical matters. [Twenty-ninth World Health Assembly.] Geneva, 1976).

physically dependent medical patient   One who continues taking the usual therapeutic dose of a drug (e.g., a benzodiazepine) over long periods without apparent problems or dose escalation. Patients typically do not abuse alcohol or other drugs, but do experience physical withdrawal or abstinence symptoms and the return of symptoms of their underlying disorder on discontinuation of the dependence-producing medicine. They are usually honest with their physicians about their use of medicines. Because physical dependence may be confused with addiction, they may label themselves as "addicted" to their medicines, but they do not exhibit the behavioral characteristics of addiction.

physical map   See **genome map.**

physiological arousal   Component of the normal anxiety response characterized by autonomic arousal, increased tension in skeletal muscles, increased ventilation of the lungs. It is part of the preparation for the increased muscular activity that accompanies approach or avoidance ("fight or flight").

physiological dependence   See **drug dependence.**

physiological tremor   See **tremor, physiological.**

Physeptine   See **methadone.**

physostigmine   (Antilirium; Eserine) Centrally active cholinesterase inhibitor that freely crosses the blood-brain barrier and increases brain adrenocorticotropic hormone levels. It also counteracts cholinergic blocking drugs. It has been used to treat anticholinergic toxicity by reducing both central and peripheral effects. Given slowly (1–2 mg intravenously or intramuscularly), physostigmine confirms suspected anticholinergic delirium if the patient's mental status improves and symptoms of muscarinic blockade subside. In treating anticholinergic toxicity due to long-acting drugs, physostigmine administration may have to be repeated every 30 minutes to 2 hours because its half life is relatively short (90–120 minutes). Although it may seem to be an ideal antidote, it can cause asystole in patients with anticholinergic syndrome, particularly if the electrocardiogram shows heart block or a prolonged QRS interval. It can be used in the treatment of the cognitive impairments associated with Alzheimer's disease. It may have antimanic properties, but it can worsen pre-existing depressive symptoms and cause transient recurrences of depressive symptoms in euthymic patients. It also can make akathisia worse. Intravenous infusion produces a behavioral syndrome characterized by anergia and fatigue, slowed and decreased thoughts, mild sedation, expressionless face, decreased spontaneous activity, and, occasionally, depression, nausea, or vomiting.

physostigmine + selegiline   Addition of selegiline (5 mg twice a day) to the regimen of Alzheimer's disease patients being treated with physostigmine was associated with significant improvement in the scores on the cognitive subscale of the Alzheimer's Disease Assessment Scale, suggesting possible additive effects of selegiline to the effects of cholinesterase inhibitors (Schneider LS, Olin JT, Pawluczyk S. A double-blind crossover pilot study of 1-deprenyl (selegiline) combined with cholinesterase inhibitor in Alzheimer's disease. *Am J Psychiatry* 1993;150:321–323).

physostigmine syndrome   Supersensitivity reaction manifested by increased heart rate, blood pressure, plasma adrenaline, adrenocorticotropic hormone, cortisol, beta-endorphin, prolactin, and possibly noradrenaline.

physostigmine toxicity   Symptoms include headache, nausea, vomiting, diarrhea, blurred vision, miosis, myopia, excessive tearing, bronchospasm, increased bronchial secretions, hypotension, incoordination, excessive sweating, muscle weakness, bradycardia, excessive salivation, restlessness or agitation, and confusion.

pica   Compulsive eating of non-nutritive unusual substances. It takes many forms and can be cultural and nonpathological; in its severest forms, it can result in serious physical pathology or death. It can mimic schizophrenic behavior. It may be caused by cancer or anemia (Parry-Jones B, Parry-Jones WLL. Pica: symptom or eating disorder? A historical assessment. *Br J Psychiatry* 1992;160:341–354; WHO. *The ICD-10 Classification of Mental and Behavioral Disorders.* Geneva: WHO, 1992).

Pick's disease Degeneration of prefrontal neurons with diagnostic inclusion bodies and inflated neurons. It is a presenile psychosis characterized by progressive dementia, personality changes, severe emotional impairment, and social and ethical aberrations. Average age of onset is mid-50s; it occurs more often in women than men, and more often in those with a family history of heredodegenerative traits. The clinical features of Pick's disease overlap those of Alzheimer's disease, but usually include language disturbance and behavioral changes early in the course of the illness. Also called "circumscribed cortical atrophy."

pickwickian Term applied to an individual who snores, is obese and sleepy, and has alveolar hypoventilation. It has been applied to many different disorders and therefore is discouraged from use.

picogram One trillionth of a gram.

picrotoxin Brain-stem stimulant that blocks the inhibitory actions of gamma aminobutyric acid (GABA) through action on a receptor linked to the GABA site.

picture recognition Cognitive task that assesses the ability to retrieve pictorial information from secondary memory.

"pier" Street name for cocaine.

Pilocar See **pilocarpine.**

pilocarpine (Pilocar) Acetylcholine receptor (muscarinic) agonist used in the form of eye drops to reduce intraocular pressure. Use of a 1% solution as a mouth rinse has been advocated to treat dry mouth.

pilot study Small test of procedures that will be used on a larger scale if they are successful.

pimozide (Opiran; Oralep Forte; Orap) Prototype diphenylbutylpiperidine neuroleptic that combines potent calcium channel blocker activity with highly selective blockade of dopamine D_1 and D_2 receptors. It has little effect on alpha$_1$, histamine H_1, or serotonin (5-HT) receptors. It is effective in the treatment of acute and chronic schizophrenia; in several trials, it was more effective than standard neuroleptics in treating negative symptoms (Opler LA, Feinberg SS. The role of pimozide in clinical psychiatry: a review. *J Clin Psychiatry* 1991;52:221–233). Pimozide is Food and Drug Administration (FDA)-approved for treating

Gilles de la Tourette's syndrome. It can be used to treat monosymptomatic hypochondriacal psychosis, delusional jealousy, and pain syndromes (postherpetic and trigeminal neuralgia). It also has a good antimanic effect and appears to be effective and well tolerated in severe Sydenham's chorea. In an open-pilot study, 3–6 mg/day decreased behavioral symptoms on all measures in eight hospitalized autistic boys (ages 4.2 to 8.3 years) over a 3-week period (Ernst M, Magee HJ, Gonzalez NM, et al. Pimozide in autistic children. *Psychopharmacol Bull* 1993;28:187–191). Because of its long half-life (50 hours), pimozide can be given less often than once daily. It is nonsedating, lacks anticholinergic effects, and is less likely to cause weight gain than phenothiazine or thioxanthene neuroleptics. Pimozide has a relatively low potential to evoke extrapyramidal reactions. Chronic use may be associated with tardive dyskinesia, but risk is low for short-term, low-dose therapy. Because of its calcium channel–blocking properties, pimozide may cause bradycardia. In dosages greater than 16 mg/day, it can cause cardiac conduction delays, prolonging the QT interval of the electrocardiogram (ECG). The manufacturer recommends limiting dosage to 10 mg/day given in the morning, particularly in patients with cardiac disease. A baseline ECG should be done at the initiation of pimozide therapy and during periods of dose adjustment. Pregnancy risk category C.

pimozide + antiarrhythmic Co-administration may have an additive effect in prolonging the QT interval.

pimozide + carbamazepine Co-administration may enhance the central nervous system depressant effects of carbamazepine (CBZ), lower seizure threshold, and decrease the anticonvulsant effects of CBZ. Dosage adjustments may be necessary to control seizures. In some patients, anticholinergic effects may be potentiated, leading to confusion and delirium.

pimozide + clomipramine Pimozide (1 mg given daily increased to 2 mg twice a day) may augment therapeutic response to clomipramine (CMI) in trichotillomania partially responsive or refractory to CMI alone (Stein DJ, Hollander E. Low-dose pimozide augmentation of serotonin reuptake blockers in the treatment of trichotillomania. *J Clin Psychiatry* 1992;53:123–126). See **trichotillomania.**

pimozide + fluoxetine Pimozide (1–4 mg/day) may augment therapeutic response in patients with trichotillomania refractory or partially responsive to fluoxetine (FLX) (Stein DJ, Hollander E. Low-dose pimozide augmentation of serotonin reuptake blockers in the treatment of trichotillomania. *J Clin Psychiatry* 1992;53:123–126). Pimozide (5 mg/day) plus FLX (20 mg/day) led to a potentially life-threatening bradycardia in a 77-year-old man (Ahmed I, Dagincourt PG, Miller LG, Shader RI. Possible interaction between fluoxetine and pimozide causing sinus bradycardia. *Can J Psychiatry* 1993;38:62–63). Co-administration may worsen extrapyramidal symptoms (Bouchard RH, Pourcher E, Vincent P. Fluoxetine and extrapyramidal side effects. *Am J Psychiatry* 1989;146:1352–1353). A patient receiving pimozide (6 mg) experienced marked mental status changes 4 days after FLX dosage was increased to 40 mg/day. Sensorium cleared completely within a week after pimozide was discontinued (Hansen-Grant S, Silk KR, Guthrie S. Fluoxetine-pimozide interaction. *Am J Psychiatry* 1993;150:1751–1752).

pimozide + fluvoxamine   Co-administration may be effective in the treatment of obsessive-compulsive symptoms with concurrent Tourette's syndrome (McDougle CJ, Goodman WK, Price LH, et al. Neuroleptic addition in fluvoxamine-refractory obsessive compulsive disorder: an open case series. *Am J Psychiatry* 1990;147:552–554; Delgado PL, Goodman WK, Price LH, et al. Fluvoxamine/pimozide treatment of concurrent Tourette's and obsessive-compulsive disorder. *Br J Psychiatry* 1990; 157:762–765).

pimozide + lithium   No interaction or additional benefit from adding lithium to pimozide has been demonstrated in clinical trials (Johnstone EC, Crow TJ, Frith CD, et al. The Northwick Park "functional" psychosis study: diagnosis and treatment response. *Lancet* 1988;2:119–125; Braden W, Fink EB, Qualls CB, et al. Lithium and chlorpromazine in psychotic inpatients. *Psychiatry Res* 1982;7:69–81).

pimozide + maprotiline   Co-administration may increase the incidence of cardiac arrhythmias and conduction defects.

pimozide + phenothiazine   Because both drugs prolong the QT interval, an additive effect may occur with co-administration.

pimozide + tricyclic antidepressant   Co-administration may result in additive prolongation of the QT interval.

pinazepam   Benzodiazepine currently available only in Italy.

pindolol   (Visken) Nonselective, lipid-soluble beta blocker with intrinsic sympathomimetic activity. In some patients with organic brain syndrome, it has reduced aggressive outbursts and assaultive episodes. It also decreases uncommunicativeness and hostility. It may benefit some patients with neuroleptic-induced akathisia (Adler LA, Reiter S, Angrist B, Rotrosen J. Pindolol and propranolol in neuroleptic-induced akathisia. *Am J Psychiatry* 1987;144:1241–1242).

pindolol + haloperidol   No significant interactions are reported (Greendyke RM, Gulya A. Effect of pindolol administration on serum levels of thioridazine, haloperidol, phenytoin and phenobarbital. *J Clin Psychiatry* 1988;49: 105–107).

pindolol + phenobarbital   Co-administration increases phenobarbital serum level (Greendyke RM, Gulya A. Effect of pindolol administration on serum levels of thioridazine, haloperidol, phenytoin and phenobarbital. *J Clin Psychiatry* 1988;49:105–107).

pindolol + phenytoin   In phenytoin (PHT)-treated patients, addition of pindolol produces no significant interactions. However, in a patient receiving haloperidol, PHT, and phenobarbital, addition of pindolol significantly increased PHT plasma level (up to 35–41%) (Greendyke RM, Gulya A.. Effect of pindolol administration on serum levels of thioridazine, haloperidol, phenytoin and phenobarbital. *J Clin Psychiatry* 1988;49:105–107).

pindolol + thioridazine   Co-administration may produce a dose-related increase in mean serum levels of thioridazine and its metabolites and an increase in serum pindolol levels. The interaction may be advantageous in some circumstances, whereas in others it could result in unacceptable elevation of serum thioridazine levels (Greendyke RM, Kanter DR. Plasma propranolol levels and their effects on plasma thioridazine and haloperidol concentrations. *J Clin Psychopharmacol* 1987;7:178–182).

"pineapple"   Street name for combination of heroin and methylphenidate.

"pink"   Street name for secobarbital.

"pink and gray"   Street name for propoxyphene hydrochloride.

"pink lady"   Street name for secobarbital.

"pink puffer"   Patient with chronic obstructive pulmonary disease who does not experience decreased oxygenation during sleep. See **"blue bloater."**

"pink wedge"   Street name for lysergic acid diethylamide (LSD).

pipamperone   (Dipiperon; Piperonil) Atypical neuroleptic that only rarely causes extrapyramidal symptoms. It has been found to be a good sleep inducer capable of regulating sleep and wakefulness rhythms that tend to be disturbed in a wide variety of psychiatric disorders. It is under investigation in Europe and elsewhere.

Pipanol   See **trihexyphenidyl.**

piperazine phenothiazine   See **phenothiazine, piperazine.**

piperidinedione   Any of a group sedative/hypnotics (e.g., chloral hydrate) biotransformed to more water-soluble compounds by hepatic enzymes.

piperidine phenothiazine   See **phenothiazine, piperidine.**

Piperonil   See **pipamperone.**

Piportil   See **pipotiazine.**

Piportil Depot   See **pipotiazine palmitate.**

Piportil L4   See **pipotiazine palmitate.**

pipotiazine   (Lonseron; Piportil) Piperidine phenothiazine neuroleptic similar in many respects to other piperidines (e.g., thioridazine). Not available in the United States. See **phenothiazine, piperidine.**

pipotiazine palmitate   (Piportil Depot; Piportil L4) Esterified depot formulation of the piperidine phenothiazine neuroleptic pipotiazine. It is administered in a sesame oil solution and released slowly from the injection site. Duration of action is about 4 weeks. Usual dosage range is 25–200 mg/month, although some patients may need up to 600 mg/month. Clinical indications and side effects are similar to those of other depot neuroleptics, except that pipotiazine palmitate causes a lower incidence of extrapyramidal reactions, which appear to be dose-related; dosage alterations (increases or decreases) may affect both incidence and severity. Not available in the United States.

PIP syndrome   (psychosis, intermittent hyponatremia, and polydipsia). See **polydipsia.**

piquindone   Pyroloisquinolone, atypical neuroleptic and selective dopamine D_2 receptor antagonist. It has a more selective action on the mesolimbic systems than typical neuroleptics, which act more generally on both the mesolimbic and the nigrostriatal pathways. Comparison trials with haloperidol indicate that piquindone is an effective antipsychotic with a low potential to evoke some side effects, but not a significantly lower incidence of extrapyramidal reactions. In both open and double-blind, placebo-controlled trials, it has been shown to effectively ameliorate the symptoms of Tourette's syndrome without evoking extrapyramidal reactions (Cohen J, Van Putten T, Marder S, et al. Treatment of the symptoms of schizophrenia with piquindone: a new atypical neuroleptic. *Psychopharmacol Bull* 1987;23:514–518).

piracetam   (Nootrop; Nootropil; Normabrain) Prototype nootropic drug used to enhance memory and cognitive function. Although well tolerated, its beneficial effects in Alzheimer's disease have been equivocal (Croisile B, Trillet M. Fondarai J, et al. Long-term and high-dose piracetam treatment of Alzheimer's disease. *Neurology* 1993;43:301–305). It may be

safe and effective for the treatment of heroin withdrawal. Marketed in Europe; not available in the United States.

piribedil   Piperazine derivative that is predominantly a dopamine agonist with little effect on the noradrenergic or serotonergic system. At low doses, it stimulates the presynaptic autoreceptors, leading to functional dopaminergic antagonism; at higher doses, it directly stimulates the postsynaptic receptors and acts as a functional dopamine agonist. In low doses, it was effective in two cases of acute mania. At higher doses, it has been found to exert an antidepressant effect (Post RM, Gerner RH, Carman JS, et al. Effects of a dopamine agonist piribedil in depressed patients. *Arch Gen Psychiatry* 1978;35:609–615; Mouret J, Lomonie P, Minuit MP. Polygraphic, clinical and therapeutic markers of dopamine dependent depressions. *Comptes Rendus De L Academie Des Sciences* 1987;305:301–306).

piribedil + selegiline   Co-administration may cause significant psychic effects (Vermersch P. Tolerability of long-term selegiline therapy in Parkinson's disease. *Therapie* 1992;47:75–78).

piroheptine + zotepine   See **zotepine + piroheptine.**

piroxicam   (Feldene) Nonsteroidal anti-inflammatory agent (NSAID) with a half-life of 48 hours. It is the only NSAID available for once-daily dosing. It may cause esophageal lesions.

piroxicam + lithium   See **lithium + piroxicam.**

"Pisa" syndrome   See **pleurothotonus.**

"pitillo"   Street name for coca paste.

pituitary gland   Small structure that rests in the sella turcica and is attached by the pituitary stalk to the ventral surface of the diencephalon. It is divided into the anterior pituitary or adenohypophysis, the posterior pituitary or neurohypophysis, and the intermediate lobe or zone. Also called "hypophysis."

pituitary, anterior   Portion of the pituitary gland that synthesizes and releases protein hormones (adrenocorticotropic hormone, beta-endorphin, follicle-stimulating hormone, growth hormone, luteinizing hormone, prolactin, and thyroid-stimulating hormone). These hormones and the endorphins are secreted in a pulsatile manner in response to several influences (e.g., sleep-wake cycles, nonrapid eye movement (NREM)/REM cycles, and circadian rhythm processes). Some of these hormones may directly affect neuroendocrine tissues or stimulate release of hormones from endocrine glands elsewhere in the body.

pituitary, posterior   Portion of the pituitary gland that secretes two hormones: vasopressin (antidiuretic hormone) and oxytocin.

PK Mez   See **amantadine.**

placebo   Any treatment that has no specific effects on the condition being treated. It is often a substance or preparation without pharmacological activity, but identical in appearance to an active drug, given as though it were pharmacologically active. Its major use is in controlled studies to determine the efficacy of medicinal preparations; any beneficial or deleterious effects of the placebo may be ascribed to psychological factors. A placebo also is used in narcotic withdrawal in a medical setting (the patient is told that some doses will be methadone and others placebo to avoid cuing withdrawal symptoms). Anything capable of affecting a patient's unconscious attitudes and expectations is capable of functioning as a placebo. Although a placebo may have no effect on organic disease, it may have an effect on the patient's subjective experience of disease (Brody H. The lie that heals: the effects of giving a placebo. *Ann Intern Med* 1982;97:112–118). See **placebo effect.**

placebo effect   Phenomenon in which a clinically significant response occurs following administration of a therapeutically inert substance. Responses include both therapeutic and side effects and are not limited to subjective reports; physiological functions may be objectively influenced. Placebo effects also may include changes stemming from the nonspecific aspects of a treatment procedure (e.g., treatment setting, caregiver, patient expectations).

placebo, impure   1. Drug of dubious efficacy. 2. Inert preparation that produces the same side effects as the active drug under study.

placebo nonreactor   Subject who does not respond therapeutically to a placebo. Placebo nonreactors may be selected for a therapeutic trial to make the comparison with an active drug more sensitive.

Placidyl   See **ethchlorvynol.**

plantar reflex   Movement of the toes when the skin on the outer aspect of the sole of the foot is stroked. In normal adults, the toes curl under; when brain damage has caused spasticity, the toes spread outward and the big toe moves upward.

plasma   Blood from which the cells have been extracted without the blood's being permitted to clot.

plasma binding   Noncovalent binding of drugs to plasma proteins, which may be a sizable fraction of drug in plasma. The bound moiety of a drug is functionally inert and unavailable for binding to sites of drug action or disposition. Generally, only the free (nonbound) portion of the drug can diffuse to pharmacologically active sites to interact with receptors.

Free drug concentration correlates more closely with drug effect than does total serum concentration. If more than 90% of a drug exists in bound form in the plasma, it is considered highly protein-bound. Psychotropic drugs that are highly protein-bound include clomipramine, diazepam, fluoxetine, haloperidol, and sertraline. The protein-bound fraction of a drug is inactive and cannot be metabolized or excreted, whereas the unbound fraction is pharmacologically active. The degree of binding is influenced by such variables as hydrogen ion concentration and the presence of drugs or endogenous compounds that compete for binding sites. Misinterpretation of total drug concentrations when binding protein concentrations are changed may lead to major errors in subsequent dose adjustment. The major drug-binding proteins are albumin and alpha$_1$-acid glycoprotein.

plasma concentration   (Cp) Bound, unbound, or total drug in plasma, usually at steady state, expressed in mass or molar units per unit of volume. Cp may serve as a guide in the selection of dosage regimen. It also helps to determine the "therapeutic range" for a drug. If the measured Cp is not within this range, dosage adjustment is warranted. When the Cp is higher than the upper limit of the therapeutic range, the drug level may be toxic. When it is lower, the drug may be at a subtherapeutic level. The therapeutic range consists of a peak or maximum level of concentration in the plasma and a trough or minimal level of concentration in the plasma. Cp determination is most useful in monitoring drugs that have a narrow range between beneficial and toxic concentrations (e.g., lithium); a close correlation between plasma concentration and beneficial effects (e.g., some tricyclic antidepressants); a close correlation between plasma concentration and adverse effects; or wide intersubject variability requiring dosage titrations to achieve therapeutic concentrations. It is often recommended that plasma levels be taken 10–14 hours after the last oral dose of the drug.

plasma concentration measurement   All drugs do not produce the same plasma concentration in all patients because of individual variation in absorption, distribution, and excretion; drug formulation; genetic variations; smoking; disease (especially renal or hepatic) effects; and drug interactions. Measurement of a drug's plasma concentration can be useful when there is difficulty in interpreting clinical evidence of therapeutic or toxic effects; a good relation between the plasma concentration of a drug and its therapeutic or toxic effects; a low toxic-to-therapeutic ratio; or no metabolism to active metabolites (Aronson JK, Hardman M. ABC of monitoring drug therapy. Measuring plasma drug concentrations. *Br Med J* 1992;305:1078–1080).

plasma homovanillic acid   See **homovanillic acid.**

plasmapheresis   Procedure to remove toxic elements from the blood by depleting the body's own plasma without depleting its cells. Whole blood is removed from the body and separated of its cellular elements by centrifugation; elements are then reinfused suspended in saline or some other plasma substitute. Also called "therapeutic plasma exchange (TPE)."

plasma protein binding   Many drugs are bound to serum albumin in the circulating blood. The extent of binding influences the drug's distribution, pharmacology, and pharmacokinetics. Only the drug fraction not bound to albumin in the bloodstream can leave the circulation, distribute in the body, and reach the site of action. See **plasma binding.**

plasmid   Extrachromosomal bacterial DNA molecule commonly used in recombinant DNA research. Many different recombinant plasmids have been engineered to contain various features useful in performing particular types of cloning experiments.

platelet   Small blood constituents formed from amine precursor, uptake, and decarboxylation (APUD) cells that are involved in blood clotting.

platelet monoamine oxidase (MAO) activity   Factor that has been related to several psychiatric and personality disorders. Low MAO activity has been suggested as a biological marker of increased vulnerability to psychopathology. Reduced activity has been reported in schizophrenia, bipolar depressive disorder, post-traumatic stress disorder, and borderline personality. Increased activity has been reported in unipolar depressive disorder.

plegia   Total weakness. Diplegia involves two limbs, hemiplegia involves one side of the body or both arms and legs, paraplegia involves both legs, and quadriplegia is total paralysis of the body from the neck down. Spastic diplegia involves motor weakness with increased muscle tone predominantly in the legs. It is the most common manifestation of cerebral palsy.

pleiotropy   Multiple, seemingly unrelated, phenotypic effects caused by one gene.

pleurothotonus   Neuroleptic-induced chronic dystonic syndrome characterized by slight rotation and tonic flexion of the trunk to one side without other concomitant dystonic symptoms. It may present with acute, subacute, or insidious tardive onset. Many clinicians considered it to be a manifestation of tardive dystonia, rather than a separate entity. It occurs in patients who have received neuroleptics for prolonged periods. It has been reported rarely in adolescents; clinical presentation is similar to that in adults, but it should not be misinterpreted as a functional disorder. It occurs in about 8% of the psychogeriatric population treated with neuroleptics. The most effective treatment is reduction or discontinuation of neuroleptics, which usually results in symptom disappearance within 24 hours (Yassa R. The Pisa syndrome: a report of two cases. *Br J Psychiatry* 1985;146:93–95). Also called "Pisa syndrome." See **dystonia, axial.**

PLM arousal index   Number of sleep-related periodic leg movements (PLMs) per hour of sleep associated with an electroencephalographic arousal.

PLM index   Number of periodic leg movements (PLMs) per hour of total sleep time. It is sometimes expressed as the number of movements per hour of non–rapid eye movement (NREM) sleep, because the movements are usually inhibited during REM sleep.

PLM percentage   Percentage of total sleep time in which recurrent episodes of periodic leg movements (PLMs) occur.

PMA   Hallucinogenic designer drug that is an analog of methamphetamine.

PMS Thioridazine   See **thioridazine.**

pneumoencephalogram   Radiograph of the skull after replacement of cerebrospinal fluid by air during a lumbar puncture. It is seldom done today.

"pocket rocket"   Street name for a marijuana cigarette.

point mutation   Mutation of a single gene due to addition, loss replacement, or change of sequence in one or more base pairs of the deoxyribonucleic acid (DNA) of that gene.

point prevalence   Proportion of the population in which a disorder is being studied at a given time. Also called "prevalence rate."

point prevalence study   See **cross-sectional design.**

polydipsia   Syndrome with serious and potentially life-threatening consequences (congestive heart failure, seizures, coma, and death) in which large amounts of water are consumed for obscure reasons unrelated to normal thirst or homeostatic needs. Whether it is a form of compulsive behavior is currently disputed; it may be due to a hippocampal ictal focus (Crapanzano KA, Casanova MF, Toro VE, Gallagher B. Drinking behavior as a result of a right hippocampal ictal focus. *Biol Psychiatry* 1994;34:889–892). It is estimated that 7% of psychiatric patients in public mental health facilities have polydipsia; of these, 75% have schizophrenia. A subgroup of patients develops water intoxication with hyponatremia. Polydipsia occurred before the use of medications and is seen in patients who are not taking medications. Patients usually come to medical attention when water seeking and water drinking are noted by the patient or observers, hyponatremia or hyposthenuria is found incidentally in laboratory testing, or medical intervention is required for symptoms of overt water intoxication. A wide range of symptoms is seen, including headache, blurred vision, anorexia, nausea, vomiting and diarrhea, muscle cramps, restlessness, confusion, exacerbation of psychosis, convulsions, coma, and death. Also called "primary polydipsia"; "psychosis-intermittent hyponatremia-polydipsia (PIP) syndrome." See **polydipsia, dipsogenic; polydipsia, psychogenic; water intoxication.**

polydipsia, dipsogenic   Excessive water consumption in medical patients, most of whom do not have psychiatric symptoms or signs of water intoxication. The pathophysiology of the disorder is unknown, although it is known to occur in association with damage to the hypothalamus. It is a rare disorder of unknown incidence. Some cases may share the pathophysiology of psychogenic polydipsia: both conditions may be related to disturbances in angiotensin II function (Verghese C, De Leon J, Simpson GM. Neuroendocrine factors influencing polydipsia in psychiatric patients: an hypothesis. *Neuropsychopharmacology* 1993;9:157–166). See **polydipsia, psychogenic.**

polydipsia, psychogenic   Primary increase in water drinking to 5 L and more daily, producing dilution of extracellular fluid, inhibition of vasopressin secretion, and a water diuresis. It may occur in patients with schizophrenia, primary affective disorder, and alcoholism. Generally, hemodilution does not occur in psychogenic polydipsia. It is important to differentiate it from both neurogenic and nephrogenic diabetes insipidus. Other known causes of polydipsia (e.g., diabetes mellitus, chronic renal failure) also should be excluded. Also called "compulsive water drinking"; "hysterical polydipsia"; "potomania."

polydrug abuse   Concomitant use of two or more psychoactive substances in quantities and with frequencies that cause the individual significant physiological, psychological, or sociological distress or impairment.

polygene   Group of genes that act together to produce quantitative variations of a particular character.

polygenic   Relating to a genetic characteristic or disease controlled by gene interaction at more than one locus.

polygenic disorder   Genetic disorder resulting from the combined action of alleles of more than one gene (e.g., heart disease, diabetes, some cancers). Although such disorders are inherited, they depend on the simultaneous presence of several alleles; thus, the hereditary patterns are usually more complex than those of single-gene disorders.

polygenic inheritance   Inheritance by many genes at different loci, with small additive effects.

polygenic trait   Blended effect of many genes.

polymerase chain reaction   (PCR) Laboratory technique that uses enzymes and highly specific primers to generate multiple copies of the original viral nucleic acid, increasing its numbers to levels that can be detected. PCR permits test-tube amplification of a target sequence of DNA between two synthesized priming oligonucleotides. There is sufficient DNA in a single cell to serve as the template for specific million-fold amplification of the target region. PCR has been widely used for the diagnosis of common recessive alleles such as sickle hemoglobinopathy and other disorders of genetic origin. It is also used to provide alternative confirmation of, or to screen selected very-high-risk groups for, human immunodeficiency virus (HIV) infection.

polymorphism   1. Occurrence together, in a population, of two or more gene structures. In humans, the nucleotide sequence of any given gene varies slightly from family to family. This variability (polymorphism) is an inherited trait (e.g., the ABO blood groups). Polymorphism usually has no biological consequence, but it occasionally can drastically alter the function of a necessary protein and thus, the organism (e.g., polymorphism present in hemoglobins that result in sickle cell anemia). 2. Occurrence of different forms, stages, or color types in individual organisms or in organisms of the same species. See **restriction fragment length polymorphism.**

polypeptide   Protein-like molecule formed by the joining together of three or more amino acids. A protein molecule may be composed of a single polypeptide chain, or of two or more identical or different polypeptides. Also called "protein chain."

polypharmacy   Use of multiple medications, effects of which may interact, clouding differentiation of desirable and side effects and putting the patient at risk for adverse reactions. In psychiatry, polypharmacy is the use of two or more drugs with similar properties to treat a single condition (e.g., use of several phenothiazine drugs to treat schizophrenia). Treatment with more than one drug is usually less effective, because drug interactions impair effectiveness and side effects may accumulate. This type of polypharmacy is usually not justified. It is more acceptable to coprescribe two or more drugs when target actions may overlap while side effects do not (e.g., use of a tricyclic plus a monoamine oxidase inhibitor for treatment-resistant depression, or lithium plus an antipsychotic or antidepressant). Also called "polytherapy."

polyploid Any multiple of the basic haploid chromosome number, other than the diploid number.

polysome immunoprecipitation Polysomes (polyribosomes) are engaged in protein synthesis; since the nascent polypeptide chain is still attached to them, they can be precipitated with a specific antiserum.

polysomnogram (PSG) Recorded results of polysomnography. It allows determination and measurement of physiological changes that occur during sleep stages. It also allows determination of sleep cycles and continuous, simultaneous recording of physiological variables during sleep (i.e., electroencephalography, electro-oculography, and electromyography, which are the three basic stage scoring parameters; electrocardiography; respiratory airflow; respiratory movements; lower limb movements; and other electrophysiological variables).

polysomnograph Biomedical instrument for the measurement of physiological parameters of sleep. Also called "hypnopolygraph."

polysomnography Synchronized recordings of electrical activity in the brain, muscles, and eyes, as well as other physiological measures during sleep. Measures include electro-oculogram, electroencephalogram, electromyogram, electrocardiogram, oxygen saturation, and nasal-oral thermocoupled air flow. The tests may help diagnosis of a variety of conditions including insomnia, nocturnal myoclonus, sleep apnea, enuresis, somnambulism, seizure disorders, impotence, vascular headache, gastroesophageal reflux, and depression. Polysomnographic studies of schizophrenic patients have revealed a number of abnormalities (reduced total sleep time, sleep continuity, and slow-wave sleep; shortened rapid eye movement [REM] latency), but their significance remains unclear. Also called "somnology."

polysomnography/major depression Extensive, all-night polysomnography studies have shown that sleep in major depression is shallow and fragmented because of a shift toward greater wakefulness, more awakenings, and lighter sleep (stage 1), and away from the deeper stages of sleep (stages 3 and 4). In addition, the onset of the first period of rapid eye movement (REM) sleep is shifted to an earlier point in the sleep cycle, and eye-movement activity in REM sleep is of greater density (Hudson JI, Lipinski JF, Keck PE Jr, et al. Polysomnographic characteristics of young manic patients. Comparison with unipolar depressed patients and normal control subjects. *Arch Gen Psychiatry* 1992;49:378–383). See **polysomnography/mania.**

polysomnography/mania Manic and depressed patients display nearly identical profiles of polysomnographic abnormalities, including disturbed sleep continuity, increased percentage of stage 1 sleep, shortened rapid eye movement (REM) latency, and increased REM density. These results are consistent with the possibility that the sleep disturbance in mania and major depression is caused by the same mechanism (Hudson JI, Lipinski JF, Keck PE Jr, et al. Polysomnographic characteristics of young manic patients. Comparison with unipolar depressed patients and normal control subjects. *Arch Gen Psychiatry* 1992;49:378–383). See **polysomnography/major depression.**

polysubstance dependence Disorder characterized by dependence on multiple categories of illicit psychoactive substances.

polytherapy See **polypharmacy.**

Ponderal See **fenfluramine.**

Ponderax See **fenfluramine.**

Pondimin See **fenfluramine.**

pons Component of the brain stem, which also is composed of the mesencephalon and the medulla oblongata. The brain stem plays a role in such basic functions as respiration, cardiovascular activity, sleep, and consciousness. It is also the site of the neuronal cell bodies for the ascending biogenic amine (dopamine, noradrenaline, serotonin) pathways (the medial forebrain bundle) to higher brain areas.

Ponstel See **mefenamic acid.**

ponto-geniculo-occipital wave (PGO) Relatively specific sign of rapid eye movement (REM) sleep. PGO waves are generated by PGO burst cells located within the region of the cholinergic/perobrachial pontine tegmentum. Continuous PGO wave activity independent of REM has been described following microinjection of the cholinergic agonist carbachol into this region. A significant dose-dependent suppression of PGO activity during eltoprazine administration supports the hypothesis that the cholinergic/PGO burst cell network is particularly sensitive to serotonergic inhibitory control (Quattrochi JJ, Mamelak AN, Binder D, et al. Dose-related suppression of REM sleep and PGO waves by the serotonin-1 agonist eltoprazine. *Neuropsychopharmacology* 1993;8:7–13).

pooled standard deviation   Method used to test when the standard deviation in two groups is equal.

poor metabolizer   See **acetylator, slow.**

"popper"   Street name for amyl nitrite used as a sexual stimulant. Amyl nitrite comes in glass ampules that make a popping sound when broken open.

"poppy"   Street name for opium.

"poppy straw"   Home-made injectable preparation made from harvested poppies that is being abused in many parts of the former Soviet Union and Poland (Chopkin K. Too many advisors, not enough aid. *Br Med J* 1992;304:1429–1432). There is concern that abuse of "poppy straw" will spread internationally.

population   Statistical term that refers to the universe of items being sampled.

population attributable risk   See **risk, population attributable.**

population pharmacokinetics   See **pharmacokinetics, population.**

population proportional attributable risk   See **risk, population proportional attributable.**

porphyria, acute intermittent   (AIP) Autosomal dominant, heritable metabolic disorder, first reported by Stokvis (1889), characterized by excessive production of porphyrins or related compounds that are excreted in the urine and feces. Freshly voided urine is clear, but on standing it turns reddish or dark. Peak age of onset is 20–30, although AIP may manifest throughout a lifetime. It occurs in attacks that are heralded by restlessness and irritability and then develop rapidly. Symptom expression depends on life style, nutrition, and alcohol and drug use. Symptoms include abdominal pain and gastrointestinal complaints that often result in unnecessary surgery; tachycardia and hypertension; visual impairment, bilateral ptosis, dilation of one pupil, and nystagmus; convulsions; and psychosis often necessitating psychiatric hospitalization. Attacks usually resolve in days or weeks; the interval between initial symptoms and correct diagnosis may range from several months to years. Attacks may be caused by low-carbohydrate and low-protein diets, fasting, smoking, and certain drugs (e.g., barbiturates, anticonvulsants, chlordiazepoxide, meprobamate, oral contraceptives, steroids, glutethimide).

Porsolt test   Laboratory procedure used preclinically to screen for antidepressant activity. Rats are placed in a water tank in which they must swim to stay afloat. They swim initially, but then give up and stop swimming. When repeatedly exposed to the test condition, rats cease swimming after shorter and shorter intervals. Antidepressants antagonize the progressive shortening of these intervals. Also called "behavior despair test."

positional cloning   See **cloning, positional.**

positive eugenics   See **eugenics, positive.**

positive predictive power   See **predictive power, positive.**

positive predictive value   See **predictive value, positive.**

positive symptoms   Florid, productive symptoms of schizophrenia that prevail in the acute stage and may signify an excessive transmission of dopamine in the brain. Prototypes include agitation, delusions, hallucinations, positive formal thought disorder manifested by incoherence, derailment, tangentiality, illogicality, conceptual disorganization, suspiciousness, unusual thought content, and disorganized or bizarre behavior. The most important clinical effect of the major antipsychotic drugs is their ability to eliminate or significantly diminish positive symptoms, which correlates highly with their ability to block dopamine D_2 receptors (Kay SR. *Positive and Negative Syndromes in Schizophrenia.* New York: Brunner/Mazel Publishers, 1991; Andreasen N, Olsen S. Negative versus positive schizophrenia: definition and validation. *Arch Gen Psychiatry* 1982;39:789–794).

positron   Positively charged particle (beta$^+$) emitted by a radionucleotide that quickly interacts with a neighboring electron and emits to 511-KeV photons 180 apart.

positron emission tomography   (PET) Imaging technique for producing cross-sectional images in which the positrons emitted from a patient (safely metabolized radioactive positron-emitting agents have been developed) are measured from multiple directions around the patient. A computer then determines the amount of radioactivity originating from each point within the patient. These values are then displayed as a gray scale "anatomical" image. Tissue contrast (ability to tell one tissue from another and whether it is normal or abnormal) is therefore due to a difference in the amount of radioactivity emitted by each tissue. Since PET agents are metabolized by the body, the images created represent a "functional" or "metabolic map." Fluorodeoxyglucose (FDG) and H_2O^{15} are the most common agents used for cerebral applications. Measurement of brain metabolism with the use of PET and FDG has been shown to be a sensitive technique to monitor regional response of the brain to acute challenge with pharmacological agents (Fowler JS, Wolf AP, Volkow ND. New directions in positron emission tomography, part II. *In*

Allen RC. Orland, FL [eds], *Annual Reports in Medicinal Chemistry*, vol 24. San Diego: Academic Press, 1990).

positron emission tomography (PET)/schizophrenia Some, but not all, PET studies have found hypofrontality of brain glucose metabolic rate in patients with schizophrenia. Other studies have found abnormalities in temporal cortical metabolism, left-right asymmetry of metabolism, and basal ganglia metabolism (Siegel BV, Buchsbaum MS, Bunney WE Jr, et al. Cortical-striatal-thalamic circuits and brain glucose metabolic activity in 70 unmedicated male schizophrenic patients. *Am J Psychiatry* 1993;150:1325–1336).

positron scanner Imaging device designed to measure the location and density of different gamma rays emitted by positron emission tomography (PET) ligands.

postconcussional syndrome Emergence and variable persistence of a cluster of symptoms following mild or minor head injury. The most common symptoms are headache, fatigue, poor concentration, and dizziness. Even after a relatively minor concussion, most patients have one or more of these symptoms in the weeks following injury. The frequency of psychiatric cases among this group was 10 times that for the control subjects and for the local community (Cairns E, Wilson R, McClelland R, et al. Improving the validity of the GHQ30 by rescoring for chronicity: a failure to replicate. *J Clin Psychol* 1990;45:793–798; Fenton G, McClelland R, Montgomery A, et al. The postconcussional syndrome: social antecedents and psychological sequelae. *Br J Psychiatry* 1993;162:493–497).

postencephalitic parkinsonism See **parkinsonism, postencephalitic.**

posterior pituitary See **pituitary, posterior.**

post hoc comparison Method for comparing means following analysis of variance. It is used to test hypotheses derived *after* an experiment is completed.

post hoc testing See **Scheffé's procedure.**

postictal Relating to the period immediately following a stroke or seizure. Duration is usually brief (seconds to minutes), but may be hours or a few days. Behavioral and/or cognitive symptoms may or may not occur. The postictal period is followed by an interictal period. See **interictal; postictal phenomena.**

postictal phenomena Physical signs and symptoms, as well as confusion, disorientation, agitation, and abnormal behavior, that occur most commonly in patients with major motor and complex partial seizures. Some patients may present with depressed mood or anxiety, or (rarely) hallucinations and paranoid ideas

that may last for a few hours but usually no longer than 2 days.

postictal psychosis See **psychosis, postictal.**

postmarketing surveillance Study of drug use and drug effects, under normal prescribing conditions, after marketing. The term is sometimes used synonymously with *pharmacoepidemiology*, which can be relevant to premarketing studies as well. Postmarketing surveillance is sometimes mistakenly thought to apply only to studies conducted after drug marketing that systematically screen for adverse drug effects. Postmarketing studies permit the study of delayed drug effects, such as tardive dyskinesia.

postmarketing surveillance study (PMS) Phase IV, cohort study in the immediate postmarketing period set up to monitor the safety and efficacy of a drug or device in common clinical practice. Such studies are commonly funded by and carried out by pharmaceutical companies. They involve a wider range of clinicians, medical centers, and countries than premarketing studies do. They give individual physicians the opportunity to compare the new drug with their own standard therapies. Careful postmarketing surveillance is the most feasible method for detecting infrequent adverse events associated with a new drug.

postmortem pharmacokinetics/tricyclic antidepressant See **pharmacokinetics, postmortem/tricyclic antidepressant.**

postoperative delirium See **delirium, postoperative.**

postpartum blues Brief mood disturbance that may occur in the first few (7–10) days after childbirth. Manifestations include mood lability, crying, anxiety, insomnia, poor appetite, irritability, and dysphoria, but there is disagreement as to whether depressed mood is characteristic. The patient also may complain about confusion and forgetfulness, but there is no evidence of cognitive impairment. The condition is brief (2–14 days) and benign; prevalence may range from 26–85% of women who have delivered recently. Symptoms resolve spontaneously within a few days and require no intervention, except for the reassurance that the experience is normal. There is little agreement on precise definition. One view is that postpartum blues is not specific to childbirth, but is a general "end reaction" that can occur after any physical stressor. Another view is that symptoms are characteristic in timing and intensity and thus differ from symptoms after other types of stressful events. Related to this view is the suggestion that postpartum blues may be induced by particular endocrine changes in the early puerperium. Studies indicate that there is a very different pattern of "blues" symptoms after childbirth than after surgery. The diagnosis is not recognized by major diagnostic systems currently in use (DSM-IV or the International Classification of Diseases). Predictors of the postpartum blues are personal and family history of depression, social adjustment, stressful life events, and levels of free and total estriol (O'Hara MW, Schlechte JA, Lewis DA, Wright EJ. Prospective study of postpartum blues. Biologic and psychosocial factors. *Arch Gen Psychiatry* 1991;48:801–806). Also called "maternity blues." See **depression, postpartum; psychosis, postpartum.**

postpartum depression See **depression, postpartum.**

postpartum psychosis See **psychosis, postpartum.**

poststroke depression See **depression, poststroke.**

poststroke pathological crying Distressing condition in which crying episodes occur in response to minor stimuli without associated mood changes. For the patient, the crying is often embarrassing and socially disabling, and may interfere with rehabilitation. Reassurance of the patient and caregivers is vital; they need to know that the reaction is a result of stroke and that the intensity of the outbursts tends to diminish with time. Pharmacological treatments reported to be effective include amitriptyline, nortriptyline, fluoxetine, and citalopram (Schiffer RB, Herndon RM, Rudick RA. Treatment of pathologic laughing and weeping with amitriptyline. *N Engl J Med* 1985;312:1480–1482; Robinson RG, Parikh RM, Lipsey JR, et al. Pathological laughing and crying following stroke: validation of a measurement scale—a double-blind treatment study. *Am J Psychiatry* 1993;150:286–293; Seliger RB, Hornstein A, Flax J, et al. Fluoxetine improves emotional incontinence. *Brain Inj* 1992;6:267–270; Sloan RL, Brown RW, Pentland B. Fluoxetine as a treatment for emotional lability after brain injury. *Brain Inj* 1992;6:315–319; Andersen G, Vestergaard K, Riis JO. Citalopram for post-stroke pathological crying. *Lancet* 1993;342:837–839). Serotonergic neurotransmission appears to play an important part in post-stroke pathological crying. Lack of response to one agent should not deter a trial of another. Patients who have failed to respond to tricyclic antidepressants have shown a prompt and sustained response to fluoxetine (Hanger HC. Emotionalism after stroke. *Lancet* 1993;342:1235–1236).

postsynaptic Relating to a part of the membrane lying adjacent to the nerve terminal that contains the postsynaptic receptors.

postsynaptic sensitivity Sensitivity of postsynaptic receptors to agonists of the particular receptor.

post-test odds In diagnostic testing, the odds that a patient has a given disease or condition after a diagnostic procedure is performed and interpreted.

post-traumatic epilepsy See **epilepsy, post-traumatic.**

post-traumatic stress disorder (PTSD) Anxiety disorder attributable to an unusual experience that would be very stressful for almost anyone (e.g., serious threat to life or physical integrity, involvement of the person or a loved one in a major catastrophe). The patient reexperiences the traumatic event by recollections, dreams, acting or feeling as if the traumatic event were recurring, and intense psychological distress on exposure to events that symbolize or resemble the traumatic event. Other manifestations include persistent avoidance of stimuli associated with the trauma, and persistent symptoms of increased arousal, neither of which were present before the trauma. To qualify for this diagnosis, a minimum of 1 month's duration of these symptoms is required (DSM-IV). This largely environmentally induced disorder has been observed frequently in combat veterans with a history of exposure to severe trauma. PTSD is more common in women than in men. Most drugs that are effective for PTSD are also useful in both major depression and in panic disorder, including tricyclics (specifically amitriptyline, imipramine, desipramine, doxepin); monoamine oxidase inhibitors (particularly phenelzine); benzodiazepines (alprazolam); lithium; carbamazepine; valproate; buspirone; fluoxetine; propanolol; and clonidine (Davidson J. Drug therapy of post-traumatic stress disorder. *Br J Psychiatry* 1992;160:309–314).

post-traumatic tremor See **tremor, post-traumatic.**

postural hypotension See **hypotension, postural.**

postural imbalance Parkinson's disease symptom that is due to impairment of the postural-righting reflexes. It makes many patients prone to falls.

postural instability Diminished response to postural displacements that results in loss of balance. It can be a symptom of both idiopathic and drug-induced parkinsonism.

postural tremor See **tremor, postural.**

postviral fatigue syndrome See **chronic fatigue syndrome**

"pot" Street name for marijuana.

potency Strength of a particular substance. It is the reciprocal of dose and is a means of comparing relative activities of drugs. The term is often used to refer to the milligram dose of a drug needed to produce a given clinical effect.

potentiated anesthesia   See **neuroleptanalgesia.**

potentiation   Special form of synergism that may occur when two drugs are co-administered in which the effect of the active drug is increased.

potentiation, long-term   (LTP) Potentiation of a neuronal response that is assumed to be associated with the encoding process for learning and memory and involving changes that persist for several days. It is believed to involve a receptor in the hippocampus.

potentiator   Drug that potentiates the effect(s) of another drug.

potomania   See **polydipsia, psychogenic.**

poverty of content of speech   Speech that is adequate in amount but conveys little information because of vagueness, empty repetitions, or use of stereotyped or obscure phrases (DSM-IV). The person may speak at some length, but give inadequate information to answer a question. Alternatively, the person may provide enough information to answer the question, but require many words to do so (i.e., the lengthy reply can be summarized in a sentence or two). Poverty of speech content generally does not refer to incoherent speech.

poverty of speech   Restriction in the amount of speech, so that spontaneous speech and replies to questions are brief and unelaborated (DSM IV). When severe, replies may be monosyllabic, and some questions may be unanswered. Poverty of speech occurs frequently in schizophrenia, major depressive episodes, and organic mental disorders (e.g., dementia).

power density   The brain's electrical potential per cycle per second.

practice guidelines   Systematically developed statements of recommendations for patient management to assist practitioner and patient decisions about appropriate health care or specific clinical circumstances (Field MJ, Lohr KN [eds]. *Clinical Practice Guidelines: Directions for a New Program.* Washington, DC: National Academy Press, 1990; Garnick DW, Hendricks AM, Brennan TA. Can practice guidelines reduce the number and costs of malpractice claims? *JAMA* 1991;266:2856–2860).

practolol   Beta$_1$ blocker that has been used in the treatment of anxiety with more effectiveness than placebo.

pramiracetam   (ci-879) Nootropic drug being tested in the treatment of cognitive impairments associated with Alzheimer's disease (Claus JJ, Ludwig C, Mohr E, et al. Nootropic drugs in Alzheimer's disease: symptomatic treatment with pramiracetam. *Neurology* 1991; 41:570–574).

praxis   Performance of an action.

praxis deficit   Symptom of mild Alzheimer's disease manifested by inability to draw a cube and difficulty in conceptualizing and drawing a rectangle or square.

Praxiten   See **oxazepam.**

prazepam   (Centrax; Entrix; Verstran) 1,4 Benzodiazepine that is a diazepam prodrug. Through hepatic first-pass metabolism, it is rapidly and completed transformed by dealkylation to N-desmethyldiazepam, its active metabolite. Neither prazepam nor its two hydroxylated metabolites, 3-hydroxyprazepam and oxazepam, can be detected in plasma in the unconjugated state. Duration of action is long; elimination half-life including metabolites is 2–4 days. Prazepam is relatively sedating. Schedule IV; pregnancy risk category D.

prazepam + alcohol   A single therapeutic dose of prazepam combined with a single low dose of alcohol appears to have a more sedating effect in healthy volunteers than the same dose of prazepam alone. Long-term effects of combined use have not been studied. Available data indicate that alcohol should be avoided during prazepam treatment, particularly when driving or performing dangerous tasks (Girre C, Hirschhorn M, Bertauz L, et al. Comparison of performance of healthy volunteers given prazepam alone or combined with ethanol. Relation to drug plasma concentration. *Int Clin Psychopharmacol* 1991;6:227–238).

prazepam + antacid   Antacids impair prazepam absorption and decrease its effects.

prazepam/breast milk   Prazepam and its metabolites are probably excreted in human milk, but whether in sufficient quantities to adversely affect a neonate is unknown. For more data, consult the manufacturer.

precursor   **1.** Early stage preceding the pathological onset of an illness or disease. **2.** Compound metabolized to a neurotransmitter (e.g., tryptophan is the precursor of 5-hydroxytryptamine). **3.** Prodrug. See **prodrug.**

prediction study   Prospective study to identify behavioral or biological precursors of a disorder in individuals who are at high risk for the disorder by virtue of their relationship to affected individuals. It is a variant of a family risk study.

predictive power, negative   Probability of not having the diagnosis given the absence of symptoms.

predictive power, positive   Probability of having the diagnosis given the presence of symptoms.

predictive value, positive   Likelihood of a positive test result being true (sensitivity is a likelihood of a patient with the disease having a positive test result). Positive predictive value diminishes as the prevalence of the disease in the population decreases.

predictor variable See **variable, independent.**

prednisone + carbamazepine See **carbamazepine + prednisone.**

prednisone + fluoxetine See **fluoxetine + prednisone.**

preferential pedophile See **pedophile, preferential.**

preferred provider organization (PPO) Organizational arrangement between providers and purchasers whereby medical/psychiatric services are purchased from providers at negotiated rates in return for referral to those providers.

prefrontal lobotomy See **lobotomy.**

pregnancy ratings Food and Drug Administration (FDA) pregnancy risk categories are based on the degree to which available information has ruled out risk to the fetus, balanced against the drug's potential benefits to the patient. Ratings range from "A" for drugs that have been tested for teratogenicity under controlled conditions without showing evidence of damage to the fetus, to "D" and "X" for drugs that are definitely teratogenic. The "D" rating is generally reserved for drugs with no safer alternatives. The "X" rating means there is absolutely no reason to risk using the drug in pregnancy.

Pregnancy Risk Category A *Controlled studies show no risk.* Adequate, well-controlled studies in pregnant women have failed to demonstrate risk to the fetus.

Pregnancy Risk Category B *No evidence of risk in humans.* Either animal findings show risk, but human findings do not; or, if no adequate human studies have been done, animal findings are negative.

Pregnancy Risk Category C *Risk cannot be ruled out.* Human studies are lacking, and animal studies are either lacking or positive for fetal risk; however, potential benefits may justify potential risks.

Pregnancy Risk Category D *Positive evidence of risk.* Investigational or postmarketing data show risk to the fetus; however, potential benefits may outweigh potential risks.

Pregnancy Risk Category X *Contraindicated in pregnancy.* Studies in animals or humans, or investigational or postmarketing reports, have shown fetal risk that clearly outweighs any possible benefit to the patient.

Prelu-2 See **phendimetrazine.**

Preludin See **phenmetrazine.**

premarketing clinical trial See **clinical trial, premarketing.**

premature morning awakening See **insomnia, terminal.**

premenstrual syndrome (PMS) Constellation of cyclical, emotional, and behavioral symptoms experienced only during the late luteal phase of the menstrual cycle. PMS does not occur before puberty, during pregnancy, or after menopause. PMS persists after hysterectomy, although it may be reduced or abolished by hysterectomy and oophorectomy. It is also abolished by drugs that suppress ovarian function (e.g., danazol, gonadotrophin releasing hormone analogs). PMS-like symptoms are reproduced in some women by gonadal steroids. In some women a single symptom, such as depression, may predominate, whereas others may have several symptoms such as headaches, depression, irritability, anxiety, mood swings, and bloating. Most women experience some premenstrual symptoms, but only about 20–40% suffer emotional, behavioral, and/or physical symptoms severe enough to cause them to seek help. In 2–6% of affected women, symptoms may be incapacitating. Cause is unclear. A genetic component has been suggested because of an increased incidence of PMS in monozygotic compared to dizygotic twins, although none of the twins studied had been brought up separately. No physiological abnormality of the luteal phase has been consistently demonstrated. The temporal association of typical PMS symptoms with an artificially induced follicular phase suggests that endocrine events during the late luteal phase do not directly generate PMS symptoms. Many features of PMS resemble major depression, and many patients have premenstrual aggravation of depression. PMS diagnosis depends on the timing of symptoms in relation to menstruation. Symptoms typically begin in midcycle and increase in number and severity to maximum intensity the day before, or at the onset of, bleeding. Symptom relief with onset of full menstrual flow is rapid and complete. A symptom-free phase lasting at least 7 days after menstruation helps to distinguish PMS from "menstrual distress," which is premenstrual exacerbation of preexisting physical or emotional problems. To help make a positive diagnosis, a woman with suspected PMS should keep a diary for at least 2 months giving daily ratings of common menstrual cycle symptoms. For many women, no medical treatment is necessary apart from an explanation of the symptoms, reassurance that they are not associated with severe underlying disease, and advice on how to cope with them. Rather than attempt to treat all PMS symptoms initially, it may be more effective to tackle the leading symptom. PMS has been treated successfully with nortriptyline, fluoxetine, evening bright light, and sleep deprivation (Wood S, Mortola JF, Chan Y-F, et al. Treatment of premenstrual syndrome with fluoxetine: a double-blind, placebo-controlled, crossover study. *Obstet Gynecol* 1992;80: 339–344). It has also been treated with high-dose (200 µg) transdermal estrogen patch (Watson NR, Studd JWW, Garnett TJ. A randomised placebo-controlled study of transdermal oestriodol for treatment of the premenstrual syndrome. *Lancet* 1989;2:730–732).

premorbid Preceding the onset of disease or illness.

premutation Repeat sequence in a gene that has a high probability of expanding to a full mutation in the next generation.

preoccupation Being absorbed with internally generated thoughts and feelings and autistic experiences to the detriment of reality orientation and adaptive behavior. It ranges from mild to severe, in which gross absorption with autistic experiences profoundly affects all major realms of behavior. The patient may constantly respond verbally and behaviorally to hallucinations and show little awareness of other people or the external milieu.

prepulse inhibition (PPI) Partially automatic involuntary inhibitory process in which a normal startle reflex is reduced when the startling stimulus is preceded 30–500 msec earlier by a weak prepulse. It provides an operational measure of sensorimotor gating. PPI is impaired in patients with three specific neuropsychiatric disorders (schizophrenia, obsessive compulsive disorder, Huntington's disease) characterized clinically by impaired ability to gate or inhibit extraneous or nonsalient cognitive, motor, or sensory information (Swerdlow NR, Auerbach P, Monroe SM, et al. Men are more inhibited than women by weak prepulses. *Biol Psychiatry* 1993;34:253–260).

Prepulsid See **cisapride.**

Presamine See **imipramine.**

prescription drug abuse Characteristics include use of prescribed drugs in therapeutically aberrant ways (e.g., taking more than the prescribed dose); reporting prescriptions as lost or stolen; filling prescriptions at different pharmacies to avoid detection; having prescriptions written by different doctors to avoid detection; report by another physician or pharmacist of additional requests for the same medicine; reports by patient, relative, or friend of prescription drug misuse; evidence or reports of adverse effects attributable to use of higher-than-usual therapeutic dose; and history of mood disorder, misuse of alcohol, and suicide attempts (Anon. Characteristics of the prescription drug abuser. *Int Drug Ther Newsl* 1988;12:16).

Prescription Event Monitoring (PEM) One of two national systems of postmarketing surveillance in operation in Britain. PEM is able to identify unique events that occur with a frequency of more than 1 in 3,000 patients. It also helps identify important events by noting higher rates of occurrence during treatment than after treatment. These act as signals that help shorten the delay in recognition of adverse drug reactions. PEM was designed to supplement the Yellow Card scheme by providing more intensive monitoring during the early period of a drug's marketed life. It allows determination of the incidence of adverse drug reactions (ADRs) by providing a denominator and by recording all adverse events, and it can identify ADRs that may not be recognized for what they are by individual physicians and therefore may not be reported to the manufacturer or to a drug regulatory agency. An event is defined as "any new diagnosis, any reason for referral to a specialist or admission to hospital, any unexpected deterioration (or improvement) in a concurrent illness, any suspected drug reaction, or any other complaint considered of sufficient import to enter into the patient's notes" (Inman WHW. *Monitoring for Drug Safety.* Lancaster, England: MTP Press, 1980). See **Yellow Card scheme.**

presenile dementia See **dementia, presenile.**

pressure of speech Speech that is increased in amount, accelerated, difficult or impossible to interrupt, and usually loud and emphatic (DSM IV). The person may talk without any social stimulation and continue to talk even though no one is listening. Pressure of speech is most often seen in manic episodes, but may also occur in some cases of organic mental disorders, major depression with psychomotor agitation, schizophrenia, other psychotic disorders, and, occasionally, acute reactions to stress.

presynaptic Relating to events or structures occurring proximal to the synapse.

presynaptic receptor See **receptor, presynaptic.**

pretend play Play in which objects are used as if they have other properties or identities. It is normally present by age 12–15 months, but is absent or abnormal in autism (Baron-Cohen S, Allen J, Gillberg C. Can autism be detected at 18 months? The needle, the haystack and the CHAT. *Br J Psychiatry* 1992;161:839–843). See **autism; joint-attention behavior.**

prevalence Frequency of cases, both old and new, in the population at a given time divided by the number of persons in that population at risk. It is distinguished from incidence, which is the frequency of new cases. See **incidence.**

prevalence, point See **point prevalence.**

prevalence rate See **point prevalence.**

prevention, dependence Social, economic, legal, or individual psychological measures aimed at minimizing the use of potentially addicting substances, or lowering the dependence risk in susceptible individuals.

prevention research Research designed to yield results directly applicable to interventions that either prevent occurrences of disease or disability or prevent the progression of detectable but asymptomatic disease (U.S. Public Health Service).

preventive aggressive device (PAD) Less restrictive method of controlling patients with a history of aggressive behavior used as an alternative to restraints. Wrist PADs allow the patient to eat, smoke, and protect himself or herself from falls; ankle PADs allow the patient to walk and participate in unit activities.

preventive therapy See **maintenance antidepressant drug therapy; maintenance psychoactive drug therapy.**

Priadel See **lithium citrate.**

priapism (Derived from the Greek god of fertility, Priapos.) Pathologically prolonged, painful erection of the penis involving the corpora cavernosa, while the corpus spongiosum and glans penis remain flaccid. The erection is usually unrelated to sexual stimulation or sexual excitation, although some cases have occurred after prolonged sexual activity. It is a urological emergency that requires immediate treatment (within 4–6 hours after onset) to decrease morbidity, the need for more invasive procedures, and impotence. It can be relieved with intrapenile injections of epinephrine or other alpha agonists. Priapism has been caused by alcohol, chlorpromazine, clozapine, flupenthixol, fluphenazine, guanethidine, haloperidol, labetalol, marijuana, phenelzine, perphenazine, prazosin, testosterone, thioridazine, thiothixene, and trazodone. The psychotropics most likely to cause priapism are trazodone and alpha-blocking neuroleptics. The risk of drug-induced priapism is greater in patients with a past history of prolonged erection with medication (Thompson JW Jr, Ware MR, Blashfield RK. Psychotropic medications and priapism: a comprehensive review. *J Clin Psychiatry* 1990; 51:430–433).

Priaxim See **flunoxaprofen.**

primary alcoholism See **alcoholism, primary.**

primary care Medical care provided by the health professional of first contact for the patient, usually a general practitioner, family practitioner, primary care internist, or primary care pediatrician, but also a nurse practitioner or paramedic. It is the nature of the contact (first compared with referred) that determines the care designation rather than the qualifications of the practitioner (Anon. Glossary of methodologic terms. *JAMA* 1992; 268:43–44).

primary care center Medical facility that offers first-contact health care only; specialized medical care is referred elsewhere, although some centers provide a mixture of primary and referred care. It is the nature of the service provided (first contact) rather than the setting that distinguishes primary care from other care levels (Anon. Glossary of methodologic terms. *JAMA* 1992;268:43–44).

primary degenerative dementia See **Alzheimer's disease; multi-infarct dementia.**

primary delusion See **delusion, primary.**

primary depression See **depression, primary.**

primary insomnia See **insomnia, primary.**

primary memory See **memory, primary.**

primary prevention Attempts to reduce the incidence of new cases (or problems) in a general population.

primary unipolar depression See **depression, primary unipolar.**

primary writing tremor See **tremor, primary writing.**

"prime" Street name for anabolic steroids.

primidone (Myidone; Mysoline) Enzyme-inducing anticonvulsant used in the treatment of generalized and partial seizures and, sometimes, other types of seizures. It is converted into phenobarbital in the body, causing barbiturate-like side effects. It also may cause megaloblastic anemia. Pregnancy risk category D.

primidone + anticoagulant Co-administration may decrease prothrombin time.

primidone + carbamazepine Co-administration may lower carbamazepine (CBZ) plasma level and reduce therapeutic efficacy. CBZ may decrease metabolism of primidone to its metabolites; increased primidone levels have been reported (Pippenger CE. Clinically significant carbamazepine drug interactions: an overview. *Epilepsia* 1987;28:S71–S76).

primidone + lamotrigine Primidone accelerates lamotrigine elimination (Jawad S, Yuen AWC, Peck AW, et al. Lamotrigine: single dose pharmacokinetics and initial one week exposure in refractory seizures. *Epilepsy Res* 1987;1: 196–201).

primidone + phenytoin Phenytoin may decrease the effects of primidone and increase its conversion to phenobarbital. Primidone plasma level should be monitored to prevent toxicity.

primidone + valproate   Co-administration may decrease valproate blood levels and reduce efficacy.

primidone + valproic acid   Valproic acid may or may not increase primidone levels (Windorfer A, Sauer W, Gaedke R. Elevation of diphenyl-hydantoin and primidone serum concentration by addition of diproplylacetate, a new anticonvulsant drug. *Acta Paediatr Scand* 1975; 64:771–772; Fincham RW, Schottelius DD. Primidone: interactions with other drugs. *In* Woodbury DM, Penry JK, Pippenger CE [eds], *Antiepileptic Drugs*, 2nd ed. New York: Raven Press, 1982, pp 421–428).

primitive reflexes   Neurological signs (e.g., snout, palmomental, and grasp reflexes) that indicate advanced cerebral damage and that are frequently seen in patients with progressive Alzheimer's disease.

"primo"   Street name for anabolic steroids.

Primonil   See **imipramine.**

Primoteston Depot   See **testosterone enanthate.**

Primperan   See **metoclopramide.**

Prinivil   See **lisinopril.**

PR interval   Electrocardiographic measure of the time from onset of atrial activation to onset of ventricular activation. It is an index of atrioventricular conduction time (normal is 100–200 ms). Greater intervals indicate some degree of conduction blockade between the atria and ventricles.

Prinzide   See **lisinopril.**

prion   See **gene, prion.**

prion disease   Transmissible, spongiform encephalopathy. In humans, there are three: kuru, Creutzfeldt-Jakob disease, and Gerstmann-Straüssler-Scheinker disease. All are central nervous system degenerative (CNS) diseases. They have long incubation periods, often measured in years, but once manifested usually progress swiftly, without remission and uninfluenced by treatment, to death within a few months (Gerstmann-Straüssler-Scheinker disease in its slower progression is an exception). Pathological features are confined to the CNS and include neuronal loss, astrocytic gliosis, and spongiform changes. There is no inflammatory reaction, which is consistent with the lack of any humoral or cellular reaction in the blood (Hughes JT. Prion diseases depend on transmissible and sometimes hereditable agents. *Br Med J* 1993:306:288).

prion gene   See **gene, prion.**

PRN orders   (Latin *pro re nata*, "as occasion arises") Orders used in almost all medical specialties that allow use or administration of medication on an as-needed basis. They can alleviate patients' suffering and relieve physicians of the need to examine a patient each time an expected treatment- or illness-related symptom occurs. Problems associated with PRN orders in psychiatric settings include (a) the majority (90%+) are written for patients already receiving psychotropic medications; (b) almost 50% lack the indication for which the drug is to be given; (c) a majority of those with a specified indication are vague (e.g., "agitation"); (d) more than two-thirds lack specification of a minimal interval between doses; (e) many lack a specified maximum dose limit per 24 hours; (f) over 50% are administered between 11:30 P.M. and 7:30 A.M., most often to patients posing a management problem; and (g) the majority are not stopped by a physician's orders, but by hospital policy or discharge from the hospital. Imprecise PRN orders delegate an inordinate amount of decision-making responsibility to the nursing staff; thus, because they are carried out by someone other than the prescriber, PRN orders should be considered carefully. Hospitals with psychiatric inpatient units should consider periodically monitoring PRN psychotropic drugs. Reasons for use of PRN psychotropic medication should be explored, and alternative methods of patient management should be considered, especially for patients with personality disorder and those over age 50. Prescription and administration of psychotropic drugs on a PRN basis preferably should be reserved for emergencies only. PRN orders should have clear and detailed instructions regarding the indications, minimum interval between doses, maximum daily dosage, monitoring of the patient's clinical condition (including therapeutic effects, side effects, and vital signs), and the duration for which the order is valid. For certain medications (e.g., neuroleptics) or certain patients (e.g., those newly admitted), PRN orders should be valid for one time only, to be followed by a physician's assessment (Craven JL, Voore PM, Voineskos G. PRN medication for psychiatric inpatients. *Can J Psychiatry* 1987;32:199–203; Ayd FJ Jr. Problems with orders for medication as needed. *Am J Psychiatry* 1985;142:939–942).

PRN orders/children   PRN orders for sedatives are commonly written for children (ages 5–13) with diagnoses of conduct disorder, attention deficit hyperactivity, and major depression. The only double-blind, placebo-controlled study designed to assess the efficacy of PRN sedative use in child psychiatric inpatients found no difference between intramuscular or oral administration of diphenhydramine (25 or 50 mg) and placebo, although intramuscular administration tended to be more effective than oral administration (Vitelli B, Riccinti AJ, Behar D. P.R.N. medication in child state hospital inpatients. *J Clin Psychiatry* 1987;48:351–354).

probable deviation   See **median deviation.**

probable error   See **median deviation.**

probability   (p) The number of times an outcome occurs in the total number of trials. It is conventionally expressed by a value between 0 (impossible event) and 1 (certain event), which is written as $p < 0.05$. By convention, it is generally conceded that the probability of error is negligible when the p value is below this arbitrary threshold. Such p values are an integral part of the statistical technique known as hypothesis testing or significance testing. They are determined by statistical tests of hypotheses that are applicable only to hypotheses fully and explicitly formed before the data are examined; if not, their value has a distinctly different meaning and a much reduced weight of inference. Although p values are a way of reporting the results of statistical tests, they do not define the practical importance of the results. A p value is the probability of obtaining a result as extreme or more extreme than the one observed as the result of chance alone. It measures surprise: the smaller the p value, the more surprising the result if the null hypothesis is true. When the p value is between 0.05 and 0.01, the result is "statistically significant;" when less than 0.01, the result is "highly statistically significant."

probability, objective   Estimate of probability from observable events or phenomena.

probability sample   See **sample probability.**

proband   **1.** Patient or family member who brings a family under study. **2.** Family member chosen as the starting point of a genealogical study, with the dominant trait. **3.** The index cases whose families are studied in genetic research. Also called "propositus."

probe   Device or agent used to enter and explore.

probe, neurobehavioral   Administration of tasks during measurement of physiological activity in the process of neuroimaging studies. Probes can show which brain regions or networks are engaged in regulatory aspects of behavior. When applied to psychiatric patients, they may link behavioral deficits to abnormalities in activating such networks. See **probe, pharmacological.**

probe, pharmacological   Substance used to examine the effects of specific agents on neuroreceptor function and regional brain activity during neuroimaging. Correlating these induced changes with behavior can help establish links between brain function and psychopathological conditions.

probenecid   (Benemid) Compound that blocks the efflux of acid metabolites (5-hydroxyin-doleacetic acid [5-HIAA] and homovanillic acid [HVA]) from cerebrospinal fluid, which does not affect neutral metabolite 3-methoxy-4-hydroxyphenylglycol (MHPG) removal. It has enabled investigators to assess the serotonin and dopamine turnover in conscious depressed and schizophrenic patients.

problem drinking   Pattern of alcohol consumption that has resulted in physical, psychological, social, family, occupational, financial, and/or legal problems. Although it does not satisfy all the criteria of alcoholism, problem drinking is characterized by an alcohol intake great enough to have generated serious consequences.

procaine   (Novocain) Local anesthetic that may induce panic attacks in patients with panic disorder.

procainamide   (Pronestyl) Type IA antiarrhythmic drug. It should not be co-prescribed with tricyclic antidepressants that have quinidine-like (IA) antiarrhythmic activity. Furthermore, because antipsychotic drugs have quinidine-like actions, arrhythmias caused by overdoses should not be treated with quinidine or related type I antiarrhythmic drugs such as procainamide.

procainamide + cyclic antidepressant   See **antidepressant, cyclic + procainamide.**

procarbazine   (Matulane; Natalin) Hydrazine derivative antineoplastic agent that exhibits some monoamine oxidase inhibitor (MAOI) activity. Patients being treated with it should avoid sympathomimetics, tricyclic antidepressants, and other drugs and foods with known high tyramine content.

Procardia   See **nifedipine.**

prochlorperazine   (Compazine; Stemetil; Vertigon) Piperazine phenothiazine derivative initially tested as a neuroleptic, but now marketed primarily as an antiemetic. It has central dopamine antagonist properties and causes early reversible extrapyramidal reactions and tardive movement disorders (tardive dyskinesia and tardive dystonia). Pregnancy risk category C.

prochlorperazine + phenytoin   Prochlorperazine may increase phenytoin plasma levels, but effects generally are insignificant (Kuth H. Interactions between anticonvulsants and other commonly prescribed drugs. *Epilepsia* 1984; 25[suppl 2]:118–131).

proconvulsant   That which favors the occurrence of a seizure.

proctalgia fugax   Disorder of the gastrointestinal tract characterized by fleeting, lightning-like, intense rectal pain that awakens patients from sleep.

procyclidine   (Kemadren; Kemadrin; Kemadrine; Osnervan) Anticholinergic drug used in the treatment of parkinsonism and early-onset neuroleptic-induced extrapyramidal reactions. It is useful for treating early tremor and rigidity, but it is not as potent as levodopa in treating akinesia and bradykinesia and their associated slowness, stooping, and falls. It helps control hypersalivation and drooling, but may cause an annoying dry mouth with its associated adverse effects. This and other anticholinergic side effects limit procyclidine's usefulness in treating moderate and advanced stages of parkinsonism. Pregnancy risk category C.

procyclidine + olanzapine   Co-administration in a patient with a tremor that pre-existed olanzapine therapy was well tolerated.

procyclidine + paroxetine   Paroxetine (30 mg/day) increases procyclidine's (5 mg every day) steady-state area under the curve (AUC) 0–24 by 35%, C_{max} by 37%, and C_{min} by 67% compared to procyclidine given alone at steady state. If anticholinergic effects occur, procyclidine dose should be reduced.

prodrome   Early warning sign or symptom of an oncoming disease. The prodromal phase connotes a time interval between the onset of prodromal symptoms and the onset of the characteristic manifestations of the fully developed illness.

prodrug   Chemical derivative of a drug that regenerates the free drug in vivo (e.g., prazepam and clorazepate are prodrugs of desmethyldiazepam; valpromide is a prodrug of valproate). It is inactive when administered and then is converted to an active metabolite. Prodrugs may be more stable, more efficiently absorbed, formulated into controlled-release preparations, or less susceptible to metabolism than the active drugs. They have been used extensively in injectable depot dosage forms (e.g., fluphenazine decanoate and haloperidol decanoate). Also called "precursor."

productive symptoms   Hallucinations and delusions in schizophrenia, and in some descriptions of autism. See **schizophrenia/deficit symptoms.**

product liability   Legal concept concerning the question of who has responsibility and what redress is available when a patient suffers injury as a result of drug therapy.

product-moment method   See **coefficient of correlation.**

prodynorphin   See **proenkephalin B.**

proenkephalin   See **proenkephalin A.**

proenkephalin A   (proenkephalin) Four met-enkephalin sequences plus one leu-enkephalin sequence that give rise to met- and leu-enkephalin as well as a variety of larger peptides containing met-enkephalin.

proenkephalin B   (prodynorphin) Three leu-enkephalin sequences that give rise to alpha- and beta-neoendorphin and dynorphin A- and dynorphin B-related peptides.

progabide   (Gabren; Gabrene) Specific gamma aminobutyric acid (GABA) agonist that is a clinically effective antidepressant (Lloyd KG, Morselli PL, Depoortere H, et al. The potential use of GABA agonists in psychiatric disorders: evidence from studies with progabide in animal models and clinical trials. *Pharmacol Biochem Behav* 1983;18:957–966; Lloyd KG, Zivkovic B, Scatton B, et al. The GABAergic hypothesis of depression. *Prog Neuropsychopharmacol Biol Psychiatry* 1989;13:341–351).

progamma-melanotropin   (progamma-MSH) Peptide that represents a portion of the N-terminal region of the pro-opiomelanocortin molecule. It has been shown, both in vivo and in vitro, to act synergistically with adrenocorticotropic hormone in stimulation of corticosteroid production.

progesterone   Major female gonadal hormone that may have a negative mood effect.

prognosis   Probable course of a disease or condition.

progressive dialysis encephalopathy   See **encephalopathy, progressive dialysis.**

progressive multifocal leukoencephalopathy   (PML) Severe, subacute demyelinating disease of the central nervous system with no known treatment. It is a rare complication of immunosuppressive therapy, but seems to be far more prevalent among acquired immunodeficiency syndrome (AIDS) patients; estimates range from 4% to 7%, which is probably low. PML may be due to the JC virus. It is characterized by foci of demyelination associated with viral infection of the oligodendrocytes, with a tendency for more mononuclear cell infiltration of white matter in AIDS patients than in others with the disorder. PML develops insidiously, with progressive limb weakness, ataxia, visual disturbance, and dementia. Death usually follows within 6 months, although a handful of "burnt out" cases have been reported. Measurement of JC virus antibody concentrations in serum and cerebrospinal fluid may assist the diagnosis and help identify patients at risk. Brain biopsy remains the definitive diagnostic procedure, from which characteristic histological changes can be observed and viral antigen and genome can be detected by immunofluorescence and in-situ hybridization, respectively. Magnetic resonance imaging (MRI) and, to a lesser extent, computed tomography (CT) are useful noninvasive procedures for detecting the specific multiple demyelinating lesions of PML

(Anon. PML: more neurological bad news for AIDS patients. *Lancet* 1992;340:943).

projection   Mechanism in which a person falsely attributes his or her own unacknowledged feelings, impulses, or thoughts to others (DSM IV). See **defense mechanism.**

projective test   Objective diagnostic instrument based on ambiguous stimuli or settings that require a relatively unstructured response. The oldest and best-known is the Rorschach inkblot test. Another example is the Thematic Apperception Test (TAT).

prokalectic therapy   Form of treatment, first described in 1969, that uses transference to achieve change. The therapist manipulates the patient into an emotionally unacceptable position that can only be avoided by two means: denouncing the therapist or giving up the symptom (Kraupi-Taylor F. Prokalectic measures derived from psychoanalytic technique. *Br J Psychiatry* 1969;115:407–419). The likelihood that the patient will chose the second alternative depends on the strength of attachment to the therapist. Once attachment is strong enough, the therapist gives a prokalectic interpretation (e.g., a sexual connotation) to the symptom which the patient finds hard to accept. The patient's dilemma between idealization of the therapist and retention of the symptom can only be avoided if the symptom disappears. This therapeutic approach may be useful in the treatment of resistant conversion symptoms when other therapies have failed (Neeleman J, Mann AH. Treatment of hysterical aphonia with hypnosis and prokalectic therapy. *Br J Psychiatry* 1993; 163:816–819).

prokaryote   Cell or organism lacking a membrane-bound, structurally discrete nucleus and subcellular compartments (e.g., bacteria).

Proketazine   See **carphenazine.**

prolactin   (PRL) Single-chain polypeptide protein hormone synthesized and released by the anterior pituitary gland. When hypothalamic receptors are stimulated by an appropriate serotonin (5-HT) agonist, serum PRL concentration increases. PRL receptors have been found in humans in the mammary glands, liver, kidney, brain, adrenal glands, ovaries, seminal vesicles, prostate, uterus, testes, and placenta. PRL induces synthesis and secretion of milk, inhibits secretion of gonadotropins, may stimulate testosterone synthesis, and is involved in the immune system. Serum PRL increases during sleep, peaks in the early morning, and declines immediately after awakening. Basal levels vary considerably; range is 5–25 ng/ml in adults and nonpregnant, nonlactating women. During pregnancy, PRL level can rise to 200 ng/ml at term and to 300 ng/ml during nursing. The principal control of PRL secretion is through the inhibitory action of dopamine (DA) acting on D_2 receptors on the surface of pituitary lactotrophs. The PRL response is a direct effect of the DA receptor blocking action of antipsychotic drugs at the hypothalamic and pituitary level. In unmedicated schizophrenic patients, PRL levels are within normal range. In normal subjects and in patients, a near maximal PRL response can be achieved with low doses of neuroleptics administered either parenterally or orally. Neuroleptics can induce hyperprolactinemia, resulting in effects on reproductive hormones, galactorrhea, and behavioral changes. A number of studies have reported a blunted PRL response to 5-HT challenge in depressed patients. Serotonergic drugs such as fluoxetine can increase PRL levels. Serum PRL levels can be used as an index of neuroleptic bioavailability, since it has been found to be a useful measure of neuroleptic activity at therapeutically relevant receptor sites (Green AI, Faraone SV, Brown WA. Prolactin shifts after neuroleptic withdrawal. *Psychiatry Res* 1990;32:213–219; Seidman LJ, Pepple JR, Faraone SV, et al. Neuropsychological performance in chronic schizophrenia in response to neuroleptic dose reduction. *Biol Psychiatry* 1993;33:575–584). Since PRL is inhibited by DA secretion, a DA deficit, such as that induced by typical neuroleptics and cocaine, produces high PRL levels. A number of studies have shown that chronic cocaine abuse results in substantially elevated PRL levels that persist for at least a month after cocaine discontinuation.

Prolixin   See **fluphenazine.**

Prolixin Decanoate   See **fluphenazine decanoate.**

Prolixin Enanthate   See **fluphenazine enanthate.**

Promaz   See **chlorpromazine**

promazine   (Prozine-50; Sparine) Aliphatic phenothiazine derivative marketed as an antipsychotic. A number of clinical studies have found it to be less effective than chlorpromazine, and others have found it no more effective than placebo. It has the pharmacological effects and therapeutic indications of other aliphatic phenothiazine neuroleptics. Pregnancy risk category C.

promethazine   (Phenergan) Piperidine phenothiazine derivative, synthesized by Charpentier in 1944, that was a predecessor of chlorpromazine. In 1950, it was used with "much success" in the therapy of psychotic patients. It was also used to potentiate anesthetic agents and was an important constituent in "lytic cocktails." Onset of action is slow (1.5–3 hours). It has antipruritic, anticholinergic, and significant sedative effects. Its hypnotic action presumably results from central histamine (H_1) receptor antagonism combined with a mild neuroleptic effect. It may cause excitement rather than sedation. It also has been reported to cause hallucinations, seizures, and dystonic reactions.

promoter gene   See **gene, promoter.**

Pronestyl   See **procainamide.**

Pronoctan   See **lormetazepam.**

pro-opiomelanocortin   (POMC) Glycoprotein precursor from which a family of peptides is derived, including adrenocorticotrophic hormone, beta-lipotropin, beta-endorphin, n-terminal pro-opiomelanocortin, and melanocyte-stimulating hormone.

propafenone   Relatively new class IC antiarrhythmic agent that is extensively metabolized with 5-hydroxylation by the hepatic cytochrome P450 isoenzyme.

propafenone + desipramine   See **desipramine + propafenone.**

propinquity   Term used by geneticists to indicate nearness of blood relationship.

propofol   (Diprivan) Intravenous anesthetic used since 1988 with electroconvulsive therapy (ECT). Its main advantages are extremely rapid recovery, reduced post-ECT hypertension compared with short-acting barbiturates, and low incidence of postanesthetic nausea or vomiting. It may also tend to decrease the hypertension associated with ECT better than methohexital does. Recent reports indicate that it reduces seizure duration, leading to concern that it may reduce ECT efficacy. Because of the widely accepted belief that most ECT-induced seizures should last approximately 25 seconds to be maximally effective, concern about decreasing seizure length may limit propofol's acceptance. Comparisons with thiopentone, however, indicate that propofol does not impair therapeutic response to ECT. Recurrent, amorous, disinhibited behavior and hallucinations with sexual connotations over a 14-hour period were reported in a 48-year-old man following intravenous administration of propofol (30 mg). He was given two intramuscular 2-mg doses of haloperidol injections. Later, he felt well and had no memory of his aggressive sexual behavior (Canaday BR. Amorous, disinhibited behavior associated with propofol. *Clin Pharm* 1993;12:449–451).

propofol + tranylcypromine   Co-administration appears to be safe (Hyde RA, Mortimer AJ. Safe use of propofol in a patient receiving tranylcypromine. *Anaethesia* 1991;46:1090).

proportion   Number of observations with the characteristic of interest divided by the total number of observations. It is a special type of ratio in which the denominator contains the numerator.

proportional attributable risk   See **risk, proportional attributable.**

propositus   See **proband.**

propoxyphene   See **dextropropoxyphene.**

propranolol   (Deralin; Inderal) Highly lipophilic, nonselective beta-adrenergic blocking agent used in the treatment of anxiety, neuroleptic-induced akathisia, hypertension, angina, and certain cardiac arrhythmias. It also has been used successfully to treat agitation, assaultiveness, and explosive rage in patients with organic brain disease of various etiologies. Duration of action is relatively short, requiring multiple dosing during the day. Therapeutic blood range is 50–200 ng/ml (190–770 mmol/L). Propranolol infrequently causes depression in anxious patients and in hypertensive patients. In patients who have been treated with high doses, discontinuation should involve tapering (60 mg/day) to avoid rebound elevated blood pressure. Propranolol is contraindicated in patients with sinus bradycardia, greater than first-degree block, and bronchial asthma. Pregnancy risk category C. See **beta-blocker/psychiatric uses; propranolol/aggression; propranolol/akathisia.**

propranolol/aggression   Propranolol has been reported effective in various types of aggressive behaviors, especially in patients with organic brain disorders due to trauma, infections, Wilson's disease, Korsakoff's psychosis, and dementias. Those with bronchial asthma, chronic obstructive pulmonary disease, insulin-dependent diabetes, cardiac diseases including angina or congestive heart failure, significant peripheral vascular disease, severe renal disease, and hyperthyroidism should not be given propranolol. Hypertensive patients should be given propranolol with caution, since sudden discontinuation may result in rebound hypertension. Propranolol should be initiated with 20 mg 3 times a day and increased by 60 mg every 3–4 days. A test dose of 20 mg may be given initially if there are clinical concerns about hypotension or bradycardia. In healthy patients, dosage may be increased until pulse rate is less than 50 or systolic blood pressure is less than 90. Dosage should be decreased if severe dizziness, wheezing, or ataxia occurs. Dosages greater than 640 mg/day are not usually required to control violent behavior. The patient should be maintained on the highest dose of propranolol for at least 1 month before concluding that there has been no response. Some patients may respond rapidly. Concurrent medications should be used with caution. Blood levels of neuroleptics and anticonvulsants should be monitored (Silver JM, Yudofsky S. Propranolol for aggression: literature review and clinical guidelines. *Int Drug Ther Newsl* 1985;20:9–12).

propranolol/akathisia   The racemic form of propranolol (but not d-propranolol, the isomer with beta-blocking properties) is effective in the treatment of akathisia. Compared with less lipophilic agents (e.g., nadolol, sotalol, atenolol), propranolol (10–80 mg/day) is more effective for akathisia, suggesting that this effect is centrally mediated. Other studies have compared propranolol, which nonselectively blocks both beta$_1$ and beta$_2$ receptors, with beta$_1$ selective blockers (e.g., low-dose metoprolol and betaxolol) and with the beta$_2$ selective agent ICI 118,551. In these studies, propranolol showed either greater or equal efficacy to the comparison drug. Thus, racemic propranolol has become the standard against which other beta-adrenergic blockers are compared in patients with neuroleptic-induced akathisia. Propranolol in low, divided doses (30–80 mg/day) does not adversely affect blood pressure and pulse rate or interact adversely with any of the known neuroleptics or antiparkinson drugs. In contrast to other drugs prescribed for akathisia (e.g., antiparkinson drugs, benzodiazepines), propranolol has fewer side effects that limit the usefulness of the other substances. As akathisia is relieved after the addition of propranolol, the antiparkinson drug often can be discontinued. Propranolol can be prescribed prophylactically to prevent recurrence of akathisia or as maintenance therapy to control or abolish akathisia induced by maintenance neuroleptic therapy. It should not be prescribed for patients with asthma, insulin-dependent diabetes mellitus, or any cardiac conduction abnormality or concurrent cardiovascular illness that requires medical treatment (Ayd FJ Jr. Propranolol therapy for neuroleptic-induced akathisia. *Int Drug Ther Newsl* 1986;21:14; Adler L, Angrist B, Peselow B, et al. Efficacy of propranolol in neuroleptic-induced akathisia. *J Clin Psychopharmacol* 1985;5:164–166; Adler L, Angrist B, Peselow E, et al. A controlled assessment of propranolol in the treatment of neuroleptic-induced akathisia. *Br J Psychiatry* 1986; 149:42–45; Adler LA, Peselow E, Rosenthal M, Angrist B. A controlled comparison of the effects of propranolol, benztropine and placebo on akathisia: an interim analysis. *Psychopharmacology Bulletin* 1993;2:284–286).

propranolol + alcohol   Alcohol impairs propranolol absorption and may affect its therapeutic effects.

propranolol/benzodiazepine withdrawal   Propranolol has been found to reduce symptom intensity during benzodiazepine (BZD) discontinuation (Tyrer P, Rutherford D, Huggett T. Benzodiazepine withdrawal symptoms and propranolol. *Lancet* 1981;1:520–522). Propranolol (20 mg every 6 hours) is started on the 5th day of gradual BZD discontinuation and continued for 2 weeks. Thereafter, propranolol is used as needed to control tachycardia, elevated blood pressure, and anxiety.

propranolol + chlorpromazine   Propranolol may retard chlorpromazine (CPZ) elimination, resulting in elevation of its serum concentration and enhancement of its therapeutic effects (Greendyke RM, Kanter DR. Plasma propranolol levels and their effects on plasma thioridazine and haloperidol concentrations. *J Clin Psychopharmacol* 1987;7:178–182; Peet M, Middlemiss DN, Yates RA. Propanolol in schizophrenia: clinical and biochemical aspects of combining propranolol with chlorpromazine. *Br J Psychiatry* 1981;138:112–117). Adverse cardiovascular changes have occurred in some patients when propranolol is added to CPZ (Miller FA, Rampling D. Adverse effects of combined propranolol and chlorpromazine therapy. *Am J Psychiatry* 1982;139:1189–1199).

propranolol + cimetidine   Co-administration increases propranolol serum concentration because of decreased clearance secondary to decreased hydroxylation.

propranolol + clomipramine   Clomipramine (CMI) (150 mg/day) + propranolol (dosage unknown) was well tolerated and effective prophylaxis for 7 years in a patient with major depression and recurrent paroxysmal tachycardia (Jouvent R, Baruch P, Simon P. *Am J Psychiatry* 1986;143:1633).

propranolol + fluoxetine   Propranolol (60–90 mg/day) produces prompt (within 36–48 hours) relief of fluoxetine (FLX)-induced akathisia (Fleischhacker WW. Propranolol for fluoxetine-induced akathisia. *Biol Psychiatry* 1991;30:531–532; Lipinski VF, Mallya G, Zimmerman P, Pope HG. Fluoxetine-induced akathisia: clinical and theoretical implications. *J Clin Psychiatry* 1989;50:339–342). There is a case report of complete heart block 2 weeks following FLX initiation in a man who had been taking propranolol for several years (Drake WM, Gordon GD. Heart block in a patient on propranolol and fluoxetine. *Lancet* 1994;343:425–426).

propranolol + fluphenazine   Delirium was reported during treatment with fluphenazine decanoate, benztropine, and propranolol (Lima BR, Vanneman D. Propranolol, benztropine, fluphenazine decanoate and delirium. *Am J Psychiatry* 1983;140:659–660).

propranolol + fluvoxamine   Co-administration increases bioavailability of oral propranolol, resulting in substantially higher propranolol serum levels (up to 5 times higher). Fluvoxamine (FVX) slightly potentiated propranolol-induced reductions in heart rate (by 3 beats/min) and exercise diastolic blood pressure, but did not interfere with its blood pressure–lowering effect. Propranolol dosage may have to be lowered if it is co-administered with FVX (Benfield P, Ward A. Fluvoxamine: a review of its pharmacokinetic properties, and therapeutic efficacy in depressive illness. *Drugs* 1986;32:313–334).

propranolol + haloperidol Co-administration has no effect on haloperidol plasma levels, but may produce serious adverse cardiovascular effects including hypotension and cardiopulmonary arrest. (Greendyke RM, Kanter DR. Plasma propranolol levels and their effects on plasma thioridazine and haloperidol concentrations. *J Clin Psychopharmacol* 1987;7:178–182; Alexander HE, McCarty K, Giffen MB. Hypotension and cardiopulmonary arrest associated with concurrent haloperidol and propranolol therapy. *JAMA* 1984;252:87–88).

propranolol + lithium Co-administration can have additive effects on the SA and AV nodes of the heart.

propranolol + maprotiline Propranolol may increase maprotiline (MAP) bioavailability by direct (inhibition of hepatic hydrolase) and indirect interference with this substance's metabolism (reduction of hepatic blood flow as a result of its cardiovascular effect). Delirium was reported in a patient treated with both drugs. In another patient who tolerated MAP (250 mg/day) without problems, addition of propranolol (120 mg/day) produced confusional symptoms and toxic MAP levels (Saiz-Ruiz J, Moral L. Delirium induced by association of propranolol and maprotiline. *J Clin Psychopharmacol* 1988;8:77–78; Tollefson G, Lesar T. Effect of propranolol on maprotiline clearance. *Am J Psychiatry* 1984;1:148–149).

propranolol + neuroleptic By competing for the same drug metabolizing enzymes, propranolol and a neuroleptic may increase each other's blood levels.

propranolol + nicotine transdermal system Because of the deinduction of hepatic enzymes on smoking cessation, a reduced dose of propranolol may be required at cessation of smoking and discontinuation of the nicotine transdermal patch.

propranolol + olanzapine Co-administration in a patient who had been receiving propranolol for over a year produced no adverse interactions.

propranolol + paroxetine No interactions have been demonstrated (Bannister SJ, Houser VP, Hulse JD, et al. Evaluation of the potential for interactions of paroxetine with diazepam, ci-metidine, warfarin and digoxin. *Acta Psychiatr Scand* 1989;80[suppl 350]:102–106).

propranolol + sumatriptan Sumatriptan does not interact with propranolol (Scott AK, Walley T, Breckenridge AM, et al. Lack of an interaction between propranolol and sumatriptan. *Br J Clin Pharmacol* 1991;32:581–584).

propranolol + thioridazine Co-administration may retard thioridazine elimination, resulting in a threefold to fivefold increase in the serum concentration of thioridazine and its metabolites and increasing the possibility of serious side effects and toxic effects (i.e., pigmentary retinopathy) (Greendyke RM, Kanter DR. Plasma propranolol levels and their effects on plasma thioridazine and haloperidol concentrations. *J Clin Psychopharmacol* 1987;7:178–182; Silver JM, Yudofsky S. Propranolol for aggression: literature review and clinical guidelines. *Int Drug Ther Newsl* 1985;20:9–12).

proprioception Sensory perception of motion. Also called "kinesthesia."

proprioreceptor Receptor sensitive to the position and movement of the body and its limbs. Some proprioreceptors (located in the vestibule of the inner ear and in the semicircular canals) are sensitive to the body's orientation in space and to body rotation. Others (located in the muscles, tendons, and joints) are sensitive to the position and movement of body members, giving rise to kinesthetic sensations.

propulsion Falling forward while walking (observed in Parkinson's disease patients) that cannot be stopped at will.

pro re nata See **PRN orders.**

Prosedar See **quazepam.**

Prosom See **estazolam.**

prosomatostatin 28-Amino-acid peptide isolated from intestine and the hypothalamus. It may be the precursor of somatostatin. It is 10 times more potent than somatostatin in inhibiting insulin secretion in rats. Its greater potency and prolonged action make prosomatostatin more useful than somatostatin in testing hormonal control mechanisms.

prosopagnosia Rare visuospatial disorder characterized by inability to recognize by sight previously familiar faces, although faces as a category are recognized and the familiar person may be recognized by voice. It is usually accompanied by a visual field defect and disturbance of color vision. These observations have spawned the hypothesis that the primary defect in prosopagnosia is not of perception, but of memory—the perception is correct, but it fails to elicit the appropriate contextual memories that usually provide the experience of familiarity. Prosopagnosia results from bilateral lesions of occipitotemporal cortex. It does not occur with unilateral lesions, and it appears that each hemisphere can recognize faces via different mechanisms. It is associated with brain injury or dementia and there is evidence of a link between it and Capgras syndrome (Bauer RM, Trobe JD. Visual memory and perceptual impairments in prosopagnosia. *J Clin Neurol Ophthalmol* 1984; 4:39–46). See **agnosia; Capgras syndrome.**

prospective study Predictive investigation in which all subjects undergoing a single event are followed to observe effects, including psychiatric illness. It usually requires many years to develop a large enough study population. Epidemiologists call a study *prospective* when the suspected cause is measured before the outcome occurs. The term should not be used without other details of the study design.

prostaglandin E₁ See **alprostadil.**

Prostep See **nicotine transdermal system.**

Prostigmin See **neostigmine.**

protective room Hospital room designed and built to provide a safe environment for a patient seriously at risk of hurting self or others.

protein Molecule consisting of chains of amino acids in a specific sequence that is determined by nucleotide sequence in the gene coding for the protein. Proteins are required for the structure, function, and regulation of the body's cells, tissues, and organs; each protein has a unique function.

protein binding See **plasma protein binding.**

protein chain See **polypeptide.**

protein, fusion See **fusion protein.**

protein, highly bound See **plasma protein binding.**

protein kinase Group of enzymes that transfer charged phosphate groups on proteins, thereby regulating intracellular processes in response to extracellular signals. Second messenger molecules (e.g., cyclic adenosine monophosphate, calcium) are the principal activators of the protein kinases.

protein kinase C (PKC) Component of the phosphoinositide (PI) second messenger system that is thought to mediate some of the actions of lithium.

protein phosphatase Substance that removes the phosphate group from substrate proteins. Abnormalities in protein phosphatase have been implicated in several neuropsychiatric conditions, including Alzheimer's disease.

protein phosphorylation Major mechanism for signal transduction in the nervous system. The three major components of protein phosphorylation are protein kinases, protein phosphatases, and substrate proteins. It is a reversible, post-translational modification of a protein. The addition or removal of a phos-

phate group from a protein changes the charge and therefore the shape of the protein, thus potentially causing a change in the functional state of that protein.

protein, regulatory Drug receptor that mediates the actions of endogenous chemical signals such as neurotransmitters, antacids, and hormones.

Prothiaden See **dothiepin.**

Protiaden See **dothiepin.**

Protiadene See **dothiepin.**

protirelin (Relefact TRH) Synthetic tripeptide believed to be structurally identical to naturally occurring thyrotropin-releasing hormone (TRH) produced by the hypothalamus. It is used as an adjunctive agent in the diagnostic assessment of thyroid function. The thyroid stimulating hormone response to protirelin has been most intensively studied in depressed patients with the finding that abnormally low responses occur in approximately 25–30%. A hyperactive response can be used to identify subclinical hypothyroidism as a cause of treatment-refractoriness in depression.

protocol Plan to be followed in a study or intervention program.

protocol violation Failure to follow a study or trial protocol correctly. Included are failure to apply selection criteria properly; failure to administer the treatment as prescribed; performance of the evaluation at the incorrect time; inclusion of a patient who does not have the illness under study; and failure of the patient to take the treatment as determined by randomization.

protodeclarative pointing See **joint-attention behavior.**

protoimperative pointing See **joint-attention behavior.**

proton Spinning charged particle that behaves as a microscopic magnet so that it tends to align when placed in the field of a magnet, giving overall magnetization of the patient. Protons (hydrogen nuclei that are bound inside large molecules such as proteins) generate signals that cannot be detected. Protein density data refer to the protons in water and free lipids and are a measure of the concentration of such protons.

proto-oncogene Gene that regulates other genes. Changes in proto-oncogenes may result in lasting alterations in neurotransmitters, neuropeptides, growth factors, and receptors.

protracted withdrawal See **withdrawal, protracted.**

protracted opioid abstinence syndrome See **opioid abstinence syndrome, protracted.**

protriptyline (Concordin; Triptil; Vivactil) Amitriptyline analog that is an effective antidepressant with clinical indications similar to those for other tricyclic antidepressants, including the treatment of nocturnal enuresis in children. It is also used for the treatment of sleep apnea. Pregnancy risk category C.

protriptyline + valproate   Co-administration may decrease valproate blood levels such that quite high doses may be needed to obtain therapeutic serum levels.

Provera   See **medroxyprogesterone.**

Prozac   See **fluoxetine.**

Prozil   See **chlorpromazine.**

Prozine-50   See **promazine.**

pseudoakathisia   Objective manifestations of akathisia (restless movements) in the absence of any subjective distress. It has been noted almost exclusively in patients with tardive dyskinesia. Stereotypes and mannerisms in chronic schizophrenia can also be confused with pseudoakathisia because the latter is often characterized by movement from foot to foot (Munetz MR. Akathisia variants and tardive dyskinesia. *Arch Gen Psychiatry* 1986;43: 1015). See **akathisia.**

pseudoautosomal region of sex chromosomes   Part of the distal ends of the short arms of the X and Y chromosomes that undergoes recombination in male meiosis. A disease allele located here will tend to be transmitted from a father to either sons or daughters depending on whether the disease is on his Y or X chromosome, respectively, with the result that affected siblings tend to be of the same sex.

pseudocholinesterase   See **butyrylcholinesterase.**

pseudocoma   See **akinetic mutism.**

pseudodelirium   Delirium-like organic cognitive disorder in the apparent absence of an organic precipitating factor; it is presumably brought about by psychosocial stress or sensory deprivation (Lipowski ZJ: Transient cognitive disorders [delirium, acute confusional states] in the elderly. *Am J Psychiatry* 1983;140: 1426–1436).

pseudodementia   Transient disturbance in high intellectual functions occurring in patients with psychiatric disorders. Approximately 20% of dementias are partially or wholly reversible. Among the causes of potentially reversible dementia are depression, drugs, normal pressure hydrocephalus, thyroid disorders, subdural hematoma, neoplasms, alcohol abuse, and metabolic disorders. It often resolves after successful treatment of the underlying disorder. Pseudodementia due to depression may be distinguished from primary dementia by subjective complaints of memory loss with little evidence of such on objective testing; inattention and slow responses to questions; answering "I don't know" rather than confabulating; and rapid onset of cognitive defects accompanied by depressive symptoms. The presence of specific depressive symptoms (e.g., early morning awakening, anxiety, impairment of libido) also help differentiate depressive pseudodementia from primary degenerative dementia. Depressed patients with reversible dementia have more delusions, motor retardation, helplessness, and hopelessness than patients with depression and irreversible dementia or patients with depression alone. Mild dementia, severe impairment in free recall, and inability to perform simple calculations correctly distinguishes the majority of patients into reversible and irreversible dementia. If pseudodementia in an older person is misdiagnosed as senile dementia, the patient may be placed in a nursing home. In many cases, electroconvulsive therapy rapidly restores the patient's health. In others, the patient may go on to develop "true" dementia. Formerly called "hysterical dementia." Also called "dementia syndrome of depression"; "reversible dementia."

pseudohallucination   Hallucination-like experience different from true hallucinations in that the person is fully cognizant of the unreality of the experience.

pseudologia fantastica   A form of lying by a person who believes in the reality of his or her fantasies and experiences these beliefs as true occurrences. Pseudologia fantastica is often a symptom exhibited by patients with a borderline personality disorder.

pseudoparkinsonism   See **parkinsonism, drug-induced.**

pseudoseizure   Seizure-like episode during which the electroencephalogram (EEG) remains normal (EEG is abnormal during an epileptic seizure). Pseudoseizures do not respond to anticonvulsant medication, except through a placebo effect. Pseudoseizure patients treated with medications are exposed to drug side effects and potential toxicity without any prospect of benefit. Also called "hysterical seizure."

pseudo-unipolar depression   See **bipolar III disorder.**

psilocybin   Substance obtained from wild mushrooms that causes hallucinations similar to those produced by lysergic acid diethylamide (LSD) and mescaline. It is usually taken orally. Onset is rapid, but hallucinations begin to wane in 2–3 hours. Physical dependence has not been reported and probably does not occur. Tolerance to it does occur, and cross-tolerance to the effects of LSD and mescaline has been demonstrated. "Magic" mushrooms were rare in the 1970s, but are now cultivated throughout the country and are readily available.

psyche Complex hierarchical structure of affective/cognitive systems of reference (or programs for feeling, thinking, and behavior) generated by repetitive concrete action.

psychedelic Term coined by Osmond (1957) for a group of drugs that have "mind-manifesting" or "mind-revealing" effects and produce hallucinations (usually visual) (Osmond H. A review of the clinical effects of psychotomimetic agents. *Ann N Y Acad Sci* 1957;66: 418). See **hallucinogen.**

psychedelic state See **"bad trip."**

psychiatric audit Systematic critical analysis of the quality of psychiatric care to improve standards of clinical care.

psychiatric ecologist See **ecology; social psychiatry.**

psychiatric life support Procedures that keep psychiatric patients alive but are not directed at ameliorating psychopathology. It involves one-to-one monitoring of suicidal patients and interventions to restrain patients from harming themselves (e.g., physical restraint, sedation). Psychopharmacotherapy, psychotherapy, and other psychosocial interventions are also used, usually to modify the course of a disorder.

psychiatrist Physician specializing in the diagnosis and treatment of mental disorders. The properly trained psychiatrist can provide a comprehensive evaluation from a psychiatric point of view, a medical differential diagnosis, treatment planning, and multiple therapeutic and health-enhancing interventions.

psychiatry, biological Study of such disciplines as biochemistry, physiology, and anatomy in relation to the genesis of psychiatric disorders.

psychiatry, consultation-liaison Work done by psychiatrists who practice as consultative assistants for diagnostic and therapeutic problems associated with other medical conditions. Psychiatrists may be consulted by medical and surgical services for problems thought to be "functional somatic" in nature, usually because no organic etiology has been determined. Consultation-liaison psychiatry addresses problems at the interface of the "organic" and the "functional."

psychic anxiety See **anxiety, psychic.**

psychic dependence See **dependence, psychic.**

psychoactive agent 1. Psychotropic drug. 2. Chemical substance that affects the mind (e.g., altering mood or states of consciousness).

psychoactive substance abuse See **drug abuse.**

psychobiology Study of the relationship between bodily functioning and human behavior and experience. The psychobiological model of disease attempts to merge biological and psychosocial approaches. It acknowledges that neither purely biological factors nor solely psychosocial influences can account for more than a minute proportion of psychiatric illnesses. The model also stresses the reciprocal nature of the environment-brain-behavior relationship; the environment can alter brain function and impinge on behavior and behavior can modify brain function and result in manipulations of the environment.

psychodermatology Study and treatment of skin disorders related to psychiatric disorders. Psychodermatological conditions can be divided into three broad subgroups: *psychophysiological disorders,* in which the severity of primary cutaneous disease is influenced by emotions; *primary psychiatry disorders,* in which the skin conditions are self-induced and reflect underlying psychiatric conditions; and *secondary psychiatric disorders,* in which psychological problems result from disfigurement associated with the skin conditions. A wide variety of clinical problems can be considered psychodermatological; some patients with a bona fide skin disorder (psoriasis, eczema) experience exacerbation of their skin condition under emotional stress; others have no dermatological condition but believe that they do (neurotic excoriations, delusions of parasitosis). Treatments may include psychotherapy, behavioral therapy, and psychopharmacotherapy. To determine which approach is most appropriate, the nature of the underlying psychopathological condition (anxiety, depression, psychosis, obsession/compulsion) should be identified.

psychodynamics Quality of interpersonal relations, recurrent conflict patterns, and, ultimately, the meaning of actions or experiences. Such meaning is understood by observing both its affective and its cognitive components.

psychodysleptic Hallucinogen that has "mind-disrupting" effects.

psychoeducation Technique that uses a didactic approach, including lectures and homework assignments, to teach coping skills.

psychoendocrinology Study of the psychological effects of neuroendocrinological activity.

psychogalvanic reflex (PGR) See **galvanic skin response.**

psychogenic That which is due to psychic, mental, or emotional factors, and not to demonstrable organic or somatic factors.

psychogenic amnesia See **amnesia, psychogenic.**

psychogenic fugue Dissociative disorder characterized by abrupt loss of personal (episodic) memory, loss of the sense of personal identity and assumption of a new one, and a period of wandering or travel. The episode usually lasts for some hours or days and is followed by amnesia for the period of the fugue. Severe precipitating stress, such as combat in wartime, is always present, and a period of depressed mood usually occurs just before onset of the fugue. Perplexity and disorientation may occur (Lipowski ZJ. *Delirium: Acute Confusional States.* New York, Oxford University, 1990). Also called "dissociative fugue." See **dissociative disorder.**

psychogenic polydipsia   See **polydipsia, psychogenic.**

psychogenic seizure   See **seizure, psychogenic.**

psychogenic urinary retention   See **paruresis.**

psychogerontology   Study of psychosocial aspects of old age. Also called "geriatric psychiatry."

psychoimmunology   Term coined by Solomon (1964) for psychological influences (experience, stress, emotions, traits, coping) on immune function and onset and course of immunologically resisted or mediated diseases.

psycholeptic   Term proposed by Jean Delay, a pioneer French psychopharmacotherapist, for psychotropic drugs with principal effects on psychomotor activity (anxiolytics and antidepressants).

psychological autopsy   Retrospective examination of a suicide death, reconstructed by examining medical, psychiatric, and social records and by interviewing family and friends (Shafii M, Carrigan S, Whittinghill JR, Derrick A. Psychological autopsy of completed suicide in children and adolescents. *Am J Psychiatry* 1985;142:1061–1064; Rich CL, Young D, Fowler RC. San Diego suicide study; I: young vs. old subjects. *Arch Gen Psychiatry* 1986;43: 577–582; Brent DA, Perper JA, Goldstein CE, et al. Risk factors for adolescent suicide. *Arch Gen Psychiatry* 1988;45:581–588; Clark DC, Horton-Deutsch SL. Assessment in absentia: the value of the psychological autopsy method for studying antecedents of suicide and predicting future suicides. *In* Maris RL, Berman A, Maltzberger JT, Yufit RY [eds], *Assessment and Prediction of Suicide.* New York: Guilford Press; 1992;144–182).

psychological dependence   See **drug dependence.**

psychological stress   Fear or anxiety associated with real or perceived threat. The so-called defense response is composed of a set of relatively well defined biological changes that help promote readiness for and execution of behaviors that will ultimately increase the probability of survival of the organism. Alterations in the cardiovascular, respiratory, and other visceral systems are adaptive and have a strong learned component to them.

psychological test   Standardized method of sampling behaviors, including feelings, thoughts, overt behavior, and intellectual functioning, in a reliable and valid way. Immediate goals are to extrapolate from representative samples of behavior in order to predict behaviors other than those being directly sampled by the test, and to measure change over time.

psychologist   Specialist, with either a masters (MA) or doctorate (PhD) degree in one or more of the various branches of psychology (analytical, behavioral, child, clinical, experimental) who is licensed to practice and/or certified to teach in one of these specialties.

psychology   Study of behavior.

psycholytic   Hallucinogen that has "mind-loosening" effects.

psychometrics   Psychological and mental testing or any quantitative analysis of an individual's psychological traits, attitudes, or mental processes (e.g., intelligence, special abilities and disabilities, manual skill, vocational aptitudes, interests, and personality characteristics).

psychometry   Science of measuring psychological processes and states.

psychomotility   Motor phenomena or habit patterns (e.g., tics, stereotypies, stammering) that are influenced by mental processes.

psychomotor   Psychically determined movement as opposed to one produced by an organic cause.

psychomotor activity   Observable behavior, verbal and nonverbal, in a given situation, including reaction time (speed of initiating movement or speech), speed of movement, flow of speech, involuntary movements, and handwriting (Lipowski ZJ. *Delirium: Acute Confusional States.* New York: Oxford University, 1990). It can be an important and often ignored sign of impending violence. When a person is unable to sit still (and does not have neuroleptic-induced akathisia) and paces in the emergency room or in hospital halls, the risk of violent behavior is high. Increased psychomotor activity of recent origin is a psychiatric emergency that warrants immediate intervention.

psychomotor agitation   Generalized physical and emotional overactivity in response to internal and/or external stimuli, as in hypomania.

psychomotor epilepsy   See **seizure, complex partial** (preferred term).

psychomotor retardation   Generalized slowing of physical, mental, and emotional reactions. Specifically, the slowing of movements such as walking and eye-blinking. It is frequently seen in depression.

psychoneuroendocrinology   Term coined by Ader (early 1980s) for a branch of medicine based on the interaction of the brain, the endocrine system, and the immune system. It encompasses the neurosciences, neurology, psychiatry, and endocrinology. The field has increasingly demonstrated hormonal influence on emotional processes.

psychoneuroimmunology   Term coined by Ader (1964) for the study of how psychological and emotional states influence disease resistance via interactions with the nervous, endocrine, and immune systems (Ader R [ed]. *Psychoneuroimmunology.* New York: Academic Press, 1981). Also called "psychobiology"; "psychoimmunology."

psycho-oncology   Study of the two major psychological dimensions of cancer: the psychological responses of patients to cancer at all stages of disease, and that of their families and their caretakers; and the psychological, behavioral, and social factors that may influence tumor initiation and progression.

psycho-organic syndrome   (POS) Irreversible change in neurological/psychological function that allegedly is induced by chronic occupational exposure to organic solvents alone or, more commonly, in mixtures. Manifestations include personality change, memory loss, fatigue, depression, loss of interest in daily activities, headache, forgetfulness, insomnia, difficulty in concentration, and loss of initiative. Whether long-term occupational exposure to solvents causes any permanent neurological dysfunction has been challenged by the results of recent studies (Sharp CW, Rosenberg NL. Volatile substances. *In* Lowenson JH, Ruiz P, Millman RB, Langrod JG [eds], *Substance Abuse. A Comprehensive Textbook,* 2nd ed. Baltimore: Williams & Wilkins, 1992).

psychopharmacology   **1.** Term coined by Macht (1918) for the study of the experimental effects of drugs by pharmacologists and psychologists. By 1955, the term included psychopharmacotherapy, psychopharmacological research, and even ethnopsychopharmacology. **2.** Medical specialty devoted to the study of medications used to treat psychiatric illnesses. Clinical psychopharmacology includes both the study of drug effects in patients and the expert use of drugs in the treatment of psychiatric conditions.

psychopharmacy   Specialty practiced by pharmacists in both private and public mental health care facilities.

psychophysics   Study of the psychological perception of the quality, quantity, magnitude, and intensity of physical phenomena.

psychophysiologic disorder   See **psychosomatic illness.**

psychophysiology   Research discipline composed of activity measures of the central, peripheral, and autonomic nervous systems (e.g., routine, ambulatory, or computerized electroencephalography, polysomnography, and evoked potentials).

psychosis   Illness characterized by major alterations in mental function, severe disturbances in cognitive and perceptual processes (e.g., hallucinations, delusions), inability to distinguish reality from fantasy, impaired reality testing, and disturbances of feeling and behavior. Psychoses may be acute or chronic and functional or organic. They can occur in children, adolescents, adults, and the elderly.

psychosis, atypical   One of a heterogenous mix of disorders whose one apparent common denominator is exclusion from other categories.

psychosis, brief reactive   A form of psychopathology, the essential characteristic of which is sudden onset of psychotic symptoms that last at least a few hours, but no more than 1 month. They appear shortly after one or more events that singly or in combination would have been markedly stressful to almost any individual in similar circumstances in the same culture. There is eventually a full return to the premorbid level of functioning.

psychosis, cannabis   See **cannabis psychosis.**

psychosis, epileptic   See **epileptic psychosis.**

psychosis, induced   See **folie a deux.**

psychosis, functional   Psychiatric illness not due to an organic cause. Functional psychoses are difficult to define as discrete entities and difficult to relate to each other and to other psychiatric disorders. Their intra- and interrelationships are poorly understood. They provide a good example of the wide range of results that can be obtained by applying various methods to the same basic material (Parshall AM, Priest RG. Nosology, taxonomy and the classification conundrum of the functional psychoses. *Br J Psychiatry* 1993;162:227–236).

psychosis, nonresponsive   Term coined by Neppe (1983) for any of a group of heterogeneous psychoses that do not improve with neuroleptic medication.

psychosis, postictal   Psychosis occurring after serial seizures, typically after a relatively lucid interval of 1 or 2 days. Duration is a few days and rarely longer than 2 weeks. The mental state is characterized by clouding of consciousness, disorientation, or delirium; delusions; hallucinations in clear consciousness; or a mixture of these symptoms. There is no evidence of extraneous factors (anticonvulsant toxicity; previous history of interictal psychosis; electroencephalographic evidence of minor status; recent history of head injury; alcohol or drug intoxication) contributing to the abnormal mental state.

psychosis, postpartum Acute psychotic illness manifested by hallucinations and agitation that occurs in the first month after childbirth. It is symptomatically indistinguishable from nonpostpartum affective psychoses. Some patients seem to have a schizophrenia-like illness. Relative risk is about 22 times greater than in any of the 24 months preceding delivery and 35 times greater after the birth of a first baby. Clinical data indicate that patients who have already begun to suffer a postpartum psychosis show virtually no response of growth hormone to challenge with apomorphine. Also called "puerperal psychosis."

psychosis, puerperal See **postpartum psychosis.**

psychosis, steroid Psychosis caused by hormones such as adrenocorticotropic hormone, cortisol, and prednisone. Depression is the major form of psychiatric disturbance induced by corticosteroids. About 15% of steroid psychoses are a hallucinatory-delusional psychosis. Steroid psychoses are more likely to (a) be due to high dosage (80+ mg/day of prednisone); (b) occur in women; (c) follow rapid increase in the dose or abrupt discontinuation of the drug; and (d) occur in patients with brain damage or disease of any etiology. Steroid psychoses are less frequent with prednisone and prednisolone than with cortisone and adrenocorticotropic hormone. Treatment should include gradual reduction of steroid dosage and haloperidol therapy for the psychosis.

psychosocial research Examination of the full array of behavioral, cognitive, emotional, sociocultural, and systems factors and interventions in health and disease.

psychosocial stress Information inputs that are personally meaningful and emotionally distressing for the individual, eliciting physiological changes that impose stress on homeostatic mechanisms.

psychosocial stressor Nonorganic factor (predisposing or precipitating) that may influence illness onset. Predisposing events generally occur early in life and apparently "sensitize" an individual to selected life situations. Precipitating events are changes in a person's life that closely precede and psychophysiologically influence the clinical onset of illness. These life changes are nonspecific and cover the entire spectrum of life adjustment.

psychosomatic illness Physical disorder in which emotional stress significantly influences pathogenesis.

psychostatic Term coined by Lehmann for the capacity of phenothiazine neuroleptics to prevent reemergence of psychotic symptoms (Lehmann HE. Drug treatment of schizophrenia. *In* Kline NS, Lehmann HE [eds], Drug treatment of schizophrenia. *Int Psychiatry Clin* 1965; 2:717–751).

psychostimulant Central nervous system stimulant drug that may be used for the treatment of depression and attention-deficit hyperactivity disorder and to counter physiological and drug-induced fatigue. Included are amphetamines, methylphenidate, and pemoline. Their major side effects are appetite suppression, insomnia, headaches, irritability and, with long-term use, weight loss and possibly growth retardation.

psychostimulant + haloperidol Haloperidol (HAL), either alone or in combination with a psychostimulant, can help control aggressive symptoms of a co-morbid conduct disorder (Shekine WO. Diagnosis and treatment of attention deficit and conduct disorders in children and adolescents. *In* Simeon JG, Ferguson HB [eds], *Treatment Strategies in Child and Adolescent Psychiatry.* New York: Plenum Press, 1993). Risks due to HAL must be considered before the combination is prescribed.

psychosurgery Surgical intervention to sever nerve fibers connecting one part of the brain with another or to remove or destroy brain tissue with the intent of modifying or altering severe disturbances of behavior, thought content, or mood. It also may be undertaken for the relief of intractable pain. Modern psychosurgery was introduced by the Portuguese neuropsychiatrist Moniz in 1935. It had been preceded by some operations on mental patients performed by the Swiss psychiatrist Burckhardt in 1890. After Moniz, Freeman and Watts in the United States standardized the operation, performing cuts in the connections between frontal lobe cortex and thalamus (lobotomy). Today, smaller, so-called stereotaxic operations using electrocoagulation or radium-like substances are aimed at circumscribed structures in the brain.

psychotherapy, confrontational Psychotherapy that stresses openness, honesty, and direct challenge to psychological defenses.

psychotherapy/depression Psychotherapy may produce some symptom remission in milder depressions. It is often unproductive in more severe depressions until symptoms remit spontaneously or through drug treatment or electroconvulsive therapy. It is appropriate for psychodynamic and interpersonal problems in depressed patients. Combination with drug therapies is highly desirable. See **cognitive therapy.**

psychotherapy, interpersonal Specific, semi-structured treatment that focuses on education about depression, depressive symptoms, and the patient's relation to the environment (especially his or her social functioning). It does not attempt to address issues related to underlying personality structures. It has not been widely used clinically, even though many of its essential elements can be adopted for clinical work (Klerman GL, Weissman MM [eds], *New Applications of Interpersonal Psychotherapy*. Washington, DC: American Psychiatric Press, 1993).

psychotic Characterized by gross impairment in reality testing and the creation of a new reality. The term may be used to describe a person at a given time or a mental disorder in which at some time during its course all people with the disorder are psychotic. When a person is psychotic, he or she incorrectly evaluates the accuracy of his or her perceptions and thoughts and makes incorrect inferences about external reality, even in the face of contrary evidence. The term does not apply to minor distortions of reality that involve matters of relative judgment (e.g., a depressed person who underestimates his achievements would not be described as psychotic, whereas one who believes that she has caused a natural catastrophe would be). Direct evidence of psychotic behavior is the presence of either delusions or hallucinations (without insight into their pathological nature). The term *psychotic* is sometimes appropriate when a person's behavior is so grossly disorganized that a reasonable inference can be made that reality testing is markedly disturbed. In DSM-IV, psychotic disorders include schizophrenia, delusional disorders, psychotic disorders not elsewhere classified, some organic mental disorders, and some mood disorders.

psychotic depression See **depression, psychotic.**

psychotic exacerbation Side effect of antipsychotic drugs that mimics the original psychosis. It consists of sudden, dramatic worsening of a pre-existing psychosis associated with subjective distress (terror) and extrapyramidal side effects, especially dystonia or akathisia. It usually can be rapidly reversed by treatment with an antiparkinsonian drug. There is a trend to replace the term *psychotic exacerbation* with *behavioral toxicity.* See **behavioral toxicity.**

psychotic relapse Resurgence of psychotic symptoms that ordinarily occurs over a period of days or weeks preceded by nonpsychotic prodromal period. Frequently reported nonpsychotic symptoms are insomnia, tension and anxiety, social withdrawal, and inability to concentrate. If intermittent antipsychotic drug therapy (i.e, use of an antipsychotic only during early signs of relapse) is to be successful, it must be instituted at the earliest signs of these prodromal symptoms.

psychotolysis See **rapid tranquilization.**

psychotomimetic Producer of psychosis (Osmond H. A review of the clinical effects of psychotomimetic agents. *Ann N Y Acad Sci* 1957;66:418). See **hallucinogen.**

psychotomystic See **hallucinogen.**

psychotoraxic See **hallucinogen.**

psychotropic drug Drug that affects psychic function, behavior, or experience. Included are neuroleptics, antipsychotics, antidepressants, stimulants (e.g, methylphenidate), and antianxiety agents.

psychotropic drug + alcohol The consumption of alcohol can be a significant modifier of the pharmacokinetics and pharmacodynamics of many, if not most, psychotropic drugs. Physicians should try to ascertain as accurately as possible a patient's true alcohol consumption, since the total grams of alcohol ingested per day affect the extent of the interactive changes. A past history of alcoholism also should be obtained, as the metabolism of some drugs is altered for prolonged periods after drinking has ceased. Abstinent alcoholics with affective or anxiety disorders are prone to relapse, and medications that have minimal interactions with alcohol may be preferred. Knowledge of the pharmacokinetic and pharmacodynamic changes produced by alcohol consumption may explain the therapeutic failure of a psychotropic drug and provide direction for dosage modification or substitution of one medication with another (Shoof SE, Linnoila M. Interaction of ethanol and smoking on the pharmacokinetic and pharmacodynamics of psychotropic medication. *Psychopharmacol Bull* 1991;27:577–594).

psychotropic drug, ideal The ideal psychotropic drug should be safe, reliable, selective, and effective. It should not demonstrate acute toxicity, cause allergic reactions, or elicit untoward physiological effects with chronic administration. It should not impair psychomotor performance or interact with central nervous system depressants. It should not induce physical or psychological dependence, cause withdrawal phenomena, or be lethal in large doses (Lehmann HE. Tranquilizers: clinical insufficiencies and needs. *In* Felding S, Lal H [eds], *Future Prospects of Anxiolytic Drugs in Industrial Pharmacology*, vol 3. Mt. Kisco, NY: Futura Publishing, 1979, p 403).

psychotropic drug + nicotine Smoking can significantly modify the pharmacokinetics and pharmacodynamics of many psychotropic drugs. Physicians should attempt to determine the true extent of a patient's smoking, since the number of cigarettes smoked per day affects the extent of these changes. Knowledge of the pharmacokinetic and pharmacodynamic changes produced by smoking may explain the therapeutic failure of a psychotropic medication and provide direction for dosage modification or substitution of one medication with another (Shoaf SE, Linnoila M. Interaction of ethanol and smoking on the pharmacokinetics and pharmacodynamics of psychotropic medications. *Psychopharmacol Bull* 1991;27:577–594).

Psytomin   See **perazine.**

publication bias   See **bias, publication.**

puerperal psychosis   See **postpartum psychosis.**

pulse voltametry   Assay technique, introduced in 1981, to estimate monoaminergic neurotransmitter activity in vivo by measuring the extraneuronal serotonin and catecholamine (metabolites) concentration.

"punch drunk syndrome"   See **dementia pugilistica.**

"punding"   See **compulsive foraging behavior.** This term is being replaced by *chasing ghosts* or *geeking.*

pupil, fixed   See **fixed pupil.**

purinergic   Neurons in the brain and heart that secrete purine neurotransmitters such as adenosine.

purine   Methylated dioxypurine that acts as a central nervous system stimulant (e.g., caffeine, theophylline).

"purple"   Street name for phencyclidine (PCP).

"purple heart"   Street name for phenobarbital.

"purple wedge"   Street name for dimethoxymethylamphetamine.

purpura   Discoloration caused by extravasation of erythrocytes into the skin or the mucous membranes, most often due to vascular lesions. Drugs may cause purpura by producing thrombocytopenia via a toxic or allergic mechanism, by damaging the blood vessel, or by affecting blood coagulation.

putamen   Area of the brain within the corpus striatum.

p value   See **probability.**

pyknolepsy   Obsolete term for a form of petit mal epilepsy characterized by frequent, brief interruptions in consciousness.

pyramidal system   Fibers that originate within pyramidal cells (Betz cells) in the motor cortex and pass to the spinal cord through the medullary pyramid. The system is responsible for precise and specific movements necessary for all fine and skillful muscular activities.

pyramidal tracts   Pathways of motor nerves that descend from the cortex into the spinal cord and regulate the activity of skeletal muscles.

pyrazolopyridine   Any of a class of novel anxiolytics that, like benzodiazepines, bind to omega sites associated with the gamma aminobutyric acid (GABA) receptor complex. These compounds have a chemical structure different from those of traditional benzodiazepine anxiolytics.

1-pyrimidinyl-piperazine   (1-PP) Metabolite of buspirone. The presence of higher brain concentrations of 1-PP than its parent following injection of buspirone suggests that 1-PP may contribute to buspirone's effects.

pyromania   Compulsive fire-setting. See **impulse control disorder.**

Q

"Q"   Street name for methaqualone.

QRS interval   Electrocardiographic measure of the time required for ventricular depolarization. It normally does not exceed 100 ms. Greater values indicate some degree of intraventricular conduction delay.

Q-sort   Personality assessment technique in which subjects (or someone observing them) indicate the degree to which a standardized set of descriptive statements actually describes them. The term reflects the "sorting" procedures occasionally used with the technique.

QTc   Electrocardiographic measure of the period from the beginning of ventricular depolarization to the end of ventricular repolarization (QT interval) corrected for heart rate, which is affected by age and sex. The cutoff point is 0.44 seconds. There may be considerable day-to-day variability in the QTc because of metabolic and autonomic factors. See **torsades de pointes.**

QT interval   Electrocardiographic measure that estimates an entire cycle of electrical depolarization and repolarization, which varies with age, gender and especially heart rate. It is often reported as QTc, which is "corrected" for the actual heart rate using a standard formula. Normal range is between 340 and 425 ms. Prolongation of the QT interval is frequently seen with tricyclic antidepressants (especially imipramine) and some phenothiazine neuroleptics (notably thioridazine). Prolongation of the QT interval prior to or during use of these drugs may be a reason for selecting an alternative medication.

Quaalude   See **methaqualone.**

qualitative observation   Characteristic measured on a nominal scale.

quality-adjusted life years   (QALY) Life expectancy adjusted for activity-limitation.

quality of life   That which makes life worth living.

quantitative electroencephalogram/evoked potential (EP)   (qEEG) Noninvasive technique for assessing brain function that involves quantitative computer analysis of the electroencephalographic signal. It may be used to study brain activity, including fluctuations that occur within milliseconds. It is complementary to computed tomography (CT) or magnetic resonance imaging (MRI), neurochemical evaluation, and behavioral examination. Its primary clinical value is in the evaluation of conditions that present with slow-wave abnormalities (strokes, dementias, deliriums, and intoxication). It can provide objective documentation for subjective complaints, allowing more appropriate intervention and more effective patient management. It is sensitive to the effects of many types of medication, including neuroleptics, antidepressants, anxiolytics, and anticonvulsants.

quantitative electrophysiological battery   See **electrophysiological test.**

quantitative genetics   See **genetics, quantitative.**

quantitative measuring instrument   Projective measures, rating scales, and self-report tests that serve two functions: (a) provide information to supplement data gathered about each patient; and (b) provide information on a number of content areas in a standard fashion to minimize clinician bias. When the instrument is based on a theoretical model, it can integrate information pertaining to broad and diverse areas.

quantitative observation   Characteristic measured on a numerical scale; resulting numbers have inherent meaning.

quantitative pharmacoelectroencephalogram (QPEEG)   Quantitative analysis of the effects of a drug on the human EEG in combination with certain statistical procedures. In the early human phase of drug development, it allows classification of psychotropic drugs as well as determination of dose- and time-efficacy relationships. It also allows objective, quantitative determination of a drug's cerebral bioavailability. The technique is painless, easy to apply, and the only noninvasive technique to investigate brain functions continuously, repetitively, and at relatively low cost. See **computerized electroencephalogram.**

quantitative trait loci   Measured polygenic markers.

quantitative trait loci mapping   Powerful device that uses animal models to detect genes involved in psychiatric disorders (e.g., substance abuse) because of the combined effects of multiple genes (Gora-Maslak G, McClearn GE, Crabbe JC, et al. Use of recombinant inbred strains to identify quantitative trait loci in psychopharmacology. *Psychopharmacology* 1991; 104:413–424).

quantitative variable   Object of observation that varies in manner or degree in such a way that it can be measured.

quartile   The 25th percentile or the 75th percentile, called the first and third quartiles, respectively.

quasi-experiment   Investigation in which the investigator lacks full control.

quazepam (Cetrane, Doral, Dormalin, Prosedar, Quazium, Quiedorm, Selepam, Temodal) Long half-life 1,4 benzodiazepine (BZD) hypnotic structurally different from other BZDs in that it has a trifluoroethyl group attached to the basic BZD ring. The first type II–selective BZD to be marketed, it has preferential affinity for BZD_1 receptors in neural centers, which are thought to induce sleep. Unlike other BZD hypnotics, quazepam has a low affinity for BZD_2 receptors, which are thought to affect cognitive, memory, and motor functions. Quazepam is highly lipophilic and rapidly crosses the blood-brain barrier. Peak plasma levels are reached within 2 hours of ingestion. Quazepam has two metabolites that also have hypnotic activity: 2-oxoquazepam (OQ), which is further biotransformed to N-desalkyl-2-oxoquazepam (DOQ). DOQ is identical to desalkylflurazepam, the major metabolite of flurazepam, which is not selective for BZD receptor subtypes. DOQ elimination half-life is 75 hours (longer in the elderly); accumulation occurs with repeated use. In healthy subjects, steady-state levels are reached by day 7 for OQ and by day 13 for DOQ. The long elimination half-life of quazepam and its metabolites accounts for the next-day sedation that can occur with quazepam. Evidence to date suggests that quazepam is as effective as any other BZD or non-BZD hypnotic. There is no evidence of rebound insomnia or rebound anxiety following withdrawal of quazepam after short-term administration. Schedule IV; pregnancy risk category X.

Quazium See **quazepam.**

questionnaire Predetermined set of questions used to collect data. The term is often applied to a self-completed survey instrument.

Quiedorm See **quazepam.**

Quiess See **hydroxyzine.**

quiet room Environment with reduced sensory stimuli for agitated patients who may or may not be in restraints. It is often used for a "time-out" to allow patients to calm down.

Quilonorm See **lithium.**

Quilonum See **lithium.**

quinidine Quinine derivative used in the treatment of malaria, atrial fibrillation, and paroxysmal ventricular tachycardia.

quinidine + imipramine See **imipramine + quinidine.**

quinolinic acid Neurotoxic convulsant metabolite of tryptophan that binds to and may down-regulate N-methyl-D-aspartate receptors, which are involved in normal neurotransmission, neural regeneration, memory, synaptic plasticity, long-term potentiation, and excitotoxicity. It is activated by interferon gamma and elevated with any infection, from a common rhinovirus to the mysterious lentivirus linked to acquired immunodeficiency syndrome (AIDS). It is a possible cause and marker of neurological damage in human immunodeficiency virus (HIV)-caused disease. It can also induce seizures and nerve cell death.

quinpirole (LY 171555; trans-[-]-4,4a,5,6,7,8,8a,9-octahydro-5-propyl-1H [or 2H]-pyrazolo [3,4g] quinoline dihydrochloride) Selective dopamine D_2 agonist.

R

rabbit syndrome Uncommon, late-onset neuroleptic extrapyramidal side effect manifested by rapid tremor of the lips and occasionally the jaw, resembling the chewing movements of a rabbit. It disappears during sleep, responds to anticholinergic drugs, and is reversible following neuroleptic discontinuation. It is related more to parkinsonism than to tardive dyskinesia (TD), with which it can coexist. Absence of dyskinesias of the tongue, jaw (apart from tremor), and limbs, and response to anticholinergics, differentiate the rabbit syndrome from TD (Jus K, Villeneuve A, Jus A. Tardive dyskinesia and rabbit syndrome during wakefulness and sleep. *Am J Psychiatry* 1972;129:765).

raclopride Atypical antipsychotic drug (substituted benzamide) that selectively blocks dopamine D_2 receptors. It is in early phase II testing in the United States. In acute schizophrenia, it is effective and well tolerated; it may cause fewer extrapyramidal side effects than classic neuroleptics such as haloperidol (Farde L, Wiesel FA, Jansson P, et al. An open label trial of raclopride in acute schizophrenia. Confirmation of D_2-dopamine receptor occupancy by PET. *Psychopharmacology* 1988;94: 1–7). Raclopride has been used as a radioligand for quantitative determination of D_2-dopamine receptors in the human brain using positron emission tomography (PET) (Nordstrom AL, Farde L, Wiesel FA, et al. Central D_2-dopamine receptor occupancy in relation to antipsychotic drug effects: a double-blind PET study of schizophrenic patients. *Biol Psychiatry* 1993;33:227–235). A statistically significant relationship between D_2-dopamine receptor occupancy and antipsychotic effect does not exclude the possibility of alternative mechanisms of action.

raclopride depot Long-acting depot formulation of raclopride.

radioimmunoassay (RIA) Antibody-mediated assay of a given substance. Labeled molecules of a known specific activity and concentration and unlabeled molecules of the same chemical species at an unknown concentration compete for antibody binding sites. At the completion of the reaction, the antibody-antigen complex can be removed, and the specific radioactivity of the unbound compound or the antibody-antigen complex can be determined. From this value, the concentration being measured can be determined. Experts advise against drawing definite conclusions about illicit drug use based on an RIA alone.

radiolabeled compound Compound synthesized to contain one or more radioactive atoms (usually ^3H or ^{14}C).

radioligand Ligand labeled with radioactive atoms.

radioligand binding Technique in which a tissue's receptors are saturated with an isotopically labeled ligand and examined radiographically to measure the number and sensitivity of receptors.

radiopharmaceutical See **ligand**.

radio receptor assay Blood level measurement in which neuroleptic activity is determined by tritiated spiroperidol displacement. It measures total dopamine receptor blocking activity rather than concentration of a particular neuroleptic or its metabolites. Dopamine receptor blockade strongly correlates with neuroleptic therapeutic potency.

rage reaction Outburst of unbridled rage evoked by little provocation, causing an abrupt change from a normal affective state to wild rage with a blindly furious impulse to violence and destruction. The person attacks whoever can be reached, striking, kicking, and biting; objects are smashed and clothes are torn while the person shouts and curses. The face is suffused with blood and heart rate is very rapid. The person seems to have the strength of five men in resisting attempts to be subdued. Rage reactions may be a manifestation of temporal lobe epilepsy or an episodic reaction without recognizable neurological etiology. Rage reactions with continuous violent activity must be differentiated from severe mania.

"rainbow" Street name for blue and red Tuinal capsules containing secobarbital and amobarbital.

Ramesin See **ondansetron**.

random Formal chance process in which occurrence of previous events is of no value in predicting future events. For example, the probability that a given subject will be assigned to a specified treatment group is fixed and constant (typically 0.50), but the subject's actual assignment is unknown until it occurs (Anon. Glossary of methodologic terms. *JAMA* 1992;268:43 44).

random allocation See **randomization**.

random assignment See **randomization**.

random error See **error, random**.

random mating See **mating, random**.

random sample See **sample, random**.

random variable See **variable, random**.

randomization   Chance allocation of study subjects to groups for experimental and control regimens. Its purpose is to eliminate bias due to investigator prejudice or subject preference and increase the likelihood that outcome differences follow from treatment differences, not inherent group differences. It is a fundamental requirement for safety and efficacy evaluation during phase I trials. Also called "random assignment."

randomized clinical trial   (RCT) Study in which the investigator controls the therapy received by each subject and allocates subjects randomly among study groups. RCTs compare treatment outcomes of patients randomized to one of at least two treatments. One therapy is declared better than another if overall trial results show a statistically significant difference between treatments on an outcome variable. Treatment effect is then often compared within subgroups. RCTs are the sine qua non for evaluating new treatments in humans, because they make it more likely that outcome differences can be attributed with high probability to treatment and not to selection biases inherent in uncontrolled or nonrandomized studies. Decisions to conduct large-scale RCTs are based on the expectation that results, positive or negative, will influence future treatment of patients. Results of well executed, clinically relevant RCTs published in highly visible clinical journals can have a measurable and prompt effect on medical practice patterns. RCT disadvantages include cost (it is the most expensive design), artificiality, and logistic difficulty. It also is the design most likely to provoke ethical objections, although part of the ethical basis for using it is that investigators are unsure about which treatment is better.

random trial   See **randomized clinical trial.**

range   Span of values, usually reported as the lowest value to the highest, within which data points or observation values fit.

range of distribution   Difference between the largest and smallest values in a distribution.

range, interquartile   Difference between the 25th percentile and the 75th percentile.

ranitidine   (Zantac) Histamine H_2-receptor antagonist used in the treatment of peptic ulcers. It binds to cytochrome P450 with less affinity than cimetidine and thus has fewer drug interactions. It has been reported to cause confusion, agitation, depression, hallucinations, and delirium, primarily in debilitated geriatric patients.

ranitidine + adinazolam   See **adinazolam + ranitidine.**

ranitidine + benzodiazepine   See **benzodiazepine + ranitidine.**

ranitidine + carbamazepine   See **carbamazepine + ranitidine.**

ranitidine + clozapine   See **clozapine + ranitidine.**

ranitidine + doxepin   See **doxepin + ranitidine.**

ranitidine + triazolam   See **triazolam + ranitidine.**

ranitidine + valproate   See **valproate + ranitidine.**

ranitidine + zolpidem   See **zolpidem + ranitidine.**

rank   Arrangement by order of magnitude of components in a series. Because the meaningfulness of any given rank depends on the number of components, rank is best expressed in terms of a percentile.

rank order   Set of numbers ranked from lowest to highest or vice versa (i.e., the lowest number is assigned the number 1, the next lowest is assigned 2, etc.).

ranking scale   Scale that arrays members of a group from high to low according to the magnitude of the observations, assigns numbers to the ranks, and neglects differences between members given the same rank. Also called "ordinal scale."

rank-order scale   Scale in which observations are arranged according to their size, from lowest to highest or vice versa.

rank-sum test   See **Mann-Whitney U test.**

rape   Forceful sexual assault, often classified according to the characteristics of the assault as well as the characteristics of the assailant. These include anger rape, power rape, and sadistic rape. Anger rape is marked by violence with the intention to hurt, debase, and express contempt for the victim. It is often opportunistic and usually in response to precipitating stress. Power rape is a means of exercising dominance, mastery, strength, authority, and control over the victim. There is little need for excessive physical force beyond that necessary to gain the victim's submission. Although less physically dangerous than anger rapists, power rapists may be more compulsive and engage in elaborate fantasies and plans. Sadistic rape represents the most severe pathology on the part of the offender and the most dangerous type of assault. The ritual of torturing the victim and the perception of her suffering and degradation become eroticized. As the assailant's arousal builds, so may the violence of his acts, progressing in some cases to lust murder.

rapid cycling   Occurrence of four or more episodes of affective illness per year, regardless of polarity; mixed affective states; frequent mood fluctuations without discrete intermorbid periods; 24- or 48-hour cycles of affective disturbance; or patients with recurrent unipolar depression with a prevalence of 1–6%, significantly less than the 29–53% found in bipolar patients. Affective states typically alternate between mania and depression, often with no intervening period of euthymia. Approximately 15–20% of bipolar disorder patients (the majority are women) have a rapid-cycling variation, 80% of whom have a late onset in the course of their illness. Some investigators believe that rapid cycling is caused by abnormalities in thyroid function. Rapid cyclers usually respond better to lithium augmented by valproate than to lithium alone (Calabrese R, Delucchi GA. Spectrum of efficacy of valproate in 55 patients with rapid cycling bipolar disorder. *Am J Psychiatry* 1990; 147:431–434). Carbamazepine and sodium valproate have been effective in the management of some rapid cyclers.

rapid information processing Task that assesses sustained processing and evaluation of rapidly presented information.

rapid neuroleptization Use of high-dose neuroleptic medication in the first several days of hospitalization to accelerate symptom remission and shorten hospital stay. Must be distinguished from rapid tranquilization.

rapid tranquilization (RT) Repeated use of moderate to high oral or intramuscular doses of high-potency, rapidly absorbed neuroleptic medication over 30–60 minutes with the specific goal of attenuating extreme agitation, hyperactivity, excitement, and combativeness. Core psychotic symptoms such as hallucinations, delusions, and disorganized thought usually are not affected. The procedure is time-limited (usually 1–4 hours). Intravenous RT is useful in intensive care units when use of oral or intramuscular medication is precluded. No cases of sudden death during RT with neuroleptics alone have been reported (Pilowsky LS, Ring H, Shine PJ, Battersby M, Lader M. Rapid tranquillisation. A survey of emergency prescribing in a general psychiatric hospital. *Br J Psychiatry* 1992;160:831–835). RT must be distinguished from rapid neuroleptization. Formerly called "digitalization," "neuroleptization," or "psychotolysis." See **rapid neuroleptization.**

rapport Intrapersonal relationship characterized by emotional affinity.

rapport, poor Lack of interpersonal empathy, openness in conversation, and sense of closeness, interests, or involvement with another. It is evidenced by interpersonal distancing and reduced verbal and nonverbal communication. In its extreme form, the patient appears to be completely indifferent and consistently avoids verbal and nonverbal interactions during an interview.

rate Measurement of the frequency of a phenomenon.

rate difference Absolute difference between two rates.

rating scale Instrument to record and quantify the estimated magnitude of a trait or quality for the case in question.

rating scale, observer Method of recording the judgment or opinion of an observer concerning a patient's condition. Observers (raters) should be familiar with the scale and the clinical phenomena to be observed to avoid having difficulty in recognizing mild symptoms. They should have sufficient skill and experience to be able to elicit information about symptoms inaccessible to the patient (e.g., delusions, hyperchondriasis, insight). Observer rating scales can have high validity and reliability because raters can overcome patients' deceptions and bias.

ratio Quotient of any two numbers; the number of observations with the characteristic of interest divided by the number without the characteristic. Ratios range from zero to infinity.

rational psychopharmacotherapy Prescribing practices to optimize efficacy, safety, and economics of treatment with psychoactive drugs.

rationalization Mechanism by which people devise reassuring or self-serving, but incorrect, explanations for their own or others' behaviors (DSM-IV).

Razepam See **temazepam.**

reaction formation Mechanism by which people substitute behavior, thoughts, or feelings that are diametrically opposed to their own unacceptable ones.

reaction time Period between application of a stimulus and appearance of a response.

reactive depression See **depression, reactive.**

reactive mania See **mania, reactive.**

reading disability Disturbance in reading ability. It may be due to or associated with lower scores on the Weschler Intelligence Scale for Children (WISC), higher Performance scale scores than Verbal scale scores on the WISC, slow vocabulary development, difficulty with auditory-visual integration and perception of auditory stimuli, visuoperceptual difficulties, difficulty with copying a visually presented standard pattern, neurological dysfunction, and inadequate resolution of internal and external conflicts.

rebound Recurrence of symptoms of the original disorder after discontinuation of pharmacotherapy, in a pattern and intensity greater than or equal to that experienced before drug treatment.

rebound anxiety See **anxiety, rebound.**

rebound hyperexcitability Withdrawal phenomenon characterized by increased psychophysiological dysphoria that occurs in a matter of hours or days following cessation of an illicit substance. There is a crescendo of distress during the immediate postcessation period followed by waning of symptoms over several days to weeks.

rebound insomnia See **insomnia, rebound.**

receptive dysphagia See **dysphagia.**

receptor Molecule geared to respond (bind) to specific molecular structures (ligands) such as neurotransmitters, hormones, or drugs. Most receptors are membrane-bound proteins on the outside surface of a cell. Binding results in an intracellular alteration of ion transport, enzyme activation, protein synthesis, or neurotransmitter release that eventuates in a biological response. During neurotransmission, the chemical neurotransmitter is released from the nerve ending. The neurotransmitter then diffuses across the synaptic cleft to stimulate the receptor. Receptors may be pre- or post-synaptic. Receptor-ligand interaction, or "binding," requires specific steric and topological properties to be present in the ligand that are complimentary to the binding site of the receptor. There are four general classes of receptors: photic receptors, which respond to light; mechanical receptors, which respond to mechanical stimuli; chemical receptors; and thermal receptors, which are sensitive to warm and cold. In addition, receptors are classified according to speed of response: fast ion channel linked receptors (e.g., nicotinic acetylcholine receptors) respond within milliseconds; G-protein linked receptors (e.g., muscarinic acetylcholine receptors) respond much slower (hundreds of milliseconds to seconds to minutes).

receptor affinity Probability of a drug occupying a receptor at any given moment.

receptor binding assay Type of assay performed in the same manner as a radioimmunoassay except that receptors are used to form complexes with labeled and unlabeled species instead of specific antibody molecules.

receptor blocker See **antagonist.**

receptor, dopamine See **dopamine receptor.**

receptor down-regulation Process in which receptors decrease in number and sensitivity in response to excessive transmitter availability in the synaptic cleft.

receptor, muscarinic See **muscarinic receptor.**

receptor, N-methyl-D-aspartate See **N-methyl-D-aspartate receptor.**

receptor occupancy Degree to which a drug shows affinity for a receptor. It is also determined by a drug's plasma concentration. The chemical effects of a drug are mediated by occupancy of that drug's receptor.

receptor, pharmacological Large proteins or glycoproteins on target cells with which many drugs must interact to induce their effects. Membrane receptors may be enzymes, ion channels, macromolecules coupled to enzymes or channels, or structural macromolecules. Cytoplasmic receptors include receptors for steroid hormones (glucocorticoids, sex hormones, vitamin D_3) and for thyroid hormones (T_3, T_4). Pharmacological receptors recognize and bind specific ligands. See **ligand.**

receptor, presynaptic Receptor on the presynaptic neuron (e.g., autoreceptors); agonist interactions decrease and antagonist interactions increase transmitter release as a homeostatic mechanism. See **autoreceptor.**

receptor site Chemical group that participates in drug-receptor combination and adjacent portions of the receptor that favor or hinder access of the drug to the active group.

receptor, "spare" Receptors are said to be "spare" for a given pharmacological response when the maximal response can be elicited by an agonist at a concentration that does not result in occupancy of all available receptors. Spare receptors are not qualitatively different from nonspare receptors. They are not hidden or unavailable, and when occupied they can be coupled to response. The spare receptor concept should help explain how the sensitivity of a cell or tissue to a particular concentration of agonist may depend not only on the affinity of the receptor for binding an agonist but also on the total concentration of receptors (Bourne HR, Roberts JM. Drug receptors and pharmacodynamics. *In* Katzing BG [ed], *Basic and Clinical Pharmacology*, 4th ed. Norwalk, CT: Appleton & Lange, 1989).

receptor subtypes Receptors with which a given neurotransmitter interacts are not identical, but exist in a variety of biochemically and functionally distinct subtypes. Receptor subtypes are usually encoded by separate genes, suggesting a possible link between synaptic activity, gene expression, and the regulation of the activity of receptor subtypes. For example, serotonin (5-HT) receptors are divided into three large receptor families: 5-HT_1, 5-HT_2, and 5-HT_3, based on differing affinities and functional effects of selective ligands. These families are also distinguished by their second messenger systems (i.e., mechanisms that mediate intracellular response to receptor activation). Hence, the 5-HT_1 receptor has been subdivided into four further subtypes, denoted by subscripts A–D.

receptor up-regulation Process in which the number and sensitivity of receptor sites increase in response to short supply of a neurotransmitter in an attempt to maintain usual levels of neurotransmitter function.

recessive Characteristic of a phenotypic trait expressed only when the responsible gene is homozygous.

recessive gene See **gene, recessive.**

recessive inheritance See **inheritance, recessive.**

recessive trait See **trait, recessive.**

rechallenge Retreatment, either accidental or deliberate, with a drug that has caused an adverse drug reaction (ADR). Accidental retreatment occurs when an ADR may not have been recognized as the result of treatment and subsequent doses of the drug are taken. The most common form of rechallenge is when the ADR occurs soon after the drug is taken and wears off before the next dose is due, so that the patient experiences the ADR each time the drug is taken. Deliberate rechallenge depends on several factors, the most important of which is avoidance of permanent harm. If the ADR is type A, rechallenge starts with a small dose that is gradually increased until the first sign of the ADR appears. Response to rechallenge is a major factor in the determination of drug causality of an ADR. This approach may enable the patient to benefit from the drug without any adverse effects. Type B ADRs are not rechallenged, because any subsequent reaction may be much more serious than the first and could have a fatal outcome. See **adverse drug reaction; adverse drug reaction, type A; adverse drug reaction, type B.**

recidivism Tendency to experience relapse of a disease, symptom, or behavioral pattern.

recklessness Any attitude or behavior that potentially endangers a person's physical health, safety, or life.

recognition site See **binding site.**

recombinant DNA that consists of two parts: a vector for propagation and an insert (often mammalian DNA).

recombinant DNA 1. DNA molecule manipulated in the lab for a specific purpose. 2. Research techniques to manipulate and clone these DNA molecules.

recombination Formation of new combinations of linked genes by crossing over between their loci.

recombination fraction Measure of the genetic distance between two loci. It is expressed as the frequency of recombination observed in offspring between parental combinations of the alleles at the loci being examined.

recombination, homologous Formation of new combinations of genes as a result of crossing over between homologous (i.e., corresponding in such ways as structure, position, origin) chromosomes.

recombination, somatic Any process by which genes are reorganized within the genome of any somatic cell. Change is heritable only in the daughter cells of the cell in which recombination occurs. A clone with a genotype different from the rest of the organism is established.

record linkage Bringing together of data from several sources on the same individual (e.g., linking a private physician's records with hospital records on the same patient).

recovering alcoholic See **alcoholic, recovering.**

recreational drugs/hypertensive crisis Rise in systolic blood pressure with a diastolic pressure above 120 mm Hg that may occur among users of crack cocaine, amphetamines, phencyclidine (PCP), lysergic acid diethylamide (LSD), and diet pills. It is an emergency requiring immediate but gradual blood pressure reduction (lowering mean arterial pressure by approximately 25% over a period of several minutes to hours). Blood pressure reduction in this situation is best accomplished by sodium nitroprusside, labetalol, phentolamine, or oral nifedipine or clonidine. Precipitous lowering of blood pressure may cause end-organ ischemia or infarction. Complications of untreated or inadequately treated hypertensive crisis often include seizures, stroke, myocardial infarction, or encephalopathy.

recreational illicit drug use Stage of substance abuse development that follows the experimental phase. The recreational user continues to use the chemical substance, usually because of a desire to repeat the psychoactive effects recalled from the experimental stage. See **experimental illicit drug use.**

recurrent brief anxiety See **anxiety, recurrent brief.**

recurrent brief depression See **depression, recurrent brief.**

recurrent unipolar depression See **depression, recurrent unipolar.**

"red" Street name for secobarbital.

"red and blue" Street name for amobarbital + secobarbital.

"red barrel" Street name for dimethoxymethylamphetamine.

"redbird" Street name for secobarbital.

"red devil" Street name for secobarbital, amphetamines, or any red pill.

"red doll" Street name for secobarbital.

"red haired lady" Street name for sinsemilla, a potent variety of marijuana.

"red leb" Street name for hashish.

"reds and blues" Street name for the blue and red capsules of Tuinal, which contain secobarbital and pentobarbital.

redistribution Passage of a drug out of the brain into the systemic circulation, from which it is distributed into tissues elsewhere in the body. The effects of many psychoactive drugs are terminated not by elimination but by redistribution. Redistribution of a drug to adipose tissue can prolong drug effects because the drug remains there longer, especially in an obese person. Since the elderly often have an increase in body fat content, drugs may have longer-lasting effects in them.

reduced drug clearance Phenomenon often associated with old age in which, after any specific dose of a given drug, an elderly person has a greater area under the plasma concentration-time curve (AUC) than a younger control subject. Thus, the elderly person receiving therapy at a specific dose and rate will have a higher steady-state plasma concentration and the possibility of greater drug response than the young control subject.

reduced haloperidol (RHAL) Major active metabolite of haloperidol that is persistent in plasma and interesting pharmacologically because it can be converted back to the parent drug by oxidative enzymes. The oxidation pathway is reportedly affected by the cytochrome P450IID6 isoenzyme. RHAL has about one-fifth to one-tenth of the dopamine-blocking potency of haloperidol. Therapeutic monitoring of HAL may not be sufficient because RHAL, which has negligible affinity to dopamine receptors, may act as a prodrug or reservoir for HAL. The ratio of RHAL/HAL can be used as an index of the activity of enzymes that metabolize HAL. Asian patients have much lower RHAL/HAL ratios than non-Asians. The lower RHAL/HAL ratio in Asians, caused either by a slower rate of reduction of HAL or a more active oxidation process converting RHAL back to HAL, could significantly affect HAL clearance and result in a higher level of HAL. Also called "hydroxyhaloperidol."

reduced penetrance See penetrance, reduced.

"reefer" Street name for a marijuana cigarette.

referred care Referral of a patient by one health professional to another with more specialized qualifications or interests. There are two levels. Secondary care is usually provided by a broadly skilled specialist such as a general surgeon, general internist, or obstetrician. Tertiary care is provided by a subspecialist such as an orthopedic surgeon, neurologist, or neonatologist (Anon. Glossary of methodologic terms. *JAMA* 1992;268:43-44).

refractory Characterized by lack of response or resistance to a therapeutic intervention.

Regibon See diethylpropion.

regimen Program, including pharmacotherapy, that regulates aspects of one's life style for a therapeutic purpose.

regional cerebral blood flow (rCBF) Amount of blood flowing in a region of the cortex is positively correlated to the metabolic activity of that region. Imaging of rCBF by scintigraphy with inhaled xenon-133 can be combined with psychological testing during the measurement of blood flow, allowing assessment of the effects of cognitive activation procedures on blood flow in specific regions of the cortex. In contrast to positron emission tomography (PET) and single photon emission computed tomography (SPECT), rCBF imaging exposes the patient to less radiation, is less expensive, and measures blood flow to the cerebral cortex and not deep brain structures that can be imaged by PET and SPECT.

regional pharmacokinetics See pharmacokinetics, regional.

Regitine See phentolamine.

Reglan See metoclopramide.

regressed pedophile See pedophile, regressed.

regression analysis Given data on a dependent variable y and one or more independent variables (x_1, x_2, etc.), the process of finding the "best" mathematical model (within some restricted class of models) to describe y as a function of the x's, or to predict y from the x's. It is performed to estimate how much one variable changes with another variable. The most common form is a linear model; in epidemiology, the logistic and proportional hazards models are also common.

regression coefficient If the linear regression of y or x is $y = mx + k$, m is the regression coefficient.

regression line Mathematical expression that allows prediction of the value of one variable if the value of the other variable is known. When data are fitted to a straight line, it is called an *estimated regression line.*

regression, linear Regression method in which a linear relationship or transformed linear relationship is constructed between a set of variables.

regressive electroshock therapy See electroshock therapy, regressive.

regulator gene See gene, regulator.

regulatory domain Region of a gene that controls its rate of transcription.

regulatory protein See protein, regulatory.

regulatory sequence Region of DNA responsible for regulating transcription of the corresponding gene. Sequences are generally found "upstream" of the start of transcription and contain specific recognition sequences for any number of DNA binding proteins. The major types of regulatory sequences are called *promotors* and *enhancers*.

rehabilitation Restoration of an optimal state of health by medical, psychological, social, and peer group support for a chemically dependent person and significant others.

reinforcement Process by which a specific stimulus appears to increase the probability that a particular behavior will occur. Reinforcement or "reward" by drugs is thought to depend on the same neuronal circuits that give rise to reinforcement by food, water, sex, and other factors essential for survival of the individual and the species. Reinforcement operates in the social drinker (or drug user) as well as in the addict, yet the former is able to abstain voluntarily.

reinforcement, negative Process by which behavior is strengthened if it leads to reduction of an unpleasant event. In cocaine users, for example, negative reinforcement is used to try to establish the behavior of repetitively self-administering cocaine or crack as a strong, enduring response.

relapse 1. Re-emergence of an illness that improved spontaneously or because of treatment. 2. Alcohol- or drug-dependent behavior in an person who previously achieved and maintained abstinence for a significant time beyond the period of detoxification. 3. Loss of therapeutic gain (deterioration during treatment discontinuation as compared with improvement during the therapeutic trial). Relapse is characterized by worsening of symptoms compared with the end of treatment.

relapse prevention Pharmacological strategy in which treatment is administered for the estimated duration of an acute episode to prevent symptom re-emergence.

relative effectiveness Efficacy, toxicity, and cost of a new drug as compared with alternative agents (Freund DA, Evans D, Henry D, Dithers R. The implications of the Australian guidelines for the United States. *Health Aff [Millwood]* 1992;11:202–206). There is a well recognized need for studies of relative effectiveness, but they are generally more complex than those now required for drug approval. They would entail larger samples, more outcome data, and longer follow-up. Requiring studies of relative effectiveness could substantially prolong premarketing tests (Ray WA, Griffin MR, Avorn J. Evaluating drugs after their approval for clinical use. *N Engl J Med* 1993;329:2029–2032).

relative (or receiver) operating characteristic analysis (ROC) Examination of the ability of a screening instrument to discriminate cases and noncases across the whole spectrum of morbidity by plotting sensitivity against the false-positive rate for all possible cutoff points.

relative potency study Study to determine the dose of a standard drug necessary to obtain an effect equivalent to that achieved by a unit dose of a test drug. Relative potency bioassays compare doses of a test drug with doses of a standard. A common design is the "four-point relative potency assay," consisting of two doses each of test and standard. A placebo may be unnecessary in such trials because demonstration of a statistically significant positive slope for the dose-response curves establishes assay sensitivity. A placebo is necessary, however, to estimate the lowest dose at which a specific efficacy might be detected.

relative risk See **risk, relative.**

release hallucination See **hallucination, release.**

Relefact TRH See **protirelin.**

reliability Extent to which the same test or procedure will yield the same result over time or with different observers. It is a desirable property of a personality inventory or trait scale. The most commonly reported reliabilities are (a) test-retest reliability (correlation between the first and second test of a number of subjects); (b) split-half reliability (correlation within a single test of two similar parts of the test); and (c) inter-rater reliability (agreement between different individuals scoring the same procedure or observations).

reliability, internal Degree to which scores for any randomly selected subtest of a test item correlate with the score obtained for all items.

reliability, inter-rater Measure of the degree of agreement by two independent raters witnessing an event. It is expressed as a percentage to which a test score obtained by one psychometrician equals the score obtained if the test is administered by another person. "Successful" can be arbitrarily defined as equal to or greater than a certain percentage. If the percentage is "successful," the results can confidently be considered an accurate description of the event.

reliability, intrarater Consistent reproducibility of measurements made by the same person at two different times.

reliability, observer Degree of agreement between two or more observers on some measure of behavior when they observe the same series of events independently.

reliance Continuing need for therapeutically prescribed doses of a medication. For example, surveys indicate that approximately

11% of patients prescribed a hypnotic still use it after 1 year under a doctor's prescription.

REM   Sleep stage characterized by rapid eye movement.

REM density   Frequency of eye movements per unit of time during sleep-stage rapid eye movement (REM).

REM latency   Time from sleep onset to rapid eye movement (REM) onset. Shortening of REM latency frequently occurs in narcolepsy and depression. Lengthening of REM latency after the start of antidepressant drug therapy may indicate that the drug will be effective in that patient.

REM rebound   Lengthened and increased frequency and density of rapid eye movement (REM)-sleep episodes that occur in subjects deprived of REM sleep for several nights once the depriving influence is removed.

REM sleep   Stage of sleep during which dreaming occurs. It is characterized by low amplitude pattern in the electroencephalogram, associated loss of muscle tone, and presence of rapid eye movements. It accounts for one-fourth to one-fifth of total sleep time. The first rapid eye movement (REM) period occurs about 90 minutes after falling asleep. REM periods recur throughout the night at approximately 90-minute intervals and lengthen as the night goes on.

REM sleep behavior disorder   Sleep-related behavior disorder that usually occurs in middle-aged or elderly men. It is associated in up to 40% of cases with organic brain disease (usually stroke or dementing illness) or with REM rebound due to prior REM sleep suppression by alcohol or drugs. Normally, a state of flaccid paralysis of the principal antigravity muscles prevails during REM sleep; muscle tone is regained when one cycles out of REM sleep and is lost on re-entering REM sleep. For reasons that are unclear, people with REM sleep behavior disorder retain normal muscle tone during REM sleep or a portion of it and can therefore act out their dreams. Patients may walk or be quite active; some have injured themselves badly, and there have been reports of assault through attempted strangulation and other violent behavior. REM sleep behavior disorder is distinct from sleepwalking, which occurs during deeper sleep stages and is not accompanied by suppression of voluntary muscle control. Tricyclic medications may suppress REM sleep behavior disorder in some patients, but more reliable results are reported with low doses of clonazepam. Low doses of other benzodiazepines also may be effective. Without sleep electroencephalographic evaluation, it may be difficult to distinguish REM sleep behavior disorder from

paroxysmal hypnogenic dystonia (Sehenck CH, Hurwitz TD, Mahowald MW. REM sleep behavior disorder. *Am J Psychiatry* 1988;145:652–654).

REM sleep episode   See **REM sleep.**

REM sleep intrusion   Brief interval of rapid eye movement (REM) sleep appearing out of its usual position in the non–rapid eye movement (NREM)-REM sleep cycle. It may be the appearance of a single dissociation component of REM sleep (e.g., eye movements or "drop-out" of muscle tone) rather than all REM sleep parameters.

REM sleep/monoamine oxidase inhibitor (MAOI)   MAOIs, especially in high dosages, suppress rapid eye movement (REM) sleep. Patients maintained on high MAOI dosages for depression completely lose REM sleep for long periods without apparently experiencing any ill effects. However, when the MAOI is discontinued, there may be marked REM rebound, often associated with vivid dreaming or nightmares for 1–2 weeks.

REM sleep onset   **1.** Commencement of an REM sleep episode. **2.** Shorthand term for a sleep-onset REM sleep episode.

REM sleep percentage   Proportion of total sleep time constituted by sleep-stage rapid eye movement (REM).

REM sleep/psychostimulant   Dextroamphetamine, methylphenidate, pemoline, and cocaine have similar effects on sleep. At first they markedly prolong sleep latency, reduce total sleep time, markedly prolong rapid eye movement (REM) sleep latency, and reduce the total amount of REM sleep. With continued use, at least partial tolerance develops with less effects on REM sleep.

REM sleep rebound   See **REM rebound.**

REM sleep/tricyclic antidepressant (TCA)   TCAs, with the exception of trimipramine, reduce rapid eye movement (REM) sleep, but to a lesser extent than monoamine oxidase inhibitors (MAOIs) do. Average REM sleep reduction with TCAs is about 30% below the normal level of REM sleep, whereas MAOI inhibition of REM sleep is greater and, at higher doses, can be complete. See **REM sleep/monoamine oxidase inhibitor.**

remission   Partial or complete abatement of the symptoms and signs of a disorder or disease.

remoxipride   (Roxiam) (RMX) Atypical benzamide antipsychotic drug that is a relatively potent and selective inhibitor of central postsynaptic dopamine (D_2) receptors and binds to sigma binding sites. It has less impact on nigrostriatal dopamine pathways and consequently fewer extrapyramidal symptoms (EPS) than standard antipsychotics. Half-life is 4–7 hours. RMX (150–600 mg/day) is as effective as haloperidol in preventing symptom recurrence after treatment of acute episodes, and significantly more effective than placebo in preventing relapse in chronic schizophrenia. RMX also may be effective in reducing both positive and negative psychotic symptoms. It has been co-administered with neuroleptics (e.g., chlorpromazine, thioridazine, haloperidol, clopenthixol) in treatment-resistant chronic schizophrenics with improvement in some and without causing significant new side effects. Long-term treatment trials indicate that RMX is effective, well tolerated, and generally safe. After marketing in Europe, cases of RMX-caused aplastic anemia led to the withdrawal worldwide of RMX by its manufacturer.

remoxipride + alcohol   Co-administration adds to the decremental effects of alcohol (Matilla MJ, Mattila ME, Korno K, et al. Objective and subjective effects of remoxipride, alone and in combination with ethanol or diazepam, on performance in healthy subjects. *J Psychopharmacol* 1988;2:138–149). Alcohol has no effects on remoxipride pharmacokinetics (Yisak W, von Bahr C, Farde L, et al. Drug interaction studies with remoxipride. *Acta Psychiatr Scand* 1990;82[suppl 358]:58–62).

remoxipride + biperiden   Neither drug influences the other's pharmacokinetics or pharmacodynamics (Yisak W, von Bahr C, Farde L, et al. Drug interaction studies with remoxipride. *Acta Psychiatr Scand* 1990;82[suppl 358]:58–62).

remoxipride C   (R-CR) Controlled-release formulation of remoxipride that produces a smoother plasma concentration profile than regular remoxipride, suggesting the possibility of once-daily dosage.

remoxipride + diazepam   Diazepam (DZ) has no effect on remoxipride pharmacokinetics, but co-administration may augment DZ's decremental effects on cognitive and neuromotor functions (Yisak W, von Bahr C, Farde L, et al. Drug interaction studies with remoxipride. *Acta Psychiatr Scand* 1990;82[suppl 358]:58–62; Matilla MJ, Mattila ME, Korno K, et al. Objective and subjective effects of remoxipride, alone and in combination with ethanol or diazepam, on performance in healthy subjects. *J Psychopharmacol* 1988;2:138–149; Mattila KN, Mattila ME. Effects of remoxipride on psychomotor performance, alone and in combination with ethanol and diazepam. *Acta Psychiatr Scand* 1990;82[suppl 358]:54–55).

remoxipride + imipramine   Neither drug influences the other's pharmacokinetics, nor does remoxipride influence the pharmacokinetics of the imipramine metabolites desipramine and 2-hydroxydesipramine.

remoxipride + phenytoin   Pharmacokinetic studies indicate no interaction.

remoxipride + warfarin   Remoxipride has no significant effect on the pharmacokinetics of either the S(–) or the R(+) warfarin, and no effect on the prothrombin time of warfarin (Yisak W, von Bahr C, Farde L, et al. Drug interaction studies with remoxipride. *Acta Psychiatr Scand* 1990;82[suppl 358]:58–62).

renal clearance (drug)   Volume of blood from which unchanged drug is removed by the kidneys in a given unit of time. For a water-soluble drug (e.g., lithium) or for water-soluble active metabolites (e.g., hydroxycyclic antidepressants), it is the rate at which the kidney removes these substances. Renal clearance is proportional to the volume of distribution of a drug and inversely related to its elimination half-life.

repeatability   See **reproducibility.**

repeated-measures design   Study design in which subjects are measured more than once.

replication   Repeating an experiment or survey several times to confirm the findings, increase precision, and obtain a closer estimation of sampling error.

replication fork   Site within a replicating duplex DNA molecule at which synthesis of complementary strands is occurring.

replicative segregation   Separation of heteroplastic mitochondrial DNAs (mtDNAs) in a progenitor cell toward homoplastic mtDNA in descendant cells during mitotic or meiotic replications.

reporter gene   See **gene, reporter.**

representative sample   See **sample, representative.**

repression   Mechanism by which a person is unable to remember or be cognitively aware of disturbing wishes, feelings, thoughts, or experiences (DSM-IV).

reproducibility   Characteristic of scientific inquiry whereby an observation or finding should be repeatable in different settings, including different geographical settings, different study designs, and different populations. A finding reported only once should be considered tentative since there may have been an error committed in the study that is not apparent to either the investigator or the reader. Also called "repeatability."

rescue medication   Nonstudy drug that can be administered to acutely ill participants in a double-blind study if, during the early days of the trial, the study medication does not sufficiently alleviate the patient's acute symptoms and thereby endangers the patient's welfare.

"rescuer"   Individual who encourages or passively permits an alcoholic to persist in drinking.

research design　Procedures and methods predetermined by the investigator that will be adhered to in the conduct of a research project.

research, experimental　Investigations in which individuals are subjected to some manipulation or predetermined condition. If the experimental factor is a drug, the subjects may be randomly assigned to treatment groups, measured at baseline before treatment, and measured again after treatment intervention.

research, quasi-experimental　Investigations in which treatment groups represent samples from different predefined populations. A study comparing the efficacy of neuroleptic drug therapy in paranoid versus nonparanoid schizophrenics is an example of this type of quasi-experimental design.

reserpine　(Serpasil) Alkaloid isolated from the rauwolfia plant that has antihypertensive and tranquilizing/antipsychotic effects. Along with chlorpromazine, reserpine contributed to the evolution of modern psychopharmacology in the early 1950s. Reserpine acts by depleting stores of catecholamines. In some patients, reserpine may be depressogenic because it depletes catecholamines at critical sites in the central nervous system. Its use in hypertension has declined because of the advent of newer effective antihypertensives, and it is rarely used as an antipsychotic. Pregnancy risk category C.

reserpine/breast milk　Reserpine is excreted in breast milk and may cause side effects in infants.

reserpine + levodopa　Co-administration may result in hyperexcitability, mania, or memory impairment.

reserpine + monoamine oxidase inhibitor (MAOI)　Co-administration may result in hyperexcitability, mania, or memory impairment.

reserve medication　Medication prescribed for a disturbed patient in whom episodic behavioral deterioration occurs before the therapeutic action of a primary drug takes effect. For example, in the early stages of lithium therapy for acute mania, a benzodiazepine such as lorazepam or clonazepam may be added as a reserve medication if behavioral deterioration is a real risk.

residual　Difference between the predicted value and the actual value of the outcome variable in regression.

residual sedation　Propensity of a hypnotic medication to produce sedation-related performance decrements after the usual sleep period. The degree of performance decrement is related to the drug's hypnotic potency, dose, and half-life. The higher the dose, the greater the degree of impairment and the longer its duration. Use of a drug with a short half-life does not necessarily protect against residual sedation. Half-lives of hypnotic drugs range from 3 to 100 hours.

resolution　Degree of molecular detail on a physical map of DNA, ranging from low to high.

resolving phase　In schizophrenia, period of varying length between manifestation of acute psychotic symptoms and development of the residual state. Patients are demoralized by the realization that they have been psychotic and are overwhelmed by interpersonal, social, employment, and economic problems.

respiratory alkalosis　See **alkalosis.**

respiratory disturbance index　(RDI) Number of apneas (obstructive, central, or mixed) plus the number of hypopneas per hour of total sleep time as determined by all-night polysomnography.

respiratory dyskinesia　See **dyskinesia, respiratory.**

respite care　Limited stays in a nursing home or hospital, not for direct therapeutic benefit for the patient, but to allow the caregiver rest and/or diversion. Respite care is a must for many caregivers for demented patients.

response rate　Number of completed or returned survey instruments divided by the total number of persons surveyed; usually expressed as a percentage.

Restas　See **flutoprazepam.**

restless legs syndrome　(RLS) Neurological syndrome characterized by an unpleasant creeping sensation that effects primarily the legs, appears only at rest, and induces an irresistible urge to keep the limbs in motion. It resembles neuroleptic-induced akathisia, which patients experience on lying down and attempting to fall asleep. It has been observed in association with heredity, pregnancy, poliomyelitis, infectious diseases, avitaminosis, different types of anemia, diabetes, and certain drugs (e.g., prochlorperazine, lithium, mianserin). Psychotropic drugs that may alleviate RLS include levodopa, bromocriptine, carbamazepine, and clonazepam. In one study, levodopa (100–600 mg/day) plus benserazide or carbidopa demonstrated therapeutic efficacy that generally persisted for at least 2 years without serious toxic effects. The side effect most commonly reported was transient insomnia. Investigators concluded that levodopa should be considered the drug of choice for RLS because of its long-term efficacy and minimal toxicity (Kaplan B, Mason NA. Levodopa in restless legs syndrome. *Ann Pharmacother* 1992;26:214–216) Also called "Ekbom's syndrome"; "tachyathetosis."

Restoril　See **temazepam.**

restraint Measures (e.g., four-point leather cufflets, cold-wet packs and camisoles, seclusion rooms) to prevent individuals from injuring themselves or others.

restriction endonuclease See **restriction enzyme.**

restriction enzyme Enzyme that recognizes short stretches of DNA (4–8 base pairs in length) in a sequence-specific manner and cleaves the DNA at specific points in a double-stranded DNA chain. Each restriction enzyme recognizes a different sequence of bases. Restriction enzymes are useful in recombinant biology. Also called "restriction endonuclease."

restriction enzyme cutting site Specific nucleotide sequence of DNA at which a restriction enzyme cuts the DNA. Some sites occur frequently in DNA, others much less frequently.

restriction fragment length polymorphism (RFLP, RIFLIP) Molecular genetic tool for direct analysis of the human genome to find undiscovered genes that predispose to genetic diseases. Basic strategy, using recombinant DNA biotechnology, is to find a DNA sequence closely associated and/or linked with a particular disease of interest. RFLPs are small variations in DNA that serve as signposts pointing out the direction to specific genes. They are scattered throughout the chromosomes, some very close to genes. When a disease is passed from generation to generation, a specific marker close to the responsible gene is also passed. Genetic linkage methods to locate genes on human chromosomes have been greatly improved by the application of RFLPs as genetic markers because they are more abundant than classic trait and protein markers. A map of the human genome (with an average interval of 10 cm between adjacent markers) is now available (Donis-Keller H, Green P, Helms C, et al. A genetic linkage map of the human genome. *Cell* 1987;51:319–337). Application of RFLP technique to heritable disorders such as Huntington's chorea has led to localization, identification, and cloning of genes responsible for a wide variety of somatic diseases. The knowledge may identify certain high-risk groups and lead to development of pharmacological agents to treat the diseases. Also called "DNA marker."

rest tremor See **tremor, rest.**

retardation, mental See **mental retardation.**

reticular formation Brain stem region consisting of the tegmental parts of the medulla, pons, and midbrain. It plays a major role in sleep and wakefulness. The reticular activating system is located in the reticular formation.

retinitis pigmentosa Degeneration of the retina due to deposition of abnormal amounts of pigment. It can occur as an isolated, usually inherited, disease of gradual onset in childhood. It can also be provoked by certain medications (e.g., thioridazine), especially in high doses.

retrocollis Hyperextension of the neck muscles with a resulting posterior orientation of the head. See **dystonia, cervical; dystonia, torsion.**

retrograde amnesia See **amnesia, retrograde.**

retropulsion Gait disturbance seen in Parkinson's disease, due to basal ganglia dysfunction, in which the patient falls backward rapidly with minimal ability to regain balance, sometimes sustaining injuries.

retrospective falsification Adding false memories to true memory. Added memories are not always entirely false, but just detractors.

retrospective research Use of informants, typically parents, as the source of data on the developmental history of adult patients. Major problems are the need to rely on the informant's long-term memory, the accuracy and details of which have decreased with time; and the possible bias of the informant's recall.

retrospective study See **case control study.**

retrotransposon Transposable element that enables RNA to be copied into DNA, a mechanism whereby a portion of the genome might become transposable: first the portion is transcribed into RNA, then a fresh DNA counterpart is produced for reinsertion elsewhere in the genome.

retroviral shuttle vector Construct with origins for replication for two hosts so that it can be used to carry a foreign sequence in prokaryotes or eukaryotes.

retrovirus Class IV eukaryotic virus that uses an RNA molecule as its genome. This RNA genome directs the synthesis of a DNA molecule that ultimately acts as the template for making mRNA. If the retrovirus contains cancer genes, the cell it infects is transformed into a tumor cell. Several human retroviruses are known. One causes a form of leukemia, and another—human immunodeficiency virus (HIV)—attacks particular lymphocytes (T_4 cells), resulting in acquired immunodeficiency syndrome (AIDS).

retrovirus vector Virus equipped to incorporate itself into host DNA. It is "ecotropic" if the host is limited to rodents or "amphotropic" if the host range is wide, including humans.

Rett's syndrome X-chromosome neurological disorder that progressively leads to decreased brain and body organ growth with autistic behavior, severe dementia, seizures, and early death.

reuptake Taking back into the presynaptic nerve terminal most of the neurotransmitter after receptor site binding, where a portion is metabolized by the enzyme monoamine oxidase (MAO), either MAO-A or MAO-B.

Revanil See **lisuride.**

reverse genetics See **genetics, reverse.**

reverse tolerance See **tolerance, reverse.**

reverse transcriptase Enzyme contained in retroviruses that converts viral RNA into a proviral DNA copy that becomes integrated into the host cell DNA.

reversible dementia See **pseudodementia.**

reversible dyskinesia See **dyskinesia, reversible.**

reversible inhibitor of monoamine oxidase type A (RIMA) Monoamine oxidase inhibitor that can be displaced by tyramine and thus requires no dietary restrictions because it does not cause hypertension. RIMAs may be efficacious in the treatment of both endogenous and nonendogenous depressive states. The most extensively studied RIMA is moclobemide (marketed in Europe). Others under investigation are befloxatone, brofaromine, and toloxatone.

reversion In genetics, a phenomenon that occurs when crosses between true-breeding varieties produce offspring that resemble a remote ancestor more than either parent.

Revimine See **dopamine HCl.**

rhabdomyolysis Breakdown of muscle cells in certain toxic conditions such as neuroleptic malignant syndrome, malignant hyperthermia, heatstroke, trauma, prolonged immobilization, seizures, strenuous exercise, and exposure to various drugs and toxins. The breakdown liberates muscle cell contents, some of which (e.g., creatinine phosphokinase [CPK]) can be detected in blood tests as a marker. Others can damage the kidneys and contribute generally to potentially fatal events. Laboratory changes include elevated urine myoglobin and serum muscle enzymes (e.g., CPK, aldolase, lactate dehydrogenase, aspartate aminotransferase) and abnormalities suggesting impaired renal function (e.g., serum creatinine and blood urea nitrogen abnormalities).

"rhapsody" Street name for methylenedioxymethamphetamine (MDMA).

Rhythm See **rimazafone.**

ribonucleic acid (RNA) Chemical substance involved in cellular protein synthesis. Its structure is coded for by DNA and may play a role in memory. There are three varieties: messenger RNA (the template upon which polypeptides are synthesized), transfer RNA (soluble RNA, which in collaboration with ribosomes brings activated amino acids into position along the messenger RNA template), and ribosomal RNA (rRNA, a component of the

ribosomes that serves as a nonspecific site of polypeptide synthesis).

ribosomal RNA (rRNA) Type of ribonucleic acid that lines up amino acids in the ribosomes to form proteins according to a particular sequence. All ribosomes have at least two rRNAs (small and large). The mitochondrial ribosomes have rRNAs of the relative sizes of 12S and 16S.

ribosome Complex structure composed of RNA and protein that is the site of protein synthesis.

Ridazin See **thioridazine.**

Rifadin See **rifampin.**

Rifampin (Rifadin) Complex macrocyclic antibiotic that inhibits mycobacterial DNA-dependent RNA polymerase. It is distributed throughout the body and cerebrospinal fluid. It is rapidly eliminated in the bile, and enterohepatic circulation ensues. Rifampin is indicated in the treatment of tuberculosis in combination with at least one other antitubercular drug. It is a recognized enzyme inducer that can affect the metabolism of other drugs.

rifampin + clozapine See **clozapine + rifampin.**

rifampin + diazepam Rifampin can hasten clearance of diazepam (DZ) and its metabolites, resulting in altered clinical or enhanced adverse effects. Dosage adjustment may be necessary during co-administration, and DZ dosage may have to be adjusted after rifampin discontinuation.

rifampin + methadone Co-administration may significantly lower methadone plasma levels and necessitate increasing the methadone dose to avert narcotic withdrawal symptoms (Kreck MJ, Gatjahr CL, Garfield JW, et al. Drug interactions with methadone. *Ann N Y Acad Sci* 1976;281:350–371).

RIFLIP See **restriction fragment length polymorphism.**

right ear advantages (REAs) In dichotic listening tests, two auditory stimuli are presented simultaneously, one to each ear. The tests yield consistent and reliable REAs for language-related stimuli, despite the fact that there are minor ipsilateral auditory afferent pathways (Wexler BE, Halwes T. Increasing the power of dichotic methods: the fused rhymed words test. *Neuropsychologia* 1983;21:59–66).

rigidity Increased muscle tone with increased resistance to passive movement. It is a common symptom of parkinsonism. It also may be manifested by cogwheeling, which is due to tremor superimposed on the rigidity.

rigidity, decerebrate State of continuous muscle spasticity due to damage to descending motor tracts. It occurs after various types of severe brain trauma and as the terminal state in several degenerative disorders, including the sphingolipidoses.

rigidity, lead pipe   Type of plastic rigidity seen in certain forms of parkinsonism and in the neuroleptic malignant syndrome. The stiffness resembles that of a lead pipe.

rigidity, severe   Rigidity manifested by dysphagia, immobility, decreased respiratory excursion, and/or myonecrosis (rhabdomyolysis), which in turn may cause serious medical complications (severe dehydration, electrolyte disturbances, pulmonary embolus secondary to deep vein thrombosis and/or venous stasis, aspiration pneumonia, and myoglobinuria with subsequent renal failure and its complications). See **rhabdomyolysis.**

RIMA   See **reversible inhibitor of monoamine oxidase type A.**

rimazafone   (Rhythm) Benzodiazepine marketed in Japan.

Riootril   See **clonazepam.**

risk   Expected frequency of occurrence of an undesirable effect of a drug or chemical.

risk, acceptable   Therapeutic intervention in which anticipated benefits are judged to outweigh potential risks.

risk assessment   Estimation of the likelihood of adverse effects resulting from exposure to a specific therapy.

risk, attributable   (AR) Rate of a disorder in exposed subjects that can be attributed to the exposure. It is derived by subtracting the rate (usually incidence or mortality) of the disorder of the nonexposed population from the corresponding rate of the exposed population. AR estimates require data from large population-based studies.

risk/benefit ratio   Results of a risk benefit analysis, expressed as the ratio of risks to benefits.

risk difference   See **excess risk.**

risk factor   Association between a characteristic of an individual, group, or the environment and increased probability of the occurrence of a particular disease or disease-related phenomenon. Identification of risk factors is important for research, public health, and clinical practice. Theoretically, risk factors offer clues to disease etiology (e.g., increased risk of affective illness among relatives of patients with bipolar disorder suggests possible genetic transmission). Identifying risk factors provides a basis for preventive and public health control measures. It is often possible to develop effective public health programs for a disorder when risk factors are known, even though exact etiology may be unknown. Clinicians can use risk factors to identify high-risk patients, determine critical periods in their clinical course, and institute appropriate medical intervention (Klerman GL. Clinical epidemiology of suicide. *J Clin Psychiatry* 1987;48[suppl 12]:33–38).

risk management   Treatment strategy with four components: (a) systematic identification of risks by internal initiatives such as incidents reported or record screening, or by detailed examination of externally initiated data such as complaints or negligence claims; (b) prevention of adverse incidents using clinical protocols, changes in technology or organization, and continuing education; (c) minimization of claims by rapid and sympathetic reactions to adverse outcomes of treatment; and (d) active management of claims, ensuring that evidence was collected promptly and informed decisions were taken about whether to resist the claim or settle.

risk, population attributable   Overall incidence of a disorder minus the incidence among those not exposed to it.

risk, population proportional attributable   Overall incidence of a disorder minus incidence among those not exposed to it divided by the overall incidence.

risk, proportional attributable   Incidence among persons exposed to a risk factor minus the incidence among those not exposed divided by the incidence of those exposed.

risk, relative   Ratio of the incidence of a disorder in those exposed to a risk factor to the rate of those not exposed to a risk factor.

Risperdal   See **risperidone.**

risperidone   (Risperdal) (RIS) Benzisoxazolyl atypical antipsychotic that is a centrally acting, potent serotonin $(5\text{-HT})_2$ and dopamine D_2 antagonist. It is postulated that blockade of these receptors can overcome the two major limitations of classic neuroleptic treatment: relative lack of effect on negative symptoms of schizophrenia and induction of extrapyramidal symptoms (EPS). RIS also substantially antagonizes $alpha_1$, $alpha_2$, and histamine (H_1) receptors. It is a potent and selective lysergic acid diethylamide (LSD) antagonist, but lacks LSD agonist properties and affinity for cholinergic receptors. Orally administered RIS is rapidly absorbed; plasma level peaks at 1 hour. It is extensively metabolized via the cytochrome P450IID6 system. Its major metabolite, 9-hydroxyrisperidone (9-OH), has pharmacological activity equivalent to that of RIS; the most pharmacologically relevant measurement is that of the active moiety (the sum of RIS plus 9-OH). In most patients, steady-state is reached within 1 day for RIS and within 5 days for the moiety. Terminal half-life of about 24 hours may permit twice- or even once-daily administration. After intravenous administration, RIS has a two-compartment disposition profile. It has a linear pharmacokinetic profile in doses between 0.5 and 25 mg, with mean peak and trough plasma concentrations increasing proportionately with increasing doses. Open and controlled trials have confirmed efficacy in the treatment of positive, negative, and affective symptoms of schizophrenia. It reduces florid symptoms in acute and chronic schizophrenic patients. It also may alleviate depression and anxiety. It has been evaluated in schizoaffective disorder, depressive type, and in psychotic major depressive disorder. Most patients derive some benefit, especially with regard to psychotic symptoms. Clinical outcomes in these patients suggest that the combination of 5-HT$_2$ and D$_2$ blocking properties results in therapeutic expansion of antipsychotic actions and minimization of neurological side effects. RIS has rapid onset of therapeutic action, often within the first treatment week and usually by the second, followed by progressive improvement without significant dosage increments. In acutely agitated patients, a benzodiazepine may be safely added. RIS initiation should be titrated over 3 days to dosages of 2, 4, and 6 mg/day, respectively; the latter dosage should be maintained as long as possible. A minimum of 1–2 weeks should be allowed to evaluate response to this dose, unless there is clinical need to adjust it. When necessary, small dosage increments/decrements of 1 mg twice a day are recommended. Most patients respond to 4–8 mg/day. Over 300 patients have been treated with RIS for over 12 months. It is well tolerated, and clinical improvement has been maintained. Benzodiazepines, chloral hydrate, and antiparkinson drugs have been co-prescribed without adverse interactions. Side effects are infrequent and generally mild, and they rarely cause treatment termination. Those causing termination include agitation, dizziness, EPS, fatigue, increased salivation, nausea, and somnolence. Although RIS is not anticholinergic, dry mouth and blurred vision, and in one case urinary retention, have occurred. Doses higher than 10 mg/day may cause difficulty in concentrating, sedation, lassitude, reduced sleep duration, and, very infrequently, erection and ejaculatory disturbance and gait disturbances. Dose-proportional weight gain, comparable to or greater than that associated with neuroleptics, may occur. Because RIS has D$_2$ receptor affinity, it may evoke early-onset EPS. Incidence is low with 4–8 mg/day and increases with doses above 10 mg/day. RIS has rarely worsened EPS and may reduce pre-existing symptoms (e.g., tremor, rigidity). It has not worsened tardive dyskinesia and in some cases has reduced its signs and symptoms. In some patients, RIS has had an antidyskinetic effect without increasing parkinsonian symptoms, such as may happen with conventional antipsychotics (Ayd FJ Jr. Risperidone (Risperdal): a unique antipsychotic. *Int Drug Ther Newsl* 1994;29:5–12).

risus sardonicus Painful-looking transverse smile caused by powerful contraction of the muscles around the mouth and the platysma of the neck. It may occur with an acute dystonic reaction.

Ritalin See **methylphenidate.**

ritalinic acid Metabolite of methylphenidate with poor lipid solubility. It may be pharmacologically inactive.

Ritalin-SR See **methylphenidate SR.**

ritanserin Highly selective, long-acting serotonin (5-HT)$_{1C}$/5-HT$_2$ receptor antagonist that is a pure and selective antagonist of lysergic acid diethylamide (LSD) discrimination in animals. Pretreatment with ritanserin attenuates anxiogenic response to intravenous metachlorphenylpiperazine (mCPP) in normal volunteers (Seibyl JP, Krystal JH, Price LH, et al. Effects of ritanserin on the behavioral, neuroendocrine, and cardiovascular responses to mCPP in healthy human subjects. *Psychiatr Res* 1991;38:227–236). Ritanserin produces dose-related increases in slow-wave sleep (Idzikowski C, Mills FJ, James RJ. A dose-response study examining the effects of ritanserin on human slow wave sleep. *Br J Clin Pharmacol* 1991;31:193–196). It improves fatigue, inhibition, lack of energy, and lack of drive in patients with anxious and/or depressive disorders. Ritanserin has been shown to be effective in the treatment of elderly depressed patients, with minimal side effects. It reduces depression severity and improves disturbed sleep and anxiety in patients with dysthymia, and has been used beneficially to treat generalized anxiety. There is some evidence that the addition of ritanserin to neuroleptic treatment can lessen persistant psychotic symptoms, attenuate extrapyramidal movement disorders, and affect neuroleptic-induced akathisia. Clinical testing has shown ritanserin to be superior to the antiparkinson drug orphenadrine in the treatment of neuroleptic-induced parkinsonism. It has had no deleterious effect on tardive dyskinesia. There is some evidence that ritanserin effectively decreases alcohol intake in chronic alcoholics without harmful side effects.

ritanserin + haloperidol In preclinical studies, co-administration did not modify the effect of haloperidol (Lappalainen J, Hietala J, Koulon M, Syvalatiti E. Neurchemical effects of chronic co-administration of ritanserin and haloperidol: comparison with clozapine effects. *Eur J Pharmacol* 1990;190:403–407). In chronic, primarily type II schizophrenia, co-administration produced improvement, especially in negative symptoms.

ritual   Elaborate, systemized compulsive behavior.

Rivotril   See **clonazepam.**

RNA   See **ribonucleic acid.**

RNA, virus   Type of messenger RNA (mRNA) that codes genetic information for virus protein in vitro and codes for more than one distinct protein.

RO 15-4513   Partial inverse benzodiazepine (BZD) agonist with a profile that is a mirror image of that of partial agonist BZDs. It acts as a selective BZD antagonist of alcohol, blocking alcohol effects on the gamma aminobutyric acid (GABA)-stimulated chloride channel. Animal studies indicate that it produces a dose-dependent suppression of alcohol intake. It is being used to probe·mechanisms that underlie the behavioral, anesthetic, and anticonvulsant properties of alcohol.

RO 16-6028   See **bretazenil.**

"roach"   Street name for chlordiazepoxide or the butt of a marijuana cigarette.

"robby"   Street name for Robitussin A-C.

Robinul   See **glycopyrrolate.**

robust   Not very sensitive to departures from the assumptions on which a statistical test or procedure is strictly predicted.

"rock"   Street term for a prepackaged, ready-to-use form of freebase cocaine that is inexpensive and has been widely available on the streets in the United States. "Rock" describes the crystalline appearance of the cocaine. It is sold in vials or foil packets and is then smoked in a pipe. Also called "crack." See **"crack."**

"rock candy"   See **"rock."**

"rocket fuel"   Street name for phencyclidine (PCP).

"rockhead"   Street term for crack abusers who smoke crack quite often in "crack houses" or "rock houses," where they not only purchase crack but also rent pipes. Rockheads may stay in rock houses for days until their money is exhausted, many prostituting themselves to support further drug use.

"rock house"   Place where cocaine users gather to smoke "crack rocks."

Ro-Diet   See **diethylpropion.**

Rohypnol   See **flunitrazepam.**

"roid"   Street name for anabolic steroids.

"roid rage"   Street term for the marked aggression and homicidal violence that can be evoked by misuse of anabolic steroids.

rolipram   Phosphodiesterase-inhibitor under investigation in Europe as an antidepressant. Results have been sufficiently encouraging to stimulate evaluation of similar compounds in the United States. Rolipram primarily affects the second messenger system by enhancing cyclic adenosine monophosphate transduction.

root mean squared deviation   See **standard deviation.**

"rope"   Street name for marijuana.

Roscommon Family Study   Epidemiological, controlled family study of severe mental illness conducted in a rural county in western Ireland (Kendler KS, McGuire M, Gruenberg AM, et al. The Roscommon Family Study, I: methods, diagnosis of probands, and risk of schizophrenia in relatives. *Arch Gen Psychiatry* 1993;50:527–540).

"rose"   Street name for central nervous system stimulants, usually amphetamine.

Roxiam   See **remoxipride.**

roxindole   (5-hydroxy-3-[4-phenyl-1,2,3,6-tetra-hydropyridil-(1)-butyl]-indol) Presynaptic dopamine D_2 autoreceptor agonist with serotonin (5-HT) reuptake inhibiting and 5-HT_{1A} agonist actions. It is being tested in Europe for treatment of positive and negative schizophrenia symptoms. Preliminary results indicate no beneficial effects for positive symptoms, although negative symptoms (e.g., affective flattening, depressed mood, alogia, avolition) are improved. Roxindole has not caused extrapyramidal symptoms, suggesting that it is an atypical neuroleptic.

rubidium   Alkali element from the Ia group of the periodic table of the elements. Closely related to lithium and potassium, it has been used experimentally in the treatment of depression with questionable therapeutic efficacy. It has a long biological half-life (50–60 days), and its preferential accumulation in intracellular fluid suggests potentially uncontrolled toxicity if safe dosage limits are inadvertently exceeded (Fieve RR, Jameson KR. Rubidium: overview and clinical perspective. *Mod Probl Pharmacopsychiatry* 1982;18:145–163; Meltzer HL. A pharmacokinetic analysis of long-term administration of rubidium chloride. *J Clin Pharmacol* 1991;31:179–184).

"rum fits"   See **alcohol withdrawal.**

"run"   Pattern of severe amphetamine abuse in which large doses are injected intravenously or smoked at relatively short intervals for as long as 6 or more days. Runs were popular in the 1960s among amphetamine abusers called "speed freaks," and are comparable to the cocaine runs or cocaine bingeing of the 1980s and 1990s. See **cocaine bingeing; cocaine run.**

"rush"   1. Street term for an over-the-counter product containing isobutyl nitrite that is used as a sex-enhancing drug. 2. Orgasm-like reaction, followed by a feeling of mental alertness and marked euphoria, that amphetamine, opiate, and cocaine abusers produce by self-administered intravenous injections of the abused drug. Total daily doses as high as 4,000 mg of amphetamine have been reported. Cocaine abusers experience a "rush" after "kicking" or "booting."

Russell's sign Abrasions and scars on knuckles of patients with bulimia nervosa caused by insertion of the fingers into the throat to stimulate the gag reflex and induce vomiting.

S

Sabril   See **vigabatrin.**

Sabrin   See **vigabatrin.**

saccade   See **saccadic eye movements.**

saccadic eye movements   (SEMs) Involuntary, rapid (up to 600–700°/sec) conjugate changes of gaze that enable the eye to center a target of interest onto the fovea. SEMs are measured by electro-oculography. They may be intensified during hallucinations and other psychotic phenomena in schizophrenia. Saccade velocity is known to be under the control of the gamma aminobutyric acid (GABA)-A receptor as it decreases with increasing doses of benzodiazepines.

S-adenosyl-L-methionine   (SAM) Active form of methionine that acts as a methyl donor and is involved in many metabolic pathways. It has beta-adrenergic and dopamine receptor agonist activity. It has been reported to be an effective antidepressant (Baldessarini RJ. Neuropharmacology of S-adenosyl-L-methionine. *Am J Med* 1987;83:95–103). Its mood-elevating effects were discovered in 1970 during an investigation of its use in schizophrenia. In double-blind studies, its antidepressant effects have been equal to or better than those of amitriptyline, imipramine, and clomipramine. It has been responsible for precipitation of mania and hypomania (Carney MWP, Chary TKN, Bottigieri EH, et al. The switch mechanism and the bipolar/unipolar dichotomy. *Br J Psychiatry* 1989;154:48–51).

sadism   Sexual deviation in which sexual pleasure is derived from the infliction of pain on others.

sadomasochism   Co-existence of sadism and masochism in the same individual.

safety profile   History of a drug's safety record.

sai/b$_{max}$ Measure of the sensitivity of the individual receptor to activation. It provides an index of changes in receptor complex responsivity, such as supersensitivity or subsensitivity.

salbutamol   Beta$_2$-adrenergic agonist used in the treatment of bronchial asthma with potential antidepressant properties that might be attributable to its capacity to increase the level of free plasma L-tryptophan or to down-regulate beta receptors.

salience   Number of household users of a substance and the degree of children's involvement in parental substance-taking behavior; a measure of salience has been found to be the best predictor of both expectations of use and actual abuse of alcohol. Salience also may be a strong predictor of children's cigarette and marijuana use (Kaminer Y. Adolescent substance abuse. *In* Frances RJ, Miller SI [eds], *Clinical Textbook of Addictive Disorders.* New York: Guilford Press, 1991, pp 320–346).

saliva drug concentration   Method of measuring drug concentration that has several advantages over the use of blood. The procedure is noninvasive, samples are easier to obtain, and frequent monitoring may be more acceptable to the patient. Because the concentration of protein-bound drug is negligible, determination of salivary drug concentration should be a good measure of the concentration of free drug, the most pharmacologically active form. However, the saliva/plasma concentration ratio varies over time and may depend on dosage schedule, absorption rate, in vivo drug release, and methods used to induce salivation. Significant correlations between salivary and plasma concentrations have been shown for chlorpromazine, haloperidol, diazepam, and lithium. In spite of the potential advantages of obtaining salivary drug concentrations, only three studies comparing haloperidol concentrations in saliva and blood have been reported. These document that saliva measurements of haloperidol and of reduced haloperidol are useful alternatives to plasma concentrations in monitoring maintenance haloperidol treatment (Dysken MW, Johnson SB, Holden L. Haloperidol and reduced haloperidol in saliva and blood. *J Clin Psychopharmacol* 1992;12:186–190).

salivary cortisol levels   Measurement of salivary cortisol levels that can be substituted for plasma cortisol in clinical studies in which the dexamethasone suppression test and hypercortisolemia are evaluated.

salsolinol   Combination of dopamine and acetaldehyde. It has opiate actions on opiate receptors. Salsolinol has been recovered in the cerebrospinal fluid of alcoholics. Salsolinol forms from a reaction of acetaldehyde and dopamine when ingested alcohol shifts acetaldehyde derived from ethanol.

sample   Selected subset of a population that may be random or nonrandom, representative or nonrepresentative. Also, an observation or a collection of observations gathered in a well-defined way.

sample, cluster random   Sampling process in which the population is divided into heterogeneous subpopulations (clusters) that should approximate each other in terms of interested variables. A random sample is then chosen from the clusters.

sample, haphazard Selection of a group of persons without concern as to whether they represent the population.

sample, nonprobability Sample selected in such a way that how a subject is selected is unknown.

sample probability Probability of an individual in the population being sampled. If the probability is well defined, the sample itself is called "probability sample."

sample, random Group of subjects selected so that each member of the population from which the sample is derived has an equal probability of being chosen for the sample.

sample, representative Sample similar in important ways to the population to which the findings of a study are generalized.

sample size Number of subjects in a trial. If the results of experimental investigations are to be convincing and statistically sound, the size of the sample chosen to represent the population must be sufficient to detect a clinically meaningful result at a certain level of statistical significance. Sample size is influenced by patient availability, expected dropout rate, definition of meaningful response by the basic study design, and the chosen method of data analysis. There are ways to calculate the desired sample size to reach such results.

sample size, small Low number of study subjects. Small sample size reduces statistical power and increases the risk of type II error.

sample, stratified random Sample consisting of random samples from each subpopulation in a population. It is used so the investigator can be sure that each subpopulation is appropriately represented in the sample.

sampled population Population from which the sample is actually selected.

sampling bias See **bias, sampling.**

sampling distribution Frequency distribution of the statistic for many samples. It is used to make inferences about the statistic from a single sample.

sampling method In population-based studies, random sampling is the ideal method of avoiding selection bias and producing a sample typical of a study population. In other studies, nonrandom sampling may be adequate.

"sandos" Street name for lysergic acid diethylamide (LSD).

Sanorex See **mazindol.**

Sansert See **methysergide.**

Sarisol No. 2 See **butabarbital.**

Saroten See **amitriptyline.**

satellite, chromosomal Small mass of chromatin attached to the short arm of the human acrocentric chromosome by a thin stalk (secondary constriction).

"sativa" Street name for marijuana (*Cannabis sativa*).

satyriasis See **compulsive sexual behavior.**

Saurat See **fluoxetine.**

savoxepine New tetracyclic cyano-dibenzoxapinoazepine derivative undergoing clinical trials in Europe. It is an antipsychotic drug exerting a potent and preferential high affinity for limbic dopamine D_2 receptors. In positron emission tomography (PET) studies, savoxepine occupied basal ganglia D_2 receptors much like classic neuroleptics do. Multicenter double-blind trials comparing savoxepine with haloperidol have provided data suggesting that savoxepine is an effective antipsychotic, causing fewer extrapyramidal side effects than haloperidol (Borison R, Haverstock S, Pathiraja A, Diamond B. Savoxepine as an atypical neuroleptic. *Biol Psychiatry* 1993;33:126A).

saw-tooth waves Form of theta rhythm that occurs during rapid eye movement sleep and is characterized by a notched appearance in the wave-form. The waves occur in bursts lasting up to 10 seconds.

scale of measurement Degree of precision with which a characteristic is measured. It is generally categorized into nominal, ordinal, and numerical scales.

"scat" Street name for heroin.

scatchard plot Relationship between applied concentrations (expressed in molar units) and the ratio of bound to free drug observed after binding of a drug, hormone, or neurotransmitter to its receptor. The x intercept reflects the number or density of binding sites (B_{max}), and the negative inverse of the slope of the line reflects the affinity for receptor (K_D). The relationship is typically used to display data from in vitro binding studies. Although the relationship initially was proposed to model binding properties of simple proteins by Scatchard in the late 1940s, it was not applied to drug- or ligand-binding experiments until 1967.

scatterplot Two-dimensional graph, ordinate and abscissa, displaying the relationship between two characteristics or variables.

SCH 23390 D_1 receptor antagonist that is an important tool for investigating the psychopharmacology of dopamine receptors. Tests in patients have shown that it lacks an acute antipsychotic effect, does not cause side effects, but does improve choreic symptoms, suggesting that D_1 receptor blockade has potential in the management of Huntington's chorea and other involuntary movement disorders.

SCH 39166 Ligand developed for D_1 dopamine receptor studies.

Scheffé's procedure   Statistical method for comparing means following a significant F test in analysis of variance. It can be used to make any comparisons among means, not simply pairwise. It is the most conservative multiple-comparison method. Also called "post hoc testing," which is used for similar purposes as Bonferroni testing.

schizoaffective psychosis   Disorder in which there is a combination of manic or major depressive symptoms along with symptoms of schizophrenia. DSM-IV includes the following criteria: (a) a disturbance during which, at some time, there is either a major depressive or a manic syndrome concurrent with symptoms that meet the A criteria of schizophrenia; (b) during an episode of the disturbance, there have been delusions or hallucinations for at least 2 weeks, but no prominent mood symptoms; (c) symptoms that meet the criteria for a mood episode are present for a substantial portion of the total duration of the active and residual periods of the illness; and (d) the disturbance is not due to the direct physiological effects of a substance (e.g., a drug of abuse, a medication) or to a general medical condition. About 10% of psychotic patients have a mixture of schizophrenic and affective symptoms, and it may be impossible to determine which is the predominant type. Although most patients make a complete recovery, a tendency to recurrence is typical of this group.

schizoid personality disorder   Personality disorder that makes the person withdrawn and socially isolated with few, if any, friends or social relationships. A percentage of schizophrenics have a premorbid schizoid personality.

schizophrenia   (SCZ) Group of psychoses, the course of which is at times chronic, at other times marked by intermittent attacks, and which can stop at any stage, but does not permit a full recovery. The term "schizophrenia" was devised in 1911 by Eugen Bleuler to replace the more awkward phrase "dementia praecox," which Kraepelin had earlier used to describe a similar group of psychotic disorders. The most common, devastating, and perplexing of the psychotic disorders, SCZ's cardinal symptoms include delusions, hallucinations, disordered cognition, and various deficits in thinking and relating to one's environment. SCZ is manifested by a "loosening of associations" and by illogical ideas, markedly inappropriate or blunted emotional responses, extreme ambivalence, and autistic withdrawal in social relations into internal fantasy. If not resolved within the first 2 years, SCZ tends to run a deteriorative course and to endure, at least in some facets, for the pa-

tient's lifetime. In the later stages, the patient may appear as a mere shell of his or her former existence, lacking a wide range of basic intellectual, emotional, social, and communicational skills. When SCZ occurs, the patient's relationship to his or her environment is radically transformed. Cognitive disabilities range widely from the elementary (such as perceptual processes) to the moderately complex (such as problem solving and verbal memory) to the highly complex (such as social perceptions, social schema, and communication). These different levels of cognitive abilities could be considered relatively independent subsystems or modules. Alien thoughts and sounds may invade the consciousness, strange ideas may take hold, and uncontrolled feelings of anger, fear, suspicion, and anxiety may dominate. Attention is usually diverted while arousal level is heightened, as though one's system is operating in constant overdrive. The ability to think clearly and rationally and to exercise sound judgment is affected, and normal social relations are typically strained as the patient becomes increasingly preoccupied and seclusive. SCZ patients often show cardinal symptoms of a depressive illness. In addition to sad mood and increased suicide risk, they frequently exhibit lack of interest in their environment, loss of energy, amotivation, and disturbed sleep. Cognitively, they can be so disabled that a significant number could be characterized as having dementia or a mental deficiency. Consequently, diagnostic confusion with mental retardation becomes a problem. SCZ is a lifelong illness for which there is no cure; like diabetes, it requires maintenance drug therapy to guard against relapse. In an untreated state, schizophrenia may fluctuate in intensity. Two patients with a confirmed diagnosis may bear little resemblance to one another, and even to themselves over the course of time. Patients can differ markedly from one another, not only in their clinical presentation, but also in their outcome with treatment. Among researchers as well as among clinicians, diagnostic concepts of SCZ differ greatly, and several sets of diagnostic criteria are widely used. Current perspectives posit a neurodevelopmental disorder, with abnormalities in brain morphology reflecting not cerebral deterioration, but a failure to attain subtle but fundamental aspects of cerebral structure and function because of etiological events occurring early in embryonic/fetal life. Postmortem and in vivo brain imaging studies have demonstrated morphological abnormalities in SCZ patients, including enlargement of the lateral and third ventricles, enlargement of the cortical sulci of the frontal, temporal, and parietal regions, and reduction in the volume of the medial temporal lobe structures. See **schizophrenia, genetics.**

schizophrenia/alcohol　In a retrospective study of 132 patients with schizophrenia or schizoaffective disorder, patients who abused alcohol were significantly more likely to relapse to a level requiring hospitalization during the course of a year than patients who did not (Frisella ME, Dufresne RL. Alcohol abuse increases relapse in outpatients with schizophrenia. *ASHP Midyear Clinical Meeting* 1993; 28:P77).

schizophrenia/deficit symptoms　Negative symptoms in schizophrenia that present as enduring traits. They include apathy and avolition. They are present during and between episodes of positive symptom exacerbation, can be observed regardless of the patient's medication status, and are not specifically responsive to anticholinergic drugs or antipsychotic drug withdrawal. Deficit symptoms are at the root of the poor social and work functions that characterize patients with chronic schizophrenia. See **schizophrenia/ negative symptoms.**

schzophrenia, disorganized type　In DSM-IV, a type of schizophrenia characterized by (a) incoherence, marked loosening of associations, or grossly disorganized behavior; (b) flat or grossly inappropriate affect; and (c) failure to meet the criteria for catatonic type.

schizophrenia, dopamine hypothesis　Hypothesis that functional overactivity at some point in mesolimbic dopamine systems is, if not the primary metabolic defect, responsible for the generation of positive psychotic symptoms (Crow TJ. Molecular pathology of schizophrenia: more than one disease process? *Br Med J* 1980;280:66–68). According to this hypothesis, D_1 receptor blockade is essential for a drug to have antipsychotic potency, and antipsychotic potency and D_2 blockade are linearly related in vitro. The demonstration of a therapeutic response to clozapine with significantly reduced D_2 blockade confirms doubts about a simple linear relationship between D_2 receptor antagonism in vivo and clinical efficacy. See **dopamine hypothesis.**

schizophrenia, first-rank symptoms　First described by Kurt Schneider in 1959, these are (a) thought insertion (experience of thoughts being put into one's mind); (b) thought broadcasting (experience of one's thoughts being known to others); and (c) feelings of passivity (experience of emotions or specific bodily movements or specific sensations being caused by an external agency or being under some external control). Psychiatrists in general often agree about the first-rank symptoms

of schizophrenia. It seems wise, therefore, to give these diagnostic priority in the absence of any external diagnostic validators.

schizophrenia, late-onset　Form of schizophrenia that first appears late in life and in which degenerative brain disorder may be implicated. An increasing number of patients are being treated with very-low-dose depot neuroleptics (3 mg of fluphenazine decanoate; 5–10 mg of haloperidol decanoate). Also called "paraphrenia."

schizophrenia, nuclear　Core symptoms of schizophrenia rather than the associated or social factors.

schizophrenia/negative symptoms　Symptom cluster in schizophrenia that depicts absence of normal function. Symptoms include alogia, affective flattening, anhedonia/asociality, depressed appearance, avolition/apathy, psychomotor retardation, and attentional impairment. Negative symptoms tend to be persistent and less responsive to neuroleptic treatment. They are associated with poor social functioning and computed tomographic evidence of cerebral atrophy. They generally predict a poor outcome. It has been hypothesized that they are largely unresponsive to neuroleptic treatment because they are manifestations of irreversible structural changes in the central nervous system (Crow TJ. Molecular pathology of schizophrenia: more than one disease process? *Br Med J* 1980;280:66–68). Negative symptoms frequently co-exist with positive symptoms. Negative symptoms of variable severity and duration are present to at least some extent in all schizophrenic patients, but are not unique to schizophrenia. Although clinical presentation may be similar, signs and symptoms may vary in etiology, course, and treatment response between patients, and even within patients, depending on illness stage and other factors. An extensive body of evidence supports the hypothesis that negative symptoms (e.g., poverty of speech and flattened affect) are associated with substantial brain abnormalities (e.g., increased ventricular/brain ratio and extensive cognitive impairment). In schizophrenia, it may be difficult to distinguish negative symptoms from depressive symptoms and drug effects, particularly bradykinesia. Negative symptoms as a manifestation of drug effects or secondary to psychotic phenomena are more likely to confuse assessment during acute psychotic episodes. Some (blunted affect and emotional withdrawal), but not all (stereotyped thinking and passive-apathetic social withdrawal), negative symptoms may be neuroleptic side effects. This may partly explain why negative symptoms occurring in acute schizophrenia may differ from persistent features of chronic schizophrenia in terms of their correlation with other clinical variables and prognostic value. Characteristic symptoms of negative schizophrenia (blunted affect, poverty of speech, motor reduction, and cognitive deficits) are also hallmarks of Parkinson's disease (Kay SR. *Positive and Negative Syndromes in Schizophrenia.* New York: Brunner/Mazel, 1991). Current (1994) thinking postulates that negative symptoms are manifestations of regional dopamine (DA) hypofunction involving mesofrontal DA projections, which occur frequently in depression as well as in schizophrenia (Chatuwedi SK, Rao GP, Mathai PJ, et al. Negative symptoms in schizophrenia and depression. *Ind J Psychiatry* 1985;27:237–241). See **schizophrenia/deficit symptoms.**

schizophrenia/serotonin hypothesis of Hypothesis that serotonin (5-HT)$_2$ receptor abnormalities have a primary role in the etiology of schizophrenia (SCZ). The serotonin hypothesis predated the dopamine hypothesis of SCZ, but was ignored for many years while the dopamine hypothesis was tested. The serotonin hypothesis was revised because of increased knowledge of the 5HT receptor chemistry, development of specific 5HT receptor agonists and antagonists, and efforts to understand the mechanism of action of the atypical antipsychotics. To date, no conclusive evidence supports the serotonin hypothesis.

schizophrenia/substance abuse Studies of patterns of substance abuse among schizophrenia patients (SCZs) have disclosed three patterns: (a) no substance abuse; (b) abuse of alcohol and cannabis; and (c) polysubstance abuse. Most studies have shown that substance-abusing SCZs tend to be young patients of low socioeconomic status who, compared with SCZs who do not abuse substances, have fewer previous hospitalizations, better premorbid personalities, and a greater likelihood of a family history of drug abuse. Other studies have found that SCZs who abuse substances have increased levels of disorganized speech, hostility, and depression; are more likely to present management problems in the hospital, in the community, and at home; have higher levels of family disturbance and noncompliance with medication; have higher rates of hospital readmission; and had their first psychiatric hospitalization at an earlier age. SCZs with substance abuse also tend to have more problems obtaining meals, managing finances, and maintaining stable housing. Other studies have suggested that SCZs who abuse substances show higher levels of sociability and fewer negative symptoms. It also has been shown that SCZs who abuse alcohol and/or cannabis, and those who are polysubstance abusers, have more depressive symptoms, but not more psychotic symptoms, than those who are not substance abusers (Cuffel BJ, Heithoff KA, Lawson W. Correlates of patterns of substance abuse among patients with schizophrenia. *Hosp Community Psychiatry* 1993;44:247–251).

schizophrenia, type I Classification proposed by Crow in 1980 for schizophrenia characterized by positive symptoms. The type I syndrome is thought to reflect an increase in dopaminergic function and to respond well to antipsychotics. Computed tomography (CT) scans are usually normal (Crow TJ. Molecular pathology of schizophrenia: more than one disease process? *Br Med J* 1980;280:66–68).

schizophrenia, type II Classification proposed by Crow in 1980 for schizophrenia characterized by negative symptoms, such as social and emotional withdrawal, apathy and loss of drive, restricted and blunted affective responsivity, narrowing of ideation, and poverty of speech. The type II syndrome is thought to be associated with structural abnormalities in the brain (cortical atrophy or ventricular enlargement), chronic course, asocial premorbid functioning, and a limited response and/or poor tolerance to antipsychotics. Some patients have computed tomography (CT) scan abnormalities. Chronic schizophrenics with a predominant type II syndrome seem to show serotonin (5-HT) abnormalities or to have a positive response to agents that influence 5-HT, thus suggesting the possible role of 5-HT dysfunction in type II schizophrenia (Crow TJ. Molecular pathology of schizophrenia: more than one disease process? *Br Med J* 1980;280:66–68).

schizophrenia/genetics Genes are now accepted as being important in the etiology of schizophrenia (SCZ). However, any adequate model for transmission must be compatible with current knowledge of neurodevelopment. It is evident from advances in the neuroimaging and neuropathology of SCZ that abnormalities exist in the temporal lobes of many schizophrenic patients and that these abnormalities originate late in the fetal development of the brain. Furthermore, several lines of evidence suggest that the pathogenic processes in SCZ are active many years before the onset of florid psychotic symptoms, during the vulnerable period when the brain is still developing.

schizophrenia, refractory Currently (1994) defined by researchers as lack of significant improvement following adequate trials with doses of at least 1,000 mg of chlorpromazine equivalents for at least 6 weeks with three or more antipsychotics from at least two chemical classes (e.g., phenothiazines, butyrophenones, or thioxanthenes) in the preceding 5 years (Kane JM, Honigfeld S, Singer J, et al. Clozapine for the treatment-resistant schizophrenic. *Arch Gen Psychiatry* 1988;45:789–796). Clinicians use less stringent criteria: trials with two or three classes of antipsychotic drugs for at least a month each, with doses of at least 500 mg of chlorpromazine equivalents (Kane JM. The current status of neuroleptic therapy. *J Clin Psychiatry* 1989;50:322–328). Some clinicians define refractory schizophrenia as (a) failure to respond "adequately" to at least two standard antipsychotic medications; and/or (b) the inability to tolerate therapeutic doses of standard antipsychotics (Risby ED, Jewart RD, Lewine RJ, et al. An association between increased concentrations of cerebrospinal fluid dopamine sulfate and higher negative symptom scores in patients with schizophrenia and schizoaffective disorder. *Biol Psychiatry* 1993;34:661–664). In controlled trials, treatments with partial success in refractory schizophrenia include electroconvulsive therapy (especially bilateral), augmentation of antipsychotics with other drugs (e.g., lithium, carbamazepine, benzodiazepines, reserpine, propranolol, and levodopa), and therapy with new atypical antipsychotics (e.g., clozapine, risperidone).

schizophrenia, refractory/electroconvulsive therapy   Some refractory schizophrenic patients may respond to a course of electroconvulsive therapy (ECT) administered during ongoing antipsychotic drug therapy. Bilateral ECT may be more efficacious than unilateral ECT. Generally, patients with refractory schizophrenia require more ECT than do those with affective disorders, and those who respond often require maintenance ECT (Gellenberg AJ. Unilateral v. bilateral ECT: grist for the mill. *Biol Ther Psychiatry* 1986;9:2–3; Remington G. Treatment options in refractory schizophrenia. Current Approaches to Psychoses. *Diagnosis and Management* 1993;2:1, 4, 5, 11).

schizophrenia, ventricular enlargement   Ventricular size in schizophrenia (SCZ) was first investigated in 1976 with computerized tomography (CT) scanning that showed significant ventricular enlargement in a group of chronic schizophrenic patients (SCZs). Subsequent investigations confirmed that lateral ventricles of SCZs are significantly larger than those of control subjects. The prevalence of ventricular enlargement varies among studies, partly because of measurement differences, differing diagnostic criteria, or the choice of control subjects. Using either CT or magnetic resonance imaging (MRI), ventricle/brain ra-

tio (VBR) has become the most widely used measurement of lateral ventricular size. Recent studies have shown a difference in VBR between SCZs and control subjects that would seem to be an indisputable characteristic of SCZ. The difference is smaller than previously thought, however, and although of theoretical interest in accounting for the etiology of SCZ, it may be too small to be of practical significance in diagnosis or differentiation of subtypes (van Horn JD, McManus IC. Ventricular enlargement in schizophrenia. A meta-analysis of studies of the ventricle/brain ratio (VBR). *Br J Psychiatry* 1992;160:687–697).

schizophreniform disorder   Schizophrenic-like illness of acute onset, somewhat atypical in form and rapid in recovery, that contrasts with "process" or "true" schizophrenia, which is regarded as having a more gradual onset and a worse prognosis. Schizophreniform patients often completely return to their premorbid level of functioning within 6 months of the onset of an episode. For this reason, DSM-IV includes in this category patients who fulfill clinical criteria for schizophrenia, but who have had the illness for less than 6 months at the time of diagnosis.

schizotypal personality disorder   Nonpsychotic personality disorder with cognitive disturbances similar to those found in schizophrenia (Kendler KS, Gruenberg AM, Strauss JS. An independent analysis of the Copenhagen sample of the Danish adoption study of schizophrenia. II. The relationship between schizotypal personality disorder and schizophrenia. *Arch Gen Psychiatry* 1981;38:982–984).

"schoolboy"   Street name for elixir terpin hydrate.

scientific misconduct   Before 1989, fabrication, falsification, and plagiarism. In August of that year the U.S. Department of Health and Human Services broadened the definition to include "deception or other practices that seriously deviate from those that are commonly accepted within the scientific community for proposing, conduction, or reporting research." The new definition has been criticized as being vague, and recommendations have been made to eliminate it. However, it is still in force.

scoliosis   Lateral curvature of the spine.

SCOPE   Acronym for an accepted set of diagnostic procedures that are systematic, complete, objective, practical, and empirical.

scopolamine   (Hyoscine) Belladonna alkaloid with central anticholinergic potency 8–9 times that of atropine. It has a long history of oral and parenteral use as part of premedication for reductions of secretions, protection against vagal overactivity, sedation, and amnesia, and for prophylaxis of motion sickness. The mechanism of action in the central nervous system is not definitely known, but may include blockade of central muscarinic receptors. Scopolamine at bedtime can produce marked rapid eye movement (REM) suppression and increased REM latency in normal volunteers. It also can produce the sleep electroencephalographic changes seen in depression without depressive mood changes. Hence, it is often used as a component of nonprescription proprietary hypnotics. Scopolamine can impair alertness and cognitive functions and may induce delirium. It produces an increased deliriogenic effect after only one night of sleep deprivation.

screening, genetic Systematic search for individuals in a population who possess certain genotypes that (a) are associated with existing disease or predisposed to future disease; (b) may lead to disease in their descendants; or (c) produce other variations of interest, but are not known to be associated with disease.

"script doctor" Physician who prescribes inordinate quantities of controlled substances (e.g., benzodiazepines, amphetamines and other psychostimulants, narcotics, analgesics) for individuals who do not have a genuine medical need for these substances. The vast majority of the "patients" for whom script doctors prescribe are substance abusers who may or may not be seen by the physician and who pay a fee for prescriptions. Many are referred to script doctors by drug dealers. Script doctors are responsible for a large segment of the illegal distribution of prescription drugs.

"scrubwoman's kick" Street name for naphtha in cleaning fluid.

SDZ 208-911 Partial D$_2$ agonist that has a "buffering" role in the dopamine system. Its high receptor affinity may prevent the effects of excessive endogenous dopamine, whereas its agonist property may be of benefit in the case of low dopaminergic activity (Coward D, Dixon K, Eng A, et al. Partial brain dopamine D$_2$ receptor agonists in the treatment of schizophrenia. *Psychopharmacol Bull* 1989;25:393–397).

SDZ 208-912 Partial D$_2$ agonist that, like SDZ 208-911, has a "buffering" role in the dopamine system. Its high receptor affinity may prevent the effects of excessive endogenous dopamine, whereas its agonist property may be of benefit in the case of low dopaminergic activity (Coward D, Dixon K, Eng A, et al. Partial brain dopamine D$_2$ receptor agonists in the treatment of schizophrenia. *Psychopharmacol Bull* 1989;25:393–397).

SDZ-912 Atypical antipsychotic drug in early phase II testing in the United States.

seasonal affective disorder (SAD) Seasonal subtype of major depressive disorder characterized by an annual pattern of symptoms (depression in fall and winter and euthymia or hypomania in spring and summer). SAD may be a variant of bipolar disorder, although it appears more frequently in unipolar patients. It occurs predominantly in women and begins in early adulthood. The recurrent episodes must occur within a particular 60-day period of the year and there must be a history of at least three episodes in 3 separate years that demonstrate a clear seasonal pattern. The depressive phases are often accompanied by atypical symptoms of enhanced appetite, carbohydrate craving, increased body weight, fatigue, and hypersomnia. For most patients, winter depression results from circadian rhythms that are abnormally delayed and respond to the corrective phase-advancing effect of morning light. A recurrent form of winter depression associated with the length of daylight or photoperiod suggests that some abnormality of photoperiod regulation may be involved in the pathogenesis of SAD (Rosenthal NE, Sack DA, Gillin JC, et al. Seasonal affective disorder: a description of the syndrome and preliminary findings with light therapy. *Arch Gen Psychiatry* 1984;41:72–80). SAD responds to treatment with bright artificial light (white, blue, green, or red); the treatment effect of green light, morning light, or evening light is superior to that of red. The time course of response to light therapy is remarkably consistent with each episode. Marked improvement can occur within 3–4 days; improvement in all depression ratings and self-rated mood, anxiety, and fatigue improve within 1 week. Serotonin uptake inhibitors such as citalopram produce improved self-rated mood within a week, but require 2 weeks for reliable decrease in depressive symptoms (Wirz-Justice A, van der Velde P, Bucher A, Nil R. Comparison of light treatment with citalopram in winter depression: a longitudinal single case study. *Int Clin Psychopharmacol* 1992;7:109–116). Neither the pathophysiology of the disorder nor the antidepressant mechanism of phototherapy is well understood. Between 40 and 50% of patients do not respond to bright light and require alternative treatments. See **seasonal affective disorder/winter type; seasonal pattern assessment questionnaire; phototherapy.**

seasonal affective disorder/diagnostic criteria The following criteria have been proposed by Rosenthal and his associates: (a) history of recurrent depressions with at least one major depressive episode according to Research Diagnostic Criteria; (b) recurrent fall or winter depressions, at least two of which have been in successive years, separated by nondepressed periods in spring or summer; (c) no other DSM-III Axis I diagnosis; and (d) absence of regularly occurring psychosocial precipitants that might account for the seasonal pattern (Rosenthal NE, Sack DA, Gillin JC, et al. Seasonal affective disorder: a description of the syndrome and preliminary findings with light therapy. *Arch Gen Psychiatry* 1984;41:72–80).

seasonal affective disorder, winter type   Affective illness characterized by the onset of a depressive syndrome in the fall or winter, and spontaneous recovery in the spring. It has been treated successfully either with antidepressant pharmacotherapy or bright light therapy.

seasonal mood disorder, type A   (SMD-A) Disorder characterized by fall-winter depression with or without spring-summer mania or hypomania. It shows consistent time of onset and remission and is distinct from SMD-B.

seasonal mood disorder, type B   (SMD-B) Disorder characterized by recurrent spring-summer depression with or without fall-winter mania or hypomania. Like SMD-A, it shows consistent time of onset and remission and is distinct from SMD-A.

"seccy"   Street name for secobarbital.

seclusion   Commonly used management technique consisting of supervised confinement of a patient alone in a locked room or other enclosed area with no means of egress to protect the patient, staff, or others from serious harm. Containment of a patient in an unlocked room does not count as seclusion.

secobarbital   (Novosecobarb; Seconal) Short-acting barbiturate that acts as a central nervous system depressant. Depending on dosage, it produces responses ranging from mild sedation to profound hypnosis. In large doses, it causes anesthesia; in overdosage, respiratory depression occurs. It is marketed as a sedative or hypnotic. Pregnancy risk category D; Schedule II.

Seconal   See **secobarbital.**

secondary amines   Tricyclic antidepressants with only one methyl group on the nitrogen atom of the side chain. Desipramine, nortriptyline, and protriptyline are secondary amines.

secondary constriction   Any constricted heterochromatic area in a chromosome other than the primary constriction, the centromere.

secondary dementia   Uncommon manifestations of conditions that often present with a different clinical picture (e.g., brain tumors,

fungal meningitis). Secondary dementias are differentiated from the primary type by their reversibility when the underlying causes are treated appropriately. Dementia syndrome of depression is a good example of secondary dementia.

secondary depression   Depressive syndrome secondary to an antecedent illness.

secondary mania   Manic symptoms associated with antecedent physical illness or drug use. It usually occurs in older patients with no family history of bipolar disorder. Thus, the term designates mania due to specific causes in patients who presumably would not otherwise develop the disease. Secondary mania has been reported in a variety of organic cerebral illnesses (toxic confusional state, postoperative psychosis, brain tumor, multiple sclerosis, influenza, encephalitis, syphilis, and epilepsy). It also can be precipitated by stimulants and other drugs, such as amphetamines, methylphenidate, antidepressants, L-dopa, bromocriptine, corticosteroids, cocaine, and phencyclidine.

secondary memory   See **memory, secondary.**

second messenger   Chemical mediator (e.g., hormones) that propagates a nerve signal or exerts the intracellular effect of receptor activation by ligands. Second messenger activity involves protein phosphorylation by enzymes called *protein kinases.* Two second-messenger systems have been well characterized. The first involves adenylate cyclase-catalyzed formation of cyclic adenosine monophosphate (cAMP). The second involves the calcium ion (Ca^{2+}) and products of the membrane phosphatidylinositol cycle. Lithium may exert its therapeutic effects by modulating the latter system. Second messengers are so named because they transduce an extracellular signal into a particular cellular response—for example, the occupation of receptors by neurotransmitters ("first messenger") into an action potential of the postsynaptic neuron. Second messengers act via the stimulation of specific protein kinases that phosphorylate a specific set of substrate proteins. Kinases are classified by the particular stimulating second messenger; for example, cAMP-dependent protein kinase, calcium/calmodulin-dependent kinases, and calcium/phospholipid-dependent kinases. Different neurons, depending on the receptors present and on the conditions, use distinct second messenger systems, resulting in the phosphorylation of specific proteins. Second messenger activity seems to involve protein phosphorylation by enzymes called protein kinases. In many cases, these reactions seem to depend on the cyclic nucleotides, 3',5'-adenosine monophosphate (cAMP) or cyclic guanine monophosphate, or on an ion such as calcium.

Sectral See **acebutolol.**

Sedabamate See **meprobamate.**

sedation Decrease in responsiveness to a constant level of stimulation, with a diminution in spontaneous activity and ideation. It is a state of being calm induced by the administration of a sedative or anxiolytic. It should not be confused with drowsiness, which would be the beginning of a hypnotic effect.

sedation threshold Point at which intravenous sodium amytal produces slurring of speech and electroencephalographic changes. This test has been used to differentiate psychotic and neurotic depressions. In the former, thresholds. are said to be low; in the latter, thresholds are high.

sedative Drug that produces a daytime calming or relaxing effect through central nervous system depression. In theory, sedatives reduce anxiety without necessarily producing sedation, but so far all have produced some sedation in a dose-dependent manner. They include the barbiturates, benzodiazepines, and azaspirones such as buspirone. Sedatives are typically used to control anxiety, but also may be used as hypnotics. They are cross-tolerant and synergistic with alcohol and with each other. Abuse of sedatives in combination with alcohol is, according to the National Institute on Drug Abuse (1987), one of the most common drug-related causes of morbidity and mortality. Also called "anxiolytic."

sedative + neuroleptic Sedatives that induce hepatic drug metabolizing enzymes may reduce neuroleptic blood levels.

sedative/hypnotics Drugs that have been used as minor tranquilizers, anxiolytics, and sleeping pills. Effects depend very much on the size of the dose given. At relatively low doses, the drugs reduce levels of anxiety and arousal; as doses are increased, they promote sleep. At very high doses they can induce unconsciousness and therefore can be used as anesthetics or to cause a fatal overdose. Initially the drugs are often effective, but if used continuously for more than 1–2 weeks, tolerance develops, dependence begins, and some users find it increasingly difficult to discontinue them.

sedative withdrawal Symptoms that emerge following abrupt discontinuation of therapeutic or higher doses of sedative-anxiolytic drugs (e.g., barbiturates, meprobamate) that have been taken continuously for at least 2–3 months. Dosage and duration affect incidence and severity. The higher the dose and the

longer it has been taken, the greater the risk and severity. Criteria for sedative withdrawal include (a) development of a substance-specific syndrome following cessation or a reduction in intake of a psychoactive drug; and (b) a clinical picture that does not correspond to any of the other specific organic mental syndromes (e.g., delirium, organic delusional syndrome, organic hallucinosis, organic mood syndrome, or organic anxiety syndrome).

Sediten See **fluphenazine.**

Sedizine See **trifluoperazine.**

"seggy" Street name for secobarbital.

segregation In an organism that is heterozygous at a given locus, the separation of the two alleles at meiosis and distribution to two different gametes.

segregation analysis Examination of the pattern of transmission, rather than the prevalence, of a trait in different classes of families. The most common way of testing a mode of inheritance, segregation analysis relies on a sample of families, segregating the disease, and aims at determining whether or not there is a factor that plays a "major role" and whether it is transmitted in a Mendelian manner. In many diseases for which the existence of a genetic component has been established, segregation analysis has not been able to demonstrate the role of a major gene. Nevertheless, it is one of the most powerful statistical methods in population genetics. It compares the observed frequency of an illness in a pedigree with a pattern that would occur if a hypothesized mode of inheritance (e.g., one of the monogenic patterns or polygenic transmission) were true. It requires systematic collection of family data and will likely play a major role in examining the genetic factors in most psychiatric disorders. Also called "complex segregation analysis."

seizure Paroxysmal spells of transitory alteration in consciousness or in other cerebral cortical functions that may result from episodic neurologic, psychiatric, or cardiovascular dysfunction. A seizure is a motor expression of uncontrolled or paroxysmal brain activity.

seizure, absence Brief (5- to 30-second) absence with a highly characteristic 3–3.5 Hz spike-wave pattern, with little motor accompaniment. Absence seizures are generalized seizures from the electroencephalographic viewpoint. They usually occur in childhood (ages 4–12) and seldom persist through adolescence into adulthood. Incidence is relatively low. Characteristics include onset between ages 2 and 15; brief lapses of consciousness without aura; slight rhythmic movements of the eyelids and hands; short duration (1–2 minutes) followed by a brief, poorly organized automatism; and rapid return to full consciousness without retrograde amnesia or confusion. Typically, the patient has no memory of what happened during an attack, and the electroencephalogram (EEG) has a characteristic pattern of paroxysms of 304/second spikes and waves. Absence seizures may or may not be the only manifestation of epilepsy. They may be an independent manifestation of primary generalized epilepsy, but they are frequently associated with tonic-clonic seizures, another manifestation of primary generalized epilepsy. Absence seizures may cease during adolescence. Until divalproex was introduced, ethosuximide was the most effective drug for treating absence seizures. Fifty percent of absence seizure patients develop generalized tonic-clonic seizures. Formerly called "petit mal." See **divalproex.**

seizure, atonic   Epileptic drop attack in which patients intermittently fall to the ground and remain unresponsive for varying periods with no associated muscular activity. Attacks are usually caused by vasovagal or orthostatic syncope in younger individuals and vertebrobasilar insufficiency in older persons. An electroencephalographic recording shows slow (less than 3 Hz) spike-wave, polyspike, and wave patterns or a rhythmic slow-wave pattern. Also called "astatic seizure."

seizure, astatic   See **seizure, atonic.**

seizure, complex partial   Ictal event with focal features and some type of impaired consciousness (in simple partial seizures, consciousness is not impaired). The majority begin in the temporal lobe; others are extrapyramidal in origin. During a complex partial seizure, patients (a) do not appear normal; (b) are not capable of performing sequential or coordinated activity; (c) may become violent. The same sequence of movements may occur each time, and lip-smacking and jerking of the mouth and face is a common accompaniment. Individuals with complex partial seizures are at risk of overactivity and behavioral abnormalities. An interictal personality disorder characterized by hypergraphia, hyper-religiosity, and circumstantiality has been associated with complex partial seizures. Infrequently, a psychosis resembling paranoid schizophrenia has been noted during interictal periods in some patients. Carbamazepine and phenytoin are considered to have the best overall combination of efficacy and freedom from adverse effects during treatment of complex partial seizures. Valproate is as effective as carbamazepine for the treatment of generalized tonic-clonic seizures, but carbamazepine pro-

vides better control of complex partial seizures and has fewer long-term adverse effects (Mattson RH, Cramer JA, Collins JF, et al. A comparison of valproate with carbamazepine for the treatment of complex partial seizures and secondary generalized tonic-clonic seizures in adults. *N Engl J Med* 1992;327:765–771). Also called "automatic epilepsy"; "psychomotor epilepsy"; "temporal lobe epilepsy."

seizure, continuous partial   Type of seizure disorder that may cause repetitive abnormal involuntary movements of one or more limbs without loss of consciousness. It may be secondary to structural or metabolic lesions in the brain. It can occur during sleep, in contrast to tardive dyskinesia movements, which disappear during sleep.

seizure, convulsive   Syncope. It is not a seizure disorder. The misleading term "convulsive" is used because the episode is manifested in part by "tonic posturing" and random clonic activity and there are no electroencephalographic spike discharges in convulsive seizures. Anticonvulsants are not warranted.

seizure, epileptic   Seizure that results from paroxysmal and abnormally synchronous discharges of cerebral cortical neurons induced by systemic or neurological disturbances. Symptoms can result from many different diseases. Epileptic seizures can be divided into primary and secondary types. Primary (idiopathic) epileptic seizures are usually inherited, often age-related, commonly benign, and unassociated with identified structural lesions. Secondary (symptomatic) epileptic seizures result from an identifiable disease or lesion of the brain. See **generalized tonic-clonic seizure; partial seizure; simple partial seizure; complex partial seizure.**

seizure, epileptiform   Convulsion of a functional nature.

seizure, feigned   Form of malingering in which seizures are consciously intended and usually consist of a more or less skilled imitation of whatever the "patient" considers to be a seizure. Grand mal attacks are most commonly imitated and even tongue bites may be found in experienced malingerers.

seizure, focal motor   The most common attacks arise in the motor cortex and consist of contralateral twitching in limited body regions (fingers, hand, arm, leg, etc.). These clonic manifestations may spread into what is known as the "Jacksonian march" and may progress into a full generalized tonic-clonic convulsion. Focal motor attacks may occur at any age and are less common than primary generalized seizures and seizures of temporal origin. Also called "simple partial seizure with motor signs." See **epilepsy, Jacksonian.**

seizure, generalized   Type of epileptic seizure which, at onset, often involves both cerebral hemispheres, consistently causes altered consciousness, and may be convulsive (tonic, clonic, and tonic-clonic seizures) or nonconvulsive (absences, myoclonic seizures, and drop attacks).

seizure, grand mal   See **seizure, tonic-clonic.**

seizure, hysterical   See **pseudoseizure.**

seizure monitoring   Prolonged video/electroencephalogram (EEG) monitoring until seizures occur to establish a more precise diagnosis. Monitoring is done for differential diagnosis if nonepileptic seizures are suspected, or for the work-up of a patient with medically intractable seizures who may be a candidate for surgical treatment.

seizure, myoclonic   Seizure manifested by brief jerks of essential bilateral character that may be quite massive. Myoclonic seizures may occur at any age but are more common in children.

seizure, nonconvulsive   Form of seizure disorder characterized by episodic disturbances of behavior ranging from brief impairment of consciousness (as in absences) to very complicated behavior. It rarely may persist over a protracted period (nonconvulsive status). The more complicated types of nonconvulsive seizures are particularly liable to be misconstrued as nonepileptic attacks.

seizure, partial   Type of epileptic seizure that begins in one part of one cerebral hemisphere and produces symptoms referable to the region of the cerebral cortex primarily involved. There are three types of partial seizures determined to some extent by the degree of brain involvement by the abnormal discharge. On the basis of many clinical trials, carbamazepine and phenytoin are considered to have the best overall combination of efficacy and freedom from adverse effects during treatment of partial epilepsy (Mattson RH, Cramer JA, Collins JF, et al. A comparison of valproate with carbamazepine for the treatment of complex partial seizures and secondary generalized tonic-clonic seizures in adults. *N Engl J Med* 1992;327:765–771).

seizure, primary generalized   Seizure in which the patient stares into space for 15–30 seconds with loss of normal responsiveness. The only motor activity is rhythmical eye blinking. There is no aura and no postictal confusion. Formerly called "nonfocal grand mal seizure."

seizure prone   Description of one who is predisposed to seizures because of conditions including (a) epilepsy; (b) alcoholism; (c) electroencephalographic abnormalities; (d) cerebral arteriosclerosis; (e) other central nervous system degenerative states; and (f) treatment with drugs that may lower seizure threshold (e.g., maprotiline).

seizure, psychogenic   Seizure characterized by a variable pattern compared to the stereotypical pattern of electrical seizures. Pelvic thrusting and truncal arching are common, but incontinence, tongue biting, loss of consciousness, pupillary changes, amnesia, or postconvulsive confusion do not occur. Such seizures, although not ictal, are real. They can be very harmful and disruptive. They may be a manifestation of hysteria.

seizure, psychomotor   Ictal event with focal features and impaired consciousness; may be of temporal lobe or (less often) of other focal origin. In simple partial seizures, consciousness is not impaired. The same sequence of movements may occur each time, and lipsmacking and jerking of the mouth and face is a common accompaniment. Individuals with complex partial seizures are at risk of overactivity and behavior problems.

seizure, secondary generalized   Type of partial seizure that begins with a simple partial or complex partial seizure and later develops into generalized tonic-clonic, clonic, or tonic seizures. Formerly called "focal onset grand mal seizure."

seizure, simple partial   Type of epileptic seizure that consists of focal neurological events with intact consciousness. It may result from a focal cortical discharge and consist of motor, sensory, autonomic, psychic, visual, and auditory types. The focal tissue abnormality may be microscopic or macroscopic. The former is not detected by computerized tomography and magnetic resonance imaging, but only by examination of a tissue specimen obtained by surgical biopsy or at autopsy. The localized seizure activity in the cerebral cortex often spreads; simple partial seizures may thus evolve into complex partial seizures, and both may evolve into secondarily generalized seizures.

seizure threshold   Conceptual term frequently used term in the medical literature, quantification of which is impossible in humans except in patients receiving electroconvulsive therapy.

seizure, tonic-clonic   the most common seizure type that can occur at any age except under 6 months. Its sequence of a tonic and clonic phase is well known. Its duration ranges from 40 to 90 seconds. Abrupt cessation of the clonic motion and temporary electroencephalographic flatness mark termination of the attack. There is a sudden loss of consciousness associated with loss of postural tone, followed by flexion and some abduction of the upper and lower extremities. The mouth is open widely and a cry or gutteral noise may be emitted. The tonic phase follows, during which the mouth clenches tightly shut, the head may be turned to one side, the arms change from flexion and abduction to extension and adduction, and the legs are in extension. Profound coma is present during the entire attack and subsides within minutes after the seizure. Tongue biting is fairly common, loss of urinary sphincter control less so, bowel incontinence is quite rare, and life-threatening complications such as asphyxia are extremely rare. Apnea, which is present throughout the seizure, may persist for several seconds after the last clonic jerk with resultant cyanosis. The pupils are fixed and unresponsive to light, and respiration returns with a deep inspiration, frequently accompanied by a gutteral sound. There is frequently excessive salivation with "frothing at the mouth." Nonfocal grand mal has been reclassified as primary generalized, and focal onset grand mal as secondary generalized tonic-clonic seizures. Formerly called "grand mal seizure."

seizure, uncinate Subjective disturbance of smell and taste produced by deep, mesial lesions of the tip of the temporal lobe. At times, the seizure is accompanied by chomping movements of the jaw, due to a lesion of the uncinate gyrus.

Selectin See **fluphenazine.**

selection Any natural or artificial process that favors the survival and propagation of individuals of a given genotype in a population.

selection bias See **sampling bias.**

selective monoamine oxidase inhibitor (MAOI) See **monoamine oxidase inhibitor, selective.**

selegiline (Eldepryl, formerly Deprenyl) Propargylamine derivative that has been reported to slow the progression of Parkinson's disease. It forms an irreversible covalent bond with the monamine oxidase subtype B (MAO-B). MAO-B is the predominant form of the enzyme in the human brain, and dopamine and phenylethylamine are its preferred substrates, whereas norepinephrine and serotonin are the preferred substrates for MAO subtype A (MAO-A). The selectivity of selegiline for MAO-B is dose-dependent; at higher doses (> 20 mg/day), selegiline becomes nonselective and also inhibits MAO-A. The overall effect of selegiline is to cause a slight but significant increase in the levels of dopamine content in the nigrostriatal system and an enhanced sensitivity of the dopaminergic neurons to physiological and pharmacological influences (Knoll J. Deprenyl [selegiline]: the history of its development and pharmacological action. *Acta Neurol Scand* 1983;95[suppl]:57–80). Major metabolites are l-amphetamine and l-meth-

amphetamine, which can exert a weak antiparkinson effect and also cause agitation in some patients (Reynolds PC. Postmortem tissue methamphetamine concentrations following selegiline administration. *J Anal Toxicol* 1990; 14:330–331) The usual therapeutic dose is 5 mg taken in the morning and again at noon with meals. No antidepressant effect of selegiline has been detected in studies that have used this dosage. Dosages greater than 10 mg/day should be avoided. Antidepressant trials have disclosed antidepressant efficacy at a selective dose (less than 15 mg/day), although others show efficacy only at nonselective doses (Mann JJ, Aarons SF, Wilner PJ, et al. A controlled study of the antidepressant efficacy and side effects of (-)-deprenyl. *Arch Gen Psychiatry* 1989;46:45–50). When prescribed in low (therapeutic) doses, no dietary restrictions are necessary. Selegiline can produce the cheese reaction (tyramine-induced hypertensive crisis) at antidepressant dosages, because at these doses it also inhibits the MAO-A enzyme. There is some preliminary research evidence that selegiline significantly improves the negative symptoms of schizophrenia and schizoaffective disorder. Selegiline is known to produce a variety of behavioral side effects, including hallucinations, nightmares, and sleep disturbances (Boyson SJ: Psychiatric effects of selegiline. *Arch Neurol* 1991;48:902). A sensation of increased energy may occur at doses greater than 10 mg/day. Hypomania has been reported in a patient who received selegiline (5 mg twice a day) (Menza MA, Golbe LI. Hypomania in a patient receiving deprenyl [selegiline] after adrenal-striatal implantation for Parkinson's disease. *Clin Neuropharmacol* 1988;11:549). Mania has also been reported in selegiline-treated patients who did not have a history of mania. Caution in the use of selegiline in patients receiving an antidepressant medication seems warranted (Kurland R, Dimitsopulos T. Selegiline and manic behavior in Parkinson's disease. *Arch Neurol* 1992;49:1231). Accumulating data indicate that selegiline may play an effective role in the treatment of Alzheimer's and other neurodegenerative diseases (Kovacs A. Growing importance of selegiline in the treatment of neurodegenerative diseases. *Acta Pharm Hung* 1992;62:259–264). Selegiline also is a powerful antioxidant that increases levels of the antioxidant enzyme superoxide dismutase in rat striatum and lowers levels of glutathione disulfide in rats treated with haloperidol, indicating a reduction on oxidative stress. Selegiline also protects against dopaminergic injury from the toxin 1-methyl-4-phenyl-1,2,3,-6-tetrahydropyridine, which produces a syndrome resembling parkinsonism in humans. Pregnancy risk category C.

selegiline/breast milk   Safety during breast feeding has not been established. For more information, contact the manufacturer.

selegiline + fluoxetine   Co-administration of fluoxetine (FLX) and selegiline (10 mg/day) may be safe for treatment of Parkinson's disease patients, many of whom have tolerated the combination well (Caley CF, Friedman JH. Does fluoxetine exacerbate Parkinson's disease? *J Clin Psychiatry* 1992;53:278–282). It has been reported to cause mania and episodes of diaphoresis and hypertension. A reaction manifested by shivering and sweating; coldness, clamminess, and vasoconstriction of the hands; blue and mottled fingers; and persistently elevated blood pressure (200/120 mmHg) was reported with selegiline (5 mg/day) plus FLX (20 mg/day). Symptoms abated a few days after both were discontinued (Suchowersky O, de Vries JD. Interaction of fluoxetine and selegiline. *Can J Psychiatry* 1990; 35:571–572). A Parkinson's disease patient treated with selegiline (10 mg/day) and FLX (20 mg/day) developed headaches, flushes, and palpitations twice a day for 4 weeks, followed by a probable generalized tonic-clonic seizure associated with hypertension (250/130 mmHg) (Montaastruc JL, Chamontin B, Senard JM, et al. Pseudophaeochromocytoma in parkinson patient treated with fluoxetine plus selegiline. *Lancet* 1993;341: 555). A 66-year-old woman with Parkinson's disease taking selegiline (10 mg/day) experienced ataxia after receiving FLX 20 (mg/day) for 1 month. Selegiline was discontinued. Six weeks later, the patient reported no depressive symptoms, and ataxia had lessened significantly. FLX was decreased to 10 mg/day and discontinued 4 weeks later. Within 1 month, the ataxia was completely resolved. This case suggests that ataxia may be the result of an interaction between FLX and selegiline (Jermain DM, Hughes PL, Follender AB. Potential fluoxetine-selegiline interaction. *Ann Pharmacother* 1992;26:1300). Despite selectivity and reversibility, selegiline and similar "new" reversible monoamine oxidase (MAO) inhibitors are not immune to the usual interactions of "old" MAO inhibitors.

selegiline + levodopa   Co-administration may reduce wearing-off phenomena and fluctuations, although the degree of improvement is modest; in some patients, selegiline may aggravate levodopa-related toxic effects such as hallucinations and dyskinesias (Standaert DG, Stern MB. Update on the management of Parkinson's disease. *Med Clin North Am* 1993; 77:169–183).

selegiline + meperidine   One of the most serious drug interactions with nonselective monoamine oxidase (MAO) inhibitors occurs with meperidine. It consists of rigidity, delirium, hyperthermia, convulsions, and death. Selegiline, even in low doses, may interact adversely with meperidine, documenting that such a reaction can occur with the inhibition of MAO-B alone. Delirium, stupor, severe agitation, muscular rigidity, sweating, and pyrexia (38.2° C; 100.76° F) occurred in a 56-year-old man taking various drugs (including selegiline) who was given meperidine postoperatively (Zornberg GL, Bodkin JA, Cohen BM. Severe adverse interaction between pethidine and selegiline. *Lancet* 1991;337:246). Despite selectivity and reversibility, selegiline and other similar "new" reversible MAO inhibitors are not immune to the usual interactions of "old" MAO inhibitors. However, it is difficult to determine if the adverse effects were due solely to an interaction between selegiline and meperidine.

selegiline + moclobemide   Co-administration leads to a supra-additive tyramine effect on sensitivity to intravenously administered tyramine. It should only be considered when accompanied by dietary restrictions with respect to tyramine-containing foods. When switching from selegiline to moclobemide, a washout period of about 2 weeks should be sufficient. When switching from moclobemide to selegiline, a washout period of 1–2 days is sufficient (Dingemanse J. An update of recent moclobemide interaction data. *Int Clin Psychopharmacol* 1993;7:167–180).

selegiline + phenylalanine   Combination that can be used effectively in patients with treatment-resistant major depressive disorder. Effects are rapid and often without side effects.

selegiline + physostigmine   Addition of selegiline (5 mg twice a day) to the regimen of Alzheimer's disease patients being treated with physostigmine was associated with significant improvement in the scores on the cognitive subscale of the Alzheimer's Disease Assessment Scale, suggesting possible additive effects of selegiline to the effects of cholinesterase inhibitors (Schneider LS, Olin JT, Pawluczyk S. A double-blind crossover pilot study of l-deprenyl (selegiline) combined with cholinesterase inhibitor in Alzheimer's disease. *Am J Psychiatry* 1993;150:321–323).

selegiline + piribedil   Co-administration may cause significant psychic effects (Vermersch P. Tolerability of long-term selegiline therapy in Parkinson's disease. *Therapie* 1992;47:75–78).

selegiline/pregnancy   Safety during pregnancy has not been established. For more information, contact the manufacturer.

selegiline + tacrine   Addition of selegiline (5 mg twice a day) to the regimen of Alzheimer's patients being treated with tacrine was associated with significant improvement in the scores on the cognitive subscale of the Alzheimer's Disease Assessment Scale, suggesting possible additive effects of selegiline to the effects of cholinesterase inhibitors (Schneider LS, Olin JT, Pawluczyk S. A double-blind crossover pilot study of L-deprenyl (selegiline) combined with cholinesterase inhibitor in Alzheimer's disease. *Am J Psychiatry* 1993;150: 321–323).

selegiline/tardive dyskinesia   A 6-week course of selegiline was ineffective in the treatment of tardive dyskinesia and in fact may have been inferior to placebo (Goff DC, Renshal PF, Sarid-Segal O, et al. A placebo-controlled trial of selegiline (L-deprenyl) in the treatment of tardive dyskinesia. *Biol Psychiatry* 1993;33:700– 706).

Selepam   See **quazepam.**

self-controlled study   Study in which subjects serve as their own controls, achieved by measuring the characteristic of interest before and after an intervention. Also called "mirror-image" design.

self-injurious behavior   (SIB) Self-destructive behavior causing obvious tissue damage, without lethal intent or severity, resulting in a temporary relief of dysphoric feelings. It is seen in a number of psychiatric disorders as well as in the context of sociocultural customs, including that seen in schizophrenia (e.g., autocastration), obsessive-compulsive disorder (e.g., compulsive hand washing), mental retardation, Lesch-Nyhan syndrome (e.g., head banging), cultural rituals (e.g., skin piercing), and sadomasochistic behavior (e.g., whipping). SIB occurs frequently in borderline personality disorder patients (Gardner DL, Cowdry RW. Suicidal and parasuicidal behavior in borderline personality disorder. *Psychiatric Clin North Am* 1985;8:389–403). Clinical manifestations and descriptions by patients of their inner experience during SIB suggest that they are complex, multidetermined behaviors that involve mood dysregulation, poor impulse control, dissociation, and abnormal physical responses (Winchel RM, Stanley M. Self-injurious behavior: a review of the behavior and biology of self-mutilation. *Am J Psychiatry* 1991;148:306–317). Research suggests that there may be subtypes of SIB borderline personality disorder patients (those who report that they do not experience pain during self-injury [BPD-NP group], and similar patients who report that they do experience pain during self-injury [BPD-P group]). These subtypes may be differentiated on the basis of

pain perception, a mood-regulating function for SIB, and, perhaps, historical factors such as severity of childhood abuse and age of onset of SIB. Patients in the BPD-NP group have an earlier onset of SIB and perhaps a more chronic course, with more lifetime episodes as well as an association between sexual and/or physical abuse during childhood and the development of SIB (Russ MJ, Roth SD, Lerman A, et al. Pain perception in self-injurious patients with borderline personality disorder. *Biol Psychiatry* 1992;32:501–511). Several studies have evaluated the effects of fluoxetine on self-injurious behavior. In the most recent, fluoxetine produced some benefit with average decreases in self-injury ranging from 20– 88% when compared with baseline levels (Ricketts RW, Goza AB, Ellis CR, et al. Fluoxetine treatment of severe self-injury in young adults with mental retardation. *J Am Acad Child Adolesc Psychiatry* 1993;32:865–869). See **eltoprazine.**

self-injurious behavior, severe   (SSIB) Self-injurious behavior in developmentally disabled children and adults that can be protracted, serious, and even life-threatening. SSIB is almost always associated with profound learning difficulties. Milder stereotyped behaviors, found in 10–15% of children and adults with severe learning difficulties, usually responds to nonaversive treatments and is prevented by the use of restraints and protective clothing. The cause of SSIB is unknown. When SSIB is not controlled by nonaversive behavioral methods, aversive therapy incorporating unpleasant tastes and smells and especially electric shock, which can act speedily and have lasting effects, may be considered in these exceptional cases. See **aversive therapy; eltoprazine.**

self-mutilation   Deliberate damage to one's own body, without conscious intent to die, associated with transient relief of tension. It is prevalent among character disorders of the borderline spectrum. Research data suggest that serotonergic dysfunction may be associated with extreme forms of self-harm (suicidal behavior and aggression). It occurs predominantly in three groups of patients: (a) the mentally retarded and those with other organic brain conditions (stereotypic self-mutilation such as head-banging); (b) the severely psychotic (major self-mutilation such as self-enucleation and autocastration); and (c) those with personality disorders (minor self-mutilation such as cutting or burning the skin). The latter are impulsive, aggressive, anxious, and angry individuals. Most frequently they have either a borderline personality disorder or an antisocial personality disorder (Simeon D, Standy B, Frances A. Self-mutilation in personality disorders: psychological and biological correlation. *Am J Psychiatry* 1992;149:221–226).

self-poisoning   Intentional self-administration of more than the prescribed dose of any drug, whether or not there is evidence that the act was intended to cause self-harm. It also includes overdoses of "drugs for kicks" and poisoning by noningestible substances and gas. Alcohol intoxication is not included unless accompanied by other types of self-poisoning or self-injury (Hawton K, Fagg J. Deliberate self-poisoning and self-injury in adolescents. a study of characteristics and trends in Oxford, 1976-89. *Br J Psychiatry* 1992; 161:816–823).

self-referral   Referral of patients to testing or treatment facilities by a physician who gains financial benefit from the referral.

self-report questionnaires   Screening instruments, the performance of which is related to a "gold standard" clinical or research diagnostic interview. Investigator-based interviews are needed when the constructs under evaluation are complex and there is no universal agreement among subjects about the meaning of terms. The Present State Examination (PSE) is an interview that is often used to assess neurotic symptoms and establish case status in hospital and community studies. The procedure is costly. The Symptom Checklist (CSL-90-R) is a suitable substitute because its subscales cover the full range of neurotic symptoms and syndromes.

self-report scale   Method to obtain comprehensive samples of a patient's behavior, feelings, or thoughts in a systematic way, based on the assumption that a patient can read and understand the items of a scale. Some patients may need to have someone read them the items in their primary language. Also called "self-report inventory, index, or test."

self-understanding   Therapeutic factor in which patients learn about the mechanisms underlying their behavior and about its origins (Bloch S, Crouch E. *Therapeutic Factors in Group Psychotherapy.* Oxford: Oxford University Press, 1985).

Semap   See **penfluridol.**

senile dementia of the Alzheimer type   (SDAT) Disease, originally described by Alzheimer, that occurred in a woman in her 50s. It was called presenile dementia. The dementia that occurs in the elderly is the same or similar to the presenile condition and is characterized by the presence of neurofibrillary tangles and senile plaques within the brain. See **Alzheimer's disease.**

senile dementia of the Lewy body type   (SDLT) Dementia characterized by a fluctuating confusional state often accompanied by hallucinations (predominantly visual) and behavioral disturbances. Mild extrapyramidal/parkinsonian features develop, and the progression of the disease is more rapid than with SDAT. SDLT accounts for 15–20% of hospitalized cases of dementias that come to postmortem examination and whose neuropathological and clinical features distinguish it from senile dementia of the Alzheimer's type (SDAT), multi-infarct dementia (MID), mixed SDAT/ MID, and Parkinson's disease (PD). The neuropathological features of SDLT include neocortical senile plaque densities similar to those reported in SDAT but with fewer associated neurofibrillary tangles and cortical Lewy bodies with a density lower than that observed in diffuse Lewy body disease but greater than that found in PD. In addition there is loss of neurons in the substantia nigra, locus ceruleus, and nucleus basalis of Meynert. Monoamine transmitter function is abnormal in SDLT (Byrne EJ, Lennox G, Godwin-Austen RB, et al. Dementia associated with cortical Lewy bodies: proposed clinical diagnostic criteria. *Dementia* 1991;2:283–284). It is the second most common form of dementia in the elderly. Patients often exhibit neuroleptic sensitivity, especially to neuroleptic extrapyramidal side effects (McKeith I, Fairbairn A, Perry R, et al. Neuroleptic sensitivity in patients with senile dementia of Lewy body type. *Br Med J* 1992;305:673–678). See **Lewy body.**

senility   Generic term for physical and mental changes that occur with advancing age.

senium   Seldom-used term for the feebleness of old age.

sensation, kinesthetic   Sensations derived from muscles, joints, and inner ear that are responsible for the perception of body weight, position, location, and movement.

sensation, proprioceptive   Ability to appreciate sensations of muscle, joint, tendon, and vibration.

sense/antisense   Polarity of the mRNA molecule. DNA is double-stranded and antiparallel so that information made from one strand is not identical with, but complementary to, that made from the opposite strand. The strand that corresponds to the mRNA is called "sense," whereas that complementary to the mRNA is the "antisense." Antisense oligonucleotides are highly specific probes (because they are directed by their DNA sequence) that will hybridize to the corresponding gene or mRNA. Upon hybridization, they can inhibit the expression of that gene or mRNA. Such antisense probes have been used experimentally to "knock out" the expression of a specific gene in cultured cells. They represent an important potential gene therapy to inhibit deleterious genes involved in disease.

sensemilla Hybrid form of marijuana that contains many more times the active ingredient (delta-9-tetrahydrocannabinol [THC]) than is found in even the most potent forms of naturally occurring cannabis. It is the seedless version of the cannabis plant that is cultivated for its high THC yield.

sensitivity 1. Probability that a symptom is present among patients given the diagnosis. 2. Ratio of the number of true positives to the sum of true positives plus false negatives. 3. Proportion of true positives correctly identified. 4. Form of validity signifying that changes in the intensity of symptoms are reflected in changes in test scores. 5. Proportion of truly affected persons in the screened population identified as affected by the screening test. 6. Ability of a test instrument to distinguish between degrees of severity throughout the full range of severity of the disorder (a scale may be sensitive in severe degrees, but unable to distinguish between milder degrees of the disorder). 7. Ability of a scale to discriminate between the effects of active drug and placebo.

sensitivity analysis In decision analysis, a method for determining the way a decision changes as a function of probabilities and utilities used in the analysis.

sensitivity testing Study of how the final outcome of an analysis changes as a function of varying one or more of the input parameters in a prescribed manner.

sensorium Consciousness; awareness of the nature of one's surroundings.

sequela Condition following, as a consequence of, a disease or illness.

sequential analysis Statistical method that allows an experiment to be terminated as soon as an outcome of the desired precision is obtained. Study and control subjects are randomly allocated in pairs or blocks. The result of the comparison of each pair, one treated and one control subject, is examined as soon as it becomes available and is added to all previous results.

sequential design Study in which data are reviewed at predetermined times during its course. After each data review, the investigator decides whether an answer of sufficient and predetermined precision to the research question has been obtained. If the answer is of sufficient precision, the study can terminate.

sequential study Study comparing different medications given to the same patient in a single clinical trial. It is a part of a longitudinal study.

sequential trial Study design in which results are analyzed as the trial proceeds whenever a case, or a case per treatment, is completed. In a sequential trial, patients are entered in pairs, one blindly receiving the experimental treatment, the other the standard or control treatment. The superiority of one treatment over the other, or the absence of a difference, is tallied for each pair, and when, as pairs accumulate, superiority in one direction or the other reaches beyond chance expectations, the trial is stopped. Sequential trials are vulnerable to an atypical run favoring one treatment early in the trial. According to Spriet and Simon, "Sequential trials entail complete examination of the data once each case has been completed, generally with breaking of the code in "blind" trials. This carries a risk of demotivating the clinician in charge of enlisting patients who may consciously or subconsciously modify the way he selects patients after seeing intermediate results which are not sufficient to draw valid conclusions. Finally, when the "limit" of significance is approached, the clinician may find himself faced with the dilemma of either discontinuing the trial too soon or continuing to prescribe a treatment which is very likely to prove the least effective" (Spriet A, Simon P. *Methodology of Clinical Drug Trials.* Basel: Karger, 1985).

Serax See **oxazepam.**

serazepine (CGS-15040A) Structurally novel serotonin receptor antagonist that may have anxiolytic potential. In a test of psychogenic stress in volunteers, it reduced cardiac output. In some studies it resembled diazepam. In a multicenter trial in patients with generalized anxiety disorder, serazapine had clinical anxiolytic effects consistent with established preclinical effects. Doses of 10 mg or higher reduced Hamilton Anxiety Scale scores; the dose-response relationship was nonlinear (Katz RJ, Landua PS, Lott M, et al. Serotonergic [5-HT$_2$] mediation of anxiety-therapeutic effects of serazapine in generalized anxiety disorder. *Biol Psychiatry* 1993;32:41–42).

sercloremine Experimental antidepressant not available in the United States.

Serenace See **haloperidol.**

serendipity Accidental discovery of new information.

serenic See **antiaggressive agent.**

Serenid-D See **oxazepam.**

"serenity" Street name for dimethoxymethylamphetamine.

Serentil See **mesoridazine.**

Sernylan Trade name for phencyclidine in veterinary practice.

Sernyl See **phencyclidine**.

Seropram See **citalopram**.

serotonergic antidepressant See **serotonin uptake inhibitor**.

serotonergic index Measurement of the serotonin system, including cerebrospinal fluid level of 5-hydroxyindoleacetic acid (5-HIAA), the prolactin response to serotonin agonists such as fenfluramine hydrochloride, and platelet scrotonin-related proteins for serotonin content. Many serotonergic indices correlate with suicidal behavior and affective disorders. See **fenfluramine challenge test**.

serotonergic neurons Major neurochemical system in the brain that helps to modulate a variety of physiological systems. The neurons are located in the median raphe nuclei of the pons from which they project to the median, temporal, and limbic cortices.

serotonin (5-hydroxytryptamine; 5-HT) Brain monoamine synthesized from tryptophan via 5-hydroxytryptophan (5-HTP) and stored in reserpine-sensitive granules in the nerve terminal. It acts as both a peripheral transmitter in the gut and a central transmitter in the brain (van Praag HM. Central monoamine metabolism in depression: serotonin and related compounds. *Compr Psychiatry* 1980;21: 30–43). Serotonin is localized to raphe neurons located in the pontine tegmental regions. Lesions that involve raphe (serotonin) nuclei may cause insomnia. It is thought that serotonin activity is increased in non–rapid eye movement sleep. After release into the synaptic cleft, the transmitter is inactivated by means of uptake into the presynaptic neuron. The intraneuronal breakdown of serotonin into its main metabolite, 5-hydroxyindole acetic acid (5-HIAA), is catalyzed by monoamine oxidase. Serotonin is involved in pain perception, aggressive and impulsive behavior, anxiety, sleep, circadian rhythms, sexual behavior, hormone secretion, thermoregulation, cardiovascular function, motor activity, food intake, and mood. It also has been implicated in a number of disorders such as anxiety, depression, migraine, and epilepsy.

serotonin$_2$ antagonists New agents being tested as novel treatments for schizophrenia, anxiety, and dysthymia/chronic depression.

serotonin$_3$ antagonists New agents being tested as antipsychotics and anxiolytics.

serotonin hypothesis of depression Theory formulated in the 1960s based on a series of pharmacological observations: (a) the antihypertensive reserpine, which causes depletion of serotonin and other brain monoamines, was observed to elicit depression in vulnerable subjects; (b) monoamine oxidase inhibitors (MAOIs), which cause an increase in brain monoamines in general, and of serotonin in particular, were found to relieve symptoms of depression; (c) tricyclic antidepressants (TCAs), which possibly increase synaptic concentrations of serotonin and noradrenaline, were found to relieve depressive symptoms; (d) para-chloramphetamine (pCPA), which inhibits serotonin synthesis, was found to antagonize the antidepressant effects of TCAs and MAOIs; and (e) the serotonin precursors tryptophan and 5-hydroxytryptophan (5-HTP) were shown to exert mild, though significant, effects in the treatment of depression.

serotonin receptor These include 5-HT$_{1A}$, 5-HT$_{1B}$, 5-HT$_{1C}$, 5-HT$_{1D}$, 5-HT$_{1E}$, 5-HT$_2$, 5-HT$_3$, 5-HT$_{3A}$, 5-HT$_{3B}$, 5-HT$_{3C}$, and 5-HT$_4$. All have been identified in the brain. The 5-HT$_1$ receptors and 5-HT$_2$ receptors are modulated by estrogens. The 5-HT$_1$ receptors are most dense in the hippocampus, the dorsal raphe, and the substantia nigra. There are lesser concentrations in the cortex. Some 5-HT$_1$ receptors are inhibitory (e.g., 5-HT$_{1B}$, 5-HT$_{1D}$). The 5-HT$_{1C}$ receptor is, however, excitatory (i.e., positively linked to phospholipase C). Consequently, the second messengers (diacylglycerol and IP$_3$) increase. 5-HT$_3$ receptors are excitatory and are localized in the area postrema. The 5-HT$_{1D}$ receptor is the most widespread receptor in the human brain, where it functions as an autoreceptor that modulates neurotransmitter release (i.e. 5-HT$_{1D}$ receptor activation inhibits release of serotonin).

serotonin receptors/cloned Three receptor subtypes have been cloned to date: the 5-HT$_{1A}$, 5-HT$_{1C}$, and 5-HT$_2$ receptors. All are members of the main neuroreceptor group: two of the G protein–coupled receptors, 5-HT$_2$ and 5-HT$_{1C}$, are closely related receptors because of their binding pharmacology, second-messenger coupling, and amino acid sequences, which has led to their classification as members of the same receptor subfamily. Another serotonin receptor is 5-HT$_{1D}$. There is evidence for at least six separate 5-HT receptors, each with unique molecular, pharmacological and anatomical profiles (Cowen PJ. Serotonin receptor subtypes: Implications for psychopharmacology. *Br J Psychiatry* 1991;159[suppl 12]:7–14).

serotonin$_{1A}$ receptor (5-HT$_{1A}$) A prime candidate for evaluating and managing clinical situations relating to aggression. The azapirone group of drugs (buspirone, gepirone) act generally as partial agonists and almost exclusively on this receptor at therapeutic doses. Buspirone and gepirone can be used as clinical probes in man. This receptor is of interest in biological psychiatry because of its involvement in the action of antidepressant drugs and in the pathophysiology of affective illnesses (Lesch KP. 5-HT$_{1A}$ receptor responsivity in anxiety disorders and depression. *Prog Neuropsychopharmacol Biol Psychiatry* 1991;15: 723–733). Administration of selective 5-HT$_{1A}$ receptor agonists produces hypothermia in both animals and humans, a response that can be used as a simple measure of 5-HT$_{1A}$ receptor sensitivity (Cowen PJ, Anderson IM, Grahame-Smith DG. Neuroendocrine effects of azapirones. *J Clin Psychopharmacol* 1990;10:21s–25s). In humans, administration of 5-HT$_{1A}$ receptor partial agonists such as buspirone, gepirone, and ipsapirone also produces hypothermic responses, although confirmatory studies of these effects are lacking (Young AH, McShane R, Park SB, Cowen PJ. Buspirone-induced hypothermia in normal male volunteers. *Biol Psychiatry* 1993;34:665–666).

serotonin (5-HT$_3$) receptor antagonists Five drugs have been synthesized (granisetron, ondansetron, tropisetron, MDL 73147EF, and RG 12915) and are in various stages of development. The first two are commercially available in various countries; the others are in phase I and II trials. They are antiemetics having side effect profiles with distinct advantages over conventional antiemetics. 5-HT$_3$ antagonists do not cause extrapyramidal side effects. Mild headaches, constipation, and transient transaminase elevations may occur, but are of little clinical consequence.

serotonin syndrome Toxic state due to increased serotonergic activity, often resulting from the combination of serotonergic agents with monoamine oxidase inhibitors (MAOIs). It is manifested by neuromuscular symptoms (e.g., restlessness, tremor, rigidity, head-shaking, and unsteady gait), elevated temperature, hyper-reflexia, myoclonic responses, cardiac arrhythmia, collapse, and death. Disseminated intravascular coagulation and acute myoglobinuric renal failure may be serious complications (Miller F, Friedman R, Tanenbaum J, et al. Disseminated intravascular coagulation and acute myoglobinuric renal failure: a consequence of the serotonergic syndrome. *J Clin Psychopharmacol* 1991;11:277–278). The syndrome usually occurs within 2 hours after the first dose of the precipitating agent. When further doses of the precipitating agent are withheld, the syndrome is self-limiting, with symptoms subsiding within 6–24 hours. All reported cases have been associated with agents that increase the availability of serotonin in the central nervous system. The serotonin syndrome has occurred in patients taking tryptophan and serotonin uptake inhibitors,

including fluoxetine and clomipramine. It also has been reported with irreversible MAOIs when co-prescribed with serotonin uptake inhibitors and tricyclic antidepressants, possibly because of release of central serotonin stores. Both sexes have been affected. Patient's ages have ranged from 20 to 68 years. The syndrome, first described by Insel and co-workers in 1982 (*Am J Psychiatry* 139:954–955), calls for clinical awareness for prevention, recognition, and prompt treatment. Discontinuation of a suspected serotonergic agent and institution of supportive measures are the primary treatment. It should not be confused with the neuroleptic malignant syndrome. Animal data suggest that the inhibition of both MAO-A and MAO-B is essential for the development of the serotonin syndrome (Marley E, Wozniak KM. Clinical and experimental aspects of interactions between amine oxidase inhibitors and amine re-uptake inhibitors. *Psychol Med* 1983;13:735–749; Sleight AJ, Marsden CA, Martin KF, Palfreyman MG. Relationship between extracellular 5-hydroxy-tryptamine and behaviour following monoamine oxidase inhibition and L-tryptophan. *Br J Pharmacol* 1988;93:303–310). Also called "central excitatory syndrome."

serotonin syndrome/drug combinations Drug combinations implicated in the serotonin syndrome include amitriptyline + phenelzine, amitriptyline + tranylcypromine, bromocriptine + levodopa/carbidopa, buspirone + fluoxetine, buspirone + trazodone, clomipramine + clorgyline, dextromethorphan + phenelzine, imipramine + isocarboxazid, fluoxetine + l-tryptophan, fluoxetine + phenelzine, fluoxetine + tranylcypromine, fluoxetine + trazodone, l-tryptophan + isocarboxazid, l-tryptophan + phenelzine, l-tryptophan + tranylcypromine, l-tryptophan + trazodone, meperidine + isocarboxazid, pentazocine + phenelzine, phenelzine + trazodone, and sertraline + tranylcypronine.

serotonin uptake inhibitor (SUI) Any of a relatively new class of clinically effective antidepressants chemically distinct from tricyclics and other heterocyclics. The group includes indalpine, citalopram, femoxetine, fluoxetine, fluvoxamine, litoxetine, paroxetine, and sertraline. SUIs selectively and potently inhibit neuronal uptake of serotonin (5-HT, 5-hydroxytryptamine) and have no or very weak effects on neuronal uptake of norepinephrine. They lack a significant affinity for various other neurotransmitter receptor systems in the brain and, in contrast to tricyclic antidepressants (TCAs), they do not have significant sedative, anticholinergic, and/or cardiovascular effects. All potentiate the pharmacological effects of serotonin and its precursor, 5-hydroxytryptophan. Like TCAs, SUIs can be divided into tertiary amines (citalopram, femoxetine), secondary amines (fluoxetine, sertraline, paroxetine), and a primary amine (fluvoxamine). Citalopram, fluoxetine, sertraline, and femoxetine are deaminated to the corresponding secondary and/or primary amines, which are also rather potent and selective SUIs. Paroxetine and fluvoxamine are biotransformed to inactive metabolites by other oxidative mechanisms. SUIs appear to be as effective as TCAs in treating a broad range of depressed patients, with some selective advantages for certain subgroups, such as those with marked anxiety or agitation. Panic disorders, obsessive-compulsive disorders, premenstrual syndrome, eating disorders (bulimarexia, exogenous obesity), chronic pain syndromes, drug abuse, disorders of impulse control (such as pathological aggression), and social phobia may respond better to SUIs than to antidepressants with weaker influence on serotonergic neurotransmission. SUIs reduce alcohol consumption in alcohol-dependent rats and heavy drinkers; their role in conjunction with psychological treatments is being examined in alcoholics. Although all SUIs act by blocking serotonin uptake, there are important differences among them. Their half-lives, for example, differ substantially, especially when their active metabolites are considered. Fluoxetine and its metabolite have a half-life of 330 hours, contrasting sharply with the half-lives of other SUIs, which range between 15 and 30 hours. Formerly called "selective serotonin reuptake inhibitors."

serotonin uptake inhibitor + fenfluramine Addition of fenfluramine (FEN) to serotonin uptake inhibitor (SUI) therapy of obsessive compulsive disorder may enhance therapeutic response (Hollander E, DeCaria CM, Schneier FR, et al. Fenfluramine augmentation of serotonin reuptake blockade antiobsessional therapy. *J Clin Psychiatry* 1990;51:119–123). Although FEN is neurotoxic in laboratory animals, an SUI may neutralize neurotoxic damage by blocking FEN entry into serotonin nerve terminals (Clineschmidt BV, Jacekei AG, Totaro JA, et al. Fenfluramine and brain serotonin. *Ann N Y Acad Sci* 1978;305:222–241).

serotonin uptake inhibitor + moclobemide Interaction studies with moclobemide have confirmed its relative safety compared to classic irreversible inhibitors of isoenzymes A and B. Moclobemide does not interact adversely with SUIs and, when switching from an SUI to moclobemide, no wash-out period is necessary. This does not apply to clomipramine, which inhibits both serotonin and noradrenaline reuptake and also exerts activity at central dopamine D_2, histamine H_1, and alpha-adrenergic receptors (Dingemanse J. An update of recent moclobemide interaction data. *Int Clin Psychopharmacol* 1993;7:167–180).

Seroxat See **paroxetine.**

Serpasil See **reserpine.**

sertindole (Lu 23-174) Potent neuroleptic with prominent selectivity for brain limbic areas and extreme selectivity on A10 and A9 dopamine neurons. Based on animal studies, sertindole is likely to have a low propensity to induce extrapyramidal side effects. This attribute, plus the lack of anticholinergic and sedative effects and a long duration of action, make sertindole a promising candidate for treating schizophrenia. It is being developed in depot form.

sertraline (Lustral, Zoloft) (SER) Naphthylamine with a unique chemical structure that is a highly selective serotonin uptake inhibitor antidepressant. It is one of the most potent serotonin-selective agents in this class of antidepressants. Its clinically inactive major metabolite is N-desmethylsertraline. SER is an effective antidepressant without sedative, anticholinergic, antidopaminergic, convulsant, or cardiotoxic effects. It has no demonstrable effects on intraventricular conduction or electrocardiographic time intervals. There is clinical evidence that in optimal doses SER improves vigilance, a considerable advantage since impairment of mental function is often a component of depressive illness. The daily dose is 50 mg, although a maximum of 200 mg may be given; half-life is 26 hours; and peak plasma concentration is attained in 6–8 hours. Thus, should SER fail, less time has to pass, by comparison with fluoxetine, before another antidepressant can be introduced. Therapeutic blood levels have not been established. In clinical trials, SER has been found to be as effective as amitriptyline and other tricyclic antidepressants. A multicenter placebo-controlled study found SER effective in obsessive-compulsive disorder (Chouinard G, Goodman W, Greist J, et al. Results of a new serotonin uptake inhibitor, sertraline, in the treatment of obsessive-compulsive disorder. *Psychopharmacol Bull* 1990;26:279–284). It has been reported to induce mania (Laporta M, Chouinard G, Goldbloom D, Beauclair L. Hypomania induced by sertraline, a new serotonin reuptake inhibitor. *Am J Psychiatry* 1987;144:1513–1514). It may be a promising medication for treating the hyperaroused, dysphoric biological and behavioral sequelae of exposure to extremely stressful life events, characterized diagnostically as post-traumatic stress disorder with co-morbid major depression (Kline NA, Dow BM, Brown SA, Matloff JL. Sertraline efficacy in depressed combat veterans with post-traumatic stress disorder. Presented at the 146th Annual Meeting of the American Psychiatric Association, San Francisco, May 1993). Pregnancy risk category B.

sertraline + alcohol   Sertraline's effects are not potentiated by alcohol, even in the elderly (Cohn CR, Shrivastava R, Mendels J, et al. Double-blind, multicenter comparison of sertraline and amitriptyline in elderly depressed patients. *J Clin Psychiatry* 1990;51[suppl B]:28–33).

sertraline + atenolol   Sertraline has no effect on the beta-adrenergic blocking ability of atenolol. Aside from an occasional mild headache, co-administration of sertraline and atenolol has evoked no serious adverse effects.

sertraline/cardiovascular effects   Effects of therapeutic doses of sertraline on electrocardiogram (ECG) were compared to those of placebo and amitriptyline in studies involving 1,048 patients with major depression. ECG findings in the elderly were essentially like those noted in nonelderly patients. Results of these analyses indicate sertraline has no significant ECG effects (Fisch C, Knoebel SB. Electrocardiographic findings in sertraline depression trials. *Drug Invest* 1992;4:305–312).

sertraline + cimetidine   Cimetidine slows sertraline clearance, increasing the area under the sertraline plasma level-time curve by about 50% following a single oral dose of sertraline. During cimetidine administration, mean sertraline plasma levels have been found to increase by about 25%, and its half-life increases as well (McGrath PJ. Preliminary information about sertraline [Zoloft]—a new, highly selective, serotonin reuptake-inhibitor. *Curr Affect Ill* 1992:11:5–14).

sertraline + clonazepam   Low-dose clonazepam has been added at bedtime for sertraline-treated patients with pressor test pretreatment insomnia. The regimen has been safe and efficacious (Kline NA, Dow BM, Brown SA, Matloff JL. Sertraline efficacy in depressed combat veterans with post-traumatic stress disorder. Presented at the 146th Annual Meeting of the American Psychiatric Association, San Francisco, May 1993).

sertraline + desipramine   Sertraline apparently has little or no effect on desipramine (DMI) plasma concentrations. Following discontinuation of sertraline, DMI level approaches baseline within 1 week. This is in contrast to the interaction of fluoxetine and tricyclic antidepressants. Concomitant administration of DMI and sertraline decreased DMI clearance 35%. This correlated modestly with sertraline and

desmethylsertraline levels. Sertraline and desmethylsertraline inhibited microsomal desipramine 2-hydroxylation, but this was less potent than that caused by fluoxetine and norfluoxetine (Preskorn SH, von Moltter L, Alderman J, et al. In vitro and in vivo evaluation of the potential for desipramine interaction with fluoxetine or sertraline. Presented at the 146th Annual Meeting of the American Psychiatric Association. San Francisco, May 1993). It has been reported that in a patient being treated with DMI (steady state 152 ng/ml), the DMI level rose to 203 ng/ml 1 week after the addition of sertraline (50 mg/day). One month later, when steady-state levels of sertraline had presumably been achieved, the DMI level was 240 ng/ml. The patient did not experience adverse effects from the combination and reported that he felt better than with prior therapy. This single case indicates a relatively modest (60%) increase in steady-state plasma DMI levels following the addition of sertraline. These data suggest that there may be a relatively limited pharmacokinetic interaction between sertraline and tricyclics (Lydiard RB, Anton RF, Cunningham T. Interactions between sertraline and tricyclic antidepressants. *Am J Psychiatry* 1993;150:1125–1126; Barros J, Asnis G. An interaction of sertraline and desipramine. *Am J Psychiatry* 1993;150:1751). See **fluoxetine + tricyclic antidepressants.**

sertraline + diazepam   Sertraline has no clinically relevant effects on the pharmacokinetics of diazepam in healthy volunteers (Gaardner MH, Ronfeld RA, Wilner KD, et al. The effects of sertraline on the pharmacokinetics of diazepam in healthy volunteers. *Biol Psychiatry* 1991;29:354S).

sertraline + digoxin   In healthy volunteers sertraline has no clinically significant effects on the plasma concentration or renal clearance of digoxin (Forster PL, Dewland PM, Muirhead D, et al. The effects of sertraline on plasma concentration and renal clearance of digoxin. *Biol Psychiatry* 1991;29:355S).

sertraline + doxepin   Low-dose doxepin (25–50 mg) has been added at bedtime for sertraline-treated patients with persistent pretreatment insomnia. The regimen has been safe and effective (Kline NA, Dow BM, Brown SA, Matloff JL. Sertraline efficacy in depressed combat veterans with posttraumatic stress disorder. Presented at the 146th Annual Meeting of the American Psychiatric Association, San Francisco, May 1993).

sertraline + electroconvulsive therapy (ECT)   There is currently (1994) insufficient experience to indicate whether co-administration is safe. Because potential interactions could include provocation of a serotonin syndrome, sertraline should be avoided during ECT (Jarvis MR, Goewert AJ, Zorumski CF. Novel antidepressants and maintenance electroconvulsive therapy. A review. *Ann Clin Psychiatry* 1992;4:275–284).

sertraline + fluoxetine   Co-administration may increase sertraline plasma level.

sertraline + glibenclamide   Administration of sertraline is not associated with any clinically important changes in the pharmacokinetics of glibenclamide.

sertraline + indapamide   Co-administration in a 54-year-old woman resulted in erythema multiforme and angioedema requiring hospitalization and treatment with intravenous corticosteroids, analgesics, and antihistamines (Gales BJ, Gales, MA. Erythema multiforme and angioedema associated with indapamide and sertraline therapy. *ASHP Midyear Clinical Meeting* 1993;28:P-28).

sertraline + lithium   Co-administration is safe and effective, although sertraline may increase lithium tremor, slightly decrease steady-state lithium levels, and slightly increase renal clearance of lithium (Apseloff G, Wilner KD, von Deutsch DA, et al. Sertraline does not alter steady-state concentrations or renal clearance of lithium in healthy volunteers. *J Clin Pharmacol* 1992;32:643–646; Dinan TG. Lithium augmentation in sertraline-resistant depression: a preliminary dose-response study. *Acta Psychiatr Scand* 1993;88:300–301). Sertraline may augment response to lithium in organic mood syndrome without causing any serious adverse effects (Workman EA, Harrington DP. Sertraline-augmented Lithium therapy of organic mood syndrome. *Psychosomatics* 1992;33: 472–473).

sertraline + nortriptyline   Co-administration can be effective in patients resistant to a standard antidepressant and a full course of electroconvulsive therapy (Seth R, Jennings AL, Bindman J, et al. Combination therapy with noradrenaline and serotonin reuptake inhibitors in resistant depression. *Br J Psychiatry* 1992;161:562–565).

sertraline + tolbutamide   Sertraline does not cause any clinically important changes in the pharmacokinetics of tolbutamide.

sertraline + tranylcypromine   A serotonin syndrome has been reported in a 46-year-old man with treatment-resistant depression who was treated with sertraline (50 mg/day), tranylcypromine (30 mg/day) and clonazepam (1.5 mg at bedtime). Sertraline initiation was associated with marked worsening of serotonergic symptoms. The patient had chills, incoordination, and mental status changes such as confusion, memory disturbance, and restlessness.

Symptoms subsided following discontinuation of sertraline and reduction of tranylcypromine dosage to 20 mg/day. Although concurrent use of sertraline and a monoamine oxidase inhibitor (MAOI) should be avoided, the quality of life of patients with severe depression refractory to standard treatment must be considered. A distinction should be drawn between the incautious combining of these drugs and their use in patients with otherwise intractable clinical depression. The above case report suggests that sertraline, like fluoxetine, should not be added without a hiatus (14 days or longer) after discontinuation of an MAOI. Concurrent use of sertraline and an MAOI should be avoided in most cases until proven safe or until effective prophylaxis has been identified. (Bhatara VS, Bandettini FC. Possible interaction between sertraline and tranylcypromine. *Clin Pharm* 1993;12:222–225; Boyer W, Feighner J. Response to letter. *J Clin Psychiatry* 1991;52:87; Peterson G. Strategies for fluoxetine-MAOI combination therapy. *J Clin Psychiatry* 1991;52:87; Rosenblatt J, Rosenblatt N. Sertraline-MAOI interaction: corrigendum cum case report. *Curr Affect Ill* 1992; 11:17 [abstract]).

sertraline + trazodone   Low-dose trazodone (25–50 mg) has been added at bedtime for sertraline-treated patients with pressor test pretreatment insomnia. The regimen has been safe and efficacious (Kline NA, Dow BM, Brown SA, Matloff JL. Sertraline efficacy in depressed combat veterans with posttraumatic stress disorder. Presented at the 146th Annual Meeting of the American Psychiatric Association, San Francisco, May 1993).

sertraline + warfarin   In a placebo-controlled trial involving healthy subjects, prothrombin time and warfarin plasma protein binding were determined after a single oral dose of warfarin. After 22 days of sertraline treatment, a second dose of warfarin was administered, and a significant increase in the prothrombin time area under the curve and a decrease in warfarin plasma protein binding were observed. Although these changes were deemed to be clinically unimportant in this study, co-administration of sertraline with anticoagulants should be accompanied by careful monitoring of prothrombin time (Wilner KD, Lazar JD, Apseloff G, et al. The effects of sertraline on the pharmacodynamics of warfarin in healthy volunteers. *Biol Psychiatry* 1991;29: 354S).

serum gamma-glutamyltransferase   (GGT) Sensitive laboratory test of early liver dysfunction useful in detecting alcohol misuse. GGT is elevated in 70% of alcoholics and heavy drinkers.

serum glutamic-oxaloacetic transaminase (SGOT) Liver enzyme often elevated in the serum of chronic alcoholics; used as a liver function test.

serum glutamic-pyruvic transaminase (SGPT) Liver enzyme that may be abnormal in alcoholics and individuals with hepatic disease; used as a liver function test.

serum level Concentration of a drug in serum. Serum is the aqueous phase of whole blood remaining after coagulation has taken place and the clot removed by centrifugation or other separation procedure. Serum level may refer to bound, free, or total drug. Expressed as units of mass (or number of moles) per unit of volume.

serum sickness Hypersensitivity reaction mediated by immune cell complexes. Main symptoms are rash, fever, myalgia, arthralgia, and lymphadenopathy. The kidneys, lungs, and heart can be involved. Rare cases of meningoencephalitis have been described. Laboratory assessment can show leukopenia or slight leukocytosis, eosinophilia, and elevated sedimentation rate. Complement levels may be low. Proteinuria and hematuria can appear, but there is no specific finding. Isolated cases of serum sickness induced by psychoactive drugs have been reported.

Servium See **chlordiazepoxide.**

setoperone Mixed serotonin (5-HT$_2$)-dopamine antagonist that lacks anticholinergic activity. Bioavailability is very poor. In chronic schizophrenics with predominantly negative symptoms, setoperone produces a 50% reduction in negative symptoms, significantly decreasing emotional withdrawal and improving blunted affect. It has been found effective in alleviating dysphoria in chronic schizophrenics with a predominant Type II syndrome. It causes fewer extrapyramidal symptoms than antipsychotics combined with antiparkinson medication.

severe self-injurious behavior See **self-injurious behavior, severe.**

sex Biological sexuality. It is defined by six component parts: chromosomes, gonads, internal and external genitalia, sex hormones, and secondary sexual characteristics.

Sexaholics Anonymous (SA) Self-help group, modeled after Alcoholics Anonymous, for individuals with a variety of sexually compulsive behaviors.

sex chromatin Chromatin mass in the nucleus of interphase cells of females of most mammalian species, including man. It represents a single X chromosome that is inactive in the metabolism of the cell. Normal females have sex chromatin, normal males lack it. See **Barr body.**

sex chromosomes Chromosomes responsible for sex determination. In humans, XX is female and XY is male.

sex determination Genetic mechanism that determines the difference between the two sexes, specifically the sex chromosomes X and Y. Under usual conditions, a fertilized egg with two XX chromosomes becomes a female; a fertilized egg with one X and one Y chromosome becomes a male.

sex-linkage Inheritance by genes on the sex chromosomes. Several neurological syndromes exhibit sex-linked transmission.

sex ratio The ratio of one sex to the other, usually defined as the ratio of males to females.

sexual abuse, early Any sexual contact before the age of 17—excluding willing contact in teenage years with nonrelated peers.

sexual addiction See **compulsive sexual behavior.**

sexual disorder One of a group of disorders that include paraphilias and sexual dysfunctions.

sexual exploitation Use of an individual who is unable to consent to, or make an informed choice because of lack of knowledge about, a sexual act by another person for his or her sexual gratification.

sexual harassment Persistent, unwanted sexual attention that is found objectionable or causes offense, operating through such things as physical contact, gestures, insults, humiliation, belittling, or ridicule. It can result in the recipient feeling threatened, humiliated, or patronized, and it can create an intimidating work environment. It is one in a range of behaviors that can be classified as "personal abuse." Assault is an extreme form of abuse, and sexual harassment is an aggressive act conveyed through words and body language. It is distinguished from flirting and sexual banter by being unwanted. Actions that may constitute sexual harassment include (a) unwanted physical contact such as unnecessary touching, patting, or pinching of another employee's body; (b) demands for sexual favors in return for promotion; (c) unwelcome sexual advances or propositions; (d) continued suggestions for social activity outside the workplace after it has been made clear that such suggestions are unwelcome; (e) offensive flirtation; (f) suggestive remarks, innuendos, or lewd comments; (g) display of sexually suggestive pin-ups or calendars; (h) leering or eyeing up a person's body; (i) derogatory remarks that are gender-related; (j) sexual assault; (k) offensive comments about appearance or dress that are gender-related; (l) sexist or patronizing behavior (NHS Management

Executive. *Harassment At Work*. London: NH-SME, 1992; *Sexual Harassment at the Workplace*. London: Industrial Relations Services, 1992 [Industrial Relations Review and Report No. 513]).

sexual masochism   Derivation of sexual pleasure from physical or psychological pain inflicted by others or by oneself. It is the opposite of sexual sadism. It is the only perversion, aside from sexual sadism, that occurs in both sexes and among heterosexuals and homosexuals. The diagnosis should be made only if the individual engages in masochistic sexual acts and not merely in fantasies. Masochism and sadism are often linked, and although an individual is usually preferentially a masochist or a sadist, he or she can occasionally enact the other role. Typical examples of masochism include the desire to be bound, the transvestic impersonation, and the desire to be beaten on the buttocks. See **sadism; sadomasochism; sexual sadism.**

sexual sadism   See **sadism.**

sexuality   Erotic excitement, genital arousal, and orgasm. It is expressed in fantasy and behavior, object choice, preferred activities, subjective desire, arousal, and actual orgasmic discharge.

"she"   Street name for cocaine.

"sheets"   Street name for phencyclidine (PCP).

"sherm"   Street name for phencyclidine (PCP). In some parts of the United States, PCP-laced cigarettes are called "sherms" because the cigarette preferred for smoking purposes was produced by a company called "Nate Sherman."

"sherman"   Street name for phencyclidine (PCP).

shift maladaptation syndrome   Disorder of the effects of long-term shift work on the health of workers who have never been able to adjust to it. Any work schedule that requires people to work when they would normally be sleeping (and to sleep when they would normally be awake) can disrupt their circadian rhythms. The result is akin to what occurs in jet lag. Although the effects of jet lag are transitory, the effects of circadian rhythm disruption associated with shift work continues unabated and interacts with other factors. Shift workers often have difficulty sleeping as a result of trying to sleep at an inappropriate time in the circadian cycle and in an environment that is not conducive to sleep (i.e., daytime sleep). Shift work can also make it difficult to fulfill domestic roles as a parent or spouse and can put a worker out of sync with the rest of society. For some shift workers, the combined stress of a desynchronized circadian system, sleep deprivation, and domestic and social disharmony may result in additional adverse effects, including health problems and diminished performance. Diminished performance can compromise the safety of the individual worker, and in some occupations, the safety of the public as well. People vary greatly in their ability to adjust to shift work, however, and some individuals suffer few, if any, problems from work schedules others find intolerable. Nonetheless, available information indicates that shift work is associated with a number of specific health problems. Gastrointestinal disorders, including general gastric discomfort and peptic ulcer disease, occur more often among shift workers. A number of cardiovascular parameters (e.g., heart rate, blood pressure) follow a circadian rhythm. There is a modestly higher incidence of cardiovascular disease among shift workers. A few studies suggest that female shift workers experience slightly increased risks for miscarriage, preterm birth, and lower-birth-weight babies. The adverse health effects of shift work are diffuse, affecting some workers' general sense of well-being. These workers frequently report sleep disturbances and fatigue, menstrual problems, increased feelings of irritation and strain, increased use of alcohol and other drugs (tranquilizers, caffeine), and a general feeling of malaise (Liskowsky DR. Biological rhythms and shift work. *JAMA* 1992;268:3047).

shift work sleep disorder   Type of dyssomnia experienced by many shift workers manifested by insomnia, sleep debt, daytime sleepiness, impaired performance, and diverse somatic complaints. To cope with the dyssomnia, many shift workers use hypnotics, stimulants, or alcohol that often do not relieve, but compound, their sleep disorder.

"shit"   Street name for heroin.

shock treatment   See **electroconvulsive therapy (ECT); insulin coma therapy (ICT).** The term *shock treatment* should be abandoned.

"shooting"   Street term for intravenous injection of drugs of abuse, including cocaine or heroin.

"shooting gallery"   Street term for a place where substance abusers inject drugs. Also called "flash house" or "galleria."

"shoot up"   Street term for injecting drugs intravenously.

short-term memory   Correct recall or appropriate performance immediately or shortly after presentation of material. Rapid decay and limited amount of remembered material distinguishes it from long-term memory.

"shroom"   Uncommon street name for psilocybin. Reportedly, it can make rituals and obsessive thoughts disappear completely for 5 or 6 hours after it is taken by an obsessive-compulsive disorder patient. Whether this is due to its effects on the serotonin system is not known.

sialorrhea Excessive salivation that may be a manifestation of parkinsonism. It is often a side effect of clozapine therapy, not related to extrapyramidal symptoms.

Sibelium See **flunarizine.**

sibship Genetic term pertaining to one series of siblings (i.e., all biological children of the same parents).

sibutramine (BTS 54-524) New antidepressant currently in clinical trials. It is a beta-adrenergic receptor agonist that induces rapid noradrenergic down-regulation.

sidedness Side of the body on which an action or behavior occurs. It does not automatically imply that the neurological substrate for the described function is located contralaterally.

side effect Unwanted and undesirable physical, emotional, and/or behavioral effects of medications that may be unrelated to their therapeutic effects. Also called "adverse effects" or "treatment-emergent events." It is essential to distinguish between the side effects of a drug and allergic reactions to it. The former are normal. They are due to the physiological and pharmacological actions of the medicine. They occur in varying intensity in all patients taking the drug and, although troublesome, most are not serious. Side effects usually remit spontaneously with continued treatment or may be modified by a temporary reduction of the dosage or the addition of other drugs. Allergic reactions, by contrast, are unexpected. Fortunately, they are infrequent, occurring usually in a low percentage of patients receiving the drug. They are potentially serious and warrant immediate discontinuation of the responsible medicine. Clinical trials before marketing discover common side effects of a drug but not those occurring rarely (less than 1 in 250 patients). New drug-related side effects may not emerge until several years after drugs have been marketed, making continual vigilance for their detection necessary. See **treatment-emergent symptoms.**

sigma 1. Symbol for one-thousandth of a second. 2. Symbol for standard deviation.

sigma antagonist Drug that blocks the effects of an opiate at opioid sigma receptors.

sigma receptor Subclass of receptors located in nonsynaptic regions of plasma membranes in the central nervous system and peripherally in endocrine and immune tissues. Stimulation of the sigma receptor results in dysphoria, psychomotor stimulation, and tachycardia. It was first identified as a binding site for [^{3}H]N-allylnormetazocine. Haloperidol has especially high affinity for the sigma receptor, and many studies use [^{3}H]haloperidol to label sigma

receptors. Several novel compounds, such as BMY 14802, bind with relative potency to sigma binding sites and show promise as antipsychotics. Remoxipride is relatively selective for the sigma site and D_2 receptors. Phencyclidine, cocaine, and anabolic steroids bind with the sigma receptor (Su TP. Review: sigma receptors. Putative links between neurons, endocrine and immune systems (*Eur J Biochem* 1991;200:633–642). Binding to the sigma receptor is thought to be the explanation for cocaine's dysphoric effects (Sharkey J, Glen K, Wolfe S, et al. Cocaine binding at sigma receptors. *Eur J Pharmacol* 1988;149:171–174). There is evidence for the existence of two sigma receptor subtypes: sigma$_1$ and sigma$_2$. These subtypes demonstrate unique ligand selectivity profiles and are differentially modulated following various treatments (Quiron R, Bowen WD, Itzhak Y, et al. A proposal for the classification of sigma binding sites. *TIPS* 1992; 13:85–86).

sign Objective manifestation of a pathological condition (DSM-IV). Signs are observed by the examiner rather than reported by the individual.

sign, bonbon One of the manifestations of the buccal-lingual-masticatory syndrome or tardive dyskinesia. It consists of the pressing of the tongue against the cheek, giving the perception of a candy (bonbon) in the mouth.

signal Reported information on a possible causal relation between an adverse event and a drug, the relation being unknown or incompletely documented previously. Usually more than a single report is required to generate a signal, depending on the seriousness of the event and the quality of the information (WHO, 1992).

signal peptides Short stretches of hydrophobic amino acid residues (20 or so) that are found at the amino terminus of membrane bound or secreted proteins prior to their insertion or transport. Generally, they contain the information used to direct their transport to a specific organelle or they target the protein for secretion. Signal peptides are generally cleaved during this process.

signal transduction General process by which a nerve impulse or electrical signal is converted into a chemical signal or neurotransmitter release by the presynaptic neuron and the process by which the postsynaptic neuron is reconverted into an electrical signal.

significance Statement that the probability of obtaining the observed effect by chance only is small and designated by the alpha error. Significance tells how likely it is that an observed difference is due to chance when the true difference is zero.

significance level Arbitrarily selected probability level for rejecting the null hypothesis, commonly .05 or .01.

significance testing Statistical technique used to determine *P* values. See *P* **values.**

significant Outcome of a formal test of a statistical hypothesis falling outside a chosen, predetermined region.

significant differences Statistical term indicating that a given difference is not likely to have occurred by chance. In many behavioral studies, the likelihood of an event occurring less frequently than 1 in 20 times (p < .05) is considered the minimal acceptable significance level. The determination that a given difference between two groups is significant can merely serve to identify the likelihood that it was not a chance event. It does not prove that the demonstrated systematic difference is necessarily due to the reasons hypothesized by the investigator. Systematic factors not considered by the investigator can sometimes be responsible for significant differences.

significant other Person with a close familial or other relationship to the patient.

Sidnocarb See **mesocarb.**

signs Phenomena observed by the physician, the patient, or others, indicating the presence of abnormal functioning of one or more bodily systems.

signs, soft Subtle signs of disability or dysfunction, such as clumsiness, often used to refer to results of neurological examinations of children who are schizophrenic and/or who have minimal brain dysfunction.

silent allele See **allele, silent.**

silent DNA See **junk DNA.**

simple phobia See **phobia, simple.**

simple random sample Group of randomly selected subjects with each having the same probability of being selected. Each pair also has the same probability of being selected. Such probabilities are the sample size over population size, and the product of sample size and sample size minus 1, divided by the product of population size and population size minus 1, respectively.

simple reaction time Task that assesses alertness, power of concentration, ability to respond rapidly.

simulation Feigning symptoms that do not exist. Also called "positive malingering."

Sinemet See **levodopa/carbidopa.**

Sinemet CR See **levodopa/carbidopa.**

Sinequan See **doxepin.**

single-blind design Study design in which subjects do not know whether they are receiving active drug or placebo.

single-compartment model Model of drug kinetics that assumes instantaneous distribution to a single compartment.

single-dose kinetics Model that describes the time course of absorption, distribution, and elimination of a given drug after a single dose.

single-gene disorders Hereditary disorders caused by a single gene.

single oral dose A drug's C_{max} is reached rapidly or slowly depending on the rate of bioavailability and clearance; its value depends on extent of bioavailability, dose, volume of distribution, and clearance.

single-patient design Study design that evolved because of the difficulty in assessing behavioral or other psychiatric interventions within the framework of traditional designs. The objective is to test within a single patient whether a particular treatment produces clinical improvement and to make the judgment within a framework that affords some statistical analysis. Also called "*n* of 1 design."

single photon Gamma radiation emitted by a radionucleotide, usually in random directions.

single photon camera Imaging device designed to measure location and density of different gamma rays emitted by single photon emission computed tomography (SPECT) ligands.

single photon emission computed tomography (SPECT) Neuroimaging technique for measuring cerebral blood flow, cerebral blood volume, cerebral metabolic rates of glucose and oxygen, and the oxygen-extraction fraction. It can also be used for imaging receptors. It uses radiochemicals present in the brain long enough to allow imaging by a rotating gamma camera. It has poor resolution but is generally more available and less expensive than positron emission tomography (PET) scans. At present, SPECT is one of the best noninvasive techniques for the study of dementia of the Alzheimer type. SPECT also has been valuable in identifying seizure foci, especially in temporal lobe seizures. Improved radiopharmaceuticals and the development of new brain SPECT equipment now provide a sensitive and valuable tool for the evaluation of abnormalities of cerebral blood flow.

Sintonal See **brotizolam.**

Sirtal See **carbamazepine.**

site-directed mutagenesis Modified proteins synthesized from mRNA that has been manipulated to alter the normal nucleotide sequence at a particular site on the molecule. Artificially synthesized versions of proteins can be produced that contain changes of single amino acids. The functional consequences of these modifications are used to understand the function of the proteins.

situational aggression See **aggression, situational.**

situational pedophile See **pedophile, situational.**

"skag" Street name for heroin.

SK-Bamate See **meprobamate.**

SK-Lygen See **chlordiazepoxide.**

SK-Pramine See **imipramine.**

skewed distribution In statistics, asymmetrical frequency distribution. A longer tail extending toward lower values (to the left) is negative skewing (i.e., the mean is lower than the mode or the median). A longer tail extending toward higher values (to the right) is positive skewing (i.e., the mean is greater than the mode or the median).

skin conductance activity See **electrodermal activity.**

skin conductance level (SCL) See **electrodermal activity.**

skin conductance response (SCR) See **electrodermal activity.**

"skin popping" Subcutaneous injections of heroin resulting in chronic, suppurative skin lesions and a persistent inflammatory state in heroin abusers. It may result in renal amyloidosis. "Skin-popping" also may be used for subcutaneous injections of other opioids. The lesions caused by skin-popping are often located in such readily accessible areas as the arm and thigh, but they may be anywhere on the body because of injections by a companion or self-injection in areas where detection is less likely.

"slamming" Street term for intravenous use of narcotics.

sleep State of decreased responsiveness to a person's surroundings. The major sleep episode occurs at night; brief periods of sleep (naps) can also occur during the day. There are two states of sleep that are as different from each other as sleep in general is different from wakefulness. They are rapid eye movement (REM) sleep and non–rapid eye movement (N-REM) sleep. REM and N-REM sleep alternate with each other in a cycle that in total lasts from 70 to 100 minutes. Usually there are 4–6 REM periods per sleep cycle. See **REM sleep; sleep-stage NREM.**

sleep, active Sleep stage considered equivalent to rapid eye movement (REM) sleep.

sleep, alpha Sleep disorder in which alpha activity occurs during slow-wave sleep, categorized as a disorder of initiating and maintaining sleep (DIMS). It is manifested by atypical polysomnographic features with the superimposition of alpha (high-voltage) waves in the sleep electroencephalogram (EEG). Alpha waves cycle 18 times/sec and are most consis-

tent and predominant during relaxed wakefulness.

sleep apnea Disorder characterized by respiratory cessations during sleep. Many physiological changes and symptoms are associated with sleep apnea, such as a drop in oxyhemoglobin saturation, cardiac arrhythmias, nocturnal hypertension, night-time confusion, and neuropsychological impairment—some of which are symptoms often found in the elderly. At the end of each apnea, the low blood-oxygen level causes an arousal response that then permits effective breathing. Chronic hypoxemia can lead to mental deterioration; some studies have demonstrated a greater incidence of sleep apnea in dementia patients. There are three types of sleep apnea: (a) obstructive apnea, which results from intermittent blockage of the upper airway; (b) central apnea, in which there is a complete absence of respiratory effort; and (c) mixed apnea, which involves a combination of obstructive and central phenomena. According to the American Sleep Disorders Association, about 1% of the population in the United States suffers from sleep apnea. Patients often present with a number of clinical symptoms, especially excessive daytime sleepiness and fatigue. Alcohol and depressive medications, such as hypnotic compounds, can increase the frequency and duration of apneic events, thereby worsening the condition. Sleep apnea should be considered a precipitating factor of or in the differential diagnosis of confusional states, heart failure, nocturnal seizures, and nocturnal bradycardia.

sleep apnea/alcohol Alcohol is a respiratory suppressant. When consumed in moderate amounts by patients with the sleep apnea syndrome, it may greatly enhance respiratory impairment.

sleep apnea, central Cessation of airflow during sleep for more than 10 seconds in the absence of any evidence of obstruction or of respiratory effort during this time. Central sleep apnea may be due to metabolic or neurological disturbances. Continuous positive airway pressure therapy is an effective treatment.

sleep apnea, obstructive (OSA) Apneic episodes characterized by upper airway closure for at least 10 seconds, causing a cessation of airflow despite the persistence of respiratory efforts. Hundreds of apneic episodes may occur during an 8-hour sleep period. OSA patients are usually obese, snore loudly, awaken several times a night and complain of excessive daytime sleepiness. Bedpartners often complain that the snoring disrupts their sleep. Continuous positive airway pressure therapy is an effective treatment. Obese OSA patients improve following weight loss. Avoidance of alcohol and sedatives prior to sleep is advisable.

sleep architecture   The different stages of sleep and their duration, including (a) total sleep time; (b) stage 1 sleep; (c) stage 2 sleep; (d) stages 3/4 sleep; (e) rapid eye movement (REM) sleep; and (f) awakenings. Sleep architecture is often plotted in the form of a hypnograph, the percentage of time spent in each of the four sleep stages.

sleep attack   Brief episode (15 minutes or less) of sleep that occurs at any time of the day. Attacks occur in patients with narcolepsy, with or without warning. Patients awake refreshed after a brief episode of sleeping. The attacks are frequently described as episodes of excessive daytime sleepiness.

sleep clinic   Clinic in which some form of sleep disorders medicine is practiced, including comprehensive work-up, evaluation, and all-night polysomnographic testing of patients with sleep-related complaints. In 1990, there were about 2,000 sleep clinics in the United States.

sleep, core   Hypothesized to be the essential first part of night sleep, mainly slow wave sleep (stages 3 and 4 of non–rapid eye movement [NREM] sleep) The other part is "optional" sleep (Horne J. *Why We Sleep.* Oxford: Oxford University Press, 1989). Core sleep occurs during the first three sleep cycles. In core sleep, NREM sleep and REM are reduced. There is also an increase in drowsiness and in the time spent awake after sleep onset. The decrease in slow wave sleep is gender-related and prevails in elderly men. REM sleep diminishes with increasing age. In the elderly, most REM sleep occurs at the beginning of the night, in contrast to the longer duration of REM sleep at the end of the night in younger persons. Core sleep is an essential and necessary part of sleep required for optimal daytime functioning (Wauquier A, van Sweden B. Aging of core and optional sleep. *Biol Psychiatry* 1992;31:866–880). See **sleep, optional.**

sleep debt   Consequence of chronic sleep deprivation resulting in next-day sleepiness, often experienced by shift workers. A few hours or nights of sleep do not repay sleep debt.

sleep, deep   Combined non–rapid eye movement (NREM) stages 3 and 4 sleep. In some sleep literature, deep sleep is applied to REM sleep because of its high awakening threshold to nonsignificant stimuli.

sleep, delta   Slow-wave sleep in the electroencephalogram (EEG). New computerized techniques, including amplitude and frequency measures and spectral analysis, have demonstrated lower delta wave intensity during the first non–rapid eye movement (NREM) period than the second one in many depressed patients. This delta sleep measure seems to be a better predictor of depression recurrence than REM latency.

sleep deprivation   (SD) Treatment for depression in which the patient is kept awake. SD for a period of 1 night has been shown to produce a marked, transient amelioration in about 60% of patients with major depressive disorder. The antidepressant effects of sleep deprivation may be state-dependent. Many patients who do respond subsequently relapse after 1 night of sleep. Relapse can be quite precipitous with no evidence of a gradual deterioration. It is unlikely that relapse results from a nonspecific effect of the disruption of sleep. This is supported by the degree of deterioration seen, with patients often returning to a moderate or severe level of depression from an essentially euthymic, or even hypomanic, state. SD combined with clomipramine or lithium has been reported to produce a rapid, sustained antidepressant effect in SD responders. SD may be used as a diagnostic aid or as a prognostic tool, and may be the only antidepressant intervention with same-day beneficial effect. SD alone may be used to treat an unmedicated depressed patient. It can be added to potentiate an ongoing antidepressant drug therapy, or be started when antidepressant drug therapy or lithium is initiated to hasten response to medication. Also, SD, either alone or in combination with antidepressants, may be useful in preventing recurrent mood cycles. However, the risk of precipitating mania in this population may be substantial. Response to adjunctive SD can be used as a diagnostic marker and a predictor of response to somatic treatment. Response to SD in geriatric patients has been used to differentiate dementia from depression. It has also been used to predict a patient's subsequent response to antidepressant medication, generally or to a particular class of antidepressants (Leibenheft E, Wehr TA. Is sleep deprivation useful in the treatment of depression? *Am J Psychiatry* 1992;149:159–168). SD is an attractive antidepressant treatment because it acts rapidly and is noninvasive, inexpensive, and well tolerated by most patients. However, a patient's response to a single night of SD may not accurately predict response to repeated treatments. A 1-day response to SD is too transient to be clinically useful. SD has been reported to be an effective treatment of depression in an elderly patient with Parkinson's disease (Perry W, Benbow C, West L, et al. Sleep deprivation in an elderly man with

Parkinson's disease. *Am J Psychiatry* 1993;150: 350). An investigation of the antidepressant effect of SD revealed that among 12 hormones measured, there was a significant rise in thyroid stimulating hormone, thyroxine, triiodothyronine, and free triiodothyronine and a significant reduction in testosterone on the morning after total sleep deprivation (Baumgartner A, Graf KJ, Kurten I, et al. Neuroendocrinology investigations during sleep deprivation in depression: I. Early morning levels. *Biol Psychiatry* 1990;28:556–568).

sleep deprivation/mania   Like other antidepressant treatments, sleep deprivation (SD) can trigger or intensify mania, at least in patients with bipolar illness who are susceptible to mania. SD-induced manias may subside after the patient returns to sleep. However, since insomnia is itself a symptom of mania, the interaction between sleep loss and mania can become self-reinforcing and escalate out of control. Thus, manias may go on for weeks or months, long after termination of the triggering event that disrupted sleep in the first place. Almost anything that disrupts sleep— stressful life events, medications (especially psychostimulants), drug withdrawal—may produce mania (Wehr TA. Improvement of depression and triggering of mania by sleep deprivation. *JAMA* 1992;267:548–551).

sleep deprivation, partial   (PSD) Treatment for depression in which the patient is kept awake for only part of the night. In early partial sleep deprivation, the patient is kept awake until 2 A.M., allowed to sleep from 2 A.M. to 7 A.M., and then kept awake until 10 P.M. In late partial sleep deprivation, the patient is awakened at 2 A.M. and kept awake until 10 P.M. Either treatment may be as effective as total sleep deprivation. Late partial sleep deprivation has been used to potentiate response to antidepressant medication; three to five treatments a week may be sufficient for this purpose.

sleep deprivation, total   Treatment for depression in which the patient is kept awake for a 36-hour period. It may be done once or twice a week, or until a predetermined maximum number of treatments is reached. Elderly patients may require a mean of 3.3 treatments, and younger patients may require a mean of 5 treatments.

sleep disorder   Disruption of normal sleep that meets accepted diagnostic criteria. The International Classification of Sleep Disorders lists 88 types of sleep disorders, in many of which insomnia is the most prominent symptom. DMS-IV divides sleep disorders into two major groups, the dyssomnias (in which the predominant disturbance is in the amount, quality, or timing of sleep) and the parasomnias (in which the predominant disturbance is an abnormal event occurring during sleep). DSM-IV dyssomnias include insomnia disorders, hypersomnia disorders, and sleep-wake schedule disorders. Sleep apnea and narcolepsy, which in some classifications are considered sleep disorders in their own right, are classified in DSM-IV as hypersomnias. DSM-IV parasomnias include nightmare disorder, sleep terror disorder, and sleepwalking disorder. The diagnosis and treatment of sleep disorders are clinically important because these disorders are very prevalent in the general population and in medical practice. The prevalence and intensity of sleep disturbances increase with advancing age. This is due to various factors: physiological, such as age-related changes in sleep patterns; medical, such as more frequent physical ailments and illnesses disturbing sleep; psychiatric, including the increased occurrence of affective and organic mental disorders associated with sleep difficulty; pharmacological, such as use, misuse, and abuse of various drugs directly or indirectly affecting sleep; and social, such as changing rest-activity schedules and, consequently, sleep-wakefulness patterns. Chronic insomnia, daytime fatigue, and tiredness impair the well-being of older individuals and increase the risk of accidents and trauma.

sleep disorder, extrinsic   Subgroup of the dyssomnias in which the sleep disturbance originates, develops, or arises from causes outside of the body.

sleep disorder, intrinsic   Subgroup of the dyssomnias in which the sleep disturbance originates, develops, or arises from causes within the body.

sleep efficiency   (SE) Percentage of time in bed spent asleep. It is usually above 90% in the young and decreases somewhat with age.

sleep electroencephalogram (EEG)   EEG recording during natural or drug-induced sleep. Sleep EEG abnormalities have been described in affective illnesses, including disturbances in sleep continuity, sleep architecture, and measures of rapid eye movement (REM) sleep. Compared with control subjects, depressed patients have more time awake during the night, longer early-morning awakening, less slow-wave sleep, a shortened latency of the first REM sleep, more REM activity, and higher REM density.

sleep episode, major   Longest sleep episode that occurs on a daily basis. It is determined by the circadian rhythm of sleep and wakefulness.

sleep episode, total   In sleep electroencephalography, the total time available for sleep during an attempt to sleep. It includes rapid eye movement (REM) and non-REM sleep as well as wakefulness. It is synonymous with and preferred to the term *total sleep period*.

"sleeper" Street name for barbiturates, central nervous system depressants.

Sleep-Eze Nonprescription proprietary hypnotic containing small quantities of scopolamine. It can cause delirium if taken in accidental or deliberate overdose.

sleep fragmentation Interruption, usually repetitive, of any sleep stage due to appearance of another stage or wakening, leading to disrupted rapid eye movement (REM)/NREM sleep cycles. The term often refers to REM sleep interruption by movement arousals or stage 2 activity.

sleep, fragmented Common sleep disturbance, especially in elderly depressives. The proportion of time asleep during time in bed is low, resulting in complaints that sleep is "inefficient" or "not restful or refreshing." Patients with fragmented sleep have frequent sleep stage changes that may be related to lowered thresholds for arousal to sound.

sleep hygiene Practices or habits that promote sleep. Sleep hygiene techniques can be used as adjuncts to treatment of the specific causes of insomnia and tried when the cause is not clear or unspecified. Sleep hygiene measures include regularization of bedtime (generally later rather than earlier); use of the bedroom primarily for sleeping and sexual activity; exercise; avoidance of alcohol and caffeine; reduced evening fluid intake; and, in the case of esophageal reflux, elevation of the head of the bed.

Sleepinal Over-the-counter preparation of 50 mg of diphenhydramine sold as a sleep aid.

sleepiness, excessive Subjective report of difficulty in maintaining the alert awake state, usually accompanied by rapid entrance into sleep when sedentary. It can be measured quantitatively with subjectively defined sleepiness rating scales or physiologically by electrophysiological tests (e.g., the multiple sleep latency test). It occurs most commonly during the daytime, but may be present at night in a person whose major sleep period is during the daytime.

"sleeping pill" **1.** Street name for barbiturates. **2.** General term for a wide variety of nighttime sedatives.

sleep interruption Break in sleep architecture resulting in arousal and wakefulness.

sleep intrusion, non-REM Interposition of non–rapid eye movement (NREM) sleep, or a component of NREM sleep physiology in REM sleep. It is a portion of NREM sleep not appearing in its usual sleep cycle position.

sleep latency Time from the beginning of the polysomnographic recording period to the onset of stage 2 sleep for at least 10 uninterrupted minutes.

sleep, light Common term for non–rapid eye movement (NREM) sleep stage 1 and sometimes stage 2.

sleep log Written daily record of an individual's sleep-wake pattern. It may include information on time of retiring and arising, time in bed, estimated total sleep time, number and duration of sleep interruptions, quality of sleep, daytime naps, use of medications or caffeine beverages, and nature of waking activities.

sleep loss Sleep loss mainly affects brain and behavior, particularly in relation to the cerebrum. The rest of the body copes well and shows little or no sign of malfunction, indicating that sleep is most necessary for the cerebrum. After sleep deprivation, only a portion of lost sleep is reclaimed. This and other evidence suggest that about the first 6 hours of a night's sleep ("CORE" sleep) is essential (to the cerebrum), with the remainder of sleep ("OPTIONAL" sleep) being more dispensable/flexible. Slow-wave delta electroencephalographic activity (SWA) is the marker for CORE sleep. During wakefulness, the cerebrum is always in a state of readiness and can only relax and recover in sleep, especially during SWA.

sleep mentation Imagery and thinking experienced during sleep. Sleep mentation usually consists of combinations of images and thoughts during rapid eye movement (REM) sleep. Imagery is vividly expressed in dreams involving all the senses in approximate proportion to their waking representations. Mentation is experienced generally less distinctly in non-REM (NREM) sleep, but it may be quite vivid in stage 2 sleep, especially toward the end of the sleep episode. Mentation at sleep onset (hypnagogic reverie) can be as vivid as in REM sleep.

sleep myoclonus See **myoclonus, nocturnal.**

sleep, nocturnal Major sleep episode related to the circadian rhythm of sleep and wakefulness.

sleep, non-REM See **sleep-stage NREM.**

sleep, normal Criteria are (a) customary total sleep time of 6.5–8.5 hours; (b) sleep latency of less than 30 minutes; (c) bed and rise time variation of no more than 1.5 hours; and (d) no evidence of any type of sleep disorder.

sleep onset Transition from awake to sleep, normally to non–rapid eye movement (NREM) stage 1 sleep (but in certain conditions, such as infancy and narcolepsy, into stage REM sleep). Most polysomnographers accept electroencephalogram (EEG) slowing, reduction, and eventual disappearance of alpha activity, presence of EEG vertex sharp transients, and slow rolling eye movements (the components of NREM stage 1 as sufficient for sleep onset; others require appearance of stage 2 patterns.

sleep onset REM (SOREM) Beginning of sleep by entrance directly into stage rapid eye movement (REM) sleep. The onset of REM sleep occurs within 20 minutes of sleep onset. It is a common feature of narcolepsy.

sleep, optional Hypothesized to be the second part of sleep, occurring after "core" sleep (Horne J. *Why We Sleep*. Oxford: Oxford University Press, 1989). It consists mainly of light sleep (stages 1–2 non–rapid eye movement [NREM] sleep). Duration is variable; prolongation (sleeping in during weekends) or decrease (getting up earlier than usual) does not necessarily affect optimal functioning and may be considered to have a safety function. Optional sleep is curtailed and disrupted in the elderly, but appears not to be associated with excessive daytime napping (Wauquier A, van Sweden B. Aging of core and optional sleep. *Biol Psychiatry* 1992;31:866–880). See **core sleep.**

sleep panic Occurrence of panic attacks during sleep in panic disorder patients. Sleep panic is not rare; it may occur in 30% of panic patients. In a subgroup of panic disorder patients, sleep panic attacks may be a frequent and dominant symptom. Preliminary clinical experience suggests that sleep panic responds to some of the pharmacological agents (e.g., tricyclic antidepressants) documented to be effective in treating "awake" panic attacks in panic disorder. Response of these nocturnal episodes to antipanic pharmacotherapy provides further evidence that they are similar to other spontaneous panic attacks. In some patients, nocturnal epilepsy must be ruled out before diagnosis of sleep panic can be established.

sleep paralysis In 1876, Weir Mitchell described a condition called "nocturnal paralysis": "The subject awakes to consciousness of his environment but is incapable of moving a muscle; lying to all appearance still asleep. He is really engaged in a struggle for movement, fraught with acute mental distress; could he but manage to stir, the spell would vanish instantly (Mitchell SW. On some of the disorders of sleep. *Virginia Med Monthly* 1876;2:769–781. *Cited in* Daly DD, Yoss RE. Narcolepsy. *In* Magnus O, Lorentz de Haas AM [eds], *Handbook of Clinical Neurology,* vol 15. Amsterdam: North Holland, 1974, pp 836–852). Sleep paralysis produces no disturbance of consciousness, and the patient has complete recall of the episode. Lasting from a few seconds to a few minutes, paralysis usually occurs at the onset of sleep or on awakening. Sleep paralysis on awakening can be very frightening because the person is aware that he or she is paralyzed and incapable of moving. It is most probably due to temporary dysfunction of the reticular activating system. Episodes of sleep paralysis are often accompanied by hypnagogic hallucinations. Current evidence suggests that sleep paralysis/excessive daytime sleepiness syndrome without cataplexy is not a subtype of the narcolepsy syndrome, but a separate disorder. Rapid eye movement (REM) sleep–suppressing serotonin uptake inhibitors (e.g., clomipramine, paroxetine, sertraline), which are useful in the treatment of cataplexy, are less effective in sleep paralysis (Dahlitz M, Parkes JD. Sleep paralysis. *Lancet* 1993;341:406–407). See **narcolepsy.**

sleep pattern An individual's clock hour schedule of bedtime and arise time as well as nap behavior; may also include time and duration of sleep interruptions.

sleep/psychostimulant Psychostimulants have profound effects on sleep, reducing total sleep duration, rapid eye movement (REM) sleep, and slow-wave sleep, and increasing the time to sleep onset and sleep fragmentation. They are indicated for the treatment of excessive daytime sleepiness. Before initiating psychostimulant therapy for this indication, a "maintenance of wakefulness" test should be done to make sure the treatment is appropriate. The test should be repeated after starting treatment to ascertain if the optimal dosage regimen has been established. Psychostimulants should be given in the recommended divided doses (highest in the morning). Methylphenidate is preferred for treating excessive daytime sleepiness because it is more rapidly absorbed and has fewer sympathomimetic side effects than amphetamines and because it is more effective than pemoline (Eisen J, MacFarlane J, Shapiro CM. Psychotropic drugs and sleep. *Br Med J* 1993;306:1331–1334).

sleep-related erections Natural periodic cycle of penile erections that occur during sleep, typically associated with rapid eye movement (REM) sleep. Sleep-related erectile activity can be characterized by four phases: T-up (ascending tumescence), T-max (plateau maximal tumescence), T-down (detumescence), and T-zero (no tumescence). Polysomnographic assessment of sleep-related erections is useful for differentiating organic from nonorganic erectile dysfunction.

sleep seizure See **narcolepsy.**

sleep, slow-wave   (SWS) Sleep characterized by electroencephalogram (EEG) waves of duration slower than 8 Hz. Synonymous with sleep stages 3 and 4 combined. SWS has been hypothesized to slow down metabolic activity as a way of dissipating the heat load incurred during wake time. A subset of depressed patients have subnormal SWS; it may be this subset that responds best to sleep deprivation. See **sleep, delta.**

sleep spindles   One of the identifying electroencephalogram (EEG) features of non–rapid eye movement (NREM) stage 2 sleep that may persist into NREM stages 3 and 4 and are generally not seen in REM sleep. They occur during the onset of true sleep. A spindle lasts less than 0.5 seconds and comprises 6 or 7 sinusoidal waves with a frequency of 13–15 Hz. Sleep spindles are generally diffuse but of highest voltage over the central regions of the head. The amplitude is generally less than 50 μV in the adult. See **K complex.**

sleep stage   Distinctive stages of sleep, best demonstrated by polysomnographic recordings of the electroencephalogram (EEG), electro-oculogram (EOG), and electromyogram (EMG).

sleep stage 1   Brief transitional stage of sleep between wakefulness and sleep, characterized by low-voltage, mixed frequency electroencephalogram (EEG) and slow eye movements. It is a stage of non–rapid eye movement (NREM) sleep that occurs at sleep onset or may follow arousal from sleep stages 2, 3, 4, or REM. Stage 1 normally accounts for 4–5% of total nocturnal sleep, but may be much higher for diurnal sleep.

sleep stage 2   Non–rapid eye movement (NREM) sleep characterized by the presence of sleep spindles and K complexes present in a relatively low-voltage, mixed-frequency electroencephalogram (EEG) background. High-voltage delta waves may account for up to 20% of stage 2 epochs. Stage 2 consists of approximately 45–75% of total sleep time. Also called "intermediary sleep stage."

sleep stage 3   Non–rapid eye movement (NREM) sleep defined by at least 20% and not more than 50% of the episode consisting of electroencephalogram (EEG) waves less than 2 Hz and more then 75 μV (high-amplitude delta waves). It is sometimes referred to as delta sleep based on the amount of delta waves in the EEG. With stage 4 it constitutes "deep" NREM sleep, so-called "slow-wave sleep" (SWS). It is often combined with stage 4 into NREM sleep stages 3 and 4 because of the lack of documented physiological differences between the two. It appears usually only

in the first third of the sleep episode and usually accounts for 4–6% of total sleep time.

sleep stage 4   All statements concerning non–rapid eye movement (NREM) sleep stage 3 apply to stage 4 except that high-voltage, electroencephalogram (EEG) slow waves persist for 50% or more of the epoch; NREM sleep stage 4 usually accounts for 12–15% of total sleep time. Sleepwalking, sleep terrors, and confusional arousal episodes generally start in stage 4 or during arousals from it.

sleep-stage demarcation   Significant polysomnographic characteristics that distinguish the boundaries of the sleep stages. In certain conditions and with drugs, sleep-stage demarcations may be blurred or lost, making it difficult to identify stages with certainty or distinguish the temporal limits of sleep stage lengths.

sleep-stage episode   Sleep stage interval that represents the stage in a non–rapid eye movement (NREM)/REM sleep cycle; easiest to comprehend in relation to REM sleep, which is a homogeneous stage (i.e., the fourth REM sleep episode is in the fourth sleep cycle unless a prior REM episode was skipped). If one interval of REM sleep is separated from another by more than 20 minutes, they constitute separate REM sleep episodes (and are in separate sleep cycles); a sleep-stage episode may be of any duration.

sleep-stage NREM   Division of sleep characterized by sleep spindles and slow wave activity in the electroencephalogram (EEG) that can be divided into four stages; stages 3 and 4 exhibit the greatest slowing and together are called "slow-wave sleep," which is the deepest stage of non–rapid eye movement (NREM) sleep. The majority of sleep is NREM. It is the form of sleep in which the individual is most deeply asleep and most difficult to arouse. If the person is awakened during NREM sleep, dreams are reported approximately 20% of the time. NREM dreams are often quite similar to thinking and speech. A person is more likely to talk during NREM sleep. Also called "synchronized sleep."

sleep-stage REM   Stage of sleep with the highest brain activity characterized by enhanced brain metabolism and vivid hallucinatory imagery or dreaming (in humans). There are spontaneous rapid eye movements (REMs), resting muscle activity is suppressed, and awakening threshold to nonsignificant stimuli is high. The electroencephalogram (EEG) is a low-voltage, mixed-frequency, nonalpha record. REM sleep usually accounts for 20–25% of total sleep time. Also called "paradoxical sleep."

sleep start   See **body jerk.**

sleep/steroid See **steroid/sleep.**

sleep structure Sleep stages and sleep cycle relationships as well as within-stage qualities of the electroencephalogram (EEG) and other physiological attributes. See **sleep architecture.**

sleep, synchronized See **sleep stage non-REM.**

sleep talking Minor parasomnia characterized by the person talking more or less incomprehensibly while sleeping. It usually occurs during rapid eye movement (REM) sleep, but also may occur during transitory arousals from non-REM (NREM) sleep. Full consciousness is not achieved, and no memory of the event remains. Sleep talking may constitute a clinical problem if it occurs in an exaggerated form.

sleep, total Time from sleep onset to final awakening as recorded by the electroencephalogram (EEG). See **sleep episode, total.**

sleep-wake cycle Clock hour relationships of the major sleep and wake episodes in the 24-hour cycle.

sleep-wake shift Reversal, in whole or in part, of customary sleep episodes and waking activity. It is common in jet lag and shift work.

sleep-wake transitional disorder Parasomnia that occurs during the transition from wakefulness to sleep or from one sleep stage to another. Not a dyssomnia.

sleep walking Disorder with a strong hereditary component in which walking and other motor acts are performed during sleep. In DSM-IV, it is called "sleepwalking disorder." The somnambulist shows no evidence of fright and will not respond to verbal commands. Episodes are usually brief (a few minutes); after they cease, the patient has no recollection of them. This sleep disorder occurs during stages 3 or 4 of non–rapid eye movement (NREM) sleep. It may affect 2.5–5% of the general population and carries a genuine risk of injury. When it occurs, the clinician should attempt to determine the causative agent and discontinue it. Sleep walking also occurs in association with night terrors in approximately 10% of cases. Diazepam (5–25 mg) may significantly reduce the frequency and intensity of the episodes. See **somnambulism.**

"sleigh ride" Street term for cocaine.

slope Amount that y changes for each unit that x changes.

slow-wave sleep See **sleep, slow-wave.**

"smack" Street name for heroin or morphine.

"smoke" Street name for marijuana.

smoking/drug metabolism Cigarette smoking increases the metabolism of a large number of drugs by induction of hepatic microsomal enzymes of the P450 system, an effect not due to nicotine but to the constituents of tar, particularly the polyaromatic hydrocarbons. It may be necessary to monitor smokers who take drugs (e.g., antipsychotics, antidepressants) chronically and to adjust medication dosage during smoking cessation. Although only drugs metabolized by microsomal enzymes are affected, quitting smoking may result in toxicity from such drugs.

smoking, passive Involuntary inhalation of tobacco smoke in the environment. Passive smoking has been established as a cause of a variety of disorders, including lung cancer in adults and children, an increased rate of respiratory infections and other symptoms, and a delayed rate of normal increase in lung function (U.S. Department of Health and Human Services. *The Health Consequences of Involuntary Smoking. A Report of the Surgeon General.* Washington, DC: Government Printing Office, 1986).

smooth-pursuit eye movement (SPEM) Voluntary, slow (up to 50°/sec) eye movements that follow targets in the visual field. Some psychoactive drugs (benzodiazepines, lithium, barbiturates) can alter SPEM measurements. SPEM impairment also has been proposed as a genetic marker for schizophrenia; it is found in up to 86% of schizophrenics and in a good number of their relatives (Iacono WG. Eye movement abnormalities in schizophrenia and affective disorders. *In* Johnston CW, Pirozzolo FJ [eds], *Neuropsychology of Eye Movements.* Hillsdale, NJ: Lawrence Erlbaum Associates, 1988). Deficits in SPEM also occur in patients with schizotypal personality disorder (Siever LJ, Keefe RR, Bernstein DP, et al. Eye tracking impairment in clinically identified patients with schizotypal personality disorder. *Am J Psychiatry* 1990;147:740–745; Lemez T, Raine A, Scerbo A, et al. Impaired eye tracking in undergraduates with schizotypal personality disorder. *Am J Psychiatry* 1993;150:152–154).

smooth-pursuit eye movement gain (SPEM gain) Measure of SPEM quality. Gain = eye velocity/target velocity.

"snapper" Street term for amyl nitrite or isobutylnitrite ampules.

"sniffer" Street term for an abuser of solvents and inhalants who inhales the material through the nose. See **huffer.**

snoring Loud upper airway breathing, without apnea or hypoventilation, caused by vibration of the pharyngeal tissues (1990 International Classification of Sleep Disorders). Snoring is classified into mild, moderate, and severe forms on the basis of frequency, body position, and disturbance to others. Snoring presents considerable problems, not only for the snorer and bed-partner, but for epidemiological studies because so much of its evaluation depends on the reports of others. Interviewing bed partners increases the reported prevalence of snoring. The prevalence of occasional snoring over the age of 50 may be as high as 80%. Obesity, cigarette smoking, and alcohol consumption increase the likelihood of snoring. In adults, associations have been found between snoring and ischemic heart disease and strokes. Clinically, it is believed that more severe snoring is likely to reflect sleep apnea. Treatment should consist of tackling obesity, smoking, and alcohol consumption first.

"snorting" Street term for nasal insufflation of cocaine or heroin.

"snow" Street name for a mixture composed of about 70% cocaine adulterated with other local anesthetics, sugar, or more dangerous "cutting agents."

"snow bird" Street name for a cocaine user.

"snow light" Visual pseudohallucination in which a cocaine user sees at the periphery of visual fields twinkling lights similar to the sparkling of cocaine crystals or frozen snow crystals.

"snow pellet" Street name for amphetamines.

"soaper" Street name for methaqualone.

sobriety State of complete abstinence from alcohol and other drugs of abuse in conjunction with a satisfactory quality of life.

Sobril See **oxazepam.**

social avoidance Diminished social involvement associated with unwarranted fear, hostility, or distrust. When extreme, the patient cannot be engaged in social activities because of pronounced fears, hostility, or persecutory delusions. To the extent possible, the patient avoids all interactions and remains isolated from others.

social phobia See **phobia, social.**

social phobia/rating scales See **phobia, social/ rating scales.**

social psychiatrist See **social psychiatry.**

social psychiatry Branch of psychiatry that deals with the relationship between disorders of the mind and the human environment. It embraces concepts such as the effects of social cohesion, shared values, economic conditions, threat by an enemy, and the expectation of survival. It is also defined as the study of "the forces which act at the interface between individuals and those around them; and which may contribute to the onset, or influence the course of mental disorders" (Henderson S. *An Introduction to Social Psychiatry*. Oxford: Oxford University Press, 1988).

social-recreational drug use World Health Organization classification based on a pattern of drug use in social settings among friends or acquaintances wanting to share an experience perceived as acceptable and pleasurable. The primary motivation for drug use is social, and the use is voluntary.

Socian See **amisulpiride.**

sodium oxybate See **gamma hydroxybutyrate.**

sodium oxybutyrate See **gamma hydroxybutyrate.**

sodium pump Mechanism that ejects intracellular sodium with the help of the enzyme NA-K ATPase.

sodium valproate See **valproate.**

sodomy Usually, anal intercourse; may be used in legal terminology to refer to a variety of sexual acts other than adult heterosexual vaginal intercourse.

Sofian See **amisulpiride.**

Soften See **etiracetam.**

soft signs Subtle signs of disability or dysfunction; often refers to results of neurological examinations of children who are schizophrenic and/or have minimal brain dysfunction.

Solazine See **trifluoperazine.**

Solfoton See **phenobarbital.**

Solian See **amisulpride.**

solvent Substance capable of dissolving another substance. Solvents usually are highly volatile liquids that evaporate easily, producing fumes that are inhaled by abusers for their central nervous system effects. Solvents are fat-soluble organic substances that easily cross the blood-brain barrier to alter consciousness, much as mild stage I or stage II anesthesia does. They include straight-chained or aliphatic hydrocarbons, the prototype of which is dexane; cyclic or aromatic hydrocarbons, the prototype of which is benzene; chlorinated hydrocarbons, of which carbon tetrachloride is the most frequently abused; and freon. Commonly abused solvents include glues containing toluene, naphtha, acetates, hexane, benzene, xylene, and chloroform; aerosols (fluorinated hydrocarbons, freon, bromochlorofluoromethane, and others); cleaning solutions (trichloroethylene, petroleum products, carbon tetrachloride); nail polish removers; lighter fluids (naphtha, aliphatic hydrocarbons); paints and paint thinners (toluene, butylacetate, acetone, naphtha, methanol); and other petroleum products such as gasoline, tetraethyl lead, benzene, toluene, and petroleum ether.

solvent abuse Inhalation (typically from a handkerchief, aerosol, or crisp pack) of fumes produced by solvents for their central nervous system (CNS) effects. Commonly abused solvents include toluene, naphtha (in model-making cement and other glues), benzene (in rubber solutions), acetone and amylacetate (nail polish remover), carbon tetrachloride, trichloroethane and trichloroethylene (typing correction fluids and dry-cleaning chemicals), benzene and naphthene compounds (gasoline), and the fluorocarbon propellants in aerosols. These substances produce CNS depression and a disinhibited, excited, confused state not unlike alcohol intoxication (many young users say they would prefer to become intoxicated with alcohol, but find the cost prohibitive). The effect wears off rapidly, but the smell remains on the breath. Inhalers may show a rash around the lips, sometimes accompanied by boils. Death from toxic effects on the brain, heart, lungs, and liver have been reported, but the most consistent causes of death are from accidents while "sniffing" in relatively isolated places. Many normal young people experiment with solvents on a transient basis, usually with a group. Persistent solvent abusers are much less numerous and often have a personality or psychiatric disorder. The clinical signs and symptoms most commonly reported in patients who, over time, have heavily abused solvents containing toluene include short-term memory loss; emotional instability; cognitive impairment; slurred and "scanning" speech; wide-based ataxic gait; staggering or stumbling in trying to walk; nystagmus, ocular flutter; tremor; optic neuropathy; unilateral or bilateral hearing loss; loss of sense of smell; diffuse slowing of the electroencephalogram (EEG); abnormal or absent brainstem auditory evoked response; diffuse cerebral, cerebellar, and brainstem atrophy; and enlarged ventricles and widening of cortical sulci, especially in the frontal or temporal cortex.

solvent toxic syndrome   Characteristic symptoms produced by inhalation of cleaning solvents and fluorinated hydrocarbons, including (a) sensory changes (light sensitivity, eye irritation, diplopia, and tinnitus); (b) respiratory symptoms (sneezing, runny nose, and coughing); (c) gastrointestinal symptoms (nausea, vomiting, diarrhea, and anorexia); and (d) miscellaneous symptoms (chest pain, abnormal cardiac rhythm, and muscle and joint aches). See **solvent abuse.**

somatic cell   Any cell in the body except reproductive cells and their precursors.

somatic concerns   Physical complaints or beliefs about bodily illness or malfunctions that may range from a vague sense of ill-being to clear-cut delusions of catastrophic physical illness. In its extreme form, numerous and frequently reported delusions, or only a few somatic delusions, of a catastrophic nature totally dominate the patient's affect and thinking.

somatic delusion   See **delusion, somatic.**

somatic hallucination   See **hallucination, somatic.**

somatic recombination   See **recombination, somatic**

somatic therapy   Biological treatment of psychiatric disorders. It includes electroconvulsive therapy and psychopharmacological treatment.

somatization   Tendency to experience and communicate somatic distress and symptoms unaccounted for by pathological findings, attribute them to physical illness, and seek medical help for them (Bass A. Psychiatry in the general hospital. *Med Int* 1991;95:3981–3982). Chronic somatization is an enduring characteristic in some individuals. It may become pronounced during periods of stress or episodes of anxiety, depression, or other psychiatric disorders.

somatization disorder   Disorder manifested by (a) multiple somatic symptoms involving several different bodily systems; (b) absence of an organic cause for the symptoms; (c) a tendency by the patient to dramatize complaints, to refuse to accept psychological explanations for them, and to manipulate the doctors; (d) menstrual and sexual complaints; (e) a history of repeated hospitalizations and multiple operations starting before age 30; and (f) a tendency to become dependent on sedatives, anxiolytics, and/or analgesics. Somatization disorder occurs predominantly in women and tends to become chronic and to run in families. Mutual hostility between somatization disorder patients and their doctors is common. Many patients complain of depressive symptoms, which may mask the somatization disorder if the clinician is not alert to somatization disorder masquerading as depression. Misdiagnosis may result in mismanagement, including treatment with a variety of antidepressant drugs that are seldom beneficial and often evoke a host of side effects about which patients complain bitterly. Also called "Briquet's syndrome." See **somatoform disorder.**

somatoform disorder   Any of a group of conditions with somatic symptoms for which no organic cause can be demonstrated and that are thought to be due to psychological or "functional" disturbances. See **somatization disorder.**

Somatomax PM   See **gamma hydroxybutyrate.**

somatosensory evoked potential   (SSEP) Electrophysiological measure of central nervous system function in which specific wave forms, recorded from the scalp, are generated as the response to a stimulus from the extremities travels through the medial tracts in the brain stem. SSEP is a simple, noninvasive method of monitoring alterations in cerebral excitability during psychopharmacological treatment. It might contribute to identification of patients especially vulnerable to potentially hazardous side effects. The predictive value of this instrument, in comparison to the electroencephalogram (EEG) or drug serum levels, remains to be investigated (Forstl H, Zagorski A, Pohlmann-Eden B. Somatosensory evoked potentials as indicators of altered cerebral excitability during psychotropic drug treatment. *Biol Psychiatry* 1991;29:397–402). See **brain stem auditory-evoked potential; brain stem evoked potential; brain stem evoked response audiometry.**

somatostatin   (SS, SRIF) Neuropeptide (tetradecapeptide) discovered in 1973 that inhibits secretion of growth hormone and many other hormones and neurotransmitters. It is widely distributed throughout the body, often in high concentration in systems and cells that are not necessarily concerned with growth hormone secretion. It is characteristically reduced in the cerebral cortex of Alzheimer patients and in patients with senile dementia of the Lewy body type (SDLT). Also called "panhibin."

Sominex   (pyrilamine maleate) Over-the-counter antihistamine preparation with anticholinergic and sedative effects used to induce drowsiness and assist in falling asleep. It also contains small quantities of scopolamine. If taken in accidental or deliberate overdose, it can cause delirium. It can interact with alcohol and other central nervous system (CNS) depressants to cause additive CNS depressant effects.

Somnafec   See **methaqualone.**

somnambulism   See **sleep walking.**

Somnatrol   See **estazolam.**

somnifacient   Drug that induces sleep.

somnogram   Addition to the techniques of monitoring electrophysiological changes in the brain during sleep.

somnolence   Excessive daytime sleepiness that can be an important symptom of several sleep disorders, most frequently obstructive sleep apnea, nocturnal myoclonus, and narcolepsy.

somnology   See **polysomnography**

Somnos   See **chloral hydrate.**

Som Pam   See **flurazepam.**

Sonazine   See **chlorpromazine.**

"sopor"   Street name for methaqualone (one proprietary name for methaqualone was Sopor).

Sopor   Trade name for methaqualone until marketing of it was discontinued.

sotalol   Beta-blocker that has been used in the treatment of anxiety.

sotalol + fluoxetine   Co-administration apparently produces no adverse interactions (Walley T, Pirmohamed M, Proudlove C, Maxwell D. Interaction of metoprolol and fluoxetine. *Lancet* 1993;341:967–968).

Southern blotting   Tool for the analysis of DNA. DNA digested with a restriction enzyme is fractionated on an agarose gel and then transferred to a solid support membrane that can be annealed to a hybridization probe. Bands of interest are revealed by autoradiography. Molecular biologists analyze genes, messenger RNA, and proteins by separating them on a gelatinous matrix with an electric current (gel electrophoresis) in which the smaller the molecule, the further down the gel it travels. Once separated on the gel, the molecules are transferred onto a piece of filter paper that exactly replicates their position in the gel (a blot). Once on the filter paper, the molecules are more readily examined with cDNA probes to specific genes and mRNA (by hybridization) and with antibodies to specific proteins. The blot is named for Ed Southern, the Scottish molecular biologist who invented the technique. For RNA, the blot is called a "northern blot," to contrast it with the Southern. For proteins, it is a western blot. There is no eastern blot yet.

"spaced out"   Street term for cognitive dysfunction induced by alcohol or drugs.

Spancap No. 1   See **dextroamphetamine.**

"Spanish fly"   See **cantharsis.**

Sparine   See **promazine.**

spasm   Involuntary contraction of a muscle or group of muscles that can be painful. Prolonged spasms sometimes occur as an extrapyramidal side effect of certain drugs. Spasms of shorter duration occur in cerebral palsy. Seizures are sometimes inappropriately referred to as spasms. A clonic spasm is a rapidly alternating contraction and relaxation of muscle, whereas a tonic spasm is a sustained, firm contraction of muscle, causing it to be rigid.

spasmodic dysphonia   See **dystonia, laryngeal.**

spasmodic torticollis   (ST) Involuntary, intermittent spasms of the neck muscles with a turning of the head to one side. It is the most common of the focal dystonias. Usual age of onset is the fourth to seventh decades of life. Etiology of ST is unknown. It may have a psychogenic or organic cause, such as drug-induced acute or tardive dystonia. It may be treated with botulinum toxin. See **botulinum toxin.**

spastic dysphonia   Severe speech impairment that is a rare symptom of tardive dyskinesia.

spatial memory   See **memory, spatial.**

Spearman's method   Nonparametric method to deal with rank data. See **rank order; Spearman rank order correlation.**

Spearman rank order correlation Nonparametric replacement for the Pearson product moment correlation. When data are not normally distributed or in some other way do not meet the assumptions of a Pearson correlation, the rank order correlation can be used. See **Pearson's correlation.**

"special L.A. coke" Street name for phencyclidine (PCP).

specificity 1. Probability a symptom is absent among those not given the diagnosis. 2. Ratio of the number of true negatives to the sum of false positives plus true negatives. 3. Proportion of true negatives correctly identified. 4. Probability of correctly identifying a nondiseased person with a screening test. 5. In psychiatric, diagnostic, or screening scales, the proportion of true cases who score above the cut-off score and/or the proportion of normals who score below the cut-off point. Specificity refers to the question of whether the cause ever occurs without the presumed effect, and whether the effect ever occurs without the presumed cause.

specific rate Rate that pertains to a specific group per segment of the observations.

spectinomycin + lithium See **lithium + spectinomycin.**

speech disorders/schizophrenia Speech abnormalities among schizophrenic patients may take the form of grunting, hawking, or other vocalizations, or delivery may be in a flat monotone, with peculiar scanning or affected intonations. In speech stereotypies and mannerisms, a word or phrase is inserted into discourse repeatedly and inappropriately; the patient may affect all kinds of accents, speak in infinitives and diminutives, add "-ism" or "-io" to every word. Other catatonic speech abnormalities include echolalia, palilalia, mutism, and verbigeration (in the original sense of the term, to denote indistinct utterances in which only a few repetitive words and phrases can be made out).

"speed" Street name for central nervous system stimulants, especially amphetamines.

"speedball" Street term for a combined injection of heroin and cocaine.

"speed freak" Term used in the 1960s for amphetamine abusers who injected intravenously large doses of amphetamine or smoked large doses of amphetamines at relatively short intervals for as long as 6 or more days. See **"run"; "speed run."**

"speed run" Single intravenous injection of a large quantity of methamphetamine (up to 1,000 mg) or repeated injections up to 5,000 mg in 24 hours.

spin lattice (T_1) Longitudinal (spin-lattice) relaxation time. It is one of the components of the signal used during magnetic resonance imaging. T_1 is the time required for net magnetization following radio frequency excitation to return to 63% of its original value.

spin-spin (T_2) Spin-spin relaxation time, or transverse relaxation time. It is one of the components of the signal used during magnetic resonance imaging. T_2 is the time required for the signal to return to 37% of its original value.

Spiperone See **spiroperidol.**

spironolactone (Aldactazide; Aldactone) A 17-spirolactone steroid that is a competitive antagonist of the sodium-retaining and potassium-secreting steroid aldosterone. It prevents sodium and potassium exchange in the distal renal tabule, producing potassium retention, natriuresis, and diuresis, and thereby lowers blood pressure. An early study (not replicated) suggested that spironolactone might substitute for lithium in the maintenance treatment of bipolar disorder.

spironolactone + lithium Co-administration may moderately increase lithium level over time; lithium serum levels should be monitored (Baer L, Platman SR, Kassir S, Fieve RR. Mechanism of renal lithium handling and their relationship to mineralocorticoids: a dissociation between sodium and lithium ions. *J Psychiatr Res* 1981;8:91–105).

spiroperidol (Spiperone) Very potent butyrophenone derivative that has been used in its radioactively labeled form as a research tool for studying dopamine receptors. It has high affinity for 5-HT_{1A} receptors, as well as the 5-HT_2 receptor. It is the most potent compound affecting the D_2 receptor and more than 1,000 times as potent as the weakest marketed neuroleptic, clozapine. Systemic administration readily blocks somatodendritic 5-HT_{1A} autoreceptors, with no immediate effect on postsynaptic 5-HT_{1A} receptors in the dorsal hippocampus (de Montigny C, Dadrava V, Ortemann C, et al. The development of selective postsynaptic 5-HT_{1A} agonists as novel antidepressant agents. *Neuropsychopharmacology* 1993;9:9S). Not available in the United States for clinical use.

splitting Rigid separation of positive and negative thoughts and feelings; keeping apart perceptions and feelings of opposite quality. Staff members are divided into "all good" and "all bad" ones, as if the patient cannot tolerate the anxiety-producing, ambivalent notion that caregivers have human limits and "good" and "bad" qualities at the same time (Groves JE. *Int J Psychiatry Med* 1975;6:337–348). See **defense mechanism.**

sponsor   Person or institution that initiates and supports, but does not conduct, an investigational study.

spontaneous reporting   Surveillance technique to monitor postmarketing drug safety and identify uncommon adverse drug reactions. It begins when a new drug is marketed, continues indefinitely, and covers the entire patient population receiving the drug. Spontaneous reports received by regulatory agencies and pharmaceutical companies come from doctors, pharmacists, nurses, published literature, coroners, lawyers, and patients. About 90% of reports to the U.S. Food and Drug Administration (FDA) come from the pharmaceutical industry. Spontaneous reporting can detect and characterize common reactions, confirm suspicions aroused during clinical trials with the drug, and identify rare reactions that premarketing studies cannot detect. Limitations include difficulty in recognizing some reactions and under-reporting of cases. Also called "voluntary reporting." See **MedWatch.**

Spontaneous Reporting System   (SRS) U.S. Food and Drug Administration (FDA) system to collect reports of adverse drug reactions (ADRs) submitted voluntarily by drug companies, clinicians, and patients. The method is particularly sensitive to unexpected side effects. Data are collected without a set of guidelines established a priori, and reporting biases are minimized because of the large numbers of reporting physicians and patients. A precise rate for the occurrence of ADRs for a given drug cannot be obtained, but a relative rate compared to other drugs can be determined by combining data on prescription rates from an independent source. Many variables, however, can affect SRS data, including time since release of the drug and media exposure. See **MedWatch.**

stabilization therapy   See **continuation therapy.**

Stablon   See **tianeptine.**

"stacking"   Mixing anabolic steroids to obtain as much of the desired effects of steroids as possible, a practice that increases the risk of complications.

"stacking the pyramid"   Term used by abusers of anabolic/androgenic steroids (AASs) to describe a pattern of raising and lowering the number and doses of AASs during an episode or "cycle" of use during which AASs are taken for 4–12 weeks. A cycle may begin by taking low doses of one or two AASs. Later, additional AASs are taken, and simultaneously the dosages are increased; toward the end of the cycle, the drugs are tapered.

Stadol   See **butorphanol.**

standard deviation   (SD) Mathematical measure of the dispersion or spread of scores clustered about the mean. It is the square root of the variance. In any distribution that approximates the normal curve in form, about 65% of the measurements will lie within 1 SD of the mean, and about 95% will lie within 2 SDs of the mean. It is applied to continuously distributed variables such as height, weight, and blood pressure, but not to percentages. It is sometimes represented by the Greek letter sigma. Also called the "root mean squared deviation."

standard error   (SE) Standard deviation of the sampling distribution of a statistic. It is a measure of how variable the mean or percentage is from one sample to another.

standard error of the estimate   Measure of the variation in a regression line based on the differences between the predicted values and the actual values of the dependent variable y.

standard error of the mean   Standard deviation of the mean(s) in a large number of samples.

standard normal distribution   Normal distribution with mean 0 and variance 1. Any other normal distribution can be transferred into standard normal distribution, which is very important in statistical analysis.

standardization   For a sample from the normal distribution, taking the observed value minus sample mean, divided by sample standard deviation. After standardization, the sample mean will be 0, and variance will be 1, so is standard deviation.

standardized mortality ratio   (SMR) Ratio of observed to expected numbers of deaths that measures the degree to which the risk of mortality is higher or lower in a cohort than in a reference population.

standardized regression coefficient   Regression coefficient that has the effect of the measurement scale removed so that the size of the coefficient can be interpreted.

"Stanley's stuff"   Street term used in the mid-1960s for a lysergic acid diethylamide (LSD) street product of high quality that many believed matched the quality of LSD legitimately manufactured by Sandoz Laboratories.

stanozolol   (Winstrol) Anabolic steroid that is a 17-alpha-methyl testosterone derivative.

startle reflex   Jerking movement produced by a loud sound or other stimuli, usually seen in a newborn infant. After infancy, it is associated with fear and anxiety, increasing in frequency with the severity of the anxiety. It is potentiated during experimentally induced anxiety (fear potentiated startle). It is also increased in various anxiety disorders. Elevated startle is a symptom of post-traumatic stress disorder and generalized anxiety disorder (Butler RW, Braff DL, Rausch JL, et al. Physiological evidence of exaggerated startle response in a subgroup of Vietnam veterans with combat-related PTSD. *Am J Psychiatry* 1990;147:1308–1312; Grillon C, Ameli R, Woods SW, et al. Fear-potentiated startle in humans: effects of anticipatory anxiety on the acoustic blink reflex. *Psychophysiology* 1991;28:588–595; Grillon C, Ameli R, Foot M, David M. Fear-potentiated startle: relationship to the level of state/trait anxiety in healthy subjects. *Biol Psychiatry* 1993;33:566–574).

state   A temporary and changeable phenomenon (e.g., state anxiety).

state dependence   Behavior that is a reflection of or a reaction to the state under which it occurs. It is not primarily determined by the subject.

state-dependent dyskinesia   See **dyskinesia, state-dependent.**

state-dependent memory   See **memory, state-dependent.**

statistic   Summary number computed from the observations in a sample, often used as an estimate of a parameter in the population. If the measurement process is not specified, the meaning of the statistic cannot be known. The specification of the measurement process is also called the "operational definition."

statistics   Science of chance. Statistics are integral to medical research.

statistics, descriptive   Statistics (e.g., mean, standard deviation, proportion, rate) used to describe attributes of a set of data.

statistical inference   Process of using a limited sample of data to infer something about a larger population of potentially obtainable data that have not been observed.

statistical significance   Arbitrarily assigned value of the level of significance by which an investigator will conclude that the observed differences are not due to chance alone. The value is often set at $P = 0.05$, meaning that there is about 1 chance in 20 that differences occurred by chance alone.

statistical table   Data summary showing the distribution of the variables according to their frequency.

statistical test   Quantification of the probability that the difference seen between two study groups could have happened simply by chance.

statistical trend   Uniform change as shown by statistics.

Statobex   See **phendimetrazine.**

status   Presence of some abnormal state or pathological condition that requires further qualification by an adjective for the particular type of condition (e.g., status epilepticus).

status epilepticus   Epileptic seizure that is so prolonged or so frequently repeated as to create a fixed or lasting epileptic condition

(persistence for at least 30 minutes without return of consciousness). Any type of seizure, either focal or generalized, that continues for more than 1 hour is called "status epilepticus." There are convulsive and nonconvulsive forms of status epilepticus. Convulsive forms include tonic-clonic status, tonic status, myoclonic status, adversive status, hemiconvulsive status, clonic status, and hemiclonic status. Nonconvulsive forms are absence status, complex partial status, and simple partial status. Whereas convulsive forms may progress to dangerous and life-threatening conditions, the nonconvulsive forms are of particular interest for the psychiatrist because they appear as abrupt behavioral changes. The most common cause of status epilepticus is abrupt discontinuation of anticonvulsant medication, and hence it is most frequent in patients with a pre-existing seizure disorder. Status epilepticus in a patient with no prior neurological disorder warrants investigation for an underlying neurological condition, after status has been controlled. Because of its relatively long duration of action, intravenously administered lorazepam is becoming the drug of choice for the initial treatment of status epilepticus (Leppik IE. Status epilepticus: the next decade. *Neurology* 1990;40[suppl 2]:4–9). Diazepam is the most effective drug for stopping generalized tonic-clonic status epilepticus. It is administered by intravenous push to a maximum total dose of 20–30 mg in adults. Intravenously administered phenytoin is the mainstay of continuing therapy for status epilepticus. If there is no response to phenytoin, intravenously administered phenobarbital in 100- to 200-mg doses to a total of 400–800 mg can be used. Benzodiazepines and diphenylhydantoin are the two preferred treatments for status epilepticus.

status epilepticus, convulsive   Most common and dangerous type of status epilepticus, characterized by symmetric tonic-clonic seizure activity associated with bilaterally symmetrical ictal discharges on the electroencephalogram (EEG). Unconsciousness plus convulsive movements are necessary for the diagnosis. It is an emergency associated with substantial morbidity and mortality, which can be reduced by prompt, appropriate pharmacological therapy. Antiepileptic drug treatment should be started whenever a seizure has lasted 10 minutes. Benzodiazepines (intravenous diazepam or lorazepam) are effective initial management. Intravenously administered phenytoin (20 mg/kg in adults and 15 mg/kg in the elderly) terminates generalized convulsive status epilepticus in 40–91% of patients (Anon. Treatment of convulsive status epilepticus. Recommendations of the Epilepsy Foundation of America's working group on status epilepticus. *JAMA* 1993;270:854–859).

status, nonconvulsive   Absence status and complex partial status of frontal or temporal origin. See **absence status; status, partial.**

status, partial   Form of epilepsy that may present in a variety of forms, but when associated with psychotic behavior is inevitably complex partial. The focus arises from either the temporal or the frontal lobes. Onset is sudden, but may follow a bout of generalized seizures. Symptoms may include confusion, automatisms, fugues, intense panic, hallucinations, delusions, and illusions.

steady state   See **steady-state plasma level.**

steady-state plasma concentration   See **steady-state plasma level.**

steady-state plasma level   (Cpss) Drug plasma level in which absorption and elimination are in equilibrium. The time to attain steady state is approximately four to five elimination half-lives after initiation of therapy at a fixed dosing rate without a loading dose. Once steady state is reached, in spite of small fluctuations, it stays fairly constant as long as the daily dose is not altered or other factors do not change clearance. For many, but not all, psychotropic drugs, behavioral response is directly related to steady-state plasma concentration. If the dosing rate remains the same, any factor that reduces clearance (e.g., old age, disease states, certain drug-drug interactions) will increase steady-state plasma concentrations of a drug.

"steam"   Street term for parachlorophenylamine (PCPA), which reputedly prolongs sexual excitement and, in high doses, can cause severe psychosis.

Stelazine   See **trifluoperazine.**

stem and leaf plot   Graphical display for numerical data that is similar to a frequency table.

Stemetil   See **prochlorperazine.**

stepwise discrimination analysis   (SDA) Under the normality assumption, performance of discriminant analysis including variables into the equation in a stepwise manner. See **discriminant analysis.**

stepwise procedure   When a number of variables are used for such procedures as predicting an outcome measure or discriminating between groups, stepwise procedure examines all other variables, discards those not useful, and synthesizes the others into weighted linear combinations. Predictive power can be inflated by chance associations.

stepwise regression   In multiple regression, a sequential method of selecting the variables to be included in the prediction equation.

stereoencephalogram   Recording of the four different physiological brain rhythms—alpha, beta, theta, and delta—from inside deep brain structures.

stereognosis   Capacity to judge the shape and form of an object by means of touch.

stereoisomerism   Two or more compounds possessing the same molecule and structural formulae but having different spatial configurations. See **isomerism.**

stereopathy   Behaviors in which there are repetitive actions or words, as in mannerisms, and some self-injurious behaviors occurring particularly in severely and profoundly mentally handicapped people. These include rocking, swaying, head-banging, eye-poking, hand waving, and finger movements. The behavior is often regarded as self-stimulation. Schizophrenic stereotypies tend to be more complex and purposeful. See **stereotypy.**

stereotactic tractotomy   See **tractotomy, stereotactic.**

stereostatic subcaudate tractotomy   See **tractotomy, stereotactic subcaudate.**

stereotaxic surgery   Neurosurgical procedure for accurately producing lesions in the brain by electrocoagulation, selective neurotoxins, or radioactive pellets.

stereotypy   Persistent repetition of gestures or movements that do not appear to be goal-directed. Often seen in certain forms of schizophrenia. See **stereopathy.**

steroid hormones   Progesterone, testosterone, estradiol, corticosterone, aldosterone, and cortisol.

steroid psychosis   See **psychosis, steroid.**

steroid/sleep   High steroid doses (e.g., 8–16 mg dexamethasone/day) may cause insomnia and vivid, frightening, or morbid dreams that seem to resolve as dosage is decreased. Insomnia may be relieved by changing dosage schedule and confining administration to early in the day. Traditionally, dexamethasone is given at regular intervals because of its short plasma half-life (3–6 hours). Its biological half-life, however is 36–45 hours, making it suitable for once-daily administration. Insomnia also may be relieved with night-time administration of a drug with sedative side effects (Turner R, Elson E. Steroids cause sleep disturbance. *Br Med J* 1993;306:1477–1478).

steroid withdrawal syndrome   Syndrome occurring in a minority of patients, usually following abrupt steroid discontinuation. It typically lasts 2–8 weeks and resolves spontaneously, although symptoms may persist and require somatic treatment. It may be manifested by depression, listlessness, anhedonia, a sense of emptiness, depersonalization, fatigue, anorexia, confusion, disorientation, impaired memory, and difficulty maintaining sequential thinking (Reus VI, Wolkowitz OM. Behavioral side effects of corticosteroid therapy. *Psychiatr Ann* 1993;23:307–308).

"stick" Street name for a marijuana cigarette.

Stilnoct See **zolpidem.**

Stilnox See **zolpidem.**

stimulant Drug that activates the central nervous system to produce increased psychomotor activity. Most act on dopaminergic and/or noradrenergic systems. Stimulants are frequently abused substances because they can produce a heightened sense of well-being, increased sense of alertness, reduced social inhibitions, and increased talkativeness. Commonly abused stimulants include amphetamine, benzphetamine, caffeine, dextroamphetamine, methamphetamine, methylphenidate, phenmetrazine, phentermine, and cocaine. Caffeine is also thought of as a stimulant, but is not as euphorigenic as dopaminergic agonists, although it does produce a form of physical dependence. Some stimulants (picrotoxin, strychnine) are convulsants with no abuse potential. See **caffeine.**

stimulant intoxication Syndrome due to excessive stimulant dosage that can be indistinguishable from mania or hypomania. Substantial depressive symptoms also can emerge during stimulant withdrawal. For these reasons, a bipolar affective disorder is diagnosed in substance-abusing patients only if the affective symptoms occurred before the onset of substance abuse or during remission from substance abuse.

stimulant toxic syndrome Syndrome caused by amphetamines, cocaine, and phencyclidine (PCP) manifested by (a) agitation, psychosis, seizures; (b) hypertension, tachycardia, arrhythmias; (c) mydriasis, and with PCP poisoning vertical and horizontal nystagmus; (d) skin warm and sweating; (e) increased muscle tone (rhabdomyolysis may occur); and (f) hyperthermia.

stimulant-type laxative withdrawal Rebound constipation following discontinuation of high-dose laxative abuse. It can be quite uncomfortable and prolonged and associated with significant fluid retention. The latter accounts for rapid weight gain (5–15 pounds in 7–10 days), a powerful stimulus for resumption of high-dose laxative abuse.

"stinkweed" Street name for marijuana.

stiripentol Experimental anticonvulsant considered the most promising of a series of ethylene alcohols. Currently undergoing controlled trials in Europe and the United States.

"stone" Street name for marijuana.

"STP" Street name for dimethoxymethylamphetamine.

straightjacket See **camisole.**

stratified random sample Sampling process in which the population is divided into internally homogeneous subpopulations called "strata" that are controlled by the characteristic factors of the population (e.g., smokers vs. nonsmokers). Units from each stratum are then chosen such that the final sample will better represent the population.

street abuser Individual who misuses/abuses illicit drugs to achieve an altered state of consciousness. Drugs may be taken orally, intravenously, subcutaneously, or by inhalation.

"street drug" Any illegally produced and sold psychoactive substance (e.g., marijuana, heroin, cocaine, crack, designer drugs).

stress Convenient but imprecise term usually used to indicate an adverse or health-threatening response in the body. See **stressor.**

stress prevention training (SPT) Training individuals to anticipate, prevent, and control stress related to human immunodeficiency virus (HIV). Four basic strategies are used: (a) education about HIV infection, risk reduction, and health-promoting behaviors; (b) enhancement of the belief in personal control and perceived self-effectiveness; (c) training to identify and rationally correct dysfunctional assumptions and images, such as exaggerated perceptions of imminent danger, unwarranted guilt and shame, and unrealistic perceptions of rejection by others and institutions; and (d) training in techniques to manage challenging situations (e.g., problem solving and assertiveness) and to prevent disruptive emotional arousal (e.g., thought diversion and cued and systematic relaxation). The "commonsense" theory and practical focus of SPT enable trainees to acquire mastery over distressful experiences, thereby increasing hope, confidence, and an interest in practicing the learned skills (Perry S, Fishman B, Jacobsberg L, Young J, Frances A. Effectiveness of psychoeducational intervention in reducing emotional distress after human immunodeficiency virus antibody testing. *Arch Gen Psychiatry* 1991; 48:143–147).

stressor External influence on the mind and the body. Stressors have widespread, subtle, and often profound effects in the body, especially on the neuroendocrine system.

striatum Area of the brain that includes the caudate and the putamen.

strict liability Legal concept indicating that a manufacturer is liable if a medicine causes an adverse reaction not identified and notified to the prescriber prior to the time of prescribing.

stroke Condition in which gross cerebral damage or softening follows acute vascular accidents, such as cerebral thrombosis, cerebral hemorrhage, and cerebral embolism. Also called "apoplexy"; "cerebrovascular accident."

strychnine   Central nervous system (CNS) stimulant that blocks the inhibitory action of glycine at several postsynaptic receptors in several CNS locations, particularly in the spinal cord.

Student's t-test   Distribution of a quotient of independent random variables, the numerator of which is a standardized normal variate and the denominator of which is the positive square root of the quotient of a chi-squared distributed variate that, under the null hypothesis, has the t-distribution, to test whether two means differ significantly, or to test linear regression or correlation coefficients. The t-distribution and the t-test were developed by W. S. Gossett, who wrote under the pseudonym "Student." Also called t-test; t-distribution.

study criterion   Standard, rule, or definitive measure stated before a study begins.

study, crossover   Study design for comparing two or more treatments given sequentially to the same patient. The investigator should be prepared to demonstrate the absence of carryover effects, guarantee low drop-out rates, and expect a stable underlying disease. Crossover designs are most appropriate in the study of treatment for a stable disease.

study, cross-sectional   Study design focusing on phenomena thought to be static over the period of interest.

study, descriptive   Study with no control group (e.g., case report, case series, analysis of secular trends).

study design   Methodology created or selected to achieve the goal(s) of an experimental trial.

study, experimental therapeutic   Study in which the investigator controls the therapy to be received by each participant. When participants are randomly allocated between or among study groups, it is called a "randomized clinical trial." See **randomized clinical trial.**

study, historical cohort   Study that uses existing records or historical data to determine the effect of a risk or exposure on a group of patients.

study, longitudinal   Prospective or retrospective study that aims to elucidate a state of nature that changes or may change.

study, parallel   Study design for comparing two or more treatments given concurrently to different groups of patients.

study, pseudolongitudinal   Cross-sectional study in which the data are collected over a brief period and treated by the investigator(s) as if they were longitudinal. A pseudolongitudinal study may be pseudoprospective or pseudoretrospective, which is determined by the mode of sampling.

study sample   Subjects selected to participate in a research study. If research is to be applicable and relevant to other populations, the study sample must represent the group from which it is drawn (study population), which, in turn, should be typical of the wider population to whom the research might apply (target population). Appropriateness of the target and study populations is usually a subjective assessment based on knowledge of the topic under investigation.

study, self-controlled   Study design in which patients serve as their own control. Self-controlled comparisons of treatment tend to be less precisely designed and conducted than crossover designs and to focus on clinical problems and patient groups that are especially difficult to study.

study validity   See **internal validity; external validity.**

stupor   State of impaired consciousness that is organically determined. Also, a psychogenic state in which there is unresponsiveness, with immobility and mutism, with retention of consciousness, and open eyes that follow external objects.

stuttering   Frequent repetitions or prolongation of sounds or syllables that markedly impair speech fluency (DSM-IV). In addition to these primary symptoms, secondary symptoms largely represent the efforts of the patient not to stutter. These include blocks or interruptions in the flow of speech sounds, tremors of the lips and jaw, rapid blinking, jerking movements of the head, arm, or upper trunk, and other manifestations of the stutterer's struggle to "get the next word out." These aspects of stuttering are often more striking to the observer than the repetitions and prolongations themselves. A great variety of pharmacological agents have been used to treat stuttering, reflecting the many theories about the origin and nature of the disorder (Brady JP. The pharmacology of stuttering: A critical review. *Am J Psychiatry* 1991;148:1309–1316). Anxiolytic agents have some use in the early treatment of stuttering by halting or reversing escalation of anxiety and associated dysfluency. Monoamine oxidase inhibitors may be useful in patients who have developed social phobias in response to their intense embarrassment in speaking situations. However, the use of either class of drug is not likely to be sufficient treatment for severe adult stutterers. The most promising approach to severe stuttering in adults is a multicomponent program that combines pharmacotherapy with individual or group psychotherapy (Brady JP. Treatment of stuttering with phenelzine. *Am J Psychiatry* 1993;150:355–356).

subaffective dysthymic disorder (SDD) Minor form of affective disorder, responsive to medication, that is a subdivision of characterological depressions. SDD patients have a short rapid eye movement (REM) latency, more continuous dysphoria, a positive family history for unipolar or bipolar depression, and depressive personality (Schneider K. *Psychopathic Personalities* [translated by M.W. Hamilton]. London: Cassell, 1958).

subclinical disease Condition in which disease is detectable by testing, but does not reveal itself by obvious signs or symptoms.

subclinical thyroid dysfunction Exaggerated release of thyroid stimulating hormone (TSH) in response to thyrotropin releasing hormone in the presence of normal or raised concentrations of circulating TSH and normal concentrations of clinical thyroxine (T_4) and triiodothyronine (T_3). Subclinical forms of hypothyroidism may occur in bipolar patients treated with lithium or carbamazepine and in a subgroup of manic depressives who are rapid cyclers. Thyroid dysfunction in patients with affective disorders is very common. In every patient suffering from a chronic or recurrent affective illness that is treatment-resistant, the function of the hypothalamic-pituitary-thyroid axis should be thoroughly investigated, and any abnormality should be corrected. Cautiously administering a small dosage (100–400 mg/day) of thyroxine, even in the absence of endocrinological evidence of thyroid dysfunction, may be worthwhile.

subcoma therapy See **insulin coma therapy.**

subcortical atherosclerotic encephalopathy See **Binswanger's disease**

subcortical dementia See **dementia, subcortical.**

subcortical hyperintensity Foci of increased T_2 signals in the subcortical white matter and gray matter nuclei detected by magnetic resonance imaging (MRI) in elderly patients with depression and in patients with bipolar disorder (Zubencko GS, Sullivan P, Nelson JP, et al. Brain imaging abnormalities in mental disorders of late life. *Arch Neurol* 1990;97:1107–1111; Figiel GS, Krishnan KRR, Rao VP, et al. Subcortical hyperintensities on brain magnetic resonance imaging: A comparison of normal and bipolar subjects. *J Neuropsychiatry Clin Neurosci* 1991;3:18–22). Inpatients referred for electroconvulsive therapy for severe depression have been found to have smaller frontal lobe volumes and a greater prevalence of subcortical hyperintensity on MRI than

control subjects do. Subcortical hyperintensity also has been observed in a population of depressed patients without age restrictions. Further studies are needed to confirm these observations and to elucidate their cause (Coffey CE, Wilkinson WE, Weiner RD, et al. Quantitative cerebral anatomy in depression. A controlled magnetic resonance imaging study. *Arch Gen Psychiatry* 1993;50:7–16). Even after controlling for age in the psychiatric population, subcortical hyperintensity is significantly associated with hypertension, history of myocardial infarction or angina, abnormal electrocardiogram (ECG), and abnormal neurological examinations. Also called "deep white matter hyperintensity" (DWMH).

subcortical structures Basal ganglia, diencephalon (thalamus and hypothalamus), mesencephalon (midbrain), and cerebellum. They have a role in arousal, attention, mood, motivation, memory, abstraction, and visuospatial skills. Subcortical nuclei are affected in Parkinson's disease, progressive supranuclear palsy, Huntington's chorea, and the acquired immunodeficiency syndrome (AIDS) dementia complex. Subcortical dysfunction slows information processing and adversely affects memory, cognition, mood, and motivation.

subcutaneous injection Route of drug administration that results in slower drug absorption. Irritating substances are particularly painful when given subcutaneously, and large volumes are not feasible unless they contain hyaluronidase, an enzyme that facilitates the spread of the injected solution through the tissue.

subdelirium Prodromal form of a full-blown delirium, manifested by restlessness, headache, hypersensitivity to auditory and visual stimuli, irritability, and emotional lability.

subictal affective disorder See **dysthymic subictal mood disorder.**

subjective measurement Rating of what a patient feels. Subjective measurements can be altered by such conditions as a patient's state of emotion, apprehension, and anxiety.

subjective probability Estimate of probability that reflects a person's opinion or best guess from previous experience.

subject as own control Comparison of an individual with him or her self before and after a given treatment. Advantages include decreasing error variance and the likelihood of showing significant differences with relatively small groups; a disadvantage is that practice effects may occur with repeated measurements. It also involves the assumption that the variable (e.g., the disease) is constant in both periods.

subject-year Product of the number of subjects under exposure factors and the number of years in the study. For example, if there are 50 subjects at the starting point, and 50 die at 6 months and the other 50 stay alive after 1 year, the total subject year is $(50 \times 0.5) + (50 \times 1) = 75$. The calculation is widely used in epidemiological studies (Berry G. The analysis of mortality by subject-years method. *Biometrics* 1983; 39:173–184).

Sublimaze See **fentanyl.**

subsensitivity Decrease of responsiveness of a tissue, organ, or receptor to a constant dose of drug. When mediated by decreases in affinity or number or density of receptors, it is called "down-regulation." See **supersensitivity; downregulation.**

substance abuse Use of a psychoactive substance in a manner detrimental to the individual or society, but not meeting criteria for substance or drug dependence. See **drug abuse; psychoactive substance abuse.**

substance-induced organic mental disorders Alcohol intoxication, alcohol idiosyncratic intoxication, uncomplicated alcohol withdrawal, alcohol hallucinosis, alcohol amnestic disorder, and dementia associated with alcoholism (DSM-IV).

substance P Neuropeptide present in peripheral afferents and in the dorsal horn. It is one of a group of naturally occurring proteins similar in structure to a portion of beta-amyloid. It is one likely candidate for the role of pain neurotransmitter for the primary sensory neurons. Reduced concentrations have been found in the brains of patients with Alzheimer's dementia. The reductions sometimes occur early in the illness and only in restricted areas; they do not correlate with the presence of plaques and tangles, but may correlate with cortical cell loss. Substance P may block the toxic effects of beta-amyloid found in the plaques in the brains of Alzheimer's disease patients and may lead to a new therapeutic intervention for Alzheimer's patients.

substances, misused These include illegal (cocaine, heroin, amphetamines), socially acceptable (alcohol, tobacco), medically prescribed (benzodiazepines) and household products (glue, lighter fluid).

substantial evidence Adequate and well controlled investigations regarding effectiveness and safety that are required by the Food and Drug Administration (FDA) to support a new drug approval or a claim for a new indication. Drug regulatory agencies in other countries have similar requirements. The FDA has described the following characteristics of an adequate and well-controlled study: (a) There is a clear statement of the objective(s) of the investigation and a summary of the proposed or actual methods of analysis in the protocol for the study. If the protocol does not contain a description of the proposed analytical methods, the study report should describe how the methods were selected. (b) The study uses a design that permits a valid comparison with a control to provide a quantitative assessment of drug effect. The protocol for the study and report of results should describe the design precisely (duration of treatment periods; whether treatments were parallel, sequential, or crossover; and whether the sample size was predetermined or based on some interim analysis). Generally, the FDA recognizes the following types of controls: (i) placebo concurrent control (usually randomized and blinded); (ii) dose comparison concurrent control (at least two doses; usually randomized and blinded); (iii) no treatment concurrent control (where objective measurements of efficacy are available and placebo effect is negligible; usually randomized); (iv) active treatment concurrent control (usually used when administration of placebo is not in the patient's interest; usually randomized and blinded; ability to detect differences between treatments needs assessing; why the drugs should be considered effective needs explaining); and (v) historical control (special circumstances, such as diseases with high and predictable mortality or effect of drugs is self-evident). Placebo and/or active treatment control are the most frequently submitted to the agency in support of a study. To a lesser extent, dose comparison controls are used. Uncontrolled or even partially controlled studies are not acceptable to the agency as the sole basis for approval of claims of effectiveness. However, such studies are considered supportive. (c) There is assurance that selected subjects have the disease or condition. (d) The method of patient assignment must minimize bias and assure comparability of treatment groups. (e) Efforts are made to minimize the required number of subjects, observers, and analysts. (f) Well-defined methods of assessment are used. (7) Analysis of results is adequate (Prettyman CW. The Food and Drug Administration's regulation of clinical studies in the United States. *In* Max M, Portenoy R, Laska E [eds], *Advances in Pain Research and Therapy*, vol 18. New York: Raven Press, 1991).

substantia nigra Neuromelanin-pigmented nuclei of the basal ganglia. The pigmented neurons of the substantia nigra contain dopamine as the major neurotransmitter; when about 80% of the dopamine in the area has been depleted, the principal motor abnormalities of Parkinson's disease occurs.

subsyndromal symptoms Symptoms of an illness that distress and impair a patient but not to a clinically significant degree. They are common in bipolar patients. Although they may seem mild to an observer, persistent subsyndromal depression symptoms may impel a patient to choose the surcease of suicide.

subtraction hybridization Method developed to take advantage of the different mRNA contents of different cells to clone a specific cDNA, particularly for those messages present in very low abundance. Different cells express differing sets of genes, depending on the cell type and conditions. By expressing different genes, cells differ in their content of mRNA. Essentially, cDNA representing mRNA species that are shared by two different cells types can be removed prior to screening a cDNA library. In this way, a great majority of the uninteresting cDNA species are eliminated, so that the chances of identifying an mRNA that is expressed in one cell type but not the other are much better. The method also can be used to characterize cell-specific expression by finding heretofore unidentified mRNA that is present in one cell but not in another—for example, in one brain region compared to others.

succinimides One of eight major groups of anticonvulsants. A prototype is ethosuximide, which is often effective in the control of absence seizures. A close analog of ethosuximide, methsuximide is more sedative than ethosuximide and has been rated as a "second-line" drug and as a useful adjunct to the treatment of refractory partial complex seizures.

succinylcholine (Anectine, Sucostrin) Depolarizing muscle relaxant frequently used during electroconvulsive therapy (ECT) induction. It is considered the muscle-relaxant of choice for ECT. It is given by rapid bolus push at a dose of 0.6 mg/kg body weight. It is a known triggering agent of malignant hyperthermia.

succinylcholine + diazepam Co-administration rarely results in intensified and prolonged respiratory depression. In most patients, diazepam has no effect on the actions of succinylcholine.

succinylcholine + lithium Lithium prolongs the neuromuscular blockade of succinylcholine and has been implicated as a cause of acute confusional states after electroconvulsive therapy. By contrast, 17 patients failed to demonstrate any interaction between lithium and succinylcholine (Martin BA, Kramer PM. Clinical significance of the interaction between lithium and a neuromuscular blocker. *Am J Psychiatry* 1982;139:1326–1328).

succinylcholine + metoclopramide Co-administration may increase and prolong succinylcholine's neuromuscular blocking effects (Kao YJ, Turner DR. Prolongation of succinylcholine blockade by metoclopramide. *Anesthesiology* 1989;70:905–908).

succinylcholine + phenelzine Co-administration may enhance succinylcholine effects (Bleaden FA, Czekanska G. New drugs for depression. *Br Med J* 1960:1:200; Bodley PO, Halwax K, Potts L. Low serum pseudocholinesterase levels complicating treatment with phenelzine. *Br Med J* 1969;3:510).

succinylcholine + tacrine Tacrine is likely to exaggerate succinylcholine-type muscle relaxation during anesthesia (Tacrine Package Insert, May 1993).

Sucostrin See **succinylcholine.**

sufentanil Derivative of fentanyl. It is an opioid analgesic that is 5–7 times more potent than fentanyl and has a somewhat shorter duration of action.

"sugar" Street name for cocaine.

"sugar cube" Street name for lysergic acid diethylamide (LSD).

suicidal act Behavior purposefully undertaken by an individual in which the outcome is reasonably likely to be self-harm, in the absence of explicit data suggesting that suicide was not intended (Hirschfeld RMA, Davidson L. Risk factors for suicide. *In* Frances AJ, Hales RE [eds], *Psychiatry Update: American Psychiatric Association Annual Review*, vol 7. Washington, DC: American Psychiatric Press 1988, pp 307–333). Also called "suicide gesture."

suicidal behavior and psychotropic medication/ ACNP consensus statement Because of publicity regarding claims that the antidepressant fluoxetine may trigger emergent suicidal and homicidal ideation and behavior, the American College of Neuropsychopharmacology appointed a task force to review evidence regarding the effect of psychotropic medications on suicidality. Conclusions of the task force, published March 2, 1992, may be summarized as follows: (a) antidepressants are effective treatments for depression. In the vast majority of patients, antidepressants substantially improve or result in total remission of suicidal ideation and impulses; (b) new-generation antidepressants, which are less likely than the older drugs to result in toxicity with overdose, may be safer in terms of suicide risk than tricyclic antidepressants; (c) there is no evidence that selective serotonin reuptake inhibitors such as fluoxetine trigger suicidal ideation over and above rates that may be associated with other antidepressants and depression itself; and (d) patients receiving antidepressant treatment should be monitored not only for clinical progress, but for suicidal ideation and impulses. Depressed patients responsive to treatment may have brief (1 or 2 days) relapses. They should be warned that suicidal ideation as well as depression may worsen during treatment and that they should contact the doctor immediately if this occurs. Emergent suicidal ideation may be due to the patient's illness, adverse changes in the life situation, or perhaps to an (unproven) adverse effect of the antidepressant.

suicidal equivalents   Behaviors, most often indulged in by men, that may be life-threatening. Examples include extreme risk-taking activities, reckless, high-speed driving, and alcohol and substance abuse.

suicidal ideation   Thoughts, ideas, or ruminations about one's suicide or overt verbal threats to kill oneself (Wheadon DE, Rampey AH, Thompson VL, Potvin JH, Masica DN, Beasley CM. Lack of association between fluoxetine and suicidality in bulimia nervosa. *J Clin Psychiatry* 1992;53:235–241).

suicidal potential   Recurrent thoughts of death (not just fear of dying), recurrent suicidal ideation without a specific plan, or a suicidal attempt or a specific plan for committing suicide.

suicidality   Suicidal ideation and acts associated with the illness depression and other affective disturbances. Treatment with antidepressants or placebo may cause worsening of, no change in, or improvement of suicidality (Mann JJ, Kapur S. Emergence of suicidal ideation and behavior during antidepressant pharmacotherapy. *Arch Gen Psychiatry* 1991;48:1027–1032; Beasley CM, Dornseif BE, Bosomworth JC, et al. Fluoxetine and suicide: a meta-analysis of controlled trials of treatment for depression. *Br Med J* 1991;303:685–692).

suicide   Killing oneself. To diagnose any death as suicide, there must be evidence that it resulted from the decedent's deliberately initiated action (or inaction) and that the person had a specific intention to cause his or her own death.

suicide, adolescent   Studies of adolescents who died by suicide indicate that (a) adolescent suicide is associated with substance abuse more often than with any other psychiatric disorder; (b) those with an affective disorder have concomitant affective and nonaffective disorders more often than do adult suicide victims; (c) acute interpersonal conflict is no more prevalent among adolescent suicide victims than among other psychiatrically ill adolescents; (d) four of five talked about their suicidal state of mind with others (usually to siblings and friends of the same age) within

the week before their suicide; and (e) only a third of adolescents who died by suicide had ever seen a mental health professional, even once.

suicide attempt   Life-threatening act requiring medical attention that is committed with a conscious intent to end one's life. Suicide attempts are associated with major depression, substance abuse disorder, schizophrenia, and borderline personality disorder. Suicidality may develop at different times during these illnesses and fluctuate in severity independently of the severity of the depression. Because patients seek treatment at different points during the illness and a significant number do not respond to treatment, the appearance or worsening of suicidality in a small number of patients receiving a medication is not sufficient to implicate the medication as a cause (Mann JJ, Kapner S. The emergence of suicidal ideation and behavior during antidepressant pharmacotherapy. *Arch Gen Psychiatry* 1991;48:1027–1033) See **suicide gesture.**

suicide, attempted   Unsuccessful, but potentially lethal action, a risk factor for future completed suicide, and a potential indicator of other biopsychosocial health problems such as alcohol and substance abuse, depression, or adjustment and stress reactions. Attempted suicide is also a morbid health event that results in personal suffering and considerable economic cost. Surveys assessing the lifetime prevalence of attempted suicide indicate that 9–14% of adolescents have attempted suicide at some time in their lives. However, the results of epidemiological surveys on attempted suicide are often difficult to interpret; they compare and provide varying estimates of the prevalence of attempted suicide. The prevalence of self-reported attempted suicide does not represent the prevalence of self-injury and provides little information concerning the seriousness of the attempt (Meehan PJ, Lamb JA, Saltzman LE, O'Carroll PW. Attempted suicide among young adults: progress toward a meaningful estimate of prevalence. *Am J Psychiatry* 1992;149:41–44).

suicide cluster   Individuals or groups committing suicide shortly after the suicide(s) of acquaintances or public figures or after publicity about suicide clusters. Clusters occur among adolescents and youth (ages 18–30) and take two forms: one influenced by local events and the other by national events. In each type, mimicking of the suicide method seems to occur. Suicide clusters have been well documented in particular communities. At the national level, social contagion contributing to cluster suicides involves the influence and power of the national media, particularly television. Klerman reported on a quasi-experimental analysis of the impact of television in West Germany, where a documentary on suicide attempts among young people featured a graphic portrayal of a young male who killed himself by throwing himself under a train. In spite of intense protest, the documentary was repeated a year later, and the research team at the Mannheim Mental Health Institute documented a significant increase in suicide by railroad trauma in the weeks following both television portrayals. The association of television portrayal and subsequent rise in suicide deaths raises difficult problems about the balance between freedom of the press and public health responsibilities of the media (Klerman GL. Clinical epidemiology of suicide. *J Clin Psychiatry* 1987;48[suppl 12]:33–38). Evidence concerning imitative suicides is contradictory, possibly as a consequence of methodological problems inherent in studies of the issue. When the news media change reporting on suicides by printing only short reports, rarely on the front page and rarely sensational, or stop reporting suicides at all, there may be a positive reduction in the incidence of imitative suicides (Etzeersdorfer E, Sonneck G, Nagel-Kuess S. Newspaper reports and suicide. *N Engl J Med* 1992;327:502–503). The Austrian Association for Suicide Prevention created media guidelines and requested that the press follow them as of June 1987. These guidelines were followed by the media, and in 1988, no subway suicide was mentioned in the press. At the same time, the number of suicides in the subway decreased abruptly from the first to the second half of 1987, and the rates have remained low for more than 3 years. The overall suicide rate in Vienna decreased steadily (by 13%) from 1987 to 1990. The authors of the report concluded that "the striking relation between the change in the style of reporting by the print media and the number of subway suicides in Vienna supports the hypothesis that press reports of suicides may trigger additional suicides" (Klerman GL. Clinical epidemiology of suicide. *J Clin Psychiatry* 1987;48[suppl 12]:33–38).

suicide, geriatric   Suicide in those over age 65 occurs predominantly in men (80%), a third of whom are married and living with their spouse. Almost two-thirds at the time of their suicide are living with family members or friends. About half explicitly mention thoughts of suicide or of dying in the last 6 months of life, yet their suicide surprises those who knew them. About 10% are terminally ill, and 25% have a severe chronic medical illness. Their rate of suicide is 15 times higher for this age group than in the general population (Lehmann HE. Recognition and treatment of depression in geriatric patients. *In* Ayd FJ Jr [ed], *Clinical Depression: Diagnostic and Therapeutic Challenges.* Baltimore: Ayd Medical Communications, 1980, pp 57–69). The majority (90%) have symptoms of major depression, but only a few have contact with a psychiatrist or a mental health professional. One-fifth of geriatric suicide patients see a physician within 24 hours before their death, and almost half see a physician within a week prior to their suicide.

suicide gesture   Behavior purposefully undertaken by an individual in which the outcome is reasonably likely to be self-harm, in the absence of explicit data suggesting that suicide was not intended (Hirschfeld RMA, Davidson L. Risk factors for suicide. *In* Frances AJ, Hales RE [eds], *Psychiatry Update: American Psychiatric Association Annual Review,* vol 7. Washington, DC: American Psychiatric Press, 1988, pp 307–333).

suicide gesture/false-positive   Engaging in suicide gestures that do not portend subsequent suicide. The behavior often occurs in females with a borderline personality disorder; one or more manipulative suicide gestures may be made before the index hospitalization. These manipulative gestures are only occasionally a harbinger of eventual suicide; those who never make gestures rarely commit suicide. Even wrist-cutting and other self-mutilative acts are often false-positive and by themselves are not predictors of suicide.

suicide, imitative   See **suicide cluster.**

suicide pact   Agreement or pledge between two or more persons to take their own lives simultaneously.

suicide, physician-assisted   Death caused by the action(s) of a physician who agreed with the patient's intent to die and acted to directly bring it about.

suicide risk factors ages 13–30   (a) Gender—male suicides are predominant; (b) race—whites commit suicide more often than blacks; (c) psychiatric illness—depression, affective disorders, and substance abuse, including alcohol; (d) positive family history of early-onset affective disorder; and (e) history of previous suicide attempts.

suicide risk factors ages 30+   (a) Family history of suicide (suggesting genetic transmission); (b) diagnosis of a major affective disorder (bipolar disease or recurrent unipolar depression), schizophrenia, and alcoholism (suicide risk is not constant in the clinical course of these disorders, but is associated with episodes of acute depressive symptoms accompanied by feelings of hopelessness, despair, pessimism, and helplessness); (c) gender—although females are more likely to become depressed than males, males are more prone to suicide, especially alcoholic males; (d) single, separated, divorced, or widowed status; (e) associated medical illness; (f) lack of support; (g) sudden change in social or economic status; (h) undesired retirement; and (i) inadequate or no treatment of the associated psychiatric disorder.

sulforidazine Extremely active metabolite of mesoridazine. It may play a role in mesoridazine's efficacy in chronic schizophrenics resistant to standard neuroleptics.

sulindac (Clinoril) Nonsteroidal anti-inflammatory drug.

sulindac + lithium See **lithium + sulindac.**

sulpiride (Dogmatyl, Dolmatil, Modal) Substituted benzamide neuroleptic with selective dopamine (D_2) antagonistic action and minimal effect on noradrenergic, cholinergic, serotonergic, histaminergic, and GABAergic systems. It preferentially blocks presynaptic autoreceptors at lower doses and inhibits feedback, resulting in an increased dopamine turnover. At higher doses it blocks postsynaptic D_2, increases prolactin levels, and functions like a classic neuroleptic (Serra G, Cullu M, D'Augila PS, et al. On the mechanism involved in the behavioral supersensitivity to DA-agonists induced by chronic antidepressants. *In* Gessa GL, Serra G [eds], *Dopamine in Mental Depression.* Oxford: Pergamon Press, 1990, pp 121–138). It has a powerful effect on prolactin release. At low dosages (150–600 mg/day), sulpiride acts as a potent antiemetic and exerts a disinhibiting action in the treatment of depression. In high doses, it can cause amenorrhea-galactorrhea. Its half-life is 8 hours. In double-blind studies, it has been shown to have antipsychotic efficacy similar to that of haloperidol and chlorpromazine. Sulpiride is considered an atypical neuroleptic because of its low propensity to elicit extrapyramidal reactions. It does not aggravate tardive dyskinesia, but may alleviate abnormal movements. It has not been known to interact adversely with other psychotropics. The antidepressant efficacy of low doses has been demonstrated in double-blind placebo-controlled trials, and in comparative trials it displays efficacy equal to that of amitriptyline (Del Zompo M, Bocchetta A, Bernardi F, et al. Clinical evidence for a role of dopaminergic system in depressive states. *In* Gessa GL, Serra G [eds], *Dopamine in Mental Depression.* Oxford: Pergamon Press, 1990, pp 177–184).

sulpiride + amitriptyline Co-administration may be useful in the treatment of severe depression (Bonceir C, Masquin A, Omieux MC. Indications psychiatriques du sulpiride. A propos de 60 observations. *J Med Lyonnais* 1971;52:519–533).

sulpiride/breast milk Sulpiride is excreted in breast milk; its safety during breast feeding has not been established.

sulpiride + clomipramine Combination reported useful in the treatment of severe depression (Masquin A. Association du Dogmatil et de l'anafranil chaus le traitement des melancolies. *Information Psychiatrique* 1972;48: 218–219)

sulpiride + fluoxetine Co-administration can evoke acute extrapyramidal reactions (Dinan TG, O'Keane V. Acute extrapyramidal reactions following lithium and sulpiride co-administration. *Hum Psychopharmacol Clin Exp* 1991;6:67–69).

sulpiride + heroin Co-treatment may cause an acute dystonic reaction secondary to sulpiride (DeMaio D, Caponeri MA, Cicchetti V, et al. Sulpiride and extrapyramidal syndromes in chronic heroin addiction. *Neuropsychobiology* 1978;4:36–39).

sulpiride + lithium Co-administration can evoke acute extrapyramidal reactions (Dinan TG, O'Keane V. Acute extrapyramidal reactions following lithium and sulpiride co-administration: two case reports. *Hum Psychopharmacol Clin Exp* 1991;6:67–69).

sulpiride/pregnancy The manufacturer recommends avoiding sulpiride use during pregnancy, particularly the first trimester.

sulthiame (Elisal; Ospolat) Sulfonamide derivative that is a weak anticonvulsant and possibly an antidepressant. Anticonvulsant activity is probably due to inhibition of the metabolism of other anticonvulsants (i.e., it is inactive by itself). Not available in the United States.

sultopride (Barnetil; Barnotil; Topral) Substituted benzamide structurally related to sulpiride. It is an atypical sedative neuroleptic with a rapid onset of action that is effective in the treatment of acute psychotic episodes. It is usually prescribed for mania and acute schizophrenia.

sumatriptan (GR 43175) (Imigran; Imitrex) Extremely potent and selective serotonin (5-H1) analog that is a specific agonist at 5-HT_{1A} and 5-HT_{1D} receptors mediating the contraction of cerebral blood vessels. It may be very effective in the acute treatment of migraine headaches and is also an effective antiemetic.

sumatriptan + fluoxetine Co-administration may increase sumatriptan effects (Anon.

Sumatriptan: a new approach to migraine. *Drug Ther Bull* 1992;30:85–87).

sumatriptan + lithium   Co-administration may increase sumatriptan effects (Anon. Sumatriptan: a new approach to migraine. *Drug Ther Bull* 1992;30:85–87).

sumatriptan + monoamine oxidase inhibitor (MAOI)   Co-administration increases sumatriptan effects (Anon. Sumatriptan: a new approach to migraine. *Drug Ther Bull* 1992;30: 85–87).

sumatriptan + propranolol   Sumatriptan does not interact with propranolol (Scott AK, Walley T, Breckenridge AM, et al. Lack of an interaction between propranolol and sumatriptan. *Br J Clin Pharmacol* 1991;32:581–584).

sum of square   Quantity calculated in analysis of variance and used to obtain the mean squares for the *F* test. For a set value, the average is subtracted from each of them, and the square of those quantities is summed.

sundowner's syndrome   Disturbance of the sleep-wake cycle common in elderly demented patients. It is characterized by drowsiness or stupor during the day and alertness and hypervigilance at night. See **sundowning.**

sundowning   Recurring confusion and increased agitation in late afternoon or early evening that is common among patients with Alzheimer's disease in nursing homes (Evans LK. Sundown syndrome in institutionalized elderly. *J Am Geriatr Soc* 1987;35:101–108). It is characterized by behavioral disturbances such as agitation, pacing, restlessness, yelling, or shouting. Sundowners often have sleep disturbances characterized by frequent daytime napping and night-time awakenings. Sensory deprivation and abnormalities of the circadian timekeeping system may contribute; behaviors may be increased during the winter months (Bliwise DL, Carroll JS, Dement WC. Apparent seasonal variation in sundowning behavior in a skilled nursing facility. *Sleep Res* 1989;18: 408). Exposure to bright light (1500–2000 lux) for 2 hours between 7 and 9 P.M. for 1 week may ameliorate sleep-wake cycle disturbances in some patients. Light therapy also may reduce sundowning behavior during the second and third posttreatment weeks (Satlin A, Volicer L, Ross V, et al. Bright light treatment of behavioral and sleep disturbances in patients with Alzheimer's disease. *Am J Psychiatry* 1992;149:1028–1032). Sundowning should not be treated with sedative-hypnotics, which have only minimal effects. If drug therapy is warranted, 10–25 mg of intramuscularly administered chlorpromazine or mesoridazine is often helpful. After administration of the drug, patients should be urged to lie down, and blood pressure should be monitored.

"sunshine"   Street name for lysergic acid diethylamide (LSD).

"superacid"   Street name for (a) phencyclidine (PCP); (b) ketamine.

"supercoke"   Street name for phencyclidine (PCP).

superego   In psychoanalysis, an outgrowth of the ego that incorporates the values and wishes of important people (e.g., parents) to form the conscience. See **ego; id.**

"supergrass"   Street name for phencyclidine (PCP).

"superjoint"   Street name for phencyclidine (PCP).

"super k"   Street name for ketamine.

supersensitivity   Increase in the physiological or biochemical effect produced by a constant dose or concentration of drug and alterations in the properties of the tissue, organ, or cell with which the drug interacts. It may be achieved through changes in drug binding or postreceptor effector mechanisms. When the changes are mediated by an increase in drug binding through either increases in affinity of drug to its receptor or an increase in the number or density of receptor sites, the process is termed "up-regulation." See **subsensitivity.**

supersensitivity psychosis   (SSP) Worsening of psychotic symptoms in association with long-term neuroleptic therapy that occurs in certain patients who relapse immediately upon reduction in neuroleptic dosage and exhibit new schizophrenic symptoms or worsening of previous psychopathology. SSP is hypothesized to result from postsynaptic dopamine receptor supersensitivity in mesolimbic pathways in the same way that tardive dyskinesia is thought to develop in the neostriatum. Incidence is estimated to be 22%. It may respond rapidly to reintroduction of neuroleptic treatment, although severe cases have an extremely poor outcome with standard neuroleptic therapy, often requiring hospitalization despite very high doses. In severe cases, increasing neuroleptic dose leads to worsened symptoms, as though reintroduction of the causative stimulus were triggering the psychosis. Anticonvulsants, chiefly valproate and carbamazepine, given in low doses producing serum levels below the conventional therapeutic range ameliorate SSP and so-called "drug-resistant" schizophrenic patients by correcting a pharmacological kindling effect in the limbic system that results from chronic neuroleptic therapy (Chouinard G, Sultan S. Treatment of supersensitivity psychosis with antiepileptic drugs: report of a series of 43 cases. *Psychopharmacol Bull* 1990;26:337–341). A small number of so-called "refractory" patients have responded to either risperidone or clozapine (Chouinard G, Beandry P, Vainer L, et al. Risperidone and clozapine in the treatment of neuroleptic-induced supersensitivity psychosis. *Biol Psychiatry* 1993;33:130A).

supersensitivity psychosis/ bipolar affective disorder   Most cases of supersensitivity psychosis have occurred in patients with schizophrenia. There is now evidence that all patients with bipolar disorder are susceptible following prolonged use of neuroleptics, even in small doses. In such patients, neuroleptics should be used sparingly (Steiner W, Laporta M, Chouinard G. Neuroleptic-induced supersensitivity psychosis in patients with bipolar affective disorder. *Acta Psychiatr Scand* 1990;81:437–440).

supersensitivity psychosis, Chouinard Research Criteria   Research diagnostic criteria developed to distinguish supersensitivity psychosis from pre-existing psychopathology. In addition to having at least a 3-month history of receiving antipsychotic medication, the patient must have at least one of the following: 1) Reappearance of psychotic symptoms upon decrease or discontinuation of medication during the last 5 years—within 6 weeks of oral medication, 3 months for intramuscular depot medication 2) Greater frequency of relapse (acute psychotic exacerbation while on continuous neuroleptic treatment) 3) Tolerance to the antipsychotic effect of the neuroleptic (overall increase in dose by 20% or more during the last 5 years) 4) Extreme tolerance: increased neuroleptic dosages no longer mask symptoms 5) Psychotic symptoms upon decrease of medication are new schizophrenic symptoms (not previously seen) *or* are of greater severity 6) Psychotic relapse occurs upon sudden decrease (< 10% of medication, but not if same decrease is gradual 7) Presence of drug tolerance in the past but presently treated with high doses of neuroleptics on at least a twice-daily regimen   If only one major criterion from the above list is present, there must also be at least one of the following: 1) Tardive dyskinesia (a standard examination must be used) 2) Rapid improvement in psychotic symptoms when the neuroleptic dose is increased after a decrease or discontinuation 3) Clear exacerbation of psychotic symptoms by stress 4) Appearance of psychotic symptoms at the end of the injection interval (for patients on long-acting intramuscularly administered medication) 5) High levels of prolactin or radioreceptor neuroleptic activity (twice normal—at least once within the last 2 years)

"super Valium"   Slang term for the benzodiazepine clonazepam, which has become a commonly abused drug among methadone-maintained heroin addicts who use it to treat opiate withdrawal symptoms.

suppression   Mechanism in which the person intentionally avoids thinking about disturbing problems, desires, feelings, or experiences. See **defense mechanism.**

suppression of zero   Misleading graph that does not have a break in the y axis to indicate that part of the scale is missing.

suppressor gene   See **gene, suppressor.**

suppressor t cell   See **T cell, suppressor.**

suprachiasmatic nucleus   (SCN) Collection of small cells in the anterior hypothalamus acting as a biological clock or oscillator that maintains the circadian rhythm of sleep-wakefulness. The SCN receives sensory input via the optic nerve and is connected through a complex egress of nerves with the pineal gland. The cells of the SCN have a circadian rhythm with a period of approximately 25 hours in man; the period is "reset" and shortened each day by external time cues (zeitgebers) to a rhythm closer to the true circadian period of the planet. In rats, SCN lesions induced early-onset transient hyperinsulinemia in response to a glucose challenge, similar to that observed in impulsive violent offenders. The SCN plays a role in the postulated "low serotonin syndrome" (Linnoila VMI, Virkkunen M. Aggression, suicidality and serotonin. *J Clin Psychiatry* 1992;53[suppl]:46–51). See **zeitgebers.**

Suprazine   See **trifluoperazine.**

suproclone   Cyclopyrrolone nonbenzodiazepine that acts at the benzodiazepine receptor–gamma aminobutyric acid receptor (BZR-GABAR)-chloride ionophore supramolecular complex.

suriclone   (RP 31264) Cyclopyrrolone nonbenzodiazepine that acts at the benzodiazepine receptor–gamma aminobutyric acid receptor (BZR-GABAR)-chloride ionophore supramolecular complex. It has been shown to have anxiolytic efficacy in generalized anxiety disorder and fewer side effects than benzodiazepines.

Surital   See **thiamylal.**

Surmontil   See **trimipramine.**

surrogate end-point   See **end-point, surrogate.**

Survector 100   See **amineptine.**

survey   Observational or descriptive, nonexperimental study in which individuals are systematically examined for the absence or presence (or degree of presence) of characteristics of interest (Anon. Glossary of methodologic terms. *JAMA* 1992;268:43–44).

survival analysis   In statistical methodology, analysis of time-to-event data. The event must be a single, well-defined event. Major interests are survival time and hazard rate. Survival analysis has been widely used in the biomedical area, and since 1992 it has been applied in psychological research with affective disorders and addictive behaviors.

suspiciousness Unrealistic or exaggerated ideas of persecution reflected in guardedness, a distrustful attitude, suspicious hypervigilance, or frank delusions that others mean one harm. In its extreme form, a network of systematized persecutory delusions dominates the patient's thinking, social relations, and behavior.

sustained release Type of drug formulation that can be divided into three basic types, single-compartment, multiparticulate, and osmotic. In single-compartment devices, the drug is incorporated into a porous wax or plastic matrix, with drug release dependent on porosity of the matrix and drug solubility. Multiparticulate devices consist of coated pellets or granules of drug contained in a gelatin capsule or compressed into a tablet. Coatings are varying thicknesses of a slowly dispersible substance, resulting in a fairly constant rate of drug release. In osmotic devices, a reservoir of drug is surrounded by a semipermeable membrane through which water may enter and drug cannot escape. As water enters, drug is forced out through a laser-drilled hole at a fairly constant rate. With single unit and osmotic devices, the spent matrix or *ghost* is excreted in feces. Ghosts can cause concern to some patients and have been reported to cause gastric outlet obstruction. Although many patients would not notice ghosts in their stools, the information should be available in patient information leaflets to prevent unnecessary patient distress and physician consultations (Janes J, Routledge PA, Rees A. The ghost of nifedipine passed. *Lancet* 1993;342: 1565).

Sustanon 100 See **testosterone propionate.**

Sustanon 250 See **testosterone propionate.**

"sweet Lucy" Street name for cannabinol.

"sweet tart" Street name for dimethoxymethylamphetamine.

switch process Change from depression to mania during treatment with electroconvulsive therapy, a heterocyclic antidepressant, or a monoamine oxidase inhibitor (Bunney WE Jr., Murphy DL, Goodwin FK. The switch process in manic depressive illness: I. A systematic study of sequential behavioral changes. *Arch Gen Psychiatry* 1972;27:295–302) The extent to which drugs exacerbate the switch process is controversial. Since 1972, National Institute of Mental Health (NIMH) researchers have contended that it has occurred in 25–60% of patients (Kennedy SH, Bradwejn J, Joffee RT, Kuslac M. Practical

issues in managing bipolar depression. *Int Clin Psychopharmacol* 1991;6[suppl]:53–72). Other investigators claim that switches are no more frequent among bipolar patients on antidepressant therapies than in those not receiving antidepressants (Lewis JL, Winokur G. The induction of mania: a natural history with controls. *Arch Gen Psychiatry* 1982;39:303–306; Angst J. The switch from depression to mania—a record study over decades between 1920–1982. *Psychopathology* 1985;18:140–154).

Symadine See **amantadine.**

symbiosis Any intimate association between two species or persons; living together.

Symmetrel See **amantadine.**

symmetric distribution Distribution that has the same shape on both sides of the mean. The mean and median are equal for this distribution. It is the opposite of a skewed distribution.

sympathetic nervous system See **nervous system, sympathetic.**

sympatholytic Agent that blocks the effects of sympathetic (adrenergic) stimulation.

sympathomimetic Drug that in usual doses stimulates central nervous system (CNS) tissues by (a) blocking the actions of inhibitory cells; (b) releasing transmitter substances; or (c) direct action of the drug itself. It increases CNS catecholamines such as dopamine and norepinephrine, raising blood pressure, heart rate, respiratory rate, and reflexes. It can interact adversely with monoamine oxidase inhibitors. Sympathomimetics include amphetamines, methylphenidate, cocaine, metaraminol, mephentermine, pemoline, phenylpropanolamine, ephedrine, phenylephrine, pseudoephedrine, naphazoline, and caffeine. Many proprietary cold and allergy remedies contain sympathomimetics. Also called "adrenergic agent."

sympathomimetic + maprotiline Co-administration may increase blood pressure.

sympathomimetic toxic syndrome Syndrome manifested by agitation, delirium, hallucinations, panic, insomnia, headache, tachycardia, and hypertension.

symptom Complaint reported by the patient or elicited by clinical history.

symptom overinterpretation Phenomenon that may occur in people discontinuing benzodiazepines (BZDs) who anticipate the development of withdrawal symptoms because of widespread publicity about BZD withdrawal. Patients may decide that any symptoms occurring after BZD discontinuation are due to its withdrawal and that they require treatment.

symptom rebound Distinct benzodiazepine discontinuation syndrome characterized by more rapid onset of symptoms than simple recrudescence. Rebound symptoms usually develop within hours to days of benzodiazepine discontinuation; the precise time course partly depends on the pharmacokinetic properties of the particular benzodiazepine. Rebound symptoms are qualitatively similar to the disorder for which the drug was originally taken, but are transiently more intense than those prior to drug treatment.

symptomatic Indicative of, or relating to, the aggregate of symptoms of a disease.

symptomatic treatment Therapy to alleviate symptoms without influencing the course of the underlying disease. Response criteria assess either the severity of the symptom, using a quantitative or qualitative scale to define absolute levels or the degree of improvement achieved, or measure the duration of the effect observed (Spriet A, Simon P. *Methodology of Clinical Drug Trials.* Basel: Karger, 1985).

symptomatic volunteer Individual with mild symptoms of an untreated anxiety disorder or depression recruited by advertisements in newspapers for participation in a clinical trial of a new drug. Because volunteers are paid for their participation in a trial, they are not ideal subjects. They frequently drop-out before the trial is completed and have a high rate of side effects. Many investigators contend that symptomatic volunteers should not be included in clinical trials.

symptoms, first-rank Group of symptoms selected and used by Kurt Schneider and his followers as a basis for making a diagnosis of schizophrenia. Signs include hallucinations, changes in thought process, delusional perceptions, somatic passivity, and other external impositions.

symptoms, productive Hallucinations and delusions in schizophrenia, or some symptoms of autism. See **deficit symptoms.**

synapse Nerve cell juncture where biochemical substances are passed. The space is contiguous with extracellular fluid between the presynaptic nerve terminal and the postsynaptic cell into which the neurotransmitter is released and diffused to act on postsynaptic receptors. The space between one axon terminal and its synaptic target neuron is termed the *synaptic gap* or *cleft.*

synapsin Closely related phosphoprotein associated with synaptic vesicles involved in the short-term regulation of neurotransmitter release.

synapsin I Phosphoprotein consisting of two polypeptides (synapsin Ia and synapsin Ib) involved in the regulation of neurotransmitter release. Its function depends on its state of phosphorylation. It is closely related to synapsin II.

synapsin II Synaptic vesicle–associated neuronal phosphoprotein that may be involved in the regulation of neurotransmitter release. It consists of two polypeptides (synapsins IIa and IIb). Variant forms of synapsin II might result in abnormalities in the regulation of neurotransmitter release. Formerly called "protein III."

synaptic cleft Space between one axon terminal and its synaptic target neuron. Also called "synaptic gap." See **synapse.**

synaptosome Pinched-off and resealed nerve ending formed following the homogenization and high-speed centrifugation of brain tissue in an isotonic medium.

synchronization Two or more rhythms recurring with the same phase relationship. In the electroencephalogram (EEG), it is indicated by an increased amplitude and usually a decreased frequency of the dominant activities.

synchronized sleep See **sleep-stage NREM.**

synchronizer Stimulus that regularizes the timing or phase of a rhythm.

syncope Fainting attack caused by transient generalized cerebral ischemia due to acute circulatory insufficiency. Because evaluation and treatment are different, syncope must be distinguished from seizures and other states of altered consciousness such as dizziness, vertigo, and narcolepsy. There should be spontaneous recovery not requiring cardioversion. There are almost no neurological causes for syncope, and an electroencephalogram (EEG) is devoid of epileptiform activity. There is no rhythmical clonic jerking activity, although there may be random clonic jerks. Incontinence, tongue biting, and postepisodic confusion are rare. Vasovagal syncope and postural hypotension are the most common causes of syncope. It also may be caused by psychoactive drugs such as phenothiazines, cyclic antidepressants, monoamine oxidase inhibitors, and barbiturates. Psychiatric illnesses that can result in syncope include (a) generalized anxiety disorder, which may produce hyperventilation and vasodepressor reaction; (b) panic disorder; (c) somatization disorder (4.5% of patients report loss of consciousness); and (d) major depression. Patients with syncope due to psychiatric disorders are generally younger and have multiple episodes. They have a lower prevalence of heart disease and may have other nonspecific complaints associated with syncope such as headache, fatigue, dizziness, and palpitations (Kapoor WN. Evaluation and management of the patient with syncope. *JAMA* 1992;268:2553–2560). See **seizure, convulsive.**

syndrome Typical roster of symptoms or complaints and signs or clinical observations. The number and severity of features may vary among people with the same syndrome; every feature need not be present to constitute the syndrome. A syndrome is not synonymous with disease and implies neither a specific etiology nor a homogeneous treatment response. The same underlying etiology may provoke a variety of syndromes, whereas the same syndrome may have differing etiologies and pathogeneses.

syndrome of inappropriate secretion of antidiuretic hormone (SIADH) Disorder occurring in hyponatremic patients who instead of conserving sodium continue to lose it in the urine as if under the influence of antidiuretic hormone (ADH) at a time when ADH release should have been suppressed. Diagnostic criteria include hyponatremia and hypo-osmolality of the serum and extracellular fluid with continued renal excretion of sodium. It is often drug-induced, particularly by drugs that impair renal excretion of free water. Psychiatric drugs that can cause hyponatremia include carbamazepine, thioridazine, amitriptyline, desipramine, fluoxetine, tranylcypromine, thiothixene, fluphenazine, haloperidol, and chlorpromazine. Although psychotropic medication is associated with SIADH, so is psychosis, and psychotropic medication is often falsely blamed for SIADH.

synergism Unpredictable pharmacodynamic drug interaction in which the effect of one drug is enhanced by the presence of another. The effect is more than would be expected from the combined amount of the two drugs.

synergy Coordination in the action of muscles, organs, or drugs.

synesthesia Condition in which experiences normally associated with one sensory modality are translated into another. Colors may be "smelled" and sounds may be "seen." Synesthesia is often produced by lysergic acid diethylamide (LSD). The perceptual aberrations have been described as pseudohallucinations, illusions, or visions, since the LSD user usually has sufficient insight to recognize that the phenomena are drug-induced.

synkinesia Contraction of unexpected muscles or voluntary facial movements that can be a sequela of Bell's palsy.

synkinesis Involuntary movement of a part of the body that automatically follows a voluntary movement of another part of the body.

syntenic Relating to loci located on the same chromosome that need not be linked.

Synthroid See **levothyroxine; thyroxine.**

Syntocinon See **oxytocin.**

systematic desensitization First widely used exposure therapy for phobic disorders. A behavioral treatment based on the classic learning theory of phobias, it uses graded imaginal exposure. Initially, a hierarchy of anxiety-producing situations related to the phobic stimulus is developed by therapist and patient. Patients are then trained in deep muscle relaxation. At the start of a session, patients are put into a state of deep relaxation, during which they are asked to visualize the first scene in the hierarchy. If this provokes anxiety, the patient stops, and immediately proceeds with a deep muscle relaxation. The scene is then revisualized. When a scene has been visualized twice without provoking anxiety, the patient proceeds up the hierarchy to the next most anxiety-provoking scene.

systematic error See **error, systematic.**

systematic random sample Sample obtained by selecting each kth subject or object.

systematized delusion See **delusion, systemized.**

systemic pharmacokinetics See **pharmacokinetics, systemic.**

T

T_1 Longitudinal or spin-lattice relaxation time, one of three components of the signal used during magnetic resonance imaging. T_1 is the time required for net magnetization following radio frequency excitation to return to 63% of its original value.

T_2 Transverse or spin-spin relaxation time, one of three components of the signal used during magnetic resonance imaging. T_2 is the time required for the signal to return to 37% of its original value.

T_3 See **triiodothyronine.**

T_4 See **thyroxine.**

tabes   Chronic, progressive nervous system disease that occurs late in the course of syphilis in a small percentage of patients. Degeneration in the posterior columns of the spinal cord produces ataxia, neuralgia, anesthesia, lancinating pains, and muscular atrophy. Also called "tabes dorsalis."

tabes dorsalis   See **tabes.**

table, life   See **life table.**

table, statistical   See **statistical table.**

"tac"   Street name for phencyclidine (PCP).

tachyathetosis   See **restless legs syndrome.**

tachykinin peptide   Any of a relatively large group of neuropeptides that are aminated at the C-terminus in the processing of the peptide prior to secretion. They arise from at least two preprotachykinins. Substance P, neurokinin A, and neuropeptide K arise from preprotachykinin I; neurokinin B arises from preprotachykinin II.

tachylogia   See **logorrhea.**

tachyphagia   Rapid eating or bolting of food, a symptom often seen in regressed, deteriorated, chronic schizophrenic patients and in some postprefrontal lobotomy patients.

tachyphylaxis   Rapid development of tolerance to a repeatedly administered drug. Also called "refractoriness" or "desensitization." See **tolerance.**

tachypnea   Rapid breathing. It may be due to a physical or psychological disorder. It is sometimes associated with a severe panic attack. See **hyperventilation.**

tacrine   (THA) (Cognex) (1,2,3,4-tetrahydro-9-acridinamine monohydrochloride monohydrate). Potent, reversible inhibitor of cholinesterase, an enzyme responsible for the breakdown of the neurotransmitter acetylcholine. THA has been marketed for treatment of early Alzheimer's disease to enhance memory. In a controlled study in Alzheimer's disease patients selected for apparent responsiveness to tacrine, there was a statistically significant reduction in the decline of cognitive function, although the reduction was not large enough to be detected by physicians' global patient assessments (Davis KL, Thal LJ, Gamzu ER, et al. A double-blind, placebo-controlled multicenter study of tacrine for Alzheimer's disease. *N Engl J Med* 1992;27:1253–1259). Tacrine's main side effect is chemically induced elevated liver enzymes in 30% of patients. Its label recommends an escalating dose regimen (80 mg/day to 160 mg/day) with frequent blood tests. For patients experiencing mild liver toxicity, dosage may be reduced or the drug stopped and later resumed at a lower dose. Hepatic injury has been reversible with treatment cessation in essentially all cases to date. Pregnancy risk category C.

tacrine/breast feeding   It is not known if tacrine is excreted in breast milk (Tacrine Package Insert, May 1993).

tacrine + cimetidine   Cimetidine increased the C_{max} and area under the curve (AUC) of tacrine by approximately 54% and 64%, respectively (Tacrine Package Insert, May 1993).

tacrine + diazepam   Tacrine has no major impact on diazepam pharmacokinetics (Tacrine Package Insert, May 1993).

tacrine + digoxin   Tacrine has no major impact on digoxin pharmacokinetics (Tacrine Package Insert, May 1993).

tacrine/pregnancy   Animal reproduction studies have not been conducted. It is not known if tacrine is teratogenic or can affect reproductive capacity (Tacrine Package Insert, May 1993).

tacrine + selegiline   Addition of selegiline (5 mg twice a day) to the regimen of Alzheimer's patients treated with tacrine was associated with significant improvement on the cognitive subscale of the Alzheimer's Disease Assessment Scale, suggesting possible additive effects of selegiline to the effects of cholinesterase inhibitors (Schneider LS, Olin JT, Pawluczyk S. A double-blind crossover pilot study of l-deprenyl (selegiline) combined with cholinesterase inhibitor in Alzheimer's disease. *Am J Psychiatry* 1993;150:321–323).

tacrine + succinylcholine   Tacrine is likely to exaggerate succinylcholine type muscle relaxation during anesthesia (Tacrine Package Insert, May 1993).

tacrine + theophylline   Co-administration increased theophylline's elimination half-life and average plasma concentrations by approximately 2 times. Monitoring of theophylline plasma concentrations and appropriate reduction of theophylline dose are recommended in patients receiving both drugs. The effect of theophylline on tacrine pharmacokinetics has not been assessed (Tacrine Package Insert, May 1993).

tacrine + warfarin Tacrine has no effect on the anticoagulant activity of warfarin (Tacrine Package Insert, May 1993).

tacrine withdrawal Worsening of cognitive function has been reported following abrupt discontinuation of tacrine or after a large reduction in total daily dose (80 mg/day or more) (Tacrine Package Insert, May 1993).

tactile hallucination See **hallucination, tactile.**

Tagamet See **cimetidine.**

"tai stick" Street term for marijuana buds wrapped in a leaf alone or the same preparation dipped in opium.

taint carrier In genetics, family members who carry a particular genetic factor in their genotypes, but do not manifest it phenotypically.

Talacen See **pentazocine.**

talbutal (Lotusate) Intermediate-acting (6–8 hours) barbiturate indicated for the short-term treatment of insomnia. Not marketed in the United States.

Talwin See **pentazocine.**

tandamine A norepinephrine reuptake inhibitor.

tandem gait Walking heel-to-toe. Inability to perform tandem gait, so that a person walks as if "drunk," indicates cerebellar dysfunction.

tandospirone Selective serotonin (5-HT)$_{1A}$ partial agonist that is a member of a new class of nonbenzodiazepine anxiolytics, the azaspirones. It is metabolized to 1-phenyl piperazine (1-PP). It may have some antidepressant activity. In a comparison of the acute effects of tandospirone and alprazolam in sedative drug abusers, both drugs produced comparable dose-related increases in subject-rated strength of drug effect. Alprazolam produced dose-related increases in subject-rated drug liking, whereas tandospirone produced dose-related increases in subject-rated drug disliking. Alprazolam produced greater impairments on psychomotor performance than tandospirone. The highest dose of alprazolam, in contrast to the highest dose of tandospirone, was predominantly classified by subjects as being a barbiturate or a benzodiazepine (71% vs. 29%, respectively). Tandospirone and alprazolam can be differentiated on the basis of subjective effects and performance measures. Current data suggest that tandospirone has a lower abuse potential than alprazolam (Evans SM, Troisi JR, Griffiths RR. Comparison of tandospirone and alprazolam: Performance impairment, subjec-

tive effects and abuse liability. Presented at the 1992 Annual Meeting of the American College of Neuropsychopharmacology).

tangentiality Thought process disturbance characterized by thought and speech that digresses readily from one topic to associated topics rather than "sticking to the point." It may be a symptom of schizophrenia and certain types of organic disorders.

"tango and cash" Street name for a form of adulterated heroin that has caused severe complications. The adulterant is probably methyl fentanyl, which makes heroin 27 times more potent. Both depress respiration by interacting with opioid receptors in the brain; the combination produces additive effects that can result in coma and respiratory arrest. In 1991, a supply of "tango and cash" created in an underground laboratory was responsible for at least 136 overdoses and 12 deaths in New York, Connecticut, and New Jersey.

tapering Gradual discontinuation of a medication by decrements in dosage over days or weeks until the drug is completely withdrawn. The purpose (essential for many drugs) is to minimize or avoid withdrawal symptoms.

"tar" Street name for opium.

Taractan See **chlorprothixene.**

Tarasan See **chlorprothixene.**

tardive Late onset of the signs and symptoms of a disorder.

tardive akathisia See **akathisia, tardive.**

tardive dyskinesia (TD) Potentially irreversible, late-onset, extrapyramidal hyperkinetic movement disorder often caused by long-term administration of neuroleptics and non-neuroleptic dopamine-blocking agents such as metoclopramide. No clear relationships, however, have emerged between TD and the lifetime antipsychotic dose or the length of exposure to antipsychotics or non-neuroleptic dopamine blockers. TD is manifested by choreiform movements of the mouth, tongue, lips, limbs, and trunk. The abnormal movements of the mouth, tongue, and lips are referred to as *bucco-lingual-masticatory syndrome.* Speech and respiration may also be affected. Symptoms fluctuate in severity with time, are transiently worse during anxiety or stress, and disappear during sleep. Patients who have acute extrapyramidal symptoms early in treatment are more likely to develop TD than those who do not. Some patients present with transient TD, others with withdrawal dyskinesia or with persistent dyskinesia, and some patients with well-established TD show reversibility several years after the discontinuation of the causative agent. It is important to note that high rates of abnormal involuntary movements have also been found among institutionalized geriatric patients never exposed to neuroleptics. TD course is characterized by repeated reactivation and remission. TD is not synonymous with irreversible dyskinesia, since TD is reversible in at least one-third of patients. An unknown number of patients lack awareness of their movement disorder and many deny awareness; they score significantly lower on a short test of cognitive function than patients who are aware of such movements. Schizophrenics, especially those with cognitive deficits and negative symptoms, are quite likely to be unaware of their TD (Macpherson R, Collis R. Tardive dyskinesia. Patients' lack of awareness of movement disorders. *Br J Psychiatry* 1992;160:110–112). In some patients, persistent dyskinetic movement may contribute to increased risk of mortality. Orofacial and lingual movements may seriously inhibit mastication and thus result in poor nutrition and weight loss. The abnormal movements may cause dysphagia and, infrequently, death due to choking. Respiratory dyskinesia and constant movement of the trunk and extremities can strain the cardiovascular system, resulting in increased morbidity (Ayd FJ Jr. Tardive dyskinesia and mortality risk. *Int Drug Ther Newsl* 1985;20:3). Although most studies on the pathophysiology of TD propose a role for hyperdopaminergic function, new hypotheses involving the gamma aminobutyric acid (GABA) neurotransmitter system, iron metabolism, and free radical damage have been advanced. The role of neurotensin in the nigrostriatal dopaminergic system has been implicated in the etiology of TD. Neurotensin increases striatal dopamine release, and striatal neurotensin is increased with neuroleptic therapy. The substantia nigra neurotensin receptor content is also increased with neuroleptic therapy, suggesting that nigral neurotensin activity results in abnormal striatal dopamine release (Uhl G. Neuropeptide systems in Parkinson's disease and tardive dyskinesia. *In* Nemeroff CB [ed], *Neuropeptides in Psychiatric and Neurological Disorders.* Baltimore: The Johns Hopkins University Press, 1988, pp 156–177). See **vitamin E.**

tardive dyskinesia, atypical   Subtype of tardive dyskinesia (TD) that includes all other manifestations of TD not fulfilling the criteria of classic TD or tardive dystonia. It includes patients with isolated gastrointestinal or respiratory dyskinesias, ballistic movements, flowing choreic movements, tardive Tourette's syndrome, and tardive akathisia (Haag H, Ruther E, Hippius H. *Tardive Dyskinesia: Vol 1. WHO Expert Series of Biological Psychiatry.* Bern: Hogrefe & Huber, 1992).

tardive   dyskinesia/calcium-channel   blockers   Studies of calcium-channel blockers in the treatment of tardive dyskinesia have yielded mixed results. Positive findings have been reported for nifedipine, verapamil, and diltiazem, with nifedipine being most efficacious. Effectiveness appears to be dose-related. Additional data are needed from double-blind, placebo-controlled studies with larger sample sizes and longer duration of therapy (Cates M, Lusk K, Wells BG. Are calcium-channel blockers effective in the treatment of tardive dyskinesia? *Ann Pharmacother* 1993;27:191–196).

tardive dyskinesia, early-onset   Tardive dyskinesia (TD) with onset in less than 2 years of neuroleptic therapy. It has been found to be associated with significantly lower maximum neuroleptic doses than late-onset TD, suggesting that it may be more closely related to increased individual vulnerability rather than to the intensity of neuroleptic therapy.

tardive dyskinesia/elderly   Elderly psychiatric patients are more at risk for tardive dyskinesia (TD) than younger patients. It is estimated that TD may develop in a short period in almost half of elderly neuroleptic-treated patients. Because spontaneous dyskinesia also may also occur in elderly psychiatric patients without prior neuroleptic therapy, the prevalence of TD among elderly psychiatric patients who had never received neuroleptic medication before their first hospitalization was investigated. Results confirmed the greater vulnerability to TD of neuroleptic-treated elderly psychiatric patients and reinforce the recommendation that caution is especially necessary when neuroleptics are prescribed for older patients with major affective disorders (Yassa R, Nastase C, Dupont D, Thibeau M. Tardive dyskinesia in elderly psychiatric patients: a 5-year study. *Am J Psychiatry* 1992;149:1206–1211).

tardive dyskinesia, late-onset   Tardive dyskinesia with an onset after 2 years of neuroleptic therapy.

tardive dyskinesia, masked   Tardive dyskinesia (TD) symptoms that are absent (masked) because of neuroleptic treatment that suppress the movements until dosage reduction or discontinuation of the neuroleptic. Masking TD symptoms with neuroleptics generally is not considered an acceptable treatment, except when used to improve the quality of life for a patient whose severe TD is refractory to other remedies.

tardive dyskinesia, mild   Low severity of dyskinesia as assessed globally by a validated scale (e.g., a score of 3 on the Simpson Rating Scale).

tardive dyskinesia, moderately severe   Intensity of dyskinesias as assessed globally using a validated rating scale (e.g., a score of 5 on the Simpson Rating Scale).

tardive dyskinesia/risk factors   Exposure to neuroleptics and non-neuroleptic dopamine-blocking agents such as metoclopramide; increasing age; female sex; affective disorder; central nervous system dysfunction; anticholinergic agents; parkinsonism; and diabetes. Other risk factors identified by Yale University researchers are race (blacks are twice as likely as whites to develop TD); dose (the higher the dose of the responsible drug, the greater the risk); duration of exposure (risk is greatest in the first 5 years of but increases with continued exposure); and handedness (left-handed patients are less likely than right-handed or ambidextrous patients to have TD) (Glazer WM, Morgenstern H, Doucette JT. Predicting the long-term risk of tardive dyskinesia in outpatients maintained on neuroleptic medications. *J Clin Psychiatry* 1993;54:133–139).

tardive dysmentia   Behavior disorder, seen in patients on long-term neuroleptic therapy, manifested by loquaciousness; intrusively loud voice; disconnected, aimless, and often inappropriate thoughts; a general euphoric mood, with occasional unpredictable explosions of hostility; and social withdrawal broken by episodes of overactivity that is often greatly invasive of others' privacy. It is a controversial diagnosis also called "tardive psychosis" (Wilson IC, Garbutt JC, Lanier CF, et al. Is there a tardive dysmentia? *Schizophr Bull* 1983;9:187–192).

tardive dystonia   Term first used by Keegan and Rajput (1973) to denote a late-onset extrapyramidal reaction characterized by sustained or slow involuntary twisting movements of the limbs, trunk, neck, or face. Tardive dystonia is related to tardive dyskinesia and may co-exist with it. It can be focal, segmental, or generalized and usually appears after an average of 3.7 years' exposure to neuroleptics and non-neuroleptic dopamine-blocking agents such as metoclopramide. Tardive dystonia produces more severe functional handicap than tardive dyskinesia. In some cases, it is accompanied by mild chorea that should prompt the clinician to obtain a detailed drug history. Some cases of tardive dystonia involving the face and neck closely resemble spontaneously occurring Meige syndrome. Tardive dystonia is quite different from acute dystonia in clinical course; co-existence with orofacial, trunk, and limb dyskinesia; time course in relation to drug exposure; resistance to anticholinergic treatment; and persistence after drug withdrawal. Response to clozapine is variable, but approximately 43% of cases, particularly those with dystonia, improve with clozapine treatment.

tardive dystonia/diagnostic criteria   The following have been proposed: (a) presence of chronic dystonia; (b) history of antipsychotic drug treatment preceding or concurrent with the onset of dystonia; (c) exclusion of known causes of secondary dystonia by appropriate clinical and laboratory evaluation; and (d) no family history of dystonia (Burke RE, Fahn S, Jankovic J, et al. Tardive dystonia: late-onset and persistent dystonia caused by antipsychotic drugs. *Neurology* 1982;32:1335–1346). Also called "dystonia tarda" (i.e., dystonia associated with prolonged exposure to antidopaminergic drugs). See **Meige syndrome.**

tardive orofacial dyskinesia   See **dyskinesia, orofacial.**

tardive psychosis   See **tardive dysmentia.**

tardive tics   Tics first appearing after neuroleptic dosage decrease or discontinuation in a patient who had been on long-term neuroleptic therapy (years). Many experts consider tardive tics to be a form of tardive dyskinesia (TD). Like TD, they may persist for months or years, and may be severe and/or irreversible. The likelihood of reversal of tardive tics after neuroleptic withdrawal decreases with age.

tardive Tourette's syndrome   Rare clinical manifestation of tardive dyskinesia (TD) first reported in 1978 as induced by chlorpromazine (Klawans HL, Falk DA, Narsieda P, Weiner WJ. Gilles de la Tourette syndrome after long-term chlorpromazine therapy. *Neurology* 1978;28:1064–1065). Produced by prolonged neuroleptic treatment, it is manifested by motor and vocal tics indistinguishable from those observed in Tourette's syndrome, rather than by the classic oro-buccal-facial dyskinetic symptoms of TD (Fog R, Pakkenberg H, Regeur L, Pakkenberg B. "Tardive" Tourette syndrome in relation to long-term neuroleptic treatment of multiple tics. *In* Friedhoff AJ, Chase TN [eds], *Gilles de la Tourette Syndrome.* New York: Raven Press, 1982, pp 419–421). Its cause is thought to be similar to that of TD. Differentiating tardive Tourette's syndrome from true Tourette's syndrome can only be based on the time of onset of the tic disorder or on a positive history of tics, compulsions, or Tourette's syndrome. See **Gilles de la Tourette's syndrome.**

target population   Population to which a study investigator wishes to generalize.

targeted pharmacotherapy   See **neuroleptic/intermittent.**

targeted steady-state concentration   (Css) Blood concentration of a drug when the amount of drug administered equals the amount eliminated in the same period.

Taroctyl　See **chlorpromazine.**

Tasedan　See **estazolam.**

tasikinesia　Term coined by Delay and Deniker (1968) to denote severe akathisia manifested by an inability to maintain a seated or lying position and a compulsion to stand up and pace about.

task-specific tremor　See **tremor, task-specific.**

TATA box　Short stretch of DNA found at about −20 to −25 base pairs relative to the start of transcription. The sequence (TA/TAA or variants thereof) is thought to be recognized by the transcription factor TFIID, which plays a role in interacting and positioning the RNA polymerase molecule.

"tau" proteins　Series of related polypeptides that are important components of paired helical filaments and appear to be the product of a single gene. Tau proteins in paired helical filaments differ from normal tau proteins. Tau proteins in paired helical filaments are found in the brains of patients with a variety of neurological diseases such as Alzheimer's disease, but not in normal brains.

Taxilan　See **perazine.**

taxonomy　Theory and practice of systematically classifying living organisms into related groups.

"t-bird"　Street name for the combination of secobarbital and amobarbital (Tuinal).

"t and blue"　Street name for the combination of the antihistamine tripelennamine and the synthetic opioid analgesic pentazocine that was used by opioid abusers. The pills were crushed and dissolved and injected intravenously, producing an effect much like that of heroin. This combination was responsible for deaths due to lung emboli caused by intravenous administration of talc, a constituent in the formulation of the tripelennamine. "Loads" have apparently replaced "t's and blues" as the heroin substitute of choice among opioid users who do not have ready access to high-quality heroin. See **"loads."**

T cell　See **T lymphocyte.**

T cell, suppressor　T cell that specifically inhibits antibody production by B cells as well as other cytotoxic T cell activities.

tc-exametazine　Intravenous ligand taken up into brain tissue in proportion to regional cerebral blood flow, thereby providing an estimate of regional metabolism.

"tcp"　Street name for an analog of phencyclidine.

t-distribution　See **Student's t-test.**

"tea"　Street name for marijuana.

technetium-99m-ethylcysteinate dimer　(Tc-99m ECD) (Neurolite) Tracer that permits single photon emission computed tomography (SPECT) measurement of cerebral blood flow.

technetium-99m-hexamethylpropylene-amine　(Tc-99m HPMAO) (Ceretec) Tracer that permits single photon emission computed tomography (SPECT) measurement of cerebral blood flow.

teciptiline　(ORG-8282) Tetracyclic antidepressant that is a mianserin analog, alpha$_2$ adrenoreceptor antagonist that also blocks 5-HT$_2$ histamine receptors. Not available in the United States.

teciptiline + lithium　Co-administration may be useful for the treatment of refractory depression without serious adverse effects.

tegmentum　Portion of an area of the brain known as the midbrain or mesencephalon.

Tegretal　See **carbamazepine.**

Tegretol　See **carbamazepine.**

Tegretol CR　See **carbamazepine CR.**

Tegretol Retard　See **carbamazepine CR.**

Teldrin　See **chlorpheniramine.**

telemedicine　Telecommunication that connects patients with a health care provider through live, two-way audio/video transmission, permitting effective diagnosis, treatment, and other health care activities. Two transmission modes are currently available, analog and digital. Analog (transmitted in the form of waves) is the technology of broadcast television; digital, the result of developments in computer science, transmits in the form of a digital bitstream of 0s and 1s. American references to telemedicine date from 1959; two projects began operating in Texas in 1991. Telemedicine advantages include (a) lower health care costs and improved quality; (b) putting specialists where needed and when; (c) bringing medical educators and primary care providers together at the electronic examining table; and (d) bedside teaching. Telemedicine may help overcome the severe shortage of medical and psychiatric expertise in rural areas (Preston J, Brown FW, Hartley B. Using telemedicine to improve health care in distant areas. *Hosp Community Psychiatry* 1992;43:25–32). Also called "interactive telemedicine."

teleradiology　See **FilmFax.**

"telescoping"　Progression to the serious complications of alcoholism after a short duration of heavy drinking (Piazza NJ, Vrbka JL, Yeager RD. Telescoping of alcoholism in women alcoholics. *Int J Addict* 1989;24:19-28).

Temaril　See **trimeprazine.**

Temaz　See **temazepam.**

temazepam　(Cerepax; Euhypnos; Levanxol; Normison; Razepam; Restoril; Temaz) Rapidly absorbed 1,4 benzodiazepine with pharmacological activity similar to that of oxazepam and diazepam. It has both anxiolytic and sedative/hypnotic activity, but is marketed as a hypnotic in doses of 15–60 mg for short-term treatment of insomnia. These doses are both safe and effective. Newer formulations are rapidly and nearly completely absorbed; peak plasma concentrations are reached in less than 1 hour. Temazepam is biotransformed mainly by direct glucuronide conjugation. It has no active metabolites. Elimination half-life is 10–20 hours, which makes temazepam useful for sleep maintenance. It does not accumulate and is less likely to produce a daytime hangover, although doses of 30 mg or higher, particularly in the elderly, may cause some hangover symptoms. The 30-mg dose has only a mild increase in efficacy over 15 mg; neither has been shown to produce significant rebound insomnia or daytime anxiety upon withdrawal. Anterograde amnesia has been reported infrequently. Temazepam is generally well tolerated. Adverse effects are usually mild and infrequent. Pregnancy risk category X; Schedule IV.

temazepam/breast milk Low levels are detected in breast milk following consumption of temazepam (10–20 mg) at bedtime for at least 2 consecutive nights (Lebedeos TH, Wojnar-Horton RE, Yapp P, et al. Excretion of temazepam in breast milk. *Br J Clin Pharmacol* 1992;33:204–206). Like other benzodiazepines, temazepam is unlikely to have serious adverse effects on the neonate.

temazepam + olanzapine Co-administration in patients who had been taking temazepam produced no adverse interactions.

Temesta See **lorazepam.**

Temgesic See **buprenorphine.**

Temodal See **quazepam.**

temperature regulation dysfunction Neuroleptics may upset hypothalamic thermoregulatory mechanisms, making schizophrenic patients and the elderly in particular vulnerable to either hyperthermia or hypothermia. See **hyperthermia; hypothermia; heat stroke.**

temporal arteritis Giant cell arteritis of the temporal artery, often associated with polymyalgia rheumatica and manifested by severe headache in the temple. Biopsy of the temporal artery may show arteritis and granuloma formation. The most serious complication is visual loss. Usual treatment is relatively high-dosage prednisone (up to 60 mg/day).

temporal disintegration Effect on short-term memory associated with smoking cannabis in which ability to undertake memory-dependent, goal-directed behavior is impaired.

temporal lobe epilepsy See **seizure, complex partial** (preferred term).

temporal lobe personality syndrome See **interictal personality disorder.**

Temposil See **calcium carbimide.**

Tempra See **acetaminophen.**

Tenex See **guanfacine.**

Tennate See **diethylpropion.**

Tenormin See **atenolol.**

tension Unpleasant increased motor and psychological activity, with overt physical manifestations of fear, anxiety, and agitation such as stiffness, tremor, profuse sweating, and restlessness. Marked tension is manifested by panic or gross motor acceleration such as rapid restless pacing and inability to remain seated longer than a minute, making sustained conversation impossible.

Tenuate See **diethylpropion.**

Tepanil See **diethylpropion.**

teratogen Substance that produces fetal abnormalities by disturbing maternal homeostasis or by acting directly on the fetus in utero. There are four major categories: *infectious agents* that attack the fetus in utero, including viruses (e.g., rubella, cytomegalovirus, herpes simplex, human immunodeficiency virus [HIV]), bacteria (syphilis, *Mycoplasma*), and parasites (*Toxoplasmosis*); *physical agents* (radiation, heat); *drugs and chemical agents* (thalidomide, organic mercury compounds); and *maternal metabolic and genetic factors.*

teratogenicity Capacity of a substance to cause malformations in the fetus.

teratogenicity, behavioral Long-term behavioral changes attributed to effects of maternally consumed drugs on the developing fetal brain (Coyle I, Wagner MJ, Singer G. Behavioral teratogenesis: a critical evaluation. *Pharmacol Biochem Behav* 1976;4:191–200).

teratological evaluation Animal studies usually required before a new drug is administered to women of childbearing age. Following drug administration, animal fetuses (rat, mouse, and rabbit) are assessed at various stages of gestation.

teratology Study of birth defects and their causes.

terbutaline + toloxatone + phenylephrine See **toloxatone + terbutaline + phenylephrine.**

terfenadine + carbamazepine See **carbamazepine + terfenadine.**

Terfluzine See **trifluoperazine.**

Terguride See **transdihydrolisuride.**

Teril See **carbamazepine.**

terminal insomnia See **insomnia, terminal.**

terminal tremor See **tremor, movement.**

"terp" Street name for terpin hydrate, or cough syrup with codeine.

tertiary amines Subgroup of tricyclic antidepressants with two methyl groups on the nitrogen atom of the side chain (imipramine, amitriptyline, clomipramine, doxepin, and trimipramine). They exert a major influence on presynaptic reuptake of serotonin. Tertiary amines tend to cause more adverse effects (sedation, orthostatic hypotension, anticholinergic effects) than do secondary tricyclic amine antidepressants. Because of their sedative effects, they potentiate alcohol central nervous system effects more than secondary amines do. See **secondary amine tricyclic antidepressants.**

tertiary care See **referred care.**

tertiary care center Medical facility that receives referrals from primary and secondary care levels and usually offers tests, treatments, and procedures not available elsewhere. See **referred care.**

tertiary memory See **memory, tertiary.**

Tertran See **iprindole.**

Teslac See **testolactone.**

Tesoprel See **bromperidol.**

Testa-C See **testosterone cypionate.**

Testadiate-Depo See **testosterone cypionate.**

Testamone 100 See **testosterone aqueous.**

Testaqua See **testosterone aqueous.**

test dose Procedure to assess the bioavailability and predict the therapeutic effects of a drug. It consists of administration of a single dose, measurement of electrophysiological response before and after the drug, and observation of clinical outcome. Also, administration of a single dose of a drug to evaluate patient tolerability.

Testex See **testosterone propionate.**

test of significance Comparison of the observed probability of an event with the predicted probability based on calculations deduced from statistical chance distributions of such events.

Testoject-50 See **testosterone aqueous.**

Testoject LA See **testosterone cypionate.**

testolactone (Teslac) Commonly abused anabolic steroid.

Testone LA See **testosterone enanthate.**

testosterone (Oreton) Androgenic steroid produced by the interstitial cells of Leydig and considered the principal testicular hormone in man. It accelerates growth in tissues on which it acts, stimulates blood flow, is required for normal sexual behavior, and is essential for normal growth and development of the male accessory sexual organs and secondary sexual characteristics (deepening of the voice as in puberty, greater muscular development, development of beard and pubic hair, distribution of fat in adults). It affects many metabolic activities and may play a role in male aggressive behaviors.

testosterone aqueous (Andro 100; Andronaq 50; Histerone; Testamone 100; Testaqua; Testoject 50) Testosterone ester derivative anabolic steroid.

testosterone cypionate (Andro Cyp; Andronaq LA; Andronate; Dep Andro; Depotest; Depo-Testosterone; Duratest; Testa-C; Testadiate Depo, Testoject LA; Virilon IM) Testosterone ester derivative anabolic steroid used primarily in androgen-deficient men for development or maintenance of secondary sex characteristics. Available as an oily solution administered (50–400 mg) every 2–4 weeks.

testosterone enanthate (Andro LA 200; Andropository 100; Delatest; Delatestryl; Durathate; Everone; Primoteston Depot; Testone LA; Testrin PA) Long-acting injectable testosterone ester derivative used primarily in androgen-deficient men for development or maintenance of secondary sex characteristics and by male athletes who use various anabolic/androgenic steroids. Long-term use could lead to hyalinization of testicular tissues. Available as an oily solution administered in strengths of 50–400 mg every 2–4 weeks. It is being tested as a possible male contraceptive.

testosterone propionate (Oreton Propionate Sustanon 100; Sustanon 250; Testex; Vivormone) Testosterone ester derivative anabolic steroid used primarily in androgen-deficient men for development or maintenance of secondary sex characteristics. Available as an oily solution for intramuscular use in strengths of 10–25 mg 2–3 times a week.

Testred See **methyltestosterone.**

test reliability Degree of stability, consistency, predictability, and accuracy of a test; the extent to which a person's test scores will be the same if tested on different occasions. Test reliability is determined in order to estimate the degree to which the test varies because of error.

test-retest reliability (stability) Test reliability coefficient determined by correlating scores on the same test taken by the same subject at two different times. If test-retest reliability has been established, the test can be used repeatedly to monitor status changes occurring between any two points in time during treatment or aftercare.

Testrin PA See **testosterone enanthate.**

test statistic Specific statistical test used to test the null hypothesis.

testing threshold Point at which the optimal decision is to perform a diagnostic test.

tetrabenazine (Nitoman) (TBZ) Short-acting reserpine analog and a nonindole benzoquinolizine that is both a presynaptic monoamine depleter and a postsynaptic dopamine receptor blocker. It has been used with limited success for treatment of tardive dyskinesia. It is now used almost exclusively to control choreas and hemiballismus. Available in the United States only on an experimental basis (Jankovic J, Orman J. Tetrabenazine therapy of dystonia, chorea, tics and other dyskinesias. *Neurology* 1988;38:391–394; Szymanski S, Manne R, Gordon MF, Lieberman J. A selective review of recent advances in the management of tardive dyskinesia. *Psychiatr Ann* 1993; 23:209–215).

tetracyclic antidepressant   Arbitrary classification for compounds formed by adding a nonplanar ring to a typical tricyclic antidepressant structure (amoxapine, mianserin). Although reputed to be a tetracyclic, maprotiline is held by most experts to be tricyclic compound. As with tricyclics, short-term administration of tetracyclics reduces norepinephrine and serotonin reuptake and blocks muscarinic and histamine receptors. Long-term administration of tetracyclics and tricyclics down-regulates beta-adrenergic receptors.

tetracycline + lithium   See **lithium + tetracycline.**

tetrahydroaminoactidine   (THA) See **tacrine.**

tetrahydrobiopterin   (BH$_4$) Rate-limiting pterin co-factor for tyrosine and tryptophan hydroxylases. Synthesized from guanacine triphosphate, it plays an important role in regulating biogenic amine synthesis (Fleischhacker WW, Levine RA, Lieberman JA, et al. Neoptrin and biopterin CSF levels in tardive dyskinesia after clozapine treatment. *Biol Psychiatry* 1993;34: 741–745).

tetrahydrocannabinol   (THC) Major chemical with psychoactive properties obtained from the Indian hemp plant, *Cannabis sativa.* It is believed to be responsible for most of the characteristic psychological effects of marijuana. Street drugs alleged to be THC frequently contain phencyclidine (PCP), which may produce extreme excitement, visual disturbances, and delirium. THC (also called "dronabinol") is marketed for treatment of nausea and vomiting associated with cancer chemotherapy. See **phencyclidine.**

tetrahydroisoquinolines   (TIQs) Condensation products of alcohol that may interact with opioid receptors to stimulate mesolimbic catecholaminergic systems. The metabolic product from alcohol, acetaldehyde, condenses noncovalently with dopamine to form TIQs. TIQs can function as opiates and provide a link between the two-carbon alcohol molecule and the more complex phenanthrene alkaloids. TIQs act as agonists at enkephalin and endorphin binding sites, further substantiating a common mechanism that links alcohol and opiates.

tetrahydropaperoline   (THP) Condensation product of dopamine and dopamine aldehyde molecules with opiate actions on opiate receptors. It is a precursor molecule in the synthesis of natural opium in poppy seeds.

tetraiodothyronine   See **thyroxine.**

"Texas shoeshine"   Street term for shoe spray containing toluene that is sniffed or inhaled by volatile substance abusers.

"Texas tea"   Street name for marijuana.

thalamic pain syndrome   Syndrome usually produced by a cerebrovascular accident that damages ventroposterior thalamic nuclei. It is manifested by autonomic changes, partial sensory loss and hemiparesis, and constant burning pain aggravated by slight stimuli to the painful area.

Thalamonal   See **fentanyl.**

thalamotomy   Psychosurgical procedure that uses thermocoagulation to produce a lesion in the thalamus. It is seldom done for psychiatric indications, but is still done in a few clinics for chronic pain.

thalamus   Part of the brain situated at the base of the cerebrum above the hypothalamus. It consists of nuclei that project to diverse areas. It comprises the anterior nucleus, the dorsomedial nucleus, the lateral and medial geniculate bodies, and the ventral nuclei. It acts as a relay station for body sensations such as pain and temperature.

thalidomide   Drug once marketed as a sleeping pill that was blamed for nearly 12,000 birth defects, particularly phocomelia, during the late 1950s. The most notorious and stigmatized drug in the recent history of drug therapy, it provoked dramatic changes in drug regulatory processes worldwide. It was removed from almost all world markets, but a few companies produce it for experimental purposes. A potent immunosuppressive that lacks the toxic side effects of steroids, it has been found useful in rheumatoid arthritis, lepromatous leprosy, Behçet's syndrome, discoid lupus erythematosus, esophageal ulcers in acquired immunodeficiency syndrome (AIDS), and chronic graft-versus-host disease, the most common cause of death following bone marrow transplant (Rejan J, Colman J, Pederrsen J, Benson E. Thalidomide to treat esophageal ulcer in AIDS. *N Engl J Med* 1992; 327:208–209).

THC   See **tetrahydrocannabinol.**

thebaine   Phenanthiane alkaloid similar to morphine that naturally occurs in opium, the milky exudate from the unripe capsule of the poppy, *Papaver somniferum.* It is converted into codeine, hydrocodone, oxycodone, oxymorphone, nalbuphine, and diacetylmorphine.

Compounds produced directly from it are called "semisynthetic" opioids.

theobramine + lithium See **lithium + theobromine.**

theophylline Indirect adrenergic agonist used therapeutically to produce bronchodilation. By inhibiting cyclic adenosine monophosphate (cAMP) metabolism, it potentiates the effects of endogenous adrenergic innervation to bronchi.

theophylline + carbamazepine See **carbamazepine + theophylline.**

theophylline + electroconvulsive therapy See **electroconvulsive therapy + theophylline.**

theophylline + fluvoxamine See **fluvoxamine + theophylline.**

theophylline + lithium See **lithium + theophylline.**

theophylline + tacrine Co-administration increased theophylline elimination half-life and average plasma concentrations by approximately 2 times. Monitoring of theophylline plasma concentrations and appropriate reduction of theophylline dose are recommended in patients receiving both drugs. Theophylline effects on tacrine pharmacokinetics have not been assessed (Tacrine Package Insert, May 1993).

"the pits" Street name for phencyclidine (PCP).

therapeutic agent Anything that produces improvement or promotes healing.

therapeutic alternative Substitute for a compound of the same class and for the same indication.

therapeutic community (TC) Significant alternative approach to treating drug abuse that uses self-help and positive peer pressure in a drug-free environment where members help manage the facility and serve as role models for each other. It emphasizes personal responsibility and advancement only through achievements. TC structure uses set behavioral limits, confrontation that provides members with social feedback on their actions, informal counseling by recovering addicts, organized recreation, and opportunities for education and formal skills training. It has applications beyond drug abuse to a variety of psychopathological disorders. See **therapeutic milieu.**

therapeutic detoxification Type of heroin detoxification in which methadone dosage is slowly reduced over a period of months (Stimmel B, Goldberg J, Rotkopf E, Cohen M. Ability to remain abstinent after methadone detoxification. *JAMA* 1977;237:1216–1220). It is considered successful if the patient can achieve abstinence without manifesting clinically significant withdrawal symptoms or a return to illicit drug use. Even with highly selected patients, failure rate is substantial. Nonetheless, the goal is worthwhile because as many as half the patients who complete methadone dose taper are able to maintain a drug-free existence for long periods (Kanof PD, Aronson MJ, Ness R. Organic mood syndrome associated with detoxification from methadone maintenance. *Am J Psychiatry* 1993;150: 423–428).

therapeutic dosage Amount of a drug determined to be effective and safe for the average patient. Important factors that influence therapeutic dose are age, body weight, sex, route of administration, time of administration, rate of inactivation and excretion, tolerance, genetic factors, and drug interactions.

therapeutic dose dependence Development of dependence, either physical, psychological, or both, on a prescribed drug of which the patient takes only the prescribed dose. It is related to rapid eye movement (REM) sleep rebound and sleep pattern deterioration.

therapeutic drug monitoring (TDM) Measurement of the plasma concentration of a drug and, if warranted, clinically pertinent metabolites, to ascertain if concentrations are above, below, or within an optimal therapeutic range. Other indications are to (a) determine absorption and compliance with medication ingestion; (b) determine if a patient is a rapid or slow metabolizer; (c) determine the impact of co-prescribing drugs A and B (e.g., acceleration or inhibition of the metabolism of each); and (d) scientifically justify prescribing higher than the usual recommended dose for a patient with a low plasma level and a partial response to treatment. Similarly, TDM could also justify using an unusually small dose by demonstrating a plasma level greater than that which would be expected. TDM is an important aid in assessing clinical response, which includes not only therapeutic but also toxic effects. For example, overall clinical response to antidepressants includes not only therapeutic response, but anticholinergic, antihistaminic, and toxic cardiac effects. Hence, the objective of TDM should be to help arrive at a correct dose while minimizing side effects.

therapeutic error Prescribing a medication at the usual dose, route, and frequency, but for an inappropriate indication, or when contraindicated.

therapeutic index 1. Ratio of the lowest drug concentration that produces toxicity to the lowest concentration that produces desired therapeutic effects. 2. Highest nonlethal drug dose divided by the usual clinical dose. It is a frequently used measure of the relative safety of a drug.

therapeutic margin   Ratio between the toxic and the therapeutic dose.

therapeutic milieu   Therapeutic setting for psychiatric patients in which all personnel are trained in interpersonal and therapeutic techniques and patients take responsibility to help each other. Frequent patient-staff group meetings are held to facilitate interpersonal communication. See **therapeutic community.**

therapeutic misadventure   Euphemism used chiefly by the British for medical interventions that harm rather than help patients.

therapeutic outcome   Status of a patient after treatment with a certain therapeutic regimen.

therapeutic plasma exchange   (TPE) See **plasmapheresis.**

therapeutic problems   Lack of a response at usual or even higher dosages or a toxic reaction at customary or lower dosages.

therapeutic range   Peak or maximum level of drug concentration in the plasma, and a trough or minimal level of concentration in the plasma, usually at steady state, within which a desirable response usually occurs.

therapeutic window   Area of a drug's plasma level below which it is ineffective and above which it may be ineffective and/or toxic. Both high and low levels are associated with suboptimal effect. For some individuals, levels above the therapeutic range may be needed to achieve therapeutic response, since a drug's therapeutic window is based on data gathered from the general population.

therapy, adjuvant   See **adjuvant therapy.**

therapy, aversion   See **aversion therapy.**

therapy, brief stimulus   See **brief stimulus therapy.**

therapy, carbon dioxide   See **carbon dioxide therapy.**

therapy, cognitive   See **cognitive therapy.**

therapy, regressive EST   See **regressive EST therapy.**

thermogenic drugs   Engodenous hormones (thyroid, insulin, and growth hormones) and sympathomimetic compounds with either alpha- or beta-stimulating properties. Some may play a role in obesity management.

theta activity   Electroencephalographic activity with a frequency of 4–8 Hz that is generally maximal over the central and temporal cortex.

theta EEG   Electroencephalogram (EEG) that predominantly has frequencies between 4 and 8 Hz (theta activity) in all recorded leads. Theta waves are typical of light sleep.

theta rhythm   One of four different physiological rhythms recorded by a scalp electroencephalogram (EEG). Theta rhythm has a frequency of 4–7 Hz. It is located in the temporal area. Amplitude is low during wakefulness and increases at sleep onset.

thiamine   Vitamin B_{12}. Thiamine deficiency may be due to failure of gastric mucosal cells to secrete the intrinsic factor necessary for normal absorption of dietary vitamin B_{12} from the ileum. Deficiency is manifested by pernicious anemia (megaloblastic anemia), mental changes (apathy, depression, irritability, encephalopathy), and neurological symptoms resulting from degenerative change in the peripheral nerves, the spinal cord, and the brain. Early, continued administration of parenteral vitamin B_{12} rapidly and completely arrests neurological manifestations of the deficiency.

thiamylal   (Surital) Rapid, ultra-short-acting barbiturate used as an intravenous anesthetic and occasionally for pre–electroconvulsive therapy anesthesia. Schedule III.

thiazide diuretic + lithium   See **lithium + diuretic.**

thiazide diuretic + monoamine oxidase inhibitor (MAOI)   Co-administration increases risk and degree of hypotension; this can be a significant interaction.

thiazolopyridines   New nonbenzodiazepine group of anxiolytics that do not bind to the gamma aminobutyric acid (GABA)-BZ-Cl-ionophore complex. Ritanserin is a member of this group of compounds.

thienodiazepines   Group of diazepines, most of which are under investigation. Brotizolam—a thienodiazepine—is currently available outside the United States. Because their pharmacological effects are comparable to those of benzodiazepines, both groups are considered "benzodiazepines" from a clinical standpoint.

thiethylperazine   (Torecan) Piperazine phenothiazine neuroleptic that blocks postsynaptic dopamine D_2 receptors. In contrast to most piperazine phenothiazines, it has weak antipsychotic properties and is used extensively for vertiginous syndromes, especially nausea. Intramuscular dose is 5–10 mg; rectal dose is 10 mg. It may cause early-onset extrapyramidal reactions, including acute dystonic reactions, akathisia, and a parkinsonian syndrome. Acute reactions are usually self-limiting and brief, and nearly all patients with extrapyramidal symptoms respond to anticholinergic therapy.

thin-fat syndrome   See **bulimia nervosa.**

thin-layer chromatography   (TLC) Chemical analysis technique used as the initial qualitative screening procedure of urine. It is a practical, economical, and sensitive method for detecting in the urine phenothiazines, heroin, morphine, barbiturates, amphetamines, codeine, cocaine, methadone, and methaqualone. It identifies parent and metabolite compounds while leaving the specimen intact for further analyses. It is inaccurate, however, relative to other analytical procedures.

thiopental (Pentothal) Thiobarbiturate that is the sulfur analog of sodium pentobarbital. It is an ultra-short-acting (usually only a few minutes) central nervous system depressant that induces hypnosis and anesthesia, but not analgesia. It is the standard for comparison in anesthesiology. Schedule III.

thioproperazine (Majeptil) Extremely potent piperazine phenothiazine neuroleptic with a high propensity to evoke acute early onset extrapyramidal reactions. Not available in the United States.

thioridazine (Apo-Thioridazine; Mellaril; Novo-Ridazine; PMS Thioridazine; Ridazin) One of the earliest piperidine phenothiazine neuroleptics, now often called an "atypical" neuroleptic. It is metabolized predominantly by sulphoxidation at both the side chain resulting in thioridazine-2-sulfoxide (mesoridazine) and thioridazine-2-sulfone (sulforidazine), and at the ring to form thioridazine-5-sulfoxide. Side chain metabolites are active, about 50% more potent than thioridazine, and contribute to its antipsychotic effect. Thioridazine-5-sulfoxide lacks psychoactive effects, but may play a role in thioridazine's cardiac side effects. Milligram per milligram, thioridazine is a low-potency, sedating neuroleptic that is very lipid-soluble and generally rapidly and completely absorbed. It has moderate anticholinergic effects (dry mouth, blurred vision, delayed micturition, constipation) that play a role in its low propensity to elicit extrapyramidal side effects. It may cause tardive dyskinesia and neuroleptic malignant syndrome. Daily doses above 800 mg may cause irreversible damage to the retina (retinitis pigmentosa) and possibly blindness. Patients being treated with high doses should have routine ophthalmological examinations to detect incipient retinitis pigmentosa and impaired vision. Thioridazine can induce abnormal T waves in the electrocardiogram (ECG), perhaps by altering potassium disposition in the myocardium, that may be responsible for life-threatening arrhythmias and sudden death. It has been implicated in causing torsades de pointes (Kemper AJ, Dunlap R, Pietro DA. Thioridazine-induced torsade de pointes. Successful treatment with isoproterenol. *JAMA* 1983;248:2931–2934). Pregnancy risk category C. See **torsades de pointes.**

thioridazine + antimuscarinic Co-administration may enhance anticholinergic effects and lower thioridazine's plasma level.

thioridazine/breast milk Thioridazine is excreted in breast milk and should not be taken by nursing mothers.

thioridazine + carbamazepine Co-administration produces no significant changes in steady state plasma levels of either carbamazepine or its metabolite, 10,11-epoxide.

thioridazine + central nervous system (CNS) depressant Thioridazine + alcohol, anesthetics, barbiturates, narcotics, or other CNS depressants increases CNS depression.

thioridazine + epinephrine Co-administration may produce severe hypotension.

thioridazine + guanethidine Co-administration use may increase guanethidine's antihypertensive effect.

thioridazine + heterocyclic antidepressant Co-administration may cause ventricular arrhythmias and additive anticholinergic toxicity effects.

thioridazine + lithium Co-administration may result in neurotoxicity (Spring G. Neurotoxicity with combined use of lithium and thioridazine. *J Clin Psychiatry* 1979;40:135–138; Bailine SH, Doft M. Neurotoxicity induced by combined lithium-thioridazine treatment. *Biol Psychiatry* 1986;21:834–837).

thioridazine + nalmefene Nalmefene plus thioridazine (300 mg/day) successfully augmented the effects of thioridazine (Rapaport MH, Wolkowitz O, Kelsoe JR, et al. Beneficial effects of nalmefene augmentation in neuroleptic-stabilized schizophrenic patients. *Neuropsychopharmacology* 1993;9:111–115).

thioridazine + paroxetine Concomitant use of paroxetine with thioridazine, which is metabolized by cytochrome P450IID6, may require use of lower doses than usually prescribed for either drug alone. A patient treated with paroxetine (up to 40 mg/day), thioridazine (30 mg/day), and trifluoperazine (10 mg/day) became oversedated, withdrawn, immobile, and unresponsive. Cessation of the neuroleptics produced no significant change. Two weeks later, paroxetine was discontinued; within 5 days, psychomotor function returned (Lewis J, Braganza J, Williams T, et al. Psychomotor retardation and semistuporous state with paroxetine. *Br Med J* 1993;306:1169).

thioridazine + phenobarbital Thioridazine may depress phenobarbital levels (Gay PE, Madsem JA. Interaction between phenobarbital and thioridazine. *Neurology* 1983;33:1631–1632).

thioridazine + phenytoin Thioridazine may increase phenytoin plasma levels. Effects are generally not significant, but there may be an increased risk of phenytoin toxicity (Kuth H. Interactions between anticonvulsants and other commonly prescribed drugs. *Epilepsia*

1984;25[suppl 2]:118–131; Aronson JK, Hordman M, Reynolds DJM. Phenytoin. *Br Med J* 1992;305:1215–1218).

thioridazine + pindolol Co-administration may produce a dose-related increase in mean serum levels of thioridazine and its metabolites and an increase in serum pindolol levels. The interaction may be advantageous in some circumstances, whereas in others it could result in unacceptable elevation of serum thioridazine levels (Greendyke RM, Kanter DR. Plasma propranolol levels and their effects on plasma thioridazine and haloperidol concentrations. *J Clin Psychopharmacol* 1987;7:178–182).

thioridazine/pregnancy Thioridazine crosses the placental barrier; after delivery, newborns may exhibit lethargy, tremor, or hyperactivity.

thioridazine + propranolol Propranolol may retard thioridazine elimination, resulting in elevation of its serum concentration (including metabolites) and enhancement of its effects (Greendyke RM, Kanter DR. Plasma propranolol levels and their effects on plasma thioridazine and haloperidol concentrations. *J Clin Psychopharmacol* 1987;7:178–182).

thioridazine + valproic acid In mentally retarded patients with nonaffective aggression (assaultive behavior not necessarily associated with dysphoria, anger, or a specific precipitant), addition of valproic acid to thioridazine may substantially reduce the number of aggressive outbursts per month without adverse interactive effects (Mattes J. Valproic acid for nonaffective aggression in the mentally retarded. *J Nerv Ment Dis* 1992;180:601–602).

thiothixene (Navane) Thioxanthene neuroleptic developed by substituting a carbon with a double bond for the nitrogen in the number 10 position of the nucleus of the phenothiazine derivative, thioproperazine. It is a high-potency neuroleptic extensively used throughout the world for the usual clinical indications for neuroleptic therapy. It has a high propensity to cause extrapyramidal reactions, is mildly sedative, and is weakly anticholinergic. Pregnancy risk category C.

thiothixene + benztropine There is a case report of esophageal atony with massive esophageal dilatation that disappeared after the drugs were discontinued and recurred when they were readministered. Esophageal dilatation was attributed to the anticholinergic effects of both drugs (Woodring JH, Martin CA, Keefer B. Esophageal atony and dilatation as a side effect of thiothixene and benztropine. *Hosp Community Psychiatry* 1993;44:686–688).

thiothixene + carbamazepine Carbamazepine increases thiothixene clearance, decreasing steady-state plasma levels and possibly interfering with therapeutic efficacy (Ereshefsky L, Jann MW, Saklad SR, Davis CM. Bioavailability of psychotropic drugs: historical perspective and pharmacokinetic overview. *J Clin Psychiatry* 1986;47[suppl]:6–15).

thiothixene + lithium Co-administration may cause the sudden appearance of extrapyramidal side effects and neurotoxicity (Fetzer J, Kader G, Dohany S. Lithium encephalopathy: a clinical, psychiatric and EEG evaluation. *Am J Psychiatry* 1981;138:1622–1623).

thioxanthenes Chemical analogs of the nucleic acids, with potent antidopaminergic properties. The three-ring nucleus of the thioxanthenes differs from the phenothiazine nucleus by the substitution of a carbon atom for the nitrogen atom in the middle ring. Thioxanthenes can be divided into aliphatic or piperazine derivatives depending on the side chain attached to the nucleus.

thioxanthene derivatives Group of antipsychotic drugs that are structurally different from other neuroleptics. They consist of aliphatic derivatives (chlorprothixene) and piperazine derivatives (clopenthixol, flupenthixol, piflutixol, and thiothixene). All are potent and effective antipsychotic agents. The cis (or alpha) isomers are the more active of the geometric isomers of thioxanthene derivatives.

Thorazine See **chlorpromazine.**

Thor-Prom See **chlorpromazine.**

thought broadcasting First-rank symptom of schizophrenia consisting of the delusion that one's thoughts can be heard by others, as though they were being broadcast into the air.

thought control Delusion that one's thoughts are being controlled by other people.

thought insertion First-rank symptom of schizophrenia consisting of the delusion that other people are implanting thoughts in one's mind.

thought withdrawal Delusion that one's thoughts are being removed by others from one's mind.

three-arm design Clinical trial design in which patients are randomly assigned to one of three groups to compare an investigational drug, a standard drug, and placebo. Separate tests of significance are done to evaluate superiority. It is the most appropriate design for proof of drug efficacy.

threohydrobupropion Pharmacologically active metabolite of bupropion.

threshold model Model for deciding when a diagnostic test should be ordered, as opposed to doing nothing or treating the patient without performing the test.

threshold, sedation See **sedation threshold.**

thrombocytes See **platelets.**

thrombocytopenia   Reduction in the number of platelets in the blood. Platelets are involved in clotting; if they are reduced, excessive bleeding and bruising can occur. Thrombocytopenia is an uncommon side effect of psychotropic drugs. It may be caused by decreased platelet production in the bone marrow or increased platelet destruction in the periphery. Thrombocytopenia is possibly the most common drug-induced blood dyscrasia, although it is associated with less mortality than aplastic anemia or agranulocytosis. The clinical picture varies with the severity of the thrombocytopenia, but onset is often abrupt with widespread minute hemorrhagic spots (petechiae), nose bleeds (epistaxes), and bleeding from the gums (the most likely presenting symptoms). The skin is the most common site of hemorrhage (purpura), but other sites include the gastrointestinal and genitourinary tracts, and, rarely, the internal organs. Cerebral hemorrhage is the most common cause of death. The mechanism of drug-induced thrombocytopenia is either selective marrow depression or an immune reaction. Drug allergy results in antibodies active against platelets that cause platelet agglutination. Drugs that can induce aplastic anemia through generalized marrow toxicity sometimes produce thrombocytopenia selectively, possibly because the platelet precursors are more vulnerable than other stem cells to cytotoxic agents. The immune mechanism of drug-induced thrombocytopenia has been widely studied. Although there appear to be some differences between drugs, the common feature is an immunoglobulin G (IgG)-mediated response with thrombocytopenia occurring weeks to years after therapy has been initiated. The patient may exhibit symptoms of allergy, with fever, chills, and like effects often preceding the purpura. On drug withdrawal, the platelet count returns to normal, supporting the diagnosis of drug-induced thrombocytopenic purpura. The drug cannot be reintroduced because the patient is sensitized, but it is possible to perform in vitro testing for platelet agglutination to determine if the patient is sensitive to drugs with similar chemical structures. Since common mechanisms are involved in drug-induced aplastic anemia, agranulocytosis, and thrombocytopenia, drugs producing these reactions are mostly the same, with either single cell lines being affected or complete marrow suppression.

thymeretic pharmaco-EEG profile   One of two main types of pharmaco-electroencephalogram (EEG) profiles for antidepressants. The thymeretic (desipramine-like) profile is characterized mainly by an alpha increase and an increase in slow and fast activities (suggesting activating properties). See **thymoleptic pharmaco-EEG profile**.

thymine   Pyrimidine base $C_5H_6N_2O_2$ that is one of the four bases coding genetic information in the polynucleotide chain of DNA.

thymoleptic   Drug that affects mood states; the term is often used to describe antidepressants.

thymoleptic pharmaco-EEG profile   One of two main types of pharmaco-electroencephalogram (EEG) profiles for antidepressants. The thymoleptic profile (imipramine or amitriptyline-like) shows a concomitant increase in slow and fast activities, and a decrease in alpha activity (which indicates sedative qualities). See **thymeretic pharmaco-EEG profile**.

thyroid dysfunction, subclinical   Exaggerated release of thyroid stimulating hormone (TSH) in response to thyrotropin releasing hormone (TRH) in the presence of normal or raised concentrations of circulating TSH and normal concentrations of clinical thyroxine (T_4) and triiodothyronine (T_3). The concept has arisen with recent refinements of endocrinological and biochemical techniques. Thyroid dysfunction is very common in patients with affective disorders. In every patient suffering from a chronic or recurrent affective illness that is treatment-resistant, hypothalamic-pituitary-thyroid axis function should be thoroughly investigated, and any abnormality should be corrected. Subclinical forms of hypothyroidism may occur in bipolar patients treated with lithium and in a subgroup of rapid cycling manic-depressive patients. In treatment-refractory, rapid cycling bipolar disorder, cautiously administering a small dosage (100–400 µg/day) of thyroxine, even in the absence of endocrinological evidence of thyroid dysfunction, may be worthwhile.

thyroid function test   Measurements of thyroid stimulating hormone (TSH), serum triiodothyronine (T_3) uptake, total serum thyroxine assay (T_4), free T_4, and serum antithyroid globulin titers. The TSH is the most valuable test for assessing thyroid function.

thyroid function/lithium   Lithium affects thyroid function in most patients, but its effects are usually not clinically significant. Circulating T_3 and T_4 are lowered and thyroid stimulating hormone (TSH) is elevated. Enlarged thyroid glands occur in a few patients, a minority of whom may develop symptoms of hypothyroidism. Baseline thyroid function should be obtained prior to or at the start of lithium therapy. If TSH becomes elevated, full thyroid function testing is warranted, and thyroid replacement therapy may be indicated.

thyroid hormone therapy, adjunctive   See **adjunctive thyroid hormone therapy.**

thyroid hormone + sympathomimetics   Co-administration is contraindicated because of the risk of cardiac decompensation.

thyroid hormone + maprotiline   Co-administration may increase the incidence of maprotiline-associated cardiac arrhythmias and conduction defects.

thyroid stimulating hormone   (TSH) For practical purposes, a normal serum THS concentration excludes hypothyroidism or hyperthyroidism. Normal concentrations may be recorded in thyrotoxicosis induced by TSH and in some patients with hypothyroidism secondary to pituitary or hypothalamic disease. These are rare conditions.

thyrotoxicosis   Condition characterized by biochemical and psychological changes resulting from a chronic excess of endogenous thyroid hormone. Laboratory testing reveals increased T_3, T_4, and free thyroxine index and increased radioactive iodine uptake. Serum T_3 is usually increased more than serum T_4. Thyroid stimulating hormone response to thyrotropin releasing hormone is blunted, a finding that must be interpreted cautiously since it may have other causes besides thyrotoxicosis. Manifestations of thyrotoxicosis may include tachycardia; gastrointestinal disturbances; hyperthermia; panic, anxiety, and agitation; and mania, dementia, and psychosis. Other symptoms are tremor, sweating, weight loss, and heat intolerance. The syndrome occurs often in women between 20 and 50 years of age. Treatment may be surgery or pharmacotherapy with antithyroid drugs, tranquilizers, or propranolol. See **hyperthyroidism.**

thyrotropin   (TSH) (Thytropar) Hormone, secreted by the adenohypophysis of the pituitary gland, that regulates formation and secretion of thyroid hormone. It is used only to test the ability of the thyroid to respond to exogenous stimulation.

thyrotropin releasing factor   (TRF) First of the hypothalamic hypophysiotropic factors to be chemically characterized and demonstrated to exert biological actions on the central nervous system.

thyrotropin releasing hormone   (TRH) Endogenous tripeptide found heterogenously throughout the central nervous system. It releases prolactin from the pituitary, an action that may be mediated through serotonin. It is the primary regulator of thyroid stimulating hormone (TSH) release from the anterior pituitary. TSH enters the systemic circulation and stimulates release of triiodothyronine (T_3) and thyroxine (T_4) hormone secretion from the thyroid gland. It also acts as a neuromodulator for a variety of neurotransmitters, including serotonin and dopamine. There is some evidence that TRH can relieve tension and anxiety in humans. In normal men, intravenous TRH administration produces maximal secretion of thyrotropin within 15–30 minutes. The TRH gene, preproTRH, has allowed studies of its regulation by hormones and factors such as cyclic adenosine monophosphate (cAMP). When administered to depressed patients, approximately 25% exhibit blunted TSH response; 15% exhibit an exaggerated response. In some studies, intravenous administration produced rapid, transient improvement in mood and other depressive symptoms in depressed patients (Lafer B, Fava M, Hammerness P, Rosenbaum JF. The influence of DST and TRH test administration on depression assessments: a controlled study. *Biol Psychiatry* 1993;34:650–653). In preclinical studies, TRH antagonized alcohol-induced sedation, motor impairment, and hypothermia. In rats, single and repeated once-daily injections of TA-0910, a centrally potent TRH analog, attenuated alcohol preference in a dose-dependent manner (Rezvani AH, Janowsky DS, Garbutt JC, Mason GA. TA-0910, a novel TRH analog, attenuates alcohol intake in alcohol preferring rats: a dopamine connection. *Neuropsychopharmacology* 1993;9:136S).

thyrotropin releasing hormone test   Intravenous injection of synthetic thyrotropin releasing hormone (TRH) and sequential monitoring of serum thyroid stimulating hormone (TSH) levels, triiodothyronine (T_3), and thyroxine (T_4). Low TSH response to TRH has been reported extensively in patients with major depression. Some patients with other disorders (alcoholism, panic disorder, dysthymic disorder, mania, anorexia nervosa, and bulimia) show blunted TSH response to TRH. The TRH test has become a common tool to assess hypothalamic-pituitary dysregulation in depressive states and is considered a useful predictor of response to pharmacotherapy. It does not have a statistically significant effect on depressive symptoms and thus does not interfere with study results and interpretation (Lafer B, Fava M, Hammerness P, Rosenbaum JF. The influence of DST and TRH test administration on depression assessments: a controlled study. *Biol Psychiatry* 1993;34:650–653).

thyrotropin releasing hormone (TRH) stimulation test   (TRH-ST) Test in which secretion of thyroid stimulating hormone (TSH) is measured following a TRH infusion. A fixed dose of TRH (200–500 µg) is administered intravenously, usually in the morning, and blood samples for TSH radioimmunoassay are obtained every 30 minutes, usually for 2–3 hours.

TSH is measured by radioimmunoassay. Most investigators consider the TRH-ST to be the most sensitive measure of hypothalamic-pituitary-thyroid (HPT) axis function because it is affected both by feedback regulation from the thyroid and feed-forward regulation from the hypothalamic release and release-inhibiting hormones TRH and somatostatin. Blunted TSH response has been defined somewhat differently in different laboratories, but a delta max TSH (the maximal increase in plasma TSH concentration after TRH minus the baseline plasma TSH concentration) of less than 5–7 mU/ml is generally considered abnormal. Although blunted TSH response to TRH in depressed patients has received considerable attention, approximately 15% of depressed patients exhibit exaggerated TSH response to TRH. This has led to the realization that many depressed patients with exaggerated TSH responses to TRH and normal baseline TSH and thyroid hormone concentrations have, by definition, grade 3 hypothyroidism (Nemeroff CB. Clinical significance of psychoneuroendocrinology in psychiatry: focus on the thyroid and adrenal. *J Clin Psychiatry* 1989;50[suppl 5]:13–20). Common factors known to yield false-positive TRH-ST blunting responses include alcoholism, age over 60, and use of corticosteroids, aspirin, and barbiturates. TRH-ST cannot be used to study affective disorders in patients with clinical thyroid disease because any abnormality of the HPT axis reflects the primary disease process (Loosen PT, Prange AJ Jr. Serum thyrotropin response to thyrotropin-releasing hormone on psychiatric patients: a review. *Am J Psychiatry* 1982; 139:405–416).

thyroxine (T$_4$; tetraiodothyronine) (Eltioxin; Euthroid; Levothroid Synthroid) Naturally occurring hormone produced by the thyroid gland, the sodium salt or natural isomer of which is levothyroxine. T$_4$ is converted to the more active hormone triiodothyronine (T$_3$) in peripheral tissues. T$_4$ level is low in patients with hypothyroidism. It is marketed for the treatment of congenital or acquired hypothyroidism, suppression of goiter, and to treat thyrotoxicosis in conjunction with antithyroid drugs. Dosages ranging from 100 to 200 μg/day are usually sufficient to maintain a euthyroid state in patients treated for hypothyroidism, resulting in increased physical and mental well-being, weight reduction, improved tolerance of cold, relief of constipation, increased heart rate, and peripheral vascular perfusion. T$_4$ is used most often by psychiatrists as an adjunct to antidepressants to enhance therapeutic response and convert a partial responder or treatment-resistant patient into a therapeutic responder. There is accumulating evidence that high doses can be very helpful in preventing rapid cycling in treatment-resistant bipolar patients when all other regimens have been maximized without stabilizing results. Optimal dose appears to be that which will bring serum T$_4$ levels to approximately 125–150% of normal. Because it takes 6–8 weeks for T$_4$ to equilibrate, treatment should be continued for 3–6 months, depending on cycle length. If no benefit is achieved after that time, T$_4$ should be slowly withdrawn. See **levothyroxine.**

thyroxine binding globulin (TBG) Acidic glycoprotein that is a major carrier of thyroid hormones. Protein binding of thyroid hormones protects them from metabolism and excretion, resulting in their long half-life in the circulation.

thyroxine/breast milk Thyroxine appears in breast milk, but has no adverse effects on the neonate of mothers taking therapeutic doses.

thyroxine + carbamazepine Use of carbamazepine in thyroxine-substituted hypothyroid children requires an increased dose of thyroxine to maintain a euthyroid state.

thyroxine + lithium High doses of thyroxine combined with lithium may decrease cycling frequency and severity in rapid cycling bipolar disorder (Bauer MS, Whybrow PC. Rapid cycling bipolar affective disorder. II. Treatment of refractory rapid cycling with high dose levothyroxine: a preliminary study. *Arch Gen Psychiatry* 1990;47:435–440).

Thytropar See **thyrotropin.**

tiagabine Anticonvulsant that appears to work in a way unlike any other anticonvulsant. It is the only anticonvulsant known to block reuptake of the inhibitory neurotransmitter gamma aminobutyric acid (GABA). By preventing return of GABA to its original cells, tiagabine can make more of GABA available and thus block the spread of abnormal electrical activity in the brain. Tiagabine may benefit epileptic patients unresponsive to other anticonvulsants.

tianeptine Novel 5-HT uptake agonist tricyclic antidepressant that acts on the hypothalamic-pituitary-adrenal axis. Its principal metabolite is MC5. It is rapidly absorbed, with peak plasma concentration (T$_{max}$) achieved in 1.59 hours. Bioavailability is high in elderly subjects. In doses of 12.5 mg 2 or 3 times daily, tianeptine has been shown to be clinically effective with fewer cardiovascular and anticholinergic side effects. It has been approved for marketing in France (Demotes-Mainard F, Galley P, Manciet G, Vinson G, Salvadori C. Pharmacokinetics of the antidepressant tianeptine at steady state in the elderly. *J Clin Pharmacol* 1991;31:174–178).

tianeptine + alcohol Alcohol decreases absorption, C_{max}, and area under the curve for tianeptine (Salvadori C, Ward C, Defrance R, Hopkins R. The pharmacokinetics of the antidepressant tianeptine and its main metabolites in healthy humans: influence of alcohol co-administration. *Fundam Clin Pharmacol* 1990;4:115–125).

Tiapridal See **tiapride.**

tiapride (Equilium; Tiapride; Tiapridex) Atypical (substituted benzamide) neuroleptic structurally related to sulpiride. It is presumed to be a specific D_2 receptor blocker without noticeable extrapyramidal side effects. Clinical experience indicates that it provides rapid relief of symptomatic agitation in the management of elderly or alcoholic patients. Experimental studies suggest that it may be helpful in some patients with tardive dyskinesia and other movement disorders such as chorea, tics, akathisia, nonparkinsonian senile tremor, and dyskinesia secondary to L-dopa (Lees AJ, Lander CM, Storn GM. Tiapride in levodopa-induced involuntary movements. *J Neurol Neurosurg Psychiatry* 1979;42:380). It also may possess anxiolytic and antidepressant properties. It is being investigated in the long-term management of alcoholics of anxious or depressive temperament.

Tiapridex See **tiapride.**

tiaspirone Buspirone analog being evaluated as a possible anxiolytic, antidepressant, or antipsychotic.

"tic" Street name for phencyclidine (PCP).

tic Brief muscle contraction (between 50 and 200 msec) that resembles myoclonus, but differs in being repetitive and stereotyped. Tics appear suddenly and intermittently; etiology remains controversial. They are often associated with dopamine excess. Motor tics can be a simple contraction of a muscle group, but are often more complex. They may be single or multiple and transient or chronic. Tics involving the diaphragm cause grunting or coughing-like sounds. Typical tics involve the face (e.g., blinking, sniffing, lip-smacking, facial grimacing, tongue darting) or the upper arms (e.g., shoulder shrugging). There is usually an irresistible urge to perform the tic; suppression by willpower leads to a build-up of internal disquiet. Tics usually appear for the first time in childhood, with a peak mean age of incidence around 7 years. They occur 3 times more often in boys than in girls. They are characterized by their situation specificity, but in general are made worse by boredom, anxiety, excitement, or fatigue. Tics are not always exacerbated by voluntary movement of an unaffected body part. Gilles de la Tourette's syndrome is characterized by chronic multiple tics, which may be treated with haloperidol or pimozide. Pimozide ordinarily should not be used to treat tics other than those due to Tourette's syndrome. See **Gilles de la Tourette's syndrome.** Also called "habit spasm."

tic douloureux See **trigeminal neuralgia.**

Tigan See **trimethobenzamide.**

tilozepine Clozapine analog that is a clinically effective atypical neuroleptic. Like clozapine, it may cause seizures.

Timelit See **lofepramine.**

time out Exclusion of a patient from certain activities developed as part of a treatment program agreed on by the patient and the clinical team. The term should not be used to describe seclusion. When time out involves the technical seclusion of a patient, the full seclusion procedure should be used.

time to relapse Time from the first day without drug treatment to the day relapse is observed.

time zero Time at which a patient enters the study group.

time zone change syndrome Condition resulting from travel across time zones, manifested by either difficulty initiating or maintaining sleep with awakening after only a few hours sleep. It is associated with daytime fatigue; sleepiness; impaired concentration, attention, memory, and performance; and gastrointestinal disturbance. At present there is no specific therapy. Some researchers are investigating use of bright light therapy, but efficacy remains to be established. Incidence of the syndrome has increased steadily since the end of World War II and the rise in number of air travelers, especially those over age 50, who pass through multiple time zones. The more rapidly time zones are crossed, the greater the likelihood the syndrome will occur and the more intense it may be. Also called "jet lag syndrome."

Timostenol See **caroxazone.**

Tindal See **acetophenazine.**

tinnitus Sound sensation in the ear or head in the absence of an external noise source. Different forms of sound have been described, such as ringing, roaring, hissing, or pulsatile clicking. The sound may be constant or intermittent, high or low in pitch, and due to multiple causes (drugs, vascular, or increased intracranial pressure). There are two types of tinnitus: objective and subjective. In objective tinnitus, the less common type, the sound produced within the head can be heard by both the patient and the examiner. Vascular and mechanical causes of objective tinnitus include arterial bruits, venous hums, palatal myoclonus, and idiopathic stapedial myoclonus. In subjective tinnitus, the sound is perceived only by the patient. Tinnitus can be caused by peripheral as well as central nervous system pathology of the auditory system anywhere along the pathway. There may be single or multiple sites of dysfunction in the middle or inner ear, primarily with hair cell damage or with retrocochlear lesions. In peripheral lesions, tinnitus is most commonly a result of noise-induced hearing loss; with age, it is most commonly due to age-related hearing deterioration. Tinnitus of central nervous system origin can be caused by acoustic neuroma or other auditory space-occupying lesions (Alster J, Shemesh Z, Ornan M, Attias J. Sleep disturbance associated with chronic tinnitus. *Biol Psychiatry* 1993;34:84–90). Salicylate, carbamazepine, propranolol, and caffeine may be responsible for tinnitus. A common cause of persistent and annoying tinnitus is long-term benzodiazepine therapy (Gordon AG. Benzodiazepines and the ear—tinnitus, hallucinations and schizophrenia. *Can J Psychiatry* 1993; 38:156–157).

tiospirone   See **neuroleptic, atypical, type A.**

tissue tolerance   Development of tolerance to opiates due to opioid receptor insensitivity.

titubating gait   Characteristic staggering gait seen in cerebellar disease.

titubation   Tremor of the neck muscles resulting in a to-and-fro movement of the head, commonly seen in patients with senile postural tremors and occasionally in Parkinson's disease.

t_{last} Area under the plasma concentration-versus-time curve up to the last time showing a measurable concentration of a drug.

T lymphocyte   (T cell) Immune cells processed by the thymus that protect against viral, fungal, and intracellular bacterial infection, and against foreign (e.g., transplanted) and malignant cells. They are released upon stimulation by an antigen. During lymphocytic activation, T lymphocytes proliferate and differentiate into effector T cell subtypes (e.g., suppressor, helper, or cytotoxic T lymphocytes) that act in concert to produce the cellular immune response. When the immune system is compromised, lymphocyte production decreases.

T lymphocyte measure   Measure of production and release of T lymphocyte cells. Degree of T cell depression is an important health assessment procedure in immunosuppressed states.

"TMA"   Street name for a designer drug made from methamphetamine.

t_{max} See **drug absorption rate.**

"TNT"   Street name for heroin.

tobacco withdrawal syndrome   Withdrawal syndrome following discontinuation of tobacco use that varies in intensity from person to person. Symptoms (tobacco craving, anger, anxiety, difficulty concentrating, hunger, weight gain, impatience, restlessness) occur in the first 2–4 weeks after tobacco withdrawal; most cease after 1 month. Hunger and weight gain may persist for at least 6 months. Difficulty concentrating and hunger do not predict the ability to remain abstinent, but increase in weight does.

tocopherol   (vitamin E) Antioxidant that traps free radicals and may cause neuronal destruction. See **vitamin E.**

Todd's paralysis   Postseizure phenomena that are transient (lasting less than 48 hours) paralytic disorders (hemiplegia, aphasia, and visual field defect) due to postictal enhanced inhibitory neurotransmitter function.

toe walking   Ambulating on the toes instead of the whole foot; may be a neuroleptic-induced extrapyramidal symptom.

tofenacin   Demethylated metabolite of orphenadrine hydrochloride. Pharmacologically, it closely resembles the antiparkinson drug orphenadrine, although there are some differences in the magnitude of the effects observed. In a double-blind comparison, tofenacin was as effective as imipramine and had a more rapid onset of antidepressant action and a low incidence of unwanted effects.

Tofranil   See **imipramine.**

"toilet water"   Street name for volatile nitrites such as amyl nitrite sold in "head" shops, pornography stores, and novelty shops and through mail order houses.

token economy   Method of behavior modification in which tokens are used to motivate patients to behave appropriately and constructively. Tokens can be exchanged for a number of different reinforcers (cigarettes, soft drinks, watching television, permission to sleep in a pleasant single room). Token economies appear to be particularly useful with long-stay, institutionalized chronic patients. Their major impact appears to be on negative symptoms. Token systems work best when there is good rapport between patients and staff. Failure to explicitly instruct patients about the contingencies is thought to be a major reason why token systems sometimes fail to work.

tolbutamide + fluoxetine   No adverse interactions have been reported (Lemberger L, Rowe H, Bosomworth JC, et al. The effect of fluoxetine on the pharmacokinetics and psychomotor responses of diazepam. *Clin Pharmacol Ther* 1988;43:412–419).

tolbutamide + sertraline   Sertraline does not cause any clinically important changes in the pharmacokinetics of tolbutamide.

tolerance Process whereby effects of initial drug doses gradually become ineffective, creating a need for dosage escalation to produce the same pharmacological effect. It may be due to changes in drug clearance, metabolism (metabolic tolerance), binding, receptor sensitivity (pharmacotolerance or tissue tolerance), or receptor populations over time. It can occur at different rates for different actions of drugs (e.g., tolerance to the euphoric effects of cocaine occurs more rapidly than tolerance to its cardiovascular effects). Tolerance is considered by many to indicate physical dependence associated with drug escalation. It can be subdivided into pharmacological and behavioral subtypes. Pharmacological tolerance is due to metabolic or receptor changes that reduce a drug's effect; behavioral tolerance is due to learned adaptation to the drug effect. No metabolic tolerance is associated with repeated benzodiazepine (BZD) use, but there are changes in receptor binding with chronic BZD administration. Behavioral tolerance to the impairing effects of BZD hypnotics also occurs (Roth T, Roehrs TA. Issues in the use of benzodiazepine therapy. *J Clin Psychiatry* 1992;53[suppl]: 14–18). Tolerance may occur with various antidepressants (e.g., phenelzine, amoxapine, fluoxetine, and tricyclic antidepressants) (Donaldson SR. Tolerance to phenelzine and subsequent refractory depression: three cases. *J Clin Psychiatry* 1989;50:33–35; Rapport DJ, Calabrese JR. Tolerance to fluoxetine. *J Clin Psychopharmacol* 1993;13:361). Also called "habituation" (nonpreferred term).

tolerance, behavioral Adaptive response that occurs when an animal or person receiving a drug learns or is conditioned to make a response that counters the drug effect or permits functioning despite drug-induced neurological impairment.

tolerance, functional Tolerance due to compensatory changes in receptors, enzymes, or membrane actions of a drug. It may be due to altered properties of critical cells, altered numbers of receptors, or recruitment of alternative neuronal systems that are otherwise labile.

tolerance, metabolic Tolerance due to increased disposition of a drug after chronic use.

tolerance, reverse Development of increased sensitivity to the effects of drugs such as psychostimulants. It may be partly related to enhanced striatal dopaminergic function (Post RM, Rubinow DR, Ballenger JC. Conditioning, sensitization, and kindling: implications for course of affective illness. *In* Post RM, Ballenger JC [eds], *Neurobiology of Mood Disor-*

ders. Baltimore: Williams & Wilkins, 1984). Both tolerance and reverse decay over time (weeks to months), and their altered responsivity occurs only while the drug continues to be administered. Also called "behavioral sensitization."

"tolly" Street name for toluene.

toloxatone (Humoryl; Perenum) First of a new generation of reversible inhibitors of monoamine oxidase type A (RIMAs), marketed in Europe as an antidepressant. It is rapidly effective and well tolerated, and has a low incidence of side effects and interactions with other drugs, including psychotropics. Almost 5 years of clinical experience indicate that it is effective and safe with tyramine-free diet. Unlike standard antidepressants, it does not modify the duration or percentage of rapid eye movement (REM) sleep. In a single-blind, placebo-controlled crossover study of pressor effects induced by 100–800 mg of tyramine, toloxatone (200 or 400 mg 3 times a day) had no significant effect on blood pressure in healthy male subjects. An interaction with tyramine in meals appears unlikely to occur during administration of therapeutic doses of toloxatone (Provost JC, Funck-Brentano C, Rovei V, et al. Pharmacokinetic and pharmacodynamic interaction between toloxatone, a new reversible monoamine oxidase-A inhibitor, and oral tyramine in healthy subjects. *Clin Pharmacol Ther* 1992;52:384–393).

toloxatone + terbutaline + phenylephrine Coadministration has been associated with a life-threatening pseudopheochromocytoma manifested by sweating, tachycardia (130 beats/min), headache, intense peripheral vasoconstriction with cyanotic extremities, hypertension (up to 230/120 mmHg), and status epilepticus (Lefebvre H, Richard R, Noblet C, et al. Life-threatening pseudopheochromocytoma after toloxatone, terbutaline, and phenylephrine. *Lancet* 1993;341:555–556). Despite selectivity and reversibility, toloxatone and other similar "new" monoamine oxidase inhibitors (MAOIs) are not immune to the usual interactions of "old" MAOIs.

toluene Constituent of some solvents/adhesives that are abused by inhaling (sniffing or huffing). Toluene is the only pure solvent that frequently has been reported to be inhaled for its euphoric effects by preteens and adolescents. It may be responsible for causing psychotic symptoms (paranoid psychosis). Adult chronic toluene abusers may exhibit severe signs of mental and physical deterioration: slow, slurred speech; tremors of hands, feet, and eyelids; and short attention span. Brain magnetic resonance imaging (MRI) studies of chronic toluene abusers show they are at risk of developing atrophy of cerebral, cerebellar, and brainstem white matter (Rosenberg NL, Spitz MC, Filly CM, et al. Central nervous system effects of chronic toluene abuse—clinical, brain stem evoked response and magnetic resonance imaging studies. *Neurotoxicol Teratol* 1988;10:489).

Tolvin See **mianserin.**

Tolvon See **mianserin.**

"tombstone" Street name for high purity heroin.

Tomography Radiographic technique that images the body in three dimensions. See **computed tomography.**

tomoxetine (LY-139603) Close structural analog to fluoxetine that is an effective antidepressant.

tongue protrusion Involuntary thrusting of the tongue to outside of the mouth. Commonly observed in tardive dyskinesia, it can occur as a clonic form (rhythmic in and out movement of the tongue), tonic form (continuous protrusion of the tongue) and "fly-catcher" form (sudden shooting out of the tongue at irregular intervals (Simpson GM, Lee JH, Zoubok B, Gardos G. A rating scale for tardive dyskinesia. *Psychopharmacology* 1979;64:171–179).

tonic-clonic seizure See **grand mal seizure.**

"tooie" Street name for Tuinal (amobarbital + secobarbital).

"toolie" Street name for Tuinal (amobarbital + secobarbital).

"toot" Street name for cocaine.

"tootie" Street name for Tuinal (amobarbital + secobarbital).

"tootsie roll" Dark, gummy version of relatively high-potency heroin. Also called "Mexican tar."

topectomy Form of psychosurgery in which selected areas of the cerebral cortex are removed for the treatment of certain types of mental illness. It is seldom done today.

topographic brain mapping Computerized analysis of electroencephalographic activity to produce a map instead of the usual electroencephalogram (EEG) recording. Multiple scalp electrodes are required. See **electroencephalographic brain mapping.**

Topral See **sultopride.**

Torate See **butorphanol.**

Torbutesic See **butorphanol.**

Torbutrol See **butorphanol.**

Torecan See **thiethylperazine.**

torpor Disorder of consciousness characterized by inactivity, sluggishness, and drowsiness.

torsades de pointes Ventricular tachyrhythmia with a characteristic electrocardiographic morphology in which points of the QRS complexes appear to twist around the isoelectric line. It is associated with delayed ventricular repolarization manifested in the electrocardiogram (ECG) by a prolonged QT interval. Episodes tend to remit and recur spontaneously, but may deteriorate to episodes of sustained ventricular tachycardia or ventricular fibrillation that require intensive treatment and that may be fatal. The disorder is frequently provoked in patients with organic heart disease receiving a type Ia antiarrhythmic medication. Various drugs have been implicated, including antiarrhythmics (quinidine, procainamide, disopyramide, aprindine, amiodarone, and sotalol); vasodilating agents (prenylamine, lidoflazine, and bepridil); antipsychotics (thioridazine, chlorpromazine, and haloperidol); hetcrocyclic antidepressants (amitriptyline, doxepin, and maprotiline); and miscellaneous drugs. Orally and intravenously administered haloperidol has rarely been reported to cause torsades de pointes. In a case report, high-dosage haloperidol (50 mg/day) was used to successfully treat a patient after recovery from thioridazine-induced torsades de pointes (Kemper AJ, Dunlap R, Pietro DA. Thioridazine-induced torsades de pointes. Successful therapy with isoproterenol. *JAMA* 1983;248:2931–2934). Patients with risk factors should have a baseline ECG measurement of the QT and QTc (corrected QT) intervals. Repeat ECGs should be done when steady state is achieved and with dosage increases. Prolongation of the QTc to greater than 450 msec, or a greater than 25% increase in the QTc over baseline, may signal development of a dangerous arrhythmia warranting consideration of a cardiology consultation and discontinuation of the psychotropic with which the patient is being treated (Tzivoni D, Keren A, Banai S, Stern S. Terminology of torsades de pointes. *Cardiovasc Drugs Ther* 1991;5:505–508; Stratmann HG, Kennedy HL. Torsades de pointes associated with drugs and toxins: recognition and management. *Am Heart J* 1987;1470-1482). See **QTc.**

torsion dystonia See **dystonia, torsion.**

torsion spasm See **dystonia, torsion.**

torticollis See **dystonia, cervical.**

total allergy syndrome See **ecologic illness.**

total clearance Assuming no other routes of drug metabolism or elimination, the sum of hepatic and renal clearances.

total cranial volume (TCV) Total cortical and subcortical gray and white matter volume plus total sulcal and ventricular cerebrospinal fluid volume. A magnetic resonance imaging (MRI) study of TCV in schizophrenic patients and control subjects revealed no significant differences between the two groups (Brier A, Buchanan RW, Elkashef A, et al. Brain morphology and schizophrenia. *Arch Gen Psychiatry* 1992; 49:921–926).

total predictive power   Total probability of correct classification.

total recording time   In sleep electroencephalography, the period from sleep onset to final awakening. In addition to total sleep time, it comprises the time taken up by wake periods and movement time until wake-up.

total sleep deprivation   See **sleep deprivation.**

total sleep episode   See **sleep episode, total.**

total sleep period   See **sleep episode, total.**

total sleep time   (TST) Amount of actual sleep time in a sleep episode; it is equal to total sleep episode less awake time. It is the total of all rapid eye movement (REM) and non-REM (NREM) sleep in a sleep episode. It is greatest in infancy, decreases in childhood, is relatively stable in young adults, and declines in old age.

Tourette's syndrome   See **Gilles de la Tourette's syndrome.**

toxic dose, median   Dose required to produce a particular toxic effect in 50% of treated animals.

toxicity   Unwanted, noxious, or deleterious drug effect.

toxicodynamics   Injurious effects on vital function of toxins and toxic doses of therapeutic agents and their metabolites.

toxicokinetics   Absorption, distribution, excretion, and metabolism of toxins and toxic doses of therapeutic agents and their metabolites.

toxicology   Study of the adverse effects of drugs and chemicals on living organisms. Forensic toxicology is devoted to the medicolegal aspects of chemicals harmful to animals and man. Clinical toxicology focuses on diseases caused by or associated with toxic substances.

toxicology screen   Test to detect high-dose recent drug abuse or toxic levels of drugs by thin-layer chromatography. It is the preferred test for emergency room use when drugs taken are unknown, concentrations are expected to be high, and quick determination of the toxic substance is the primary task.

toxic psychosis   Psychosis caused by exogenous or endogenous toxic substances. See **delirium, anticholinergic.**

T-Quil   See **diazepam.**

tracazolate   Nonbenzodiazepine, pyrazolopyridine derivative being tested as an anxiolytic drug.

"tracer"   Small amount of a substance that is added to a drug and easy to detect in the urine. Tracers allow detection of therapeutic noncompliance. To be truly helpful, a tracer must (a) be indiscernible to the subject; (b) be pharmacologically inert; (c) be safe; and (d) not react chemically with the study drug. Disadvantages include (a) provision of information only about the most recent dose taken; (b) possible need for a special drug formulation, entailing the risk of altered bioavailability.

"track marks"   Marks in the arms and/or elsewhere in the body of drug abusers where drugs have been repeatedly injected intravenously. There is a tattoo effect at the injection site produced by carbon from heating the drugs. Tracks are an uncommon finding in cocaine and methamphetamine abusers (Wetle C. Fatal reactions to cocaine. *In* Washington AM, Gold MS [eds], *Cocaine: A Clinician's Handbook.* New York: Guilford Press, 1987).

tractotomy, stereotactic   Modification of psychosurgery in which radioactive yttrium-90 seeds are implanted in the substantia innominata below the head of the caudate nucleus. The procedure has been reported to be of benefit in intractable depression, anxiety, and obsessional states (Knight GD. Stereotactic tractotomy in the surgical treatment of mental illness. *J Neurol Neurosurg Psychiatry* 1965;28:304–310).

tractotomy, stereostatic subcaudate   (SST) Psychosurgical procedure used in the United Kingdom for patients with treatment-resistant affective disorder. Therapeutic outcome is sufficiently successful to offer hope of improvement for affective disorders that persist despite treatment with antidepressant drugs alone or combined, one or more courses of electroconvulsive therapy, and lithium, L-tryptophan, and anticonvulsants (e.g., carbamazepine).

trait   1. Inherited or acquired characteristic that is consistent, persistent, and stable. A trait associated with an illness in a family may represent a specific genetic susceptibility factor that may help identify relatives at risk. 2. Combination of motives and habits that is a principal unit of personality structure. It is a neuropsychic system that determines to a great extent which stimuli will be perceived (selective perception) and what kind of response will be given (selective action). Each individual's traits determine behavior in a unique way.

trait, carrier   In genetics, family member actually exhibiting the hereditary characteristic under observation.

trait, dominant   In genetics, a gene that will produce the same effect in heterozygote or homozygote. A trait is dominant if it is expressed in the heterozygote when the allele of the gene that determines the trait is not expressed.

trait, recessive   Genetically controlled trait that remains latent or subordinate to a dominant trait except when both members of the gene pair are recessive.

trance   Altered state of consciousness such as seen in hypnosis, catalepsy, or ecstasy.

Trandate   See **labetalol.**

traneptine   New tricyclic antidepressant (TCA) with a unique mechanism of action. In contrast to fluoxetine, sertraline, paroxetine, and fluvoxamine, which inhibit serotonin (5-HT) uptake, traneptine increases it. Its properties also are different from those of classic TCAs, which inhibit 5-HT and/or norepinephrine (NE) neuronal uptake, thereby increasing the amount of 5-HT and/or NE molecules available to postsynaptic receptors. Traneptine enhances 5-HT uptake but does not affect NE uptake processes or monoamine oxidase activity.

Tranmep   See **meprobamate.**

"tranq"   Street name for (a) central nervous system depressants; (b) phencyclidine (PCP).

"tranquility"   Street name for dimethoxymethylamphetamine.

tranquilizer   Term coined in 1953 by Dr. F. F. Yonkman at Ciba in Summit, New Jersey, to characterize the psychotropic effects of reserpine; adopted in English-speaking countries shortly after the importation of chlorpromazine in 1954. With the introduction of meprobamate, tranquilizers were classified as major (now called "neuroleptics") or minor (now called "anxiolytics" or "antianxiety drugs"). The term *tranquilizer* may now denote any psychotropic drug that induces tranquility by decreasing anxiety or agitation, usually without clouding consciousness.

tranquilizer, major   See **major tranquilizer.**

tranquilizer, minor   See **minor tranquilizer.**

Tranquilizer Recovery and New Existence (TRANX) British self-help organization that provides national telephone and mail counseling and support to members withdrawing from benzodiazepines (BZDs). It is a realistic alternative and adjunct to orthodox health care for those wishing to withdraw from BZDs (Tattersall ML, Halstrom C. Self-help and benzodiazepine withdrawal. *J Affect Dis* 1992; 24:193–198).

transcerebral electrotherapy   See **electrosleep.**

transcranial Doppler ultrasonography   (TCD) New method for continuous long-term computer-aided registration of cerebral perfusion in human sleep. It permits noninvasive monitoring of the direction and velocity of blood flow in the large intracranial arteries in a time course of seconds.

transcribed domain   Part of a gene that is copied into nRNA.

transcription   Process whereby RNA is transcribed from a DNA template by the enzyme RNA polymerase. Information present in the DNA is retained in the RNA molecule produced (they are complementary).

transcription, reverse   Copying a gene with enzymes that can make DNA from RNA.

transcutaneous electrical nerve stimulation (TENS) Pain relief method in which the patient carries a small, portable, battery-powered stimulator connected via wires to electrodes. The electrodes are self-adhering, or applied to the skin with adhesive tape with an intervening layer of conductive gel. Dual-output machines allow two sites to be stimulated simultaneously. The stimulator produces a pulsatile output that can be of different wave-forms and delivered either continuously or in bursts. Patients can alter the output by adjusting the current intensity, pulse frequency, and width to produce a tingling sensation. TENS has been tried in numerous conditions, most often for chronic low back pain. How it works is unclear. It has a placebo effect as powerful as other pain-relieving methods, especially at the start of treatment. About 30% of patients are helped by sham stimulation with little risk.

transdermal administration   Application of drugs to the skin for transfer into the systemic circulation. Prolonged blood levels of some drugs can be achieved because the drugs are slowly absorbed. An increasing number of drugs are being administered transdermally.

transdihydrolisuride   (Terguride) Ergot-derived neuroleptic in use in Czechoslovakia. It is a mixed dopamine agonist/antagonist that appears to exhibit variable activity at different dopamine receptors. It reduces prolactin, unlike standard neuroleptics, which typically have the opposite effect. In a controlled trial of 57 chronic schizophrenic patients (SCZs), it was statistically equivalent in efficacy to prochlorperazine. It has been reported to significantly improve both tardive dyskinesia and psychotic symptoms in some SCZs also receiving neuroleptic drugs (Filip V. Treatment of extrapyramidal side effects with Terguride. *J Psychiatry Res* 1992;41:9–16). It is also used in the treatment of Parkinson's disease.

***trans*-doxepin**   One of the two geometric isomers of doxepin.

transducer   Device that converts a biological activity into an electrical voltage.

transduction (gene)   Acquisition and transfer of eukaryotic genetic material by retroviruses.

transduction (signal)   Transfer and processing of growth factor or other genetic signals via cytoplasmic messengers to influence nuclear events.

transfection   Process of introducing DNA into a eukaryotic cell for experimental purposes. The DNA is usually in the form of a recombinant plasmid and is introduced into the cells by coprecipitation with calcium phosphate, electroporation, or by liposome fusion. The cells are then monitored according to the needs of the researcher. For example, an electrophysiologist may want to determine the properties of a particular receptor of interest that has been cloned. He can transfect the plasmid containing the receptor cloned into an appropriate expression vector. This allows him to patch the cells and determine various physical properties of the receptor that is generated. A transient transfection is the time frame in which the measurements can be made. In general, the transfected DNA remains in the nucleus of the cell as a plasmid molecule that is stable for only a period of days. It soon becomes diluted out during cell division or is degraded by the cell's DNAs, which digest nonchromosomal DNA. Stable transfection is the small percentage of time that the plasmid DNA will stably integrate into the host cell's genome and propagate when the cell divides. Using special techniques, researchers can select for those stable transformants and propagate them after isolating single cells. The advantage is that because the cell is stably transformed, the researcher has a continuous supply of cells expressing the transfected DNA.

transferase   See **conjugating enzyme.**

transfer RNA   (tRNA) RNA that associates specific three base codon sequences in the mRNA with their cognate amino acids during protein synthesis.

transformation   **1.** In genetics, process by which a cell, generally a lymphocyte, is "immortalized" to a lymphoblast that can be grown indefinitely in cell culture for a continuing source of the DNA from the individual donating the lymphocyte. The usual method involves incubation of the isolated lymphocytes with Epstein-Barr virus. The cells are then referred to as transformed or immortalized and may be cultured or stored in a frozen state. **2.** In statistics, change in the scale for the values of a variable. Major purposes are to obtain a more accurate quantitative relation between variables and to meet certain statistical assumptions required by the analysis itself.

transgenic animal   Animal manipulated into producing foreign gene products that they normally cannot produce. Such manipulation enables determination of the normal biological function of a gene and creation of a biological system in which a specific perturbation occurs. Both mice and rats have now been so manipulated. Because these animals are made up of so many cells, it is impossible to give each cell the gene directly. Therefore, the gene is given to the animal's fertilized egg. With each cell division, the new gene becomes transferred, along with all the other natural DNA of the cell, to each new cell. As the organism develops, every cell gets the foreign DNA. Selective expression has been achieved by using a part of the gene called the "promoter," a master switch of the gene, that tells the gene when to be expressed. Different genes have different promoters. By giving a gene the promoter sequence from a gene expressed in the brain (such as neurofilament), the foreign gene will be expressed only in the brain of the transgenic animal. The foreign gene will be taken up by the fertilized egg and incorporated into its chromosome in such a way that the new gene will be expressed by the cells, and the promoter will direct the expression so that only specific tissues will make the new protein. Transgenic animals are models of altered gene expression. If a gene is identified to be responsible for Alzheimer's disease, it can be used to produce transgenic animals as models to investigate the pathogenesis of the disease.

transient global amnesia   See **amnesia, transient global.**

transient ischemic attack   (TIA) Temporary cerebral impairment of rapid onset and brief duration (less than 24 hours) due to an insufficient supply of blood to part of the brain. Most common symptoms are slurred or impaired speech, weakness, dizziness, and nausea, but the clinical presentation depends on the brain area affected.

transient tardive dyskinesia–like reaction   See **dyskinesia, withdrawal.**

transitional tremor   See **tremor, movement.**

translation   Entire process by which the base sequence of an RNA molecule is used to order and join the amino acids in a protein. The linear sequence of the RNA is retained in the linear sequence of amino acids found in the protein.

translocation   Breaking of a chromosome and its rejoining at a different site on a different chromosome. For example, in a variant of Down syndrome, translocation occurs between chromosome 21 and one of the D group, such as chromosome number 15. If two nonhomologous chromosomes exchange places, translocation is reciprocal.

transmethylation   Biochemical process in which one or more methyl groups are added to the structure of a compound. One hypothesis of schizophrenia posits that hallucinogenic agents are made within the body via transmethylation of catecholamines or indolamines.

transmitter substance   Chemical released from one brain cell to stimulate the next cell.

***trans*-n-desmethyldoxepin**   Active metabolite of *trans*-doxepin.

transposition   Transfer of a segment of DNA from one site to another in the genome either between chromosomal sites or between an extrachromosomal site and a chromosome.

transposon   Fragment of DNA capable of changing its position within the genome of the organism that carries it, or in some bacteria capable of undergoing transfer between an extrachromosomal plasmid and a chromosome. Transposons are sometimes used to introduce genes into an organism from an exogenous source.

trans-sexualism   Condition marked by persistent discomfort about one's sex assignment, preoccupation with a desire to be rid of one's sex characteristics, and a wish to obtain the characteristics of the opposite sex. Described in nearly every race and culture, it occurs worldwide with a prevalence of 1/30,000 males and 1/100,000 females. Since the 1960s, reassignment surgery has been used to treat the disorder. It is frequently accompanied by depression, and there has been a high rate of suicide in trans-sexual patients following surgery. See **gender dysphoria.**

transthyretin   Serum transport protein for T_4 and retinol synthesized in abundance in the nervous system and secreted by the choroid plexus. It accounts for 10–25% of total ventricular cerebrospinal fluid (CSF) protein. Evidence strongly suggests that transthyretin transports thyroxine from the blood to the brain. Measurement of CSF transthyretin in eight inpatients with major depression and nine neurological patients showed that the depressed patients had significantly lower transthyretin levels than comparison subjects, suggesting that central hypothyroidism, with normal peripheral thyroid concentrations, occurs in some depressed patients (Hatterer JA, Herbert J, Hidaka C, et al. CSF transthyretin in patients with depression. *Am J Psychiatry* 1993; 150:813–815).

transversion mutation   Mutation resulting from the substitution in DNA or RNA of a purine for a pyrimidine or vice versa.

transvestism   Heterosexual cross-dressing in which the clothing is used fetishistically to promote sexual excitement that can lead to either masturbation or heterosexual intercourse. Cross-dressing may begin in childhood, but usually becomes sexualized in adolescents. It is sporadic at first and in most transvestites remains so. In some, however, it becomes a daily occurrence. Transvestites are invariably preferential heterosexuals who characteristically spend a considerable portion of their cross-dressing sessions in rapt contemplation of their appearance in the mirror (mirror complex).

TRANX   See **Tranquilizer Recovery and New Existence.**

Tranxal   See **clorazepate.**

Tranxene   See **clorazepate.**

Tranxilium   See **clorazepate.**

tranylcypromine   (TCP) (Eskapar; Parnate) First-generation nonhydrazine irreversible nonselective monoamine oxidase (MAO)-A and -B inhibitor with a close structural similarity to amphetamine. It is the only nonhydrazine MAO inhibitor currently in use in psychiatry. It is an efficacious antidepressant also used in refractory and electroconvulsive therapy–resistant depression, panic, and some phobic disorders. Well-executed trials have established that 70–80% of depressed patients with fatigue, psychomotor retardation, and/or reversed neurovegetative features respond well to MAO inhibitors such as TCP, even if they first fail to benefit from treatment with standard tricyclics (Thase ME, Mallinger AG, McKnight D, Himmelhoch JM. Treatment of imipramine-resistant recurrent depression, IV: a double-blind crossover study of tranylcypromine for anergic bipolar depression. *Am J Psychiatry* 1992;149:195–198). Although TCP is generally regarded as a psychostimulant, daytime fatigue/somnolence is increasingly recognized as a possible adverse drug effect, which study data suggest could be counteracted by evening dosing. The interaction between MAO inhibitors and indirectly acting sympathomimetic amines (the "cheese reaction") is important, but the danger may be exaggerated. Before 1970, 3.5 million patients took TCP, and there were fewer than 100 reports of intracranial hemorrhage and fewer than 20 reported deaths. Although the morbidity and mortality rates compare favorably with those of tricyclic antidepressants, the severe toxicity of MAO inhibitors has resulted in an overly cautious attitude toward their use (Belknap SM, Nelson JE. Drug interactions in psychiatry. *In* Musa MN [ed], *Pharmacokinetics and Therapeutic Monitoring of Psychiatric Drugs.* Springfield, IL: Charles C Thomas, 1993, pp 57–112). Pregnancy risk category C.

tranylcypromine abuse   Tranylcypromine (TCP) is involved in more cases of tolerance and dependence than any other monoamine oxidase inhibitor (MAOI), but abuse has been reported infrequently. TCP abusers usually have histories of alcohol, and sometimes polysubstance, abuse. Stimulant abuse also may be a predisposing factor. TCP's capacity to exert amphetamine-like effects presynaptically, and its minor metabolic pathway to amphetamine, may help to explain its abuse potential. Like amphetamine, TCP used chronically may result in habituation and a withdrawal reaction. High dosages (up to 300 mg/day) invariably cause marked central nervous system stimulation and delirium (Brady KT, Lydiard RB, Kellner C. Tranylcypromine abuse. *Am J Psychiatry* 1991;148:1268–1269).

tranylcypromine + alcohol-free beer Tyramine content of de-alcoholized beer is similar to that of regular beer. Severe vascular and acute generalized headache followed by a right hemiplegia and expressive dysphagia have occurred in tranylcypromine-treated patients who drank alcohol-free beer (Draper R, Sandler M, Walker PL. Chemical curio: monoamine oxidase inhibitors and non-alcoholic beer. *Br Med J* 1984;289:308; Murray JA, Walker JP, Doyle JB. Tyramine in alcohol-free beer. *Lancet* 1988;1:1167–1168).

tranylcypromine + alprazolam Co-administration has been reported to be effective in treatment-resistant panic disorder, without serious adverse drug interactions.

tranylcypromine + amitriptyline Co-administration may cause a hypertensive crisis, significant increase in heart rate, and significant lengthening of the PR interval.

tranylcypromine + amphetamine Co-administration is generally considered contraindicated because of the risk of a hypertensive crisis or hyperthermia. Some investigators have suggested that combined use could be safe and effective for treatment-resistant depression (Sovner R. Amphetamine and tranylcypromine in treatment-resistant depression. *Biol Psychiatry* 1990;28:1011–1013). A transient response to dextroamphetamine in treatment-resistant depression may predict response to the combination of dextroamphetamine and tranylcypromine. Although some patients have been safely treated with this combination, in view of the potentially fatal adverse reactions that have occurred, it should be reserved for patients with truly drug-resistant depressive disorders.

tranylcypromine/breast milk Tranylcypromine is excreted in canine breast milk. Because there is no evidence for its safety in human neonates, tranylcypromine should not be prescribed for nursing mothers.

tranylcypromine + buspirone See **buspirone + monoamine oxidase inhibitor.**

tranylcypromine + clomipramine Clomipramine (CMI) should not be prescribed during tranylcypromine therapy or within 14 days after tranylcypromine discontinuation. Tranylcypromine should not be added to CMI therapy. Either regimen may cause hypotension, collapse, convulsions, coma, and death. Disseminated intravascular coagulation along with agitated delirium, hyperpyrexia, tachycardia, and rigidity occurred in a patient when CMI was added to chronic tranylcypromine therapy (Tackley RM, Tregaskis B. Fatal disseminated intravascular coagulation following a monoamine oxidase inhibitor/tricyclic interaction. *Anesthesia* 1987;42:760–763). However, a combination of CMI plus tranylcypromine plus trifluoperazine has been used safely and effectively in some patients with treatment-resistant depression (Schmauss M, Kapfhammer HP, Meyr P, Hoff P. Combined MAO-inhibitor and tri (tetra) cyclic antidepressant treatment in therapy resistant depression. *Progr Neuropsychopharmacol* 1988;12:523–532).

tranylcypromine + electroconvulsive therapy (ECT) Data are sparse, but no adverse side effects or any enhancement of ECT by tranylcypromine have been reported.

tranylcypromine + fluoxetine Death was reported following initiation of tranylcypromine shortly after fluoxetine (FLX) treatment was discontinued (*Physicians' Desk Reference* ["Prozac"]. Oradell, NJ: Medical Economics; 1990, pp 905–908). A serotonin-like syndrome manifested by fevers, chills, flushes, disorientation, diplopia, memory loss, confusion, incoordination, abdominal cramping and diarrhea, paraesthesias, insomnia, and a hypomanic mood occurred in a patient who was started on tranylcypromine (20 mg/day) 6 weeks after discontinuing FLX. Symptoms remitted 48 hours after tranylcypromine was discontinued 3 weeks later. The reaction is attributed to interaction between tranylcypromine and residual norfluoxetine (Coplan JD, Gorman JM. Detectable levels of fluoxetine metabolites after discontinuation: an unexpected serotonin syndrome. *Am J Psychiatry* 1993;150:837; Sternbach H. Danger of MAOI therapy after fluoxetine withdrawal. *Lancet* 1988;2:850–851).

tranylcypromine + ketamine There is a single case report of co-administration precipitating an adrenergic crisis. Another report described safe anesthesia induction with ketamine in a patient treated with tranylcypromine (20 mg/day for 7 weeks), although the author conceded that the absence of ill effects may have been "due more to good luck and careful anesthetic management than to the lack of interaction" (Doyle DJ. Ketamine induction and monoamine oxidase inhibitors. *J Clin Anesthesiol* 1990;2:324–325).

tranylcypromine + lithium Lithium has been co-administered with tranylcypromine to potentiate its antidepressant effects without adverse reactions in depressed patients refractory to other antidepressant regimens (Nolan WA, Haffmans J, Bouvy PF, Duivenvoorden HJ. Monoamine oxidase inhibitors in resistant major depression. A double-blind comparison of brofaromine and tranylcypromine in patients resistant to tricyclic antidepressants. *J Affect Dis* 1993;28:189–197; Price LH, Charney DS, Heninger GR. Efficacy of lithium-tranylcypromine treatment in refractory depression. *Am J Psychiatry* 1985;142:619–623). Two cases of tardive dyskinesia (bucco-lingual-masticatory type) have been reported after long-term treatment with tranylcypromine and lithium (Stancer HC. Tardive dyskinesia not associated with neuroleptics. *Am J Psychiatry* 1979; 136:727).

tranylcypromine + maprotiline Tranylcypromine (10–30 mg/day) may augment therapeutic response to maprotiline (MAP) without producing any more side effects than occur with MAP alone (Ayd FJ Jr. Combined maprotiline-MAOI therapy. *Int Drug Ther Newsl* 1982; 17:4).

tranylcypromine + monosodium glutamate Co-administration resulted in hypertensive episodes in two of five healthy men (Balon R, Pohl R, Yeragani VK, et al. Monosodium glutamate and tranylcypromine administration in healthy subjects. *J Clin Psychiatry* 1990; 51:303–306).

tranylcypromine + paroxetine Animal data indicate that co-administration can cause symptoms of the serotonin syndrome. In healthy volunteers, single paroxetine doses (30 mg) increased the maximum plasma concentration of single tranylcypromine doses (20 mg) by 15% (data on File, SmithKline Beecham). The manufacturer recommends waiting at least 2 weeks after paroxetine therapy is stopped before a monoamine oxidase inhibitor is initiated.

tranylcypromine + propofol Co-administration appears to be safe (Hyde RA, Mortimer AJ. Safe use of propofol in a patient receiving tranylcypromine. *Anaesthesia* 1991;46:1090).

tranylcypromine + sertraline Serotonin syndrome was reported in a 46-year-old man with treatment-resistant depression treated with sertraline (50 mg/day), tranylcypromine (30 mg/day), and clonazepam (1.5 mg at bedtime). The start of sertraline therapy was associated with marked worsening of serotonergic symptoms. The patient had chills, incoordination, and mental status changes such as confusion, memory disturbance, and restlessness. Symptoms subsided following discontinuation of sertraline and reduction of tranylcypromine dosage to (20 mg/day). Although concurrent use of sertraline and a monoamine oxidase inhibitor (MAOI) should be avoided, the quality of life of patients with severe depression refractory to standard treatment must be considered. A distinction should be drawn between the incautious combining of these drugs and their use in patients with otherwise intractable clinical depression. The above-cited case report suggests that sertraline, like fluoxetine, should not be added without a hiatus (14 days or longer) after discontinuation of an MAOI. Concurrent use of sertraline and an MAOI should be avoided in most cases until proven safe or until effective prophylaxis has been identified. (Bhatara VS, Bandettini FC. Possible interaction between sertraline and tranylcypromine. *Clin Pharm* 1993;12:222–225; Boyer W, Feighner J. Response to letter. *J Clin Psychiatry* 1991;52:87; Peterson G. Strategies for fluoxetine-MAOI combination therapy. *J Clin Psychiatry* 1991;52:87; Rosenblatt J, Rosenblatt N. Sertraline-MAOI interaction: corrigendum cum case report. *Curr Affect Ill* 1992;11:17 [abstract]).

tranylcypromine + trifluoperazine (Jatrosom; Parstelin) Combination product marketed outside the United States as an antidepressant.

tranylcypromine/withdrawal Gradual or abrupt withdrawal of tranylcypromine in patients taking 40 mg+/day may result in syndromes ranging in severity from mild discomfort to incapacitation due to severe depression or impaired cognition. Withdrawal phenomena may begin within 2–3 days of dosage reduction or discontinuation (Dilsaver SC. Heterocyclic antidepressant, monoamine oxidase inhibitor and neuroleptic withdrawal phenomena. *Prog Neuropsychopharmacology Biol Psychiatry* 1990;14:137–161; Halle MT, Del Medicao VJ, Dilsaver SC. Symptoms of major depression: acute effects of withdrawing antidepressants. *Acta Psychiatry Scand* 1991;83:238–239; Halle MT, Dilsaver. Tranylcypromine withdrawal phenomena. *J Psychiatry Neurosci* 1993;18:49–50).

TRAP Acronym for the major components of the parkinsonian syndrome: T (tremor), R (rigidity), A (akinesia), and P (postural disturbances).

traumatic affect Maximally aversive state often accompanying the experience of catastrophic stressors. It partly fuels the symptoms of posttraumatic stress and related disorders.

traumatic stress See **posttraumatic stress disorder.**

Trazodil See **trazodone.**

trazodone (Depyrel; Desyrel; Dotazone; Molipaxin; Trazodil; Trialodine) (TRA) Complex heterocyclic triazolopyridine derivative used primarily as an antidepressant. It has an unusual pharmacological profile. Since it has both agonist and antagonist activity in the cerebral serotonin (5-HT)-mediated pathways, it reduces the sensitivity of central beta-adrenoreceptors. Trazodone down-regulates 5-HT$_2$ receptors and slightly inhibits 5-HT reuptake. It also has substantial alpha$_2$ receptor antagonism which may be responsible for its hypnotic effects. Animal and clinical studies indicate that it does not have substantial anticholinergic or cardiotoxic effects compared to tricyclic antidepressants. TRA is metabolized to m-chlorophenylpiperazine, a potent and specific serotonergic receptor agonist. Other major metabolites are trazodone-N-oxide and oxatriazolepyridine propionic acid (OPTA), which are inactive as 5-HT reuptake inhibitors or 5-HT agonists. Many patients have difficulty tolerating therapeutic dosages of TRA because of undue sedation, lightheadedness, or confusion. Its potent alpha-adrenergic blocking properties can cause troublesome orthostatic hypotension. It also may cause priapism and exacerbate ventricular arrhythmias in patients with pre-existing heart disease. However, trazodone has minimal adverse cardiovascular effects and it can safely benefit depressed patients with a variety of cardiovascular disorders by alleviating depression, which can have its own adverse cardiac effects. Food may influence the rate of TRA absorption, resulting in delayed and/or lower peak concentration. Although food may decrease absorption rate, the total amount of TRA absorbed may remain the same. Pregnancy risk category C.

trazodone + alcohol Combined use may result in enhanced sedative and central nervous system effects. Patients should be advised of the potential adverse interaction and counseled to limit or avoid alcohol use, especially when taking more than 250 mg/day of trazodone (Warrington SJ, Ankier SI, Turner P. Evaluation of possible interactions between ethanol and trazodone or amitriptyline. *Neuropsychobiology* 1986;15[suppl 1]:31–37).

trazodone + antihypertensive Co-administration with an antihypertensive (e.g., clonidine, methyldopa) may cause more hypotension than either drug alone. Adjustment of both drugs' dosages may be warranted to avert serious hypotension.

trazodone/breast milk Small quantities of trazodone (approximately 10% of maternal plasma concentration) are excreted in human breast milk. The safety of breast-feeding during trazodone treatment has not been established, and nursing should be avoided if at all possible (Verbeeck RK, Ross SG, McKenna EA. Excretion of trazodone in breast milk. *Br J Clin Pharmacol* 1986;22:367–370).

trazodone + buspirone Co-administration has been associated with the serotonin syndrome (Goldberg RJ, Huck M. Serotonin syndrome from trazodone and buspirone. *Psychosomatics* 1992;33:235–236).

trazodone + clonidine Trazodone may affect blood pressure response to clonidine (van Zwieten PA. Inhibition of the central hypotensive effect of clonidine by trazodone: a novel antidepressant. *Pharmacology* 1977;15:331–335).

trazodone + clozapine No significant adverse interactions between therapeutic doses have been reported.

trazodone + digoxin Co-administration can result in toxic digoxin serum levels (up to 50%) with clinical symptoms of digoxin toxicity (nausea and vomiting). Trazodone should be used cautiously in combination with digoxin and digoxin levels should be closely monitored (Rauch PR, Jenike MA. Digoxin toxicity possibly precipitated by trazodone. *Psychosomatics* 1984;25:334–335).

trazodone + electroconvulsive therapy (ECT) Co-administration has been reported to cause prolonged seizures to the point of status epilepticus that required intravenous diazepam intervention (Kaufman KR, Finstead B, Kaufman ER. Status epilepticus following electroconvulsive therapy. *Mt Sinai J Med* 1986;53:119–122). Thus, some clinicians feel that trazodone should be withheld in patients while they are receiving ECT. However, since during a series of ECT, the seizure threshold is increased secondary to the anticonvulsant properties of ECT itself, the therapist must use either increased power settings or epileptogenic agents in order to assure therapeutic treatments. The first option results in increased morbidity (cognitive defects); the second possesses other complications when caffeine is utilized. In the latter case, trazodone can be utilized as the epileptogenic agent without complications (Kaufman KR, Finstead B, Kaufman ER. Electroencephalography and electroconvulsive therapy. *Electroencephalography and Clinical Neurophysiology* 1985;61:S178).

trazodone + fluoxetine Trazodone may augment the antidepressant effect of fluoxetine (FLX), counteract its stimulant effect, and overcome its delayed sleep onset effect (Jacobsen FM. Low-dose trazodone as a hypnotic in patients treated with MAOIs and other psychotropics: a pilot study. *J Clin Psychiatry* 1990;51:298–302; Nierenberg AA, Cole JO, Glass L. Possible trazodone potentiation of fluoxetine. A case series. *J Clin Psychiatry* 1992;53:83–85). In some patients, the combination may cause intolerable headaches, dizziness, or daytime sedation and fatigue possibly due to FLX reducing trazodone clearance (Aranow RB, Hudson JI, Pope HG, Jr., et al. Elevated antidepressant plasma levels after addition of fluoxetine. *Am J Psychiatry* 1989;46:911–913; Metz A, Shader RI. Adverse interactions encountered when using trazodone to treat insomnia associated with fluoxetine. *Int Clin Psychopharmacol* 1990;5:191–194). In 4 of 13 obsessive-compulsive disorder patients, rating scale scores dropped by more than 20% when trazodone was added to ongoing FLX treatment, but trazodone caused excessive daytime sedation (Jenike MA. Approaches to the patient with treatment-refractory obsessive-compulsive disorder. *J Clin Psychiatry* 1990;51[suppl 2]:15–21; Jenike MA. Management of patients with treatment-resistant obsessive-compulsive disorder. *In* Pato MT, Zohar J [eds], *Obsessive-Compulsive Disorders.* Washington, DC: APA Press, 1991, pp 135–156).

trazodone + L-tryptophan   Combined used may cause the serotonin syndrome (Patterson BD, Srisopark MM. Severe anorexia and possible psychosis or hypomania after trazodone-tryptophan treatment of aggression. *Lancet* 1989; 1:1017).

trazodone/mania   There have been a number of reports of trazodone-induced mania since 1972. A study of the time to onset of mania for patients on trazodone showed that it was 16 days average, with individual patients relapsing on days 70, 30, 28, 17, 14, 7, 7, 5, 4, 4, 4, and 4. The study found that trazodone induces a manic or hypomanic state more rapidly than fluoxetine (Terao T. Comparison of manic switch onset during fluoxetine and trazodone treatment. *Biol Psychiatry* 1993;33: 477–478).

trazodone + monoamine oxidase inhibitor (MAOI)   It is not known if interactions occur. If an MAOI is discontinued shortly before or is given with trazodone treatment, therapy should be initiated cautiously with gradual dosage increases until optional response is achieved.

trazodone overdose   Trazodone (TRA) was among the first antidepressants that appeared to be relatively safe in overdosage, a major advantage for the treatment of suicidally depressed outpatients. Its low incidence of anticholinergic and cardiovascular side effects make it less toxic than tricyclic and tetracyclic compounds when taken in overdose. Hyponatremia and seizures occurred in a 72-year-old woman 10 hours after she took 350 mg. Serum sodium dropped to 118 mmol/L. She was treated with fluid restriction and recovered. Profound hyponatremia in this case suggests inappropriate secretion of antidiuretic hormone (Balestrieri G, Cerudelli B, Ciaccion S, et al. Hyponatremia and seizure due to trazodone overdose. *Br Med J* 1992;304: 686).

trazodone + pergolide   Co-administration has been used to treat patients refractory to traz-

odone alone. Response is usually rapid (within a week) and without incremental improvement over the next month. Some patients tolerate the combination well; others develop nausea and vomiting that may or may not respond to lowering pergolide dose (Bouckoms A, Mangini L. Pergolide: an antidepressant adjuvant for mood disorders. *Psychopharmacol Bull* 1993;29:207–211).

trazodone + phenytoin   Co-administration may raise phenytoin serum levels by as much as 50%, increasing the risk of adverse phenytoin effects (Dorn JM. A case of phenytoin toxicity precipitated by trazodone. *J Clin Psychiatry* 1986;47:P89–P90).

trazodone/pregnancy   There are no controlled studies documenting safety during pregnancy. Until more data are available, trazodone should not be prescribed for pregnant or nursing women if at all possible.

trazodone/screaming   Trazodone (TRA) has been reported to produce improvement in a demented elderly woman with repetitive screaming and head banging (Greenwald BS, Marin DB, Silverman SM. Serotonergic treatment of screaming and banging in dementia. *Lancet* 1986;1:464–465). TRA alleviated continuous repetitive screaming in an 84-year-old mentally retarded woman who would scream 10–12 hours each day, often until exhausted and soaked with sweat. Her screaming lasted 10–30 seconds, with gasps for breath between each scream. TRA was gradually escalated over 2 weeks to 300 mg/day with no significant adverse effects. Two weeks after starting her on TRA, the screaming stopped and verbal outbursts were limited to intermittent calls for assistance. One-year follow-up showed no return of screaming with a dosage of 300 mg/day (Pasion RC, Kirby SG. Trazodone for screaming. *Lancet* 1993;341:970).

trazodone/seizures   Trazodone overdose may be associated with seizures in patients with a history of epilepsy, neurological disease, or an abnormal electroencephalogram (EEG) (Lefkowitz D, Kilgo G, Lee S. Seizures and trazodone therapy. *Arch Gen Psychiatry* 1985;42: 523). There is one report of a trazodone-associated seizure in a patient with no history of seizures (Himmelhoch JJ. Cardiovascular effects of trazodone in humans. *J Clin Psychopharmacol* 1981;1:76S–81S).

trazodone + sertraline   Low-dose trazodone (25–50 mg) has been added at bedtime for sertraline-treated patients with pressor test pretreatment insomnia. The regimen has been safe and effective (Kline NA, Dow BM, Brown SA, Matloff JL. Sertraline efficacy in depressed combat veterans with posttraumatic stress disorder. Presented at the Annual Meeting of the American Psychiatric Association, San Francisco, May 1993).

trazodone + triiodothyronine (T₃) T_3 (25 µg/day) has been reported to augment trazodone's antidepressant effect, possibly because of stimulation of trazodone's weak noradrenergic effects or facilitation of the hypothalamic-pituitary-thyroid axis (Browne JL, Rice JL, Rice DL, et al. Triiodothyronine augmentation of the antidepressant effect of the nontricyclic antidepressant trazodone. *J Nerv Ment Dis* 1990;178:598–599).

trazodone + tryptophan Co-administration may cause the serotonin syndrome (Patterson BD, Srisopark MM. Severe anorexia and possible psychosis or hypomania after trazodone-tryptophan treatment of aggression. *Lancet* 1989; 1:1017). See **serotonin syndrome.**

trazodone + warfarin In a warfarin-treated patient, a significant decrease in prothrombin time and partial prothrombin time occurred after trazodone was started, necessitating an increased warfarin dose. Warfarin requirements decreased after trazodone discontinuation (Hardy JL, Sirois A. Reduction of prothrombin and partial prothrombin times with trazodone. *Can Med Assoc J* 1986;135:1372). Combined use also results in decreased anticoagulant effect.

treatment adherence Suggested replacement for the term *compliance*, since it implies a voluntary effort by the individual to adhere to the prescribed treatment regimen.

treatment emergent events See **side effects; treatment emergent signs and symptoms.**

treatment-emergent signs and symptoms (TESS) Any events during treatment that are new or worsened compared to the baseline period. Whenever TESS are discussed, it is very important to remember that many symptoms during treatment can emerge spontaneously and can be unrelated to ongoing drug therapy. TESS are best determined in placebo-controlled studies. Also called "side effects."

treatment outcome prospective study (TOPS) Major treatment evaluation research effort from 1979 to the early 1980s supported by the U.S. government. TOPS collected a broad array of data on more than 11,000 patients undergoing various forms of drug abuse treatment.

treatment resistance Characteristic of a patient who, despite compliance, fails to respond to adequate therapeutic intervention with known therapeutic doses of a drug administered for the usual period established for the drug to ordinarily be therapeutically effective.

treatment-resistant depression See **depression, treatment-resistant.**

treatment-resistant depression/reserpine See **depression, treatment-resistant/reserpine.**

treatment response Outcome during the course of a therapeutic regimen. To avert an erroneous conclusion about the cause of a treatment response, the term must be qualified by the fact that this outcome encompasses spontaneous remission and placebo response as well as a more specific response to an active treatment. Failure to achieve a treatment response to the first treatment modality for a depressive episode after an appropriately maximal trial (e.g., 6–8 weeks for pharmacotherapy and 12–16 weeks for psychotherapy) should prompt the clinician to consider an alternative treatment.

treatment threshold In diagnostic testing, point at which the decision is to treat the patient without first performing a diagnostic test.

treatment use investigational new drug (IND) Mechanism by which a physician, under an IND, can use an unapproved new drug product in a desperately ill patient. It provides accessibility to promising drugs prior to completion of more formal studies necessary to obtain marketing approval.

Tremen See **trihexyphenidyl.**

tremor Regular, rhythmic movement of a body part resulting from contractions of agonist and antagonist muscles. Usual frequency is 3–12 Hz/second. It occurs most often in the fingers, toes, head, and tongue. Tremors may be classified into fine and coarse types, tremors at rest, postural tremors, kinetic tremors, task-specific tremors, and hysterical tremors. Fine tremors may be a manifestation of an anxiety state, alcohol withdrawal, thyrotoxicosis, or lithium therapy. Coarse tremors may be either static or active. The former occurs when the affected part is at rest; the latter occurs during voluntary movements. Tremor often accompanies dystonia, improvement in which is often associated with an improvement in the tremor. In patients with disabling tremors of the head, neck, and hand, treatment with botulinum toxin results in a marked to moderate functional improvement and a reduction in the amplitude of the tremor in 67% of patients.

tremor, essential Tremor that often occurs in families as an autosomal dominant trait. Frequency ranges from about 4 to 9 Hz. It may occur in childhood or late in life and typically runs a slowly progressive course. It is usually postural, but in some patients it increases with kinetic movement. When primarily associated with kinetic movement, it is called "essential intentional tremor." It rarely persists at rest. Although all parts of the body can be affected, it most commonly occurs in the distal upper extremities. Individual fingers can be affected; side-to-side finger tremor is characteristic. The head can be affected, with flexion and extension or rotational movements. The vocal tract can be affected, giving a tremorous quality to the voice. Essential tremor interferes with daily activities (shaving, cutting food, drinking from a cup, using tools or utensils). Alcohol is very effective in suppressing essential tremor, but it worsens when the alcohol wears off. Beta-blockers (e.g., propranolol 60–240 mg/day) are beneficial in about 70% of cases. Metoprolol, a relatively selective beta-blocker, is sometimes useful in patients with concomitant pulmonary disease that contraindicates use of propranolol. Other effective treatments include phenobarbital and primidone (Mysoline). Diazepam, chlordiazepoxide, and antiparkinson agents are generally worthless.

tremor, flapping See **asterixis.**

tremor, hysterical Tremor can be a conversion symptom. Hysterical tremor can take many forms, but most common are tremors with movement. Tremors may be of irregular frequency or variable intensity and may have a tendency to diminish or disappear when the patient's attention is distracted. Distinguishing features of hysterical tremor are (a) tremor is often not sustained at a fixed frequency; (b) behavioral characteristics may change from moment to moment; (c) distraction of the patient's attention may result in abrupt suppression of the tremor; and (d) performance of a manual task with one hand may suppress tremor in the other.

tremor, initial See **tremor, movement.**

tremor, intention Large-amplitude, low-frequency tremor at the termination of goal-directed movement seen in cerebellar disease. It is absent at rest and during the first parts of a voluntary movement (the term *intention tremor* can be misleading since any form of muscular activity is intentional). Frequency is not finely tuned, and amplitude varies greatly. Intention tremor sometimes occurs as a toxic manifestation of alcohol or drugs such as phenytoin or divalproex. There is no satisfactory pharmacological treatment because of other neurological disorders.

tremor, kinetic Tremor characterized by rhythmic oscillations about the target. Amplitude may increase as the target is approached, but once it is attained, the tremor will cease. Postural tremor continues once the target is reached if posture is maintained on the target. Frequency varies from about 3 to 5 Hz. Kinetic tremor without postural tremor is usually ascribed to cerebellar dysfunction.

tremor, movement Tremor provoked by any form of movement. It may occur at movement initiation (initial tremor), during movement (transitional tremor), or at movement termination (terminal tremor). It may only become apparent or exacerbated during one of these phases. Also called "initial tremor."

tremor, orthostatic Rapid tremor of the legs and trunk that appears only on standing and is alleviated or abolished by walking or leaning against support. It is not known whether it is a distinct entity or a variant of benign essential tremor. Support for the suggestion that orthostatic tremor is separate from essential tremor includes lack of (a) family history; (b) response to alcohol or beta-blockers; and (c) tremor in other limbs. Orthostatic tremor is benefited by treatment with clonazepam and phenobarbital (Heilman KM. Orthostatic tremor. *Arch Neurol* 1984;41:880–881).

tremor, parkinsonian Patients with parkinsonism can have tremor with movement, or tremor at rest. The latter is more specific. It can involve all parts of the body and be markedly asymmetrical, but it is most typical with a flexion-extension movement at the elbow, pronation and supination of the forearm, and movements of the thumb across the fingers ("pill rolling"). Frequency is usually 4–5 Hz, but ranges from 3 to 7 Hz. Tremor typically disappears with onset of movement but, later in the course of the disease, may return with maintained posture. The tremor usually improves with the dopaminergic therapy given for Parkinson's disease. When the tremor is isolated or refractory to dopaminergic agents, anticholinergic therapy should be considered.

tremor, physiological Tremor that normally occurs with the attempt to maintain a posture. In certain circumstances and with specific drugs, it increases and becomes symptomatic, resulting in a condition known as "exaggerated physiological tremor." In the hands, frequency is 8–12 Hz, but may be as slow as 6.5 Hz in other parts of the body. It can be treated either by removing the precipitating cause or by low doses of a beta-adrenergic blocker such as propranolol.

tremor, posttraumatic Late consequence of severe head trauma, usually appearing a few months after the event. Frequency ranges from 4 to 6 Hz. Tremor is typically proximal, may worsen with kinetic movement, and resembles severe cerebellar postural tremor. Tremor resembling essential tremor can result from mild head trauma and may respond to clonazepam or propranolol.

tremor, postural Tremor provoked predominantly by maintenance of a posture. It is characterized by rapid, low-amplitude oscillations that are made worse with action or holding a posture. It can be caused by drugs that drive central beta-adrenergic receptors (e.g., caffeine, lithium, exogenous thyroid, tricyclic antidepressants, theophylline, and beta-adrenergic agonists) It can be treated with beta-adrenergic antagonists such as propranolol therapy. Also called "action tremor"; "essential tremor"; "familial tremor"; "senile tremor." See **tremor, essential.**

tremor, primary writing Prototype of task-specific tremors that appears only with handwriting or a few other skilled manual tasks, but not with all skilled tasks; often misdiagnosed as essential tremor. It is not produced by posture or goal-directed movement in general. It is asymmetrical and often focal. It responds to anticholinergic agents, alcohol, and beta-blockers.

tremor, rest Tremor most commonly encountered in Parkinson's disease that is often complex, involving several muscle groups and producing oscillation at more than one joint (e.g., the classic pill-rolling of parkinsonism). It typically disappears with the intention to move and during the movement itself, but may become re-established with maintenance of posture. Neuroleptics may produce a rest tremor similar to that seen in Parkinson's disease, though more often, an action tremor is produced.

tremor, task-specific Tremor appearing only with specific tasks. It is similar to both essential tremor and writer's cramp. The tremor responds favorably to anticholinergic agents, alcohol, or beta-blockers. See **tremor, primary writing.**

tremor, terminal See **tremor, movement.**

tremor, transitional See **tremor, movement.**

trend Long-term movement in an ordered series (e.g., a time series). An essential feature is that the movement, although possibly irregular in the short term, is consistently in the same direction over the long term. Movement also loosely refers to an association that is consistent in several samples or strata, but is not statistically significant.

trend, temporal In epidemiology, variation in rate (age, period, cohort trends) over time. Age trends refer to changes in age-specific rates of illness, usually the age at first onset of the disorder. Period trends refer to changes in the rates of illness associated with a demarcated period. Cohort trends refer to changes in rates of illness among individuals who are defined by some shared, continual temporal experience, usually the year or decade of birth.

Trental See **pentoxifylline.**

Trexan See **naltrexone.**

TRH See **thyrotropin-releasing hormone.**

Triadapin See **doxepin.**

triage Process of screening patients to determine relative treatment priority. Often patients are divided into three groups: (a) those not expected to survive even with treatment; (b) those who will recover without treatment; and (c) the highest-priority group, those who need treatment for survival.

trial An experiment involving humans; replication of an experiment, commonly called a "clinical trial."

trial, clinical See **clinical trial.**

Trialodine See **trazodone.**

trial, open-label Trial in which both the investigator(s) and the patient(s) know the identity of the treatment.

triamterene/hydrochlorothiazide (Dyazide) Diuretic/antihypertensive drug product combining natriuretic and antikaliuretic effects that can be administered once daily. Each component compliments the action of the other.

triamterine + lithium See **lithium + triamterene.**

Triavil See **amitriptyline + perphenazine.**

triazolam (Halcion; Novodorm) (TZL) High-potency, low-dose triazolobenzodiazepine hypnotic with half-life (including metabolites) of 1.5–5 hours. It has a very rapid absorption phase followed by a rapid elimination phase. In humans, it is metabolized by hepatic oxidation to two major hydroxylated metabolites, alpha-hydroxytriazolam and 4-hydroxytriazolam, that are rapidly glucuronidated and excreted in the urine. TZL has potent affinity for the benzodiazepine receptor and can have pharmacological effects at a very low level that is difficult to detect by the conventional chemical method. However, TZL can be measured in serum by radioreceptor assay, which indicates total benzodiazepine receptor binding activity. Present data show that TZL kinetics are affected by age, which affects the drug's metabolic pathway and not its half-life. Central nervous system sensitivity to benzodiazepines, including TZL, increases in the elderly. TZL accumulation in the elderly after prolonged use has been reported. Of all benzodiazepine hypnotics, it produces, by far, the greatest degree of memory impairment and episodes of anterograde amnesia. Schedule IV; pregnancy risk category X.

triazolam + alcohol There is a paucity of data on any interaction between triazolam and alcohol. Nevertheless, it is prudent to assume that their co-consumption would have some additive effect, a fact about which patients should be warned, especially when they drive or operate dangerous machinery. Triazolam combined with alcohol may increase the likelihood of "blackouts" with smaller amounts of alcohol than are usually required (Morris HH, Estes ML. Traveler's amnesia. *JAMA* 1987;258: 945–946).

triazolam/anterograde amnesia Nocturnal motor behavior, anxiety, and suicidal ideation followed by amnesia regarding the incidents are reported in 22 of 44 psychiatric patients taking triazolam (2 mg at night) for 1–19 days for insomnia. Most common occurrence was nocturnal bulimia in 13 patients, with other motor behaviors observed in another 6. Six patients expressed anxiety with typical panic attacks; 5 expressed suicidal ideation, 4 of whom made suicide attempts. None of the patients recalled the events during an interview the next morning. The adverse events stopped in 21 patients when triazolam was stopped. Dosage given was much higher than that currently recommended; the report indicates that dosage is a crucial factor in the incidence of amnestic reactions (Anssequ M, Poncelet PF, Schmitz D. High dose triazolam and anterograde amnesia. *Br Med J* 1992;304: 1178).

triazolam/breast milk Not studied in humans; animal studies (rats) indicate triazolam and its metabolites are excreted in milk. Administration of triazolam to nursing mothers is not recommended.

triazolam + cimetidine Co-administration decreases triazolam hydroxylation, which decreases its clearance and increases its serum concentration (Abernethy DR, Greenblatt DJ, Divoll M, et al. Interaction of cimetidine with the triazolobenzodiazepines alprazolam and triazolam. *Psychopharmacology* 1983;80:275–278).

triazolam + fluoxetine No pharmacokinetic interactions occur (Wright CE, Lasher-Sisson TA, Steenwyck RC, Swanson CN. Pharmacokinetic evaluation of the combined administration of triazolam and fluoxetine. *Pharmacotherapy* 1992;12:103–106).

triazolam/pregnancy It is not known whether triazolam has teratogenic effects. Prescription during any stage of pregnancy is not recommended. Transplacental distribution may occur following ingestion of therapeutic doses during the last weeks of pregnancy, resulting in neonatal central nervous system depression.

triazolam + ranitidine Ranitidine significantly increases the area under the serum drug concentration-time curve of oral triazolam. Ranitidine pretreatment has no effect on triazolam's terminal disposition rate constant or on the time to reach maximum serum triazolam concentration. Ranitidine pretreatment increases systemic availability of triazolam by increasing its absorption.

triazolobenzodiazepine One of a group of benzodiazepines (BZDs) that differ structurally from the classic 1,4-benzodiazepines (e.g., diazepam) in that the triazolo ring is incorporated into the benzodiazepine nucleus, resulting in more rapid clearance, decreased half-life elimination, and shorter duration of action. The triazolobenzodiazepine family consists of alprazolam, its demethylamino derivative adinazolam, triazolam, and the investigational compound U-43,465. Triazolobenzodiazepines have high affinity for the BZD receptor. Alprazolam and adinazolam are anxiolytic, antipanic, and possibly antidepressant. Triazolam is primarily a hypnotic. U-43,465 is being investigated as an anxiolytic and antipanic drug.

tribulin Endogenous monoamine oxidase inhibitor (EMAOI) of indole origin that was isolated from human urine by Sandler and his colleagues. It is a relatively low-molecular-weight compound with acidic or neutral properties. Tribulin excretion increases following stress and in anxiety states and agitation. It has been found to inhibit binding of benzodiazepines to their binding sites. It may be related to the endogenous anxiogenic factor and structurally related to the beta-carbolines (Sandler M. The emergence of tribulin. *Trends in Pharmacological Sciences* 1982;3:471–472).

trichloroethanol (TCE) Pharmacologically active metabolite of all chloral derivatives. It is detoxified to trichloroacetic acid (TCA), which is tightly protein-bound and can displace other drugs bound to serum albumin. TCE is an active sedative hypnotic. Half-life is 6–10 hours.

trichloroethylene Inhalant anesthetic abused by habitual abusers of volatile solvents and sometimes by medical personnel who have access to it. It is usually sniffed, which can produce cardiac arrhythmias, myocarditis, and heart failure.

trichophagia Hair eating; an activity often engaged in by trichotillomania patients. It may cause significant medical complications.

trichotillomania Disorder characterized by impulses to pull out one's hair; listed in DSM-IV under *Impulse Control Disorders Not Elsewhere Classified*. Numerous controversies exist on how best to classify it. Some clinicians believe it is a variant of obsessive compulsive disorder because of similarities in phenomenology, family history, and response to treatment. Originally thought to occur more frequently in females, it is now known to affect males as often. Latest prevalence estimate is 2% (Swedo SE, Rapoport JL. Annotation: trichotillomania. *J Child Psychol Psychiatry* 1991;32:401–409). Two types have been identified. One often begins in adolescence, is associated with greater psychopathology (Orange J, Peereboom-Wynia J, De Raeymaeker K. Trichotillomania in childhood. *J Am Acad Dermatol* 1986; 15:614–619), and has been described as an impulse-control disorder or obsessive-compulsive disorder (George MS, Brewerton TD, Chochrane C. Trichotillomania (hair pulling). *N Engl J Med* 1990;322:470–471). The other typically begins in preschool years, is generally considered benign, and has been described as a habit disorder (Watson TS, Allen KD. Elimination of thumb-sucking as a treatment for severe trichotillomania. *J Am Acad Child Adolesc Psychiatry* 1993;32:830–834). Trichotillomania often involves multiple hair sites; most common are scalp, eyebrows, and eyelashes. Others include pubic, axillary, chest, and rectal areas. Many patients have histories beginning in childhood with refractoriness to all attempted remedies. Co-morbidity of trichotillomania with affective, anxiety, substance abuse, and eating disorders is common. It also may co-exist with mental retardation and psychotic disorders. Currently, all treatments are considered experimental, including pharmacological interventions, behavior therapies, hypnosis, 12-step programs, psychoanalysis, and intensive psychotherapy. Pharmacotherapy is considered preferable. Clomipramine and fluoxetine may reduce frequency and intensity of the disorder. In addition, clomipramine and a topical steroid have been reported effective (Black DW, Blum N. Trichotillomania treated with clomipramine and a topical steroid. *Am J Psychiatry* 1992;149: 842–843; Gupta S, Freimer M. Trichotillomania, clomipramine, topical steroids. *Am J Psychiatry* 1993;150:524). An effective adjunctive agent in some cases of obsessive-compulsive disorder, fenfluramine also may be effective in the treatment of trichotillomania (Judd FK, Chua P, Lynch C, et al. Fenfluramine augmentation of clomipramine treatment of obsessive-compulsive disorder. *Aust N Z J Psychiatry* 1991;25:412–414; Mahr G. Fenfluramine and trichotillomania. *Psychosomatics* 1993;34:284). Lithium has been reported to lead to decreased hair-pulling and mild to marked hair regrowth. For children, such treatments should be reserved for severe refractory forms of trichotillomania. Cases responsive to a monoamine oxidase inhibitor, tricyclic antidepressants, or trazodone have been reported (Sunkureddi K, Markovitz P. Trazodone treatment of obsessive-compulsive disorder and trichotillomania. *Am J Psychiatry* 1993;150:523–524). Relapse after initial improvement has also been reported. Behavioral techniques are considered a second choice when drug therapy is ineffective or has bothersome side

effects. Follow-up has indicated a 40% (moderate) reduction in symptom severity. Interim treatments included psychotherapy, behavior therapy, and a variety of medications (alone or in combination with other drugs). Adverse effects during drug therapy included weight gain, dry mouth, and sedation. No subject reported reduced sexual response. These results suggest that pharmacotherapy with serotonin reuptake blockers may be of long-term benefit to some patients (Swedo SE, Leonard HL, Rapoport JL, et al. A double-blind comparison of clomipramine and desipramine in the treatment of trichotillomania [hair pulling]. *N Engl J Med* 1989;321:497–501; Swedo SE, Lenane MC, Leonard HL. Long-term treatment of trichotillomania [hair pulling]. *N Engl J Med* 1993;329:141–142). A combination of drug treatment and behavior therapy may provide maximal benefit (Swedo SE, Leonard HL. Trichotillomania: an obsessive compulsive spectrum disorder? *Psychiatr Clin North Am* 1992;15:777–790).

triclofos　(Tricloryl; Triclos) Sedative/hypnotic agent with actions similar to those of chloral hydrate. Not marketed in the United States.

Tricloryl　See **triclofos.**

Triclos　See **triclofos.**

tricyclic antidepressant　(TAD, TCA) One of a group of antidepressants classified as tricyclic because of their structure. TCAs were the first heterocyclic antidepressants. They are subdivided into tertiary amines (imipramine, amitriptyline, trimipramine, and doxepin) and secondary amines (desipramine, nortriptyline, protriptyline). All inhibit neuronal uptake of norepinephrine to varying degrees. They are broad-spectrum antidepressants effective across a wide range of depressions. They are indicated in the presence of an established depressive syndrome of all but very mild severity. They also have uses beyond depression, including treatment of post-traumatic stress disorder, panic disorders, obsessive-compulsive disorder, pain, enuresis, and leishmaniasis.

tricyclic antidepressant + alcohol　Co-consumption can enhance sedation and impair psychomotor skills and other tricyclic antidepressant (TCA) central nervous system effects. Synergistic effects are more pronounced with the more sedative TCAs (e.g., amitriptyline). Chronic alcohol use increases TCA metabolism, reducing its therapeutic efficacy.

tricyclic antidepressant + amphetamine　Coadministration may produce therapeutic effects, but because of release of norepinephrine may also potentiate cardiovascular effects including arrhythmias, tachycardia, severe hypertension, or hyperpyrexia.

tricyclic antidepressant + antiarrhythmic Tricyclics have additive effects with quinidine and other antiarrhythmics.

tricyclic antidepressant/anticholinergic effects All have anticholinergic effects (dry mouth, visual disturbances, constipation, delayed micturition, and other atropine-like effects) due to their antimuscarinic properties. Thus, administration may be hazardous for patients with untreated glaucoma, intestinal sluggishness, and prostate hypertrophy.

tricyclic antidepressant + antihistamine Tricyclics have additive effects with antihistamines such as diphenhydramine, resulting in more sedation and more anticholinergic effects.

tricyclic antidepressant + antipsychotic See **tricyclic antidepressant + neuroleptic.**

tricyclic antidepressant + barbiturate Barbiturates effectively lower tricyclic antidepressant plasma levels (Alexanderson B, Price-Evans DA, Sjoqvist F. Steady-state plasma levels of nortriptyline in twins: influence of genetic factors and drug therapy. *Br Med J* 1969;4:764–768).

tricyclic antidepressant + carbamazepine Carbamazepine (CBZ) induces metabolism of tricyclic antidepressants (TCAs), resulting in lower plasma levels and possible depressive relapse (Preskorn SH, Burke MJ, Fast GA. Therapeutic drug monitoring: principles and practice. *Psychiatr Clin North Am* 1993;16:611–645). If patients fail to respond to standard TCA doses or develop adverse effects, CBZ, TCA, and TCA metabolite levels should be checked (De la Fuente JM. Carbamazepine-induced low plasma levels of tricyclic antidepressants. *J Clin Psychopharmacol* 1992;12:67–68).

tricyclic antidepressant/cardiovascular effects These are among the more frequent and potentially more serious adverse effects of tricyclic antidepressants (TCAs), especially in the elderly and patients with pre-existing cardiac disease. They include orthostatic (postural) hypotension due to blockade of alpha$_1$ adrenoceptors, cardiac arrhythmias, and exacerbation of pre-existing arrythmias and heartblock. Sudden death has occurred in patients treated with a TCA. Adverse cardiovascular effects are dose-related; they may occur with therapeutic doses, but more often with doses above the drugs' usual maximum therapeutic dose. TCA overdoses are often fatal because of the cardiotoxic effects. Risk of cardiac arrhythmia may persist for several days after a patient has recovered from a TCA overdose, even though drug plasma levels have dropped into the therapeutic range.

tricyclic antidepressant + chlorpromazine Co-administration may elevate chlorpromazine plasma levels and tricyclic antidepressant plasma concentration, causing additive anticholinergic effects and excessive sedation.

tricyclic antidepressant + clozapine Co-administration may increase incidence of delirium, possibly because of additive central cholinergic activity. Agranulocytosis has been reported (Grohmans R, Schmidt LG, Spieb-Kiefer C, Ruther E. Agranulocytosis and significant leukopenia with neuroleptic drugs. Results from the AMUP program. *Psychopharmacology* 1989;99:109–112).

tricyclic antidepressant + disulfiram Co-administration decreases TCA clearance, necessitating reduced TCA dosage to prevent toxicity.

tricyclic antidepressant + electroconvulsive therapy (ECT) Although there is hope that a beneficial additive or synergistic effect could lead to faster, more complete recovery, co-administration could result in adverse interactions, mainly cardiovascular, between a tricyclic antidepressant and ECT or anesthetic agents used during ECT. Most experts recommend that antidepressants be stopped prior to ECT (American Psychiatric Association Task Force on Electroconvulsive Therapy. *The Practice of Electroconvulsive Therapy: Recommendations for Treatment, Training, and Privileging.* Washington, DC: American Psychiatric Press, 1990).

tricyclic antidepressant + fluoxetine Co-administration may benefit patients unresponsive to either drug alone (Weillburg JG, Rosenbaum JF, Biedermann J, et al. Fluoxetine added to non-MAOI antidepressants converts non-responders to responders: a preliminary report. *J Clin Psychiatry* 1989;50:447–449). Fluoxetine (FLX) inhibits hepatic metabolism of tricyclic antidepressants (TCAs) and may cause a twofold increase in TCA plasma level. If a TCA overdose is taken by an FLX-treated patient, side effects are consistent with TCA toxicity (Bergstrom RF, Peyton AL, Lemberger L. Quantification and mechanism of fluoxetine and tricyclic antidepressant interaction. *Clin Pharm Ther* 1992;51:239–248). FLX also can prolong TCA elimination so that TCA levels may remain elevated for a prolonged period following overdose. Recent treatment with FLX may significantly influence metabolism of subsequently prescribed TCAs, requiring dosage adjustments over time to establish and maintain TCA therapeutic levels and clinical response. It has been suggested that TCA dosage should be reduced by 75% when FLX is added and that about 3 months must be allowed for a new steady-state TCA blood concentration to be reached. Co-administration without monitoring TCA plasma levels may be associated with more side effects and/or poor response. TCA levels may fall as FLX's inhibition of TCA metabolism dissipates; thus, TCA dosage may need to be increased to maintain therapeutic plasma levels and achieve clinical response. Failure to increase TCA dosage may lead to some patients being falsely labeled as TCA nonresponders (Westermeyer J. Fluoxetine-induced tricyclic toxicity: extent and duration. *J Clin Pharmacol* 1991;31: 388–392; Suckow RF, Roose SP, Cooper TB. Effect of fluoxetine on plasma desipramine and 2-hydroxydesipramine. *Biol Psychiatry* 1992;31:200–204).

tricyclic antidepressant + fluvoxamine Fluvoxamine can increase previously stable tricyclic antidepressant plasma levels (Bertschy G, Vandel S, Vandek B, et al. Fluvoxamine-tricyclic antidepressant interactions: an accidental finding. *Eur J Clin Pharmacol* 1991;40:119–120).

tricyclic antidepressant + guanfacine The antihypertensive effect of guanfacine may be inhibited by tricyclic antidepressants (Buckley M, Feely J. Antagonism of antihypertensive effect of guanfacine by tricyclic antidepressants. *Lancet* 1991;337:1173–1174).

tricyclic antidepressant/high-fiber diet Three patients treated with tricyclic antidepressants (two with doxepin, one with desipramine) reportedly became refractory after eating a high-fiber diet. The diet resulted in decreased serum antidepressant levels. When fiber was reduced, there was improvement in depression and a concomitant rise in serum tricyclic levels (Stewart DE. High-fiber diet and serum tricyclic antidepressant levels. *J Clin Psychopharmacol* 1992;12:438–440).

tricyclic antidepressant + lithium Co-administration has been used successfully in treatment-resistant depression (Schou M. Lithium and treatment-resistant depression. A review. *Lithium* 1990;1:3–8). It may decrease the metabolism of each drug, resulting in increased plasma concentrations of both. Central nervous system depressant and hypotensive effects may be additive. Addition of lithium to TCAs may cause emergence or exacerbation of myoclonus (Devanand DP, Sackeim HA, Brown RP. Myoclonus during combined tricyclic antidepressant and lithium treatment. *J Clin Psychopharmacol* 1988;8:446–447). A comparison of electroconvulsive therapy (ECT) with a combination of lithium and a TCA in depressed tricyclic nonresponders showed that lithium augmentation is comparable with ECT in severely depressed patients (Dinan TG, Barry S. A comparison of electroconvulsive therapy with a combined lithium and tricyclic combination among depressed tricyclic nonresponders. *Acta Psychiatr Scand* 1989; 80:97–100).

tricyclic antidepressant + moclobemide Co-administration is associated with minimal risk of adverse drug-drug interactions (Korn A, Eichler HG, Fischbach R, Gasic S. Moclobemide, a new reversible MAO inhibitor—interaction with tyramine and tricyclic antidepressants in healthy volunteers and depressive patients. *Psychopharmacology* 1986;88:153–157; Carl G, Laux G. Moclobemide in long-term treatment of depression. *Psychiatr Prac* 1990; 17:26–29).

tricyclic antidepressant + monoamine oxidase inhibitor (MAOI) Since 1966, several thousand patients with mixed depression, anxiety, phobic, and somatic symptoms not relieved by other therapies have been treated successfully with combined tricyclic-MAOI therapy. Candidates are depressed/anxious patients of good previous personality who, regardless of age, sex, or severity and duration of illness, are not and never have been psychotic; do not have symptoms of a classic endogenous depression; have never had a hypomanic or manic episode; have not responded to or possibly have been made worse by separate, adequate trials of a tricyclic, MAOI, or electroconvulsive therapy (ECT); refuse or have a physical contraindication to ECT or to very high doses of a tricyclic or MAOI; have not benefited from prophylactic lithium therapy for depression; have considerable overt anxiety not relieved substantially by a benzodiazepine alone or in combination with an MAOI or beta-blocker; are not a serious suicidal risk; and are likely to adhere faithfully to dietary and other precautions while taking an MAOI. Most side effects are mild and usually can be relieved by dosage reduction of one or both drugs. Speed of improvement and individual dosage requirements are unpredictable; some patients respond in a few days to low doses, but most require weeks of the usual therapeutic dosages, and some may require even higher dosages to achieve benefit. Medications should not be stopped as soon as improvement occurs; they should be continued for some weeks thereafter and then gradually withdrawn. Some patients relapse unless kept on maintenance therapy. Before treatment is started, patients and responsible relatives should receive clear, firm instructions about dietary and other precautions, which should be explicit but not too stringent (Stewart MM. MAOIs and food: fact and fiction. *Adverse Drug Reaction Bull* 1976;58:200–203). They should be told to inform any physician, dentist, or pharmacist whose services may be required that the patient is taking an MAOI to obviate any potential adverse drug-drug interaction. They should receive an explanation of expected and infrequent side effects and what should be done if they occur.

tricyclic antidepressant + morphine Tricyclics may exaggerate and prolong morphine's central nervous system depressant effects.

tricyclic antidepressant/neonatal withdrawal Tricyclics cross the placenta and accumulate in the fetus, setting the stage for neonatal withdrawal shortly after birth. Symptoms include tachypnea, tachycardia, cyanosis, irritability, diaphoresis, hypertonia, tremor, clonus, spasm, and seizures (Webster PAC. Withdrawal symptoms in neonates associated with maternal antidepressant therapy. *Lancet* 1973;2:318–319; Calabrese JR, Gulledge AD. Psychotropics during pregnancy and lactation: a review. *Psychosomatics* 1985;26:413–426).

tricyclic antidepressant + neuroleptic Co-administration may decrease the metabolism of each drug, resulting in increased plasma concentrations of both. Anticholinergic, central nervous system depressant, and hypotensive effects of the drugs may be additive (Gram LF, Overo KF, Kirk L. Influence of neuroleptics and benzodiazepines on metabolism in tricyclic antidepressants in man. *Am J Psychiatry* 1974;131:863–866).

tricyclic antidepressant + neuroleptic + lithium Several case reports indicate that lithium may potentiate response to tricyclic/neuroleptic therapy failures (Nelson JC, Maguire CM. Lithium augmentation in psychotic depressions refractory to combined drug therapy. *Am J Psychiatry* 1986;143:363–366; Pai M, White AC, Deane AG. Lithium augmentation in the treatment of delusional depression. *Br J Psychiatry* 1986;148:736–738; Price LH, Yeates C, Nelson JC. Lithium augmentation of combined neuroleptic-tricyclic therapy in delusional depression. *Am J Psychiatry* 1983;140:318–322).

tricyclic antidepressant/overdose Tricyclic antidepressant (TCA) overdose affects the heart, respiratory system, and parasympathetic and central nervous systems. Parasympathetic effects include dry mouth, blurred vision, dilated pupils, constipation, retention of urine, and pyrexia. They are most common in mild poisoning, but may be absent in severe poisoning. Central nervous system complications include agitation and delirium (which may be particularly troublesome on recovery from the overdose), muscle twitching, convulsions (patients may present in status epilepticus), hallucinations, both pyramidal and, less frequently, extrapyramidal neurological signs, and varying degrees of coma ranging from mild drowsiness to total unresponsiveness. Respiratory effects include respiratory depression and aspiration of stomach contents lead-ing to pneumonitis, intrapulmonary shunts, shock lung, and apnea, which in severe poisoning may be sudden. In serious poisoning, TCAs have exactly the same effect on respiration as do barbiturates. Cardiac complications have attracted the most attention from clinical investigators. There is usually sinus tachycardia, but in severe poisoning, the heart rate may be normal or slow. All manner of arrhythmias have been described. Blood pressure may be slightly raised in mild poisoning, but is usually low in severe poisoning. On the electrocardiogram (ECG), both the PR and QRS intervals become progressively longer. The P wave decreases in size, and the ECG may resemble either a supraventricular or a ventricular arrhythmia. In massive poisoning, there may be atrioventricular block. The pharmacological basis of TCA cardiotoxicity is complex. Initially, it was believed that ECG changes are due to anticholinergic effects and potentiation of circulating catecholamines. It is now believed that the most important factor is the quinidine-like or membrane-stabilizing properties of the TCAs (Crome P. Antidepressant poisoning. *Acta Psychiatry Scand* 1983; [suppl 302]:95–101).

tricyclic antidepressant + paroxetine Paroxetine, a potent inhibitor of the CYP450IID6 isoenzyme in the liver responsible for metabolism of drugs such as tricyclic antidepressants (TCAs), may increase TCA plasma concentrations (van Harten J. Clinical pharmacokinetics of selective serotonin reuptake inhibitors. *Clin Pharmacokinet* 1991;24:203–220).

tricyclic antidepressant/postmortem pharmacokinetics Postmortem blood values of some drugs may be affected by a phenomenon called "postmortem release" or "redistribution" of drugs. Tricyclic antidepressants (TCAs) have a high protein binding affinity and are stored in specific binding sites in the body. At death, these drugs are released from their antemortem sites because of a variety of mechanisms, including decompensation of circulating proteins and membrane macromolecules that bind drugs, and the destruction of biological membranes that delineate drug compartments in the body. Postmortem release can lead to massive increases (to 150,000 ng/ml or higher) in TCA blood levels during the hours following death, especially if there has been a delay between death and the autopsy. TCA levels rise 2–8 times over the first 15 postmortem hours and continue to rise over at least another 15 hours. The longer the postmortem interval, the greater the difference in the heart/femoral drug concentration ratio (Popper C, Elliott GR. Postmortem pharmacokinetics of tricyclic antidepressants. Are some deaths during treatment misattributed to overdose? *J Child Adolesc Psychopharmacol* 1993;3:x–xii; Apple FS, Brandt CM. Liver and blood postmortem TCA concentrations. *Am J Clin Pathol* 1988;89:794–796; Prouty RW, Anderson WH. The forensic science implications of site and temporal influences on postmortem blood-drug concentrations. *J Forens Sci* 1990;35:243–270). Thus, postmortem drug redistribution can create difficulties in the interpretation of how much drug the decedent took (Hilberg T, Bugge A, Beylich KM, et al. An animal model of postmortem amitriptyline redistribution. *J Forens Sci* 1993;38:81–90). Although postmortem levels greater than 1,000 ng/ml may be viewed as consistent with death secondary to TCA ingestion, pathologists now emphasize that high postmortem blood levels *cannot* be assumed to indicate overdose or even intoxication (Hebb JH, Caplan YH, Crooks CR, Mergner WJ. Blood and tissue concentrations of TCAs in post-mortem cases: literature survey and a study of 40 deaths. *J Anal Toxicol* 1982;6:209–216; Hanzlick RL. Postmortem blood concentrations of parent tricyclic antidepressant [TCA] drugs in 11 cases of suicide. *Am J Forens Med Pathol* 1984;5:11–13; Hanzlick RL. Postmortem tricyclic antidepressant concentrations: lethal vs. nonlethal levels. *Am J Forens Med Pathol* 1989;10:326–329). Following fatal TCA overdose, there are significant differences in TCA levels in the body (Bailey DN, Shaw RF. Tricyclic antidepressants: interpretation of blood and tissue levels in fatal overdose. *J Anal Toxicol* 1979;3:43–46). Release of drug from drug-rich tissue (heart, lung, liver) increases drug concentration in the blood adjacent to the tissue. Blood concentrations in the central vessels (abdominal and thoracic) are much higher (50–60%) than in the peripheral vessels (femoral and subclavial veins); highest concentration is in blood from the pulmonary vein and artery. Drugs with the widest concentration in blood are most highly concentrated in organ tissues, particularly the lungs and liver. This is probably due to (a) postmortem release of drugs from tissue sites of high concentration into blood contained within those tissues or in connecting vessels; (b) drugs concentrated in the lungs being released from organ parenchyma into the pulmonary arterial and venous blood and ultimately to the heart; (c) drugs concentrated in the liver being diffused into the hepatic venous blood and then only a few centimeters into the inferior vena cava in the right atrium of the heart; (d) blood within the aorta having high TCA concentrations because of its intimate relationship to the heart and lungs; and (e) arterial venous differences in drug concentration if death occurs before steady-state has been reached (Jones GR, Pounder DJ. Site dependence of drug concentrations in postmortem blood—a case study. *J Anal Toxicol* 1987;11:186–190). Recent data on postmortem TCA levels and ratios in adults suggest that samples obtained from the liver are more reliable than blood samples for differentiating acute overdose from therapeutic use (Apple FS. Post-mortem TCA concentration: assessing cause of death using parent drug to metabolite ratio. *J Anal Toxicol* 1989;13:197–198). The assumption that postmortem blood concentrations mirror blood concentrations at the time of death cannot be considered valid. Findings of postmortem pharmacokinetics document that there is a risk of attributing the cause of death to overdose (whether acute or chronic, medical or self-inflicted, intentional or accidental) when the culprit may be the toxicity of the drug itself.

tricyclic antidepressant + pimozide Co-administration may result in additive prolongation of the QT interval.

tricyclic antidepressant + prazosin Tricyclics have additive effects with anti–alpha$_1$-adrenergics such as prazosin.

tricyclic antidepressant/seizures All tricyclic antidepressants (TCAs) lower seizure threshold, some more than others. For TCAs as a group, seizure risk is about 1/1,000.

tricyclic antidepressant/teratogenicity No major teratogenic effects have been identified.

tricyclic antidepressant + triiodothyronine (T$_3$) In most, but not all, open and controlled studies, T$_3$ augments response to tricyclic antidepressants (TCAs). Up to 50% of patients who fail to respond to a TCA benefit from addition of T$_3$ (Extein IL, Gold MS. Thyroid hormone potentiation of tricyclic antidepressants. *In* Extein IL [ed], *Treatment of Tricyclic-Resistant Depression.* Washington, DC: American Psychiatric Press, 1989, pp 1–27; Joffe R, Singer W, Levitt AJ, MacDonald C. A placebo-controlled comparison of lithium and triiodothyronine augmentation of tricyclic antidepressants in unipolar refractory depression. *Arch Gen Psychiatry* 1993;50:387–393). Available data indicate that T$_3$ is more effective than thyroxine (T$_4$) in augmenting TCA antidepressant response (Joffe RT, Singer W. Thyroid hormone potentiation of antidepressants. Abstract of paper presented at the 141st Annual Meeting of the American Psychiatric Association, May 1988).

tricyclic antidepressant + trimeprazine Co-administration produces more anticholinergic effects than either drug alone and may result in anticholinergic toxicity.

tricyclic antidepressant + valproic acid Valproic acid inhibits hepatic enzymes and may elevate tricyclic plasma concentrations (Bertschy G, Vandel S, Jounet JM, Allers G. Valpromide-amitriptyline interaction. Increase in the bioavailability of amitriptyline and nortriptyline caused by valpromide. *Encephale* 1990;16:43–45).

tricyclic antidepressant/withdrawal Withdrawal reactions after discontinuation of tricyclic antidepressants (TCAs) have been reported in neonates, children, adolescents, and adults. They usually begin within a day or two after the last dose of an antidepressant that has been taken in low or therapeutic doses for a minimum of 6–8 weeks. The longer the antidepressant has been taken, and the higher its daily dose, the greater the risk of withdrawal phenomena. Onset usually begins by 48 hours after abrupt discontinuation in some, but not all, patients. Symptoms usually subside within 2 weeks, or earlier if the drug is resumed. They include malaise, muscle aches, anergia, sweating, flashes of feeling hot or cold, nausea, vomiting, anorexia, abdominal pains, diarrhea, insomnia, drowsiness, agitation, irritability, apathy, withdrawal, and recurrence of depressed mood or hypomania or mania. There also may be vivid dreams, akathisia, bradykinesia, and cogwheel rigidity. Cardiac arrhythmia has occurred after discontinuation of imipramine, amitriptyline, and clomipramine. Antidepressant and anticholinergic withdrawal symptoms are similar. Withdrawal symptoms may be related to the anticholinergic potency of the tricyclic. Drug discontinuation produces a state of muscarinic receptor supersensitivity resulting in cholinergic overdrive, which can be successfully treated with anticholinergic agents such as atropine (Dilsaver SC, Greden JF, Michael S. Antidepressant withdrawal syndromes: phenomenology and pathophysiology. *Int Clin Psychopharmacol* 1987;2:1–19). Abrupt discontinuation of antidepressant medication can be associated with mood shifts, including the precipitation of mania or hypomania (Ghadirian AM. Paradoxical mood response following antidepressant withdrawal. *Biol Psychiatry* 1986;21:1298–1300). Significant mood shifts to either euthymia or hypomania may occur upon the withdrawal of antidepressant drugs because of lack of efficacy more frequently than upon the withdrawal of placebo. It is important for clinicians and researchers to be aware of this possibility (McGrath PJ, Stewart JW, Tricamo E, et al. Paradoxical mood shifts to euthymia or hypomania upon withdrawal of antidepressant agents. *J Clin Psychopharmacol* 1993;13:224–225). If abrupt tricyclic discontinuation should be necessitated by a switch to hypomania or mania, temporary benztropine therapy should be initiated to minimize risk of abstinence symptoms. All antidepressants should be discontinued by gradual taper whenever possible.

Tridione See **trimethadione.**

trifluoperazine (Apo-Trifluoperazine; Eskazine; Novo-Flurazine; Sedizine; Solazine; Stelazine; Suprazine; Terfluzine) (TFP) Piperazine phenothiazine derivative that is a high-potency neuroleptic. It is a well established, therapeutically effective antipsychotic. It has minimal sedative and hypotensive effects but a high propensity to evoke acute, early onset extrapyramidal reactions and various late-onset extrapyramidal reactions such as tardive dyskinesia and tardive dystonia. It can also induce the neuroleptic malignant syndrome. Pregnancy risk category C.

trifluoperazine + alcohol Trifluoperazine potentiates the central nervous system depressant effects of alcohol; simultaneous consumption may be hazardous.

trifluoperazine + anticoagulant Co-administration may decrease anticoagulant effects.

trifluoperazine/breast milk Trifluoperazine is excreted in breast milk in small quantities that are unlikely to have serious adverse effects on the neonate.

trifluoperazine + clozapine Agranulocytosis has been reported (Adams CE, Riccio M, McCarthy D, et al. Agranulocytosis induced by clozapine with the early addition of trifluoperazine: a case report. *Int Clin Psychopharmacol* 1990;5:287–290).

trifluoperazine + paroxetine See **thioridazine + paroxetine.**

trifluoperazine + tranylcypromine (Jatrosom; Parstelin) Combination product marketed outside the United States as an antidepressant.

trifluperidol (Triperidol) Butyrophenone neuroleptic.

triflupromazine (Vesprin) Aliphatic phenothiazine neuroleptic that, milligram per milligram, is the most potent of the aliphatic phenothiazines. It is an effective antipsychotic and antiemetic. It is quite sedative and hypotensive and slightly more likely than chlorpromazine to induce early and tardive extrapyramidal reactions. Its use has declined since the advent of more potent piperazine phenothiazines and other potent nonphenothiazine neuroleptics.

trigeminal neuralgia Condition characterized by excruciating paroxysmal pain of short duration (15–30 seconds) located in the mandibular branch of the trigeminal nerve (which differentiates it from atypical facial pain), flushing of the face, watering eyes, and rhinorrhea. It is usually unilateral (affecting the fifth cranial nerve), more common after age 40, and more frequent among women. Cause is unknown. Carbamazepine is considered a pharmacological treatment of choice. Baclofen also may be effective. In prolonged episodes, intravenous phenytoin may be warranted. Also called "tic douloureux."

Trihexane   See **trihexyphenidyl.**

Trihexidyl   See **trihexyphenidyl.**

Trihexy-2   See **trihexyphenidyl.**

Trihexy-5   See **trihexyphenidyl.**

trihexyphenidyl   (Aparkane; Apo-Trihex; Artane; Artane Sequels; Benzhexol; Novohexidyl; Partane; Pipanol; Tremen; Trihexane; Trihexidyl; Trihexy-2; Trihexy-5) Anticholinergic compound very similar to benztropine that is used in the treatment of Parkinson's disease. It has been abused by patients and illicit drug users. Pregnancy risk category C. See **benzhexol.**

triiodothyronine   (T_3) Thyroid hormone that is low in patients with hypothyroidism. It may potentiate the clinical effects of antidepressants or lithium in partially responsive or refractory patients (Stein D, Avni A. Thyroid hormones in the treatment of affective disorders. *Acta Psychiatr Scand* 1988;77:623–636). Doses of 25–50 µg/day are usually sufficient, especially in women. T_3 potentiation is usually evident within 3–5 days; if it has not helped by 2 weeks, it should be discontinued.

triiodothyronine (T_3) + clomipramine   In patients partially responsive to clomipramine, addition of triiodothyronine (T_3) did not improve therapeutic response (Pigott TA, Pato MT, L'Heureux F, et al. A controlled comparison of adjuvant lithium carbonate or thyroid hormone in clomipramine-treated patients with obsessive-compulsive disorder. *J Clin Psychopharmacol* 1991;11:242–248).

triiodothyronine (T_3) + fluoxetine T_3 has been reported to augment fluoxetine's antidepressant effect (Crowe D, Collins JP, Rosse RB. Thyroid hormone supplementation of fluoxetine treatment. *J Clin Psychopharmacol* 1990; 10:150–151; Jaffe R. Triiodothyronine potentiation of fluoxetine in depressed patients. *Can J Psychiatry* 1992;37:48–50).

triiodothyronine (T_3) + fluoxetine + lithium   Lithium may act synergistically (perhaps via separate mechanisms) with fluoxetine and T_3 to enhance mood (Geracioti TD, Loosen PT, Gold PW, Kling MA. Cortisol, thyroid hormone, and mood in atypical depression: A longitudinal case study. *Biol Psychiatry* 1992;31: 515–519).

triiodothyronine + lithium   Open and controlled studies indicate that a substantial pro-

portion of tricyclic antidepressant nonresponders may have a therapeutic response with the addition of small amounts of liothyronine (Joffe R, Singer W, Levitt AJ, MacDonald C. A placebo-controlled comparison of lithium and triiodothyronine augmentation of tricyclic antidepressants in unipolar refractory depression. *Arch Gen Psychiatry* 1993;50: 387–393).

triiodothyronine (T_3) + monoamine oxidase inhibitor (MAOI) T_3 may augment response to MAOIs (Joffe RT. Triiodothyronine potentiation of the antidepressant effect of phenelzine. *J Clin Psychiatry* 1988;49:409–410).

triiodothyronine resin uptake   (T_3RU) Indirect measure of thyroid binding protein. Elevated levels occur in hyperthyroidism and illnesses that cause protein depletion (e.g., malnutrition, liver disease); decreased levels occur in hypothyroidism and pregnancy and sometimes in patients taking oral contraceptives.

triiodothyronine (T_3) + trazodone T_3 (25 µg/day) has been reported to augment trazodone's antidepressant effect. Augmentation has been attributed to stimulation of trazodone's weak noradrenergic effects or facilitation of the hypothalamic-pituitary-thyroid axis (Browne JL, Rice JL, Rice DL, et al. Triiodothyronine augmentation of the antidepressant effect of the nontricyclic antidepressant trazodone. *J Nerv Ment Dis* 1990;178:598– 599).

triiodothyronine (T_3) + tricyclic antidepressant   In most, but not all, open and controlled studies, T_3 has been found to augment response to tricyclic antidepressants (TCAs). Up to 50% of patients who fail to respond to a TCA will benefit from addition of T_3 (Extein IL, Gold MS. Thyroid hormone potentiation of tricyclic antidepressants. *In* Extein IL [ed], *Treatment of Tricyclic-Resistant Depression.* Washington, DC: American Psychiatric Press, 1989, pp 1–27; Joffe R, Singer W, Levitt AJ, MacDonald C. A placebo-controlled comparison of lithium and triiodothyronine augmentation of tricyclic antidepressants in unipolar refractory depression. *Arch Gen Psychiatry* 1993;50: 387–393). Available data indicate that T_3 is more effective than thyroxine (T_4) in augmenting antidepressant response to a TCA (Joffe RT, Singer W. Thyroid hormone potentiation of antidepressants. Abstract of paper presented at the 141st Annual Meeting of the American Psychiatric Association, May 1988).

Trilafon   See **perphenazine.**

Trilafon Enanthate   See **perphenazine enanthate.**

Trileptal   See **oxcarbazepine.**

Trilisate   See **magnesium choline trisalicylate.**

trimeprazine   (Temaril) Aliphatic phenothiazine derivative that is not an antipsychotic drug. In contrast to chlorpromazine, the prototype phenothiazine derivative neuroleptic, trimeprazine is an H_1-receptor antagonist used primarily because of its central sedative actions in the treatment of pruritus. Therapeutic indications include urticaria and pruritus, premedication for anesthesia, and nighttime sedation. Like other aliphatic phenothiazine derivatives, it can cause early-onset extrapyramidal reactions, especially akinesia and parkinsonism, even though it has anticholinergic effects.

trimeprazine + tricyclic antidepressant   Co-administration produces more anticholinergic effects than either drug alone and may result in anticholinergic toxicity.

trimethadione   (Tridione; Troxidone) Commonly used anticonvulsant for treatment of refractory absence seizures. It has a long half-life metabolite, dimethadione, which is a major therapeutic advantage in achieving steady blood levels. Pregnancy risk category D.

trimethobenzamide   (Tigan) Benzamide derivative marketed for treatment of nausea and vomiting. It can be administered orally, intramuscularly, or in suppository form. Like other benzamide derivatives, it can evoke a variety of acute early-onset extrapyramidal reactions. Pregnancy risk category C.

trimethoprim-sulfamethoxazole + lithium   See **lithium + trimethoprim-sulfamethoxazole.**

2,4,5-trimethoxy-amphetamine   (TMA) Methoxylated amphetamine that has more psychoactive potency than mescaline. It produces the same effects as mescaline, but has a lower therapeutic index. The amount of TMA required to cause hallucinatory or psychedelic experiences is not very different from that needed to produce toxicity (Chesher G. Designer drugs—the "whats and the whys." *Med J Aust* 1990;153:157–161).

trimipramine   (Surmontil) Tricyclic antidepressant (TCA) that is a hybrid of two other compounds. Its nucleus is that of imipramine; its side chain is that of levomepromazine, a phenothiazine neuroleptic with some antidepressant and analgesic properties. It is an effective tertiary amine antidepressant with anxiolytic, sedative, anticholinergic, and analgesic properties. It has numerous active and inactive metabolites responsible for its rather long half-life. Extensive worldwide clinical use for over 32 years has documented the relative safety and efficacy of trimipramine (100–300 mg/day). Unlike other TCAs, which may be hazardous when co-prescribed with monoamine oxidase inhibitors (MAOIs), trimipramine has been co-administered with MAOIs without

adverse consequences (Settle EC, Jr., Ayd FJ, Jr. Trimipramine: twenty years' worldwide clinical experience. *J Clin Psychiatry* 1980;41:266–274). Pregnancy risk category C.

Trioldene   See **trazodone.**

"trip"   Street name for lysergic acid diethylamide (LSD).

tripelennamine   Antihistamine combined with pentazocine by substance abusers because the combination, known on the street as "t's and blues," appears to be more euphorigenic than either agent alone. See **"t's and blues."**

Triperidol   See **trifluperidol.**

triple-blind study   Study in which identity of the treatment is concealed from those who organize and analyze study data and from subjects and investigators.

triple repeat   Mutation that leads to multiple repeated copies of three base pair sequences appearing in DNA.

triplet codon   Three nucleotides needed to "code" for a specific amino acid (at a particular position in a sequence).

triple-X syndrome   Sex chromosome anomaly, often associated with mental retardation, in which the patient is anatomically female but has the sex chromosome complement XXX.

triploid   Cell with three times the normal haploid chromosome number, or an individual made up of such cells.

"tripper"   Slang term for an individual who has an acute adverse reaction to an hallucinogen or other pharmacological agents taken for pleasure. During a "bad trip," "trippers" are awake and usually responsive, manifesting a variety of signs, symptoms, and alterations of mental status. See **"bad trip."**

"tripping"   Street term for the taking of an hallucinogen.

Triptil   See **protriptyline.**

triptorelin   Depot gonadotropin luteinizing releasing hormone analog (GnRHa) used to treat severe male paraphilia. It can produce reversible castration with no other side effects than those related to hypoandrogenism. It is given intramuscularly (3.75 mg/month). It represents a new trend in the pharmacological treatment of sex offenders and may favor the possibility of concurrent psychotherapy (Thibaut F, Cordier B, Kuhn J-M. Effect of a long-lasting gonadotropin hormone-releasing hormone agonist in six cases of severe male paraphilia. *Acta Psychiatr Scand* 1993;87:445–450).

"trip weed"   Street name for marijuana.

trismus   Firm closing of the jaw secondary to tonic spasm of masticatory muscles from disease of the motor branch of the trigeminus. A common symptom of tetanus, it also can be a manifestation of a drug-induced extrapyramidal reaction, especially acute dystonic reactions, which are one of the more common causes of trismus. Also called "lockjaw." See **dystonia.**

trisomic syndrome   Disorder characterized by the presence in triplicate of one of the chromosomes of a complimentary pair.

trisomy   State of having three of a given chromosome instead of the usual pair.

trisomy 21   (Down syndrome) The most common chromosomal abnormality among children and the most common genetic cause of mental retardation. Since the early 1970s, inherited morphological variations of the short arms of chromosomes seen in karyotypes (i.e., chromosomal heteromorphisms) have been studied in families with a Down syndrome child to determine the parental origin of the extra chromosome. After the introduction of analytical techniques involving DNA polymorphisms, it became possible to determine parental origin in most cases. Using these techniques, investigators have shown that in trisomy 21, the extra chromosome 21 is maternal in origin in about 95% of the cases and paternal in only about 5%— considerably less than reported with cytogenic methods. DNA polymorphic analysis is now the method of choice for establishing the parental origin of nondisjunction. See **Down syndrome.**

trisomy, partial   Rare chromosome disorder in which there is an extra part of a chromosome in each body cell that may be a duplication of part of a long arm or a short arm of a chromosome.

Trivastal   See **piribedil.**

Trofan   See **tryptophan.**

Trolone   See **sulthiame.**

Tropamine   Trade name for a nutritional supplement or pharmacological adjunct for the treatment of cocaine abusers. It allegedly reduces drug craving or drug hunger because it includes precursors for each of the affected neurotransmitters in chronic cocaine users (dopamine, norepinephrine, and serotonin) that are usually depleted in the drug-dependent. Tropamine is a prototypical nutrient product that helps to realize the first goal of treatment, which is to keep the patient in the facility. Preliminary data suggest that it may be a promising pharmacological adjunct insofar as it permits approximately 95% of patients to manage drug hunger and complete inpatient detoxification.

tropisetron $5-HT_3$ antagonist marketed as an antiemetic in several countries (not in the United States). It has good bioavailability and does not cause extrapyramidal side effects. Mild headache, constipation, and transient

transaminase elevations are often associated with $5-HT_3$ antagonists, but are of little consequence.

Troxidone   See **trimethadione.**

"truck driver"   Street name for central nervous system stimulants.

true-negative   Negative test result in a person who does not have the disease. See **false-positive.**

true-positive   Positive test result in a person who has the disease. See **false-negative.**

truncal dyskinesia   See **hyperkinesia, axial.**

Truxal   See **chlorprothixene.**

Tryptal   See **amitriptyline.**

tryptamine   Trace amine synthesized from tryptophan by L-aromatic amino acid decarboxylase. Tryptamine is converted by monoamine oxidase and aldehyde dehydrogenase to indoleacetic acid.

Tryptizol   See **amitriptyline.**

Tryptocin   See **tryptophan.**

tryptophan   (Trofan; Tryptocin) (TRP) Essential amino acid that is the precursor of serotonin (5-HT). Oral administration affects 5-HT synthesis in and release from 5-HT neurons. It can influence synthesis of other neurotransmitters as it competes with other neutral amino acid precursors to gain access from the blood into the brain. There is some evidence that the mental symptoms of postcardiotomy delirium are the consequence of reduced cerebral tryptophan availability due to a catabolic state. Tryptophan has been tested as an antidepressant with equivocal results. It can potentiate the antidepressant effects of monoamine oxidase inhibitors and clomipramine. It has been taken off the market because of its association with the eosinophilia-myalgia syndrome. See **tryptophan + monoamine oxidase inhibitor.**

tryptophan/breast milk   There appears to be no contraindication to the use of tryptophan during lactation.

tryptophan + clomipramine   Co-administration augments antiobsessional response to clomipramine.

tryptophan depletion   In the majority of depressed patients who improve with serotonin uptake inhibitor (SUI) therapy, depression reemerges following acute tryptophan depletion induced by a low-tryptophan diet. It usually consists of a transient return of symptoms. Acute tryptophan depletion also can lower mood in some normal subjects.

tryptophan depletion test   Twenty-four-hour, 160-mg/day tryptophan (TRP) diet (Day 1) with placebo capsules 3 times a day, followed the next morning by a TRP-free, 15-amino-acid drink (Day 2). Control testing consists of a 24-hour, 160-mg/day TRP diet supplemented with capsules containing 500 mg L-tryptophan (L-TRP) 3 times a day, followed the next morning by a 16-amino-acid drink containing 2.3 g of L-TRP. Patients are rated and plasma for free and total TRP is obtained at 9:00 A.M. before starting the diet (Day 1) and 15 minutes prior to, and 5–7 hours after, the drink (Day 2). Ratings are obtained again between 11:00 A.M. and 1:00 P.M. the day after each amino acid drink (Day 3).

tryptophan + fluoxetine   Fluoxetine increases tryptophan blood level and may result in toxicity. A serotonin-like syndrome manifested by agitation, restlessness, insomnia, nausea, and abdominal cramps was reported with the combination (Steiner W, Fontaine R. Toxic reaction following the combined administration of fluoxetine and L-tryptophan: five case reports. *Biol Psychiatry* 1986;21:1067–1071). See **serotonin syndrome.**

tryptophan + lithium   Tryptophan may potentiate the therapeutic effects of lithium in bipolar patients partially responsive to lithium.

tryptophan + monoamine oxidase inhibitor (MAOI)   Co-administration potentiates the antidepressant effect of an MAOI and may induce hypomania. In normal subjects it induces an lysergic acid diethylamide (LSD)-like syndrome and worsens psychotic symptoms among schizophrenic patients (van Praag HM. Serotonergic mechanisms in the pathogenesis of schizophrenia. *In* Lindenmayer JP, Kay SR [eds], *New Biological Vistas on Schizophrenia.* New York: Brunner/Mazel, 1992, pp 187–206). It can result in the serotonin syndrome, manifested by myoclonus, hyper-reflexia, ataxia, ocular muscle oscillation, and drowsiness. See **serotonin syndrome.**

tryptophan + paroxetine   Co-administration may produce increased agitation, restlessness, gastrointestinal effects, and other manifestations of the serotonin syndrome.

tryptophan + phenelzine   Several cases of myoclonus have developed after the serotonin precursor tryptophan was added to phenelzine. Symptoms included ataxia, ocular movements, dysarthria, hyper-reflexia, and spontaneous jerking movements of the legs. They usually disappeared within 24 hours after stopping tryptophan (Levy AB, Bucher P, Votolato N. Myoclonus, hyperreflexia and diaphoresis in patients on phenelzine-tryptophan combination therapy. *Can J Psychiatry* 1985;30: 434–436). Theoretically, co-administration also could predispose to development of serotonin syndrome. See **tryptophan + monoamine oxidase inhibitor.**

tryptophan/pregnancy   Pregnant women should not be given very high doses of tryptophan (Young SN. The clinical pharmacol-

ogy of tryptophan. *In* Wurtman RJ, Wurtman JJ [eds], *Nutrition and the Brain,* vol. 7. New York: Raven Press, 1986).

tryptophan + trazodone   Co-administration may cause the serotonin syndrome (Patterson BD, Srisopark MM. Severe anorexia and possible psychosis or hypomania after trazodone-tryptophan treatment of aggression. *Lancet* 1989; 1:1017). See **serotonin syndrome.**

tryptophan test   Administration of tryptophan to normal and depressed patients increases prolactin levels, which may reflect changes in the activity of 5-hydroxytryptamine neurons projecting from the raphe to the hypothalamus. Response to tryptophan is reported to be blunted in depressed patients (Charney DS, Heninger GR, Sternberg DE. Serotonin function and mechanism of action of antidepressant treatment. *Arch Gen Psychiatry* 1984;41: 359–365). Administration of antidepressants enhances the reduced response (Heninger GR, Charney DS, Sternberg DE. Serotonergic function in depression. *Arch Gen Psychiatry* 1984;41:398–402).

t-test   Statistical procedure to compare two means, used with continuous unpaired data. A modification is the paired t-test, used for continuous paired data. See **Student's t-test.**

Tubarine   See **d-tubocurarine.**

tuberoinfundibular system   System that connects the hypothalamus and the pituitary. It originates in the arcuate nucleus of the hypothalamus, projecting from there and the periventricular nuclei into the intermediate lobe of the pituitary and median eminence. The tract regulates production and release of prolactin, a hormone associated with sexual function and lactation. Altered dopamine levels in the tract influence breast growth and milk production in men and women.

Tuinal   See **amobarbital + secobarbital.**

Tukey's honestly significant difference test   Post hoc test for making multiple pairwise comparisons between means following a significant F test in analysis of variance.

tumescence (penile)   Hardening and expansion of the penis that may be a normal response to sexual stimulation, a natural occurrence during sleep, or the beginning of priapism. Penile erection is usually associated with rapid eye movement (REM) sleep and referred to as nocturnal penile tumescence in sleep electroencephalogram (EEG) recordings. See **priapism.**

tumor virus   Virus that causes neoplastic or cancerous growth.

"turp"   Street name for elixir of terpinhydrate with codeine.

Tutran   See **buspirone.**

"tweaking" Slang term for the severely paranoid, hallucinatory behaviors and hypervigilant thinking, as well as suicidal depression and addictive use, prolonged by "ice" or dextroamphetamine. See **"ice."**

twentieth century disease See **ecological illness.**

twilight state Faint or indistinct mental perception, or a transitory disturbance of consciousness, during which complicated and noncomplicated acts may be performed without the patient's conscious volition or memory of them. It can be a postepileptic phenomenon; it also is often induced by alcohol.

twins There are two different types of twin pairs determined by the nature of the zygote from which the individuals are derived: monozygous (monozygotic, MZ, identical), wherein both members of a pair are derived from a single fertilized egg and can therefore be presumed to be genetically identical; and dizygous (dizygotic, DZ, fraternal), wherein members of the pair develop from different fertilized eggs and are thus comparable to normal siblings. Differences between members of a monozygous pair are nongenetic (environmental) in origin, whereas differences between members of a dizygous pair are due to a combination of genetic and environmental influences.

twins, fraternal (dizygous twins) Twins that develop from two separate ova fertilized at the same time; they can be of the same or of a different sex, since they have different genetic structures.

twins, identical (monozygous twins) Twins that develop from a single fertilized ovum in the same chorionic sac and consequently are of the same sex and same genetic structure.

twin study Study using twins to determine the influence of heredity. It may compare identical and fraternal twins, or identical twins who are discordant for a disease.

twitch (body twitch) Very small body movement such as a local foot or finger jerk that is not usually associated with arousal.

two-by-two factorial design See **factorial design, two-by-two.**

two-compartment model Model characterized by "fast" initial drug distribution followed by a "slower" redistribution/equilibrium with less well-perfused tissues such as lipoidal tissue. In this and other multicompartment models, the distribution process is progressively more lengthy and complex, and significant amounts of drug are eliminated before equilibrium is established (Gibaldi ML. *Biopharmaceutics and Clinical Pharmacokinetics,* 3rd ed. Philadelphia: Lea & Febiger, 1984, pp 1–235).

two-sample t-test Statistical test for the null hypothesis that two independent groups have different means.

two-tail test Statistical significance test based on the assumption that data are distributed in both directions from some central value(s). It tests for the hypothesis that the parameter(s) is/are equal to certain values, or the populations being studied are identical. It is so named because the statistic needs to be compared with two sides of the probability distribution. Also called a "two-side test."

two-way analysis of variance ANOVA with two independent variables. See **analysis of variance.**

Tylenol See **acetaminophen.**

Tylox See **oxycodone.**

Tymelyt See **lofepramine.**

Tymium See **febarbamate.**

type I adverse drug reaction See **adverse drug reaction, type A.**

type II adverse drug reaction See **adverse drug reaction, type B.**

type I error See **error, alpha.**

type II error See **error, beta.**

type I schizophrenia See **schizophrenia, type I.**

type II schizophrenia See **schizophrenia, type II.**

type A adverse reaction See **adverse drug reaction, type A.**

type A personality Individual who is intensely competitive, aggressive, and impatient, with a high sense of urgency and a strong need for recognition and advancement. There is a certain degree of association between coronary artery disease and type A behavior patterns. See **type B personality.**

type B adverse reaction See **adverse drug reaction, type B.**

type B personality Individual who is relaxed, less aggressive, less time-pressured, and less apt to compete to achieve goals than persons with type A personality. See **type A personality.**

typological study Study used to research or look at the different types of a disease.

typological validity Type of a disease that is at once relevant and meaningful to the main disease of study.

typology Study of types.

tyramine First known substrate of monoamine oxidase and a sympathomimetic substance that is a constituent of most diets. When monoamine oxidase inhibitors block tyramine metabolism, dietary tyramine will enter the blood, from which it can be taken up by adrenergic nerves. There it displaces stored noradrenaline, leading to a hypertensive response that can be fatal.

tyramine + moclobemide   Co-administration poses minimal risk of adverse drug-drug interactions (Korn A, Da Prada M, Raffesberg W, et al. Tyramine absorption and pressure response after MAO-inhibition with moclobemide. The Second Amine Oxidase Workshop, Uppsala, August 1986. *Pharmacol Toxicol* 1987; 60:30; Gieschke R, Schmid-Burgk W, Amrein R. Interaction of moclobemide, a new reversible monoamine oxidase inhibitor, with oral tyramine. *In* Youdin MBH, Da Prada M, Amrein R [eds], The cheese-effect and new reversible MAO-A inhibitors. *J Neural Transmission* 1988;26[suppl]:97–104; Schmid-Burgk W, Gieschke R, Allen SR, Amrein R. Moclobemide, a new reversible monoamine oxidase inhibitor, and tyramine interaction studies. *Curr Ther Res* 1988;42:5; Burkard WP, Bonetti EP, Da Prada M, et al. Pharmacological profile of moclobemide, a short-acting and reversible inhibitor of monoamine oxidase type A. *J Pharmacol Exp Ther* 1989;248:391–399; Simpson GM, Gratz SS. Comparison of the pressor effect on tyramine after treatment with phenelzine and moclobemide in healthy male volunteers. *Clin Pharmacol Ther* 1992;52:286–291).

tyramine pressor test   Clinical tool to assess the risk that a monoamine oxidase inhibitor will cause a hypertensive crisis produced by tyramine. Intravenous and oral tests have been used. Oral tests more closely approximate clinical reality, especially when tyramine is administered with a full meal. The tests are more sensitive when both tyramine sensitivity (dosage of tyramine needed to increase the systolic blood pressure by 30 mmHg) and delay of systolic pressure return to normal are measured (Ghose K. Tyramine pressor test: implications and limitations. *Methods Find Exp Clin Pharmacol* 1984;6:455–464).

tyramine test   Well-established trait marker for endogenous depression. Although the biochemical basis remains unclear, low output of the tyramine sulfate conjugate after an oral tyramine load distinguishes endogenous from neurotic depression. Such low output also seems to correlate with a response to tricyclic antidepressant therapy (Hale AS, Sandler M, Hannah P, et al. Tyramine conjugation for production of treatment response in depressed patients. *Lancet* 1989;1:234–236).

tyrosine   Precurser of the catecholamines dopamine and norepinephrine (NE). It significantly increases 3-methoxy-4-hydroxyphenylglycol (MHPG), the principal metabolite of NE, in cerebrospinal fluid (CSF). It also increases CSF concentration of homovanillic acid.

tyrosine hydroxylase   Important enzyme that converts tyrosine to 3,4-dihydroxyphenylalanine (dopa) and subsequently to dopamine, norepinephrine, and epinephrine. It is the rate limiting enzyme in catecholamine biosynthesis. Its blockade via alpha-methyl-p-tyrosine has putative antipsychotic actions.

ubiquitin   Cell stress protein, one of the most conserved proteins in evolution. It has a role in directing damaged or abnormal proteins for proteolysis. Ubiquitin is a major component of many of the neurofibrillary tangles in Alzheimer's disease and appears to be present at a late stage of tangle maturation. It is also a major component of cortical Lewy bodies seen in cases of diffuse Lewy body disease. Immunocytochemical staining of sections with antibodies to ubiquitin is now the gold standard for detection of this disorder.

ultradian rhythm   Biological rhythm with a cycle of less than 24 hours.

ultrasound   High-frequency sound waves that are absorbed and reflected to different degrees by various body tissues. The reflections may be seen as pictures. Ultrasound is useful for diagnostic and treatment procedures. High-powered doses of ultrasound can be used to destroy abnormalities such as gallstones.

Umbrium   See **diazepam.**

Unakalm   See **ketazolam.**

unanticipated beneficial effect   Desirable treatment effect that could not have been predicted on the basis of preclinical and premarketing clinical data.

unanticipated harmful effect   Unwanted treatment effect that could not have been predicted on the basis of preclinical and premarketing clinical data.

unbiasedness   Statistic whose mean from a large number of samples is equal to the population parameter.

unblinded study   Study in which investigators, subjects, and others associated with the study know the identity of the treatment and when it is being administered. Also called an "open-label study."

uncinate seizure   See **seizure, uncinate.**

uncooperativeness   Active refusal to comply with the will of significant others. It may be associated with distrust, defensiveness, stubbornness, negativism, rejection of authority, hostility, or belligerence. In its extreme form, active resistance seriously affects virtually all major areas of functioning. The patient may refuse to join in any social activities, tend to personal hygiene, converse with family or staff, or participate briefly in an interview.

uncontrolled study   Experimental study that has no control subjects.

undoing   Mechanism in which the person engages in behavior designed to symbolically make amends for or negate previous thoughts, feelings, or actions (DSM-IV).

unequal crossover   Study design in which the order of administering drugs or procedures varies on an unequal basis so as to balance out any possible disturbing time trend.

unequal randomization   Procedures that unbalance the allocation of subjects into treatment and control groups. It may be used to increase the number of patients exposed to a test intervention without increasing the overall sample size.

unidentified bright object   In neuroimaging, small area of focal signal hyperintensities suggesting larger ventricular size and abnormal tissue. Focal signal hyperintensities are found infrequently in normal control subjects, more often in schizophrenics, and most often in bipolar patients. They also have been observed in elderly depressed patients, in patients with multi-infarct dementia, and in patients with Alzheimer's disease. Common predisposing factors include hypertension and diabetes. The pathophysiological significance of these findings is unclear. The number of focal signal hyperintensities detected by neuroimaging depends in part on the sensitivity of the screening technique used (Swayze VW, Andreasen NC, Allizer RJ, Ehrhardt JC, Yuh WTC. Structural brain abnormalities in bipolar affective disorder. Ventricular enlargement and focal signal hyperintensities. *Arch Gen Psychiatry* 1990;47:1054–1059).

unifactorial disorder   Genetic disease resulting from the presence of a single mutant gene.

Unified Medical Language System   Method developed at the National Library of Medicine to facilitate retrieval and integration of information from many machine-readable sources, including descriptions of the biomedical literature, clinical records, factual databanks, and medical knowledge bases. It is not an attempt to impose a single standard vocabulary; but a thesaurus or vocabulary and a set of computer programs that can compensate for differences in the vocabularies or coding systems used in different computer-based information sources.

unilateral electroconvulsive therapy (ECT)   See **electroconvulsive therapy, unilateral.**

uniparental disomy   Two chromosomes from the same parent.

unipolar depression   See **depression, unipolar.**

unipolar II depression   See **bipolar III disorder.**

unipolar mania   See **mania, unipolar.**

unit character   Single-gene trait that is transmitted independently of other unit characters.

Univer   See **verapamil.**

universality   Phenomenon occurring in group therapy when patients perceive that other group members have similar problems and feelings, thus reducing the sense of uniqueness (Bloch S, Crouch E. *Therapeutic Factors in Group Psychotherapy*. Oxford: Oxford University Press, 1985).

unreality, feeling of   See **depersonalization.**

unusual thought content   Thinking characterized by strange, fantastic, or bizarre ideas, ranging from the remote or atypical to the distorted, illogical, and patently absurd. In its extreme form, thinking is replete with absurd, bizarre, and grotesque ideas.

"up"   Street name for central nervous system stimulants.

"uphead"   Slang term for drug abusers who use primarily amphetamines or other central nervous system stimulants.

"upper"   Street name for amphetamines or Dexedrine.

up-regulation   Repeated overexposure of receptors to the endogenous transmitter, producing supersensitive responses that are accompanied by increases (up-regulation) in the density of receptors mediating the responses. See **down-regulation.**

Urbanyl   See **clobazam.**

Urecholine   See **bethanechol.**

urinary incontinence   Loss of ability to prevent release of urine. It can be divided into four basic types: urge, stress, overflow, and functional. Urge incontinence is the most common type in the elderly and is caused by involuntary contractions of the detrusor muscle of the bladder. It is often seen in patients with stroke, Parkinson's disease, Alzheimer's disease, and detrusor hyperactivity. Stress incontinence occurs in elderly women with weakness of the pelvic floor, resulting in urine loss with increases in intra-abdominal pressure induced by coughing, sneezing, and laughing. Overflow incontinence may be due to obstruction of urinary outflow or atony of the bladder. Obstruction may be caused by anticholinergic drugs, benign prostate hypertrophy, prostate cancer, and urethral strictures. An atonic bladder cannot empty properly. Neurological disorders, detrusor-sphincteric dyssynergy, and medications may cause bladder atony and overflow incontinence. Functional incontinence may be due to inability or unwillingness to get to the toilet. The former may be due to restraints; the latter to physical or psychiatric illness. Medications (e.g., diuretics, anticholinergics, psychotropics, narcotics, alpha-adrenergic blockers and agonists, and beta-adrenergic agonists) may cause iatrogenic functional incontinence.

urinary retention, psychogenic   See **paruresis.**

urine screening test   Inexpensive procedure that can identify in urine a variety of drugs, including amphetamines, antidepressants, antihistamines, carbamazepine, ephedrine, phencyclidine, ethchlorvynol, flurazepam, meprobamate, methaqualone, phenothiazine, codeine, morphine, heroin, methadone, meperidine, propoxyphene, benzodiazepines, ethanol, phenytoin, and salicylates. The urine sample must be collected under direct observation to ensure its validity (Green S. The use of the toxicology laboratory. *Crit Care Q* 1982; 2:19–23).

urticaria   Hives. A common pruritic skin disorder manifested by the development of wheals. It may be acute or chronic. It has been attributed to anxiolytics (diazepam, meprobamate, and oxazepam); antidepressants (amitriptyline, amoxapine, desipramine, fluoxetine, nortriptyline, and trimipramine); antihistamines (cyproheptadine and diphenhydramine); neuroleptics (chlorpromazine, fluphenazine, perphenazine, thioridazine, thiothixene, and trifluoperazine); carbamazepine; and methylphenidate.

"user"   Slang term for a morphine or heroin addict who takes small daily doses for years to keep comfortable.

utility   Value of the different outcomes in a decision tree; also, the ease of use of a measurement instrument in the disorder for which it was designed. For example, obscure phrasing will diminish comprehension and so decrease the utility of the instrument.

utilization management   System directed by a fourth party or a hospital to manage health-care costs and monitor the appropriateness of treatment. Techniques include preadmission certification, continued stay review, prepayment certification, and retrospective review.

utilization review   Function of utilization management through which payment decisions are made.

V

"V"   Slang term for Valium (diazepam).

Vaben   See **oxazepam**.

"val"   Slang term for Valium (diazepam).

Valcote   See **valproate semisodium**.

validation   Process of establishing that a method is sound and reliable. The objective of validation is to determine, from a number of vantage points, whether an instrument is measuring precisely what it purports to assess.

validity   Extent to which the measures used accurately reflect the phenomenon under investigation. The psychometric evaluation of validity involves examining four aspects: face validity, content validity, construct validity, and predictive validity. *Face validity* is determined by whether or not the system or category "makes sense" in that it describes conditions or patients that experienced clinicians find familiar or acceptable. *Content validity* is assessed by exploring coverage; the nosological categories are examined to determine whether patients will in fact fall into one of the categories. *Construct validity* refers to the extent to which a diagnostic system is consistent with some theoretical system or construct such as the catecholamine hypothesis or behavioral theories of reinforcement. The strength of construct validity rests on establishing the construct itself as valid. *Predictive validity* is the ability to predict some future reaction or outcome, such as prognosis or response to treatment.

validity, study   See **study validity**.

Valium   See **diazepam**.

Valmed   See **ethinamate**.

Valmid   See **ethinamate**.

Valporal   See **valproic acid**.

valproate   (Apilepsin; Depakote, Depakene, Epilim; Epival) (2-propylpentanoate) Simple branched chain carbolic acid marketed for the treatment of epilepsy. It can enhance gamma aminobutyric acid (GABA)-mediated inhibition and reduce excitatory membrane currents, making it useful in a variety of seizure disorders (tonic-clonic seizures, simple and complex absence seizures, myoclonic seizures, infantile spasms, and photosensitive epilepsy). Since 1966, published reports have indicated that valproate and its amide prodrug valpromide may be effective in psychiatric disorders, particularly the manic phase of bipolar disorder. In acute mania, valproate is as effective as lithium with regard to length of hospitalization, need for adjunctive medications, and antimanic efficacy. Onset of antimanic effect occurs within 7 days of achieving therapeutic serum concentrations (50–120 µg/ml). Rapid cyclers, patients with dysphoric or mixed mania, and patients with electroencephalogram (EEG) abnormalities are likely to respond favorably. Valproate's acute antidepressant effects are less pronounced than its antimanic effects, but open trials have shown that it may reduce the frequency and intensity of recurrent manic and depressive episodes over extended periods. Preliminary evidence suggests that valproate may also be useful in treatment-resistant depressions, post-traumatic stress disorder, anxiety disorders (particularly panic disorder), alcohol and sedative/hypnotic withdrawal states, and behavioral dyscontrol syndrome (Keck PE Jr, McElroy SL, Friedman LM. Valproate and carbamazepine in the treatment of panic and post-traumatic stress disorders, withdrawal states and behavioral dyscontrol syndromes. *J Clin Psychopharmacol* 1992;12:36S–41S). Valproate is commercially available in the United States in four orally administered preparations: divalproex sodium (Depakote), an enteric-coated, stable coordinated complex containing equal proportions of valproic acid and sodium valproate in a 1:1 molar ratio; valproic acid (Depakene and others); sodium valproate (Depakene syrup); and divalproex sprinkle capsules (Depakote Sprinkle Capsules) containing coated particles of divalproex sodium that can be ingested intact or pulled apart and sprinkled on food. Valproate is also available in suppository form for rectal administration. An intravenous preparation is currently under development. The rate of absorption of valproate depends on the formulation. In general, rapid-release formulations such as syrup, capsules, and tablets are absorbed with peak times of less than 2 hours. Enteric-coated tablets exhibit variable absorption rates that are usually delayed by 3 or more hours. The sprinkle capsule has the most favorable absorption profile. Valproate has a narrow therapeutic range requiring careful attention when prescribed. Side effects are dose-related and tend to occur during periods of rapid rise of the serum levels. Common side effects are gastrointestinal problems (nausea, stomach cramps, diarrhea), tremors, lethargy, weight gain, and hair thinning. Taking valproate with meals may minimize the risk of persistent nausea. Because valproate can cause liver problems, which can be fatal if missed, and because liver disease may alter valproate's metabolism, its use is discouraged in patients with liver disease. Valproate can also cause thrombocytopenia and altered platelet aggregation. There is some evidence of an increased risk of birth defects if valproate is taken during the first 3 months of pregnancy. A 1–1.5% incidence of neural tube defects (spina bifida) has been reported. Minor dysmorphic syndromes have also been reported. For a patient unable to function because of chronic illness, valproate benefits may outweigh risks (McElroy SL, Keck PE, Pope HG, Hudson JI. Valproate in the treatment of bipolar disorder: literature review and clinical guidelines. *J Clin Psychopharmacol* 1992;12:42S–52S). Valproate has activity against both absence and generalized tonic-clonic seizures. Since 50% of absence seizure patients later develop generalized tonic-clonic seizures, valproate is an important broad-spectrum anticonvulsant. It is as effective as carbamazepine for the treatment of generalized tonic-clonic seizures, but carbamazepine provides better control of complex partial seizures and has fewer long-term adverse effects (Mattson RH, Cramer JA, Collins JF, et al. A comparison of valproate with carbamazepine for the treatment of complex partial seizures and secondary generalized tonic-clonic seizures in adults. *N Engl J Med* 1992;327:765–771). Two types of liver toxicity may occur with valproate: (a) transient asymptomatic transaminase elevation, which may occur within 3 months; and (b) an idiosyncratic fatal hepatitis. The latter is more common in patients taking valproic acid in combination with other anticonvulsants and can be minimized by using valproate monotherapy. Valproate is likely to cause intention tremor. Pregnancy risk category D. See **valproic acid.**

valproate + amitriptyline Amitriptyline (100 mg/day) increased valproate half-life, but the change was not clinically significant (Pisani F, Primerano G, D'Agostino AA, et al. Valproic acid amitriptyline interactions in man. *Ther Drug Monit* 1986;8:382–383).

valproate + aspirin Co-administration may result in higher valproate blood levels and clinical toxicity. If aspirin is taken regularly, valproate doses may need to be lowered (Goulden KJ, Dooley JM, Camfield PR, et al. Clinical valproate toxicity induced by acetylsalicylic acid. *Neurology* 1987;37:1392–1394).

valproate + barbiturate Sodium valproate inhibits metabolism of phenobarbital by the liver, resulting in its accumulation in the body. Co-administration should be well monitored, and suitable phenobarbital dosage reductions should be made when necessary to avoid excessive sedation and lethargy (de Gatta MRF, Gonzales ACA. Effect of sodium valproate on phenobarbital serum levels in children and adults. *Ther Drug Monitor* 1986;8:416–420).

valproate + benzodiazepine See **valproate + diazepam.**

valproate + benzodiazepine + neuroleptic Combination frequently used when manic patients have psychotic symptoms such as hallucinations, threats to others, and insomnia not responsive to benzodiazepines (BZDs). Concomitant use of valproate, a neuroleptic, and a BZD (clonazepam, lorazepam) as clinically indicated is safe and effective and reduces drop-outs. Furthermore, a BZD can enhance sedation and reduce the amount of neuroleptic needed. As the manic episode comes under control, dosage of the neuroleptic and the BZD is reduced gradually until they have been totally discontinued. See **benzodiazepine/adjunctive therapy; neuroleptic + benzodiazepine.**

valproate/breast milk Small amounts of valproate are secreted in breast milk, but are unlikely to adversely affect the baby.

valproate + bupropion Bupropion may increase sodium valproate plasma levels (Popli AP, Tanquary JF, Lamparella V, Masand P. Bupropion revisited: how much is too much? Presented at the 146th Annual Meeting of the American Psychiatric Association, San Francisco, May 1993).

valproate + buspirone Buspirone is of particular benefit as an adjunct to valproate in the treatment of psychosis associated with temporal lobe injuries. It also has been used with partial success in the treatment of post-traumatic akathisia, a frequent element of the postconcussion syndrome.

valproate + carbamazepine Valproate inhibits metabolism of carbamazepine (CBZ), increasing its blood concentration. Conversely, CBZ increases metabolism of valproate, decreasing its blood level over 60%, so that quite high doses may be needed to obtain therapeutic serum levels (Jann MW, Fidone GS, Israel MK, et al. Increased valproate serum concentrations upon carbamazepine cessation. *Epilepsia* 1988;29:578–581; Keck PE Jr, McElroy SL, Vuckovic A, et al. Combined valproate and carbamazepine treatment of bipolar disorder. *J Neuropsychiatry Clin Neurosci* 1991;4:319–322). Both drugs compete for protein binding sites and, when they are prescribed together, the concentration of the free fraction (bioactive component) of the drug may increase. Thus, dosages previously tolerated with a single agent may result in enhanced central nervous system effects and even toxicity when different drugs are co-administered. Adding valproate to ongoing CBZ therapy can result in a decrease in CBZ concentration and increase the CBZ metabolite 10,11-epoxide; CBZ in turn may induce oxidation of valproate through a microsomal P450-mediated process. Acute psychosis occurred in a patient on long-term valproate therapy following addition of CBZ, even though CBZ levels were "nontoxic" (McKee RJW, Larkin JG, Brodie MJ. Acute psychosis with carbamazepine and sodium valproate. *Lancet* 1987;1:167). Co-administration requires monitoring of drug serum levels and awareness of clinical signs and symptoms of toxicity. Data indicate that co-administration is safe for bipolar and schizoaffective patients, but more effective in the former. Bipolar patients refractory to carbamazepine or valproate alone are likely to respond, suggesting a possible synergistic effect (Token M, Castillo JM, Pope HG, Jr. Concurrent use of valproate and carbamazepine in bipolar disorder. Presented at the 146th Annual Meeting of the American Psychiatric Association, San Francisco, May 1993).

valproate + chlorpromazine   Co-administration may decrease valproate blood level and necessitate quite high doses to obtain therapeutic serum levels (Ishizaki T, Chiba K, Saito M, et al. The effect of neuroleptics [haloperidol and chlorpromazine] on the pharmacokinetics of valproic acid in schizophrenic patients. *J Clin Psychopharmacol* 1984;4:254–261).

valproate + clofibrate   Co-administration increases valproate clearance (Heinemeyer G, Nau H, Hildebrandt AG, Roots I. Oxidation and glucuronidation of valproic acid in male rats—influence of phenobarbital, 3-methylcholanthrene, beta-naphthofarone and clofibrate. *Biochem Pharmacol* 1985;34:133–139).

valproate + clomipramine   Co-administration may have beneficial effects in the treatment of pain. In some patients, especially the elderly, it may cause undesirable drowsiness.

valproate + clonazepam   Co-administration may induce absence status in patients subject to absence seizures. See **absence status.**

valproate + clozapine   Some manic, mixed manic, or schizoaffective patients with manic symptoms, particularly those unresponsive to lithium or anticonvulsants alone, may respond to co-administration with no adverse interactions. It also has been used to decrease risk of clozapine-induced seizures. No data are available on valproate effects on clozapine plasma levels (Meltzer HY. New drugs for the treatment of schizophrenia. *Psychiatr Clin North Am* 1993;16:365–385).

valproate + diazepam   Co-administration, even using a lower-than-normal dose of valproate, may produce a 1.4-fold increase in the serum concentration of free valproate. Valproic acid also displaces diazepam (DZ) from binding sites, increasing DZ plasma levels. Since valproate has a low therapeutic index, a dose lower than the standard 1,500 mg/day should be used to avoid toxicity (Monfort S-C. Diazepam increases the serum level of free valproate. Presented at the 146th Annual Meeting of the American Psychiatric Association, San Francisco, May 27, 1993).

valproate + electroconvulsive therapy (ECT)   Since valproate may prevent seizure induction, many experts advise stopping it during ECT therapy (Roberts MA, Attah JR. Carbamazepine and ECT. *Br J Psychiatry* 1988;153: 418).

valproate + erythromycin   Erythromycin should not be co-prescribed with valproic acid. Addition of erythromycin may lead to an increase in serum levels of valproic acid causing toxicity manifested by anxiety, confusion, and dysarthria. Discontinuation of erythromycin is followed by prompt recovery and a gradual fall in serum valproic acid (Redington K, Wells C, Petitio F. Erythromycin and valproate interaction. *Ann Intern Med* 1992;116:877–878).

valproate + felbamate   Felbamate (FBM) increases valproate plasma concentration by about one-third (Wagner ML, Graves NM, Leppik IE, et al. The effect of felbamate on valproate disposition. *Epilepsia* 1991;32[suppl 3]:15). Valproate does not seem to influence FBM clearance (Ward DL, Wagner ML, Perlach JL, et al. Felbamate steady-state pharmacokinetics during co-administration of valproate. *Epilepsia* 1991;32[suppl 3]:8).

valproate + fluoxetine   Sodium valproate may augment fluoxetine (FLX) in the treatment of refractory depression (Corrigan FM. Sodium valproate augmentation of fluoxetine or fluvoxamine effects. *Biol Psychiatry* 1992;31:1178–1179). FLX-mediated inhibition of hepatic valproic acid metabolism may increase valproate plasma level as much as 50%, exposing the patient to increased risk of drug-related side effects (Sovner R, Davis JM. A potential drug interaction between fluoxetine and valproic acid. *J Clin Psychopharmacol* 1991;11: 389).

valproate + fluvoxamine   Sodium valproate may augment fluvoxamine effects in the treatment of refractory depression (Corrigan FM. Sodium valproate augmentation of fluoxetine or fluvoxamine effects. *Biol Psychiatry* 1992;31: 1178–1179).

valproate + haloperidol   Co-administration may decrease valproate plasma levels and may require quite high valproate doses to obtain therapeutic serum levels (Ishizaki T, Chiba K, Saito M, et al. The effect of neuroleptics (haloperidol and chlorpromazine) on the pharmacokinetics of valproic acid in schizophrenic patients. *J Clin Psychopharmacol* 1984; 4:254–261).

valproate/hepatotoxicity Valproate therapy has been associated with a rare, but severe and often fatal, hepatotoxicity that develops rapidly with lethargy and lassitude in almost all patients. Anorexia, vomiting, and rapid progression to coma follow. Liver histopathology is characterized by steatosis with and without necrosis. Several hypotheses have been postulated, but none entirely explains the diverse characteristics of the disorder (Stephens JR, Levy RH. Valproate hepatotoxicity syndrome: hypothesis of pathogenesis. *Pharm Weekbl [Sci]* 1992;14:118–121).

valproate + lamotrigine Small doses of lamotrigine combined with valproate may be useful in refractory idiopathic generalized epilepsies with typical absence seizures, potentially avoiding serious dose-related adverse effects (Panayiotopoulos CP, Ferrie CD, Knott C, Robinson RO. Interaction of lamotrigine with sodium valproate. *Lancet* 1993;341:445). It also has benefited children and adults with refractory partial seizures. In all cases, addition of valproate caused a striking increase in serum lamotrigine concentrations (Pisani F, DiPerri R, Perucca E, Richens A. Interaction of lamotrigine with sodium valproate. *Lancet* 1993; 341:1224). Sodium valproate, which inhibits liver enzyme metabolism, may double the half-life of lamotrigine (Jawad S, Yuen WC, Peck AW, et al. Lamotrigine: single-dose pharmacokinetics and initial 1 week experience in refractory epilepsy. *Epilepsy Res* 1987;1:194–201; Yuen AWC, Land G, Weatherly BC, Peck AW. Sodium valproate acutely inhibits lamotrigine metabolism. *Br J Clin Pharmacol* 1992; 33:511–513). The rise in serum lamotrigine concentrations may result in toxic symptoms (sedation, ataxia, fatigue) that remit after lamotrigine dosage reduction. Tremors also may occur, especially at higher doses (Reutens DC, Duncan JS, Patsalos PN. Disabling tremor after lamotrigine with sodium valproate. *Lancet* 1993;342:185–186).

valproate + lithium Lithium has been shown to augment the antidepressant effect of valproate. In rapid cyclers, co-administration decreases rapid cycling, especially in patients refractory or only minimally responsive to lithium and neuroleptics (Sharne V, Persad E. Augmentation of valproate with lithium in a case of rapid cycling affective disorder. *Can J Psychiatry* 1992;37:384–385; Sharma V, Persad E, Mazmanian D, Kaarunaratne K. Treatment of rapid cycling bipolar disorder with combination therapy of valproate and lithium. *Can J Psychiatry* 1993;38:137–139).

valproate + neuroleptic + benzodiazepine See **valproate + benzodiazepine + neuroleptic.**

valproate + paroxetine Co-administration in patients with well-controlled epilepsy was well tolerated in one single-blind, placebo-controlled study. No clinically relevant changes in valproate plasma concentration were noted (Mikkelsen M, Anderson BB, Dam M, et at: Paroxetine: no interaction with anti-epileptic drugs. *Psychopharmacology* 1991;103:B13).

valproate + phenobarbital Co-administration may lower valproate blood level (Heinemeyer G, Nau H, Hildebrandt AG, Roots I. Oxidation and glucuronidation of valproic acid in male rats—influence of phenobarbital, 3-methylcholanthrene, beta-naphthofarone and clofibrate. *Biochem Pharmacol* 1985;34:133–139). See **valproate/polypharmacy.**

valproate + phenytoin Co-administration may decrease valproate blood level and possibly its therapeutic efficacy.

valproate/polypharmacy The influence of co-administration of multiple drugs on the disposition of valproate can be significant. Its more toxic metabolites are produced through the microsomal P450 pathway, which tends to be enhanced or inhibited by other drugs. Normally the concentration of toxic metabolites is quite low. However, when the P450 pathway is enhanced by dosing with another enzyme-inducing drug such as carbamazepine or phenobarbital, the production of the toxic metabolites can be increased, thereby causing adverse effects. When significant concentrations of these metabolites accumulate, they may result in microvesicular steatosis, liver necrosis and, at times, death. Microvesicular steatosis and liver necrosis are extremely rare in patients on valproate monotherapy (Wilder BJ. Pharmacokinetics of valproate and carbamazepine. *J Clin Psychopharmacol* 1992;12:64S–68S).

valproate/pregnancy Valproate may cause spina bifida (Robert E, Guibaud P. Maternal valproic acid and congenital neural tube defects. *Lancet* 1982;2:937) According to published and unpublished reports, valproic acid may produce teratogenic effects in the offspring of women who take it during pregnancy. Multiple reports in the clinical literature indicate that use of antiepileptic drugs during pregnancy results in an increased incidence of birth defects. The incidence of neural tube defects in the fetus may be increased in mothers receiving valproate during the first trimester. The Centers for Disease Control (CDC) estimates the risk of valproic acid-exposed women having children with spina bifida to be approximately 1–2%. This risk is similar to that for nonepileptic women who have had children with neural tube defects, anencephaly, and spina bifida. Animal studies also have demonstrated valproate-induced teratogenicity (*Physician's Desk Reference*. Odell, NJ: Medical Economics Co., 1993, pp 512–516).

valproate + primidone   Co-administration may decrease valproate blood levels and reduce efficacy.

valproate + protriptyline   Co-administration may decrease valproate blood levels such that quite high doses may be needed to obtain therapeutic serum levels.

valproate + ranitidine   Ranitidine does not inhibit the hepatic microsomal enzyme oxidase system and hence does not alter the levels of hepatically metabolized anticonvulsants such as valproate (Webster LK, Mihaly GW, Jones DB, et al. Effect of cimetidine and ranitidine on carbamazepine and sodium valproate kinetics. *Eur J Clin Pharmacol* 1984;27:341–343).

valproate semisodium   (Valcote) Enteric-coated product containing equal proportions of valproic acid and sodium valproate. It causes less gastrointestinal discomfort than valproic acid.

valproate + tricyclic antidepressant   Combined use may increase tricyclic antidepressant blood levels and induce clinically significant neurotoxicity (Mathews NT, Ali S. Valproate in the treatment of persistent chronic daily headache: an open label study. *Headache* 1991;31: 71–74).

valproate + warfarin   Valproate may interact adversely with warfarin and increase the risk of bleeding.

valproic acid   (Depakene, Valporal, Convulex) (VPA) (N-dipropylacetic acid) Anticonvulsant agent, chemically different from other anticonvulsants, that increases gamma aminobutyric acid (GABA)-ergic transmission. It is commercially available in three preparations; valproic acid, sodium valproate, and divalproex sodium. The common compound in plasma is valproic acid. Valproic acid is used less often than valproate because it causes a somewhat higher incidence of side effects, including gastrointestinal disturbance, initial lethargy, tremor, increased liver enzymes, weight gain, and hair loss. Valproic acid also may cause the following idiosyncratic reactions: coagulopathy, hepatotoxicity, agranulocytosis, and pancreatitis. Pregnancy risk category D. See **valproate**.

valproic acid + antacid   Taking an antacid shortly before or after a dose of valproic acid increases bioavailability of the latter by 3–28% (mean 12%), resulting in a possible toxic blood level. Antacids should be given 1 hour before or 2 hours after a dose of valproic acid.

valproic acid + aspirin   Co-administration may increase the risk of valproic acid toxicity.

valproic acid + carbamazepine   Co-administration has been used in epileptic patients without problems. It also may result in sustained prophylactic response in bipolar patients inadequately responsive to CBZ or VPA alone (Ketter TA, Pazzaglia PJ, Post RM. Synergy of carbamazepine and valproic acid in affective illness: case report and review of literature. *J Clin Psychopharmacol* 1992;12:276–281; Keck PE Jr, McElroy SL, Vuckovic A, Friedman LM. Combined valproate and carbamazepine treatment of bipolar disorder. *J Neuropsychiatry Clin Neurosci* 1992;4:319–322). Although not an enzyme inducer, valproic acid (VPA) inhibits carbamazepine (CBZ) metabolism and displaces it from plasma proteins, increasing the free CBZ fraction that is active and available to be metabolized. Depending on which effect predominates, total CBZ level can rise, fall, or not change. VPA inhibits epoxide hydrolase, increasing the plasma level of CBZ-epoxide (CBZ-E), at times without altering total plasma CBZ level (Sovner R. A clinically significant interaction between carbamazepine and valproic acid. *J Clin Psychopharmacol* 1988;8:448–449). Because of their complex pharmacokinetics, it may be useful to monitor plasma levels of both CBZ and VPA during combined therapy. VPA serum concentrations have been reported to increase in some patients following CBZ discontinuation (Jann MW, Fidone GS, Israel MK, Bonadero P. Increased valproate serum concentrations upon carbamazepine cessation. *Epilepsia* 1988;29:578–581). The combination should probably be avoided in pregnancy because of the possibility of increased risk of congenital malformations.

valproic acid + chlorpromazine   Chlorpromazine may competitively inhibit metabolism of valproic acid, decrease its clearance, and result in valproic acid toxicity.

valproic acid + clobazam   Clobazam (CLB) has been reported to have no significant effect on the blood level/dose ratio (LDR) of valproic acid (VPA). However, VPA significantly decreased LDR of the CLB metabolite N-desmethylclobazam (NCLB), thereby increasing the NCLB/CLB ratio (Sennome S, Mesdjian E. Interactions between clobazam and standard antiepileptic drugs in patients with epilepsy. *Ther Drug Monit* 1992;14:269–274).

valproic acid + clozapine   Co-administration is used to decrease risk of clozapine-induced seizures.

valproic acid + dicumarol   Co-administration may increase bleeding time and alter the serum levels of both drugs. Plasma level monitoring is warranted.

valproic acid + ethosuximide   Co-administration results in a decrease of ethosuximide clearance and higher steady-state concentrations of ethosuximide. The interaction is due to inhibition of ethosuximide metabolism (Mattson RH, Cramer JA. Valproic acid and ethosuximide interaction. *Ann Neurol* 1980;7: 583–584; Pisani F, Narbone MC, Trunfio C, et al. Valproic acid—ethosuximide interaction: a pharmacokinetic study. *Epilepsia* 1984;25:229–233). Valproic acid plus ethosuximide is effective in controlling atypical absence seizures refractory to either drug used alone (Rowan AJ, Meijer JWA, de Beer-Pawlikowski N, et al. Valproate—ethosuximide combination therapy for refractory absence seizures. *Arch Neurol* 1983;40:797–802).

valproic acid + isoniazid   Co-administration has been associated with toxicity; no toxic effects occurred when each drug was used alone (Olanow CW, Finn AL, Prussak C. The effect of salicylate on the pharmacology of phenytoin. *Neurology* 1981;31:341–342).

valproic acid + lithium   Valproic acid may produce fewer central nervous system effects when combined with lithium (Calabrese JR, Delucchi GA. Phenomenology of rapid cycling manic depression and its treatment with valproate. *J Clin Psychiatry* 1989;50[suppl]:30–34).

valproic acid + nimodipine   Co-administration may decrease plasma nimodipine concentrations and necessitate increased nimodipine dosage to achieve adequate therapeutic levels (Tartara A, Galimberti CA, Manni R, et al. Differential effects of valproic acid and enzyme-inducing anticonvulsants on nimodipine pharmacokinetics in epileptic patients. *Br J Clin Pharmacol* 1991;32:335–340).

valproic acid + oxcarbazepine   Oxcarbazepine (OXC) may decrease valproic acid (VPA) serum levels. When OXC is discontinued, there is an average 30% increase in the level/dose ratio of total VPA at the end of a study, preceded by an average 50% increase in the level/dose ratio of free VPA. This leads to VPA-related side effects, requiring retitration of VPA daily doses (Batino D, Croci D, Granata T, et al. Changes in unbound and total valproic acid concentrations after replacement of carbamazepine with oxcarbazepine. *Ther Drug Monit* 1992;14:376–379).

valproic acid + oxiracetam   Valproic acid lowers the half life of oxiracetam, necessitating its more frequent administration. No adverse interactions have been reported.

valproic acid + perphenazine   Addition of valproic acid to perphenazine has been reported to substantially reduce the number of aggressive outbursts per month, with no adverse interactive effects, in mentally retarded patients with nonaffective aggression (assaultive behavior not necessarily associated with dysphoria, anger, or a specific precipitant) (Mattes J. Valproic acid for nonaffective aggression in the mentally retarded. *J Nerv Ment Dis* 1992;180:601–602). Valproic acid has no effect on perphenazine plasma levels (Ellenore GL, Kodsi AB. Drug interactions: case report of carbamazepine vs valproic acid with perphenazine. *ASHP Midyear Clinical Meeting* 1993;28:P–169).

valproic acid + phenobarbital   Valproic acid may impair phenobarbital metabolism and increase its plasma levels. In 20 epileptic patients receiving 900 mg/day of valproate sodium plus 100 mg/day of phenobarbital, valproate plasma levels were significantly lower during concomitant phenobarbital therapy. Maximum plasma concentrations after a single dose of valproate alone were 61–98 mg/L, compared with 45.5–79 mg/L in patients on combined therapy. Area under the concentration-time curve, plasma clearance, and elimination rate constant were significantly higher in patients on combined therapy, whereas the elimination half-life was significantly lower. Phenobarbital may have a clinically significant effect on the pharmacokinetics of valproate (Pokrajac M, Miljkovic B, Varagic VM, Levic Z. Pharmacokinetic interaction between valproic acid and phenobarbital. *Biopharm Drug Dispos* 1993;14:81–86).

valproic acid + phenytoin   Valproic acid may increase phenytoin (PHT) metabolism and decrease serum PHT levels. Co-administration may require PHT dosage adjustment according to the clinical situation (Pisani F, Perucca E, Di Perri R. Clinically relevant anti-epileptic drug interactions. *J Int Med Res* 1990;18:1–15).

valproic acid + primidone   Valproic acid may or may not increase primidone levels (Windorfer A, Sauer W, Gaedke R. Elevation of diphenylhydantoin and primidone serum concentration by addition of diproplylacetate, a new anticonvulsant drug. *Acta Paediatr Scand* 1975; 64:771–772; Fincham RW, Schottelius DD. Primidone: interactions with other drugs. *In* Woodbury DM, Penry JK, Pippenger CE [eds], *Antiepileptic Drugs*, 2nd ed. New York: Raven Press, 1982, pp 421–428).

valproic acid + salicylates   Co-administration of aspirin, bismuth subsalicylate (Pepto-Bismol), or other salicylates displaces valproic acid from binding sites, resulting in increased blood levels and possible toxicity. In addition, there can be an increase in valproic acid metabolism, leading to a greater formation of epitotoxic metabolites.

valproic acid + thioridazine Addition of valproic acid to thioridazine has been reported to substantially reduce the number of aggressive outbursts per month, with no adverse interactive effects, in mentally retarded patients with nonaffective aggression (assaultive behavior not necessarily associated with dysphoria, anger, or a specific precipitant) (Mattes J. Valproic acid for nonaffective aggression in the mentally retarded. *J Nerv Ment Dis* 1992;180: 601–602)

valproic acid + tricyclic antidepressant Combined use has been reported to increase tricyclic antidepressant blood levels and induce clinically significant neurotoxicity in tricyclic-treated patients (Mathews NT, Ali S. Valproate in the treatment of persistent chronic daily headache. An open label study. *Headache* 1991; 31:71–74).

valproic acid + warfarin Valproic acid may potentiate the anticoagulant effects of warfarin.

valpromide Amide prodrug of valproate.

Valrelease See **diazepam.**

vanillylmandelic acid (VMA; 3-methoxy-4-hydroxy mandelic acid) Norepinephrine (NE) metabolite and marker in blood or urine for the rate of NE turnover.

Vaposole See **amyl nitrate.**

variable 1. Factor whose quantity can be increased or decreased in either discrete steps or along a continuum without any other concomitant change in that factor. 2. Anything that can change or take on different characteristics appropriate to specified conditions.

variable, confounding Study variable, the effect(s) of which cannot be distinguished from the effect(s) of another variable. Alcohol consumption and high benzodiazepine use, for example, can be confounding variables in a study of children born of mothers who drink and take high benzodiazepine doses during pregnancy.

variable, control Independent variable that has a potential effect on the dependent variable.

variable, dependent (DV) Study variable measured after manipulation of the independent variable and assumed to vary as a function of the independent variable.

variable, design Study variable, the distribution of which in subjects is determined by the investigator.

variable, dichotomous Nominal measure that has only two possible outcomes (e.g., gender; survival).

variable, independent Study variable under the experimenter's control and regarded as a cause, predictor, or correlate of the outcome or dependent variable. Examples include: preceding experimental presentations of the stimuli; previous occurrences of the behavior; instances of reinforcement of the behavior; drive level or deprivation level of the organism; appropriateness of the goal object; types of stimuli; types of responses required; and experimental apparatus. Also called "predictor variable."

variable, input Selection variable that may be a determinant of outcome.

variable, intermediate Variable that occurs in the course from an independent to a dependent variable.

variable, intervening Something occurring between an antecedent circumstance and its consequence that modifies the relation between the two. For example, appetite can be an intervening variable determining whether or not a given food will be eaten. The intervening variable may be inferred rather than empirically detected.

variable, outcome Dependent or criterion variable in a study.

variable, output Selection variable that may be a determinant of the status of treatment subjects or follow-up.

variable, predictor See **variable, independent.**

variable, random Study variable in which subjects are randomly selected or randomly assigned to treatments.

variable, uncontrolled Confounding variable that has not been brought under control.

variance Measure of the variability of any characteristic that changes from sample to sample. It is calculated in square units. Its square root is called either a "standard deviation" or a "standard error." See **analysis of variance.**

variation Changes in measurements of the same object or subject that may occur naturally or may represent an error in measurement.

variation, observer Error due to failure of the observer to measure accurately.

Vasculoflex See **flunarizine.**

vasoactive intestinal peptide Peptide associated with nerve terminals in the brain and gastrointestinal tract that activates specific pre- or post-synaptic receptors and thereby modulates the responsiveness of the membrane to the action of neurotransmitters such as acetylcholine or noradrenaline. In the human brain, acetylcholine co-localizes with vasoactive intestinal peptide.

vasoconstriction Narrowing of the blood vessels.

vasopressin (VP) Posterior pituitary peptide important in the regulation of learning, memory, and water diuresis. See **antidiuretic hormone.**

vasopressin + lithium See **lithium + vasopressin.**

Vasotec See **enalapril.**

vector DNA molecule from which other genetic material can be introduced. Vectors introduce foreign DNA into host cells, where it can be reproduced in large quantities.

vegetative symptoms Certain symptoms of a major depressive disorder, especially sleep and appetite disturbances, weight change, fatigue, and low energy.

velnacrine (Mentane) Maleate salt of an alcohol derivative of the cholinesterase inhibitor tetrahydroaminoacridine. It possesses central cholinergic activity and enhances memory in animals. In patients with Alzheimer's disease, there is some evidence of memory improvement in about half of the subjects (Pomara N, Deptula D, Singh R. Pretreatment postural blood pressure drop as a possible predictor of response to the cholinesterase inhibitor velnacrine [HP 029] in Alzheimer's disease. *Psychopharmacol Bull* 1991;27:301–307; Cutler NR, Sramek J J, Murphy MF, Nash RJ. Implications of the study population in the early evaluation of cholinesterase inhibitors for Alzheimer's disease. *Ann Pharmacother* 1992;26:1118–1122).

venlafaxine (Effexor) (VEN) Structurally novel tricyclic compound with an antidepressant biochemical profile. It inhibits or blocks the neuronal uptake of serotonin, norepinephrine, and dopamine. Venlafaxine induces noradrenergic down-regulation after acute and chronic administration. It does not have monoamine oxidase inhibitor activity and shows no affinity for rat brain muscarinic, cholinergic, histaminergic, or noradrenergic receptors. Unlike all other agents, venlafaxine has a rapid onset of noradrenergic subsensitivity. Clinical trials to date indicate that it may have antidepressant activity within the first 2 weeks of treatment. Venlafaxine has been shown to be effective in patients with rigorously defined treatment-resistant depression (no response to at least three adequate trials of antidepressants from at least two different classes of antidepressants, electroconvulsive therapy, and at least one attempt at augmentation). About one-third of such patients treated with venlafaxine were considered to be full responders as measured by the 21-item Hamilton Depression Rating Scale, the Montgomery-Asberg Depression Rating Scale, and the Clinical Global Impressions Scale. In addition, 80% of responders remained well for at least 6 months (Nierenberg AA, Feighner JF, Rudolph RR, et al. Venlafaxine for treatment-resistant depression. Presented at the 146th Annual Meeting of the American Psychiatric Association, San Francisco, May 1993). Dosages of 25, 75, and 125 mg 3 times a day

have been well tolerated. The most common side effect is nausea.

ventral noradrenergic bundle Part of the central noradrenergic system that is located caudally and ventrally to the locus ceruleus. It terminates in the hypothalamus and the subcortical limbic regions.

ventral tegmental area Dopamine-rich region of the mesocortical system. Parkinsonism patients have a reduced dopamine content in this area.

ventricular brain ratio (VBR) Ratio (usually expressed as a percentage) of the area of the lateral ventricle to the intracranial area on the computerized axial tomography (CT) section in which the ventricles are the largest. Measurements are done either by a planimeter from the CT scan film, by computer-assisted methods in which the outline of the relevant structures are traced with a cursor, or determination of thresholds that demarcate boundaries of cerebrospinal fluid (CSF)/brain and CSF/cranium with subsequent automated measurements by the computer. The sensitivity of detection of ventricular enlargement has recently improved by using area measurements on successive CT sections and multiplying them by the slice thickness to obtain a volume measurement. In 1962, Hang reported ventricular enlargement in schizophrenia, an observation confirmed repeatedly by CT studies demonstrating cortical atrophy with enlarged lateral and third ventricles, as well as widening of cerebral nuclei and cerebellar atrophy in as many as 40–50% of schizophrenics. Magnetic resonance imaging (MRI) has documented that many schizophrenics have enlarged ventricular and associated cortical atrophy, especially in the temporal lobe and hippocampal nuclei (Hang JO. Pneumoencephalographic studies in mental disorders. *Acta Psychiatry Scand* 1962;[suppl 165]:1–114; Shelton RC, Weinberger DR. Brain morphology in schizophrenia. *In* Meltzer HY [ed], *Psychopharmacology: The Third Generation of Progress.* New York: Raven Press, 1987). These changes may be related to negative symptoms, intellectual deterioration, poor performance on neuropsychological tests, the presence of soft neurological signs, and poor response to antipsychotic drugs. Similar, less marked cortical atrophy also has been observed in normal control subjects and in patients with a wide variety of other psychiatric disorders. See **schizophrenia, ventricular enlargement.**

veralipride Benzamide derivative with dopamine antagonistic activity widely used in Europe. Although initially claimed to be free of extrapyramidal side effects, it has been reported to cause segmental tardive dystonia.

verapamil (Calan, Cordilox, Isoptin, Univer; Verelan) Calcium channel blocker effective in the treatment of moderately severe manic states. Generally, dosages of 160–240 mg/day have antimanic effects. For severe manic symptoms, however, it is less effective than clonidine, lithium, or carbamazepine. It may not be effective in lithium-resistant patients. Also, since it is not sedating, verapamil, like lithium, is less suitable for highly active manic patients. A controlled trial comparing verapamil with neuroleptics showed that it was as effective as neuroleptics alone or a neuroleptic-lithium combination, without producing the sedative, hypnotic, or cataleptic effects associated with neuroleptics (Hoschel C, Kozeny J. Verapamil in affective disorders: a controlled, double-blind study. *Biol Psychiatry* 1989;25:128–140). Verapamil also is effective in the treatment of migraine and cluster headaches. The suggested dose for migraine prophylaxis is 120 mg 3 times a day. Verapamil binds with moderate affinity to 5-HT$_2$ receptors on cerebral blood vessels and brain neurons, suggesting that it may act via mechanisms similar to those of other antimigraine drugs. Side effects are relatively benign, but include hypotension and bradycardia (Garza-Trevino ES, Overall JE, Hollister LE. Verapamil versus lithium in acute mania. *Am J Psychiatry* 1992;149:121–122). Pregnancy risk category C.

verapamil + alcohol Verapamil may significantly inhibit alcohol elimination, resulting in a rise in blood alcohol levels that may remain elevated for a longer period than usual (Schumock G, Bauer LA, Horn J, Opheim K. Verapamil inhibits ethanol elimination. *Pharmacotherapy* 1989;9:184–185; Bauer LA, Schumock G, Horj J, Opheim K. Verapamil inhibits ethanol elimination and prolongs the perception of intoxication. *Clin Pharmacol* 1992;42:6–10).

verapamil + carbamazepine Co-administration may result in elevated carbamazepine (CBZ) plasma levels and sometimes in CBZ toxicity. To compensate for increased CBZ plasma level, CBZ dose should be reduced or nifedipine should be used as an alternative to verapamil (Macphee GJA, McInnes GT, Thompson GG, Brodie M. Verapamil potentiates carbamazepine neurotoxicity: a clinically important inhibitory interaction. *Lancet* 1986;1:700–703; Price WA, DiMarzio LR. Verapamil-carbamazepine neurotoxicity. *J Clin Psychiatry* 1988;49:80). CBZ dosage should be readjusted when verapamil is discontinued.

verapamil + lithium With careful monitoring, co-administration can be used in patients intolerant of lithium side effects. In eight normal male volunteers, controlled-release verapamil (200 mg/day) added to lithium (600 mg/day) for 7 days did not alter previously established pharmacokinetics of lithium alone in any measure of clearance, half-life, or volume of distribution (Myers CW, Perry PJ, Kathol RG. Plasma and erythrocyte lithium concentrations before and after oral verapamil. *Lithium* 1990;1:49–53). Co-administration has been reported to cause cardiotoxicity, neurotoxic side effects, and decreased serum lithium levels (Price WA, Giannini AJ. Neurotoxicity caused by lithium-verapamil. *J Clin Pharmacol* 1986;26:717–719; Price WA, Shalley JE. Lithium-verapamil toxicity in the elderly. *J Am Geriatr Soc* 1987;35:177–179; Weinrauch LA, Belok S, D'Elia JA. Decreased serum lithium during verapamil therapy. *Am Heart J* 1984;108:1378–1379).

verapamil + phenytoin Phenytoin, an inducer of hepatic-drug metabolizing enzymes, can interfere with verapamil absorption and markedly reduce its steady-state concentration (Woodcock BG, Kirsten R, Nelson K, et al. A reduction in verapamil concentrations with phenytoin. *N Engl J Med* 1991;325:1179).

verapamil/pregnancy Oral (up to 480 mg/day in divided doses) and intravenous (up to 10 mg over 2 minutes) administration of verapamil to pregnant women has had no adverse effects on the fetus. Three women previously diagnosed as bipolar were started and maintained on verapamil (180–240 mg/day) throughout pregnancy with good symptom control. All delivered healthy infants after 36–40 weeks' gestation (Goodnick P. Verapamil prophylaxis in pregnant women with bipolar disorder. *Am J Psychiatry* 1993;150:1560).

verbal intelligence Ability to understand and use spoken and sometimes written language. Some intelligence tests measure verbal intelligence separately from nonverbal performance skills.

verbigerate To repeat the same word, phrase, or sentence over and over again.

verbigeration Manifestation of stereopathy consisting of the morbid repetition of words, phrases, or sentences.

Verelan See **verapamil.**

Versed See **midazolam.**

Verstran See **prazepam.**

Vertex See **flunarizine.**

vertex sharp transient Sharp negative potential, maximal at the vertex, occurring spontaneously during sleep or in response to a sensory stimulus during sleep or wakefulness. Amplitude varies but rarely exceeds 250 µV (Thorpy MJ. *Handbook of Sleep Disorders.* New York: Marcel Dekker, 1990). The term *vertex sharp wave* is discouraged from use.

vertigo Sensation of motion, frequently called "dizziness" by patients, that is due to disturbances of vestibular function secondary to peripheral or central disorders. The former include vestibular neuronitis, labyrinthitis, benign positional vertigo, Meniere's disease, and post-traumatic vertigo. The latter include brainstem ischemia/infarct, posterior fossa tumors, and multiple sclerosis. Vertigo must be distinguished from ill-defined lightheadedness. The latter, a common diagnosis among patients referred to dizziness clinics, is usually due to psychiatric disorders, especially the hyperventilation syndrome, and less frequently to anxiety disorders and hysterical neurosis.

vertigo, drug-induced Drugs that may cause vertigo include (a) anticonvulsants (barbiturates, carbamazepine, phenytoin); (b) sedatives/anxiolytics (benzodiazepines, meprobamate); (c) alcohol; (d) cinchona alkaloids (quinine, quinidine); (e) salicylates; (f) nonsteroidal anti-inflammatory drugs (ibuprofen); and (g) aminoglycoside antibiotics (e.g., streptomycin, kanamycin).

Vertigon See **prochlorperazine**.
Victoril See **dibenzepin**.
video task Computerized technique for measuring affect-related behavior. It may provide a sensitive measure of negative features in schizophrenia.
vigabatrin (Sabril; Sabrin) Gamma-vinyl-GABA, a structural analog of gamma aminobutyric acid (GABA) that irreversibly inhibits GABA transaminase (GABA-T), increasing the concentration of GABAergic synapses in the brain. At therapeutic doses in humans, vigabatrin produces dose-related increases in cerebrospinal fluid (CSF) concentrations of free and total GABA. Data to date (1993) indicate that vigabatrin is useful as an "add-on" therapy in patients with chronic refractory epilepsy who are either unresponsive to or intolerant of other antiepileptic drugs. Epileptic patients with complex partial seizures who respond to vigabatrin have higher CSF increases in total GABA than do nonresponders. Since there are no differences in plasma or CSF concentrations of vigabatrin in responders and nonresponders, plasma levels are not suitable as a guide to therapy, because the action of vigabatrin long outlasts its presence in plasma. In epileptic patients not responding to vigabatrin, plasma GABA was not increased compared with control subjects. By contrast, vigabatrin responders (patients showing more than 50% reduction in seizure frequency) had significantly increased plasma GABA, compared with both control subjects and nonresponders. There were no significant differences in dose or plasma concentrations of vigabatrin or duration of treatment with vigabatrin between responders and nonresponders. Plasma GABA may reflect differences in CSF GABA increases previously found between vigabatrin responders and nonresponders. Thus, plasma GABA measurement might be useful for therapeutic monitoring in vigabatrin-treated patients (Loscher W, Gram L, Stefan H. Plasma GABA and seizure control with vigabatrin. *Lancet* 1993;341:117). Vigabatrin's side effect profile is similar to that of other anticonvulsants, especially in the early phases of treatment. Behavior changes associated with the initiation of vigabatrin therapy have been reported. Behavior has been variously documented as improved or deteriorating. In some patients, severe agitation and psychosis have occurred, necessitating withdrawal of vigabatrin. There have been an increasing number of reports of major depressive episodes associated with vigabatrin treatment. No long-term hazards have been identified. There is some evidence that vigabatrin may also be a spasmolytic drug useful in the symptomatic treatment of spasticity due to metabolic diseases in children.

vigabatrin + carbamazepine No significant changes in carbamazepine (CBZ) plasma levels have been reported. Two patients developed acute encephalopathy after vigabatrin was added to CBZ. Both had stupor and slowed electroencephalographic background activity, dysphoria, and irritability. One developed a novel type of seizure; the other developed myoclonic status epilepticus. In the first case, serum CBZ was slightly raised, but clinical symptoms could not be related to intoxication with CBZ or its epoxide. It is unknown whether an interaction between vigabatrin and CBZ caused acute encephalopathy, which has been reported with vigabatrin monotherapy (Salke-Kellerman A, Baier H, Rambeck B, Boenigk HE, Wolf P. Acute encephalopathy with vigabatrin. *Lancet* 1993;342:185).

vigabatrin + lamotrigine Co-administration has marked benefits in some patients with intractable seizures partially or fully refractory to either drug alone. Patients had clinical and electroencephalographic evidence of frequent secondary generalization that improved after lamotrigine was added to vigabatrin (Stewart J, Hughes E, Reynolds EH. Lamotrigine for generalized epilepsies. *Lancet* 1992;340:1223).

vigabatrin + phenytoin Vigabatrin may reduce phenytoin's (PHT) steady state by 20–40%, possibly resulting in loss of PHT efficacy. Vigabatrin discontinuation may increase PHT serum level and risk of PHT intoxication

(Rimmer RM, Richens A. Interaction between vigabatrin and phenytoin. *Br J Clin Pharmacol* 1989;27[suppl 1]:27S–33S). During co-administration, PHT plasma levels should be monitored and dosage should be adjusted to assure therapeutic levels and maintenance of seizure control.

Vigorex   See **methyltestosterone.**

viloxazine   (Catatrol, Vivalen) Bicyclic drug with antidepressant and anticonvulsant properties introduced in Europe in the mid-1970s. Unlike conventional tricyclic antidepressants, it inhibits the neuronal uptake of noradrenaline without affecting serotonin uptake. It has little effect on adrenoceptors, dopamine receptors, or cholinergic receptors, and has little sedative or cardiac depressant activity. Viloxazine use has declined because of doubts about its efficacy and the high incidence of nausea it causes. Also available in a sustained-release form.

viloxazine + carbamazepine   Co-administration may increase serum carbamazepine (CBZ) levels up to 50%, but only slightly increase CBZ epoxide levels. There may be symptoms of CBZ intoxication (fatigue, dizziness, ataxia). Viloxazine discontinuation produces symptom remission and return of serum CBZ level to initial value (Pisani F, Fazio A, Oteri G, et al. Elevation of plasma carbamazepine and carbamazepine 10,11-epoxide levels by viloxazine in epileptic patients. *Acta Pharmacol* 1986;59,[suppl 5/II]:109; Pisani F, Fazio A, Oteri G, et al. Carbamazepine-viloxazine interaction in patients with epilepsy. *J Neurol Neurosurg Psychiatry* 1986;49:1142–1145).

viloxazine + phenytoin   Co-administration may increase phenytoin (PHT) serum levels and risk of PHT intoxication. PHT plasma levels should be monitored and its dosage should be adjusted to avoid toxicity.

violence   Any act of aggression involving physical contact, irrespective of outcome. Often categorized according to the target of the assault: fellow patients, staff, the self, and property. Violent behavior may respond to beta-blockers and lithium. There is preliminary evidence that violence also can be managed with buspirone, carbamazepine, and valproate.

viqualine   (PK-5078) A serotonin uptake inhibitor that in clinical trials has decreased mean alcohol drinking by 10–18% in low dependent drinkers. These results suggest that viqualine acts by decreasing both the desire to drink and the reinforcing properties of alcohol. It may be an important treatment for substance abuse and dependence.

Virilon   See **methyltestosterone.**

Virilon IM   See **testosterone cypionate.**

virus   Smallest type of organism that infects another type of cell and takes over in order to replicate itself.

visceral epilepsy   See **epilepsy, visceral.**

Viscoleo   See **zuclopenthixol.**

viscosity   Interictal behavior syndrome symptom in which patients show a striking preoccupation with detail and concerns over moral or ethical issues.

viscosity, ideational   Perseveratory thoughts, either grandiose or self-deprecatory. It is a temporal lobe symptom sometimes manifested in bipolar disorder.

viscosity, interpersonal   Interictal behavioral symptom in temporal lobe epilepsy manifested by inability to bring a conversation to an appropriate end; insensitivity to temporal or spatial cues regulating social interactions; or prolonged clinical interviews followed by frequent attempts to reestablish contact with phone calls, letters, notes, or messages. It tends to be associated with circumstantiality. Also called "clinging."   See **circumstantiality.**

Visken   See **pindolol.**

Vistacon   See **hydroxyzine.**

Vistaject   See **hydroxyzine.**

Vistaquel   See **hydroxyzine.**

Vistaril   See **hydroxyzine.**

Vistazine   See **hydroxyzine.**

visual analog scale   Self-rating instrument composed of opposite words or phrases and horizontal or vertical lines, generally 10 cm long, the ends of which represent the extreme states of the criterion under consideration (for example, no pain at one end and pain as bad as it can be at the other end). Patients situate their status somewhere between the two extremes.

visual aphasia   See **alexia.**

visual evoked potential   (VEP) Test used extensively in the evaluation of visual disturbances and function of posterior cortex. VEP may be recorded in response to either unpatterned stimuli (e.g., simple flashlight) or pattern stimuli (e.g., checkerboard pattern). Reversal of a checkerboard pattern (white checks turning black, and black checks turning white) normally produces a predictable wave form. Also called "visual evoked response."

visual hallucination   See **hallucination, visual.**

visual-spatial agnosia   Syndrome characterized by failure to analyze spatial relationships and the inability to perform simple constructional tasks under visual control. It is usually associated with lesions of the occipitoparietal portions of the right cerebral hemisphere in right-handed patients.

visual tracking   Task that assesses eye-hand coordination.

vital statistics Mortality and morbidity rates used in epidemiology and public health.

vitamin B$_{12}$ deficiency Condition that may be manifested as dementia, depression, or anergia before the onset of pernicious anemia. An estimated 70—75% of pernicious anemia patients have objective memory impairment, and 60% have abnormal electroencephalograms (EEGs). Elderly patients with unexplained dementia, especially those with persistent fatigue or a history of gastric surgery, should be tested for megaloblastic anemia, and their serum B$_{12}$ levels should be checked.

vitamin E (Alpha-tocopherol) Free-radical scavenger reported to improve symptoms of tardive dyskinesia (TD) in patients who have had TD for 5 years or less. Improvement was not due to increased blood levels of neuroleptic medications (Egan MF, Hyde TM, Albert GW, et al. Treatment of tardive dyskinesia with Vitamin E. *Am J Psychiatry* 1992;149:773–777). Vitamin E significantly improved TD during short-term (8 weeks) treatment and also up to 36 weeks (Adler L, Peselow E, Angrist B, et al. Vitamin E in tardive dyskinesia: effects of longer term treatment. Presented at the 1992 Annual Meeting of the American College of Neuropsychopharmacology, San Juan, Puerto Rico, December 1992). The most recent study found vitamin E improved TD scores compared to placebo (Adler LA, Peselow E, Rotrosen J, et al. Vitamin E treatment of tardive dyskinesia. *Am J Psychiatry* 1993;150:1405–1407). Although vitamin E in daily doses of 400–1200 mg/day has been reported to improve TD of relatively short duration without any noticeable adverse effects aside from diarrhea, its true efficacy requires large-scale and longer-term studies (*Tardive Dyskinesia: A Task Force Report of the American Psychiatric Association*. Washington, DC: American Psychiatric Association, 1992, pp 13–120). An analysis of trials of the vitamin E in the treatment of TD suggests questionable efficacy. Conflicting evidence and problems in methodology and inclusion criteria in the available trials complicate the issue (Schneiderhan ME. Vitamin E in tardive dyskinesia. *Ann Pharmacother* 1993;27:311–313). Vitamin E is generally safe with few side effects; abdominal pain, headaches, muscle cramps, nausea, and fatigue are reported rarely. It may elevate triglycerides and cholesterol, and decrease thyroid indices.

These abnormalities and symptoms disappear after discontinuation of the drug.

vitamin E + warfarin Vitamin E may interact with warfarin to prolong bleeding time.

"vitamin K" Street name for ketamine.

Vivactil See **protriptyline.**

Vivalen See **viloxazine.**

Vivol See **diazepam.**

Vivormone See **testosterone propionate.**

Volital See **pemoline.**

volition disturbance Changes in willful initiation and control of one's thoughts, behavior, movements, and speech. In its extreme form, there is almost complete failure of volition manifested by immobility and/or mutism.

Voltaren See **diclofenac.**

volume of distribution (V$_d$) Unit of volume that reflects the degree to which a drug is distributed in the body. It is calculated by dividing the amount of drug in the body by its plasma concentration. V$_d$ is often referred to as the apparent volume of distribution, since V$_d$ is a hypothetical volume at equilibrium under certain pharmacokinetic models. Factors that affect distribution of drugs throughout the body include nature of the drug, characteristics of the various organs, and individual patient variation. A drug highly bound by tissues that accumulates to a high degree in tissue has a large apparent V$_d$. Larger V$_d$ is also associated with a longer elimination half-life. The larger the V$_d$, the more rapidly the drug will disappear from plasma, and the shorter its duration of action. V$_d$ for a given drug can vary widely among individuals because of variability in drug binding to blood components and tissues.

volunteer bias See **bias, volunteer.**

voyeurism Sexual deviation in which sexual gratification is derived from secretly watching sexual activity or by looking at others in situations construed as sexual (e.g. spying on a woman who is undressing). It may include preferring to masturbate while observing nude women rather than having heterosexual intercourse. Voyeurism is reported only in men.

vulnerability factor Any condition that renders a person more susceptible than average to stress, stimulation, or disease.

vulnerability, genetic See **genetic vulnerability.**

W

"wack"   1. Street name for marijuana alone or marijuana dipped in phencyclidine (PCP), insect spray (Raid), turpentine, or formaldehyde, then dried and smoked. 2. Street name for phencyclidine.

"wafer"   Street name for methadone.

wakefulness   State of not being asleep (Kleitman N. *Sleep and Wakefulness.* Chicago: University of Chicago Press, 1963). Wakefulness is not identical to consciousness; the terms refer to distinct yet overlapping states.

wakefulness after sleep onset   (WASO) Sleep study term for wake time after sleep onset. It usually increases with age, in part because older people are more easily aroused by either internal or external stimuli.

wake time   Total time scored as wakefulness between sleep onset and final wake-up in a polysomnogram.

"wakeup"   Street name for amphetamine sulfate (Benzedrine).

walking the chromosome   Genetic technique to identify a specific gene whose approximate location has been determined.

wandering   Frequent, disturbing symptom of dementia manifested by a tendency to move about in a seemingly aimless fashion, or in pursuit of an unattainable goal. The person may get lost, leave a safe environment, or inadvertently intrude where unwanted. The goal of management is to ensure safety while allowing the wandering individual a measure of autonomy. Restraint can be harmful and can increase the risk of injury.

warfarin   (Coumadin; Panwarfin) Oral anticoagulant that is an indirect antagonist of vitamin K. It reduces hepatic synthesis of the vitamin K–dependent clotting factors (II, VII, IX, and X protein). It has a narrow therapeutic index, and monitoring of prothrombin time is necessary. Hemorrhage due to excessive anticoagulant effect is the most important adverse reaction to warfarin. Because of the actions of nicotine on the liver, smokers may induce enzymes, resulting in increased warfarin metabolism. Since many psychiatric patients, especially schizophrenics, are heavy smokers, prescribers should consider the impact of nicotine on the metabolism of a variety of drugs.

warfarin + alcohol   Co-administration may result in either an increase or a decrease in prothrombin time.

warfarin + Bactrim   Co-administration can result in an increase in prothrombin time.

warfarin + benzodiazepine   Benzodiazepines have been used extensively and safely with warfarin (Stockley IH. *Drug Interactions: A Source Book of Drug Interactions, Their Mechanisms, Clinical Importance and Management,* 2nd ed. Oxford: Blackwell Scientific, 1991).

warfarin + carbamazepine   Carbamazepine (CBZ), a powerful inducer of hepatic microsomal enzymes, can decrease warfarin's effectiveness; dosage adjustments based on monitoring of prothrombin time may be necessary during and after CBZ (Hansen J, Siersbaek-Nielsen K, Skovsted L. Carbamazepine-induced acceleration of diphenylhydantoin and warfarin metabolism in man. *Clin Pharmacol Ther* 1971;12: 539–543).

warfarin + chloral hydrate   Co-administration may displace warfarin from its plasma protein binding sites, resulting in increased anticoagulation effects and risk of bleeding.

warfarin + cimetidine   Cimetidine can increase prothrombin time in subjects taking warfarin, apparently by inhibiting the metabolism of the less-active R-enantiomer in a stereospecific manner (Serlin MJ, Sibeon RG, Mossman S, et al. Cimetidine interaction with oral anticoagulants in man. *Lancet* 1979;2:317–319; Niopas I, Toon S, Rowland M. Further insight into the stereoselective interaction between warfarin and cimetidine in man. *Br J Pharmacol* 1991; 32:508–511).

warfarin + clomipramine   Co-administration may increase the plasma concentrations of these drugs, resulting in adverse effects.

warfarin + dextroamphetamine   Co-administration decreases dextroamphetamine metabolism, resulting in increased plasma levels of dextroamphetamine.

warfarin + fluoxetine   Co-administration may alter warfarin serum concentration, resulting in increased bleeding time, a coagulation disorder, or increased coagulation time manifested by severe bruising and other complications (Claire RJ, Servis ME, Cram DL: Potential interaction between warfarin sodium and fluoxetine. *Am J Psychiatry* 1991;148:1604; Woolfrey S, Gammack NS, Dewar MS, Brown PJE. Fluoxetine-warfarin interaction. *Br Med J* 1993;307:241).

warfarin + fluvoxamine   Fluvoxamine inhibits warfarin metabolism, increasing warfarin serum levels (about 65%) and lengthening prothrombin time (Benfield P, Ward A. Fluvoxamine: a review of its pharmacokinetic properties and therapeutic efficacy in depressive illness. *Drugs* 1986;32:481–508). Warfarin dosage may have to be adjusted (*British National Formulary Number 24*. London: British Medical Association and the Royal Pharmaceutical Society of Great Britain, 1992; 5-Hydroxytryptamine reuptake inhibitors. *MeReC Bull* 1991;2:29–32).

warfarin + imipramine Co-administration can increase hypothrombinemic effect.

warfarin + maprotiline Co-administration may increase prothrombin time and cause bleeding.

warfarin + methylphenidate Co-administration may increase prothrombin-time (PT) response. It also may decrease metabolism of methylphenidate, resulting in increased methylphenidate plasma levels. When methylphenidate is added to warfarin, PT should be monitored more frequently.

warfarin + monoamine oxidase inhibitor (MAOI) Co-administration may increase prothrombin-time (PT) response. When an MAOI is added to warfarin, PT should be monitored more frequently.

warfarin + neuroleptic Neuroleptics decrease warfarin blood concentration, resulting in decreased bleeding time.

warfarin + other drugs Many drug interactions with warfarin have been reported. Whenever a new drug is prescribed for a warfarin-treated patient, prothrombin time must be monitored closely for the first month unless the added drug is known *not* to interact with warfarin.

warfarin + paroxetine Co-administration may increase bleeding tendency. Despite paroxetine's lack of significant effect on prothrombin time, mild but clinically significant bleeding occurred in 5 of 27 healthy volunteers given both drugs; 3 were withdrawn from the study (Bannister SJ, Houser VP, Hulse JD, et al. Evaluation of the potential for interactions of paroxetine with diazepam, cimetidine, warfarin and digoxin. *Acta Psychiatry Scand* 1989; 80[suppl 350]:102–106; *British National Formulary Number 24*. London: British Medical Association and the Royal Pharmaceutical Society of Great Britain, 1992; 5-Hydroxytryptamine reuptake inhibitors. *MeReC Bull* 1991;2:29–32). Careful monitoring of prothrombin time is advisable when warfarin and paroxetine are co-prescribed.

warfarin + pemoline Co-administration decreases pemoline metabolism, resulting in increased pemoline plasma levels.

warfarin + phenytoin Co-administration may increase phenytoin (PHT) blood levels and risk of PHT toxicity.

warfarin/pregnancy Warfarin should be avoided during the first trimester of pregnancy because of the risk of teratogenicity (mainly chondrodysplasia punctata). Warfarin also should be avoided during the last 4 weeks because it crosses the placental barrier and may cause hemorrhage at birth.

warfarin + remoxipride Remoxipride has no significant effect on the pharmacokinetics of either the S(–) or the R(+) warfarin. It also has no effect on the prothrombin time of warfarin (Yisak W, von Bahr C, Farde L, et al. Drug interaction studies with remoxipride. *Acta Psychiatry Scand* 1990;82[suppl 358]:58–62).

warfarin + sertraline In a placebo-controlled trial involving healthy subjects, prothrombin time and warfarin plasma protein binding were determined after a single oral dose of warfarin. After 22 days of sertraline treatment, a second dose of warfarin was administered and a significant increase in the prothrombin time area under the curve and a decrease in warfarin plasma protein binding were observed. Although the changes were considered clinically unimportant in this study, co-administration of sertraline with anticoagulants should be accompanied by careful monitoring of prothrombin time (Wilner KD, Lazar JD, Apseloff G, et al. The effects of sertraline on the pharmacodynamics of warfarin in healthy volunteers. *Biol Psychiatry* 1991;29:354S).

warfarin + trazodone In a warfarin-treated patient, a significant decrease in prothrombin time and partial prothrombin time occurred after trazodone was started, necessitating an increased warfarin dose. Warfarin requirements decreased after trazodone discontinuation (Hardy JL, Sirois A. Reduction of prothrombin and partial prothrombin times with trazodone. *Can Med Assoc J* 1986;135:1372). Combined use also results in decreased anticoagulant effect.

warfarin + valproate Co-administration may increase the risk of bleeding.

warfarin + valproic acid The hematological effects of valproic acid may potentiate the anticoagulant effects of warfarin.

warfarin + vitamin E Co-administration may prolong bleeding time.

warfarin + zolpidem Concurrent administration does not alter the pharmacokinetics of either drug.

washer Patient with a form of obsessive-compulsive disorder characterized by fear of dirt or contamination. Patients avoid "contaminated" objects such as door knobs, light switches, telephones, and money, but still may spend hours every day washing their hands.

washout Initial phase of a clinical drug trial, preceding administration of the study drug, during which other active substances (and their metabolites) are discontinued and excreted. A washout period minimizes the influence of other substances on subsequent drug therapy. See **carryover effect.**

water intoxication Potentially fatal syndrome, often seen in polydipsic patients, that may follow very large intakes of fluid. It is manifested by headache, ataxia, tremor, nausea, vomiting, confusion, lethargy, psychosis, seizures, or death. In psychiatric patients, it may exacerbate the underlying mental disorder. It ensues when hyponatremia is severe (serum sodium concentration < 120 mEq/L) or occurs very rapidly. Long-standing hyponatremia has been associated with hypertension and atherosclerosis. Overcorrection or overly rapid correction of hyponatremia by infusion of hypertonic saline can cause the irreversible and potentially fatal neurological syndrome called "central pontine myelinolysis." See **polydipsia.**

waxing and waning "Crescendo-descrescendo" pattern of electroencephalographic activity.

waxy flexibility See **catalepsy.**

wearing off See **akinesia, end of dose.**

"weed" Street name for marijuana.

"weight phobia" Morbid fear of becoming fat. It is an essential characteristic of both bulimia nervosa and anorexia nervosa.

weighted average Number formed by multiplying each number in a set of numbers by a constant and then averaging the resulting products.

weighting Determination of the relative influence any one element should have in the total by the assignment of a relative constant by which that element is multiplied.

Wellbutrin See **bupropion.**

Wernicke's encephalopathy See **Wernicke's syndrome.**

Wernicke-Korsakoff syndrome Co-existence of Wernicke's syndrome and alcohol amnestic disorder (Korsakoff's syndrome), occurring in less than 5% of alcoholics. Treatment of choice is thiamine administration for up to 2 months. See **alcohol amnestic disorder; Wernicke's syndrome.**

Wernicke's syndrome Condition frequently occurring in alcoholics due to thiamine deficiency resulting from poor nutritional intake, alcohol-induced malabsorption in the small bowel, and decreased production of the thiamine-dependent enzyme transkalose. Resulting malnutrition leads to neurological symptoms including ataxia, ophthalmoplegia, nystagmus, a global confused state, and coma. It is a medical emergency. Failure to treat the coma can increase the risk of mortality; the longer the coma remains untreated, the poorer the prognosis. Recommended treatment is 100 mg/day of thiamine administered

intramuscularly for at least 3 days. If ocular motor signs do not improve within several hours of receiving thiamine, 1–2 ml of magnesium sulfate in a 50% solution should be administered intramuscularly. See **alcohol amnestic disorder.**

Western blotting Test in which viral antigens are separated on a gel, transferred to a blotting strip, and exposed to a patient's serum. Uses include detection of the presence of antibodies to human immunodeficiency virus (HIV) rather than the HIV antigen itself. Also called "immunoblot." See **Southern blotting.**

"whack" Street name for phencyclidine (PCP).

"whippets" Street name for whipped cream propellants that are abused by volatile substance abusers.

"white" Street name for amphetamines.

"white cross" Street name for amphetamines.

"white horse" Street name for heroin.

"white lady" Street name for cocaine.

"white stuff" Street name for morphine.

"white wedge" Street name for dimethoxymethylamphetamine.

"whiz bang" Street name for heroin.

Wilcoxon rank-sum test Nonparametric test for comparing two independent samples with ordinal data or with numerical observations that are not normally distributed.

Wilcoxon signed-rank test See **Wilcoxon test.**

Wilcoxon test Analytic test devised by Wilcoxon (1945) to compare two sets of results that are combined and then scored in terms of an ordered classification (Wilcoxon F. Individual comparisons by ranking methods. *Biometrics* 1945;1:80–83). It concerns differences between two groups in paired samples, examining only differences for each pair. It is the nonparametric analog of the paired sample t-test. In 1947, Mann and Whitney devised a different, but exactly equivalent, version of the test that may or may not be more convenient to use. The Mann-Whitney version compares each individual in the first group with each individual in the second group, recording how many times the comparison favors the individual in the second group (Mann HB, Whitney DZ. One test of whether one of two random variables is statistically larger than the other one. *Ann Math Stat* 1947;18:50–60). Also called "Mann-Whitney-Wilcoxon test"; "Wilcoxon Signed Rank test."

wild type Genetic locus or allele that specifies a phenotype that predominates in natural populations or that is designated as "normal."

Wilpowr See **phentermine.**

Wilson's disease (WD) Rare autosomal recessive disorder of copper metabolism in which copper is deposited in the liver, brain, and other tissues. Symptoms usually appear between the ages of 10 and 25 (range, 5–50 years). WD presents with hepatic cirrhosis or neuropsychiatric symptoms. Neurological manifestations are highly variable; extrapyramidal signs usually predominate, but cerebellar symptoms may occasionally be in the foreground (e.g., parkinsonian, intention and/or flapping tremors, torticollis or other dystonias, rigidity, postural instability, dysarthria). Psychiatric symptoms include emotional lability, progressive intellectual deterioration, schizophrenic-like illness, and auditory hallucinations. About half of WD patients exhibit psychiatric symptoms; most common is incongruous behavior (typically aggressive, childish, disinhibited, or reckless with loss of impulse control). There may also be personality changes, depression, and cognitive impairment. Psychiatric symptoms are more strongly associated with neurological symptoms (such as dysarthria or dystonia) than with hepatic symptoms. WD figures prominently in the differential diagnosis of tardive dystonia; diagnosis is based on a family history of neurological and/or hepatic disease, progressive extrapyramidal symptoms, presence of Kayser-Fleischer ring (greenish-brown pigmentation of the limbus of the eye), cirrhosis of the liver (biopsy), and laboratory findings (cupriuria, aminoaciduria, abnormal liver function tests, mostly decreased serum levels of ceruloplasmin) (Haag H, Ruther E, Hippius H. *Tardive Dyskinesia.* Seattle: Hogrefe & Huber, 1992). The WD patient presenting to a general psychiatrist is likely to be a young adult with minor neurological complaints or signs, or with Kayser-Fleischer signs. A neurological examination, careful family history, ceruloplasmin level (if indicated), 24-hour urine copper excretion, and referral to an ophthalmologist may result in a life-saving diagnosis (Akil M, Schwartz JA, Dutchak D, et al. The psychiatric presentations of Wilson's Disease. *J Neuropsychiatry Clin Neurosci* 1991;3:377–382). Treatment is with the copper-chelating agent penicillamine, which may produce dramatic improvements in neurological and psychological symptoms. Also called "hepatolenticular degeneration."

"window pane" Street name for lysergic acid diethylamide (LSD).

window, therapeutic See **therapeutic window.**

Winstrol See **stanozolol.**

winter depression Form of seasonal affective disorder identified in the early 1980s and observed primarily in women. It occurs most often in the second or third decade of life, but several cases in children have been reported. Episodes are characterized by hypersomnia, hyperphagia, anergia, carbohydrate craving, and weight gain. Other symptoms of depression—decreased libido, hopelessness, social withdrawal, suicidal thoughts—also may be present. Winter depression begins in the fall and usually ends in March, to be followed by normal mood, hypomania, or mania. See **seasonal affective disorder.**

withdrawal Symptoms following drug discontinuation. With benzodiazepines, for example, "new," time-limited symptoms occur that were not present as part of the original anxiety state. Symptoms begin and end depending on the pharmacokinetics of the discontinued benzodiazepine. Withdrawal also refers to signs and symptoms after cessation of illicit drug or alcohol use by an individual in whom dependence is established. See **withdrawal syndrome.**

withdrawal akathisia See **akathisia, withdrawal.**

withdrawal attenuation Use of pharmacological strategies (e.g., phenobarbital, propranolol, clonidine, carbamazepine) to block or minimize physiological withdrawal during active discontinuation of a central nervous system substance.

withdrawal dyskinesia See **dyskinesia, withdrawal.**

withdrawal-emergent syndrome See **dyskinesia, withdrawal.**

withdrawal insomnia See **insomnia, withdrawal.**

withdrawal, protracted Continuation of subjective and physiological disturbances for weeks or months after initiation of abstinence from alcohol, opiate, stimulant, or benzodiazepine use. A consistent feature of the syndrome is that it follows the acute withdrawal syndrome. It is almost always associated with craving for the relinquished substance and has important clinical relevance because it may contribute to relapse. Protracted withdrawal occurs infrequently and is often unrecognized or attributed to other psychiatric disorders. Examples include prolonged depression following withdrawal from opioids, alcohol, or cocaine, and irritability and anxiety following cessation of alcohol, benzodiazepine, opiate, or nicotine use.

withdrawal syndrome Predictable constellation of symptoms that may develop in any individual who gradually or abruptly discontinues or abruptly decreases dosage of any central nervous system active drug taken daily in therapeutic or, more often, excessive doses for more than a few weeks. Specific clinical features are characteristic for the particular drug. The key clinical discriminator between withdrawal and relapse (a return of the original symptoms for which the drug was prescribed) is that withdrawal symptoms are more intense and present new features. Also called "abstinence syndrome."

Wolfram syndrome   Autosomal, recessive, neurodegenerative syndrome manifested by diabetes mellitus and progressive optic atrophy, usually associated with diabetes insipidus, deafness, atonic bladder, and diverse neurological abnormalities. Twenty-five percent of the individuals who are homozygous for the condition have severe psychiatric symptoms that lead to suicide attempts or psychiatric hospitalizations. Since heterozygous carriers of the gene for the Wolfram syndrome are 50 times more common among blood relatives than among spouses, the larger proportion among blood relatives is evidence that heterozygous carriers of the gene are predisposed to significant psychiatric illness.

Women for Sobriety   Self-help group developed specifically for women alcoholics.

word blindness   See **alexia.**

word recall   Task that assesses un-cued recall from secondary verbal memory.

word recognition   Task that assesses cued ability to retrieve stored verbal information from secondary memory.

word salad   Type of speech consisting of a jumble of words, meaningless phrases, groups of neologisms, etc., seen most frequently in the advanced stages of schizophrenia.

writer's cramp   Hand symptoms brought on by writing; probably one of the oldest known forms of focal dystonia. Age of onset is younger than with the other focal dystonias, with the highest incidence between 20 and 50 years of age. Initial complaints are often vague, usually a recognition of a change in handwriting. Tremor is present in up to 50% of cases. Writing even single words may become impossible.

WY-45,233   The major metabolite of venlafaxine, a combined norepinephrine and serotonin uptake inhibitor antidepressant. WY-45,233 also has antidepressant effects and a favorable side effect profile. Its pharmacological profile is similar to venlafaxine since it inhibits norepinephrine and serotonin uptake and produces noradrenergic desensitization. It does not appear to add any side effect liability beyond that of the parent drug. See **venlafaxine.**

Wyamine   See **mephentermine.**

X

X^2 See **chi squared.**

Xanax   See **alprazolam.**

xanthene   Potent central nervous system stimulant with many peripheral actions, represented primarily by caffeine and theophylline, which are chemically related plant alkaloids. Xanthenes are well absorbed from the intestines and metabolized by the liver. Caffeine is devoid of any therapeutic uses. Most habitual users like its stimulant effects. See **caffeine.**

X chromosome   The larger and longer of the sex-determining chromosomes. In males, the X chromosome, inherited from the mother, is paired with the tiny Y chromosome, inherited from the father. In women, an X chromosome, inherited from the mother, is paired with a second X chromosome, inherited from the father. Like all chromosomes, the X chromosome has a short and a long arm. The short arm of any chromosome is designated the "p" arm, and the long arm the "q" arm.

Xemovan   See **zopiclone.**

xenobiotic   Substance that is pharmacologically, endocrinologically, and toxicologically active, but is not endogenously produced. Xenobiotics may be absorbed through the lungs or skin, but most often are ingested unintentionally as agents in food or drink, or deliberately as therapeutic or illicit drugs. Some xenobiotics are innocuous, but many can have pharmacological or toxic effects depending on conversion of the absorbed substance into an active metabolite.

xenophobia   Fear of strangers.

xerostomia   Dry mouth secondary to reduced or absent salivary secretions. It can occur in states of fear, anxiety, or depression, and is a common side effect of many psychoactive drugs, especially tricyclic antidepressants and other compounds with anticholinergic effects.

Ximovane   See **zopiclone.**

X linkage   Genes on the X chromosome, or traits determined by such genes, are X-linked. If a disorder is X-linked, with a gene on the X chromosome, differential sex incidence will be found. X-linked dominant disorders are more common in women. An X-linked recessive condition such as hemophilia occurs almost solely in men, but is transmitted to offspring only via women. Although some evidence indicates X-linkage in bipolar disorder, there is no good evidence for X-linkage in unipolar disorders.

"XTC"   Street name for 3,4-methylenedioxymethamphetamine (MDMA).

XXX syndrome   Chromosome abnormality in which there is one extra X chromosome. Women with the syndrome usually appear normal, may be of normal intelligence or only mildly mentally handicapped, and are likely to be fertile. They may have some characteristics of the XXXX syndrome.

XXXX syndrome   Chromosome abnormality in which there are two extra X chromosomes. Women with the syndrome are usually mildly mentally handicapped and may have a slightly unusual facial appearance with wide-set eyes (hypertelorism). Fusion of the bones in the forearm, congenital dislocation of the hips, incurving of the fifth finger and several other congenital abnormalities have been reported. Menstruation may be irregular or normal.

XXXY syndrome   Chromosome abnormality in which there are two extra X chromosomes. Men with the syndrome have similar features to men with the XXYY syndrome but are usually more mildly affected. Height is in the normal range and mental handicap is generally mild. Mild breast enlargement is common after puberty.

XXYY syndrome   Chromosome abnormality in which there is an extra X and an extra Y chromosome. Men with the syndrome are mildly to severely mentally handicapped. Neck webbing, breast enlargement, and reduced facial hair are usually seen. The testes are small. There is a tendency to have varicose veins. Many men with this condition are excessively tall, and a few have been reported to have had aggressive or bizarre behavior.

Xylocaine   See **lidocaine.**

XYY syndrome   Common chromosome abnormality in which there is an extra Y chromosome. It has been associated with unusually tall stature, dull normal intelligence, delayed speech, and some learning problems. It is also manifested by prominent glabella, facial asymmetry, long ears, radioulnar synostosis, and increased length vs. breadth in the skeletal structures. Minor abnormalities of the nervous system have also been detected on neurological examination. The condition was originally associated with criminal behavior because of its high rate of detection in surveys of prisons and secure hospitals. More recent studies have confirmed a tendency to impulsive behaviors, temper outbursts, and problems in dealing with aggression. Any association with mental handicap is slight.

Y

Yates' correction   Process of subtracting 0.5 from the numerator at each term in the chi-squared statistic for 2 × 2 tables prior to squaring the term.

Y chromosome   The shorter sex chromosome. See **X chromosome.**

"yellow"   Street name for pentobarbital.

"yellow bullet"   Street name for pentobarbital.

Yellow Card scheme   In the United Kingdom, a method for spontaneous reporting of adverse drug reactions by physicians, dentists, coroners, and others, including the pharmaceutical industry, to the Committee on Safety on Medicines. See **prescription event monitoring.**

"yellow doll"   Street name for pentobarbital.

"yellow football"   Street name for pentobarbital.

"yellow jacket"   Street name for pentobarbital.

"yellow sunshine"   Street name for lysergic acid diethylamide (LSD).

"yellow wedge"   Street name for dimethoxymethylamphetamine.

"yesca"   Street name for marijuana.

Yocon   See **yohimbine.**

yohimbine   (Actibine; Aphrodyne; Corynine; Yocon) (YOH) Indolalkylamine chemically similar to reserpine. It is an alpha$_2$-adrenergic antagonist that prevents inhibition of norepinephrine release, resulting in increased synaptic availability. YOH is used as a sympathicolytic and mydriatic. It has been used to treat sexual impotence and can be used to test the functional sensitivity of certain adrenergic systems (Heninger GR, Charney DS. Monoamine receptor systems and anxiety disorders. *Psychiatr Clin North Am* 1988;11:326) In young panic disorder patients, but not in patients with generalized anxiety disorder, obsessive-compulsive disorder, depression, or schizophrenia, YOH causes increased anxiety, elevated blood pressure, and elevated levels of peripheral cortisol and methoxyhydroxyphenylglycol (MHPG). It stimulates moods, may increase anxiety, and has been found to precipitate manic episodes in predisposed individuals.

yohimbine + bupropion   Marked and persistent improvement in mood occurred in a patient with treatment-resistant major depression when yohimbine was added to counteract anorgasmia associated with bupropion therapy (Pollack MH, Hammerness P. Adjunctive yohimbine for treatment in refractory depression. *Biol Psychiatry* 1993;33:220–221).

yohimbine challenge test   Test that demonstrates significantly elevated cortisol responses and other measures of arousal to yohimbine in post-traumatic stress disorder patients compared to control subjects.

yohimbine challenge test/panic patients   Because yohimbine has been shown to precipitate anxiety in a variety of subjects, yohimbine challenge has been tried in a number of panic patients. Results indicate that it may be a nonspecific anxiogenic that can precipitate panic symptoms in vulnerable patients.

yohimbine + clomipramine   In a double-bind crossover placebo study, the effect of low-dosage (4 mg 3 times a day) yohimbine was tested in 12 depressed patients with orthostatic hypotension induced by clomipramine. Yohimbine significantly increased systolic blood pressure, possibly because of a pharmacodynamic and pharmacokinetic interaction between yohimbine and clomipramine or desmethylclomipramine (Lacomblez L, Bensimon G, Isnard F, et al. Effect of yohimbine on blood pressure in depressed patients with orthostatic hypotension induced by clomipramine. *Fundam Clin Pharmacol* 1989;3:579).

yohimbine + fluoxetine   Yohimbine (5.4 mg 3 times a day) may produce partial or complete relief of fluoxetine (FLX)-induced sexual dysfunction in up to 90% of those treated. Favorable response occurs within the first treatment week and persists as long as yohimbine is continued. It is usually well tolerated; most common side effects are nausea, anxiety, insomnia, and urinary frequency (Jacobsen FM. Fluoxetine-induced sexual dysfunction and an open trial of yohimbine. *J Clin Psychiatry* 1992; 53:119–122). Combined use has been reported to negate FLX's antidepressant effect. See **fluoxetine/sexual dysfunction.**

yule statistic   Mathematically similar to the kappa statistic, but stable over a wider range of base rates (Spitznagel EL, Helzer JE. A proposed solution to the base-rate problem in the kappa statistic. *Arch Gen Psychiatry* 1985;42: 725–728). Also called the "coefficient of colligation."

Z

Z-10-hydroxynortriptyline Minor metabolite of nortriptyline that occurs in about one-fifth the concentration of the active metabolite hydroxynortriptyline, but is equally potent in noradrenergic uptake inhibition. See **hydroxynortriptyline.**

zacopride Serotonin$_3$ antagonist being investigated as a possible therapy for schizophrenia (Tricklebank MD. Interaction between dopamine and 5-HT$_3$ receptors suggest new treatments for psychosis and drug addiction. *Trends Pharmacol Sci* 1989;10:127–128). It may have antidopaminergic activity in the limbic system.

Zamanol See **ondansetron.**

Zantac See **ranitidine.**

Zapex See **oxazepam.**

z approximation z-Test used to test the equality of two independent proportions.

Zarontin See **ethosuximide.**

z distribution Normal distribution with mean 0 and standard deviation 1. Also called the "standard normal distribution."

zeitgeber From the German *zeit* (time) *geber* (giver). Term coined in 1954 by Archoff, a German physiologist, for synchronizing agents or periodic environmental time cues (e.g., sunlight, noise) that usually help entrainment to the solar day. They do not create circadian rhythms, but strongly influence them. In the absence of zeitgebers, it is difficult for a person to know about the time of day (Archoff Z. Circadian systems in man and their implications. *Hosp Pract* 1976;11:51–57).

Zestoretic See **lisinopril.**

Zestril See **lisinopril.**

zetidoline Low-potency neuroleptic, chemically unrelated to any available antipsychotic, with selective dopamine receptor blocking properties and only weak muscarinic receptor, and alpha$_1$ noradrenergic receptor blocking activity. It produces significantly fewer extrapyramidal symptoms than most other neuroleptics.

zidovudine Thymidine analog commonly used in the treatment of acquired immunodeficiency syndrome (AIDS) and human immunodeficiency virus (HIV) infection. It blocks viral replication by inhibiting reverse transcriptase. It is virustatic but not virucidal (i.e., it blocks replication of the virus but does not kill it). Studies have shown that zidovudine increases survival time in HIV infection. Originally called "azidothymidine" (AZT).

zidovudine + acetaminophen Concern that concomitant use might cause increased hema-

tological toxicity has not been substantiated (Richman DD, Rischl MA, Gueco MH, et al. The toxicity of azidothymidine [AZT] in the treatment of patients with AIDS and AIDS-related complex. *N Engl J Med* 1987;317:192–197). Serum levels of zidovudine and its glucuronidated metabolite are not increased by acetaminophen administration; leading to the conclusion that the moderate use of acetaminophen in patients on zidovudine therapy need not be avoided (Steffe EM, Krug JH, Inciardi FJ, et al. The effect of acetaminophen on zidovudine metabolism in HIV-infected patients. *J AIDS* 1993;5:691–694).

zidovudine + lithium See **lithium + zidovudine.**

zidovudine/mania Episodes of secondary mania induced by zidovudine therapy in acquired immunodeficiency syndrome (AIDS) patients have been reported. Symptoms resolved with cessation of zidovudine therapy, but recurred with its reinstitution (Maxwell S, Scheftner W, Kessler H, et al. Manic syndrome associated with zidovudine treatment. *JAMA* 1988;259:3406–3407). See **lithium + zidovudine.**

zidovudine + methadone See **methadone + zidovudine.**

zidovudine/pregnancy No teratogenic abnormalities or pattern of serious hematological toxicity in infants or any pattern of observable adverse pregnancy outcomes has been directly attributed to zidovudine (Sperling RS, Stratton P, O'Sullivan MJ, et al. A survey of zidovudine use in pregnant women with human immunodeficiency virus infection. *N Engl J Med* 1992;326:857–861).

Zimovane See **zopiclone.**

ZK 112-119 See **abecarnil.**

ZK-93426 Benzodiazepine (BZD) inverse agonist that has cognitive-enhancing effects in volunteers similar to effects of drugs that facilitate central cholinergic transmission. There also is experimental evidence suggesting that ZK-93426 facilitates acetylcholine release. In this respect it resembles some of the centrally acting angiotensin-converting enzyme inhibitors such as captopril, which has been shown to exhibit cognitive-enhancing properties in experimental studies, possibly by stimulating acetylcholine release (Leonard BE. *Fundamentals of Psychopharmacology*, New York: John Wiley & Sons, 1992).

Zofran See **ondansetron.**

Zoloft See **sertraline.**

zolpidem (Ambien, Bikalm, Niotal, Stilnoct, Stilnox) Nonbenzodiazepine hypnotic that has been shown to be effective in inducing and maintaining sleep in adults. Its pharmacological profile is different from that of the benzodiazepines in that it has no muscle relaxant, anxiolytic, or anticonvulsant effects at sedative doses. Zolpidem is thought to bind specifically to the benzodiazepine type 1 receptor and to have very low affinity for other receptor subtypes. It is rapidly absorbed after oral administration, reaching peak blood levels in approximately 2.2 hours, and is highly bound to plasma protein. Half-life is 2.4 hours in adults and 2.9 hours in the elderly. In normal young adults, doses up to 90 mg have been safe and effective, especially in doses between 10 and 20 mg. In doses of 5 mg and above, zolpidem is effective in inducing and maintaining sleep in the elderly. Compared to older hypnotic drugs, zolpidem has similar sleep enhancing properties, but like zopiclone, it is less likely to alter sleep architecture. Compared to triazolam, zolpidem is equieffective as a hypnotic, but more strongly affects stages 3 and 4 (slow-wave sleep). Studies to date (1994) indicate that zolpidem is devoid of residual effects on high cerebral functions on the morning after administration and may have advantages over short-acting benzodiazepines. Single oral doses of zolpidem and diazepam produce similar, but not identical, effects in substance abusers. Zolpidem has some potential for abuse of the diazepam type. Whether patients are less likely to develop tolerance or dependence on zolpidem remains to be determined. A case of zolpidem intoxication characterized by development of a profound but short-lasting coma associated with pinpoint pupils and respiratory depression has been reported. Symptoms were not influenced by naloxone but responded clearly and rapidly to flumazenil (Lheureux P, Debailleul G, De-Witte O, Ashkenasi R. Zolpidem intoxication mimicking narcotic overdose: response to flumazenil. *Hum Toxicol* 1990;9:105–107). Two cases of amnestic psychotic reactions with zolpidem have been reported (Ansseau M, Pitchot W, Hansenne M, et al. Psychotic reactions to zolpidem. *Lancet* 1992;339:809). A third psychotic reaction was reported in a 20-year-old woman with restrictive anorexia nervosa. Twenty minutes after taking zolpidem (10 mg), she was terrified, began to see persons and objects in her room, saw her arm become gigantic, and saw serial multiplication of furniture. The episode lasted a few minutes, following which she slept for several hours and awoke with a "hangover." She remembered all the episode's characteristics, during which her level of consciousness had been normal. Physical and neurological examina-

tions, an electroencephalogram (EEG), and computed tomography (CT) scan were normal. A similar, less intense episode occurred a week later when she took 5 mg of zolpidem. A week later, 2.5 mg of zolpidem produced macropsia, during which the patient remained calm (Iruela LM, Ibanez-Rojo V, Baca E. Zolpidem-induced macropsia in anorexic woman. *Lancet* 1993;342:443–444).

zolpidem + chlorpromazine   Co-administration may increase sedation without altering pharmacokinetics of either drug.

zolpidem + cimetidine   Co-administration does not alter the pharmacokinetics of either drug.

zolpidem + haloperidol   Co-administration does not alter the pharmacokinetics of either drug.

zolpidem + imipramine   Co-administration does not alter the pharmacokinetics of either drug, although there may be increased sedation.

zolpidem + ranitidine   Co-administration does not alter the pharmacokinetics of either drug.

zolpidem + warfarin   Concurrent administration does not alter the pharmacokinetics of either drug.

zonisamide   (ZNS) Anticonvulsant originated in Japan and now marketed there for the treatment of simple and complex partial seizures, partial-onset generalized tonic-clonic seizures, generalized tonic-clonic seizures, tonic seizures, atypical absence seizures, and combinations of these. A substituted 1,2-benzisoxazole, zonisamide has been shown to have clinical and preclinical profiles similar to those of carbamazepine. It also may have a moderate antimanic effect. Trials in the United States have been halted because the drug has been associated with renal calculi (Yagi K, Seino M. Methodological requirements for clinical trials in refractory epilepsies. Our experience with zonisamide. *Prog Neuropsychopharmacol Biol Psychiatry* 1992;16:79–85).

"zoom"   Street name for cocaine or a mild stimulant that is a cocaine "substitute."

zoophilia   Condition in which an individual gains sexual satisfaction from sexual contact with animals.

Zophran   See **ondansetron.**

Zophren   See **ondansetron.**

zopiclone   (Amoban, Datolan, Datovane, Foltran, Imovane, Limovane, Xemovan, Ximovane, Zimovane) Cyclopyrrolone derivative, nonbenzodiazepine hypnotic with a high affinity for benzodiazepine receptors. It is chemically unrelated to other sedative-hypnotics currently available for clinical use. It competes directly with benzodiazepines at receptor sites. Zopiclone is rapidly absorbed after oral administration and extensively metabolized. Its half-life is 4–6 hours, with mostly inactive metabolites, N-desmethyl zopiclone and an N-oxide derivative. It is effective in improving sleep onset latency, sleep quality, sleep duration, and frequency of nocturnal awakenings. Optimal dose is 7.5 mg. Hangover effects are infrequent with 7.5 mg and undetectable after 3.75 mg. Since zopiclone has a short elimination half-life, its hypnotic effect may not be followed by performance impairment the next day and it causes less daytime rebound anxiety than triazolam. Side effects include a metallic taste. It is claimed to be safe in overdose, which can be counteracted by flumazenil. Its use should be restricted to short-term treatment, since most controlled clinical studies have involved short-term or intermediate-term administration. Compared to older hypnotic compounds, zopiclone seems to have similar sleep-enhancing properties, but it is less likely to alter sleep architecture. It may, however, increase the amount of slow wave sleep or reduce both the quality and quantity of slow wave sleep. Evidence is limited regarding tolerance and withdrawal.

zopiclone + alcohol   Combined use produces immediate, enhanced impairment of the psychomotor effects of zopiclone without altering its pharmacokinetics. The reaction is short-lived, usually lasting no more than 8 hours (Kuitunen T, Mattila MJ, Seppala T. Actions and interactions of hypnotics on human performance: single doses of zopiclone, triazolam, and alcohol. *Int Clin Psychopharmacol* 1990;5[suppl 2]:115–130). Co-administration also decreases rapid eye movement (REM) sleep duration during the first half of the night (Misaki K, Kishi H, Koshino Y, et al. The influence on sleep by zopiclone or ethanol alone or in combination: a polysomnographic study. *Jpn J Psychiatry Neurol* 1991;45:915–916).

zopiclone + carbamazepine   Although co-administration reduces plasma concentrations of each drug, it also produces clear additive impairment of psychomotor performance (Kuitunen T, Mattila MJ, Seppala T, et al. Actions of zopiclone and carbamazepine, alone and in combination, on human skilled performance in laboratory and clinical tests. *Br J Clin Pharmacol* 1990;30:453–461).

zopiclone + erythromycin   In healthy volunteers, co-administration results in a rapid and slight increase in the plasma level of zopiclone that is rapidly dissipated. The interaction is of minor clinical significance.

zopiclone + metoclopramide   Co-administration may decrease zopiclone plasma levels (O'Toole DP, Carlisle RJT, Howard PJ, Dunkee JW. Effects of altered gastric motility on the pharmacokinetics of orally administered zopiclone. *Irish J Med Sci* 1986;155:136).

zopiclone + trimipramine   In volunteers given simultaneous oral doses of trimipramine (50 mg) and zopiclone (7.5 mg), the pharmacokinetics of both drugs remained unchanged. Although a trend has been seen toward a decreased area under the curve, which might lead to a lessened antidepressant effect of trimipramine, the clinical importance of this and other interactions remains undetermined (Caille G, DuSouich P, Spenard J, et al. Pharmacokinetics and clinical parameters of zopiclone and trimipramine when administered simultaneously to volunteers. *Biopharmaceutics and Drug Disposition* 1984;5:117–125).

Zopran   See **ondansetron.**

zotepine   (Engramon, Lodopin, Nipolept) (ZOT) Atypical dibenzothiepine antipsychotic with antidopaminergic, anticholinergic, adrenolytic, and strong antiserotonergic effects. Blood levels peak 1–4 hours after administration; elimination half-life is roughly 8 hours. Clinical trials in Japan and Europe indicate that ZOT has good antipsychotic properties in acute schizophrenia and can effectively alleviate negative symptoms in chronic schizophrenia. It is more sedative than clozapine, does not cause extrapyramidal side effects, and in trials to date has not had any adverse hematological effects (Barnas C, Stuppack CH, Miller C, et al. Zotepine in the treatment of schizophrenic patients with prevailing negative symptoms. A double-blind trial vs. haloperidol. *Int Clin Psychopharmacol* 1992;7:23–27). It also may have antimanic effects.

zotepine + biperiden   Biperiden does not affect zotepine serum level.

zotepine + piroheptine   Piroheptine does not affect zotepine serum level.

z ratio   Statistic, used in the z-test, formed by subtracting the hypothesized mean from the observed mean and dividing by the standard error of the mean.

z score   Deviation of x from the mean divided by the standard deviation.

z-test   Statistical test for comparing a mean with a norm or comparing two means for large samples.

z-track technique   Injection method for depot neuroleptics to prevent drug leakage that involves sliding the skin to the side and then back after the injection.

z transformation   Transformation that changes a normally distributed variable with mean x and standard deviation s to the z distribution with mean 0 and standard deviation 1.

zuclopenthixol   (Acuphase; Ciatyl; Cisordinal; Cisordinal Acutard; Clopixol; Viscoleo) (ADD) A thioxanthene neuroleptic that is available in oral tablet form, intramuscular depot form (decanoate), and a shorter-acting intramuscular form (acetate). The efficacy and side effects of each form are similar to those of other neuroleptics, and thus zuclopenthixol is another treatment option rather than a superior treatment. Only the acetate form is a new treatment method that offers the advantage of a simpler regimen, providing the initial dose is prudently chosen. Zuclopenthixol is the *cis* isomer of clopenthixol (i.e., clopenthixol is the racemic mixture [contains both isomers]). The *cis* isomers of thioxanthene neuroleptics are more active at dopamine receptors than the *trans* isomers are. *Trans*-clopenthixol and *trans*-flupenthixol are considered inactive (Anon. Zuclopenthixol: profile. *Pharmabulletin* 1994;18:29–31; Gravem A, Elgen K. *Cis*(Z)-clopenthixol: the neuroleptically active isomer of clopenthixol. A presentation of five double-blind clinical investigations and other studies with *cis*(Z)-clopenthixol. *Acta Psychiatr Scand* 1981; 64[suppl 294]:5–120).

zuclopenthixol acetate (ZPT-A) (Clopixol Acuphase; Clopixol Acutard; Cisordinal Acutard) Thioxanthene neuroleptic formulation with a duration of action of 2–3 days and proven effectiveness in the initial treatment of acute psychotic episodes. Clinical experience indicates that acute psychotic episodes can be controlled with a minimal number of injections of ZPT-A. It contains 50 mg/ml of zuclopenthixol acetate in thin vegetable oil. The usual dose is 50–150 mg by deep intramuscular injection, repeated if necessary after 1, 2, or 3 days. Maximum accumulated dosage should not exceed 400 mg. Sedation is quickly achieved, and maintenance treatment easily instituted. It can be mixed in a syringe with the depot formulations of zuclopenthixol or flupenthixol to initiate maintenance treatment.

zuclopenthixol + clonazepam Co-administration is safe and effective in acute mania (Gouliaev G, Licht RW, Vestergaard P. Treatment of acute mania with lithium and clonazepam or zuclopenthixol and clonazepam. *Clin Neuropharm* 1992;15[suppl 1]:210B).

zuclopenthixol decanoate (Clopixol Decanoate) Formulation containing zuclopenthixol decanoate (200 mg/ml) in thin vegetable oil. Dosage is 200–500 mg every 2–4 weeks by deep intramuscular injection.

zygosity determination Determination of whether twins are monozygotic (MZ; all blood factors are identical) or dizygotic (DZ; one or more blood factors are different). Accurate zygosity diagnosis is based on a battery of tests: most importantly, tissue typing, blood factor analysis (e.g., red blood cell antigens, serum proteins, and enzymes) using electrophoresis and isoelectric focusing, or DNA testing. Genetic testing points to "real" zygosity. "Perceived" zygosity is usually determined by interviews or questionnaires that focus on physical similarity, frequency of confusion by the family and social environment, and twins' beliefs regarding their zygosity. Some data suggest that perceived zygosity corresponds with real zygosity in 80–90% of twin pairs, provided interviews and questionnaires are thorough and meticulous throughout, with high reliability for scoring zygosity status (Kendler KS, Neale MC, Kessler RC, et al. A test of the equal-environment assumption in twin studies of psychiatric illness. *Behav Genet* 1993; 23:21–28).

zygote Either the fertilized egg resulting from the union of two cells to form one single cell in sexual reproduction, or the organism that develops from a fertilized egg.

Index

agranulocytosis, 141
arrhythmias after withdrawal, 653
central anticholinergic syndrome, 124
hyponatremia, 328
neonatal, 145, 146
sulpiride and, 146, 611
sympathomimetic and, 146
thiothixene and, 146
thyroid drug and, 146
tranylcypromine and, 146, 640
triiodothyronine and, 146, 654
tryptophan and, 146, 656
valproate and, 146, 664
warfarin and, 146, 674
yohimbine and, 146–147, 680
Clomipramine challenge test, 142
Clonazepam, 147, 613
biotransformation of, 71
in breast milk, 147
carbamazepine and, 108, 110, 147
chemical structure of, 70
clomipramine and, 142
clozapine and, 147, 154
desipramine and, 147, 203
dosage of, 69, 147
fluoxetine and, 147–148, 271–272
half-life of, 67, 70, 147
haloperidol and, 309
indications for, 147
adjunctive therapy, 68
blepharospasm, 84
catatonia, 121
juvenile myoclonic epilepsy, 250
mania, 49, 71
nonfearful panic disorder, 484
oneiric behavior, 474
periodic movements in sleep, 499
psychotic agitation, 148
restless legs syndrome, 558
social phobia, 515
tremor, 645
isocarboxazid and, 148, 346
lithium and, 148, 366
metabolites of, 147
neuroleptic and, 72, 148, 447, 448
valproate and, 663
phenelzine and, 148, 507
phenobarbital dosage equivalent for, 510
phenytoin and, 148, 513
in pregnancy, 147, 148
sertraline and, 148, 584
side effects of, 147
absence status, 1, 148
valproate and, 148, 664
zuclopenthixol and, 148, 684
Clone, 148
Clonex. See Clonazepam
Clonidine, 149
abuse of, 149
amphetamine and, 38, 149
in breast milk, 149
clomipramine and, 142, 150
fluoxetine and, 150, 272
indications for, 149
autism, 60
delirium tremens, 189
methadone withdrawal, 150
opioid withdrawal, 149, 150, 476
post-traumatic stress disorder, 527
methylphenidate and, 150, 410
naltrexone and, 149, 150, 439
diazepam and, 150, 211, 439
in pregnancy, 149
side effects of, 149

trazodone and, 642
use in children, 149
withdrawal from, 149, 150
Clonidine challenge test, 149–150, 446
Clonidine skin patch, 150
for clozapine-induced hypersalivation, 155
Cloning
gene, 296
molecular, 150
positional, 150–151
Cloning vector, 151
cosmid, 177
Clonopin. See Clonazepam
Clonus, 151
Clopenthixol, 684
moclobemide and, 420
Clopenthixol decanoate, Clopixol decanoate. See Zuclopenthixol decanoate
Clopixol. See Zuclopenthixol
Clopixol Acuphase, Clopixol Acutard. See Zuclopenthixol acetate
Clorazepate, 52, 151, 205, 534
alcohol and, 151
antacid and, 151
in breast milk, 151
chemical structure of, 70
cimetidine and, 151
dosage of, 69
erythromycin and, 70
fluoxetine and, 70, 268–269
half-life of, 67, 70, 151
isoniazid and, 71
nicotine and, 458
phenobarbital dosage equivalent for, 510
in pregnancy, 151
Clorgyline, 151, 429
clomipramine and, 142–143, 151, 582
lithium and, 151, 366, 372
Clostebol, 151
Clotiazepam, 71
Clouding of consciousness, 151
Clovoxamine, 151
alcohol and, 151
digoxin and, 151
Cloxazepam. See Loxapine
Cloxazolam, 151
Clozapine, 49, 151–152, 447
anticholinergic drug and, 45, 153
antihypertensive drug and, 153
atenolol and, 57, 153
benzodiazepine and, 69, 153–154
benztropine and, 77, 154
in breast milk, 154
bromocriptine and, 91, 154
buspirone and, 99, 154
captopril and, 154
carbamazepine and, 110, 154
chloral hydrate and, 126, 154
cimetidine and, 154
clonazepam and, 147, 154
diazepam and, 154
diphenhydramine and, 154
divalproex and, 154, 218
dopamine receptor occupancy by, 220–221
dosage of, 151–152
electroconvulsive therapy and, 154, 240
fluoxetine and, 155, 272
indications for, 152
akathisia, 153
mania, 451
Parkinson's disease, 152, 156–157

polydipsia, 157
schizophrenia, 151–152
supersensitivity psychosis, 613
tardive dyskinesia, 158
lack of response to, 152
levodopa/carbidopa and, 155, 357
lithium and, 155, 366–367
lorazepam and, 155–156, 381
mechanism of action of, 151–152
metabolite of, 466
methylphenidate and, 156, 410
moclobemide and, 420
nicotine and, 156, 458–459
nortriptyline and, 156, 468
overdose of, 156
perazine and, 157, 498
pergolide and, 157, 498
phenytoin and, 157, 513
in pregnancy, 157
ranitidine and, 157
reinitiation of, 157
rifampin and, 157
side effects of, 152
agranulocytosis, 14, 54, 85, 152–153, 155, 367–368
diarrhea, 155
fever, 155
hypersalivation, 155
hyponatremia, 155, 328
myoclonic jerks and drop attacks, 156
neuroleptic malignant syndrome, 155, 156
neutropenia, 457
orthostatic hypotension, 478–479
pancytopenia, 482
priapism, 157, 531
seizures, 156, 157–158
trazodone and, 158, 642
tricyclic antidepressant and, 158, 649
trifluoperazine and, 158, 653
valproate and, 158, 664
valproic acid and, 158, 666
withdrawal from, 158
dyskinesia and, 158
Clozapine-N-oxide, 156
Clozapine syndrome, 158
Clozaril. See Clozapine
Cluster, 158
homicide/suicide, 319
Cluster analysis, 158
Cluster headache, 313–314
Cluttering, 158
"Coast to coast," 158
Co-beneldopa, 158
Cocaethylene, 159
Cocaine, 124, 159, 176, 604, 614
abuse of, 159
extrapyramidal susceptibility and, 160
fluoxetine for, 267, 272
addiction to, 7
adverse effects of
acute psychotic agitation, 5
cardiovascular, 161
choreoathetoid movements, 161
compulsive foraging behavior, 171, 295
corneal changes, 161
hallucinosis, 162
hepatotoxicity, 316
hypertensive crisis, 553
intravenous use, 160
mania, 572
neonatal, 160, 162

709

Index

aberrant, 296
allele of, 25, 296
amplification of, 296
APP, 296
candidate, 105
carrier of, 120
C-fos, 125–126
cloning of, 296
  positional, 150–151
cocaine, 162
contiguous gene syndrome, 175
conversion of, 296
dominant, 219, 296
dopamine receptor, 221
expression of, 296
globin, 297
immediate early, 297
lethal, 297
locus of, 297, 379
major, 297
modifying, 297
mutation of, 297
  detected by ligand chain reaction,
    359–360
oncogene, 473
operator, 474
polygene, 523
prion, 297
promoter, 297
proto-oncogene, 539
quantitative trait loci mapping of, 547
recessive, 297
recombination of, 553
regulation of, 297
regulator, 297
regulatory domain of, 554
reporter, 297
sequencing of, 297
splicing of, 297
suppressor, 297
transcribed domain of, 637
transfer of, 298
Gene therapy, 297–298
Genetically engineered drug, 300
Genetic analysis, 298
Genetic code, 298
Genetic counseling, 298
Genetic cross, 298
Genetic disorder, 298
Genetic drift, 298–299
Genetic engineering, 299
Genetic heterogeneity, 299, 317
Genetic marker, 299
Genetic probe, 299
Genetic recombination, 299
Genetic redundancy, 299
Genetics, 299
  behavioral, 299
  biochemical, 82
  biometrical, 299
  clinical, 299
  community, 299
  cytogenetics, 184
  forward, 299
  human, 299
  medical, 299–300
  molecular, 296
  quantitative, 300
  reverse, 300
Genetic screening, 299, 571
Genetic sequence, 299
Genetic trait, 299
Genetic variance, 299
Genetic vulnerability, 299
Genogram, 300
Genome, 300

Genome map, 300
Genomic library, 300
Genotype, 300, 511
Gepirone, 53, 62, 300
  hypothermia induced by, 582
  as probe for serotonin$_{1A}$ receptor
    sensitivity, 581–582
Gerontology, 300
Geropsychiatry, 300
Gerstmann-Straüssler-Scheinker disease,
  532
Gesell Developmental Examination, 505
Gesture, 300
Gewacalm. See Diazepam
Ghosts, 614
Giant cell arteritis, 622
Giddiness, 300
Gilex. See Doxepin
Gilles de la Tourette's syndrome, 300–
  301
  after long-term neuroleptic therapy,
    620
  desipramine for, 202
  eye blink rate in, 257
  haloperidol and nicotine for, 459
  obsessive-compulsive disorder and,
    471
  palilalia in, 482
  pimozide for, 518
  piquindone for, 520
  tics of, 300, 632
Ginkgo biloba, 301
"Girl," 301
"Girls & boys," 301
Gland, 301
  adrenal, 301
  pituitary, 301, 328, 520
Glasgow Coma Scale, 294
"Glass," 301
Glia, 301
Gliatilin. See Choline alfoscerate
Glibenclamide, 301
  moclobemide and, 418, 419–420, 421
  sertraline and, 585
Gliclazide, moclobemide and, 418, 421
Global introspection, 301
Global rating, 301
Globus hystericus, 301
Globus pallidus, 64, 301
Glorium. See Medazepam
Glossopharyngeal contraction, 301
Glucocorticoid, 301
Glucose-6-phosphate dehydrogenase
  deficiency, 301
Glucuronidation, 70
Glue sniffing, 301
Glutamate, 301–302
Glutamate receptor, 302, 464
Glutamic acid, 302, 457
Glutamic acid decarboxylase, 302
Glutamic oxaloacetate transferase. See
  Aspartate aminotransferase
Glutethimide, 124, 302, 326
  in breast milk, 302
  liver enzyme induction due to, 379
  phenobarbital dosage equivalent for,
    510
Glycine, 302, 456, 457
Glycopyrrolate, 302
Godot syndrome, 302
Goiter, carbamazepine-induced, 108
"Gold," 302
"Gold dust," 302
Gold standard, 179–180
Gonadal hormone, 302
Gonadotropic hormone, 302

Gonadotropin-releasing hormone, 302,
  355
"Good shit," 302
"Goofball," 302
"Goofer," 302
"Goon," 302
Goosebumps, 302
G proteins, 303
GR 43175. See Sumatriptan
Gradient. See Flunarizine
Grammatic Comprehension, 353
Grandiosity, 303
Granisetron, 303, 582
  haloperidol and, 303, 310
Granulocyte colony-stimulating factor,
  168, 320
Granulocyte-macrophage colony-
    stimulating factor, 168, 303–304
Graph, 304
"Grass," "grasshopper," 304
Grateful Med, 304
"Green," 304
"Green and black," 304
"Green and clear," 304
"Green and white," 304
"Greenie," 304
Grief, 431
Grimace, 304
Group therapy, 167
Growth hormone, 304, 483, 520, 626
Growth hormone releasing factor, 304
Growth hormone stimulation test, 304,
  446
Guanethidine, 228
  priapism due to, 531
  thioridazine and, 627
Guanfacine, 304
  amitriptyline and, 34
  imipramine and, 334
  tricyclic antidepressant and, 650
Guanine, 304
Guanylate cyclase, 304
"Guerrilla," 304
Guidance, 305
Guillain-Barré syndrome, 305, 434
Guilt feelings, 305
Gyrectomy, 305
"H," 306
Habilitation, 306
Habit, 306
Habitrol. See Nicotine transdermal
    system
Habit spasm, 632
Habitual body manipulation, 306
Habituation, 634
Hair drug analysis, 306
Hair pulling, 647–648
Halazepam, 205, 306
  dosage of, 69
  erythromycin and, 70
  fluoxetine and, 70, 268–269
  isoniazid and, 71
  phenobarbital dosage equivalent for,
    510
Halcion. See Triazolam
Haldol. See Haloperidol
Half-life, 306
  alpha, 306
  beta, 306
  biphasic, 83
  elimination, 227
  metabolite, 306
Halfway house, 306
Hallucination(s), 306, 534, 567
  antiparkinson drug-induced, 49–50
  auditory, 306